Clinical Nuclear Cardiology

*State of the Art
and Future Directions*

Clinical Nuclear Cardiology

State of the Art and Future Directions

FOURTH EDITION

Barry L. Zaret, MD

Robert W. Berliner Professor of Medicine
Professor of Diagnostic Radiology
Section of Cardiovascular Medicine
Yale University School of Medicine
New Haven, Connecticut

George A. Beller, MD

Ruth C. Heede Professor of Cardiology
Professor of Medicine
Cardiovascular Division
Department of Medicine
University of Virginia Health System
Charlottesville, Virginia

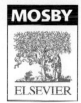

MOSBY

ELSEVIER

MOSBY
ELSEVIER

1600 John F. Kennedy Blvd.
Ste 1800
Philadelphia, PA 19103-2899

Clinical Nuclear Cardiologty

ISBN: 978-0-323-05796-7

Library of Congress Cataloging-in-Publication Data

Clinical nuclear cardiology: state of the art and future directions/[edited by] Barry L. Zaret, George A. Beller. — 4th ed.
      p. ; cm.
   Includes bibliographical references and index.
   ISBN 978-0-323-05796-7 (alk. paper)
   1. Heart—Radionuclide imaging. I. Zaret, Barry L. II. Beller, George.
   [DNLM: 1. Heart—radionuclide imaging. 2. Myocardial Ischemia—radionuclide imaging.
   3. Radionuclide Imaging—instrumentation. 4. Radionuclide Imaging—methods. WG 141.5.
   R3 C6415 2010]
   RC683.5.R33N833 2010

616.1'207575–dc22
2009022837

Executive Publisher: Natasha Andjelkovic
Developmental Editor: Julie Goolsby
Project Manager: Nayagi Athmanathan
Design Direction: Ellen Zanolle

Printed in China

Last digit is the print number: 9 8 7 6 5 4 3 2 1

To Myrna Zaret, my wife of almost 50 years, my muse, my companion, my love.

Barry Zaret

To my wonderful and supportive wife, Katherine Brooks, and my six delightful grandchildren, Max, Pietro, Giacomo, Emily, Colin and Grace.

George Beller

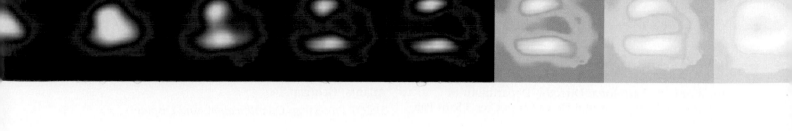

CONTRIBUTORS

· · · · · · · · · ·

NIKOLAOS ALEXOPOULOS, MD
Research Scholar, Division of Cardiology, Department of Medicine, Emory University, Atlanta, Georgia; Researcher, 1st Cardiology, University of Athens Medical School, Athens, Greece

Coronary Artery Computed Tomography Angiography

TIMOTHY M. BATEMAN, MD
Professor, Department of Medicine, University of Missouri School of Medicine; Co-Director, Cardiovascular Radiologic Imaging, Department of Cardiovascular Disease, Mid America Heart Institute of Saint Luke's Hospital, Kansas City, Missouri.

Radiation Considerations for Cardiac Nuclear and Computed Tomography Imaging

JEROEN J. BAX, MD, PhD
Cardiology, Leiden University Medical Center, Leiden, The Netherlands

Stress Myocardial Perfusion Imaging in Patients with Diabetes Mellitus

Myocardial Viability: Comparison with Other Techniques

ROB S. BEANLANDS, MD, FRCPC
Professor, Medicine (Cardiology)/Radiology, Department of Medicine, University of Ottawa, Chief, Cardiac Imaging; Director, National Cardiac PET Centre, Cardiology Department, University of Ottawa Heart Institute, Ottawa, Ontario, Canada

Diagnosis and Prognosis in Cardiac Disease Using Cardiac PET Perfusion Imaging

GEORGE A. BELLER, MD
Ruth C. Heede Professor of Cardiology and Professor of Medicine, Cardiovascular Division, Department of Medicine, University of Virginia Health System, Charlottesville, Virginia

Comparison of Noninvasive Techniques for Myocardial Perfusion Imaging

FRANK M. BENGEL, MD
Associate Professor of Radiology and Medicine, Director of Cardiovascular Nuclear Imaging, Division of Nuclear Medicine, Department of Radiology, Johns Hopkins University School of Medicine, Baltimore, Maryland

Cardiac Neurotransmission Imaging: Positron Emission Tomography

DANIEL S. BERMAN, MD
Professor of Medicine, David Geffen School of Medicine at University of California, Los Angeles, Chief, Department of Cardiac Imaging, Cedars-Sinai Medical Center, Los Angeles, California

Digital/Fast SPECT: Systems and Software

Regional and Global Ventricular Function and Volumes from SPECT Perfusion Imaging

Prognostic Implications of MPI Stress SPECT

ROBERT O. BONOW, MD
Goldberg Distinguished Professor of Cardiology, Division of Cardiology, Northwestern University Feinberg School of Medicine; Chief, Division of Cardiology, Co-Director, Bluhm Cardiovascular Institute, Northwestern Memorial Hospital, Chicago, Illinois

Assessment of Myocardial Viability with Thallium-201 and Technetium-Based Agents

KENNETH A. BROWN, MD, FACC, FAHA, FASNC
Director, Nuclear Cardiology and Cardiac Stress Laboratory, Department of Cardiology, University of Vermont College of Medicine, Burlington, Vermont

Nuclear Imaging in Revascularized Patients with Coronary Artery Disease

MATTHEW M. BURG, PhD
Associate Clinical Professor of Medicine, Yale University School of Medicine, New Haven; VA-CT Healthcare System, West Haven, Connecticut

Mechanistic and Methodological Considerations for the Imaging of Mental Stress Ischemia

DENNIS A. CALNON, MD, FACC, FASE, FASNC
Director, Nuclear Cardiology, McConnell Heart Hospital at Riverside Methodist Hospital, Columbus, Ohio

Atlas of Cases

JOHN M. CANTY, JR, MD
Albert and Elizabeth Rekate Professor of Medicine, Chief, Division of Cardiovascular Medicine, Department of Medicine, University at Buffalo; Staff Cardiologist, VA Western New York Healthcare System at Buffalo, Buffalo, New York

Pathophysiologic Basis of Hibernating Myocardium

IGNASI CARRIÓ, MD
Chair and Professor, Nuclear Medicine, Universitat Autònoma de Barcelona; Director, Department of Nuclear Medicine, Hospital De La Santa Creu I Sant Pau, Barcelona, Spain
Cardiac Neurotransmission Imaging: Single-Photon Emission Computed Tomography

JAMES A. CASE, PhD
Associate Professor, Director of Physics, University of Missouri, Kansas City, Missouri
Attenuation Correction and Scatter Correction of Myocardial Perfusion SPECT Images

JI CHEN, PhD
Assistant Professor, Department of Radiology, Emory University, Atlanta, Georgia
SPECT Processing, Quantification, and Display

S. JAMES CULLOM, PhD
Director, Research and Development, Cardiovascular Imaging Technologies, LLC, Kansas City; Adjunct Professor, Department of Nuclear Engineering and Sciences, University of Missouri, Columbia; Technical Director, ASPIRE Foundation, Kansas City, Missouri
Radiation Considerations for Cardiac Nuclear and Computed Tomography Imaging

SETH T. DAHLBERG, MD
Associate Professor, Medicine and Radiology, University of Massachusetts Medical School; Director of Nuclear Cardiology, Divisions of Nuclear Medicine and Cardiology, UMass Memorial Medical Center, Worcester, Massachusetts
Imaging for Preoperative Risk Stratification

ROBERT A. DEKEMP, PhD
Associate Professor, Medicine and Engineering, University of Ottawa; Head Imaging Physicist, National Cardiac PET Centre, University of Ottawa Heart Institute, Ottawa, Ontario, Canada
Diagnosis and Prognosis in Cardiac Disease Using Cardiac PET Perfusion Imaging

E. GORDON DEPUEY, MD
Professor, Department of Radiology, Columbia University College of Physicians and Surgeons; Director of Nuclear Medicine, Radiology, St. Luke's-Roosevelt Hospital, New York, New York
Single-Photon Emission Computed Tomography Artifacts

MARCELO F. DI CARLI, MD
Associate Professor of Radiology and Medicine, Harvard Medical School; Director of Noninvasive Cardiovascular Imaging Program, Chief of Nuclear Medicine and Molecular Imaging, Departments of Radiology and Medicine, Brigham and Women's Hospital, Boston, Massachusetts
PET/CT and SPECT/CT Hybrid Imaging
Assessment of Myocardial Viability with Positron Emission Tomography

TRACY L. FABER, PhD
Professor, Department of Radiology, Emory University, Atlanta, Georgia
SPECT Processing, Quantification, and Display

JAMES A. FALLAVOLLITA, MD
Professor, Department of Medicine, University at Buffalo; Staff Cardiologist, VA Western New York Healthcare System at Buffalo, Buffalo, New York
Pathophysiologic Basis of Hibernating Myocardium

ANTONIO B. FERNANDEZ, MD
Cardiovascular Imaging Fellow, Yale University School of Medicine, VA-CT Healthcare System, West Haven, Connecticut
Mechanistic and Methodological Considerations for the Imaging of Mental Stress Ischemia

ALBERT FLOTATS, MD
Associate Professor, Department of Nuclear Medicine, Universitat Autònoma de Barcelona; Consultant, Nuclear Medicine, Hospital De La Santa Creu I Sant Pau, Barcelona, Spain
Cardiac Neurotransmission Imaging: Single-Photon Emission Computed Tomography

OLIVER GAEMPERLI, MD
Department of Cardiac Imaging, University Hospital Zurich, Zurich, Switzerland
Hybrid Cardiac Imaging

SANJIV SAM GAMBHIR, MD, PhD
Professor, Department of Radiology and Bioengineering; Director, Molecular Imaging Program at Stanford (MIPS); Chief, Division of Nuclear Medicine, Stanford Hospital and Clinics, Stanford University, Stanford, California
Molecular Imaging of Gene Expression and Cell Therapy

ERNEST V. GARCIA, PhD
Professor of Radiology, Emory University, Atlanta, Georgia
SPECT Processing, Quantification, and Display

GUIDO GERMANO, PhD, MBA
Professor, Department of Medicine, University of California School of Medicine, Los Angeles; Director, Artificial Intelligence Program, Department of Medicine, Cedars-Sinai Medical Center, Los Angeles, California
Digital/Fast SPECT: Systems and Software
Regional and Global Ventricular Function and Volumes from SPECT Perfusion Imaging

RAYMOND J. GIBBONS, MD
Professor of Medicine, Department of Cardiovascular Diseases, Mayo Clinic, Rochester, Minnesota
Appropriate Use of Nuclear Cardiology

DAVID K. GLOVER, ME, PhD
Associate Professor, Department of Medicine and
Cardiovascular Division, University of Virginia,
Charlottesville, Virginia
*Overview of Tracer Kinetics and Cellular Mechanisms of
Uptake*
*State-of-the-Art Instrumentation for PET and SPECT Imaging
in Small Animals*

DENNIS A. GOODMAN, MD, FACP, FACC, FCCP
Clinical Associate Professor, Medicine, University of
California, San Diego, La Jolla, California; Past Chief
of Cardiology, Scripps Memorial Hospital, La Jolla,
California; Senior Cardiologist, Tisch/Bellvue
Hospital, New York, New York; Clinical Associate
Professor, Medicine, New York University, New York,
New York
*Coronary Artery Calcification: Pathogenesis, Imaging, and
Risk Stratification*

ROBERT J. GROPLER, MD
Professor of Radiology, Medicine, and Biomedical
Engineering; Lab Chief, Cardiovascular Imaging
Laboratory, Mallinckrodt Institute of Radiology,
Washington University School of Medicine; Attending
Physician, Radiology and Medicine, Barnes-Jewish
Hospital, St. Louis, Missouri
Imaging of Myocardial Metabolism

RORY HACHAMOVITCH, MD, MSC
Department of Medicine and Division of Cardiovascular
Medicine, Kech School of Medicine of the University of
Southern California, Los Angeles, California
Prognostic Implications of MPI Stress SPECT

GARY V. HELLER, MD, PhD
Professor of Medicine, University of Connecticut School
of Medicine, Farmington; Director, Nuclear Cardiology,
Associate Director, Cardiac Division, Hartford Hospital,
Hartford, Connecticut
Imaging in Women

THOMAS A. HOLLY, MD
Associate Professor of Medicine and Radiology,
Northwestern University Feinberg School of Medicine;
Medical Director, Nuclear Cardiology, Northwestern
Memorial Hospital, Chicago, Illinois
*Assessment of Myocardial Viability with Thallium-201 and
Technetium-Based Agents*

**AMI E. ISKANDRIAN, MD, MACC, FAHA,
FASNC**
Distinguished Professor of Medicine and Radiology,
Department of Medicine, University of Alabama at
Birmingham, Birmingham, Alabama
*Coronary Artery Disease Detection: Pharmacologic Stress
SPECT*

DIWAKAR JAIN, MD, FACC, FRCP, FASNC
Professor of Medicine, Department of Cardiology;
Director of Nuclear Cardiology Laboratory, Drexel
University College of Medicine; Attending Physician,
Cardiology, Hahnemann University Hospital,
Philadelphia, Pennsylvania.
Atlas of Cases

PHILIPP A. KAUFMANN, MD
Professor and Director of Cardiac Imaging, Zurich
Center for Integrative Human Physiology, University of
Zurich, Zurich, Switzerland
Hybrid Cardiac Imaging

SANJIV KAUL, MD
Professor of Medicine, Division Chief, Division of
Cardiovascular Medicine, Oregon Health Science
University, Portland, Oregon
*Myocardial Perfusion Imaging with Contrast
Echocardiography*

JANUSZ K. KIKUT, MD
Assistant Professor of Radiology and Nuclear Medicine,
University of Vermont; Director of Nuclear Medicine
and PET/CT, Department of Radiology, Fletcher Allen
Health Care, Burlington, Vermont
*Nuclear Imaging in Revascularized Patients with Coronary
Artery Disease*

MICHAEL A. KING, PhD
Professor, Department of Radiology, University of
Massachusetts Medical School, Worcester, Massachusetts
Attenuation/Scatter/Resolution Correction: Physics Aspects

JUHANI KNUUTI, MD, PhD
Professor, Turku PET Centre, University of Turku, Turku,
Finland
*Assessment of Myocardial Viability with Positron Emission
Tomography*

MICHAEL C. KONTOS, MD
Associate Professor, Internal Medicine (Division of
Cardiology, Pauley Heart Center), Radiology and
Emergency Medicine; Associate Director, Acute Cardiac
Care; Co-Director, Stress Laboratory; Associate Professor,
Internal Medicine, Department of Cardiology,
Radiology, and Emergency Medicine, Virginia
Commonwealth University, Richmond, Virginia
*Imaging Patients with Chest Pain in the Emergency
Department*

CHRISTOPHER M. KRAMER, MD
Professor, Departments of Medicine and Radiology;
Director, Cardiovascular Imaging Center, University of
Virginia Health System, Charlottesville, Virginia
Myocardial Perfusion: Magnetic Resonance Imaging

BIJOY KUNDU, PhD
Assistant Professor, Department of Radiology, University of Virginia, Charlottesville, Virginia
State-of-the-Art Instrumentation for PET and SPECT Imaging in Small Animals

AVIJIT LAHIRI, MBBS, MSC, MRCP, FACC, FESC
Consultant Cardiologist and Director, Clinical Imaging and Research Centre (CIRC), The Wellington Hospital, St John's Wood, London; Medical Director, British Cardiac Research Trust; Honorary Professor, Middlesex University; Honorary Senior Lecturer, Imperial College, London, United Kingdom
Coronary Artery Calcification: Pathogenesis, Imaging, and Risk Stratification

JEFFREY A. LEPPO, MD
Professor, Department of Medicine and Radiology, University of Massachusetts, Worcester; Chief of Cardiology, Department of Medicine, Berkshire Medical Center, Pittsfield, Massachusetts
Imaging for Preoperative Risk Stratification

JONATHAN R. LINDNER, MD
Professor of Medicine, Associate Chief for Education, Division of Cardiovascular Medicine, Oregon Health Science University, Portland, Oregon
Myocardial Perfusion Imaging with Contrast Echocardiography

JOHN J. MAHMARIAN, MD
Professor of Medicine, Department of Cardiology, Weill Cornell Medical College, New York, New York; Director, Nuclear Cardiology and CT Services, Methodist DeBakey Heart and Vascular Center, The Methodist Hospital, Houston, Texas
Risk Stratification for Acute ST-Segment Elevation and Non-ST-Segment Elevation Myocardial Infarction

DALTON S. McLEAN, MD
Cardiology Fellow, Division of Cardiology, Department of Medicine, Emory University, Atlanta, Georgia
Coronary Artery Computed Tomography Angiography

TODD D. MILLER, MD
Professor of Medicine, Department of Cardiovascular Diseases, Mayo Clinic, Rochester, Minnesota
Appropriate Use of Nuclear Cardiology

ALAN R. MORRISON, MD, PhD
Cardiovascular Medicine Fellow, Department of Internal Medicine, Yale University School of Medicine, New Haven, Connecticut
Molecular Imaging Approaches for Evaluation of Myocardial Pathophysiology: Angiogenesis, Ventricular Remodeling, Inflammation, and Cell Death

LAURA FORD-MUKKAMALA, DO, FACC
Clinical Cardiologist, Department of Cardiology, Billings Clinic, Billings, Montana
Imaging in Women

JAGAT NARULA, MD, PhD
Professor of Medicine and Chief of Cardiology; Medical Director, Memorial Heart and Vascular Institute; Medical Director, Edwards Life Sciences Center for Advanced Cardiovascular Technology, University of California, Irvine, Irvine, California
Radionuclide Imaging of Inflammation in Atheroma

TINSU PAN, PhD
Associate Professor, Department of Imaging Physics, The University of Texas, MD Anderson Cancer Center, Houston, Texas
Attenuation/Scatter/Resolution Correction: Physics Aspects

AMIT R. PATEL, MD
Director of Cardiac Magnetic Resonance, Assistant Professor of Medicine, Department of Medicine, University of Chicago, Chicago, Illinois
Myocardial Perfusion: Magnetic Resonance Imaging

JAMES A. PATTON, PhD
Professor, Department of Radiology and Radiological Sciences, Vanderbilt University Medical Center, Nashville, Tennessee
Digital/Fast SPECT: Systems and Software

LINDA R. PETERSON, MD
Associate Professor of Medicine and Radiology, Cardiovascular Division and Division of Geriatrics and Nutritional Sciences, Department of Medicine, Washington University School of Medicine, St. Louis, Missouri
Imaging of Myocardial Metabolism

DON POLDERMANS, MD, PhD, FESC
Professor, Department of Medicine, Erasmus Medical Centre, Department of Vascular Surgery, Rotterdam, The Netherlands
Myocardial Viability: Comparison with Other Techniques

DONNA M. POLK, MD, MPH
Director, Preventive Cardiology, Department of Cardiology, Hartford Hospital, Hartford, Connecticut
Imaging in Women

P. HENDRIK PRETORIUS, PhD
Associate Professor, Department of Radiology, University of Massachusetts Medical School, Worcester, Massachusetts
Attenuation/Scatter/Resolution Correction: Physics Aspects

PAOLO RAGGI, MD
Associate Professor of Medicine, Division of Cardiology, Department of Medicine, Emory University, Atlanta, Georgia
Coronary Artery Computed Tomography Angiography

RAYMOND R. RUSSELL, MD, PhD
Associate Professor, Departments of Medicine and Diagnostic Radiology, Yale-New Haven Hospital, New Haven, Connecticut
Principles of Myocardial Metabolism as They Relate to Imaging
Coronary Artery Disease Detection: Exercise Stress SPECT

ANTTI SARASTE, MD, PhD
Research Fellow, Nuklearmedizinische Klinik und Poliklinik, Klinikum rechts der Isar der Technische Universität München, Munich, Germany
Cardiac Neurotransmission Imaging: Positron Emission Tomography

HEINRICH R. SCHELBERT, MD, PhD
The George V. Taplin Professor, Department of Molecular and Medical Pharmacology, University of California, Los Angeles, California
State-of-the-Art Instrumentation for PET and SPECT Imaging in Small Animals
Myocardial Blood Flow Measurement: Evaluating Coronary Pathophysiology and Monitoring Therapy

THOMAS HELLMUT SCHINDLER, MD, PhD
Assistant Professor, Department of Medicine and Cardiology, Cardiovascular Center, School of Medicine at the University Hospitals of Geneva, Geneva, Switzerland
Myocardial Blood Flow Measurement: Evaluating Coronary Pathophysiology and Monitoring Therapy

AREND F.L. SCHINKEL, MD, PhD
Cardiology, Thoraxcenter, Erasmus Medical Center, Rotterdam, The Netherlands
Myocardial Viability: Comparison with Other Techniques

MARKUS SCHWAIGER, MD, FACC, FA
Professor, Nuclear Medicine, Technische Universität München; Director, Nuclear Medicine, Klinikum rechts der Isar, Munich, Germany
Cardiac Neurotransmission Imaging: Positron Emission Tomography

LESLEE J. SHAW, PhD
Professor of Medicine, Department of Medicine, Emory University, Atlanta, Georgia
Cost Effectiveness of Myocardial Perfusion Single-Photon Emission Computed Tomography

HOSSAM M. SHERIF, MD
Post-Doctoral Nuclear Cardiology Research Fellow, Nuclear Medicine, Technical University of Munich, Munich, Germany; Assistant Professor, Cardiovascular Critical Care Medicine, Cairo University Hospitals, Cairo, Egypt
Cardiac Neurotransmission Imaging: Positron Emission Tomography

ALBERT J. SINUSAS, MD
Professor, Department of Internal Medicine and Diagnostic Radiology, Yale University School of Medicine; Director, Department of Cardiovascular Nuclear Imaging and Stress Laboratory, Yale-New Haven Hospital, New Haven, Connecticut
Role of Intact Biological Models for Evaluation of Radiotracers
Molecular Imaging Approaches for Evaluation of Myocardial Pathophysiology: Angiogenesis, Ventricular Remodeling, Inflammation, and Cell Death

PIOTR SLOMKA, PhD
Professor, Department of Medicine, University of California, Los Angeles; Research Scientist, Department of Medicine and Imaging, Cedars-Sinai Medical Center, Los Angeles, California
Digital/Fast SPECT: Systems and Software

PREM SOMAN, MD, PhD, FRCP (UK), FACC
Assistant Professor of Medicine, Department of Medicine, University of Pittsburgh Medical Center, Pittsburgh, Pennsylvania
Radionuclide Imaging in Heart Failure

ROBERT SOUFER, MD
Professor of Medicine, Chief of Cardiology, VA-CT Healthcare System, Yale University School of Medicine, West Haven, Connecticut
Mechanistic and Methodological Considerations for the Imaging of Mental Stress Ischemia

H. WILLIAM STRAUSS, MD
Professor of Radiology (Nuclear Medicine), Weill Cornell Medical College; Attending Physician, Nuclear Medicine, Memorial Sloan Kettering Cancer Center, New York, New York
Radionuclide Imaging of Inflammation in Atheroma

RAGHUNANDAN DUDDA SUBRAMANYA, MBBS, MD
Fellow in Cardiology, Drexel University College of Medicine, Philadelphia; Fellow in Cardiology, Hahnemann University Hospital, Philadelphia; Fellow in Cardiology, Abington Memorial Hospital, Abington, Pennsylvania
Atlas of Cases

INES VALENTA, MD
Research Fellow, Department of Medicine and
Cardiology, Cardiovascular Center, School of Medicine
at the University Hospitals of Geneva, Geneva,
Switzerland
*Myocardial Blood Flow Measurement: Evaluating Coronary
Pathophysiology and Monitoring Therapy*

SERGE D. VAN KRIEKINGE, PhD
Assistant Professor, Department of Medicine, University
of California, Los Angeles, School of Medicine; Research
Scientist, Artificial Intelligence Program, Department of
Medicine, Cedars-Sinai Medical Center, Los Angeles,
California
*Regional and Global Ventricular Function and Volumes from
SPECT Perfusion Imaging*

SHREENIDHI VENURAJU, MBBS, MRCP
Clinical Research Fellow in Cardiology, Cardiac Imaging,
Clinical Imaging and Research Centre, Wellington
Hospital, London, United Kingdom
*Coronary Artery Calcification: Pathogenesis, Imaging, and
Risk Stratification*

JOHAN W.H. VERJANS, MD
Cardiology, University Medical Center Utrecht, Utrecht,
Netherlands; Cardiology, University of California,
Irvine, Irvine, California
Radionuclide Imaging of Inflammation in Atheroma

FRANS J.TH. WACKERS, MD, PhD
Professor Emeritus of Diagnostic Radiology and
Medicine, Senior Research Scientist, Departments of
Diagnostic Radiology and Internal Medicine, Yale
University School of Medicine, New Haven, Connecticut
Coronary Artery Disease Detection: Exercise Stress SPECT
*Stress Myocardial Perfusion Imaging in Patients with
Diabetes Mellitus*

ERNST E. VAN DER WALL, MD, PhD
Department of Cardiology, Leiden University Medical
Center, Leiden, The Netherlands
Myocardial Viability: Comparison with Other Techniques

DENNY D. WATSON, PhD
Professor of Radiology, Director of Nuclear Cardiology,
University of Virginia Health System, Charlottesville,
Virginia
*Overview of Tracer Kinetics and Cellular Mechanisms of
Uptake*

JOSEPH C. WU, MD, PhD, FACC
Assistant Professor, Medicine (Cardiology) and
Radiology, Stanford University School of Medicine,
Stanford, California
Molecular Imaging of Gene Expression and Cell Therapy

AJAY KUMAR YERRAMASU, MBBS, MRCP
Clinical Research Fellow in Cardiology, Cardiac Imaging,
Clinical Imaging and Research Centre, Wellington
Hospital, London, United Kingdom
*Coronary Artery Calcification: Pathogenesis, Imaging, and
Risk Stratification*

KEIICHIRO YOSHINAGA, MD, PhD
Associate Professor, Molecular Imaging, Hokkaido
University Graduate School of Medicine, Sapporo,
Hokkaido, Japan
*Diagnosis and Prognosis in Cardiac Disease Using Cardiac
PET Perfusion Imaging*

BARRY L. ZARET, MD
Robert W. Berliner Professor of Medicine and Professor
of Diagnostic Radiology, Department of Internal
Medicine, Section of Cardiovascular Medicine, Yale
University School of Medicine; Attending, Internal
Medicine/Cardiovascular Medicine, Yale-New Haven
Hospital, New Haven, Connecticut
Cardiac Performance
Imaging in Patients Receiving Cardiotoxic Chemotherapy
Radionuclide Imaging of Inflammation in Atheroma

MARIA CECILIA ZIADI, MD
Clinical Research Fellow in Molecular Function and
Imaging, Nuclear Cardiology, University of Ottawa Heart
Institute, Ottawa, Ontario, Canada
*Diagnosis and Prognosis in Cardiac Disease Using Cardiac
PET Perfusion Imaging*

GILBERT J. ZOGHBI, MD, FACC, FSCAI
Assistant Professor of Medicine, Department of
Medicine, University of Alabama at Birmingham;
Birmingham Veterans Association Medical Center,
Birmingham, Alabama
*Coronary Artery Disease Detection: Pharmacologic Stress
SPECT*

CONTENTS

· · · · · · · · · · ·

PREFACE

. . . .

INTRODUCTION: INTEGRATED CARDIOVASCULAR IMAGING— THE FUTURE

This book first appeared in 1993; the preceding third edition was published in 2005. Each new edition has been associated with significant expansion, revision, and updating, as well as significant changes in orientation that reflect new advances in the field. At the time of this fourth edition, nuclear cardiology is firmly established as a key noninvasive modality for the clinical evaluation of patients with cardiovascular disease. Concomitantly, there have been further advances in instrumentation, radiopharmaceutical development, and new clinical research, leading to additional understanding of clinical utility, cost-effectiveness, appropriateness, and relationship of imaging findings to patient outcomes. Nuclear cardiology has been incorporated into major large multicenter clinical trials. In addition, as other modes of cardiovascular imaging have approached maturity, there has been movement toward integrating the various imaging modalities under the broad umbrella of cardiovascular multimodality imaging. The cardiovascular imager of the future will likely be trained in more than one modality and will be housed in dedicated imaging centers that offer a variety of imaging approaches. It will be the imager's job to determine the study most appropriate for answering the posed clinical question. In recognition of this trend, new chapters are included in this edition that provide additional focus on non-nuclear cardiovascular imaging modalities such as computed tomography, magnetic resonance imaging, and contrast echocardiography.

The fourth edition continues to focus on nuclear cardiology and represents a major effort to incorporate new advances in clinical nuclear cardiology, thereby providing a road map for up-to-date clinical use. In addition, we seek to point out the new directions in which nuclear cardiology as well as integrated cardiovascular imaging are headed. Our goals in the fourth edition continue to be twofold: first, to present the most up-to-date and comprehensive clinically applicable data available in the field, thereby offering both the practitioner and student/trainee the current clinical state of the art; and second, to present the newest and most exciting directions in the field that reflect both technologic and biological

advances. To meet these combined goals, the book has once again expanded—now to a total of 45 chapters—and also includes a totally new and expanded atlas of case presentations to provide concrete examples of the clinical relevance of nuclear cardiology. Once again, the book is grouped into nine specific sections. Twenty of the 45 chapters, as well as the atlas, are totally new. An almost equal number of chapters have been eliminated, and, all remaining chapters have been revised, updated, and, in certain instances, consolidated.

Section 1 addresses issues related to radiopharmaceuticals and tracer kinetics. The three chapters in this section provide information concerning tracer kinetics and cellular mechanisms of uptake, principles of myocardial metabolism as they relate to imaging, and the role of intact biological models in evaluating radiotracers.

Section 2 deals with instrumentation. The eight chapters in this section address issues relating to processing, quantification, and display of single-photon emission tomography (SPECT) data, SPECT artifacts, attenuation/scatter/resolution and correction from both physics and clinical standpoints, hybrid imaging, digital/fast SPECT imaging, radiation considerations of imaging technologies, and small-animal imaging.

Section 3, as in the previous edition, contains two chapters dealing with cardiac function and performance, as evaluated by blood-pool imaging and gated SPECT imaging.

Section 4 addresses major issues that relate to perfusion imaging and detection of coronary disease. The 12 chapters in this section address the issues of coronary artery disease detection by exercise and pharmacologic stress, their prognostic implications, assessment of myocardial perfusion imaging by magnetic resonance imaging, echocardiography, and positron emission tomography (PET), and hybrid imaging. Specific chapters deal with computed tomography angiography and use of computed tomography to assess coronary artery calcification. Chapters also address cost-effectiveness as well as the appropriate use criteria for nuclear cardiology. A chapter also compares the various noninvasive approaches for assessment of myocardial perfusion.

Section 5 focuses on disease- and gender-specific issues. Specific chapters focus on imaging in women, imaging for preoperative risk assessment, revascularized patients, patients with diabetes mellitus, imaging in the heart failure population, imaging of patients receiving cardiotoxic chemotherapy, mental stress imaging, and the use of PET measurements of myocardial blood flow to evaluate cardiovascular pathophysiology and therapeutic efficacy.

Section 6 addresses acute coronary syndromes. The two chapters in this section deal with imaging in the emergency department and risk stratification of patients with acute myocardial infarction, based on new data from a multicenter randomized trial.

Section 7 contains four chapters focusing on myocardial viability. Viability assessment with SPECT studies, PET, and other techniques is addressed in three specific chapters, while an additional chapter focuses on the pathophysiologic basis of hibernating myocardium.

Section 8 contains three chapters on tracer-specific imaging techniques. These three chapters deal with imaging of myocardial metabolism and cardiac neurotransmission imaging with either SPECT or PET.

Section 9 deals with new molecular approaches and contains three chapters dealing with molecular imaging of angiogenesis matrix metalloproteases and cell death, vascular abnormalities, and imaging of gene expression and cell therapy. Such techniques are primarily being evaluated in preclinical experimental models but have already shown promise in early clinical studies.

The Atlas of Cases is the final section of the book and is designed to provide complementary information to the numerous clinical issues discussed in the text. It exemplifies the substantial clinical utility of nuclear cardiology and shows a variety of images set in their clinical context. This atlas is significantly expanded from the one included in the third edition.

Barry L. Zaret and George A. Beller

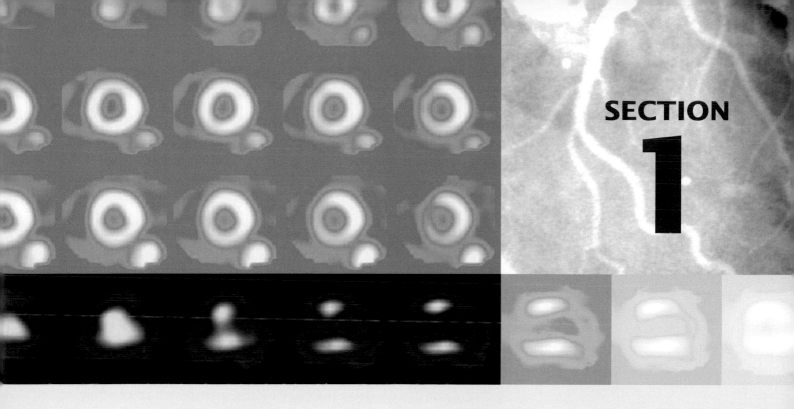

Radiopharmaceuticals/ Tracer Kinetics

Chapter 1

Overview of Tracer Kinetics and Cellular Mechanisms of Uptake

DENNY D. WATSON AND DAVID K. GLOVER

INTRODUCTION

The kinetics of tracer transport provides a skeletal framework that supports the body of clinical imaging using radionuclide tracers. This underlying framework provides an essential basis for understanding and clinical interpretation of tracers, including the sensitivity of different tracers to indicate reduction of coronary flow reserve, the use and limitations of redistribution and reinjection, and the applications of tracers for indication of myocardial viability and prediction of recovery of myocardial contractile function.

Tracer transport kinetics are most compactly and simply understood in terms of "models." A *model* is a mathematical function that defines a relationship. An example would be the curve that relates tracer uptake as a function of myocardial blood flow. There are certain basic relationships that govern the extraction, washout, and recirculation of tracers. These basic generic relationships facilitate the understanding of many different tracers used in various ways.

As an introduction to perfusion tracers, the first part of this chapter will review the basic properties and cellular uptake mechanisms of a few of the single-photon emission computed tomography (SPECT) myocardial perfusion agents. Next, we will present the "bare bones" of tracer extraction, retention, and recirculation. We will employ a common solute absorption model to help understand the relationship of tracer extraction to capillary perfusion and use a simplified compartmental exchange model to help understand tracer redistribution. Comparing model predictions to experimental data will add some fascinating light to the mechanism of myocardial vasoregulation. Following this introduction, and in the light of our improved understanding of tracer kinetics, we will discuss specific clinical applications of the tracers commonly used for myocardial imaging.

CELLULAR UPTAKE OF MYOCARDIAL PERFUSION AGENTS

Before delving into a modeling approach to better understand the complex behavior of a myocardial perfusion imaging agent after intravenous injection, we will briefly review the physical and/or chemical properties of a few classes of these agents that play a role in their cellular uptake in the myocardium.

Thallium-201

Thallium-201 (^{201}Tl) is a radioactive potassium analog. The initial myocardial uptake of ^{201}Tl is dependent upon myocardial blood flow and its first-pass extraction fraction, which is approximately 85% under resting flow conditions.[1,2] At higher flow rates, such as those obtained during pharmacologic vasodilation, the extraction of ^{201}Tl is not linear with respect to flow.[3] The plateau in extraction results in an underestimation of the true maximal flow. This phenomenon is true of all diffusible flow tracers and will be discussed in detail in the next section of this chapter.

The intracellular uptake of ^{201}Tl predominantly involves active exchange across the sarcolemmal membrane of the myocytes via the Na^+/K^+ adenosine triphosphate (ATP) transport system.[4] Because this system is energy dependent, thallium transport can only occur in viable myocardium. Once inside the myocyte, ^{201}Tl is not bound intracellularly and can diffuse back out into the circulation. As will be discussed in detail later, these uptake and redistribution kinetic properties form the basis of clinical assessment of myocardial perfusion and viability using ^{201}Tl. Although the introduction of ^{201}Tl in the mid-1970s represented a major advance in nuclear cardiology, its physical properties are not ideal for gamma camera imaging. The low-energy 69- to 80-keV x-ray photopeak can result in attenuation artifacts and the relatively long 73-hour half-life limits the maximal dose that can be safely administered.

Monovalent Cationic Technetium-99m-Labeled Tracers

Technetium-99m (^{99m}Tc) is a generator-produced isotope that is readily available and has a number of advantages over ^{201}Tl for gamma camera imaging. The higher-energy 140-keV principle photopeak is ideal for detection using standard collimated gamma cameras with less attenuation, and its short 6-hour half-life allows for a higher administered dose yielding improved count statistics.

Over the years, there have been a number of ^{99m}Tc-labeled myocardial perfusion imaging agents that have been investigated as replacements for ^{201}Tl. The most successful ones to date are the lipophilic monovalent cationic agents, ^{99m}Tc-sestamibi (sestamibi, Cardiolite) and ^{99m}Tc-tetrofosmin (tetrofosmin, Myoview), that are now widely used for clinical studies. Following an intravenous injection, the first-pass extraction fractions of sestamibi and tetrofosmin are approximately 65% and 54%, respectively, under basal resting flow conditions.[5,6] Because of their lower extraction fractions compared with ^{201}Tl, the plateau in tracer uptake observed during hyperemia occurs at lower flow rates. The effect of this "roll-off" in extraction at lower flow rates is to diminish the relative difference in tracer activities between high-flow regions and those myocardial regions subtended by a coronary stenosis, making it more difficult to detect milder stenoses.

Although these agents are members of two distinct chemical classes of compounds, isonitriles and diphosphines, respectively, they share several common properties. Unlike ^{201}Tl, which utilizes a specific membrane-active transporter, these tracers are passively drawn across the sarcolemmal and mitochondrial membranes along a large electronegative transmembrane potential gradient, owing to their lipophilicity and positive charge.[7] Once inside the mitochondria, these cationic tracers are tightly bound by the potential gradient such that there is a very slow net efflux resulting in prolonged myocardial retention times. Although ATP is not directly required for the intracellular sequestration of cationic tracers, as it is for ^{201}Tl, the influx and retention of these tracers are energy dependent because the presence of a normal electronegative transmembrane gradient is required. With irreversible injury, the mitochondrial and sarcolemmal membranes are depolarized, and the uptake of these cationic tracers is impaired.[8] Accordingly, like ^{201}Tl, the cationic ^{99m}Tc-labeled agents can be used to assess myocardial viability.

In addition to the lower plateau in extraction mentioned, another disadvantage to both sestamibi and tetrofosmin is the problem of photon scatter from the adjacent liver that can interfere with the interpretation of myocardial perfusion defects, particularly in the inferior left ventricular wall. Accordingly, there has been renewed interest in recent years to design improved

cationic ^{99m}Tc-labeled tracers that exhibit more rapid liver clearance. ^{99m}Tc-(N)(PNP5)(DBODC5)$^+$ (DBODC5) is a lipophilic nitride that is rapidly taken up and retained by the myocardium in a manner that is mechanistically similar to sestamibi and tetrofosmin. However, studies in both rats and dogs demonstrated that DBODC5 cleared more rapidly from the liver than either of these other cationic tracers, with virtually no liver activity observed after only 1 hour.[9,10] The first-pass extraction fraction of DBODC5 is intermediate to that of sestamibi and tetrofosmin.[10] Although there is no improvement in the ability of DBODC5 to track myocardial blood flow at hyperemic flow rates, its more favorable biodistribution properties offer a potential advantage that warrants further investigation.

Another new lipophilic cationic tracer with improved biodistribution and very rapid liver clearance is ^{99m}Tc-[N(MPO)(PNP5)]$^+$ (MPO). The myocardial uptake of MPO in Sprague Dawley rats was reported to be between that of sestamibi and DBODC5 over 2 hours.[11] Interestingly, the heart-liver ratio of MPO at 30 minutes after injection was more than twice that of DBODC5 and approximately 4 times higher than that of sestamibi.[11] With such rapid liver clearance, clinically useful images might be obtainable as early as 15 minutes post injection. At the present time, the first-pass extraction fraction studies have not been conducted using MPO.

Neutral Lipophilic Tracers

^{99m}Tc-teboroxime (teboroxime) is a member of a class of neutral lipophilic molecules known as *BATOs* (*B*oronic acid *A*dducts of *T*echnetium di*O*xime). After intravenous injection, the initial instantaneous uptake of teboroxime is high, with a first-pass extraction fraction of approximately 90%—higher than even ^{201}Tl.[12,13] However, unlike the cationic ^{99m}Tc-labeled myocardial perfusion tracers discussed earlier that are retained in the myocardium, teboroxime exhibits rapid flow-dependent myocardial clearance in under 10 minutes. Thus, although the myocardial extraction fraction that is observed immediately after injection is very high, the rapid clearance of this tracer results in a loss of defect contrast within the first 5 minutes post injection.[14] Additionally, because the myocardial clearance rate of teboroxime is flow dependent, with slower clearance from ischemic versus normally perfused zones, the differential clearance rates give the scintigraphic equivalent of "redistribution," with an apparent filling-in of the initial perfusion defects over time, as is observed with ^{201}Tl.[15] The mechanism for such rapid clearance is that teboroxime is believed not to cross the sarcolemmal membrane into the intracellular space of the myocyte, remaining instead within the intravascular space in association with the endothelial layer.[16] Furthermore, its myocardial uptake is passive, not dependent on either active transport or other energy-dependent processes. Thus, teboroxime is considered to be a pure perfusion tracer.

Although teboroxime was approved for clinical imaging at the same time as sestamibi, its rapid dynamic myocardial clearance kinetics proved difficult to image using the relatively slow, single-head gamma cameras that were standard in the early 1990s. With the exciting new generation of fast cardiac SPECT instrumentation that has recently become available on the market, there may be renewed interest in this tracer in the future.

Another neutral lipophilic perfusion tracer that has undergone Phase III clinical testing is ^{99m}Tc-N-NOET (NOET). Like teboroxime, NOET exhibits a first-pass extraction fraction that is higher than either sestamibi or tetrofosmin, with flow-dependent differential clearance of the tracer from the myocardium.[17,18] Because of the differential clearance from ischemic versus normal zones, NOET has been shown to undergo apparent redistribution like teboroxime, albeit at a slower rate.[18,19] Another similarity between NOET and teboroxime involves their mechanism of localization in the myocardium. NOET is also believed to remain within the intravascular space in association with the endothelial layer.[20] Because of its accessibility, NOET clearance can be affected by a host of intravascular factors. Experimental studies demonstrated that the myocardial clearance rate of NOET could be accelerated not only by increasing the flow rate but also by elevating the blood lipid concentration.[16,21] Like teboroxime, the uptake and retention of NOET does not involve active or energy-dependent processes, and thus it would also be considered a pure perfusion tracer.

In summary, the advent of the ^{99m}Tc-labeled myocardial perfusion imaging agents, particularly the lipophilic cationic tracers, sestamibi and tetrofosmin, represented a major advance by virtue of their superior imaging properties compared with [201]Tl. Some aspects of these tracers may not be ideal, but in general they have shown excellent diagnostic accuracy and have fueled the growth of the field of nuclear cardiology for nearly 20 years. New SPECT perfusion tracers that exhibit both improved myocardial first-pass extraction fraction and more favorable biodistribution properties are clearly warranted.

MODELING TRACER EXTRACTION

If a tracer is injected intravenously, the number of tracer atoms passing through a capillary bed will be proportional to the fraction of total cardiac output passing through the capillary bed. If all the tracer atoms were extracted in a single pass through the capillary bed, the number of tracer atoms per unit volume of tissue would then be proportional to the fraction of cardiac output perfusing the unit volume of tissue. The only tracers that approximate this ideal are microspheres.

The tracers used for clinical imaging of myocardial blood flow are not completely extracted. For these tracers, the fraction of tracer extracted on passing through a capillary bed depends on the blood flow through the capillary bed. A model based on the work of Gosselin and Stibitz [22] provides insight into this process. The model is that of a diffusible tracer traveling through a cylindrical capillary. The tracer can diffuse outward from the blood across the capillary endothelium, but it can also diffuse back into the blood from outside the capillary endothelium. The outward and back-diffusion coefficients can be different. The extraction coefficient reflects the net loss in tracer concentration between the arterial and venous ends of the capillary. This leads to a tracer "extraction fraction" of the form:

$$1 - e^{-\frac{PS}{b}} \qquad (1)$$

where PS is a product of capillary permeability and surface area, and b is the capillary blood flow. The relationship between blood flow and tracer extraction predicted by this model is shown graphically in Figure 1-1. The top curve with $PS = 2$ would represent a tracer with high first-pass extraction, such as [201]Tl. The lower curve with $PS = 1$ would represent a tracer with lower first-pass extraction, similar to sestamibi and tetrofosmin. The term *first-pass extraction* is often used to characterize radionuclide tracers, but it is not often carefully defined. Since the extracted fraction of tracer is flow dependent, the *first-pass extraction* indicates the fraction of extracted tracer measured at baseline resting blood flow. In Figure 1-1, the first-pass extraction of the two tracers shown would be about 86% for the upper line and about 64% for the lower line.

The amount of tracer taken up by the myocardium shortly after bolus injection is the product of extraction fraction and myocardial blood flow per unit volume, denoted by the letter b. This product is:

$$\textit{Myocardial Extraction} \propto b\left(1 - e^{-\frac{PS}{b}}\right) \qquad (2)$$

Although the equation was derived for solute exchange in a single capillary, it can be shown that the functional form remains unchanged for a generalized distribution of capillaries if the parameters are taken to represent the averages over the entire capillary distribution. The curve with the functional form shown has been ubiquitous in representing myocardial uptake as a function of myocardial blood flow. Figure 1-2 shows

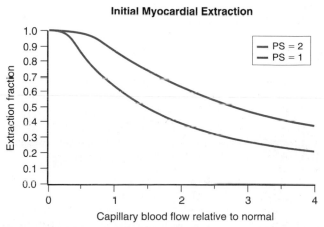

Initial Myocardial Extraction

Figure 1-1 Tracer extraction fraction as predicted by the Gosselin and Stibitz model. Curves are shown for PS = 1, representing a tracer with first-pass extraction similar to the molecular Tc-99 m tracers, and PS = 2, representing a tracer with first-pass extraction of Tl-201.

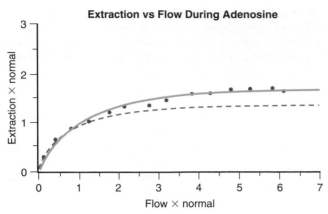

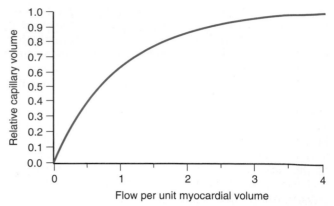

Figure 1-2 The *solid curve* shows the basic Gosselin and Stibitz model using the value of PS that produces the best fit for the extraction-versus-flow data. The *dashed curve* uses the value of PS that produces the best prediction of first-pass extraction. The model cannot simultaneously predict both sets of data using the same PS value. This indicates a flaw in the model.

Figure 1-3 Relationship between the fraction of open capillary volume and myocardial blood flow per unit of myocardial volume.

some experimental data of sestamibi extraction versus blood flow. The solid line of Figure 1-2 has the functional form of Equation 2. It fits the experimental data quite well if the PS coefficient is chosen empirically to best fit the data. However, if we substitute the PS coefficient that best agrees with the first-pass extraction data, it results in the dashed line of Figure 1-2 and produces a poor fit for the flow-versus-extraction curve. The dashed line predicts a more extreme reduction of tracer extraction with increasing myocardial blood than experimentally observed.

The same PS product should predict both the measured first-pass extraction coefficient and the flow-versus-extraction curve. The fact that it does not indicates that something is wrong with the model. A possible problem with the simple Gosselin and Stibitz model is that it does not account for myocardial flow regulation by opening and closing of capillary channels. Selective opening and closing of parallel capillary channels is thought to be an important mechanism to regulate capillary resistance and myocardial blood flow. This has been experimentally demonstrated.[23,24] Further evidence for the role of capillary closure has been more recently found in the context of contrast echocardiography[25] and for sestamibi perfusion measurements in the dog model.[26]

To account for the effect of variable capillary volumes, we wish to extend the basic model as follows: The first factor in Eq. 2 is replaced by F, which represents flow per unit myocardial volume. The term b in the exponential represents flow per unit of *open* capillary volume. We now introduce a new relationship:

$$\frac{F}{b} = 1 - e^{-F} \qquad (3)$$

Equation 3 allows for flow in the open capillaries to be different from flow per unit myocardial volume determined by the arterial supply vessels. Equation 3 further introduces the assumption that capillary blood volume

decreases with decreasing flow due to capillary closure, and it increases to some maximum value when all the capillary channels are fully utilized at high flow. Figure 1-3 shows the relative capillary volume assumed by Eq. 3. This is in qualitative accord with the observations of Wu et al.[23] The exact way that capillary volume changes in the course of vasoregulation is unknown. Our purpose here is limited to that of showing what effect variable capillary volume would have on tracer extraction.

The effect of capillary closure can be seen in Figure 1-4. The curves of first-pass extraction become less blood-flow dependent. The first-pass extraction fraction at low flow is less than would be predicted by the basic model of Gosselin and Stibitz,[22] and the decrease of extracted fraction with increasing blood flow is less severe. The curves of Figure 1-4 are plotted for PS = 1.6 and 3.1, which represent the values that fit the experimentally measured extraction fractions of 0.64 and 0.86 for sestamibi and ^{201}Tl, respectively. These values, obtained from first-pass extraction data, were used to compute the myocardial uptake-versus-flow curves, and

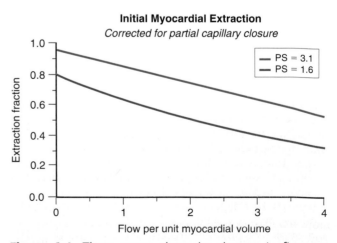

Figure 1-4 These curves show the changes in first-pass extraction caused by the introduction of variable capillary volume as assumed in Figure 1-2. Curves are for values of PS = 1.6 and 3.1, which predict first-pass extractions of 0.64 and 0.86, respectively, for Tc-sestamibi and Tl-201.

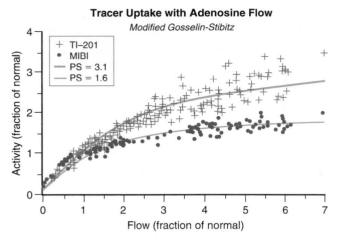

Figure 1-5 Tracer uptake versus myocardial blood flow using the modified model for Tc-sestamibi (PS = 1.6) and Tl 201 (PS = 3.1). Data obtained from an animal model. The curves now fit the experimental data, using the same PS values as needed to predict the first-pass extraction. The modified model is self-consistent.

those curves are plotted with experimental data from Glover in Figure 1-5. The predicted curves fit quite well to the experimental data. Thus, by including the effect of variable capillary blood volume, we are able to simultaneously predict all the experimental data from the same PS coefficient. The modified model is self-consistent, indicating that it is a better representation of reality.

The curves of Figure 1-5 represent a transition from a low-flow state, where tracer extraction is flow limited and therefore proportional to flow, to a high-flow state, where extraction is membrane-diffusion limited and therefore not dependent on flow. Another way of thinking of this is that the tracer spends less time in the capillary at higher flows and consequently has a lower probability of being extracted in a single pass through the capillary. At sufficiently low flows, most of the tracer atoms are extracted, and the tracer acts more like an ideal microsphere. If there is substantial closure of capillary pathways as flow decreases, the increased extraction at low flow is less marked, and tracer extraction remains linear over a somewhat wider range of flow. The introduction of capillary closure was essential in order that the model could simultaneously predict the first-pass extraction fractions and fit the uptake-versus-flow data. We note, however, that if we had modeled the system by having flow entirely controlled by the fraction of open capillaries, the flow-extraction curves would have been linear, and this is clearly not so. Thus, we conclude that there is both capillary flow modulation and partial capillary closure at work simultaneously.

The flow dependence of myocardial tracer uptake has more than theoretical relevance. It limits the sensitivity for a given tracer to detect coronary artery disease (CAD). It has significant implications for pharmacologic stress agents and may be the determining factor in choosing the best tracer for a given circumstance. The flattening of the curves of tracer uptake versus

myocardial blood flow means that the tracer defect will be much less than the actual blood-flow disparity. Underestimation of flow disparity will be particularly severe when we compare a viable myocardial region with limited flow reserve with an assumed normal myocardial region. The study by Glover et al.[3] showed that obstructions that only limit flow reserve can give minimal tracer defect contrast despite maximum vasodilatation with adenosine. Tracers with higher first-pass extraction will track blood flows over a wider range compared to tracers of lower first-pass extraction. This does not apply to scar. Tracers with different extraction coefficients will indicate myocardial scar with equal contrast.

TRACER RETENTION

All tracers used for myocardial perfusion imaging are extracted in a blood-flow-dependent manner similar to that described. Generally, the tracer must also be retained in the myocardium long enough to acquire an image of the tracer distribution. As reviewed in detail earlier, myocardial perfusion tracers differ greatly in their mechanism of retention. [201]Tl, being a potassium analog, enters myocardial cells through active channels and equilibrates with the intracellular cytosolic potassium pool. However, because it is not bound intracellularly, ^{201}Tl is free to back-diffuse out of the myocardial cells and reenter the circulating blood pool where it can undergo further exchange in the myocardium or other tissue beds. Because 60% of the intracellular transport of ^{201}Tl requires ATP,[4] only viable myocardial cells that maintain a transmembrane potassium gradient will retain [201]Tl. This feature makes [201]Tl a useful myocardial cell viability marker.

In contrast to ^{201}Tl, the lipophilic monovalent cationic compounds are taken up and bound intracellularly within the mitochondrial compartment because of their net positive charge. Accordingly, the net efflux of these tracers is very slow, and they exhibit prolonged myocardial retention and minimal redistribution. By virtue of being bound by the mitochondrial membrane potential, these agents share with ^{201}Tl the property of being retained only in viable myocardium.

The neutral class of agents represented by teboroxime and NOET are highly diffusible and highly extracted in passing through a capillary bed. However, because there is no active mechanism of retention, and because these molecules are believed to remain within the intravascular (or possibly interstitial) spaces, they can rapidly diffuse back into the bloodstream and be carried away. Because washout is so rapid, these tracers are not good for static imaging. Owing to the flow dependence of the myocardial washout rate of these neutral diffusible tracers, both exhibit differential washout rates from ischemic versus normally perfused myocardium; this results in an apparent "redistribution" whereby defects appear to resolve over time. Furthermore, because of differential washout, it may be possible to employ dynamic imaging to measure regional washout rates that may provide additional blood-flow information for diagnosis of CAD. Finally, because the uptake and retention mechanisms of these neutral tracers do not require active transport or energy-dependent processes, they are expected to be pure perfusion markers.

REDISTRIBUTION

The Mechanism

Most myocardial tracers are not fixed in the myocardium but have some intrinsic rate of washout. If the tracer were injected only in the myocardium, its washout rate would reflect myocardial blood flow, with higher blood flow encouraging more rapid tracer washout.[15,21,27] Unfortunately, the tracer washout following intravenous systemic injection will have no simple relationship to myocardial blood flow. Following a systemic tracer injection, no more than 3% to 5% of the tracer is delivered to the myocardium. The rest is distributed through all of the other body compartments. After initial extraction, the tracer will start to exchange between the various compartments. The amount of "washout" from the myocardium depends not only on how much tracer is leaving the myocardium but also on how much is being continuously accumulated by exchange from other compartments. The net washout, which is all we can observe, cannot be expected to be simply related to myocardial blood flow.

The process of redistribution has been a central issue in the detection of myocardial ischemia and viability. A compartmental exchange model will help to gain a better understanding of the redistribution process. We will tailor the model specifically for ^{201}Tl for two reasons. First, it is the most important example of using redistribution as part of clinical practice. Second, it is an unusually simple example for multicompartmental models. It is simple by virtue of the fact that the extraction process is rapid, the membrane exchange process is intermediate (about 1 hour), and the systemic excretion process is long (greater than 10 hours). Under these circumstances, the differential equations describing the process can be effectively decoupled to result in a very simple closed analytic solution of multiple exponentials with coefficients that can be intuitively understood. In keeping with our desire to not get bogged down in mathematics, let us again provide some graphic solutions.

Figure 1-6 shows the myocardial uptake and washout of an exchangeable tracer that is injected intravenously. The curves are based on parameters that reflect ^{201}Tl. Specifically, a blood clearance half-time of 1 to 5 minutes is assumed, a systemic excretion of about 10 hours is assumed, and the intrinsic myocardial membrane transport coefficient is taken as 0.01, representing a half-time of 69 minutes, in accordance with experimental data.[28] In words, the curves show rapid early myocardial uptake roughly proportional to myocardial perfusion. Blood levels of the tracer fall rapidly as it is extracted by the heart as well as all the other systemic compartments. After initial extraction, the tracer molecules are slowly released back into the blood, maintaining a nearly constant low-level blood concentration of tracer. The subsequent exchange of tracer between blood

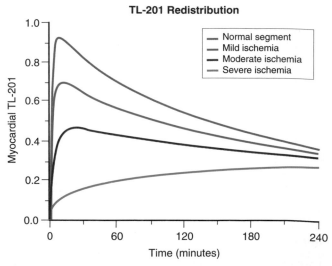

Figure 1-6 Multicompartmental model of Tl-201 including extraction, redistribution, and systemic excretion. Myocardial tracer uptake is shown for normal flow and transiently reduced flows to 75%, 50%, and 25% of normal, respectively.

and myocardial cells continues until an equilibrium point is reached, where the myocardium loses one tracer molecule for each new molecule it picks up from the blood. This exchange equilibrium is not dependent on blood flow, but only on the relative concentrations of intravascular and extravascular tracer molecules. The level of net tracer uptake at equilibrium is determined by the residual blood concentration and by the magnitude of the intracellular/extracellular concentration gradient supported by the membrane potentials or by active membrane transport.

We can summarize the clinically relevant parts of this process as follows: (1) The initial myocardial extraction reflects the distribution of blood flow at the time of injection, and (2) the delayed uptake after equilibrium is reached is flow independent but reflects an intact myocardial cell membrane and membrane potential and is thus a marker of cell viability. This is the principle behind redistribution imaging. The fact that delayed uptake is flow independent means that if a myocardial segment is chronically hypoperfused, even when injection is performed at rest, redistribution can still occur. Redistribution in chronically hypoperfused regions is a clinically useful feature of ^{201}Tl.[29] Sestamibi and tetrofosmin are more tightly bound, so myocardial washout is slower and systemic blood clearance is also greater with these tracers. Therefore, while there is the potential for some redistribution, it is too slow and of too little magnitude to be clinically useful.

Redistribution Versus Persistent Defect

Flow tracers that are trapped by membrane potentials are not retained by infarcted myocardium, and the infarcted tissue will have a negligible tracer concentration. However, most perfusion defects are not samples of totally infarcted myocardium but consist partly of infarcted myocardium mixed with normal (or ischemic) myocardium. In addition, the infarct borders are usually

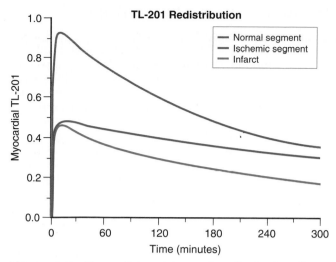

Figure 1-7 Myocardial uptake and redistribution for a normal segment, a segment mixed with half normal myocardium and half scar, and a viable segment with flow reduced to 50% of normal.

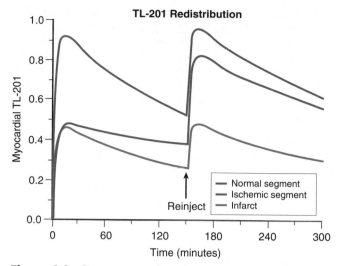

Figure 1-8 Compartmental exchange model of myocardial tracer activity showing redistribution and the effect of reinjection at 150 minutes.

ragged and ill-defined. Since the resolution of our imaging systems is not high enough to resolve the details of the infarct, the infarct will usually be sampled along with noninfarcted tissue.

Consider the tracer uptake and washout curves in Figure 1-7, comparing one myocardial segment, which is a mixture of half infarct and half normal, to another myocardial segment, which is all viable but has 50% reduced blood flow. The half-infarcted defect will continuously have half the uptake of the normal sample. The ischemic segment starts with half-normal uptake but returns to normal by redistribution. Examination of the curves in Figure 1-7 shows that at any one time, the difference between the fixed defect and the redistributing defect is surprisingly small. The "signal" (representing the difference between the two curves) is weak and comparable to the "noise" (representing the error of measurement) involved in real clinical imaging. This means that under the best of circumstances, differentiation of partly infarcted from moderately ischemic myocardium will be a subtle differentiation subject to some uncertainty. We will return to this point when we discuss reinjection.

Reinjection (See Chapter 37)

Redistribution of ^{201}Tl is a marker of myocardial viability, but in some cases there appears to be little or no reversibility in viable segments.[30] It has been reported that reinjection of ^{201}Tl at rest will expose more redistribution than delayed imaging alone and that this will enhance viability detection.[31] We can model this process. Figure 1-8 shows the same comparison of a myocardial segment, half normal and half infarct, with another myocardial segment that is transiently ischemic with half-normal tracer uptake at stress. We have assumed that the blood flow returns to normal following stress, and reinjection of half the initial dose takes place at 150 minutes following stress injection. Figure 1-8 points out that tracer reinjection does two things: First, it adds

more tracer to both the normal and abnormal segments. Second, it adds more redistribution—the sudden equivalent of about 2 more hours of redistribution. Figure 1-9 summarizes data from an animal study in which a very severe perfusion defect (resulting from mild subendocardial infarction and surrounding ischemia) was followed for 3 hours of redistribution and then imaged again after reinjection. We see in this experiment a severe defect with slow redistribution and a sudden addition of a bit more reversibility upon reinjection. The change following reinjection is predictable—the equivalent of about 2 more hours of redistribution—but the amount of additional redistribution induced by reinjection is not dramatic.

Neither the model in Figure 1-8 nor the animal data of Figure 1-9 show an absence of redistribution in a defect that reverses upon reinjection. However, the juxtaposition of initial and delayed images with reinjection

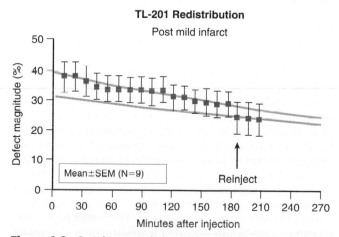

Figure 1-9 Serial myocardial uptake measurements of defect to normal ratio following Tl-201 injection in an animal model of severe ischemia with small subendocardial infarction. Reinjection was performed after 180 minutes.

images sometimes creates the appearance of a patently fixed defect that suddenly reverses upon reinjection. There is no physiologically logical model for that and no quantitative measurements that confirm that a truly fixed defect would spontaneously become reversible upon reinjection. Scintiphoto images, however, do occasionally appear to show a fixed defect that reverses only after reinjection.

There are two reasons that scintiphoto images can give an amplified perception of reversibility following reinjection. Most images, particularly those of SPECT slices, have some background suppression. Severe defects that have some tracer uptake and some redistribution may have too little tracer to be visible above the background suppression level. The addition of more tracer activity by reinjection can lift the level of activity in these regions over the suppression level, resulting in the abrupt appearance of significant activity in these regions that previously appeared devoid of significant tracer uptake. A second reason we might miss redistribution has to do with sampling statistics. The amount of "tracer activity" in a sampled myocardial segment is not the ground truth. Rather, it is an estimate based on a sample, and this estimate is represented as an intensity level in an image. In SPECT images, the intensity level of a pixel representing myocardial tracer uptake is computed from a large number of statistically noisy samples. The presence of statistical noise means that if we acquire two images while the myocardial tracer uptake is identical, the uptake represented to us by the images will be different to the extent of the statistical sampling uncertainty. In comparing images from only two samples, the amount of redistribution will be underestimated half the time simply by virtue of sampling error. If we set aside all of the image examples for which redistribution was shown (including the statistical overestimates) and select those examples for which redistribution was not demonstrated (including the statistical underestimates), then a third sample will have a high statistical probability (around 50%) of showing "reversibility" upon resampling, without reinjection. If we had performed reinjection in the interim, we would have attributed the additional reversibility to reinjection. This is a classic example of a statistical phenomenon called *regression to the mean*. The indication of additional redistribution is real but not caused by reinjection.

In the last paragraph, we have argued that additional reversibility upon reinjection will be observed as a result of nonlinear count representation in images and also as a result of sampling statistics. For the most part, however, these situations arise from underestimates of redistribution (either by imaging problems or sampling error), and an additional imaging procedure following reinjection will tend to correct the problem. Thus, reinjection followed by additional imaging can identify more viable segments than were identified by delayed imaging alone. There are logical reasons for this that do not require us to postulate that the ischemic muscle has some mysterious affinity for freshly reinjected tracer after refusing to extract that which had been previously injected, or that redistribution becomes physiologically suspended and then restarted by reinjection.

Tracers That Do Not Redistribute

All tracers must redistribute to some extent; it is a question of degree. The ^{99m}Tc-labeled tracers that employ a cationic lipophilic molecule are more firmly trapped by membrane potentials after they diffuse out of the vascular bed. This means the intrinsic transmembrane transport half-time is long, and the time to reach exchange equilibrium is correspondingly long. This time for ^{201}Tl is on the order of 1 hour. That means that half of all the remaining possible redistribution will take place each hour. Thus, redistribution times of 2 to 4 hours represent two to four half-times in the equilibration process and are adequate for us to see most of the significant redistribution. The lipophilic cationic molecules as represented by sestamibi and tetrofosmin appear to be bound well enough that the exchange times are an order of magnitude longer. This puts the intrinsic transport half-time on the order of 10 hours, and the corresponding time for redistribution from a systemic injection would be 20 to 40 hours. Since the ^{99m}Tc decay half-time is 6 hours, these isotopes decay before they redistribute. We should expect some redistribution, but the amount is probably not enough to be clinically useful within the time frame during which there is enough tracer remaining for adequate imaging.

Reverse Redistribution

We occasionally see a focal defect in a stress image that appears to be more severe on rest images. Additionally, we sometimes see a defect on rest images that was not seen on stress images. This phenomenon has been called *reverse redistribution*. The kinetic transport models leave us with no logical explanation for a defect to grow larger in delayed images. It is not logical for the myocardium to initially extract a normal amount of tracer (implying normal blood flow and normal metabolic extraction) and then excessively lose tracer to grow a defect in the delayed images. There is no model for tracer uptake and washout curves that cross each other. This leaves us with a puzzle: explaining the observations of "reverse redistribution." There are a number of ways to create the appearance of reverse redistribution. For example:

1. Motion artifact on the rest images.
2. Tissue attenuation artifact on the rest images caused by position shifts.
3. Misalignment on SPECT slices such that the rest image slice cuts through the edge of a fixed defect, whereas the stress slice misses the edge of the defect.
4. Mild fixed defects can appear more severe on rest images if the image scale factor is changed. This can happen due to tracer washout or because of higher visceral activity in rest images that can set the maximum image scale to a higher value and reduce the relative intensity of uptake in the defect region.

All of these situations are common, so the appearance of reverse redistribution must be at least partly the result of image artifact. One possible situation that may create the appearance of reverse redistribution is the result of comparing an infarct to an ischemic segment, with the mistaken assumption that there is a normal myocardial segment for reference. Suppose that we had an ischemic segment and a segment that was partly infarcted as shown in Figure 1-7. Now suppose further that the normal segment (the solid line) was not visible. This could happen in a case of diffuse multiple-vessel disease so severe that there is no normally perfused segment for reference. The tracer then redistributes into the ischemic segments so that they have more uptake than the partly infarcted segments. This can create the appearance of a defect (the infarct) in the delayed or rest images that was not apparent in the stress images.

When there is no physiologically reasonable explanation for the appearance of reverse redistribution, our experience has been that it is one of the several artifacts mentioned. We have found no convincing evidence for a more mysterious explanation and indeed find that the vast majority of apparent reverse redistribution (or "reverse reversibility" in the case of sestamibi and tetrofosmin) is caused by one of the several artifacts.

DETECTION OF CORONARY ARTERY DISEASE

We have shown that highly extractable tracers are extracted in proportion to the fraction of total cardiac output passing through the capillary bed. Once the tracer leaves the capillary bed, it must be trapped by some mechanism, or it will rapidly diffuse back out of the myocardium. ^{201}Tl is an example of a potassium-like tracer that will be retained within the myocyte. At equilibrium, the tracer will be concentrated within the cytosolic compartment relative to the blood pool, so that the intracellular concentration will be much greater than the blood pool concentration. There is a continuous exchange between intracellular and extracellular ions, giving rise to the process of redistribution. The cationic molecular tracers labeled with ^{99m}Tc behave in a similar manner, except that they are bound more firmly, purportedly within the mitochondria. These tracers are exchanged more slowly, and because they decay more rapidly than they exchange, redistribution is insignificant.

None of these tracers is completely extracted in a single capillary passage. The first-pass extraction coefficients vary from about 54% for tetrofosmin,[6] to about 65% for sestamibi,[5] and about 85% to 88% for ^{201}Tl.[1] Tracers with lower extraction fraction are more blood-flow dependent, with lower extraction at higher blood flow. The blood-flow dependence of tracer extraction places a limitation on our ability to detect CAD at the level where it causes only moderate reduction of the coronary reserve capacity. When comparing a myocardial segment with greatly enhanced flow due to stress or vasodilator to another segment with less enhanced flow due to a flow-limiting stenosis, the tracers will greatly underestimate the flow disparity. This effect is related to the extraction coefficient, and thus a tracer with higher extraction coefficient will be more sensitive for

detection of mild flow-limiting stenoses. Detection of myocardial infarction or myocardial regions with severe reduction of flow will be similar for tracers having different extraction fractions.

MYOCARDIAL VIABILITY (See Chapters 37–39)

The cationic tracers that are retained by membrane potentials will be viability agents in the sense that significant tracer uptake requires both delivery, implying perfusion, and retention, implying enough cellular integrity to generate membrane potentials. This includes ^{201}Tl, sestamibi, and tetrofosmin. In fact, these tracers could be viewed as nearly ideal "viability" markers. Substantial tracer uptake is equivalent to substantial residual myocardial viability. Viability alone, however, is not enough to answer the clinical question of whether improved perfusion can improve myocardial function. When myocardial function is depressed, the demonstration of resting ischemia leads to the logical assumption that function is depressed due to ischemia and should improve if adequate perfusion is restored. Rest ischemia can be demonstrated by redistribution of ^{201}Tl following injection at rest. It should be understood that reinjection will not be helpful following a rest injection. Following a rest injection, any redistribution that had taken place would simply be obscured by a second rest injection. Sestamibi and similar compounds do not redistribute sufficiently for redistribution to be of clinical value.

We can, however, use both ^{201}Tl and sestamibi equally to demonstrate substantial tracer uptake by a myocardial segment. Substantial uptake of these tracers indicates viability. If a segment is deemed viable by evidence of tracer uptake but is not contracting, we may reasonably expect that the myocardium is stunned or hibernating and that improving perfusion to the myocardium could improve its function. Thus, we are led to another viability tool. If we observe significant tracer uptake in a myocardial region that has discordantly poor contractile function, this suggests a favorable outcome following repair of obstructed supply arteries.

The absence of uptake of these tracers indicates the absence of membrane function or mitochondrial membrane potential. This essentially is equivalent to the absence of restorable myocardial viability. Thus, the absence of myocardial uptake of monovalent cationic tracers is a reliable predictor of non-recovery of function.

ACUTE CORONARY SYNDROME

One additional situation of clinical importance might well be considered in the light of kinetic models. Acute myocardial infarction and possibly acute coronary syndrome that allows reperfusion following severe ischemic insult may induce partial capillary closure, either due to mechanical pressure of intracellular edema or by disabling normal vasoregulatory function. It is certainly conceivable in this case that total myocardial blood flow through an epicardial vessel can return to normal but be non-uniformly distributed through capillary channels, so that some capillaries have very high blood flow while blood flow in other capillary channels is severely decreased.

In the situation described, the actual capillary tracer extraction will be less than predicted by the relationship of capillary extraction to epicardial flow as predicted in cases of normal vasoregulation and normal capillary flow distribution. Therefore, there will be a relative tracer deficit even after the myocardial blood flow in epicardial vessels has been restored to normal values. This could account for the exaggeration of a tracer defect or the appearance of a "fixed" defect in the region of myocardium that has been recently ischemic but retains significant residual viability and potential for recovery of perfusion and function.

REDUCED FLOW RESERVE AND "BALANCED ISCHEMIA" (See Chapter 23)

Most myocardial tracer imaging performed today is limited to the determination of relative myocardial blood flow. The infusion of a coronary vasodilator works only if it can increase flow in normal myocardial segments. Then, myocardial segments supplied with partially obstructed vessels and impaired flow reserve will have less tracer uptake and appear as "defects" relative to myocardial segments with normal flow reserve. Exercise stress as well is expected to cause flow differential due to increased flow to myocardium served by normal vessels and failure to increase flow in regions served by vessels compromised by flow-limiting lesions.

Myocardial flow reserve may be decreased, however, by several mechanisms other than discrete atherosclerotic plaques. Flow resistance in major coronary vessels could be increased due to diffusely distributed disease. Left ventricular hypertrophy is known to decrease flow reserve. In fact, anything that impairs the mechanical efficiency, increases oxygen demand, or impairs the vasoregulatory function will reduce myocardial reserve capacity. Patients with metabolic syndrome have various degrees of reduced flow reserve. In such cases, the ability to detect discrete lesions by observing defects in relative blood flow may be reduced or eliminated. The cause of this is simply that while stress does not cause increased flow in vessels with discrete flow-limiting lesions, neither does it cause increased flow to other parts of the heart served by vessels without discrete flow-limiting lesions. Thus, the flow differential that we use as indicator of a flow-limiting lesion is reduced or eliminated.

Another possible failure to detect CAD is the case of balanced multivessel disease, often noted as *balanced ischemia*. This situation is well known and often quoted. However, situations of discrete plaques that reach a truly balanced state of flow obstruction uniformly throughout the entire myocardium are statistically improbable and probably are not encountered frequently in clinical practice. Alternatively, the situations of diffusely reduced myocardial flow reserve for all the other reasons suggested in the previous paragraph are quite common and undoubtedly exist in a significant fraction of today's referral population. These limitations could be obviated by adding the ability to measure relative coronary flow reserve or by measurements of absolute blood flow. The absence of currently available techniques for doing this attests to the difficulty of developing and perfecting these measurements.

SUMMARY

In the preceding, we examined a model of tracer extraction. The model shows very nonlinear extraction of tracers that are not completely extracted, with higher extraction at low flow and extraction becoming nearly independent of flow when myocardial blood flow is elevated. This basic model was in qualitative accord with experimental data, but in order to make the model consistently fit the available experimental data, it was necessary to add the assumption of capillary recruitment with increasing flow and capillary decruitment with decreasing flow. With that addition, the model is in excellent agreement with experimental data and allows us to extend our understanding of tracer kinetics and additionally sheds some light on the mechanisms of myocardial flow regulation.

The clinical implication of flow-dependent tracer extraction is that most existing flow tracers significantly underestimate the actual amount of myocardial flow impairment. Tracers with higher extraction coefficients give a better representation of actual flow impairment. The extent to which capillary recruitment is involved in flow regulation is an important determinate of tracer uptake in regions of subnormal flow. Changes in capillary volume apparently occur when there is an upstream stenosis with a significant pressure gradient. A better understanding of this process could lead to improved methods to detect and quantify the loss of coronary flow reserve.

Tracer washout and redistribution also play an important role in the use of myocardial blood-flow tracers. The compartmental exchange model gives us a compact way to study temporal changes in myocardial tracer activity following initial extraction. Tracer retention needs to be long enough to allow imaging after stress. ^{201}Tl has been a good example. If retention is too long, then the amount of redistribution will become insignificant. This seems to be the case with sestamibi and tetrofosmin. However, these tracers can give a good indication of regional wall thickening. Therefore, the best viability marker for these tracers may be the observation of disparity between regional perfusion and function.

Redistribution is determined by membrane transport, not by blood flow. This gives us a clinical tool to determine membrane viability in chronically underperfused myocardium. Redistribution is a gradual process and the "signal" indicating redistribution is very subtle if there is scar mixed in the myocardial region being sampled. It can therefore be difficult to detect. Reinjection can be helpful to enhance the detection of redistribution; however, reinjection would diminish the detection of redistribution in chronically hypoperfused (hibernated) regions. Reverse redistribution can be modeled in cases of multivessel disease where we are comparing a partly scarred region with an ischemic region. We have neither a model nor experimental evidence for reverse redistribution associated with simple transient ischemia.

Better understanding of tracer kinetics leads to an appreciation of clinically important limitations. The maldistribution of blood flow following severe acute ischemic insult can lead to the underestimation of viability and failure of the tracer to indicate residual ischemia. Balanced ischemia cannot be detected by tracer heterogeneity. More important to common clinical usage, uniformly decreased myocardial blood-flow reserve capacity can reduce or eliminate the sensitivity of relative tracer distribution to indicate significantly compromised myocardial blood flow.

There is a growing arsenal of myocardial perfusion tracers, but better methods to quantify absolute flow or at least relative flow reserve, are still needed. We may soon have access to molecular tracers with a rich variety of metabolic properties. All tracers exhibit patterns of uptake, retention, and redistribution that seem complex but have the potential to yield more detailed clinical information. It seems unlikely that we now understand the full potential clinical value of radionuclide tracers. Continued study and deeper understanding of these tracers should be fruitful.

REFERENCES

1. Weich HF, Strauss HW, Pitt B: The extraction of thallium-201 by the myocardium, *Circulation* 56(2):188–191, 1977.
2. Strauss HW, Harrison K, Langan JK, Lebowitz E, Pitt B: Thallium-201 for myocardial imaging. Relation of thallium-201 to regional myocardial perfusion, *Circulation* 51(4):641–645, 1975.
3. Glover DK, Ruiz M, Edwards NC, et al: Comparison between ^{201}Tl and ^{99m}Tc sestamibi uptake during adenosine-induced vasodilation as a function of coronary stenosis severity, *Circulation* 91(3):813–820, 1995.
4. McCall D, Zimmer LJ, Katz AM: Kinetics of thallium exchange in cultured rat myocardial cells, *Circ Res* 56(3):370–376, 1985.
5. Mousa SA, Cooney JM, Williams SJ: Relationship between regional myocardial blood flow and the distribution of ^{99m}Tc-sestamibi in the presence of total coronary artery occlusion, *Am Heart J* 119(4):842–847, 1990.
6. Glover DK, Ruiz M, Yang JY, Smith WH, Watson DD, Beller GA: Myocardial ^{99m}Tc-tetrofosmin uptake during adenosine-induced vasodilatation with either a critical or mild coronary stenosis: comparison with ^{201}Tl and regional myocardial blood flow, *Circulation* 96(7):2332–2338, 1997.
7. Piwnica-Worms DP, Kronauge JF, LeFurgey A, et al: Mitochondrial localization and characterization of 99Tc-SESTAMIBI in heart cells by electron probe x-ray microanalysis and 99Tc-NMR spectroscopy, *Magn Reson Imaging* 12(4):641–652, 1994.
8. Piwnica-Worms D, Kronauge JF, Delmon L, Holman BL, Marsh JD, Jones AG: Effect of metabolic inhibition on technetium-99m-MIBI kinetics in cultured chick myocardial cells, *J Nucl Med* 31(4):464–472, 1990.
9. Hatada K, Riou LM, Ruiz M, et al: ^{99m}Tc-N-DBODC5, a new myocardial perfusion imaging agent with rapid liver clearance: comparison with ^{99m}Tc-sestamibi and ^{99m}Tc-tetrofosmin in rats, *J Nucl Med* 45(12):2095–2101, 2004.
10. Hatada K, Ruiz M, Riou LM, et al: Organ biodistribution and myocardial uptake, washout, and redistribution kinetics of Tc-99m N-DBODC5 when injected during vasodilator stress in canine models of coronary stenoses, *J Nucl Cardiol* 13(6):779–790, 2006.
11. Kim YS, Wang J, Broisat A, Glover DK, Liu S: Tc-99m-N-MPO: novel cationic Tc-99m radiotracer for myocardial perfusion imaging, *J Nucl Cardiol* 15(4):535–546, 2008.
12. Leppo JA, Meerdink DJ: Comparative myocardial extraction of two technetium-labeled BATO derivatives (SQ30217, SQ32014) and thallium, *J Nucl Med* 31(1):67–74, 1990.
13. Beanlands R, Muzik O, Nguyen N, Petry N, Schwaiger M: The relationship between myocardial retention of technetium-99m teboroxime and myocardial blood flow, *J Am Coll Cardiol* 20(3):712–719, 1992.
14. Glover DK, Ruiz M, Bergmann EE, et al: Myocardial technetium-99m-teboroxime uptake during adenosine-induced hyperemia in dogs with either a critical or mild coronary stenosis: comparison to thallium-201 and regional blood flow, *J Nucl Med* 36(3):476–483, 1995.
15. Stewart RE, Heyl B, O'Rourke RA, Blumhardt R, Miller DD: Demonstration of differential post-stenotic myocardial technetium-99m-teboroxime clearance kinetics after experimental ischemia and hyperemic stress, *J Nucl Med* 32(10):2000–2008, 1991.
16. Johnson G 3rd, Nguyen KN, Pasqualini R, Okada RD: Interaction of technetium-99m-N-NOET with blood elements: potential mechanism of myocardial redistribution, *J Nucl Med* 38(1):138–143, 1997.
17. Vanzetto G, Calnon DA, Ruiz M, et al: Myocardial uptake and redistribution of ^{99m}Tc-N-NOET in dogs with either sustained coronary low flow or transient coronary occlusion: comparison with ^{201}Tl and myocardial blood flow, *Circulation* 96(7):2325–2331, 1997.
18. Petruzella FD, Ruiz M, Katsiyiannis P, et al: Optimal timing for initial and redistribution technetium-99m N-NOET image acquisition, *J Nucl Cardiol* 7(2):123–131, 2000.
19. Jeetley P, Sabharwal NK, Soman P, et al: Comparison between Tc-99m N-NOET and Tl-201 in the assessment of patients with known or suspected coronary artery disease, *J Nucl Cardiol* 11(6):664–672, 2004.
20. Uccelli L, Giganti M, Duatti A, et al: Subcellular distribution of technetium-99m N-NOET in rat myocardium, *J Nucl Med* 36(11):2075–2079, 1995.
21. Riou LM, Unger S, Toufektsian MC, et al: Effects of increased lipid concentration and hyperemic blood flow on the intrinsic myocardial washout kinetics of [99m]TcN-NOET, *J Nucl Med* 44(7):1092–1098, 2003.
22. Gosselin RE, Stibitz GR: Rates of solute absorption from tissue depots: theoretical considerations, *Pflugers Arch* 318(2):85–98, 1970.
23. Wu XS, Ewert DL, Liu YH, Ritman EL: In vivo relation of intramyocardial blood volume to myocardial perfusion. Evidence supporting microvascular site for autoregulation, *Circulation* 85(2):730–737, 1992.
24. Lindner JR, Kaul S: Insights into the assessment of myocardial perfusion offered by different cardiac imaging modalities, *J Nucl Cardiol* 2(5):446–460, 1995.
25. Wei K, Le E, Bin JP, Coggins M, Jayawera AR, Kaul S: Mechanism of reversible ^{99m}Tc-sestamibi perfusion defects during pharmacologically induced vasodilatation, *Am J Physiol Heart Circ Physiol* 280(4):H1896–1904, 2001.
26. Jayaweera AR, Wei K, Coggins M, Bin JP, Goodman C, Kaul S: Role of capillaries in determining CBF reserve: new insights using myocardial contrast echocardiography, *Am J Physiol* 277(6 Pt 2):H2363–2372, 1999.
27. Beller GA, Holzgrefe HH, Watson DD: Effects of dipyridamole-induced vasodilation on myocardial uptake and clearance kinetics of thallium-201, *Circulation* 68(6):1328–1338, 1983.
28. Grunwald AM, Watson DD, Holzgrefe HH Jr, Irving JF, Beller GA: Myocardial thallium-201 kinetics in normal and ischemic myocardium, *Circulation* 64(3):610–618, 1981.
29. Sansoy V, Glover DK, Watson DD, et al: Comparison of thallium-201 resting redistribution with technetium-99m-sestamibi uptake and functional response to dobutamine for assessment of myocardial viability, *Circulation* 92(4):994–1004, 1995.
30. Yang LD, Berman DS, Kiat H, et al: The frequency of late reversibility in SPECT thallium-201 stress-redistribution studies, *J Am Coll Cardiol* 15(2):334–340, 1990.
31. Dilsizian V, Rocco TP, Freedman NM, Leon MB, Bonow RO: Enhanced detection of ischemic but viable myocardium by the reinjection of thallium after stress-redistribution imaging, *N Engl J Med* 323(3):141–146, 1990.

Principles of Myocardial Metabolism as They Relate to Imaging

RAYMOND R. RUSSELL

INTRODUCTION

The metabolic cost on the heart of maintaining an adequate cardiac output is extremely high. Based on measurements of myocardial oxygen consumption[1] and the degree of coupling between oxygen consumption and mitochondrial adenosine triphosphate (ATP) synthesis,[2] the heart of a 70-kg individual would produce (and consume) 4.6 kg of ATP per day. As a result, the total content of ATP in the heart turns over approximately 8 times per minute to meet this high rate of flux. While the majority of this ATP expenditure is utilized for contractile activity, ATP is also required for maintaining cellular ionic homeostasis and supporting protein synthesis.

To meet these metabolic demands, the heart can utilize a wide variety of substrates, including fatty acids, glucose, lactate, ketone bodies, and amino acids. Because of the importance of myocardial metabolism in supplying the energy needs of the heart, evaluation of key aspects of substrate utilization provides important information concerning the (mal)adaptation of the heart to a variety of disease states. Furthermore, metabolic evaluation currently provides important diagnostic and prognostic information, specifically for patients with heart failure, but may also provide important information in the future to help guide therapy in a variety of disease states.

OVERVIEW OF METABOLIC REGULATION IN THE NORMAL HEART

To understand the merits and drawbacks of various metabolic radiotracers, it is important to understand how cardiac metabolism is regulated. As noted above, the heart is an "omnivore," synthesizing ATP through the metabolism of a variety of fuel substrates.[3] Furthermore, the relative contribution of the different substrates varies, and the heart must adapt rapidly to changing sources of substrate. A good example of this plasticity of substrate selection by the heart is reflected in the changes that occur during different physiologic states based on nutritional status and degree of physical activity (Fig. 2-1). The relative contribution of a given substrate to myocardial ATP production is dependent on a variety of selection pressures, including the arterial concentration of the substrate, the availability of oxygen, hormonal stimulation, the workload imposed upon the heart, and the presence of pathologic conditions that affect myocardial utilization of substrates (e.g., coronary artery disease, heart failure, diabetes) through changes in the cardiac myocyte's expression of regulatory proteins and enzymes.

The metabolism of the primary fuels in the heart is graphically depicted in Fig. 2-2 and illustrates three major phases of metabolism. The first phase is involved in converting fatty acids, glucose, and lactate into a common substrate for entry into the tricarboxylic acid (TCA) cycle in the mitochondria. In the second phase, reducing equivalents in the form of reduced nicotinamide adenine dinucleotide ($NADH_2$) and reduced flavin adenine dinucleotide ($FADH_2$) are produced in the TCA cycle and provide electrons for the electron transport chain that ultimately are used to convert oxygen to water. In the third phase, a proton gradient across the inner mitochondrial membrane, which is generated by the proteins of the electron transport chain, drives ATP synthesis.

Fatty Acid Metabolism

Under normal conditions, fatty acids and triglycerides are the preferred substrate for the normal heart. Fatty acids are taken up by the cardiac myocyte through

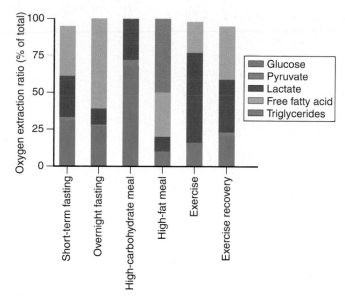

Figure 2-1 Relative contributions of carbohydrate (glucose, lactate, and pyruvate) and lipids (free fatty acids and triglycerides) to energy production as assessed by the oxygen extraction ratio. *(Based on data from Opie LH, Lopaschuk GD: Fuels: Aerobic and anaerobic metabolism. In Opie LH (ed): Heart Physiology: From Cell to Circulation, 4th ed. Philadelphia: Lippincott Williams & Wilkins, 2004, pp 306-354.)*

facilitative transport via fatty acid translocase (FAT/CD36).[4] Once inside the myocyte, fatty acids are esterified to fatty acyl-CoA derivatives through a reaction mediated by fatty acyl-CoA synthetase, which utilizes the hydrolysis of ATP to adenosine monophosphate (AMP) to drive the reaction. This energy-requiring step may be of great importance in understanding the decrease in accumulation of the fatty acid analog, [^{123}I]β-methyl-iodophenyl pentadecanoic acid (BMIPP), seen in ischemic myocardium. After this activation, fatty acyl-CoA may be transported into the mitochondria following transesterification with carnitine by carnitine palmitoyltransferase 1 (CPT-1). This step represents the

rate-limiting step of fatty acid oxidation and is regulated by cytosolic concentrations of malonyl-CoA; this important regulatory step of fatty acid metabolism is discussed in detail later in the chapter. Once inside the mitochondria, CPT-2 converts the fatty acylcarnitine back into fatty acyl-CoA for entry into the β-oxidation pathway. Another metabolic fate of the cytosolic fatty acyl-CoA is incorporation into triglycerides. It is this fate that predominates for BMIPP because the β-methyl group inhibits it entry into β-oxidation in the mitochondria.[5]

β-Oxidation represents a cycle of reactions that remove sequential 2-carbon acetyl-CoA units from the long-chain fatty acyl-CoA for entry into the TCA cycle. Not only is this set of four reactions necessary for breaking long-chain fatty acids up into smaller units, it also produces reducing equivalents in the form of $NADH_2$ and $FADH_2$ with each turn of the β-oxidation spiral. Along with $NADH_2$ and $FADH_2$ produced by the TCA cycle, these reducing equivalents drive the electron transport chain of the inner mitochondrial membrane, which is coupled to ATP synthesis and is discussed in detail later. The β-oxidation cycle is regulated by feedback inhibition through the accumulation of $NADH_2$ and $FADH_2$, and therefore the activity of this pathway is decreased by ischemia because the $NADH_2$ and $FADH_2$ cannot be oxidized to NAD and FAD, owing to decreased flux through the electron transport chain.

Glucose Metabolism

Glucose represents the other major fuel of the heart. The initial transport of glucose across the cell surface membrane represents the rate-limiting step of glucose metabolism and is mediated by facilitative glucose transporters (GLUTs).[6] Of the 13 described GLUTs, only two, GLUT1 and GLUT4, are expressed to a significant degree in the heart. GLUT1 is present mostly on the cardiomyocyte cell surface and is responsible for basal glucose uptake. In contrast, GLUT4 exists both on the cell surface and in an intracellular pool of membrane vesicles that can

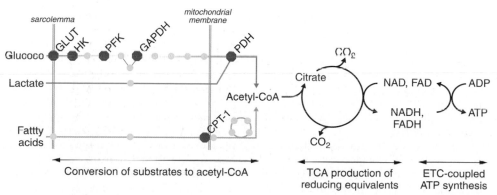

Figure 2-2 Metabolic pathways for the main fuels for the heart. Metabolism can be conceptually compartmentalized into three processes: (1) the conversion of substrates into acetyl-CoA, (2) the entry of acetyl-CoA into the tricarboxylic acid cycle, with the production of reducing equivalents, and (3) the production of adenosine triphosphate (ATP), which is coupled to the electron transport chain. The *red "stop signs"* represent key enzymes that regulate the conversion of substrates to acetyl-CoA. CPT-1, Carnitine palmitoyltransferase-1; GAPDH, glyceraldehyde 3-phosphate dehydrogenase; GLUT, facilitative glucose transporters 1 and 4; HK, hexokinase; PDH, pyruvate dehydrogenase; PFK, phosphofructokinase.

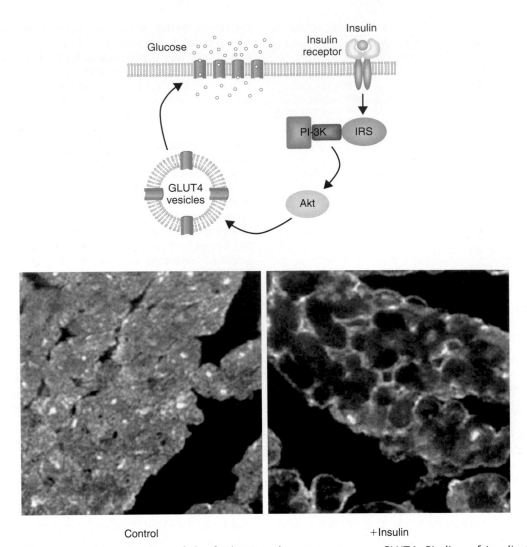

Control

+Insulin

Figure 2-3 Insulin-stimulated translocation of the facilitative glucose transporter, GLUT4. Binding of insulin to the insulin receptor results in activation of insulin receptor substrates (IRS) 1 and 2. Activation of IRS increases the association of phosphatidylinositol-3 kinase (PI-3 K), which results in the phosphorylation and activation of Akt, ultimately resulting in translocation of GLUT4 from intracellular storage vesicles to the cell surface, increasing the transport of glucose into the cell *(top panel)*. Immunofluorescent microscopy in heart muscle demonstrates diffuse intracellular distribution of GLUT4 under basal (Control) conditions; however, with insulin stimulation (+Insulin), there is redistribution of immunofluorescence to the cell surface *(bottom panel)*.

translocate to the cell surface in response to insulin (Fig. 2-3). It is therefore GLUT4 translocation that is responsible for insulin-stimulated glucose uptake in the insulin-sensitive tissues of the heart, skeletal muscle, and adipose tissue. The translocation of GLUT4 is also responsible for the enhanced glycolysis observed during ischemia, although the mechanism of this translocation is independent of the insulin signaling pathway as described later in this chapter.[7–9]

Once inside the cardiac myocyte, glucose enters into the glycolytic pathway. Although the glycolytic pathway includes 10 separate enzymatic reactions, three reactions play critical roles in regulating glycolytic flux in the heart. The first is the phosphorylation of glucose by hexokinase; glucose-6-phosphate cannot be transported back out of the cell by the glucose transporters and therefore is trapped in the cell. This initial step in the glycolytic pathway requires energy from the hydrolysis of ATP to

Adenosine diphosphate (ADP). It is also this reaction that is at the center of viability assessment, which is discussed later in detail. The glucose-6-phosphate that is produced by the hexokinase reaction sits at a branch point and either may continue in the glycolytic pathway or may be shunted into glycogen synthesis. In times of adequate provision of myocardial substrates, glycogen is synthesized for use during metabolic and hemodynamic stress.

The second regulatory step of glycolysis is catalyzed by phosphofructokinase 1 (PFK-1), which converts fructose 6-phosphate to fructose 1,6-bisphosphate and, as with the hexokinase reaction, requires the hydrolysis of ATP to ADP. The activity of PFK-1 is decreased by increases in the cytosolic content of ATP. Therefore, when the energy charge of the cytosol is high, that is, there is abundant ATP, PFK-1 inactivation will decrease glycolysis. The end result is a shunting of glucose to storage as glycogen for use when ATP stores fall.

PFK-1 is also inhibited by citrate, which increases when there is sufficient TCA cycle flux to meet the energetic needs of the cell. This inhibition of glycolysis at the level of PFK-1 by ATP and citrate is the basis of a critical aspect of myocardial metabolism that regulates substrate selection: the glucose/fatty acid, or Randle, cycle. The oxidation of fatty acids in the mitochondria results in an increase in both ATP and citrate, which inhibits PFK-1 and thereby reduces glucose uptake.[10] The operation of the Randle cycle has important implications with respect to myocardial substrate utilization under physiologic conditions such as the transition from the postprandial state, in which insulin stimulation and abundant circulating glucose lead to increased reliance on glucose, to the fasting state, in which the greater concentration of free fatty acids increases fatty acid metabolism, and disease states such as diabetes, in which there is a persistent increase in the free fatty acid concentration.

PFK-1 is also inhibited by decreases in the intracellular pH, which is important in the setting of myocardial ischemia. Specifically, with profound myocardial ischemia (i.e., a > 95% reduction in myocardial blood flow), the lactate and hydrogen ions produced by anaerobic glycolysis cannot be washed out of the myocyte, and the intracellular pH drops dramatically, resulting in cellular damage. The inhibition of PFK-1 by such a drop in pH during severe ischemia slows the production of hydrogen ions. However, this comes at the cost of diminished generation of ATP by anaerobic glycolysis. Because ATP cannot be generated by oxidative metabolism in this setting, this degree of ischemia represents a critical metabolic state in which irreversible myocyte damage can occur if adequate blood flow is not restored.

The third step of glycolysis that contributes to the regulation of glucose uptake and its ultimate conversion to pyruvate is catalyzed by glyceraldehyde 3-phosphate dehydrogenase, which converts glyceraldehyde 3-phosphate to 1,3-bisphosphoglycerate through an oxidation-reduction reaction. While glyceraldehyde 3-phosphate is oxidized to 1,3-bisphosphoglycerate, NAD is reduced to $NADH_2$. Like many of the reactions of the glycolytic pathway, the reaction catalyzed by glyceraldehyde 3-phosphate dehydrogenase can be inhibited by the accumulation of its end products. Under normal conditions, the majority of $NADH_2$ that is formed is transported to the mitochondria through the malate/aspartate shuttle to drive the electron transport chain and does not cause inhibition of glyceraldehyde 3-phosphate dehydrogenase. With ischemia, in which glycolysis is enhanced but the $NADH_2$ that is produced by the glyceraldehyde 3-phosphate dehydrogenase reaction is not utilized by the mitochondria, cytosolic $NADH_2$ can accumulate. With mild to moderate ischemia, when there is sufficient blood flow to remove the end products of glycolysis, lactate dehydrogenase will convert pyruvate to lactate with the concomitant oxidation of $NADH_2$ back to NAD. Under these conditions, glyceraldehyde 3-phosphate dehydrogenase will not be inhibited. However, with severe ischemia, there is insufficient washout of metabolic end products, and pyruvate cannot be converted to lactate. The resulting accumulation of $NADH_2$ will inhibit glyceraldehyde

3-phosphate dehydrogenase and thereby inhibit anaerobic glycolysis.

Once glucose is metabolized to pyruvate, it is transported into the mitochondria, where it is converted to acetyl-CoA through the action of pyruvate dehydrogenase (PDH). PDH is a multienzyme complex that is regulated by the metabolic status of the cell. Specifically, PDH is inhibited by increased $[NADH_2]/[NAD]$ and $[acetyl-CoA]/[CoASH]$ ratios, both of which occur when there is a relative overabundance of $NADH_2$ and acetyl-CoA that outstrips the ability of the mitochondria to utilize these metabolites.[11] This regulation of PDH activity is mediated by PDH kinase, which phosphorylates and thereby inactivates the PDH complex. In the setting of enhanced fatty acid oxidation, flux through PDH is inhibited by increased PDH kinase activity,[12] providing another level of regulation of substrate selection in the heart. Conversely, PDH activity can be increased by dephosphorylation, which occurs in response to insulin stimulation.[13] In addition, PDH can be activated by increases in workload through a calcium-dependent mechanism.

In addition to fatty acids and glucose, lactate can be a significant source of ATP production in the myocardium. This is especially true during exercise because the lactate that is released by exercising muscle is avidly taken up by myocardium through the monocarboxylic acid transporter. This exogenous lactate is converted to pyruvate through the action of lactate dehydrogenase, which now will produce additional $NADH_2$ through the reverse of the reaction described earlier. Because of the high content of lactate dehydrogenase in the myocardium, this enzyme is not rate limiting for lactate metabolism. Rather, it is the regulation of PDH that determines the utilization of lactate by the heart.

Tricarboxylic Acid Cycle Metabolism and the Electron Transport Chain

β-Oxidation of fatty acids, glycolysis of both exogenous glucose and endogenous glycogen, and uptake of exogenous lactate result in the conversion of these fuels to a common energetic currency, namely acetyl-CoA, which enters the TCA cycle by condensing with oxaloacetate to form citrate. The citrate that is formed undergoes subsequent oxidative and decarboxylating reactions in the TCA cycle, which results in the generation of five important compounds that not only help to drive mitochondrial ATP synthesis but are also important with respect to metabolic imaging. The first is the ultimate conversion of the 6-carbon citrate to the 4-carbon oxaloacetate, which is then available for another "turn" of the TCA. This is linked to the second important product, carbon dioxide (CO_2), which is produced through two decarboxylation steps, one mediated by isocitrate dehydrogenase and the other mediated by α-ketoglutarate dehydrogenase. This CO_2 is released from the cell and ultimately leaves the body through the lungs. The third is the production of $NADH_2$ by isocitrate dehydrogenase, α-ketoglutarate dehydrogenase, and malate dehydrogenase. This $NADH_2$ is used by the electron transport chain to generate the mitochondrial

OMM

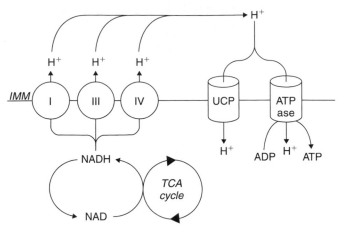

Figure 2-4   Coupling of tricarboxylic acid (TCA) cycle flux with adenosine triphosphate (ATP) synthesis. Reducing equivalents in the form of nicotinamide adenine dinucleotide ($NADH_2$) and flavin adenine dinucleotide ($FADH_2$) are generated by the TCA cycle and provide electrons for complexes of the electron transport chain. This results in an oxidation back to NAD and FAD and transport of protons from the mitochondrial matrix to the space between the inner (IMM) and outer mitochondrial membrane (OMM), creating a membrane potential. This membrane potential drives ATP synthesis by F_0F_1-ATPase, although the membrane potential can also be dissipated by uncoupling proteins (UCPs), without the production of ATP.

membrane potential required to power the mitochondrial F_0F_1-ATPase that converts ADP to ATP (Fig. 2-4). In addition, $FADH_2$ is produced by succinate dehydrogenase and also contributes electrons to the electron transport chain for the conversion of oxygen to water, but because of the location of succinate dehydrogenase in the inner aspect of the inner mitochondrial membrane, it does not contribute to the mitochondrial membrane potential. Finally, the high-energy phosphate, guanosine triphosphate (GTP), is generated through substrate-level phosphorylation by succinyl-CoA synthetase, a reaction that becomes important to energy production during ischemia because, like glycolysis, it does not require oxygen to produce high-energy phosphates.[14]

Of great importance to the evaluation of myocardial mitochondrial function by nuclear methods is the fact that there is a direct relationship between the entry of acetyl-CoA into the tricarboxylic acid cycle and the conversion of oxygen to water through the electron transport chain. Because of this coupling of acetyl-CoA metabolism to oxygen consumption, it is possible to determine rates of myocardial oxygen consumption noninvasively using the positron emission tomography (PET) tracer [1-^{11}C]-acetate.[15] Furthermore, a coupling between energy demand and energy production translates to the coupling of TCA flux to ATP synthesis. Specifically, increases in workload result in an increase in cytosolic calcium; this increased cytosolic calcium concentration increases mitochondrial calcium content, which activates not only PDH but the calcium-dependent enzymes, isocitrate dehydrogenase and α-ketoglutarate dehydrogenase, that are part of the TCA cycle.

METABOLIC TRACERS

Radiotracers of metabolic pathways fall into two categories: those that are radioisotopes of the parent compound (e.g., [1-^{11}C]glucose and [1-^{11}C]palmitate) or those that are analogs of the parent compound (e.g., [2-^{18}F]-2-fluoro-2-deoxyglucose [FDG] and BMIPP). The quantitative evaluation of metabolic pathways generally utilizes the former tracers because they follow the same metabolic fate of the parent compound, whereas the latter compounds are utilized for qualitative assessments of metabolism because they generally are retained by the tissue, making imaging easier. For example, because the PET tracer [1-^{11}C]glucose is biochemically indistinguishable from glucose, it will follow the exact fate of glucose, including the eventual release from the cardiomyocyte as $^{11}CO_2$. As a result, there is uptake, retention, and ultimately disappearance of radiotracer from the heart (Fig. 2-5). In contrast, FDG is taken up and phosphorylated by hexokinase, but it is not further metabolized in the cardiomyocyte because of the modification of the carbohydrate structure from glucose to deoxyglucose. As a result, FDG becomes trapped in the cell. Kinetic analysis of the time activity curves for FDG can be used to estimate the initial uptake and phosphorylation of glucose,[16,17] but it offers no information about the oxidative fate of glucose.

Although the kinetic analysis of a tracer such as FDG that demonstrates irreversible trapping would appear to be more straightforward than the analysis required for tracers that demonstrate accumulation and disappearance, there are two issues that must be kept in mind in translating information gained from irreversibly trapped radiotracers to conclusions about myocardial substrate utilization. First, as demonstrated earlier, these tracers only provide information about a portion of a given metabolic pathway. Second, differences in the structure of the parent compound and the radiotracer will alter the fidelity with which the tracer measures utilization of the parent compound, and this relationship between tracer and tracee can vary under different metabolic conditions.[18]

In addition to categorizing metabolic radiotracers based on their ability to trace metabolic pathways accurately and completely, they can also be grouped according to whether they are single photon–emitting or positron-emitting radiotracers (Table 2-1). Because of the coincidence detection of the two 511-keV photons produced by positron annihilation combined with the attenuation correction that is required for PET, kinetic analysis can be performed with the positron-emitting metabolic radiotracers, providing quantitative measurements of rates of substrate uptake and metabolism. In contrast, single photon–emitting metabolic radiotracers can only provide qualitative assessments of metabolic processes but have the advantage in that they do not require an on-site cyclotron, which is necessary for the production of short-lived C-11 and O-15 compounds. Because of this advantage, there is growing interest not only in the established I-123-labeled fatty acid analog, BMIPP, but newer Tc-99 m-labelled fatty acid analogs for metabolic imaging.[19]

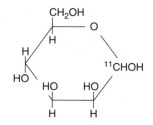

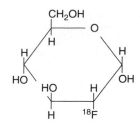

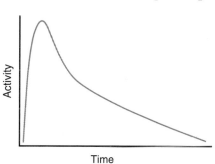

[1−^{11}C]glucose → → → → 5CO$_2$ + ^{11}CO$_2$

FDG → FDG-6-phosphate

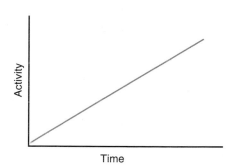

Figure 2-5 Comparison between the structure, metabolic fate, and time activity curves of [1-^{11}C]glucose and [2-^{18}F]-2-deoxyglucose (FDG). Because of the F-18 substitution for a hydroxyl group in the C-2 position of glucose in FDG, the radiotracer is metabolically trapped after transport into the cell and phosphorylation by hexokinase. As a result, there is linear accumulation of FDG under steady-state conditions, but it only allows for the evaluation of the initial uptake of glucose. In contrast, [1-^{11}C]glucose is metabolically identical to glucose and has a complex time activity curve. However, kinetic modeling of the [1-^{11}C]glucose time activity curve allows for the determination of glucose uptake and oxidation.

Table 2-1 Radiotracers Used in Metabolic Imaging

Radiotracer	Modality	Half-Life	Quantitative	Metabolic Process Evaluated
^{18}F-fluorodeoxyglucose	PET	110 min	Yes	Glucose uptake
[1-^{11}C]glucose	PET	20 min	Yes	Glucose utilization and oxidation
[1-^{11}C]lactate	PET	20 min	Yes	Lactate uptake and oxidation
[1-^{11}C]palmitate	PET	20 min	Yes	Fatty acid utilization, esterification, and oxidation
^{18}F-fluoro-6-thia-heptadecanoic acid	PET	110 min	Yes	Fatty acid oxidation
^{123}I-iodophenyl pentadecanoic acid	SPECT	13 hours	No	Fatty acid uptake and oxidation
^{123}I-β-methyl-iodophenyl pentadecanoic acid	SPECT	13 hours	No	Fatty acid uptake
[1-^{11}C]acetate	PET	20 min	Yes	Oxygen consumption
^{15}O$_2$	PET	2 min	Yes	Oxygen extraction and consumption

METABOLIC RESPONSES TO DISEASE STATES

Cardiac metabolism is a dynamic process that adapts both acutely and chronically to physiologic changes and pathologic conditions. The acute adaptations generally occur through the regulation of metabolic proteins through covalent modifications, such as phosphorylation and dephosphorylation, or by noncovalent regulation, such as by feedback inhibition by a downstream metabolite. In contrast, chronic alterations in metabolism generally are due to changes in the expression of proteins based on transcriptional regulation of metabolic genes. Although each of the disease entities discussed here have both an acute and a chronic phase of metabolic regulation, most of the research on the metabolic changes associated with congestive heart failure and diabetes has focused on the chronic metabolic changes. In contrast, both the acute and chronic metabolic changes in response to myocardial ischemia have been studied extensively.

Myocardial Ischemia

With a decrease or cessation of blood flow, the cardiac myocyte rapidly switches from oxidative metabolism of fatty acids and glucose to a greater reliance on anaerobic glycolysis with the production of lactate (Fig. 2-6). The increase in glucose uptake is due in large part to the translocation of the facilitative glucose transporter, GLUT4, from intracellular storage vesicles to the surface of the cardiac myocyte.[20] As discussed previously, GLUT4 translocates to the cell surface in response to stimulation of the insulin signaling pathway, which

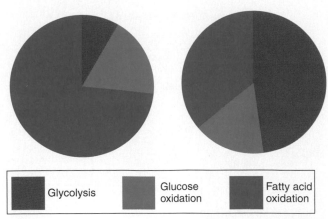

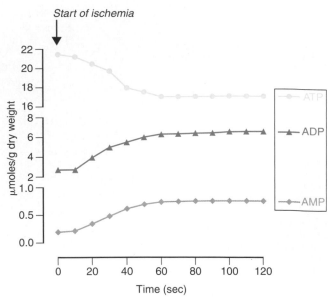

Figure 2-6 Relative contributions to adenosine triphosphate (ATP) synthesis in the nonischemic and ischemic perfused mouse heart. *(Based on data from Russell RR III, Li J, Coven DL, et al: AMP-activated protein kinase mediates ischemic glucose uptake and prevents postischemic cardiac dysfunction, apoptosis, and injury. J Clin Invest 114:495-503, 2004.)*

Figure 2-7 Changes in high-energy phosphates during ischemia. With the onset of ischemia, there is a rapid hydrolysis of adenosine triphosphate (ATP) to meet the energetic demands of the heart. However, the adenosine diphosphate (ADP) and adenosine monophosphate (AMP) are not converted back to ATP because of the lack of oxygen and accumulate. *(From Williamson JR: Glycolytic control mechanisms. II. Kinetics of intermediate changes during the aerobic-anoxic transition in perfused rat heart. J Biol Chem 241:5026-5036, 1966.)*

involves activation of key proteins that include phosphoinositidyl 3-kinase and Akt. However, the translocation of GLUT4 in response to myocardial ischemia is independent of the insulin signaling pathway.[8,21]

The molecular mechanisms responsible for the translocation of GLUT4 have recently been elucidated and start with the rapid hydrolysis of ATP to ADP and AMP that occurs with the onset of ischemia (Fig. 2-7). This change in the energy charge of the cell activates the metabolic stress protein, AMP-activated protein kinase (AMPK), both through phosphorylation of AMPK by upstream kinases and through noncovalent activation by binding of AMP to a regulatory subunit of AMPK.[8,22]

AMPK activation is a critical response to cellular metabolic stress, not only increasing GLUT4 translocation and thereby enhancing glucose uptake but also increasing the uptake and oxidation of fatty acids.[23] The increase in fatty acid oxidation by AMPK is mediated indirectly through phosphorylation of acetyl-CoA carboxylase (ACC), which decreases the conversion of acetyl-CoA to malonyl-CoA. Malonyl-CoA is an inhibitor of CPT-1, the enzyme that regulates the entry of fatty acids into the mitochondria, thereby regulating fatty acid oxidation. Therefore, inactivation of ACC by AMPK relieves malonyl-CoA inhibition of CPT-1 to increase fatty acid oxidation. AMPK inhibition of ACC has no impact on fatty acid oxidation during ongoing ischemia, because the limitation of oxygen delivery to the myocyte inhibits β-oxidation of fatty acids and TCA cycle flux, AMPK remains activated during early reperfusion, which can result in enhanced postischemic fatty acid oxidation.[23] This increase in fatty acid oxidation in the reperfused myocardium has been hypothesized to increase the production of lipid-derived free radicals and uncouple glucose uptake from glucose oxidation.

Another target of regulation by AMPK is PFK-1, one of the enzymes regulating glycolytic flux. Recent studies have demonstrated that PFK-1 activity is increased by fructose 2,6-bisphosphate, which is synthesized from fructose 6-phosphate by PFK-2. Furthermore, PFK-2 is activated through phosphorylation by AMPK.[24] Therefore, the increase in glucose utilization in the ischemic heart is due to increased glucose uptake through GLUT4 translocation to the cell surface and increased glycolytic flux through activation of PFK-1, both of which are mediated by AMPK.

At the same time that AMPK activation increases the synthesis of ATP, it also decreases the consumption of ATP in energy-requiring cellular processes such as protein synthesis and cholesterol synthesis (Fig. 2-8). Because of these diverse actions, AMPK has been thought of as a metabolic fuel gauge for cells.[25] Loss of AMPK function in transgenic mice has demonstrated the critical role of the protein in the heart's response to ischemia, with loss of AMPK function resulting in a lack of an ischemia-mediated increase in glycolysis and increased myocyte damage and apoptosis resulting in decreased postischemic recovery of contractile function.[9]

The duration of the acute translocation of GLUT4, and the concomitant increase in glucose uptake in response to myocardial ischemia, is variable and has been suggested to persist as much as 24 hours.[26] As a result, there has been some interest in whether FDG could be used as a metabolic memory agent in patients presenting with a history of chest pain that has resolved. This concept is supported by the finding that increased FDG accumulation can be detected in patients with exercise-induced ischemia if they are injected with

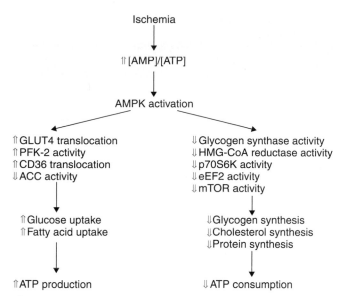

Figure 2-8 Role of adenosine monophosphate–activated protein kinase (AMPK) in regulating the metabolic response to myocardial ischemia. Ischemia results in an increase in the adenosine monophosphate/adenosine triphosphate (AMP/ATP) ratio, which activates AMPK. The activation of AMPK enhances energy-producing pathways and inhibits energy-consuming pathways to restore the AMP/ATP ratio.

FDG either at the time of exercise or 1 hour after exercise.[27,28] However, it is not known how long increased myocardial FDG uptake will persist after the resolution of ischemia. This is further complicated by the fact that GLUT4 translocation and increased glucose uptake can be mediated by insulin stimulation, making it difficult to identify increased FDG uptake in a patient who has either eaten or received insulin around the time of an ischemic episode. Given the fact that AMPK is not activated by insulin, this metabolic stress protein may be a better target for molecular imaging of a prior ischemic event, although the time course for the deactivation of AMPK requires further evaluation.

Another radiotracer that can be used to evaluate acute myocardial ischemia or a prior ischemic event is BMIPP. BMIPP has been in clinical use in Japan for more than a decade for the detection of myocardial ischemia. However, in contrast to FDG, which is a "hot-spot" imaging agent for myocardial ischemia, BMIPP is a "cold-spot" imaging agent. As a fatty acid analog, BMIPP is taken up and undergoes thioesterification with CoA, which requires a significant energy expenditure, with the hydrolysis of ATP to AMP. It has been demonstrated that the intracellular trapping of BMIPP is dependent on ATP content.[29] Unlike dietary fatty acids that do not have a β-methyl substitution, BMIPP does not undergo significant mitochondrial β-oxidation. Rather, it is incorporated in the cytosolic triglyceride pool.[30,31] However, the rate-determining enzyme of triglyceride synthesis, glycerol 3-phosphate acyltransferase, which esterifies fatty acyl-CoA to the glycerol backbone of triglycerides, is inhibited by ischemia.[32] As a result of ATP depletion and decreased triglyceride synthesis in the

setting of ischemia, free BMIPP can back-diffuse out of ischemic myocardium.[33]

Based on the decrease in BMIPP uptake in the ischemic myocardium, it has recently been shown that BMIPP defects may be seen from 4 to 30 hours after exercise-induced ischemia.[34] Given this rather large window in which a prior ischemic insult may be detected, BMIPP may be superior to FDG for late imaging of ischemia. In addition, BMIPP does not require an on-site cyclotron for production, so its clinical use is more practical. Further studies defining the effects of patient characteristics such as diabetes and heart failure, duration of BMIPP defects, and prognostic impact of the results of BMIPP imaging of a previous ischemic insult remain to be defined.

Chronic myocardial ischemia results in metabolic remodeling of the heart to increase glucose utilization and decrease fatty acid utilization.[35–38] This alteration in substrate utilization is due chiefly to the greater reliance on anaerobic glycolysis in the setting of reduced oxygen delivery. However, there is also a theoretical advantage to the oxidation of glucose over fatty acid oxidation, owing to the fact that a greater amount of ATP is produced per mole of oxygen consumed for glucose oxidation compared to fatty acid oxidation (Table 2-2). These changes in myocardial metabolism are due in part to increased expression of key proteins involved in glucose metabolism, including GLUT1, hexokinase, pyruvate kinase, lactate dehydrogenase, and pyruvate dehydrogenase.[39–42] The increase in expression of the GLUT1 and lactate dehydrogenase genes may be due to chronic AMPK activation[43] and is mediated by the transcription factor, hypoxia inducible factor (HIF)-1α.[44]

Congestive Heart Failure

The development of heart failure is associated with a variety of alterations in the expression of proteins involved in contraction, metabolism, ionic homeostasis, and transcriptional regulation.[45,46] In general, these alterations result in a reversion to a more fetal pattern of gene expression.[47–49] The metabolic implications of these changes in gene expression in the setting of heart failure include a greater reliance on glucose utilization and a decrease in fatty acid oxidation, which has been

Table 2-2 Energetic Yields of the Primary Myocardial Substrates

Substrate	ATP/ Molecule	ATP/Carbon Atom	P/O Ratio
Palmitate	105	6.7	2.33
Glucose	32	5.2	2.58
Lactate	14.75	4.9	2.46
Pyruvate	12.25	4.1	2.50

P/O ratio: ATP produced per oxygen atom consumed. Based on Opie LH, Lopaschuk GD: Fuels: Aerobic and anaerobic metabolism. In Opie LH (ed): Heart Physiology: From Cell to Circulation, 4th ed. Philadelphia: Lippincott Williams & Wilkins; 2004, pp 306-354.

Table 2-3   Alterations in Myocardial Substrate Utilization in Humans Based on PET Kinetic Studies

Condition	Oxygen Consumption	Fatty Acid Utilization	Fatty Acid Oxidation	Glucose Utilization
Women[95]	⇑	⇔	⇔	⇓
Dobutamine[96]	⇑	⇑	⇑	⇑
Aging[1]	⇑	⇓	⇓	⇔
Left ventricular hypertrophy[97]	⇔	⇔	⇓	ND
Obesity[98]	⇑	⇔	⇔	⇔
Type 1 diabetes (replacement insulin)[75]	⇑	⇑	⇑	⇓
Type 1 diabetes (hyperinsulinemic/ euglycemic)[84]	⇑	⇔	⇔	⇔
Type 1 diabetes (dobutamine)[99]	⇔	⇔	⇔	⇓
Heart failure[50]	⇔	⇓	⇓	⇑

ND: not determined

demonstrated in both animal models of heart failure and patients with nonischemic cardiomyopathy (Table 2-3).[50–52]

These changes are due in part to alterations in the expression of the key transcriptional regulators, peroxisome proliferator activated receptor (PPAR)-α and peroxisome proliferator activated receptor-γ coactivator (PGC)-1α. PPAR-α and PGC-1α interact in the nucleus to increase the transcription of a variety of genes that are primarily involved in mitochondrial biogenesis and fatty acid metabolism (Fig. 2-9).[53,54] In the setting of heart failure, the expression and activity of these regulators of metabolic gene transcription are decreased in association with decreased expression of key proteins involved in fatty acid metabolism.[55,56] In transgenic mice lacking PPAR-α, stimulating glucose utilization improves left ventricular function.[57] Interestingly, overexpression of PPAR-α has been demonstrated to cause a cardiomyopathy, likely related to excessive utilization of fatty acids.[58]

Metabolic imaging in patients with heart failure is already a standard of care for the identification of viable myocardium based on the uptake of FDG in hypoperfused but viable myocardium. As discussed previously,

FDG is transported into intact cells and phosphorylated by hexokinase in a manner similar to glucose. The phosphorylation of FDG to FDG-6-phosphate by hexokinase requires ATP, which is only found in viable cells. In the setting of persistent low-flow ischemia under resting conditions, perfusion defects may appear fixed, suggesting the presence of scar tissue. However, viable cardiac myocytes in the region utilize anaerobic glycolysis to generate ATP to maintain survival and will therefore take up FDG, producing the classic mismatch pattern between blood flow, determined by PET blood flow tracers such as N-13 ammonia or Rb-82, and metabolism. Numerous studies have demonstrated that regions of the heart with flow/metabolism mismatch will benefit from revascularization, with improvement in left ventricular function.[35,59–68]

In addition to the identification of viable myocardium in patients with presumed ischemic myocardium using FDG, metabolic imaging may provide insights into the metabolic efficiency of the failing myocardium.[69] Using [1-¹¹C]acetate to evaluate myocardial oxygen consumption, abnormalities in mitochondrial function can be evaluated[70] and may be used to evaluate the response to therapies such as cardiac resynchronization therapy.[71]

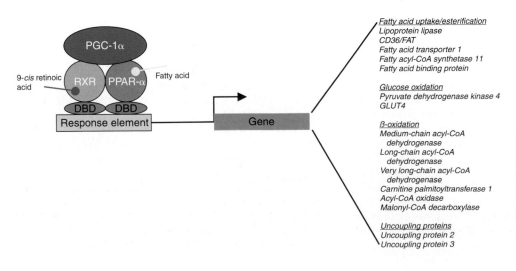

Figure 2-9   Regulation of metabolic genes by peroxisome proliferator-activated receptor-α (PPAR-α) and PPAR-γ coactivator-1α (PGC-1α). DBD: DNA binding domain; RXRα: retinoic acid receptor. (*Based on Huss JM and Kelly DP: Nuclear receptor signaling and cardiac energetics, Circ Res 95:568–578, 2004.*)

Because congestive heart failure is an increasingly common entity, understanding the basic pathophysiology, including the metabolic (mal)adaptations of the failing heart, becomes increasingly important. Specifically, is the switch to a greater reliance on glucose a protective response in the failing heart? It has been demonstrated that β-blocker treatment of heart failure patients, a therapy that has been demonstrated to reduce mortality, is associated with increased myocardial glucose utilization and decreased fatty acid oxidation.[72] Furthermore, treatment with the fatty acid oxidation inhibitor, ranolazine, has been shown to improve left ventricular performance.[73] In contrast, increased activation of PPAR-α with fenofibrate in a canine model of heart failure increases fatty acid metabolism but does not result in a significant improvement in left ventricular function.[74] Based on the metabolic changes that occur in the failing heart, combined with potential metabolically based therapies, there may be a greater role for metabolic imaging for the assessment of patients with congestive heart failure and evaluation of the response to therapeutic interventions.

Diabetes

The growing worldwide problems of obesity, insulin resistance, and diabetes have helped to draw greater attention to the cardiac manifestations of these metabolic disorders and the alterations in myocardial energetics. Diabetes, especially type 2 diabetes, represents not only an abnormality of glucose homeostasis but also an abnormality of fatty acid metabolism. The diabetic heart is characterized by increased fatty acid utilization and decreased glucose utilization (see Table 2-3).[75-77] This increased reliance on fatty acids is due to a variety of factors. First, increases in circulating concentrations of free fatty acids and triglycerides in diabetic individuals result in greater uptake and utilization of fatty acids in the cardiac myocyte. While circulating glucose concentrations are also increased in the setting of diabetes, there is down-regulation of GLUT1 and GLUT4 protein expression so that basal glucose uptake is decreased.[78] Furthermore, because of the defects in the insulin signaling cascade that are responsible for insulin resistance, the translocation of GLUT4 to the cardiomyocyte surface is blunted, resulting in decreased insulin-stimulated glucose uptake.[79,80] In addition to the decreased uptake of glucose in the diabetic heart, the conversion of glucose to pyruvate through the glycolytic pathway and the oxidation of pyruvate are inhibited by the enhanced fatty acid oxidation through the effects of the Randle cycle discussed earlier.

Just as the decreases in glucose utilization are determined in part by changes in protein expression, the enhanced fatty acid metabolism is due to altered expression of genes involved in fatty acid metabolism. Fatty acids regulate the expression of key enzymes involved in fatty acid transport and β-oxidation through PPAR-α-mediated changes in gene expression.[58,81] Therefore, in the diabetic patient, the elevated plasma concentrations of free fatty acids increase the expression of PPAR-α-regulated genes.

These alterations in the utilization of fatty acids have been hypothesized to cause lipotoxicity in the diabetic heart and may in part be responsible for the entity of diabetic cardiomyopathy.[82] In fact, triglyceride accumulation in the myocardium precedes the development of left ventricular systolic dysfunction in patients with diabetes,[83] although it remains to be established if it is triglyceride or another fatty acid metabolite that is responsible for alterations in contractile function. However, measures that normalize myocardial utilization of substrates may be beneficial in preventing changes in cardiac function in patients with diabetes, and studies using PET assessment of glucose utilization have been able to demonstrate improvements in myocardial glucose utilization in diabetic patients in response to insulin, sulfonylureas, and thiazolidinediones.[84-87] As with future therapies for heart failure, metabolic imaging may play an important role in identifying diabetic patients at risk of developing cardiomyopathy and may also play a role in guiding therapy and determining the response to metabolic interventions.

Renal Disease

Patients with renal disease are at increased risk for left ventricular dysfunction and cardiac death.[88] This is certainly attributable in large part to the development of atherosclerosis due to factors such as the cause of renal impairment (e.g., diabetes) and the development of hypertension in the setting of renal disease. However, renal failure and uremia have also been shown to alter cardiac metabolism in both in vivo and in vitro animal studies,[89-92] which may contribute to the cardiac manifestations of renal disease. Recent studies have demonstrated that BMIPP imaging can identify hemodialysis patients who are at high risk for cardiac death.[93] Interestingly, this finding extends to hemodialysis patients who have undergone coronary revascularization.[94] It was hypothesized that such patients most likely have extensive microvascular disease and repetitive ischemia, but metabolic derangements may also contribute to the abnormalities in fatty acid imaging using BMIPP and to cardiovascular morbidity and mortality.

FUTURE TARGETS FOR METABOLIC IMAGING

With the advent of molecular imaging, nuclear cardiology is undergoing a paradigmatic shift. Specifically, molecular imaging provides tools to evaluate alterations in cardiomyocyte biology rather than observing the end result of those changes. Radioligands that identify unique processes would also provide specificity that might not be available with current metabolic tracers. A case in point is the enhanced FDG uptake that can be observed following an ischemic insult. As mentioned previously, ischemia increases glucose uptake through AMPK-dependent translocation of GLUT4. However, because insulin also causes translocation of GLUT4 and increased glucose uptake, FDG uptake as a marker of ischemia would not be specific in a patient who had eaten a meal or received insulin. In contrast, because AMPK is not activated by insulin, it might provide a more reliable target for molecular imaging of a prior ischemic event. Similarly, development of radioligands based on the actions of PPAR-α may help provide important insights into derangements in fatty acid metabolism by supplying vital information concerning the regulation of metabolic gene transcription.

These are just two possible targets for molecular imaging of important metabolic processes in the heart. The identification of other potential targets will be informed by an in-depth understanding of the regulation of metabolic processes in the heart in both healthy and diseased states. Progress will rely on translational studies utilizing many models ranging from transgenic animals to patients and will utilize techniques ranging from classic biochemical assays to genomics and proteomics. Furthermore, imaging of these processes will rely on hybrid imaging modalities such as single-photon emission computed tomography/computed tomography (SPECT/CT) and PET/CT.

REFERENCES

1. Kates AM, Herrero P, Dence C, et al: Impact of aging on substrate metabolism by the human heart, *J Am Coll Cardiol* 41(2):293–299, 2003.
2. Kingsley-Hickman PB, Sako EY, Ugurbil K, et al: 31P NMR measurement of mitochondrial uncoupling in isolated rat hearts, *J Biol Chem* 265(3):1545–1550, 1990.
3. Taegtmeyer H: Energy metabolism of the heart: From basic concepts to clinical applications, *Curr Prob Cardiol* 19:57–116, 1994.
4. Schaffer JE: Fatty acid transport: the roads taken, *Am J Physiol* 282(2):E239–E246, 2002.
5. Morishita S, Kusuoka H, Yamamichi Y, et al: Kinetics of radioiodinated species in subcellular fractions from rat hearts following administration of iodine-123-labelled 15-(p-iodophenyl)-3-(R,S)-methylpentadecanoic acid (123I-BMIPP), *Eur J Nucl Med* 23(4):383–389, 1996.
6. Mueckler M: Facilitative glucose transporters, *Eur J Biochem* 219 (3):713–725, 1994.
7. Sun D, Nguyen N, DeGrado T, et al: Ischemia induces translocation of the insulin-responsive glucose transporter GLUT4 to the plasma membrane of cardiac myocytes, *Circulation* 89:793–798, 1994.
8. Russell RR, Bergeron R, Shulman GI, Young LH: Translocation of myocardial GLUT4 and increased glucose uptake through activation of AMP-activated protein kinase by AICAR, *Am J Physiol* 277: H643–H649, 1999.
9. Russell RR III, Li J, Coven DL, et al: AMP-activated protein kinase mediates ischemic glucose uptake and prevents postischemic cardiac dysfunction, apoptosis, and injury, *J Clin Invest* 114(4):495–503, 2004.
10. Newsholme E, Randle P, Manchester K: Inhibition of the phosphofructokinase reaction in perfused rat heart by respiration of ketone bodies, fatty acids and pyruvate, *Nature* 193:270–271, 1962.
11. Olson M, Dennis S, DeBuysere M, Padma A: The regulation of pyruvate dehydrogenase in the isolated perfused rat heart, *J Biol Chem* 253:7369–7375, 1978.
12. Holness MJ, Smith ND, Bulmer K, et al: Evaluation of the role of peroxisome-proliferator-activated receptor alpha in the regulation of cardiac pyruvate dehydrogenase kinase 4 protein expression in response to starvation, high-fat feeding and hyperthyroidism, *Biochem J* 364(Pt 3):687–694, 2002.
13. Sugden MC, Holness MJ: Therapeutic potential of the mammalian pyruvate dehydrogenase kinases in the prevention of hyperglycaemia, *Curr Drug Targets Immune Endocr Metabol Disord* 2(2):151–165, 2002.
14. Taegtmeyer H, Russell R: Glutamate metabolism in rabbit heart: Augmentation by ischemia and inhibition with acetoacetate, *J Appl Cardiol* 2:231–249, 1987.
15. Dence CS, Herrero P, Schwarz SW, et al: Imaging myocardium enzymatic pathways with carbon-11 radiotracers, *Methods Enzymol* 385:286–315, 2004.
16. Reivich M, Kuhl D, Wolf A, et al: Measurement of local cerebral glucose metabolism in man with [18-F]-2-fluoro-2-deoxy-D- glucose, *Acta Neurol Scand* 56(Suppl 64):190–191, 1977.
17. Patlak C, Blasberg R, Fenstermacher J: Graphical evaluation of blood-to-brain transfer constants from multiple-time uptake data, *J Cereb Blood Flow Metab* 3:1–7, 1983.
18. Russell R, Mrus J, Mommessin J, Taegtmeyer H: Compartmentation of hexokinase in rat heart. A critical factor for tracer kinetic analysis of myocardial glucose metabolism, *J Clin Invest* 90:1972–1977, 1992.
19. Heintz AC, Jung CM, Stehr SN, et al: Myocardial uptake and biodistribution of newly designed technetium-labelled fatty acid analogues, *Nucl Med Commun* 28(8):637–645, 2007.
20. Young LH, Renfu Y, Russell R, et al: Low flow ischemia leads to translocation of canine heart GLUT-4 and GLUT-1 glucose transporters to the sarcolemma in vivo, *Circulation* 95:415–422, 1997.
21. Egert S, Nguyen N, Brosius F III, Schwaiger M: Effects of wortmannin on insulin- and ischemia-induced stimulation of GLUT4 translocation and FDG uptake in perfused rat hearts, *Cardiovasc Res* 35(2):283–293, 1997.
22. Baron SJ, Li J, Russell RR III, , et al: Dual mechanisms regulating AMPK kinase action in the ischemic heart, *Circ Res* 96(3):337–345, 2005.
23. Kudo N, Barr AJ, Barr RL, et al: High rates of fatty acid oxidation during reperfusion of ischemic hearts are associated with a decrease in malonyl-CoA levels due to an increase in 5′-AMP-activated protein kinase inhibition of acetyl-CoA carboxylase, *J Biol Chem* 270(29):17513–17520, 1995.
24. Marsin AS, Bertrand L, Rider MH, et al: Phosphorylation and activation of heart PFK-2 by AMPK has a role in the stimulation of glycolysis during ischaemia, *Curr Biol* 10(20):1247–1255, 2000.
25. Hardie D, Carling D: The AMP-activated protein kinase: Fuel gauge of the mammalian cell?*Eur J Biochem* 246:259–273, 1997.
26. McNulty PH, Jagasia D, Cline GW, et al: Persistent changes in myocardial glucose metabolism in vivo during reperfusion of a limited-duration coronary occlusion, *Circulation* 101(8):917–922, 2000.
27. Abbott BG, Liu YH, Arrighi JA: [18F]Fluorodeoxyglucose as a memory marker of transient myocardial ischaemia, *Nucl Med Commun* 28(2):89–94, 2007.
28. He ZX, Shi RF, Wu YJ, et al: Direct imaging of exercise-induced myocardial ischemia with fluorine-18-labeled deoxyglucose and Tc-99 m-sestamibi in coronary artery disease, *Circulation* 108(10):1208–1213, 2003.
29. Fujibayashi Y, Yonekura Y, Takemura Y, et al: Myocardial accumulation of iodinated beta-methyl-branched fatty acid analogue, iodine-125–15-(p-iodophenyl)-3-(R,S)methylpentadecanoic acid (BMIPP), in relation to ATP concentration, *J Nucl Med* 31(11):1818–1822, 1990.
30. Yamamichi Y, Kusuoka H, Morishita K, et al: Metabolism of iodine-123-BMIPP in perfused rat hearts, *J Nucl Med* 36(6):1043–1050, 1995.
31. Nohara R, Hosokawa R, Hirai T, et al: Basic kinetics of 15-(p-iodophenyl)-3-R,S-methylpentadecanoic acid (BMIPP) in canine myocardium, *Int J Card Imaging* 15:11–20, 1999.
32. Heathers GP, Brunt RV: The effect of coronary artery occlusion and reperfusion on the activities of triglyceride lipase and glycerol 3-phosphate acyl transferase in the isolated perfused rat heart, *J Mol Cell Cardiol* 17(9):907–916, 1985.
33. Hosokawa R, Nohara R, Fujibayashi Y, et al: Myocardial kinetics of iodine-123-BMIPP in canine myocardium after regional ischemia and reperfusion: implications for clinical SPECT, *J Nucl Med* 38:1857–1863, 1997.
34. Dilsizian V, Bateman TM, Bergmann SR, et al: Metabolic imaging with β-methyl-p-[123I]-iodophenyl-pentadecanoic acid identifies ischemic memory after demand ischemia, *Circulation* 112(14):2169–2174, 2005.
35. Gerber BL, Vanoverschelde JL, Bol A, et al: Myocardial blood flow, glucose uptake, and recruitment of inotropic reserve in chronic left ventricular ischemic dysfunction. Implications for the pathophysiology of chronic myocardial hibernation, *Circulation* 94(4):651–659, 1996.
36. McFalls EO, Baldwin D, Palmer B, et al: Regional glucose uptake within hypoperfused swine myocardium as measured by positron emission tomography, *Am J Physiol* 272(1 Pt 2):H343–349, 1997.
37. Kim SJ, Peppas A, Hong SK, et al: Persistent stunning induces myocardial hibernation and protection: flow/function and metabolic mechanisms, *Circ Res* 91(11):1233–1239, 2003.
38. Liedtke A, DeMaison L, Eggelston A, et al: Changes in substrate metabolism and effects of excess fatty acids in reperfused myocardium, *Circ Res* 62:535–542, 1988.
39. Brosius F III, Liu Y, Nguyen N, et al: Persistent myocardial ischemia increases GLUT1 glucose transporter expression in both ischemic and non-ischemic heart regions, *J Mol Cell Cardiol* 29(6):1675–1685, 1997.
40. Hammond GL, Nadal-Ginard B, Talner NS, Markert CL: Myocardial LDH isozyme distribution in the ischemic and hypoxic heart, *Circulation* 53(4):637–643, 1976.
41. Liedtke A, Lynch M: Alteration of gene expression for glycolytic enzymes in aerobic and ischemic myocardium, *Am J Physiol* 277:H1435–H1440, 1999.
42. Feldhaus LM, Liedtke AJ: mRNA expression of glycolytic enzymes and glucose transporter proteins in ischemic myocardium with and without reperfusion, *J Mol Cell Cardiol* 30(11):2475–2485, 1998.

43. Abbud W, Habinowski S, Zhang JZ, et al: Stimulation of AMP-activated protein kinase (AMPK) is associated with enhancement of Glut1-mediated glucose transport, *Arch Biochem Biophys* 380(2):347–352, 2000.

44. Chen C, Pore N, Behrooz A, et al: Regulation of glut1 mRNA by hypoxia-inducible factor-1. Interaction between H-ras and hypoxia, *J Biol Chem* 276(12):9519–9525, 2001.

45. Hwang JJ, Allen PD, Tseng GC, et al: Microarray gene expression profiles in dilated and hypertrophic cardiomyopathic end-stage heart failure, *Physiol Genomics* 10(1):31–44, 2002.

46. Chen Y, Park S, Li Y, et al: Alterations of gene expression in failing myocardium following left ventricular assist device support, *Physiol Genomics* 14(3):251–260, 2003.

47. Depré C, Shipley GL, Chen W, et al: Unloaded heart in vivo replicates fetal gene expression of cardiac hypertrophy, *Nat Med* 4(11):1269–1275, 1998.

48. Razeghi P, Young ME, Alcorn JL, et al: Metabolic gene expression in fetal and failing human heart, *Circulation* 104(24):2923–2931, 2001.

49. Sack MN, Rader TA, Park S, et al: Fatty acid oxidation enzyme gene expression is downregulated in the failing heart, *Circulation* 94(11):2837–2842, 1996.

50. Davila-Roman VG, Vedala G, Herrero P, et al: Altered myocardial fatty acid and glucose metabolism in idiopathic dilated cardiomyopathy, *J Am Coll Cardiol* 40(2):271–277, 2002.

51. Osorio JC, Stanley WC, Linke A, et al: Impaired myocardial fatty acid oxidation and reduced protein expression of retinoid X receptor-alpha in pacing-induced heart failure, *Circulation* 106(5):606–612, 2002.

52. Stanley WC, Recchia FA, Lopaschuk GD: Myocardial substrate metabolism in the normal and failing heart, *Physiol Rev* 85(3):1093–1129, 2005.

53. Huss JM, Kelly DP: Nuclear receptor signaling and cardiac energetics, *Circ Res* 95(6):568–578, 2004.

54. Lehman JJ, Barger PM, Kovacs A, et al: Peroxisome proliferator-activated receptor gamma coactivator-1 promotes cardiac mitochondrial biogenesis, *J Clin Invest* 106(7):847–856, 2000.

55. Barger PM, Brandt JM, Leone TC, et al: Deactivation of peroxisome proliferator-activated receptor-alpha during cardiac hypertrophic growth, *J Clin Invest* 105(12):1723–1730, 2000.

56. Garnier A, Fortin D, Delomenie C, et al: Depressed mitochondrial transcription factors and oxidative capacity in rat failing cardiac and skeletal muscles, *J Physiol* 551(Pt 2):491–501, 2003.

57. Luptak I, Balschi JA, Xing Y, et al: Decreased contractile and metabolic reserve in peroxisome proliferator-activated receptor-{alpha}-null hearts can be rescued by increasing glucose transport and utilization, *Circulation* 112(15):2339–2346, 2005.

58. Finck BN, Han X, Courtois M, et al: A critical role for PPARα-mediated lipotoxicity in the pathogenesis of diabetic cardiomyopathy: Modulation by dietary fat content, *Proc Natl Acad Sci U S A* 100(3):1226–1231, 2003.

59. Tillisch J, Brunken R, Marshall R, et al: Reversibility of cardiac wall-motion abnormalities predicted by positron tomography, *N Engl J Med* 314(14):884–888, 1986.

60. Marwick TH, MacIntyre WJ, Lafont A, et al: Metabolic responses of hibernating and infarcted myocardium to revascularization. A follow-up study of regional perfusion, function, and metabolism, *Circulation* 85(4):1347–1353, 1992.

61. Tamaki N, Yonekura Y, Yamashita K, et al: Positron emission tomography using fluorine-18 deoxyglucose in evaluation of coronary artery bypass grafting, *Am J Cardiol* 64(14):860–865, 1989.

62. Gropler RJ, Geltman EM, Sampathkumaran K, et al: Comparison of carbon-11-acetate with fluorine-18-fluorodeoxyglucose for delineating viable myocardium by positron emission tomography, *J Am Coll Cardiol* 22(6):1587–1597, 1993.

63. Maes AF, Borgers M, Flameng W, et al: Assessment of myocardial viability in chronic coronary artery disease using technetium-99m sestamibi SPECT. Correlation with histologic and positron emission tomographic studies and functional follow-up, *J Am Coll Cardiol* 29(1):62–68, 1997.

64. Tamaki N, Kawamoto M, Tadamura E, et al: Prediction of reversible ischemia after revascularization. Perfusion and metabolic studies with positron emission tomography, *Circulation* 91(6):1697–1705, 1995.

65. Knuuti MJ, Saraste M, Nuutila P, et al: Myocardial viability: fluorine-18-deoxyglucose positron emission tomography in prediction of wall motion recovery after revascularization, *Am Heart J* 127(4 Pt 1):785–796, 1994.

66. Baer FM, Voth E, Deutsch HJ, et al: Predictive value of low dose dobutamine transesophageal echocardiography and fluorine-18 fluorodeoxyglucose positron emission tomography for recovery of regional left ventricular function after successful revascularization, *J Am Coll Cardiol* 28(1):60–69, 1996.

67. Lucignani G, Paolini G, Landoni C, et al: Presurgical identification of hibernating myocardium by combined use of technetium-99m hexakis 2-methoxyisobutylisonitrile single photon emission tomography and fluorine-18 fluoro-2-deoxy-D-glucose positron emission

tomography in patients with coronary artery disease, *Eur J Nucl Med* 19(10): 874–881, 1992.

68. Carrel T, Jenni R, Haubold-Reuter S, et al: Improvement of severely reduced left ventricular function after surgical revascularization in patients with preoperative myocardial infarction, *Eur J Cardiothorac Surg* 6(9):479–484, 1992.

69. Bengel FM, Permanetter B, Ungerer M, et al: Non-invasive estimation of myocardial efficiency using positron emission tomography and carbon-11 acetate: comparison between the normal and failing human heart, *Eur J Nucl Med* 27(3):319–326, 2000.

70. Kronenberg MW, Cohen GI, Leonen MF, et al: Myocardial oxidative metabolic supply-demand relationships in patients with nonischemic dilated cardiomyopathy, *J Nucl Cardiol* 13(4):544–553, 2006.

71. Lindner O, Sorensen J, Vogt J, et al: Cardiac efficiency and oxygen consumption measured with 11C-acetate PET after long-term cardiac resynchronization therapy, *J Nucl Med* 47(3):378–383, 2006.

72. Stanley WC, Chandler MP: Energy metabolism in the normal and failing heart: potential for therapeutic interventions, *Heart Fail Rev* 7(2):115–130, 2002.

73. Chandler MP, Stanley WC, Morita H, et al: Short-term treatment with ranolazine improves mechanical efficiency in dogs with chronic heart failure, *Circ Res* 91(4):278–280, 2002.

74. Labinskyy V, Bellomo M, Chandler MP, et al: Chronic activation of peroxisome proliferator-activated receptor-alpha with fenofibrate prevents alterations in cardiac metabolic phenotype without changing the onset of decompensation in pacing-induced heart failure, *J Pharmacol Exp Ther* 321(1):165–171, 2007.

75. Herrero P, Peterson LR, McGill JB, et al: Increased myocardial fatty acid metabolism in patients with type 1 diabetes mellitus, *J Am Coll Cardiol* 47(3):598–604, 2006.

76. Chatham JC, Forder JR: Relationship between cardiac function and substrate oxidation in hearts of diabetic rats, *Am J Physiol* 273(1 Pt 2):H52–58, 1997.

77. Belke DD, Larsen TS, Gibbs EM, Severson DL: Altered metabolism causes cardiac dysfunction in perfused hearts from diabetic (db/db) mice, *Am J Physiol* 279(5):E1104–E1113, 2000.

78. Depre C, Young ME, Ying J, et al: Streptozotocin-induced changes in cardiac gene expression in the absence of severe contractile dysfunction, *J Mol Cell Cardiol* 32(6):985–996, 2000.

79. Fischer Y, Thomas J, Rosen P, Kammermeier H: Action of metformin on glucose transport and glucose transporter GLUT1 and GLUT4 in heart muscle cells from healthy and diabetic rats, *Endocrinology* 136(2):412–420, 1995.

80. Voipio-Pulkki LM, Nuutila P, Knuuti MJ, et al: Heart and skeletal muscle glucose disposal in type 2 diabetic patients as determined by positron emission tomography, *J Nucl Med* 34(12):2064–2067, 1993.

81. Brandt JM, Djouadi F, Kelly DP: Fatty acids activate transcription of the muscle carnitine palmitoyltransferase I gene in cardiac myocytes via the peroxisome proliferator-activated receptor alpha, *J Biol Chem* 273(37):23786–23792, 1998.

82. Young ME, McNulty P, Taegtmeyer H: Adaptation and maladaptation of the heart in diabetes: Part II: potential mechanisms, *Circulation* 105(15):1861–1870, 2002.

83. McGavock JM, Lingvay I, Zib I, et al: Cardiac steatosis in diabetes mellitus: a 1H-magnetic resonance spectroscopy study, *Circulation* 116(10):1170–1175, 2007.

84. Peterson LR, Herrero P, McGill J, et al: Fatty acids and insulin modulate myocardial substrate metabolism in humans with type 1 diabetes, *Diabetes* 57(1):32–40, 2008.

85. Yokoyama I, Inoue Y, Moritan T, et al: Myocardial glucose utilisation in type II diabetes mellitus patients treated with sulphonylurea drugs, *Eur J Nucl Med Mol Imaging* 33(6):703–708, 2006.

86. Lautamaki R, Airaksinen KE, Seppanen M, et al: Rosiglitazone improves myocardial glucose uptake in patients with type 2 diabetes and coronary artery disease: a 16-week randomized, double-blind, placebo-controlled study, *Diabetes* 54(9):2787–2794, 2005.

87. Hallsten K, Virtanen KA, Lonnqvist F, et al: Enhancement of insulin-stimulated myocardial glucose uptake in patients with Type 2 diabetes treated with rosiglitazone, *Diabet Med* 21(12):1280–1287, 2004.

88. Parfrey PS, Foley RN, Harnett JD, et al: Outcome and risk factors for left ventricular disorders in chronic uraemia, *Nephrol Dial Transplant* 11(7):1277–1285, 1996.

89. Scheuer J, Stezoski W: The effects of uremic compounds on cardiac function and metabolism, *J Mol Cell Cardiol* 5(3):287–300, 1973.

90. Penpargkul S, Scheuer J: Regulation of glycogen metabolism in acute uremic hearts, *Metabolism* 23(7):631–644, 1974.

91. Williams ES, Luft FC: The effect of chronic uremia on fatty acid metabolism in the heart, *J Lab Clin Med* 92(4):548–555, 1978.

92. Smogorzewski M, Perna AF, Borum PR, Massry SG: Fatty acid oxidation in the myocardium: effects of parathyroid hormone and CRF, *Kidney Int* 34(6):797–803, 1988.

93. Nishimura M, Tsukamoto K, Hasebe N, et al: Prediction of cardiac death in hemodialysis patients by myocardial fatty acid imaging, *J Am Coll Cardiol* 51(2):139–145, 2008.

94. Nishimura M, Tokoro T, Nishida M, et al: Myocardial fatty acid imaging identifies a group of hemodialysis patients at high risk for cardiac death after coronary revascularization, *Kidney Int* 74(4):513–520, 2008.

95. Peterson LR, Soto PF, Herrero P, et al: Sex differences in myocardial oxygen and glucose metabolism, *J Nucl Cardiol* 14(4):573–581, 2007.

96. Soto PF, Herrero P, Kates AM, et al: Impact of aging on myocardial metabolic response to dobutamine, *Am J Physiol* 285(5):H2158–H2164, 2003.

97. de las Fuentes L, Soto PF, Cupps BP, et al: Hypertensive left ventricular hypertrophy is associated with abnormal myocardial fatty acid metabolism and myocardial efficiency, *J Nucl Cardiol* 13(3):369–377, 2006.

98. Peterson LR, Herrero P, Schechtman KB, et al: Effect of obesity and insulin resistance on myocardial substrate metabolism and efficiency in young women, *Circulation* 109(18):2191–2196, 2004.

99. Herrero P, McGill J, Lesniak DS, et al: PET detection of the impact of dobutamine on myocardial glucose metabolism in women with type 1 diabetes mellitus, *J Nucl Cardiol* 15(6):791–799, 2008.

Role of Intact Biological Models for Evaluation of Radiotracers

ALBERT J. SINUSAS

INTRODUCTION

The development of radiolabeled tracers for clinical application in humans has been critically dependent on evaluation and testing in biological models. Although in vitro models have been important in the evaluation of radiotracers, this chapter will focus only on the use of intact models. Initial evaluation of a radiotracer generally focuses on assessment of in vivo organ selectivity as determined by biodistribution and pharmacokinetics.[1] Often, radiolabeled compounds are evaluated in various species to ensure that behavior of a compound does not demonstrate important species differences. More important, radiotracers must be evaluated for specific organ pharmacokinetics in different disease processes.[2]

This chapter will define the role of intact biological models in the evaluation of radiotracers for use in the diagnosis and management of cardiovascular disease. Important species differences will be defined as they relate to cardiovascular disease. The selection of short-term versus long-term animal models will be discussed, with particular attention to the need for conscious or sedated models. Approaches for determination of myocardial radiotracer kinetics will be reviewed, including dynamic imaging (planar imaging, single-photon emission computed tomography [SPECT],[3] or positron emission tomography [PET]), miniature detectors, serial biopsies, and postmortem tissue well counting or autoradiography. Special consideration will be given to imaging in small animals and the utilization of transgenic models. Approaches for evaluation of radiotracer biodistribution and myocardial radiotracer uptake and clearance will be reviewed briefly, with emphasis on the effect of cellular viability, flow, metabolic inhibitors, and pharmacologic stress on radiotracer kinetics.

Animal models are often used to validate specific clinical applications of radiolabeled tracers. This chapter will also focus on the use of small- and large-animal models for evaluation of radiotracers for detection of coronary artery disease, assessment of the extent of myocardial ischemia or infarction, evaluation of congestive heart failure, and risk stratification for atrial and ventricular arrhythmias. For these clinical applications, radiotracers must provide measures or indices of myocardial flow and coronary flow reserve, myocardial metabolism, tissue oxygenation, and regional and global ventricular function. In the future, targeted radiotracers may provide insight into other biological processes, including atherosclerosis, inflammation, thrombosis, apoptosis, angiogenesis, and postinfarction remodeling. To understand the underlying physiology and evaluate potential future clinical applications, specific pathophysiologic states must be modeled. The additional use of transgenic models opens the doors for the evaluation of a myriad of radiotracers targeted at many other biological processes involved in cardiovascular health and disease.

SELECTION OF ANIMAL MODEL

Use of Small Mammals for Definition of Biodistribution

The first step in the evaluation of any radiopharmaceutical involves determination of the normal biodistribution of a radiotracer over time. These initial screening studies are usually performed in mice, rats, or rabbits to minimize cost. A measured dose is injected intravenously, and the percentage of uptake per gram of tissue is determined for critical organs.[4–7] Uptake in the heart, the target organ, is compared with adjacent background structures at multiple time points after injection. Blood clearance can be easily derived by serial sampling of blood for gamma well counting. Tissue clearance curves can be derived either by sacrificing animals at different time points or by performing serial imaging. Segregation of tissue into cell fractions can provide information on tracer localization in specific cellular fractions.[8] This information may offer insight into the mechanism of uptake and retention. The smaller hearts in these animals lend themselves to microautoradiography.

Use of Small Mammals for Evaluation of Specific Disease Processes (See Chapter 11)

A limited number of natural biological models are currently available in smaller mammals for evaluation of specific cardiovascular disease processes. The Syrian hamster model is an example of a small model for evaluation of radiotracer kinetics under cardiomyopathic conditions. Other researchers have developed rabbit models of congestive heart failure.[9,10] Investigators have also created a chronic volume-overloaded condition by mechanically disrupting the aortic valve, instigating aortic insufficiency.[11] It is more difficult to create a small-animal model of regional ischemia or infarction. However, this has been accomplished by placing a ligature or small clamp around a proximal coronary artery. In the mouse and rat, this occlusion can be done blindly with a small needle and suture through a thoracotomy.[12,13] Unfortunately, this approach generally necessitates disruption of both venous drainage and arterial inflow. Regarding rat models of infarction, the use of Lewis rats may be preferable over other strains because of the improved survival and greater uniformity of myocardial injury.[14] Several investigators have used a rabbit model of regional myocardial ischemia.[15,16] In the rabbit, it is possible to selectively isolate and occlude a proximal coronary artery. Fujita et al. recently established a chronic rabbit model of myocardial infarction without the need for endotracheal intubation, which significantly improves survival.[16] Production of graded ischemia in smaller animals is nearly impossible. The use of radiolabeled microspheres for independent assessment of regional myocardial blood flow is more difficult in these preparations. In addition, these preparations do not permit regional arterial-venous balance measurement for the independent assessment of regional metabolism. However, with the advent of dedicated small-animal imaging systems, quantitative evaluation of radiotracers in these physiologic small-animal models will become more feasible.[17,18]

Use of Genetically Engineered Small Mammals for Evaluation of Specific Biological Processes and Radiotracers (See Chapter 45)

The ability to selectively alter gene expression permits the evaluation of the significance of certain gene products for structure-function studies of cardiac proteins and their role in cardiovascular disease. These transgenic models facilitate the evaluation of targeted radiotracers in relevant biological models. Hundreds of mutant mouse strains and also a few mutant rat and rabbit strains have been generated. The number of genetically engineered

mouse lines for cardiovascular research is continuously growing. Recent reviews have provided a summary of important new genetically modified animals with cardiovascular disease.[19–27] Transgenic mice are most frequently used for this purpose, since mice breed rapidly, the maintenance costs are lower, and our knowledge of mouse genetics is far more advanced. Although the small size of these animals leads to significant challenges in the evaluation of radiotracers, there have been significant advances in small-animal SPECT and PET instrumentation that make imaging of mice feasible.[17,18]

Approaches for creation of transgenic animals are nicely reviewed by Williams and Wagner in their application for evaluation of integrative biology.[28] However, the use of transgenic animals will be equally useful for the development and testing of biologically targeted radiotracers. Once targeted radiotracers, are established, they could also be used to evaluate new transgenic strains in conjunction with radiotracers which provide information about physiologic processes (i.e., perfusion, metabolism). Thus, the use of radiotracer imaging would also permit phenotyping of transgenic animals.

There are two basic approaches to mouse genomic manipulation: random chromosomal integration, which can be used for addition of an exogenous transgene, and homologous recombination of foreign DNA, which leads to targeted mutation of an endogenous gene.[28]

Random chromosomal integration is based on addition of DNA into fertilized oocytes in order to generate "gain-of-function" mutations, in which the transgene is overexpressed.[28] Another common application of random chromosomal integration of transgenes is to identify transcriptional control elements that respond to physiologic stimuli. In this application, the coding region of a so-called reporter gene is linked to the regulatory elements of interest. By definition, reporter genes encode biologically innocuous proteins that are easily detected. The goal of this approach is to avoid perturbation of the cell in which the reporter is expressed while assessing the function of transcriptional regulatory sequences that are attached to the reporter gene. For application with radiotracer imaging, these reporter genes are linked with a radiolabeled "reporter probe" that can be detected in vivo in mice with microPET or microSPECT imaging systems.

Gambhir et al. reported methods for monitoring reporter gene expression by using herpes simplex virus type I mutant thymidine kinase (HSV1-sr39tk) as a PET reporter gene and 9-(4-[^{18}F]-fluoro-3 hydroxymethylbutyl) guanine ([^{18}F]-FHBG) as a PET reporter probe in animal models.[29] Wu et al. applied this technology using microPET imaging to noninvasively monitor cardiac reporter gene expression in rats.[30] More recently, Wu et al. applied this approach for the noninvasive assessment of myocardial response to cell therapy using embryonic cardiomyoblasts expressing HSV1-sr39tk and/or firefly luciferase.[31] The location, magnitude, and survival duration of the transplanted cells were monitored noninvasively using PET and bioluminescence optical imaging.

Gene targeting via homologous recombination in embryonic stem cells is frequently used to create "loss-of-function" mutations, known as knockouts. Targeted inactivation can be accomplished by introducing a positive selection marker, which will disrupt gene structure. A conditional gene targeting approach is preferred, since this approach provides cell-type-specific and/or inducible gene targeting. One conditional gene targeting approach involves Cre/*loxP*-mediated targeted mutagenesis.[32] This approach is based on the ability of Cre recombinase to recognize a unique nucleotide sequence (*loxP* site), allow the introduction of mutations in the gene of interest, and by the controlled expression of Cre also control the expression during different time points and avoid germline mutations that may be lethal. Alternatively, temporal or cell-type-specific transcriptional control can be accomplished using a tetracycline-responsive promoter.[33]

We are at the beginning of a new era for radiopharmaceutical testing with the development of transgenic models for many cardiovascular disease processes. However, the full impact of testing radiopharmaceuticals in transgenic models still remains undefined.

Use of Large Mammals for Evaluation of Specific Disease Processes

Dogs, pigs, and sheep are the large mammals most commonly used for the evaluation of cardiovascular physiology. These models have been used for many years, and the methodologies of their use are well established. The higher cost of large-animal models almost precludes their use for simple biodistribution studies; rather, they are mostly used to evaluate radiotracer kinetics in specific disease processes. In the evaluation of radiotracers, dogs and pigs have been most commonly used. Important interspecies differences in radiotracer uptake have been observed over the years. The most notable example is the uptake of technetium-99m (^{99m}Tc) 1,2-*bis* (dimethylphosphino)ethane. This ^{99m}Tc-labeled perfusion tracer showed favorable uptake characteristics in rats, dogs, rabbits, and monkeys; however, in phase I trials, no appreciable uptake was noted in the hearts of pigs or humans. Although there was transient uptake of this radiotracer by human heart, trapping was not observed because of a reductive mechanism that is prominent in human myocardium.[34]

Canine models have been used for many years in fundamental cardiac physiologic studies. All of the important physiologic conditions (ischemia, infarction, stunning, and even hibernation) have been modeled in dogs, and all of the currently approved radiotracers have been evaluated in canine models. Thus, the characteristics of new tracers can be easily compared with existing data on older tracers. However, it is becoming prohibitively expensive to use dogs in these types of studies.

The dog has a dominant left coronary system. In almost all cases, the left circumflex coronary leads to the posterior descending coronary artery; very rarely does the right coronary artery provide any of the blood supply to the left ventricle. The coronary vascular tree in the dog is also highly collateralized. Therefore, some investigators claim that the dog is the ideal model of chronic coronary artery disease in humans, because patients with longstanding critical coronary disease frequently are highly collateralized. In addition, the dog

is very tolerant of ischemic injury. In contrast, pigs and sheep have limited native collaterals and tolerate ischemic insults less reliably. When conducting radioisotope experiments in the dog, it may sometimes be necessary to tie off superficial epicardial collaterals to minimize the nearly instantaneous opening of epicardial collateral circuits. Dogs can also be trained to walk on a treadmill, providing an effective model for evaluation of pharmacologic stress agents.[35]

The pig has a coronary circulation that is more similar than that of the dog to human coronary circulation in that both the right and left coronary artery supply the left ventricle with blood. Pig coronary circulation systems have less native coronary collaterals, a characteristic akin to normal coronaries in humans. Therefore, the pig may be a better model of acute coronary occlusion in humans, because under conditions of acute occlusion, coronary collaterals may not have yet developed. In recent years, porcine models of ischemia, infarction, stunning, and hibernation have been established. However, sheep may provide the best model for studying chronic infarction and left ventricular remodeling.[36]

In all of these large-animal models, acute coronary occlusion may be created surgically[37] or with a balloon angioplasty catheter under fluoroscopic guidance.[38,39] In acute and chronic models, partial occlusions can be created with the aid of a hydraulic occluder or partially occluding ligature. A better way to achieve chronic partial or total occlusion may be placement of an ameroid occluder.[40,41] An ameroid occluder is a small ring that is surgically placed around a vessel. This device slowly swells over 3 to 4 weeks. A complete or partial coronary occlusion is thus created very gradually, allowing for the development of coronary collaterals.

Large-animal models offer important advantages over studies in smaller animals. First, studies in larger animals allow for more complete instrumentation and regional interventions.[42–47] Second, the distribution of a radiotracer can be easily evaluated with standard radionuclide imaging equipment.[48,49] Finally, independent regional measures of flow, function, and metabolism are much easier to obtain in larger animals.[50]

Many physiologic issues can be addressed by using acute animal models. However, to evaluate changes over an extended period of time, chronic models must be used. Chronic models also offer the ability to evaluate radiotracer behavior under conscious conditions. Animals are usually surgically instrumented and allowed to recover for at least 1 week after surgery. After full surgical recovery, an ischemic insult is implemented or stress is applied while the animal is conscious.[35,51]

SELECTION OF ANESTHESIA

Selection of the method of anesthesia may have a greater effect on radiotracer uptake than many investigators realize. Uptake of perfusion and metabolic tracers can be substantially affected by heart rate, contractile state, systemic pressures, and loading conditions. All of these hemodynamic variables are altered by anesthesia.

The cardiovascular effects of anesthesia in experimental animals have been previously reviewed.[52] These effects vary with different species and with dosages. Opioids tend to decrease preload, contractility, afterload, and heart rate.[52] Benzodiazepines induce taming effects in animals, facilitating imaging of chronically instrumented animals. These drugs may affect the cardiovascular system as a result of their central nervous system effects. Narcotic analgesics tend to have less cardiovascular effects than do general anesthetics. However, these agents require additional use of neuromuscular blocking agents. Inhalant anesthetics tend to decrease contractility, aortic pressure, and cardiac output and cause a compensatory increase in heart rate. Halothane is the most commonly used inhaled anesthetic for research purposes. Halothane at low end-tidal concentrations (1%) has little effect on the coronary circulation.

METHODS OF MEASUREMENT

Dynamic Imaging

Pharmacodynamics can be evaluated noninvasively with serial planar imaging, SPECT, and dynamic PET immediately after injection of a radiotracer. Dynamic imaging sequences allow determination of blood clearance and clearance of a radiotracer from the heart and other critical noncardiac structures. All of these imaging approaches can be easily applied to both open-chest and long-term models.

Planar Imaging

Planar imaging offers some advantages for evaluation of radiotracer pharmacodynamics, including high temporal and spatial resolution. Planar imaging of the heart is complicated by superimposition of activity in adjacent extracardiac structures. This can be obviated in open-chest models by isolation of the heart from other structures by using a flexible lead sheet. It is critical that the shielding material is placed directly under the heart, thereby completely isolating the beating heart from extracardiac structures. Time-activity curves can be derived for determination of blood and regional myocardial pharmacodynamics. In this type of kinetic analysis, placement of the regions of interest is critical. We have found that moving the myocardial region of interest one pixel toward or away from the blood pool can greatly alter the myocardial clearance curves. To facilitate optimal placement of the myocardial region of interest, we generate a reference image by subtracting an early blood-pool image from a later image (Fig. 3-1). An initial left ventricular blood-pool image can be derived by reconstruction of the left ventricular phase of the first-pass list mode acquisition. A myocardial perfusion image can be derived by summing the last 1 minute of the dynamic image sequence. The initial blood-pool image is then subtracted from the final perfusion image, providing an index myocardial image that is minimally contaminated by blood pool. The myocardial clearance curves generated by using this planar imaging approach can provide useful information on myocardial uptake and clearance of radiotracer in carefully controlled experimental models of regional ischemia or infarction. This model allows for selective arterial and venous sampling for simultaneous determination of regional metabolism or radiotracer extraction. Figure 3-2 shows a dynamic image series and corresponding clearance curves that can be derived from it.

In 1979, it was recognized that distortion of global and regional left ventricular geometry could cause artifact defects in perfusion images obtained with thallium-201 (^{201}Tl) or intracoronary administration of ^{99m}Tc-labeled albumin microspheres.[53] Sinusas et al. subsequently demonstrated that changes in regional function may confound analysis of planar ^{99m}Tc-sestamibi images.[44] Thus, changes in regional myocardial thickening may lead to misinterpretation of myocardial tracer uptake or clearance because of partial volume effects.[44] *Partial volume effects* refers to the underestimation of count density from a structure that is thinner than twice the resolution of the imaging system (usually 12 to 20 mm for a gamma camera).[54] In models of regional ischemia, systolic thinning may occur in ischemic or postischemic stunned regions.

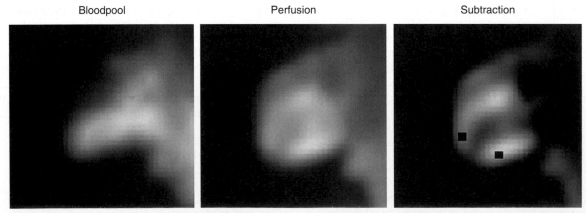

Bloodpool   Perfusion   Subtraction

Figure 3-1   Generation of myocardial uptake and clearance curve from serial planar images. An early blood-pool image *(left)* can be subtracted from the last perfusion image *(middle)* to define the myocardial regions within the image that were relatively devoid of blood-pool contamination. A typical subtraction image is shown *(right)*. Regional myocardial uptake and clearance can be derived from regions of interest placed on the subtraction image.

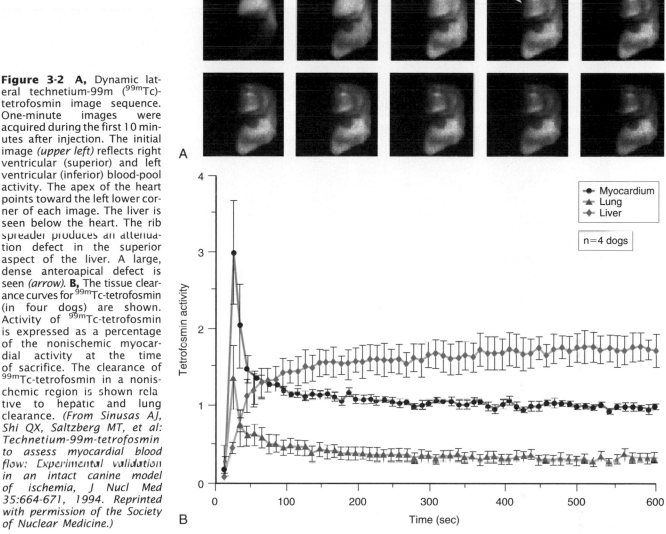

Figure 3-2 A, Dynamic lateral technetium-99m (^{99m}Tc)-tetrofosmin image sequence. One-minute images were acquired during the first 10 minutes after injection. The initial image *(upper left)* reflects right ventricular (superior) and left ventricular (inferior) blood-pool activity. The apex of the heart points toward the left lower corner of each image. The liver is seen below the heart. The rib spreader produces an attenuation defect in the superior aspect of the liver. A large, dense anteroapical defect is seen *(arrow).* **B,** The tissue clearance curves for ^{99m}Tc-tetrofosmin (in four dogs) are shown. Activity of ^{99m}Tc-tetrofosmin is expressed as a percentage of the nonischemic myocardial activity at the time of sacrifice. The clearance of ^{99m}Tc-tetrofosmin in a nonischemic region is shown relative to hepatic and lung clearance. *(From Sinusas AJ, Shi QX, Saltzberg MT, et al: Technetium-99m-tetrofosmin to assess myocardial blood flow: Experimental validation in an intact canine model of ischemia, J Nucl Med 35:664-671, 1994. Reprinted with permission of the Society of Nuclear Medicine.)*

Differences in wall thickness would be most prominent at end systole. The potential impact of these partial volume errors are illustrated in Figure 3-3. We found that analysis of end-diastolic images may compensate somewhat for the partial volume effect associated with regional dyskinesis.

Dynamic planar imaging has been used by several investigators to establish the clearance kinetics of ^{201}Tl,[55] ^{99m}Tc-sestamibi,[56] ^{99m}Tc-tetrofosmin,[45] and ^{99m}Tc-teboroxime.[57] Serial planar imaging permits nontraumatic serial assessment of changes in regional activity. However, dynamic planar imaging is limited by camera resolution, partial volume effects, and potential motion artifacts and may be influenced by background scatter and tissue cross-talk.

Dynamic planar images can also be obtained in animals as small as a mouse using high-resolution pinhole collimators.[58] Figure 3-4 illustrates a series of planar pinhole images in a mouse injected with a ^{99m}Tc-labeled compound targeted at the $\alpha_v\beta_3$ integrin, and corresponding tissue clearance curves. Using an external radioactive reference source (~10 μCi), the regional

counts within selected organs can be converted to μCi and expressed as a percentage of injected dose.

Single-Photon Emission Computed Tomography

High-quality tomographic images can be acquired to evaluate the biodistribution of a radiotracer. Imaging by SPECT provides better separation of organs than planar imaging. Dynamic SPECT imaging has only recently become feasible with the development of multidetector cameras. Several investigators have used dynamic SPECT imaging for kinetic modeling.[59–61] Stewart et al. performed dynamic tomographic imaging with ^{99m}Tc-teboroxime in closed-chest dogs by using a single-photon ring tomographic system.[61] These investigators demonstrated monoexponential clearance of ^{99m}Tc-teboroxime with this approach. By using a triple-detector SPECT system, Smith et al. demonstrated the feasibility of acquiring dynamic 10-second tomographic data with a continuous acquisition protocol.[60] Analysis of wash-in of ^{99m}Tc-teboroxime in myocardial tissue measured with this dynamic SPECT approach, in

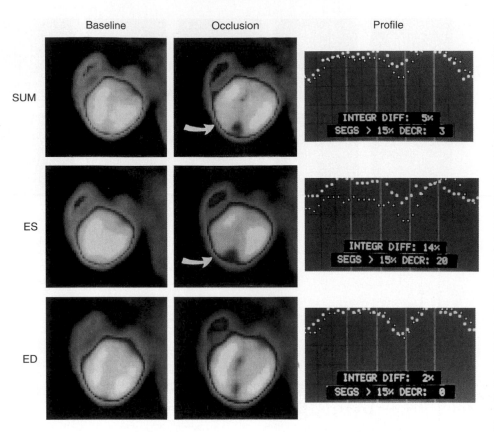

Baseline · Occlusion · Profile

SUM

ES

ED

INTEGR DIFF: 5%
SEGS > 15% DECR: 3

INTEGR DIFF: 14%
SEGS > 15% DECR: 20

INTEGR DIFF: 2%
SEGS > 15% DECR: 0

Figure 3-3 Images showing that regional left ventricular dysfunction creates an artifactual perfusion defect. Technetium-99m labeled sestamibi was injected during baseline conditions before coronary occlusion and reperfusion. Shown are lateral planar images obtained at baseline *(left)* and during coronary artery occlusion *(middle)*. A large anteroapical defect *(arrow)* is seen both on summed (SUM) and end-systolic (ES) images during coronary artery occlusion. This artifact is less evident on the end-diastolic (ED) image. The corresponding baseline and occlusion quantitative profiles are superimposed on the right. *White dots* represent the circumferential profile derived from each baseline image. *Black-and-white dots* represent the corresponding occlusion profile. Changes in defect scores are also shown. *(From Sinusas AJ, Shi QX, Vitols PJ, et al: Impact of regional ventricular function, geometry, and dobutamine stress on quantitative ^{99m}Tc-sestamibi defect size, Circulation 88:2224-2234, 1993. Reprinted with permission.)*

conjunction with compartmental modeling, provided an index of regional myocardial blood flow. Smith et al. also demonstrated that the use of attenuation correction in conjunction with dynamic SPECT was critical for compartmental analysis of ^{99m}Tc-teboroxime. Figure 3-5 provides an example of a series of high-quality images and corresponding clearance curves derived from dynamic SPECT in a dog. The potential advantage of kinetic modeling with SPECT over PET is the greater availability of SPECT equipment and reduced cost. However, the accuracy of the dynamic SPECT approach is not established.

Pinhole SPECT systems have been developed to evaluate regional properties of radiopharmaceuticals in small animals.[62,63] Unfortunately, the ten-fold gain in resolution of these systems is at the expense of a 100-fold loss in sensitivity.[64] This limitation has been overcome by using multidetector SPECT systems.[62] Optimal reconstruction of the pinhole images will probably require more computer-intensive, three-dimensional, maximum-likelihood expectation-maximization (ML EM) algorithms.[64] Although these systems cannot compete with the high resolution of microautoradiography, they may provide an alternative to macroautoradiography or well counting. Hirai et al. demonstrated the feasibility of serial SPECT with pinhole collimators for estimation of flow and metabolism in vivo in rat hearts.[65] Wu et al. performed myocardial perfusion imaging of mice using ^{99m}Tc-sestamibi and demonstrated the feasibility for measurement of perfusion defect size from pinhole SPECT images (Fig. 3-6).[31] Other investigators recently

demonstrated the feasibility of electrocardiographic (ECG)-gated pinhole SPECT imaging in mice[66] and rats[67] for the evaluation of regional left ventricular function by applying standard clinical image analysis software to reconstructed ECG-gated microSPECT images.

High-speed and high-sensitivity SPECT cameras have recently become available that employ cadmium zinc telluride (CZT) detectors and novel schemes for reconstruction and collimation.[68,69] The novel design of these new systems significantly increases sensitivity and reduces imaging time while providing higher spatial resolution than the conventional Anger camera approach.[70,71] These systems will permit dynamic SPECT imaging, facilitating evaluation of the biodistribution and uptake and the clearance kinetics of new radiotracers under evaluation. They also offer the potential for absolute quantification of radiotracers. The increased sensitivity is at the cost of the size of the field of view, but for experimental imaging, these systems may be ideally suited for dynamic imaging of rabbits or focused imaging of larger animals. These systems should expand the horizons of SPECT imaging in experimental animal models.

Positron Emission Tomography
(See Chapter 11)

Dynamic PET imaging in large-animal models plays an important role in evaluation of the kinetics of positron-emitting radiopharmaceuticals. However, this chapter will not review this topic. Technetium-94m (^{94m}Tc), a positron emitter with a 53-minute

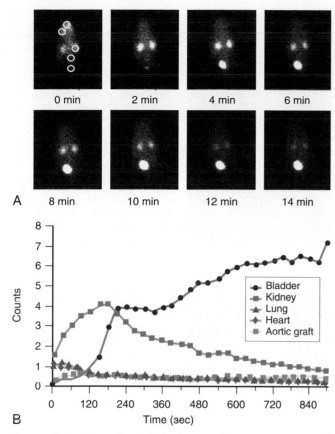

Figure 3-4 Dynamic pinhole images in a mouse injected with ^{111}In-labeled RP748, a radiotracer targeted at the $\alpha_v\beta_3$ integrin. **A,** Dynamic gamma camera images of RP748 clearance in ApoE$^{-/-}$ mouse at various time points after tracer administration, acquired with large field of view gamma camera and 1-mm pinhole aperture. *Circles* represent different regions of interest. **B,** Time-activity curve derived from dynamic image series, demonstrating rapid renal clearance of the tracer. *(From Sadeghi MM, Krassilnikova S, Zhang J, et al: Detection of injury-induced vascular remodeling by targeting activated $\alpha_v\beta_3$ integrin in vivo, Circulation 110:84-90, 2004. Reprinted with permission.)*

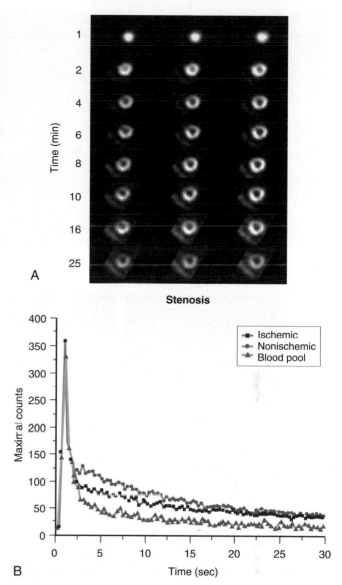

Figure 3-5 Dynamic SPECT technetium-99m (^{99m}Tc)-teboroxime images were acquired (20 seconds per image) over 30 minutes in an open-chest dog after creation of a partial occlusion of the left anterior descending region. **A,** Short-axis ^{99m}Tc-teboroxime images are shown from mid-ventricle over time. A perfusion defect is seen in the anteroapical region. Blood-pool and myocardial clearance curves were generated from this dynamic image set. **B,** Maximum counts from ischemic, nonischemic, and blood-pool regions are plotted over time. Differences in regional ^{99m}Tc-teboroxime clearance are evident.

half-life, can be used to evaluate the biodistribution and pharmacokinetics of ^{99m}Tc radiopharmaceuticals for SPECT.[72,73] Performing PET in animal models with Tc-labeled compounds allows in vivo evaluation of regional myocardial uptake and clearance kinetics. Figure 3-7 provides an example of ^{94m}Tc-sestamibi PET images. Imaging with PET offers great advantages in the evaluation of SPECT tracers: It provides high temporal and spatial resolution and reliable attenuation correction. Labeling of SPECT tracers with ^{94m}Tc allows the direct comparison of SPECT radiotracers with PET compounds.

Recently, several microPET imaging systems have become commercially available and are capable of performing dynamic PET imaging in mice and rats.[74] However, accurate kinetic modeling with microPET requires a reliable arterial input function, which is difficult to obtain in mice. Some investigators have attempted to derive an input function using high-sensitivity detectors placed over an extracorporeal circuit, while others are designing precision devices for serial blood sampling.

Serial microPET imaging was recently applied in rats following myocardial infarction and transient ischemia, as well as in control rats, to (1) evaluate the biodistribution and uptake and the clearance kinetics of a new ^{18}F-labeled pyridazinone analog (18F-BMS-747158-02) under a range of physiologic conditions, and (2) define the changes in the uptake ratio of heart to adjacent organs (Fig. 3-8A-B). Serial microPET imaging was also used to define the regional uptake and clearance of normal myocardium and myocardium following permanent (see Fig. 3-8C) and transient (see Fig. 3-8D) coronary occlusion.

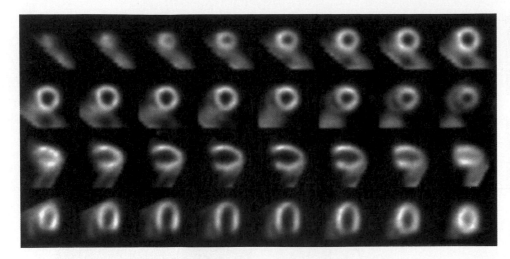

Figure 3-6 Pinhole ^{99m}Tc-sestamibi SPECT images of a mouse heart. Short-axis *(first two rows)*, vertical long-axis *(third row)*, and horizontal long-axis *(fourth row)* slices are shown from a myocardial perfusion study in a normal mouse. Image quality is excellent, with the left ventricle well resolved and the right ventricle clearly visible. *(From Wu MC, Gao DW, Sievers RE, et al: Pinhole single-photon emission computed tomography for myocardial perfusion imaging of mice, J Am Coll Cardiol 42:576-582, 2003. Reprinted with permission of the American College of Cardiology.)*

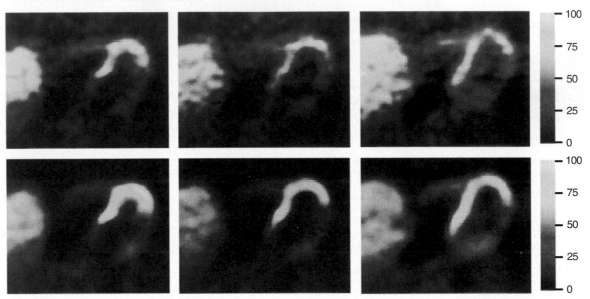

Figure 3-7 Technetium-94m (^{94m}Tc)-sestamibi and nitrogen-13 (^{13}N)-ammonia PET images in a 66-year-old woman with previous posterolateral wall myocardial infarction. Shown are transaxial ^{94m}Tc-sestamibi images *(top row)* and ^{13}N-ammonia images *(bottom row)*. Greater hepatic uptake is seen on the ^{94m}Tc-sestamibi images. *(From Stone CK, Christian BT, Nickles RJ, Perlman SB: Technetium 94m-labeled methoxyisobutyl isonitrile: Dosimetry and resting cardiac imaging with positron emission tomography, J Nucl Cardiol 1:425-433, 1994. Reprinted with permission of the American Society of Nuclear Cardiology.)*

Miniature Detectors

Myocardial radiotracer kinetics can also be derived in large open-chest animal preparations with the use of miniature radiation detectors. In many studies by Okada et al., miniature cadmium telluride radiation detectors were used to evaluate myocardial uptake and clearance of several radiopharmaceuticals, including ^{201}Tl- and ^{99m}Tc-sestamibi.[56,75,76] These probes allow continuous monitoring and display of regional myocardial activity.[77] High-quality myocardial clearance curves derived by using a cadmium telluride detector are shown in Figure 3-9. The use of these probes can be complicated by changes in myocardial thickness and underlying blood pool beneath the probe and in the stability of

the instrumentation. In some studies, probes have been placed on the myocardium in combination with a device to measure wall thickening. This system allows online correction of changes in counts associated with cyclic wall thickening. More recently, Stewart et al. measured myocardial clearance of ^{99m}Tc-teboroxime with a 1-inch collimated sodium-iodine (Tl) probe.[57] The first component of ^{99m}Tc-teboroxime washout derived by using this probe was related to microsphere blood flow. This miniature probe approach allows continuous monitoring of regional myocardial activity under different ischemic conditions or during pharmacologic stress. Despite the potential limitations of these miniature probes, much insight into the in vivo

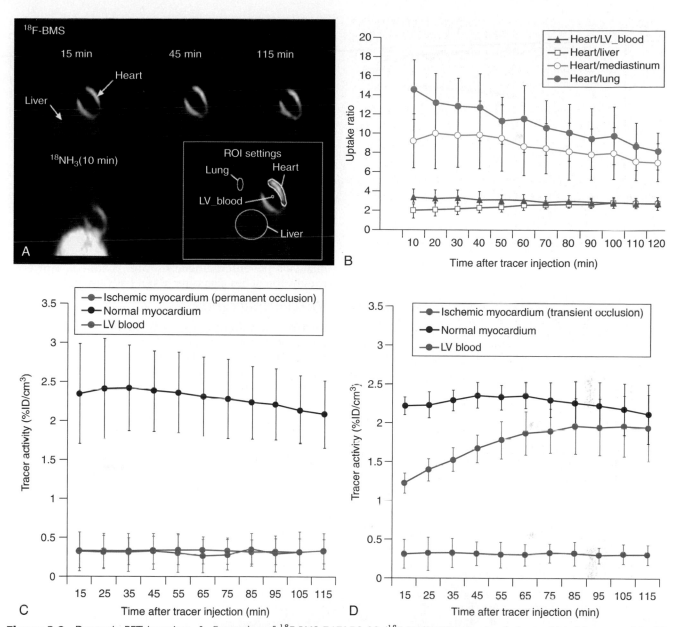

Figure 3-8 Dynamic PET imaging. **A,** Examples of ^{18}F-BMS-747158-02 (^{18}F-BMS) PET images of chest of healthy rat at 15, 45, and 115 minutes after tracer injection and ^{13}N-ammonia PET image at 10 minutes in coronal view. Example of regions of interest for measurement of tracer activity is displayed in *white box.* **B,** Ratio of ^{18}F-BMS uptake between myocardium and surrounding organs. **C-D,** Mean values are shown for tracer activity in induced defect and normally perfused myocardium after permanent (**C**) and transient (**D**) occlusion. Tracer activity in defect increased over time after reperfusion in transient coronary occlusion. *(Modified from Higuchi T, Nekolla SG, Huisman MM, et al: A new ^{18}F-labeled myocardial PET tracer: Myocardial uptake after permanent and transient coronary occlusion in rats, J Nucl Med 49:1715-1722, 2008. Reprinted with permission.)*

behavior of ^{201}Tl-labeled and newer ^{99m}Tc-labeled compounds has been derived from probe studies.

Serial Myocardial Biopsy

Investigators have obtained serial myocardial biopsy specimens after injection of a radiotracer to evaluate changes in absolute myocardial activity over time.[78-80] This approach is the most accurate method to serially determine changes in absolute myocardial counts per gram. However, serial myocardial biopsy results in myocardial injury, necessitates the analysis of very small pieces of tissue, and has a potential sampling error.

Postmortem Imaging

Imaging of excised organs or tissues can be very useful to establish the final distribution of a radiotracer that has been injected in vivo under a specific physiologic condition. Some investigators have acquired high-resolution, tomography-like images by placing slices of the heart on the surface of a gamma camera (Fig. 3-10).[43] Images acquired by using this method are similar to those obtained using macroautoradiography. The gamma camera approach enables the simultaneous acquisition of high-resolution images by using multiple energy windows. Investigators have used this method to compare

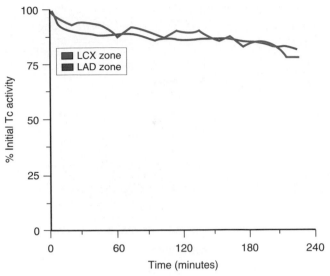

Figure 3-9 Typical decay-corrected myocardial time-activity clearance curves derived from miniature cadmium telluride probes for an ischemic left circumflex (LCX) and control left anterior descending (LAD) region in a dog with a critical coronary stenosis. Both probes were positioned on the epicardial surface of the left ventricle. In this example, there was minimal and equal washout from the two regions. *(From Okada RD, Glover D, Gaffney T, et al: Myocardial kinetics of technetium-99-m hexakis-2-methoxy-2-methylpropyl-isonitrile, Circulation 77:491-498, 1988. Reprinted with permission.)*

the distribution of perfusion and metabolic tracers labeled with different radioisotopes. Effective application of this method necessitates sectioning the heart in slices of uniform thickness, which requires an automated slicing device. Alternatively, a complete three-dimensional set of short-axis images of the intact heart can be acquired ex vivo with a SPECT camera (Fig. 3-11).

This eliminates the need for precision slicing of the heart and avoids the problems of attenuation and motion. To simulate the in vivo geometry of the heart, hearts are generally stuffed with gauze, frozen in a distended state, or filled with inert dental molding material. All methods of postmortem imaging eliminate partial volume errors associated with cardiac deformation. Images derived using this method can be easily quantified and readily compared with postmortem histochemical stains.

Autoradiography

Microautoradiology and macroautoradiography have been critical in the development and evaluation of radiopharmaceuticals.[11,43,81,82] One of the major limitations of this approach is that each animal provides data for only a single experimental time point, possibly two if dual-isotope autoradiographs are acquired. However, these approaches also offer several advantages.

Microautoradiography

Microautoradiography permits high-resolution assessment of the distribution of radioactivity within an organ. This approach allows several isotopes to be compared directly if they can be separated on the basis of differences in half-life. The appropriate use of this technique requires preparation of tissue standards for each isotope in exponentially increasing activity concentrations.[82,83] Tissue standards are necessary to convert autoradiographic intensity into tracer activity. Digitized autoradiographs can be quantitatively analyzed if the appropriate standards are used; the details of this approach have been reported elsewhere.[81] Figure 3-12 provides an example of digitized dual-isotope microautoradiographs and quantitative profiles comparing the myocardial distribution of ^{201}Tl- and ^{99m}Tc-

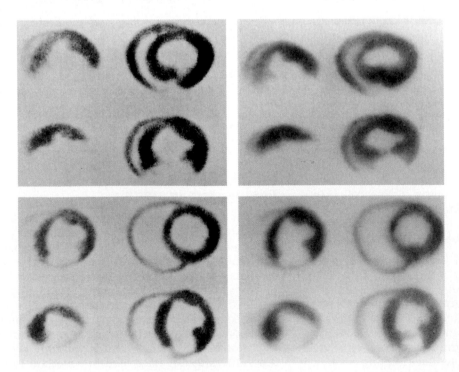

Figure 3-10 Comparability of technetium-99m-sestamibi gamma camera ex vivo slice images *(left)* and macroautoradiographs *(right)*. Shown are images from two dogs that underwent 3 hours of left anterior descending coronary artery occlusion followed by 3 hours of reperfusion. ^{99m}Tc-sestamibi was injected during coronary occlusion *(top)* in one dog and after 90 minutes of reperfusion in the second dog *(bottom)*. *(From Sinusas AJ, Trautman KA, Bergin JD, et al: Quantification of area at risk during coronary occlusion and degree of myocardial salvage after reperfusion with technetium-99m-methoxyisobutyl-isonitrile, Circulation 82: 1424-1437, 1990. Reprinted with permission.)*

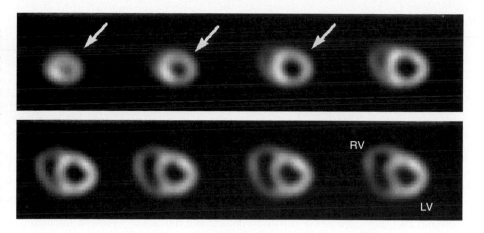

Figure 3-11 Postmortem ex vivo technetium-99m-sestamibi SPECT images oriented in standard short-axis format. ^{99m}Tc-sestamibi was injected during inotropic stress in the presence of a partial stenosis of the left anterior descending coronary artery. Short-axis images (5 mm thick) are shown from apex to base. The right ventricle (RV) is seen on the left and the left ventricle (LV) on the right of each image. A mild perfusion defect is seen in the anteroapical region *(arrows).*

teboroxime in a rabbit model of acute coronary occlusion. Figure 3-13 provides another example of dual-isotope microautoradiography using ^{99m}Tc-sestamibi and an ^{111}In-labeled agent (^{111}In-RP748) targeted at the $\alpha_v\beta_3$ integrin in a rat following occlusion and reperfusion resulting in nontransmural infarction. Uptake of ^{111}In-RP748 demonstrates increased expression and activation of the $\alpha_v\beta_3$ integrin in angiogenic vessels within the infarct region as defined by ^{99m}Tc-sestamibi.

Digital microautoradiography can also be performed with ^{18}F-labeled PET radiotracers using 20-μm thick frozen sections placed in a specimen imaging system capable of detecting either beta or gamma radiation.[7,84,85] Higuchi et al. used a specimen imaging system to obtain digital microautoradiographs in rat hearts to determine the time course of an [^{18}F]galacto-RGD compound for targeted imaging of the $\alpha_v\beta_3$ integrin following myocardial infarction (Fig. 3-14).[7]

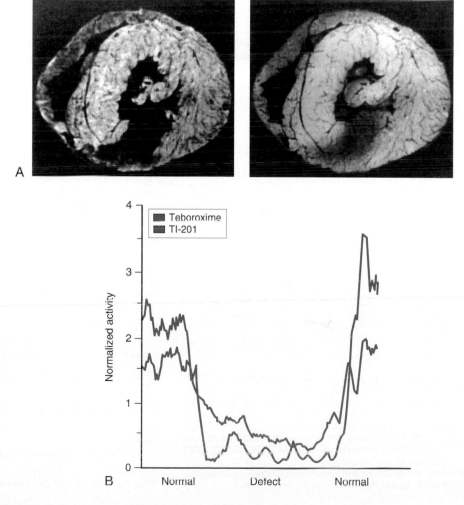

Figure 3-12 A, Dual-isotope microautoradiographs showing technetium-99m (^{99m}Tc)-teboroxime *(left)* and thallium-201 (^{201}Tl) *(right)*. Myocardial activity distributions in the same rabbit heart during coronary artery occlusion. Microautoradiographs were obtained from 30-μm thick short-axis slices. Note the increased contrast and clearer delineation of normal and low-flow zones produced by ^{99m}Tc-teboroxime compared with ^{201}Tl-simultaneously injected. **B,** A representative pair of dual-isotope ^{99m}Tc-teboroxime and ^{201}Tl profiles across the defect. Normal-to-defect contrast was increased and normal-to-defect transition was sharper for ^{99m}Tc-teboroxime compared with ^{201}Tl. *(From Weinstein H, Reinhardt C, Leppo J. Teboroxime, sestamibi and thallium-201 as markers of myocardial hypoperfusion: comparison by quantitative dual isotope autoradiography in rabbits. J Nucl Med. 1993;34:1510-1517.)*

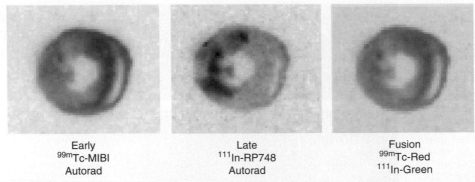

Early
^{99m}Tc-MIBI
Autorad

Late
^{111}In-RP748
Autorad

Fusion
^{99m}Tc-Red
^{111}In-Green

Figure 3-13 **A,** Dual-isotope ^{99m}Tc-sestamibi (early) and (^{111}In-RP748) (late) microautoradiographs (autorad) from a short-axis section (10-μ thick) from rat heart following 45 minutes of occlusion and 3 hours of reperfusion. The early ^{99m}Tc-sestamibi microautoradiography *(left)* demonstrates a perfusion defect, and the late ^{111}In-RP748 microautoradiograph *(middle)* demonstrates focal retention of ^{111}In-RP748, which is targeted at the $\alpha_v\beta_3$ integrin (a marker of angiogenesis) within the infarct region. A color-fused image is shown *(right)* demonstrating clear localization of ^{111}In-RP748 with the perfusion defect.

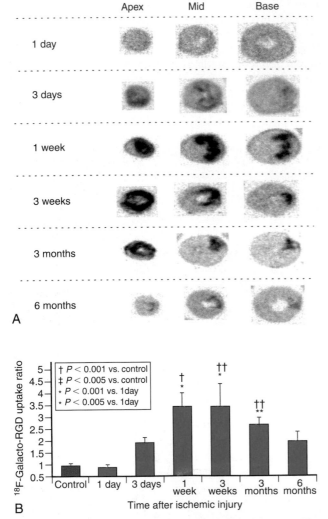

Figure 3-14 **A,** Representative autoradiographs of [^{18}F]-galacto-RGD uptake in the heart after ischemia and reperfusion with three slices (apex, middle, and base) studied at different time points. **B,** The bar graph depicts the changes in the myocardial [^{18}F]galacto-RGD uptake ratio (versus remote myocardium) after coronary occlusion and reperfusion as defined by autoradiography. *(From Higuchi T, Bengel FM, Seidl S, et al: Assessment of $\alpha_v\beta_3$ integrin expression after myocardial infarction by positron emission tomography, Cardiovasc Res 78:395-403, 2008. Reprinted with permission.)*

The resolution of autoradiographs depends on the energy level of the tracers and the thickness of the sections.[86] Hearts are typically cut into sections that are 10 to 50 μm thick. For quantitative analysis, a high-precision cryotome is required, and the thickness of the specimen must be uniform. Spatial resolution is improved if the specimen is firmly pressed onto the film. This technique is relatively economical because a gamma well counter is not required.

Macroautoradiography

Lower-resolution macroautoradiographs can be more easily obtained in larger animal hearts.[43] This approach does not even require a cryotome. Thin slices (2 to 5 mm) can be obtained with an inexpensive meat slicer. These myocardial slices are laid flat on cardboard, covered in plastic wrap, and inverted on x-ray film. Macroautoradiographs obtained in this manner can provide information on the spatial distribution of a radiotracer under experimental conditions of low-flow ischemia, myocardial stunning, or infarction. As shown in Figure 3-15, macroautoradiographs can be directly compared with postmortem stains to relate radiotracer uptake to myocardial viability.

Postmortem Tissue Well Counting

Postmortem tissue well counting is the most widely applied approach for assessment of myocardial uptake and clearance of a radiotracer. This technique is applied in larger-animal models in which specific physiologic states can be modeled. In general, the radiotracer under evaluation is injected during a specific physiologic condition; the activity retained in the myocardium is determined by doing gamma well counting of the excised tissue. If hearts are excised within minutes of injection, the initial myocardial distribution of a radiotracer can be determined. Hearts excised hours after injection provide information about the relative late retention of a radiotracer.

The initial uptake of a tracer is dependent on flow or delivery of the radiotracer to the tissue and the extraction of the tracer by the tissue. Retention of a tracer

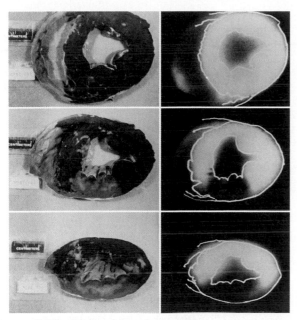

Figure 3-15 Postmortem dual-perfusion maps *(left)* and technetium-99m (⁹⁹ᵐTc)-sestamibi macroautoradiographs *(right)* from a dog undergoing 3 hours of left anterior descending coronary artery occlusion followed by 3 hours of reperfusion. ⁹⁹ᵐTc-sestamibi was injected 90 minutes into the reperfusion period. Shown are three slices oriented with the right ventricle on the left and the anterior wall on the bottom. The risk area is stained brick-red with triphenyltetrazolium chloride (TTC). The infarct area is the pale, unstained region within the risk area. Defects seen on the unenhanced macroautoradiographs with superimposed overlay *(right)* correlate closely with the area of infarction defined by TTC staining. No significant ⁹⁹ᵐTc-sestamibi activity is seen in the central necrotic region, whereas some activity is seen in the perinecrotic area. This approach allows for direct comparison of macroautoradiographs with postmortem stains to evaluate radiotracer uptake to myocardial viability. *(From Sinusas AJ, Trautman KA, Bergin JD, et al: Quantification of area at risk during coronary occlusion and degree of myocardial salvage after reperfusion with technetium-99m-methoxyisobutyl-isonitrile, Circulation 82:1424-1437, 1990. Reprinted with permission.)*

may be influenced by perturbations in regional metabolism, cellular viability, or flow. Frequently the distribution of a radiotracer under evaluation is compared with independent measures of regional myocardial blood flow determined using the radiolabeled microsphere technique.

Tissue is counted in a gamma well counter, which has excellent energy discrimination and permits simultaneous evaluation of as many as six radiotracers if each one has gamma emissions at distinguishable energy ranges. Activity spillover from the energy window of one radiotracer to another can be corrected with a matrix derived from counting pure specimens of each radiotracer. This approach has been described in detail by Heymann et al.[87] and has been applied by many other investigators.[88] Identification of ²⁰¹Tl redistribution was accomplished using this approach (Fig. 3-16).[89]

Gamma well counting in postmortem tissue has obvious advantages and disadvantages. A major disadvantage is that the myocardial distribution of a radiotracer can only be determined at discrete time points. In addition, a given animal can be examined only once.

Finally, the resolution of this approach is dependent on how finely the heart is sectioned, usually in 0.3-gm samples. The tissue counting approach is very reproducible and avoids interference of background activity. To facilitate comparisons of results between animals, myocardial radiotracer activity is usually normalized. One way to normalize activity is to express activity in each segment as a percentage of a predefined normal region.[42] This method enables evaluation of the myocardial activity within an ischemic or infarcted region relative to a normal region in a manner analogous to the interpretation of clinical images. Alternatively, regional myocardial activity can be normalized by the computed average activity for each heart, as proposed by Yipintsoi et al.[90] A less desirable approach normalizes activity in each myocardial segment according to the segment with the highest activity.[91]

Evaluation of Tracer Kinetics and Kinetic Modeling

Regional myocardial uptake of a diffusible tracer is dependent on flow and myocardial extraction. The simplest approach to kinetic modeling assumes a monoexponential clearance. Under these conditions, dynamic image data are fitted to a monoexponential equation, $A = A_0 e^{-kt}$, where A_0 represents initial activity, K the decay constant in the elapsed time. Myocardial clearance half-time can be derived from the slope of the linear regression of the natural logarithmic transformation of the raw counts over time ($t_{1/2} = \ln 2/k$). To further simplify the analysis, the initial data from 0 to 2 minutes after injection may be excluded to avoid potential blood pool contamination. More sophisticated compartmental modeling is often required. The dynamic data can be derived from both planar imaging and SPECT; this topic is covered in detail in other sections of the book.

PHYSIOLOGIC MODELS

To define the behavior of a new radiopharmaceutical under different clinical cardiovascular conditions, the myocardial kinetics of a radiotracer is evaluated in animal models. Clinical applicability can be evaluated by testing a radiotracer under specific pathophysiologic states or using specific genetic models. Important ischemic conditions include acute and chronic low-flow ischemia (hibernation), postischemic dysfunction (stunning), and transmural or nontransmural myocardial infarction. A major goal of radionuclide imaging in the evaluation of patients with ischemic heart disease is noninvasive discrimination of stunned, hibernating, and infarcted myocardium. Important nonischemic conditions include myocardial hypertrophy and dilated cardiomyopathy. These disease states may involve a host of biological processes, including necrosis, apoptosis, and inflammation. Newer biologically targeted radiotracers offer the potential to evaluate atherosclerosis, angiogenesis, and thrombosis. These topics are the focus of other chapters in the book.

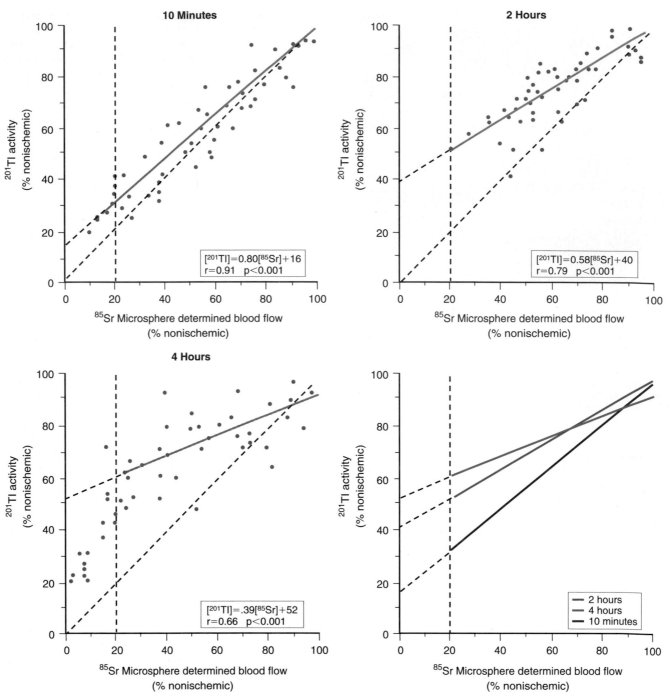

Figure 3-16 Relationship of myocardial thallium-201 (^{201}Tl) activity and radiolabeled microsphere regional myocardial blood flow as determined by gamma well counting. ^{201}Tl- was injected in the presence of a fixed coronary stenosis. The myocardial distribution of ^{201}Tl was compared with the strontium-85-microsphere–determined blood flow at the time of radiotracer injection in animals sacrificed at 10 minutes *(upper left)*, 2 hours *(upper right)*, and 4 hours *(lower left)* after radiotracer injection. The left ventricle was cut into 1-gm to 3-gm pieces for gamma well counting. Regional myocardial ^{201}Tl activity and flow were expressed as a percentage of nonischemic region. The *solid line* represents the line of regression; the *dashed line* represents the line of identity. Linear regression analysis was performed only on the 20% to 100% flow range. The graph in the *lower right* shows the superimposed regression lines for each subset of animals. The regression lines become progressively lower between 10 minutes, 2 hours, and 4 hours, with a ^{201}Tl excess relative to the ischemic flow region. This is consistent with an relative increase in ^{201}Tl in the ischemic region relative to the nonischemic region and represents ^{201}Tl redistribution. *(From Pohost GM, Okada RD, O'Keefe DD, et al: Thallium redistribution in dogs with severe coronary artery stenosis of fixed caliber, Circ Res 48:439-446, 1981. Reprinted with modification and permission.)*

The most frequently used short-term and long-term physiologic models are reviewed in the following discussions. Many of these models are experimental, although some models of cardiovascular disease occur naturally or are genetically engineered.

Myocardial Infarction

It has been well established in canine models of coronary occlusion that myocardial necrosis progresses from the subendocardium to the subepicardium in a wavefront manner.[37,92] Advancing myocardial necrosis can be halted by coronary reperfusion. In canine models, permanent cellular injury begins after approximately 40 minutes of occlusion. The extent of necrosis depends on the area at risk and the duration of occlusion. In dogs, the maximum degree of infarction occurs after about 6 hours of occlusion. However, the extent of infarction may be affected by heart rate and left ventricular loading conditions. Thus, in anesthetized models, the method of anesthesia may affect infarct size. Myocardial flow following reperfusion varies and is critically dependent on timing after reperfusion, because a period of hyperemic flow is often seen following release of an occlusion.

Connelly et al. reported that complete coronary occlusion in the rabbit produced an expanding necrotic wavefront from the subendocardium.[93] This effect is similar to the phenomenon first described by Reimer and Jennings in the canine model of occlusion.[92] In the rabbit, mild subendocardial necrosis can be detected by nitroblue tetrazolium staining as early as 15 minutes after occlusion; 1 hour of coronary occlusion consistently produces completed transmural infarction.

Coronary occlusion can be produced by various noninvasive and invasive methods.[52] Noninvasive closed-chest approaches include sustained coronary occlusion with angioplasty catheters[38,39]; selective coronary embolization[94]; and deployment of intracoronary copper coils,[95] which promote thrombosis. Some of these approaches permit subsequent reperfusion. More invasive surgical approaches involve acute occlusion with a surgical ligature[37,92] or more gradual occlusion after implantation of an ameroid occluder.[96]

Small-rodent models of surgical myocardial infarction are now widely used in the evaluation of the pathophysiology of infarction and postinfarction remodeling[97–101] and have only recently been used for evaluation of targeted radiotracers following infarction.[12,13,18,102] These small-animal imaging studies will be facilitated by the availability of high-resolution microSPECT and microPET imaging systems. Larger experimental models of coronary occlusion and reperfusion are more frequently used to assess the behavior of radiolabeled perfusion tracers under conditions of reduced flow and in the presence of myocardial necrosis. The myocardial uptake and retention of a perfusion tracer is critically dependent on the timing of injection relative to reperfusion.[79,103] Appropriate use of experimental occlusion-reperfusion models allows analysis of the uptake and clearance characteristics of a radiotracer in relation to

cellular viability independent of flow.[43] These models have also been used to evaluate sympathetic innervation of the heart after coronary occlusion and reperfusion with iodine-123 (^{123}I) meta-iodobenzyl guanidine[39] or to examine myocardial metabolism with radiolabeled tracers of aerobic or anaerobic metabolism.[38,104–106]

A model of chronic congestive heart failure can be produced by repeated coronary embolization[94,107] or by surgery.[108] Animals with extensive infarction producing extensive myocardial necrosis can be created by repetitive transmyocardial direct current shocks.[109]

Myocardial Stunning

Myocardial stunning is characterized by a condition of postischemic mechanical dysfunction that persists after reperfusion despite the absence of irreversible injury. In the dog, a coronary occlusion lasting less than 20 minutes does not result in any myocardial necrosis; however, it produces regional dysfunction that may persist for hours.[110,111] Myocardial stunning can also be produced by repeated brief (5- or 10-minute) coronary occlusions.[112] In other species with fewer coronary collaterals, much briefer periods of coronary occlusion result in myocellular necrosis. Myocardial stunning can also occur after a prolonged partial coronary occlusion,[113] in association with nontransmural infarction,[114] or with exercise-induced ischemia.[115]

We recently developed a long-term canine model of ameroid-induced gradual subtotal coronary occlusion resulting in regional myocardial dysfunction (Fig. 3-17). Although resting flow was normal in these animals, on PET imaging with nitrogen-13 ammonia, coronary flow reserve was markedly impaired in response to adenosine. This model matches the clinical scenario reported by Vanoverschelde et al. in which reversible left ventricular dysfunction was identified in patients with viable collateralized occluded coronary arteries with preserved resting flow.[116] In our canine model, dysfunctional regions with impaired coronary flow reserve also demonstrate increased fluorine-18 deoxyglucose uptake, similar to the clinical condition reported by Camici et al.[117] These observations support the contention that the chronic regional dysfunction may be caused by repetitive stress-induced ischemia in the setting of normal resting flows and impaired flow reserve. This chronic model should prove useful in the evaluation of radiolabeled fatty acids such as [^{123}I]β-methyl-iodophenyl pentadecanoic acid (BMIPP), which are reportedly "memory" markers of reversible ischemic injury.[106]

All radiopharmaceuticals directed at evaluating myocardial metabolism should be evaluated in one of these pure experimental models of myocardial stunning. These models allow evaluation of a radiotracer under conditions of predominantly altered metabolism. As in infarct models of occlusion-reperfusion, the timing of radiotracer injection during conditions of post-reperfusion stunning is critical because of a transient period of hyperemic flow. The reperfusion hyperemia observed following a brief period (<15 minutes) of ischemia tends to be more intense but shorter in duration.

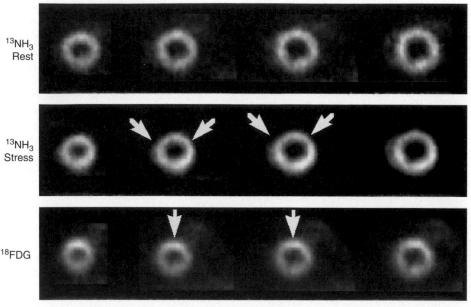

Figure 3-17 Long-term canine model of ischemic dysfunction. PET, perfusion, and metabolic imaging were performed in dogs 5 weeks after implantation of an ameroid occluder. Images from PET with nitrogen-13 ammonia *(top row)* demonstrate normal resting flow. Nitrogen-13 ammonia images during adenosine stress *(middle row)* demonstrate reduced flow in the anterior wall *(between arrows)*. Increased accumulation of fluorine-18 deoxyglucose *(arrow)* is seen in the area of impaired flow reserve *(bottom row)*. A coronary angiogram at 4 weeks showed 90% stenosis of the left anterior descending coronary artery at the site of the ameroid occluder. Magnetic resonance imaging and serial echocardiography showed profound regional dysfunction; however, postmortem examination revealed no significant necrosis in this region. This animal model seems to be analogous to the condition observed clinically in patients with collateralized viable myocardium subtended by a subtotal occlusion. Regional dysfunction can be attributed to repeated myocardial stunning.

Myocardial Hibernation (See Chapter 36)

The term *myocardial hibernation* has generally been applied to patients with coronary artery disease who have chronically depressed left ventricular function in the absence of myocardial infarction that improves after coronary revascularization. It is unclear whether chronic left ventricular dysfunction in humans represents an adaptive response to chronic reduction in coronary blood flow.[118] Impairment of left ventricular function under these conditions has been regarded as a protective mechanism by which the heart down-regulates its energy requirements, thereby preventing irreversible myocardial injury.

Short-term canine and porcine studies have successfully demonstrated sustained (1- to 5-hour) matching of reduced flow and function.[113,119,120] We also developed a short-term canine model of sustained low-flow ischemia (Fig. 3-18).[42,47,121] A hydraulic occluder is placed around a proximal coronary artery, allowing for the creation of a variable stenosis. The distal coronary artery is cannulated with a non–flow-obstructing catheter, which permits accurate regulation of the stenosis severity on the basis of measurement of distal coronary artery pressure and transstenotic pressure gradient. The degree of ischemic dysfunction can be assessed by measuring regional myocardial thickening with epicardial Doppler thickening probes.

Changes in regional metabolism can also be assessed in this model by selective venous sampling for arterial-venous balance measurements. Additional application

of atrial pacing or intravenous administration of inotropic agents can provide a model of stress-induced ischemia as it may occur in patients with critical coronary artery disease.[47] Many investigators have used this type of low-flow model to evaluate radiolabeled tracers of perfusion, myocardial metabolism, and tissue hypoxia.[42,47,89,122] Using this experimental model of sustained low flow, the perfusion tracer ^{99m}Tc-NOET (bis[N-ethoxy, N-ethyl dithiocarbamato]-nitrido ^{99m}Tc) demonstrates substantial redistribution,[122] as was previously observed for ^{201}Tl[89]- and ^{99m}Tc-sestamibi.[46]

The condition of chronic low-flow perfusion-contraction matching has been more difficult to model experimentally. Recently, investigators succeeded in producing regional dysfunction over extended periods in pigs and dogs.[123–125] In each of these studies, the severity of regional dysfunction was out of proportion to the reduction in regional myocardial blood flow. In a clinical study, Vanoverschelde et al. suggested that chronic regional myocardial dysfunction in the presence of relatively preserved resting coronary flow may be attributed to repetitive stunning associated with intermittent stress-induced ischemia.[116] The presence of ^{201}Tl rest redistribution in patients with reversible left ventricular dysfunction supports the idea that true myocardial hibernation with chronic resting reduction in flow can and does occur.[126] Whereas a resting defect may be attributed to partial volume errors, the presence of ^{201}Tl redistribution suggests differential myocardial clearance that is most likely secondary to reduced resting myocardial flow. Additional imaging studies in

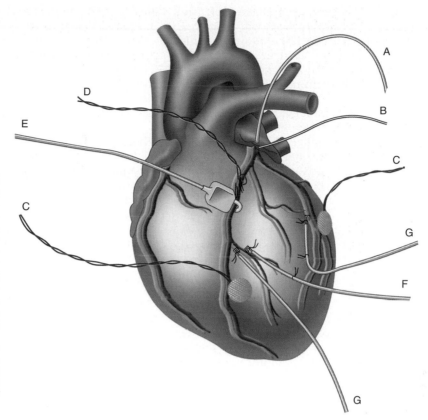

Figure 3-18 Heart surgical preparation and instrumentation of a model of partial coronary occlusion and pacing-induced demand ischemia. **A,** Left atrial catheter; **B,** atrial pacing wire; **C,** Doppler thickening crystals; **D,** Doppler flow probes; **E,** hydraulic occluder; **F,** distal coronary artery catheter; and **G,** coronary venous catheters. *(From Shi CQX, Sinusas AJ, Dione DP, et al: Technetium-99m-nitroimidazole [BMS 181321]: A positive imaging agent for detecting myocardial ischemia. J Nucl Med 36:1078-1086, 1995. Reprinted with permission of the Society of Nuclear Medicine.)*

animal models of chronic hibernation are needed to establish the pathophysiology of reversible ischemic dysfunction in the presence of coronary artery disease. In an excellent recent review, Canty and Fallavollita suggest that chronic stunning and chronic hibernation represent the extremes of a continuum.[127] They present the recent experimental studies that demonstrated that there is a progression from chronic stunning with normal flow to hibernating myocardium with reduced resting flow. The application and evaluation of new metabolic radiotracers in these models will be critical for advancing our understanding of this important clinical condition. These low-flow models also will be invaluable in assessing new radiolabeled perfusion tracers.

Dilated Cardiomyopathy

The value of animal models in the evaluation of cardiomyopathies was recently reviewed by Yarbrough and Spinale.[128] Although several landmark discoveries regarding the pathophysiology of cardiomyopathies have arisen from small-animal models, the proof of concept must ultimately be reproduced in animal species that more closely mimic human physiology, function, and anatomy.[128] While small-animal models allow the identification of potential novel imaging targets, larger-animal models facilitate the direct translation of radiotracer imaging approaches to applications in patients with cardiomyopathies.

Many canine species are known to have idiopathic dilated cardiomyopathies.[52] This is seen almost exclusively in the larger breeds of dogs and is characterized by biventricular cardiac dilation. Dilated cardiomyopathies have also been seen in domestic cats, and there is a cardiomyopathic strain of Syrian hamsters. Several investigators have developed experimental models of congestive heart failure associated with ventricular dilation. Chronic rapid atrial or right ventricular pacing in the dog or pig produces dilated cardiomyopathy.[129–131] Chronic mitral insufficiency also results in dilated cardiomyopathy. This can be accomplished surgically or noninvasively by cutting chordae tendineae of the mitral valve with a urologic forceps.[88,132] Other investigators have created a volume-overloaded state by creating aortic insufficiency.

Magid et al. developed a rabbit model of chronic aortic insufficiency.[133] The regurgitant fraction and resulting left ventricular dilation and hypertrophy produced by this rabbit model are similar to those reported in severe aortic insufficiency in human beings. Lu et al. used this model to evaluate the value of ^{111}In-labeled antimyosin antibody Fab fragment imaging for identification of myocyte necrosis associated with chronic aortic insufficiency.[11] These types of experimental studies help to generate hypotheses about the potential role of radionuclide imaging in the evaluation and management of patients with acute or chronic aortic insufficiency.

Atherosclerosis (See Chapter 44)

Several recent reviews have summarized the many models of atherosclerosis that are available for testing of radiotracers targeted at critical components of the atherosclerotic process.[134,135] Animal models of atherosclerosis generally involve use of a high-fat diet in combination with endothelial injury. Vascular injury can be produced by direct physical injury, chemical injury, or immunologic injury. Some animals develop atherosclerosis as a naturally occurring disease: The Watanabe heritable hyperlipidemic rabbit, for example, has a natural LDL-receptor deficiency and provides a natural model for homozygous familial hypercholesterolemia.[136] The St. Thomas' Hospital (STH) strain of rabbits resembles human triglyceridemia and combined hyperlipidemia and also develops advanced atherosclerotic lesions.[137] The most commonly used animal model of atherosclerosis is the high-cholesterol-diet-fed rabbit.[52] The pig is also commonly used as a model of atherosclerosis. Vallabhajosula et al. developed a novel porcine model of complex coronary atherosclerosis that employs balloon injury followed by an injection of cholesterol esters into the coronary arteries of healthy pigs, creating coronary lesions (15 mm in length).[138] These investigators demonstrated that the uptake of [18F]fluorodeoxyglucose (FDG) in the coronary lesions was dependent on the progression of the lesion. Within the first 2 to 3 months after the induction of lesion, FDG uptake was seen in some of the lesions. But after 4 months, most of the lesions were clearly identified by FDG. To reduce the problems associated with use of this large species, miniaturized breeds of swine have been developed. Nonhuman primates are considered to provide a model of atherosclerosis that is most similar to the atherosclerosis seen in humans. Limitations of the nonhuman primate include expense and the rapid development of atherosclerotic lesions.

The transgenic/knockout animal models have greatly enhanced our understanding of atherosclerosis. The most widely used mouse models of atherosclerosis are apolipoprotein E–deficient (ApoE[−/−]), LDL receptor–deficient (LDLr[−/−]), and ApoE*3Leiden (E3L).[26] These models may differ strikingly from one another in their response to specific experimental manipulations. The ApoE[−/−], mouse has become an established model of hypercholesterolemia and spontaneous atherosclerotic lesion development.[139,140] ApoE mice demonstrate lesions of all phases of atherosclerosis throughout the arterial tree.[141] Williams et al. more recently demonstrated that the brachiocephalic lesion that develops in ApoE-deficient mice is characteristic of the unstable plaque seen in human patients.[142] The brachiocephalic lesions that develop in the ApoE-deficient mice are characterized by large plaques with a thin fibrous cap and increased lipid core. These are all features associated with plaque rupture. Lesions in this region are also characterized by multiple buried caps, suggesting repeated rupture, and support a higher rupture rate of the brachiocephalic region compared with other vascular segments in these mice. The ApoE mouse fed a high-fat diet develops lesions similar to those in humans. Therefore, the ApoE model provides an excellent approach for evaluation of radiotracers targeted at unstable components of the atherosclerotic plaque. Figure 3-19 illustrates the gross atherosclerotic lesions that develop in ApoE-deficient mice.

The LDLr[−/−] mouse model develops atherosclerosis, particularly following feeding with a lipid-rich diet. E3L mice have a mutant form of the human *apoE3* gene and develop atherosclerosis when fed a high-cholesterol diet. These E3L mice are more sensitive to lipid-lowering drugs then either the ApoE[−/−] or LDLr[−/−] mice.[26]

Mouse models have proved useful in the study of atherosclerosis, but differences in anatomy, lipid metabolism, and gene expression complicate translation of experimental results obtained in mice to humans.[26]

Models of atherosclerosis have been used to evaluate a number radiotracers targeted at the vulnerable plaque.[143,144] As outlined earlier, plaques vulnerable to rupture typically have a large, necrotic lipid core and an attenuated fibrous cap that are significantly infiltrated by macrophages and lymphocytes. There is emerging evidence that apoptosis contributes to the instability of the atherosclerotic lesion. Apoptosis of macrophages contributes substantially to the size of the necrotic core,[145] whereas apoptosis of smooth muscle cells results in thinning of the fibrous cap.[146] Annexin V can be radiolabeled with [99mTc] and has been previously used for the noninvasive detection of apoptosis in myocardial infarction and inflammatory myocardial diseases. Kolodgie et al. applied annexin V planar in vivo and ex vivo imaging in experimental atherosclerotic lesions in hypercholesterolemic rabbits for noninvasive detection of atherosclerosis.[143] They demonstrated that annexin V targeted apoptotic macrophages within the atherosclerotic plaque and may provide an attractive imaging agent for the noninvasive detection of unstable atherosclerotic plaques. Narula et al. also demonstrated the feasibility of noninvasive visualization of experimental atherosclerotic lesions with a mouse/human chimeric antibody Z2D3 F(ab')$_2$ directed against proliferating smooth-muscle cells.[147] Narula et al. subsequently demonstrated that [111In]-Z2D3 antibody imaging could be used for noninvasive assessment of the rate of smooth-muscle cell proliferation after coronary angioplasty.[148] Other investigators using a rabbit model of atherosclerosis demonstrated that radiolabeled MCP-1 may also be a useful tracer for imaging monocyte/macrophage-rich experimental atherosclerotic lesions.[144]

MODELS OF PLAQUE RUPTURE

There is no single experimental model that perfectly replicates plaque rupture in man.[149] Some of the available small- and large-animal models of plaque rupture are summarized in Table 3-1. The large-animal models are essentially models of atherosclerosis. The small-animal models of induced or spontaneous plaque rupture have the limitation that the lesions formed are usually in non-coronary vessels. Despite these limitations, genetically modified mice—particularly apolipoprotein E knockout mice—are routinely used to develop and evaluate radiotracers for identification of vulnerable plaque.

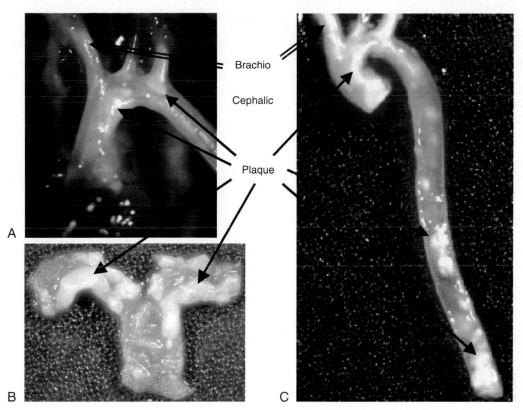

Figure 3-19 Illustration of the gross atherosclerotic lesions that develop in ApoE-deficient mice after prolonged feeding on a high-fat diet. **A,** Aorta isolated within animal demonstrates location of the brachiocephalic artery *(open arrow)*, which is a common site for atherosclerotic lesions that have many of the characteristics of unstable plaque. **B,** Entire aorta dissected free, demonstrating atherosclerosis throughout the aorta. **C,** Aorta opened for better visualization of the endocardial lesions that are present in the aortic arch. *Arrows* indicate location of atherosclerotic plaques. *(Figure provided courtesy of Paula J. Silva, Bristol-Myers Squibb Medical Imaging, Billerica, MA.)*

Table 3-1 Summary of Animal Models of Unstable Plaque

Species	Manipulation	Refs
Mouse	ApoE$^{-/-}$, mechanical injury	Reddick[159]
	ApoE$^{-/-}$, non-constrictive carotid collar, p53 adenovirus	von der Thusen[160]
	ApoE$^{/}$, constrictive carotid collar	Cheng[161]
		Johnson & Jackson[162]
	ApoE$^{-/-}$, high-fat diet plus cholesterol	Williams[163]
		Johnson[164]
	ApoE$^{-/-}$, SR-BI$^{-/-}$	Braun[165]
Rat	Heritable inducible hypertension	Herrera[166]
Rabbit	Cholesterol diet, viper venom, histamine	Conastantinides[167]
		Abela[168]
	Cholesterol diet, implanted balloon catheter	Rekhter[169]
Pig	Injection into arterial tunica media	Granada[170]
	Heritable hyperlipidemia	Prescott[171]

Modified from Jackson CL, Benbow U, Galley DJ, Karanam S: Models of plaque rupture. Drug Discov Today Dis Models 4:171-175, 2007 (reprinted with permission).

MODELS OF AORTIC ANEURYSMS

Many mouse models of aortic aneurysms have been developed that use a diverse array of methods for producing the disease, including genetic manipulation and chemical induction.[150] A common chemical-induced model involves the periaortic application of calcium chloride, which results in aortic dilation over a 2- to 4-week period. These models could provide insight into potential mechanisms in the development of this disease and in the process of vascular remodeling.[151] These models have been used to evaluate radiotracers targeted at investigation of vascular remodeling.[152]

There are also large-animal models of aortic aneurysms. Hynecek et al. have developed a novel porcine model of abdominal aortic aneurysm.[153] This porcine model has been shown to replicate the gene expression patterns that have been observed in human studies as well as in rodent models of aneurysms.[154] These large-animal models may offer advantages for investigating the interrelationship of vascular remodeling, aneurysm expansion, and regional shear and vascular mechanics.

SHORT-TERM AND LONG-TERM MODELS

Short-term and long-term models have important practical and physiologic differences, some of which have already been outlined. Whereas long-term models are much more expensive and labor intensive to maintain, they offer the important advantage of evaluating a physiologic state at multiple time points with multiple radiotracers. Long-term models also offer the option of evaluating a radiotracer under conscious, unsedated conditions, which may be particularly important in the evaluation of metabolic tracers or pharmacologic stressors. Radiotracer kinetics can be evaluated even during treadmill exercise in permanently instrumented animals. To facilitate the injection of diffusible radiotracers and radiolabeled microspheres in conscious animals during different physiologic conditions, indwelling vascular access devices can be implanted. These devices are implanted under the skin between the scapula; the end of the device can be tunneled subcutaneously for insertion in the left atrium through a small thoracotomy. They can also be implanted in the neck for direct and repeated access to the carotid artery.

EVALUATION OF PHARMACOLOGIC STRESSORS

Radiotracers are often used in conjunction with pharmacologic stressors, particularly for the detection of coronary artery disease. Recent evidence suggests that radiotracer pharmacokinetics may be influenced by the type of pharmacologic stress applied.[155-158] Therefore, biological models have an important role in evaluation of pharmacologic stressors.

The effects of pharmacologic stress on radiotracer kinetics can be initially evaluated in short-term anesthetized models. However, the effects of inotropic agents such as dobutamine and arbutamine on global hemodynamics, regional myocardial flow, and function may be greatly influenced by the type of anesthesia. For example, the anesthetized dog is more sensitive to inotropic stimulation; in contrast, it requires much higher doses of adenosine to elicit the same effect on coronary flow. These differences must be taken into consideration when designing experimental protocol involving a pharmacologic stressor. Ultimately, pharmacologic stressors must be evaluated in long-term, conscious experimental models to define their true effects on radiotracer kinetics.

CONCLUSIONS

Intact biological models play a critical role in the evaluation of radiotracers for application in the diagnosis and management of cardiovascular disease. The toxicity, biodistribution, and dosimetry of a radiotracer can be determined effectively with small-animal models. Larger-animal models permit evaluation of myocardial radiotracer kinetics under control and ischemic conditions. This kinetic analysis can be accomplished by using dynamic imaging (planar, SPECT, or PET), miniature detectors, serial biopsies, postmortem tissue well counting, or autoradiography.

Animal models are often used to validate specific clinical application of radiolabeled tracers. To understand the underlying physiology and evaluate these potential clinical applications, specific physiologic states must be modeled. This chapter described short-term and long-term models of ischemia, infarction, stunning, hibernation, and congestive heart failure. The development of more advanced instrumentation and image reconstruction may permit kinetic analysis of new radiotracers in smaller animals. These advances may allow for application of transgenic models in our evaluations of radiotracers in specific diseases.

In the future, study of radiotracers by using intact animal models may provide fundamental insight into our understanding of the pathophysiology of the cardiovascular system. We may be better able to define such processes as atherosclerosis or ischemic injury. Radiotracer studies will certainly provide insight into membrane transport and receptor binding and regulation in the heart and vasculature. Study of intact biological models will be necessary for optimal development of diagnostic approaches that use radioisotopes. These diagnostic approaches can ultimately be used to assess the efficacy of new pharmacologic or mechanical therapies. Through application of radiotracers in physiologic models, we will learn more about metabolic regulation of the cardiovascular system and the interrelation of cardiovascular structure and function.

REFERENCES

1. Lambrecht R, Eckelman W: *Animal models in radiotracer design*, New York, 1983, Springer-Verlag.
2. Lambrecht R: *Biological models in radiopharmaceutical development*, Dordrecht, The Netherlands, 1996, Kluwer Academic Publishers.
3. Bader M, Ganten D: Transgenic rats: tools to study the function of the renin-angiotensin system, *Clin Exp Pharmacol Physiol Suppl* 3:S81–87, 1996.
4. Pasqualini R, Duatti A, Bellande E, et al: Bis(dithiocarbamato)-nitrido technetium-99m radiopharmaceuticals: A class of neutral myocardial imaging agents, *J Nucl Med* 35:334–341, 1994.
5. Hatada K, Riou LM, Ruiz M, et al: 99mTc-N-DBODC5, a new myocardial perfusion imaging agent with rapid liver clearance: Comparison with 99mTc-sestamibi and 99mTc-tetrofosmin in rats, *J Nucl Med* 45(12):2095–2101, 2004.
6. Higuchi T, Nekolla SG, Huisman MM, et al: A new 18F-labeled myocardial PET tracer: Myocardial uptake after permanent and transient coronary occlusion in rats, *J Nucl Med* 49(10):1715–1722, 2008.
7. Higuchi T, Bengel FM, Seidl S, et al: Assessment of {alpha}v{beta}3 integrin expression after myocardial infarction by positron emission tomography, *Cardiovasc Res* 78(2):395–403, 2008.
8. Morishita S, Kusuoka H, Yamamichi Y, Suzuki N, Kurami M, Nishimura T: Kinetics of radioiodinated species in subcellular fractions from rat hearts following administration of iodine-123-labeled 15-(p-iodophenyl)-3-(R,S)-methylpentadecanoic acid (123I-BMIPP), *Eur J Nucl Med* 23:383–389, 1995.

9. Kubota K, Som P, Oster Z, Brill A, Goodman M, Knapp FJ, et al: Detection of cardiomyopathy in animal model using quantitative autoradiography, *J Nucl Med* 29:1697–1703, 1988.
10. Takatsu H, Uno Y, Fujiwara H: Modulation of left ventricular iodine-125-MIBG accumulation in cardiomyopathic Syrian hamster using the renin-angiotensin system, *J Nucl Med* 36:1055–1061, 1995.
11. Lu P, Zanzonico P, Goldfine S, et al: Antimyosin antibody imaging in experimental aortic regurgitation, *J Nucl Cardiol* 4:25–32, 1997.
12. Lindsey ML, Escobar GP, Dobrucki LW, et al: Matrix metalloproteinase-9 gene deletion facilitates angiogenesis after myocardial infarction, *Am J Physiol Heart Circ Physiol* 290(1):H232–239, 2006.
13. Su H, Spinale FG, Dobrucki LW, et al: Noninvasive targeted imaging of matrix metalloproteinase activation in a murine model of postinfarction remodeling, *Circulation* 112(20):3157–3167, 2005.
14. Liu Y-H, Yang X-P, Nass O, Sabbah H, Peterson E, Carretero O: Chronic heart failure induced by coronary ligation in Lewis inbred rats, *Am J Physiol Heart Circ Physiol* 272:H722–H727, 1997.
15. Reinhardt C, Weinstein H, Marcel R, Leppo J: Comparison of iodine-125-BMIPP and thallium-201 in myocardial hypoperfusion, *J Nucl Med* 36:1645–1653, 1995.
16. Fujita M, Morimoto Y, Ishihara M, et al: A new rabbit model of myocardial infarction without endotracheal intubation, *J Surg Res* 116(1):124, 2004.
17. Sinusas A, Bengel F, Nahrendorf M, et al: Multimodality cardiovascular molecular imaging, Part I, *Circ Cardiovasc Imaging* 1.244–256, 2008.
18. Nahrendorf M, Sosnovik D, French B, et al: Multimodality cardiovascular molecular imaging, Part II, *Circ Cardiovasc Imaging* 2:56–70, 2009.
19. Bader M, Bohnemeier H, Zollmann F, Lockley-Jones O, Ganten D: Transgenic animals in cardiovascular disease research, *Exp Physiol* 85:713–731, 2000.
20. Carmeliet P, Collen D: Transgenic mouse models in angiogenesis and cardiovascular disease, *J Pathol* 190(3):387–405, 2000.
21. Fazio S, Linton MF: Mouse models of hyperlipidemia and atherosclerosis, *Front Biosci* 6:D515–525, 2001.
22. Olgin JE, Verheule S: Transgenic and knockout mouse models of atrial arrhythmias, *Cardiovasc Res* 54(2):280–286, 2002.
23. de Winther MP, Hofker MH: New mouse models for lipoprotein metabolism and atherosclerosis, *Curr Opin Lipidol* 13(2):191–197, 2002.
24. Daugherty A: Mouse models of atherosclerosis, *Am J Med Sci* 323(1):3–10, 2002.
25. Xu Q: *A handbook of mouse models of cardiovascular disease*, Chichester, England; Hoboken, NJ, 2006, John Wiley & Sons.
26. Zadelaar S, Kleemann R, Verschuren L, et al: Mouse models for atherosclerosis and pharmaceutical modifiers, *Arterioscler Thromb Vasc Biol* 27(8):1706–1721, 2007.
27. Moon A, Robert SK: Chapter 4 Mouse models of congenital cardiovascular disease, *Curr Top Dev Biol* 84:171, 2008.
28. Williams RS, Wagner PD: Transgenic animals in integrative biology: approaches and interpretations of outcome, *J Appl Physiol* 88(3):1119–1126, 2000.
29. Gambhir S, Bauer E, Black M, et al: A mutant herpes simplex virus type I thymidine kinase reporter gene shows improved sensitivity for imaging of reporter gene expression with positron emission tomography, *Proc Natl Acad Sci U S A* 97:2785–2790, 2000.
30. Wu J, Inubushi M, Sundaresan G, Schelbert H, Gambhir S: Positron emission tomography imaging of cardiac reporter gene expression in living rats, *Circulation* 106:180–183, 2002.
31. Wu JC, Chen IY, Sundaresan G, et al: Molecular imaging of cardiac cell transplantation in living animals using optical bioluminescence and positron emission tomography, *Circulation* 108(11):1302–1305, 2003.
32. Rajewsky K, Gu H, Kuhn R, et al: Conditional gene targeting, *J Clin Invest* 98(3):600–603, 1996.
33. Furth P, Onge L, Boger H, et al: Temporal control of gene expression in transgenic mice by a tetracycline-responsive promoter, *Proc Natl Acad Sci U S A* 91(20):9302–9306, 1994.
34. Deutsch E, Ketring A, Libson K, Vanderheyden J, Hirth W: The Noah's Ark experiment: Species dependent biodistributions of cationic 99mTc complexes, *Int J Nucl Med Biol* 16:191–232, 1989.
35. Ball RM, Bache RJ, Cobb FR, Greenfield JC: Regional myocardial blood flow during graded treadmill exercise in the dog, *J Clin Invest* 55:43–49, 1975.
36. Gupta KB, Ratcliffe MB, Fallert MA, Edmunds LH Jr, Bogen DK: Changes in passive mechanical stiffness of myocardial tissue with aneurysm formation, *Circulation* 89(5):2315–2326, 1994.
37. Reimer K, Lowe J, Rasmussen M, Jennings R: The wavefront phenomenon of ischemic cell death. I. Myocardial infarct size vs duration of coronary occlusion in dogs, *Circulation* 56:786–794, 1977.
38. Buxton D, Schelbert H: Measurement of regional glucose metabolic rates in reperfused myocardium, *Am J Physiol* 261:H2058–H2068, 1991.
39. Dae M, O'Connell J, Botvinick E, Chin M: Acute and chronic effects of transient myocardial ischemia on sympathetic nerve activity, density and norepinephrine content, *Cardiovasc Res* 30:270–280, 1995.
40. Sinusas AJ: Targeted imaging offers advantages over physiological imaging for evaluation of angiogenic therapy, *JACC Cardiovasc Imaging* 1(4):511–514, 2008.
41. Johnson LL, Schofield L, Donahay T, Bouchard M, Poppas A, Haubner R: Radiolabeled arginine-glycine-aspartic acid peptides to image angiogenesis in swine model of hibernating myocardium, *JACC Cardiovasc Imaging* 1(4):500–510, 2008.
42. Sinusas A, Watson D, Cannon J, Beller G: Effect of ischemia and postischemic dysfunction on myocardial uptake of technetium-99m-labeled methoxyisobutyl isonitrile and thallium-201, *J Am Coll Cardiol* 14(7):1785–1793, 1989.
43. Sinusas A, Trautman K, Bergin J, et al: Quantification of area at risk during coronary occlusion and degree of myocardial salvage after reperfusion with technetium-99m methoxyisobutyl isonitrile, *Circulation* 82:1424–1437, 1990.
44. Sinusas A, Shi Q, Vitols P, et al: Impact of regional ventricular function, geometry, and dobutamine stress on quantitative 99mTcSestamibi defect size, *Circulation* 88:2224–2234, 1993.
45. Sinusas A, Shi Q, Saltzberg M, et al: Technetium-99m-tetrofosmin to assess myocardial blood flow: Experimental validation in an intact canine model of ischemia, *J Nucl Med* 35:664–671, 1994.
46. Sinusas A, Bergin J, Edwards N, et al: Redistribution of 99mTc-sestamibi and 201Tl in the presence of a severe coronary artery stenosis, *Circulation* 89:2332–2341, 1994.
47. Shi C, Sinusas A, Dione D, et al: Technetium-99m-nitroimidazole (BMS181321): A positive imaging agen for detecting myocardial ischemia, *J Nucl Med* 36:1078–1086, 1995.
48. Meoli DF, Sadeghi MM, Krassilnikova S, et al: Noninvasive imaging of myocardial angiogenesis following experimental myocardial infarction, *J Clin Invest* 113(12):1684–1691, 2004.
49. Kalinowski L, Dobrucki LW, Meoli DF, et al: Targeted imaging of hypoxia-induced integrin activation in myocardium early after infarction, *J Appl Physiol* 104(5):1504–1512, 2008.
50. Shi CQ, Young LH, Daher E, et al: Correlation of myocardial p-(123)I-iodophenylpentadecanoic acid retention with (18)F-FDG accumulation during experimental low-flow ischemia, *J Nucl Med* 43(3):421–431, 2002.
51. Mays A, Cobb F: Relationship between regional myocardial blood flow and thallium-201 distribution in the presence of coronary artery stenosis and dipyridamole-induced vasodilation, *J Clin Invest* 73:1359–1366, 1984.
52. Gross D: *Animal models in cardiovascular research*, ed 2, Dordrecht, The Netherlands, 1994, Kluwer Academic Publishers.
53. Gewirtz H, Grote G, Strauss H, et al: The influence of left ventricular volume and wall motion on myocardial images, *Circulation* 59:1172–1177, 1979.
54. Kojima A, Matsumoto M, Takahashi M, Hirota Y, Yoshida H: Effect of spatial resolution on SPECT quantification values, *J Nucl Med* 30:508–514, 1989.
55. Okada R, Pohost G: The use of preintervention and postintervention thallium imaging for assessing the early and late effects of experimental coronary arterial reperfusion in dogs, *Circulation* 69:1153–1160, 1984.
56. Okada RD, Glover D, Gaffney T, Williams S: Myocardial kinetics of technetium-99m-hexakis-2-methoxy-2-methylpropyl-isonitrile, *Circulation* 77(2):491–498, 1988.
57. Stewart R, Heyl B, O'Rourke R, Blumhardt R, Miller D: Demonstration of differential post-stenotic myocardial technetium-99m-teboroxime clearance kinetics after experimental ischemia and hyperemic stress, *J Nucl Med* 32:2000–2008, 1991.
58. Sadeghi MM, Krassilnikova S, Zhang J, et al: Detection of injury-induced vascular remodeling by targeting activated alphavbeta3 integrin in vivo, *Circulation* 110(1):84–90, 2004.
59. Nakajima K, Taki J, Bunko H, et al: Dynamic acquisition with a three-headed SPECT system: application to technetium-99m-SQ30217 myocardial imaging, *J Nucl Med* 1991:1273–1277, 1991.
60. Smith A, Gullberg G, Christain P, FL D: Kinetic modeling of teboroxime using dynamic SPECT imaging of a canine model, *J Nucl Med* 35:484–495, 1994.
61. Stewart R, Schwaiger M, Hutchins G, et al: Myocardial clearance kinetics of technetium-99m-SQ30217: A marker of regional myocardial blood flow, *J Nucl Med* 31:1183–1190, 1990.
62. Ishizu K, Mukai T, Yonekura Y, et al: Ultra-high resolution SPECT system using four pinhole collimators for small animal studies, *J Nucl Med* 36:2282–2287, 1995.
63. Weber D, Ivanovic M, Franceschi D, et al: An approach to in vivo high-resolution SPECT imaging in small laboratory animals, *J Nucl Med* 35:342–348, 1994.
64. Weber D, Ivanovic M: Pinhole SPECT: Ultra-high resolution imaging in small animal studies [editorial], *J Nucl Med* 36:2287–2289, 1995.
65. Hirai T, Nohara R, Hosokawa R, et al: Evaluation of myocardial infarct size in rat heart by pinhole SPECT, *J Nucl Cardiol* 7(2):107, 2000.
66. Constantinesco A, Choquet P, Monassier L, Israel-Jost V, Mertz L: Assessment of left ventricular perfusion, volumes, and motion in mice using pinhole gated SPECT, *J Nucl Med* 46(6):1005–1011, 2005.

67. Vanhove C, Lahoutte T, Defrise M, Bossuyt A, Franken PR: Reproducibility of left ventricular volume and ejection fraction measurements in rat using pinhole gated SPECT, *Eur J Nucl Med Mol Imaging* 32 (2):211, 2005.

68. Sharir T, Ben-Haim S, Merzon K, et al: High-speed myocardial perfusion imaging: Initial clinical comparison with conventional dual-detector Anger camera imaging, *JACC Cardiovasc Imaging* 1 (2):156–163, 2008.

69. Berman DS, Kang X, Tamarappoo B, et al: Stress thallium-201/rest technetium-99m sequential dual isotope high-speed myocardial perfusion imaging, *JACC Cardiovasc Imaging* 2(3):273–282, 2009.

70. Wagenaar D, Parnham K, Sundal B, et al: *Advantages of semiconductor CZT for medical imaging*, Paper presented at: Penetrating Radiation Systems and Applications VIII, 2007.

71. Montemont G, Bordy T, Rebuffel V, Robert C, Verger L: *CZT pixel detectors for improved SPECT imaging*, Paper presented at: Nuclear Science Symposium Conference Record, 2008. NSS '08. IEEE, 2008.

72. Nickles R, Nunn A, Stone C, Christian B: Technetium-94m-teboroxime: Synthesis, dosimetry and initial PET imaging studies, *J Nucl Med* 34:1058–1066, 1993.

73. Stone C, Christian B, Nickles R, Perlman S: Technetium 94m-labeled methoxyisobutyl isonitrile: Dosimetry and resting cardiac imaging with positron emission tomography, *J Nucl Cardiol* 1:425–433, 1994.

74. Berger F, Yu-Po L, Loening A, et al: Whole-body skeletal imaging in mice utilizing microPET: optimization of reproducibility and applications in animal models of bone disease, *Eur J Nucl Med* 29:1225–1236, 2002.

75. Okada R: Kinetics of thallium-201 in reperfused canine myocardium after coronary artery occlusion, *J Am Coll Cardiol* 3:1245–1251, 1984.

76. Okada R, Jacobs M, Daggett W, et al: Thallium-201 kinetics in nonischemic canine myocardium, *Circulation* 65:70–77, 1982.

77. Jacobs M, Okada R, Daggett W, Fowler B, Strauss H, Pohost G: Regional myocardial radiotracer kinetics in dogs using miniature detectors, *Am J Physiol* 242:H849–854, 1982.

78. Gerson M, Millard R, Roszell N, et al: Kinetic properties of 99mTc-Q12 in canine myocardium, *Circulation* 89:1291–1300, 1994.

79. Granato J, Watson D, Flanagan T, GAscho J, Beller G: Myocardial thallium-201 kinetics during coronary occlusion and reperfusion: Influence of method of reflow and timing of thallium-201 administration, *Circulation* 73:150–160, 1986.

80. Li QS, Solot G, Frank TL, Wagner HJ, Becker LC: Myocardial redistribution of technetium-99m-methoxyisobutyl isonitrile (SESTAMIBI), *J Nucl Med* 31(6):1069–1076, 1990.

81. Weinstein H, Reinhardt CP, Leppo JA: Teboroxime, sestamibi and thallium-201 as markers of myocardial hypoperfusion: Comparison by quantitative dual-isotope autoradiography in rabbits, *J Nucl Med* 34:1510–1517, 1993.

82. Weinstein H, Reinhardt CP, Wironen JF, Leppo JA: Myocardial uptake of thallium-201 and technetium 99m-labeled sestamibi after ischemia and reperfusion: Comparison by quantitative dual-tracer autoradiography in rabbits, *J Nucl Cardiol* 1:351–364, 1994.

83. Ito T, Brill A: Validity of tissue paste standards for quantitative whole-body autoradiography using short-lived radionuclides, *Appl Radiat Isot* 41:661–667, 1990.

84. Crumeyrolle-Arias M, Jafarian-Tehrani M, Cardona A, et al: Radioimagers as an alternative to film autoradiography forin situ quantitative analysis of125I-ligand receptor binding and pharmacological studies, *Histochem J* 28(11):801, 1996.

85. Barthe N, Chatti K, Coulon P, Maîtrejean S, Basse-Cathalinat B: Recent technologic developments on high-resolution beta imaging systems for quantitative autoradiography and double labeling applications, *Nucl Instrum Methods Phys Res A* 527(1–2):41, 2004.

86. Tomoike H, Ogata I, Maruoka Y, Sakai K, Kurozumi T, Nakamura M: Differential registration of two types of radionuclides on macroautoradiograms for studying coronary circulation: Concise communication, *J Nucl Med* 24:693–699, 1983.

87. Heymann M, Payne B, Hoffman J, Rudolph A: Blood flow measurements with radionuclide-labeled particles, *Prog Cardiovasc Dis* 20:55–79, 1977.

88. Morais D, Richart T, Fritz A, Acree P, Davila J, Glover R: The production of chronic experimental mitral insufficiency, *Ann Surg* 145:500–508, 1957.

89. Pohost G, Okada R, O'Keefe D, Gewirtz H, Beller G, Strauss H, Chaffin J, Leppo J, Daggett W: Thallium redistribution in dogs with severe coronary stenosis of fixed caliber, *Circ Res* 48:439–446, 1981.

90. Yipintsoi T, Dobbs W, Scalon P, Knopp T, Bassingthwaighte J: Regional distribution of diffusable tracers and carbonized microspheres in the left ventricle of isolated dog hearts, *Circ Res* 33:573–587, 1973.

91. Meleca M, McGoron A, Gerson M, et al: Flow versus uptake comparisons of thallium-201 with technetium-99m perfusion tracers in a canine model of myocardial ischemia, *J Nucl Med* 38:1847–1856, 1997.

92. Reimer K, Jennings R: The "wavefront phenomenon" of myocardial ischemic cell death. II. Transmural progression of necrosis within the framework of ischemic bed size (myocardium at risk) and collateral flow, *Lab Invest* 40:633–644, 1979.

93. Connelly C, Vogel W, Hernandez Y, Apstein C: Movement of necrotic wavefront after coronary occlusion in rabbit, *Am J Physiol* 243: H682–H690, 1982.

94. Stone H, Bishop V, Guyton A: Cardiac function after embolization of coronaries with microspheres, *Am J Physiol* 204:16–27, 1963.

95. Kordenat R, Kezdi P, Stanley F: A new catheter technique for producing experimental coronary thrombosis and selective coronary visualization, *Am Heart J* 83:360–367, 1972.

96. Roth D, Maruoka Y, Rogers J, White F, Longhurst J, Bloor C: Development of coronary collateral circulation in left circumflex ameroid-occluded swine myocardium, *Am J Physiol* 253:H1279–H1288, 1987.

97. Ducharme A, Frantz S, Aikawa M, et al: Targeted deletion of matrix metalloproteinase-9 attenuates left ventricular enlargement and collagen accumulation after experimental myocardial infarction, *J Clin Invest* 106(1):55–62, 2000.

98. Creemers EEJM, Davis JN, Parkhurst AM, et al: Deficiency of TIMP-1 exacerbates LV remodeling after myocardial infarction in mice, *Am J Physiol Heart Circ Physiol* 284(1):H364–H371, 2003.

99. Hayashidani S, Tsutsui H, Ikeuchi M, et al: Targeted deletion of MMP-2 attenuates early LV rupture and late remodeling after experimental myocardial infarction, *Am J Physiol Heart Circ Physiol* 285(3): H1229–H1235, 2003.

100. Chen J, Song S-K, Liu W, et al: Remodeling of cardiac fiber structure after infarction in rats quantified with diffusion tensor MRI, *Am J Physiol Heart Circ Physiol* 285(3):H946–954, 2003.

101. Chung G, Sinusas AJ: Imaging of matrix metalloproteinase activation and left ventricular remodeling, *Curr Cardiol Rep* 9(2):136–142, 2007.

102. Morrison AR, Sinusas AJ: New molecular imaging targets to characterize myocardial biology, *Cardiol Clin* 27(2):329, 2009.

103. Beller G, Glover D, Edwards N, Ruiz M, Simanis J, Watson D: 99mTc-sestamibi uptake and retention during myocardial ischemia and reperfusion, *Circulation* 87:2033–2042, 1993.

104. Buxton D, Vaghaiwalla Mody F, Krivokapich J, Phelps M, Schelbert H: Quantitative assessment of prolonged metabolic abnormalities in reperfused canine myocardium, *Circulation* 85:1842–1856, 1992.

105. Miller D, Gill J, Livni E, et al: Fatty acid analogue accumulation: A marker of myocyte viability in ischemic-reperfused myocardium, *Circ Res* 63:681–692, 1988.

106. Nishimura T, Sago M, Kihara K, et al: Fatty acid myocardial imaging using 123I-B-methyl-iodophenyl pentadecanoic acid (BMIPP): Comparison of myocardial perfusion and fatty acid utilization in canine myocardial infarction (occlusion and reperfusion model), *Eur J Nucl Med* 15:341–345, 1989.

107. Young D, Cholrin N, Roth A: Pressure drop across artificially induced stenosis in the femoral arteries in dogs, *Circ Res* 36:735–743, 1975.

108. Anversa P, Loud A, Leviscky V, Guideri G: Left ventricular failure induced by myocardial infarction. I. Myocyte hypertrophy, *Am J Physiol* 248:H876–H882, 1985.

109. McDonald K, Francis G, Carlyle P, et al: Hemodynamic, left ventricular structural and hormonal changes after discrete myocardial damage in the dog, *J Am Coll Cardiol* 19:460–467, 1992.

110. Bolli R, Zhu W, Thornby J, O'Neill P, Roberts R: Time-course and determinants of recovery of function after reversible ischemia in conscious dogs, *Am J Physiol* 254:H102–H114, 1988.

111. Heyndrickx G, Millard R, McRitchie R, Maroko P, Vatner S: Regional myocardial functional and electrophysiological alterations after brief coronary artery occlusion in conscious dogs, *J Clin Invest* 56:978–985, 1975.

112. Nicklas J, Becker L, Bulkley B: Effects of repeated brief coronary occlusion on regional left ventricular function and dimension in dogs, *Am J Cardiol* 56:473–478, 1985.

113. Matsuzaki M, Gallagher K, Kemper W, White F, Ross JJ: Sustained regional dysfunction produced by prolonged coronary stenosis: Gradual recovery after reperfusion, *Circulation* 68:170–182, 1983.

114. Lavallee M, Cox D, Patrick T, Vatner S: Salvage of myocardial function by coronary artery reperfusion 1,2, and 3 hours after occlusion in conscious dogs, *Circ Res* 53:235–247, 1983.

115. Homans D, Sublett E, Dai X, Bache R: Persistence of regional left ventricular dysfunction after exercise-induced myocardial ischemia, *J Clin Invest* 77:66–73, 1986.

116. Vanoverschelde J-L, Wijns W, Depre C, et al: Mechanism of chronic regional postischemic dysfunction in humans: New insights from the study of noninfarcted collateral dependent myocardium, *Circulation* 87:1513–1523, 1993.

117. Camici P, Araujo L, Spinks T, et al: Increased uptake of 18F-fluorodeoxyglucose in postischemic myocardium of patients with exercise-induced angina, *Circulation* 74:81–88, 1986.

118. Vanoverschelde J, Wijns W, Borgers M, et al: Chronic myocardial hibernation in humans: From bedside to bench, *Circulation* 95:1961–1971, 1997.

119. Arai A, Pantely G, Anselone C, Brislow J, Brislow J: Aicve down regulation of myocardial energy requirements during moderate ischemia in swine, *Circ Res* 69:1458–1469, 1991.

120. Fedele F, Gewirtz H, Capone R, Sharaf B, Most A: Metabolic response to prolonged reduction of myocardial blood flow distal to a severe coronary artery stenosis, *Circulation* 78:729–735, 1988.

121. Edwards N, Sinusas A, Bergin J, Watson D, Ruiz M, Beller G: Influence of subendocardial ischemia on transmural myocardial function, *Am J Physiol* 31:H568–H576, 1992.

122. Vanzetto G, Calnon DA, Ruiz M, et al: Myocardial uptake and redistribution of 99mTc-N-NOET in dogs with either sustained coronary low flow or transient coronary occlusion: Comparison with 201Tl and myocardial blood flow, *Circulation* 96(7):2325–2331, 1997.

123. Fallavollita JA: Spatial heterogeneity in fasting and insulin-stimulated 18F-2-deoxyglucose uptake in pigs with hibernating myocardium, *Circulation* 102(8):908–914, 2000.

124. Gerber B, Laycock S, Melin J, Flameng W, Vanoverschelde J: Perfusion-contraction matching, inotropic reserve and vasodilatory capacity in a canine model of dysfunctional collateral-dependent myocardium, *Circulation* 92(suppl):I–314, 1995.

125. Shen Y, Vatner S: Mechanism of impaired myocardial function during progressive coronary stenosis in conscious pigs: Hibernation versus stunning?*Circ Res* 76:479–488, 1995.

126. Berger B, Watson D, Burwell L, et al: Redistribution of thallium at rest in patients with stable and unstable angina and the effects of coronary artery bypass graft surgery, *Circulation* 60:1114–1125, 1979.

127. Canty J, Fallavollita J: Chronic hibernation and chronic stunning: A continuum, *J Nucl Cardiol* 7:509–527, 2000.

128. Yarbrough W, Spinale F: Large animal models of congestive heart failure: A critical step in translating basic observations into clinical applications, *J Nucl Cardiol* 10:77–86, 2003.

129. Packer D, Bardy G, Worley S, et al: Tachycardia-induced cardiomyopathy: a reversible form of left ventricular dysfunction, *Am J Cardiol* 57:563–570, 1986.

130. Spinale F, Fulbright B, Mukherjee R, et al: Relations between ventricular and myocyte function with tachycardia-induced cardiomyopathy, *Circ Res* 71:174–187, 1992.

131. Spinale F, Zellner J, Tomita M, Tempel G, Crawford F, Zile M: Tachycardia induced cardiomyopathy: Effects on blood flow and capillary structure, *Am J Physiol* 261:H140–H148, 1991.

132. Zile M, Tomita M, Nakano K, et al: Effects of left ventricular volume overload produced by mitral regurgitation on diastolic function, *Am J Physiol* 261:H1471–H1480, 1991.

133. Magid N, Opio G, Wallerson D, Young M, Borer J: Heart failure due to chronic experimental aortic regurgitation, *Am J Physiol* 267: H226–H233, 1994.

134. Brousseau ME, Hoeg JM: Transgenic rabbits as models for atherosclerosis research, *J Lipid Res* 40(3):365–375, 1999.

135. Moghadasian MH: Experimental atherosclerosis: A historical overview *Life Sci* 70(8):855–965, 2002.

136. Watanabe Y: Serial inbreeding of rabbits with hereditary hyperlipidemia (WHHL-rabbit): Incidence and development of atherosclerosis and xanthoma, *Atherosclerosis* 36:261–268, 1980.

137. Nordestgaard B, Lewis B: Intermediate density of lipoprotein levels are strong predictors of the extent of aortic atherosclerosis in the St. Thomas's Hospital rabbit strain, *Atherosclerosis* 87:39–46, 1992.

138. Vallabhajosula S, Granada J, Kothari P, et al: Porcine model of complex coronary atherosclerosis (CCA) or vulnerable plaque: Role of FDG-PET to study the disease progression and assess lesion macrophage activity, *J Nucl Med* 48(Suppl 2):104, 2007.

139. Piedrahita J, Zhang S, Hagaman J, Oliver P, Maeda N: Generation of mice carrying a mutant apolipoprotein E gene inactivated by gene targeting in embryonic stem cells, *Proc Natl Acad Sci U S A* 89:4471–4475, 1992.

140. Zhang S, Reddick R, Burkey B, Maeda N: Diet-induced atherosclerosis in mice heterozygous and homozygous for apolipoprotein E gene disruption, *J Clin Invest* 94:937–945, 1994.

141. Nakashima Y, Plump A, Raines E, Breslow J, Ross R: ApoE-deficient mice develop lesions of all phases of atherosclerosis throughout the arterial tree, *Arterioscler Thromb* 14:133–140, 1994.

142. Williams II, Johnson J, Carson K, Jackson C: Characteristics of intact and ruptured atherosclerotic plaques in brachiocephalic arteries of apolipoprotein E knockout mice, *Arterioscler Thromb Vasc Biol* 22:788–792, 2002.

143. Kolodgie FD, Petrov A, Virmani R, et al: Targeting of apoptotic macrophages and experimental atheroma with radiolabeled annexin V: A technique with potential for noninvasive imaging of vulnerable plaque, *Circulation* 108(25):3134–3139, 2003.

144. Ohtsuki K, Hayase M, Akashi K, Kopiwoda S, Strauss HW: Detection of monocyte chemoattractant protein-1 receptor expression in experimental atherosclerotic lesions: An autoradiographic study, *Circulation* 104(2):203–208, 2001.

145. Bjorkerud S, Bjorkerud B: Apoptosis is abundant in human atherosclerotic lesions, especially in inflammatory cells (macrophages and T cells), and may contribute to the accumulation of gruel and plaque instability, *Am J Pathol* 149(2):367–380, 1996.

146. Geng Y-J, Henderson LE, Levesque EB, Muszynski M, Libby P: Fas is expressed in human atherosclerotic intima and promotes apoptosis

147. Narula J, Petrov A, Bianchi C, et al: Noninvasive localization of experimental atherosclerotic lesions with mouse/human chimeric Z2D3 F (ab')2 specific for the proliferating smooth muscle cells of human atheroma: Imaging with conventional and negative charge–modified antibody fragments, *Circulation* 92(3):474–484, 1995.

148. Narula J, Petrov A, Pak K-Y, Ditlow C, Chen F, Khaw B-A: Noninvasive detection of atherosclerotic lesions by 99mTc-based immunoscintigraphic targeting of proliferating smooth muscle cells, *Chest* 111:1684–1690, 1997.

149. Jackson CL, Benbow U, Galley DJ, Karanam S: Models of plaque rupture, *Drug Discov Today Dis Models* 4(4):171, 2007.

150. Daugherty A, Cassis LA: Mouse models of abdominal aortic aneurysms, *Arterioscler Thromb Vasc Biol* 24(3):429–434, 2004.

151. Kuivaniemi H, Platsoucas CD, Tilson MD III, : Aortic aneurysms: An immune disease with a strong genetic component, *Circulation* 117 (2):242–252, 2008.

152. Nie L, Razavian M, Zhang J, et al: Imaging matrix metalloproteinase activation to predict aneurysm expansion in vivo, *J Nucl Med* 2009 (in press).

153. Hynecek RL, DeRubertis BG, Trocciola SM, et al: The creation of an infrarenal aneurysm within the native abdominal aorta of swine, *Surgery* 142(2):143, 2007.

154. Sadek M, Hynecek RL, Goldenberg S, Kent KC, Marin ML, Faries PL: Gene expression analysis of a porcine native abdominal aortic aneurysm model, *Surgery* 144(2):252, 2008.

155. Calnon DA, Glover DK, Beller GA, et al: Effects of dobutamine stress on myocardial blood flow, 99mTc sestamibi uptake, and systolic wall thickening in the presence of coronary artery stenoses: Implications for dobutamine stress testing, *Circulation* 96(7):2353–2360, 1997.

156. Wu JC, Yun JJ, Heller EN, et al: Limitations of dobutamine for enhancing flow heterogeneity in the presence of single coronary stenosis: implications for technetium-99m-sestamibi imaging, *J Nucl Med* 39(3):417–425, 1998.

157. Calnon DA, Ruiz M, Vanzetto G, Watson DD, Beller GA, Glover DK: Myocardial uptake of 99mTc-N-NOET and 201Tl during dobutamine infusion: Comparison with adenosine stress, *Circulation* 100(15): 1653–1659, 1999.

158. He Z-X, Cwajg E, Hwang W, et al: Myocardial blood flow and myocardial uptake of 201Tl and 99mTc-sestamibi during coronary vasodilation induced by CGS-21680, a selective adenosine A2A receptor agonist, *Circulation* 102(4):438–444, 2000.

159. Reddick RL, Zhang SH, Maeda N: Aortic atherosclerotic plaque injury in apolipoprotein E deficient mice, *Atherosclerosis* 140(2):297, 1998.

160. von der Thusen JH, van Vlijmen BJM, Hoeben RC, et al: Induction of atherosclerotic plaque rupture in apolipoprotein E-/- mice after adenovirus-mediated transfer of p53, *Circulation* 105(17):2064–2070, 2002.

161. Cheng C, Tempel D, van Haperen R, et al: Atherosclerotic lesion size and vulnerability are determined by patterns of fluid shear stress, *Circulation* 113(23):2744–2753, 2006.

162. Johnson JL, Jackson CL: Atherosclerotic plaque rupture in the apolipoprotein E knockout mouse, *Atherosclerosis* 154(2):399, 2001.

163. Williams H, Johnson JL, Carson KGS, Jackson CL: Characteristics of intact and ruptured atherosclerotic plaques in brachiocephalic arteries of apolipoprotein E knockout mice, *Arterioscler Thromb Vasc Biol* 22(5):788–792, 2002.

164. Johnson J, Carson K, Williams H, et al: Plaque rupture after short periods of fat feeding in the apolipoprotein E-knockout mouse: Model characterization and effects of pravastatin treatment, *Circulation* 111(11):1422–1430, 2005.

165. Braun A, Trigatti BL, Post MJ, et al: Loss of SR-BI expression leads to the early onset of occlusive atherosclerotic coronary artery disease, spontaneous myocardial infarctions, severe cardiac dysfunction, and premature death in apolipoprotein E-deficient mice, *Circ Res* 90 (3):270–276, 2002.

166. Herrera V, Didishvili T, Lopez L, et al: Hypertension exacerbates coronary artery disease in transgenic hyperlipidemic Dahl salt-sensitive hypertensive rats, *Mol Med* 7:831–844, 2001.

167. Constantinides P, Chakravarti R: Rabbit arterial thrombosis production by systemic procedures, *Arch Pathol* 72:197–208, 1961.

168. Abela GS, Picon PD, Friedl SE, et al: Triggering of plaque disruption and arterial thrombosis in an atherosclerotic rabbit model, *Circulation* 91(3):776–784, 1995.

169. Rekhter MD, Hicks GW, Brammer DW, et al: Animal model that mimics atherosclerotic plaque rupture, *Circ Res* 83(7):705–713, 1998.

170. Granada J, Moreno P, Burke A, Schulz D, Raizner A, Kaluza G: Endovascular needle injection of cholesteryl linoleate into the arterial wall produces complex vascular lesions identifiable by intravascular ultrasound: early development in a porcine model of vulnerable plaque, *Coron Artery Dis* 16:217–224, 2005.

171. Prescott M, McBride C, Hasler-Rapacz J, Von Linden J, Rapacz J: Development of complex atherosclerotic lesions in pigs with inherited hyper-LDL cholesterolemia bearing mutant alleles for apolipoprotein B, *Am J Pathol* 139:139–147, 1991.

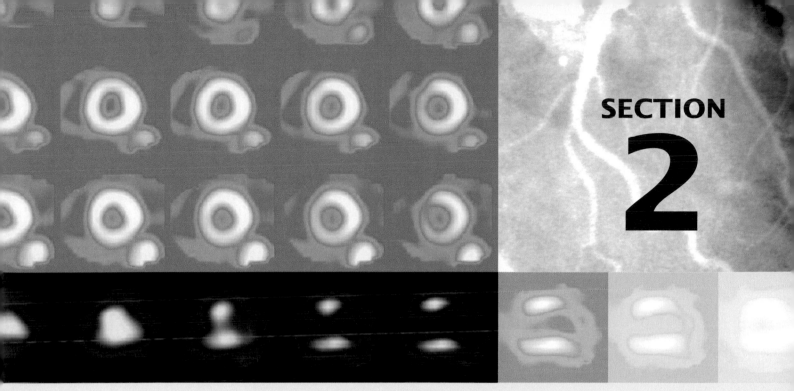

Instrumentation

Chapter 4

SPECT Processing, Quantification, and Display

TRACY L. FABER, JI CHEN AND ERNEST V. GARCIA

INTRODUCTION

Myocardial perfusion imaging with single-photon emission computed tomography (SPECT) is the most frequently performed study in nuclear cardiology, and utilization is actually increasing. One important reason for this is that vast improvements in image quality and processing sophistication have brought about the ability to perform completely automatic motion correction, reconstruction, reslicing, quantification, and high-level analysis of the results. New databases consistent with the new studies being performed, including dual-isotope protocols and attenuation-corrected images, are commercially available. Three-dimensional (3D) displays of quantitated perfusion are now commonly used in conjunction with the original slices for patient evaluation. Automated interpretation of the quantitative information in the form of expert systems is available to help train new nuclear medicine physicians, aid in the analysis of complex cases, or act as a second opinion. Explicit automatic comparisons of serial studies are improving the assessment of changes in perfusion so that a patient's condition can be more easily tracked. Integration of perfusion images with those obtained from other modalities is becoming more and more common as a way to combine and compare all available image information for a given patient. Finally, recently developed software methodologies allow phase analysis of gated myocardial perfusion SPECT images to quantitatively measure left ventricular dyssynchrony. These and other

similar advances will continue to improve the quality of information obtained from nuclear myocardial perfusion imaging, so that in the future, there will be more automation applied to more types of studies to further objectify and standardize analysis, display, integration, and interpretation.

OBLIQUE REORIENTATION AND RESLICING

Although the original tomograms obtained by reconstructing raw data from positron emission tomography (PET) and SPECT scanners are in a transaxial orientation, cardiac images are generally viewed in different formats consisting of short-axis, horizontal long-axis, and vertical long-axis slices. Short-axis slices are also necessary for some automatic perfusion quantification algorithms, and determination of functional parameters can depend upon accurate reorientation.[1] Generation of these standard sections from the original transaxial images used to be performed interactively, requiring the user to mark the location of the left ventricular (LV) axis. In the past few years, automatic techniques for performing this task have been described and are commercially available.[2–4]

Two approaches[2,3] for automatic reorientation start by identifying the LV region in the transaxial images, using a threshold-based approach that includes knowledge about expected position, size, and shape of the LV. Once isolated, the approach described by Germano et al.[2] uses the original data to refine the estimate of the myocardial surface. Normals to an ellipsoid fit to the LV region are used to resample the myocardium; a Gaussian function is fit to the profiles obtained at each sample. The best fit Gaussian is used to estimate the myocardial center for each profile, and after further refinement based on image intensities and myocardial smoothness, the resulting mid-myocardial points are fitted to an ellipsoid whose long axis is used as the final

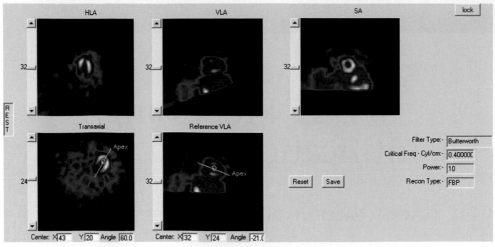

Figure 4-1 Example of oblique reorientation. Bottom row shows automatically detected long axis on the original transaxial *(left)* and resliced sagittal *(right)* slices. Horizontal long-axis, vertical long-axis, and short-axis sections resulting from this automatically determined long axis are displayed from *left to right on the top row.*

LV long axis. The method was tested on 400 patient images and the result compared to interactively denoted long axes. Failure of the method was described as either not localizing the LV, presence of significant hepatic or intestinal activity in the LV region of the image, or greater than 45 (o) difference between automatically and interactively determined axes. With these criteria, the method was successful in 394 of the 400 cases.

Faber et al.[3] also use the expected size and location of the heart in the image to isolate the ventricles. They then use a search algorithm to find the best axis of symmetry in the transaxial plane by reflecting the image about this axis and subtracting the result from the original slices. To improve comparisons in the case of reduced perfusion, the image is normalized separately on each side of the axis being tested. Once the best axis on the transaxial slice is located, the image is resliced parallel to this axis, and the process is repeated using the resulting near-sagittal images. This method was applied to 25 rest and stress studies; automatic center and axis angles were compared to those chosen by an expert, and the difference in quantitative results resulting from the automatic and interactive reorientation were evaluated. The average absolute mean difference between the interactively and automatically chosen horizontal long-axis angles was 6.3 ± 5(o). The average absolute mean difference between the interactively and automatically chosen veritcal long-axis angles was 5.7 ± 4.2(o). In addition, using the quantitation following interactively chosen reorientation angles as the gold standard, the automatic reorientation resulted in an accuracy of 92% for diagnosing coronary artery disease (CAD). Example results from this method can be seen in Figure 4-1.

Slomka et al.[4] take a different approach entirely to automated reorientation. Their method registers the original image data to a "template" image in which the orientation of the LV is known and standardized. The template is created by averaging a large number of registered, normal patient data sets, and a separate template is created for males and females. The registration is done by first translating and scaling the image based on

principal axes; the match is refined by minimizing the sum of the absolute differences between the template and the image being registered. This method was not compared to interactively reoriented images, but it was evaluated visually for 38 normal and 10 abnormal subjects and found to be successful for all.

MOTION CORRECTION (See Chapter 5)

Patient or organ motion during SPECT scanning can cause small image artifacts in the best case and make the scan unreadable in the worst case. A good overview of the effects of motion and how to detect them are given by Fitzgerald and Danias.[5] Most manufacturers now provide automatic motion correction algorithms that account for a patient moving during the acquisition. One early approach by Cooper et al.[6] attempted to determine the position change of the heart in the sinograms and correct for this. This method, along with manual correction, was found by O'Conner et al.[7] to be particularly effective in removing various kinds of patient movement in a phantom study. More recently, a motion correction technique has been introduced that is based on the operation of making projections or sinograms more consistent with the reconstruction.[8] From the original data, a reconstruction is created. New projections are computed using the original reconstruction and compared to the original projections. Each original projection is aligned with the new projections created from the reconstruction. The registered projections are reconstructed again to create a new starting reconstruction, and the process is iterated until the registered original projections match the reprojections of the reconstruction created from them. This occurs when the data sets are consistent (i.e., when the motion artifacts are removed from the projections through the iterative alignment). An evaluation of this approach was published by Matsumoto et al.[9] The importance of motion correction on both slices and quantitative results is demonstrated in Figure 4-2.

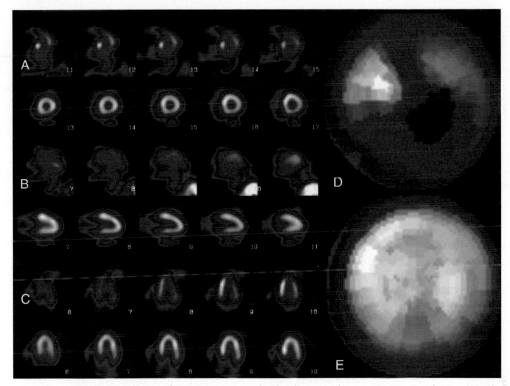

Figure 4-2 Automatic motion correction software improves both slices and quantitative analysis. (**A**) Short-axis sections, (**B**) vertical long-axis sections, and (**C**) horizontal long-axis sections. In each of A, B, and C, the original resting study is shown on the *top*, and the motion-corrected study is shown on the *bottom*. (**D**) Original blackout map showing resting perfusion defects. (**E**) Blackout map from the motion-corrected slices. Note the significant changes between **D** and **E**.

AUTOMATED PERFUSION QUANTIFICATION

Data based methods for identifying a patient's myocardial perfusion abnormalities from thallium (Tl)-201 SPECT studies have been previously developed and commercialized by investigators at Cedars-Sinai Medical Center[10] and Emory University[11] and reported as early as 1985. More recently, these methods have been widely used by various investigators to quantify myocardial perfusion SPECT studies imaged using technetium ^{99m}Tc-based agents. These methods utilize a statistically defined database of normal (and abnormal) patients to be used as a pattern to compare prospective CAD patients. These methods have been extensively validated[12] and proven to be clinically valuable[12] in standardizing and objectifying[13] myocardial perfusion scans. These validations have shown that in stable patients having serial perfusion studies, quantification is more reproducible than the visual interpretation of experts for determining the magnitude of the perfusion abnormality.[13] This improved reproducibility of quantitative techniques over visual analysis promotes the need for the use of quantification in randomized clinical trials and in monitoring the effects of therapy in an individual patient.[13]

Five major limitations of initial quantification approaches had to be overcome to reach the present high level of accuracy and reproducibility. One limitation had been the extensive operator interaction that results in reduced objectivity and reproducibility of the program. By automating the process, this limitation has been overcome, as was partially addressed in the previous section. A second limitation had been the failure to sample the count distribution perpendicular to the myocardial wall, particularly at the apex. This usually results in artifactually increasing the counts from the apical region. A third limitation had been the lack of databases for specific perfusion tracer/acquisition protocol combinations. Comparison of patients acquired with different tracers and/or different protocols to a normal database often leads to incorrect identification of abnormalities. A fourth limitation had been the inability of these data-based approaches to compensate for attenuation in a patient whose attenuating tissue (such as breast and diaphragm) is significantly more than those of the normal patients selected for the normal database. This almost always leads to artifactually defining these photopenic regions as hypoperfused myocardium. The fifth limitation had been the inability of the polar map display to represent accurately the true extent and location of an abnormality. This is due to the warping created by transforming a 3D distribution into a two-dimensional (2D) polar map. This limitation results in underestimating the extent of hypoperfused apical regions and overestimating the extent of hypoperfused basal regions. Details about how these limitations have been overcome are provided in the following discussion.

Myocardial Isolation and Sampling

Newer quantitative methods have been developed to overcome the major limitations described. These methods use several automatic image-identification techniques for isolation of the left myocardium from the remainder of the image.[14] Once the left myocardium is identified, the apex and base, the coordinates of the central axis of the ventricular chamber, and a limiting radius for count profile search are determined automatically. In the majority of cases, operator interaction is required only for verification of automatically determined parameters. If at any time these automated programs fail to locate any of the features, they will branch to an interactive mode and require the operator to select the parameters manually.

Once the LV has been isolated from the myocardial perfusion scan, these automated programs extract the 3D LV myocardial count distribution. This sampling is done using either a hybrid, two-part, 3D sampling scheme of stacked short-axis slices[15] or an ellipsoidal sampling of the 3D distribution inside the ellipsoid.[16] In the hybrid sampling approach used in the CEqual program, the apical region of the myocardium is sampled using spherical coordinates, and the rest of the myocardium is sampled using cylindrical coordinates. This approach promotes a radial sampling that is mostly perpendicular to the myocardial wall for all points and thus results in a more accurate representation of the perfusion distribution with minimal sampling artifacts. Following operator verification of the automatically derived features, the 3D maximum count myocardial distribution is extracted from all stacked short-axis tomograms.[16] During cylindrical sampling, maximum count circumferential profiles, each composed of 40 points, are automatically generated from the short-axis slices. During spherical sampling, maximal counts are extracted from the apical region, with the number of samples proportional to the apical area from which they are extracted. The combination of the cylindrical and spherical coordinates forms a set of 3D count profiles representing the myocardial tracer uptake. In the approach used by the QPS program, the sampling geometry is performed using an ellipsoidal rather than a hybrid model, and count profiles from endocardium to epicardium are used rather than maximal counts. Other methods used variations of these approaches, including a slice-by-slice maximal count circumferential profile extraction.[17,18]

These 3D count distributions are generated for the stress and the rest myocardial perfusion distributions. A normalized percent change between stress and rest is also calculated as a reversibility distribution.[19] The most normal region of the stress distribution is used for normalizing the rest to the stress distribution.

Normal Databases and Criteria for Abnormality

Once the stress and rest count distributions have been extracted from a patient's LV myocardium and the reversibility distribution determined, they are compared to normal patterns found in computerized databases. These normal databases are usually generated from patients with a low likelihood of CAD. Although there is variation among methods as to how best to define these patients, in general, patients with less than 5% probability of CAD are used. This probability is based on the Diamond and Forester[20] criteria that uses a Bayesian analysis of the patient's age, sex, symptoms, and the results of other noninvasive tests such as stress EKG.

The stress, rest, and reversibility distributions from males and females are separately combined to produce gender-matched normal files. This is done to help account for differences in body habitus that cause changes in the expected normal patterns between men and women due to photon attenuation. The distributions from these normal patients are statistically combined to provide the mean normal regional LV normalized count distribution and its corresponding regional standard deviation for the stress, rest, and reversibility distributions.[11,21]

The next step in this process is to determine the criteria for abnormality. These criteria are usually determined as the number of standard deviations below the mean for each region in the stress and rest distributions and above the mean for the reversibility distribution. These numbers then represent the cutoff points between a normal and an abnormal region. Here also there is variation between methods. Some methods always use two standard deviations below the mean, some always use 2.5, some allow it to vary from patient to patient by the interpreter, and others determine the optimal cutoff criteria.

Determination of the optimal cutoff criteria for each region requires that perfusion studies from both normal and abnormal patients be used. In the normal databases used by the CEqual processing program, for example, the optimal cutoff point is determined using receiver operator curve (ROC) analysis.[21] By varying the standard deviation (and/or any other quantitative parameter used, such as the extent of the abnormality) the determination of "normal" or "abnormal" by the program is compared to a gold standard such as expert visual analysis or catheterization results. ROC curves are then generated by plotting the true-positive rate versus the false-positive rate. The best cutoff is then determined as the desired tradeoff between the expected sensitivity and specificity for the detection and localization of CAD. Depending on the developers' strategy, optimal criteria could mean the best tradeoff between sensitivity and specificity, or high-sensitivity with lower specificity, or higher specificity with lower sensitivity. These results can and do vary between methods, but they can also vary between normal databases used by the same program. It is imperative that the physician using these programs has reviewed published validations performed against prospective populations to understand the true performance characteristics of the quantitative software/normal database combination they are using.

Quantitative Parameters

The programs for quantifying LV myocardial perfusion report findings in terms of quantitative parameters. One typical parameter used is the extent of the perfusion abnormality. This extent is expressed either as a percentage of the total LV epicardial area that is hypoperfused or, in systems that calculate total LV mass, as the mass in grams that is hypoperfused. Usually in these systems, the extent of the hypoperfused region that reverses is also reported.

Quantitative parameters that take into account both the extent and severity of the abnormality are also determined. The total severity score is calculated as the total number of standard deviations below the mean normal distribution for regions exhibiting perfusion defects.[22] The sum stress score is the sum of segmental scores in a (17 or 20) segmental model of the LV where each segment is scored from 0 (normal) to 4 (perfusion absent).[23] These scores are either manually or automatically assigned. Automatic assignment is performed by comparison to the normal database, with the scores calibrated to interpretations by human experts.

It is important to understand the thresholds that are used for differentiating normal from hypoperfused regions and how these thresholds are used to validate the various commercial programs. This knowledge will prevent the interpreter from misinterpreting small statistical fluctuations as abnormal hypoperfusion. For example, in the Emory Cardiac Toolbox (ECTb) program that uses the CEqual algorithm for quantification of myocardial perfusion, the key quantitative parameter used for identifying abnormality is the extent of the abnormality expressed as percent of the abnormal area. With this technique, at least 3% of the entire LV myocardium has to be hypoperfused before the patient is deemed to be abnormal. Similarly, at least 10% of the left anterior descending (LAD) region, 10% of the left circumflex (LCx) region, and 12% of the right coronary artery

(RCA) region must be hypoperfused before CAD is localized to that vascular territory. Similarly, the extent of the stress perfusion defect has to reverse (improve) by at least 5% at rest for the region to be deemed partially reversible and at least 15% for it to be considered to improve post revascularization.

Commercial Implementations

Variations of the methods described thus for have been commercialized in at least eight separate products at the time of this writing. Three of these methods have become the most popular. These are the ECTb developed at Emory University,[24,25] Corridor 4DM developed at the University of Michigan,[26,27] and QPS/QGS developed at Cedars-Sinai in Los Angeles.[16,28] A fourth method also used commercially is the Wackers-Liu CQ software developed at Yale University.[17,29]

These software packages have become popular because (1) they are automated; (2) they (usually) integrate image display, perfusion quantification, and functional quantification in one package; and (3) they are well validated.[25,30,31] Examples of applying three commercial programs to quantify the same patient are shown in Figures 4-3 through 4-5. It is important to understand that the implementation of these programs varies from vendor to vendor. Thus, even though one should expect that the same program will yield the same results given the same perfusion study, the case and speed of obtaining and displaying results may vary not only between the packages but also from vendor to vendor and between versions of the same program.

Figure 4-3 Perfusion quantification results obtained from processing a patient with ECTb. The *top row* shows the quantitated stress *(left)* and rest *(middle)* perfusion and the difference between the two *(right)*. The *middle row* shows the stress blackout map *(left)*, the rest blackout map *(middle)*, and the whiteout reversibility map *(right)*. The *bottom left* map displays the number of standard deviations (SD) below normal of each myocardial sample of the stress *(left)* and rest *(middle)* perfusion, and the number of SDs above normal for reversibility *(right)*. This patient had a completely reversible anteroseptal perfusion defect.

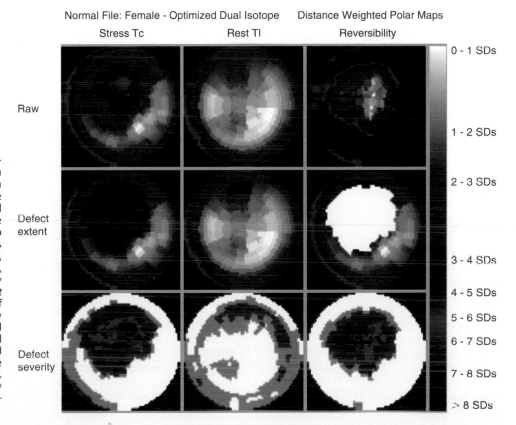

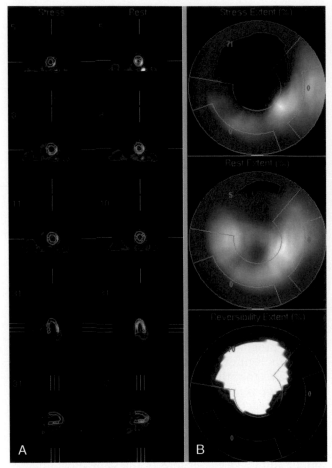

Figure 4-4 Perfusion quantification results obtained from processing the same patient as in Figure 4-3 with QPS. The *left side* of the figure (**A**) shows slices from the patient; the *top three rows* contain short-axis slices, and the *bottom two rows* show horizontal long-axis and vertical long-axis slices, respectively. The *right side* of the figure (**B**) shows the results of quantitation: the stress blackout map *(top)*, the rest blackout map *(middle)*, and the whiteout reversibility map *(bottom)*. Note the similarities of these results compared with those of Figure 4-3.

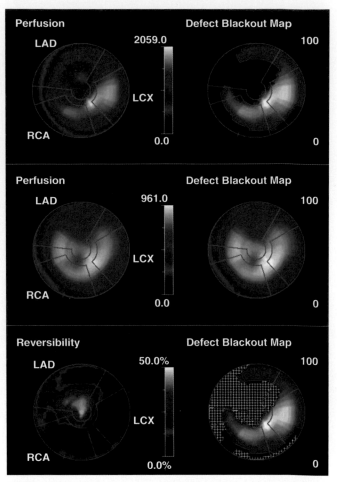

Figure 4-5 Perfusion quantification results obtained from processing the same patient as in Figure 4-3 with Corridor 4DM. The *top row* shows the quantitated stress *(left)* and stress blackout map *(right)*. The *middle row* shows the quantitated rest *(left)* and rest blackout map *(right)*. The *bottom row* shows the difference between rest and stress perfusion *(left)* along with the whiteout reversibility map *(right)*. Note the similarities of these results with those of Figures 4-3 and 4-4.

To date, no definitive study has been performed to compare the relative ease of operation, robustness, and accuracy of these programs. It is well accepted that in general the automation in these programs is quite robust, and they yield similar diagnostic accuracy.

New Databases

As new acquisition protocols and/or new perfusion tracers become popular, new normal databases must be developed. For example, for ECTb, gender-matched normal databases have been defined[21] and validated for the following SPECT protocols:

1. Low-dose rest, high-dose stress, 1-day [99mTc]-sestamibi (Cardiolite) protocol[32]
2. High-dose stress and rest 2-day [99mTc]-sestamibi protocol
3. Stress-redistribution [201Tl]-protocol
4. Rest [201Tl]-/stress [99mTc]-sestamibi dual-isotope protocol[32]

5. Low-dose stress, high-dose rest [99mTc]-tetrofosmin (Myoview) 1-day protocol

All protocols used treadmill exercise to stress the patients.

The choice of which radiopharmaceutical and/or protocol should be used is more of a clinical question or a question of laboratory logistics and is beyond the scope of this chapter. However, there are a number of questions related to these normal databases that are very often asked and merit further discussion.

One concern is whether the normal databases developed using patients stressed with exercise can be used for patients undergoing pharmacologic stress. It is evident by looking at these studies that patients imaged after pharmacologic stress have more background activity and more myocardial activity than patients undergoing treadmill exercise. Nevertheless, the relative distributions in normal and CAD patients are similar enough that when the same normal database is used for both forms of stress, it results in similar diagnostic accuracy.[33] Although it would be ideal to have separate databases for protocols using pharmacologic stress, the development cost would be prohibitive.

A second concern is whether the normal database developed for ^{201}Tl-stress/redistribution studies may be used for stress/reinjection protocols. The stress protocol is the same for both studies, so no new errors should be introduced. However, the reinjection images do appear different from the redistribution images. Nevertheless, in the CEqual program used by ECTb, the resting distribution is not quantified, but rather the reversibility or change between rest and stress is analyzed. Since reinjection is supposed to result in a more marked difference between the two physiologic states, it is actually easier for the program to detect this difference in the form of defect reversibility. Thus, the stress/redistribution ^{201}Tl-normal database may be used to quantify stress/reinjection studies.

The last concern is whether the normal database for the ^{99m}Tc-sestamibi protocols may be used for ^{99m}Tc-tetrofosmin studies and vice versa. Although there are some subtle differences in how these two radiopharmaceuticals are distributed in the body, the main parameters driving the final count distributions in the images are the type of collimators and filters used for a given count distribution. It appears that these normal databases are interchangeable, but additional studies are required to confirm these observations.

DISPLAY

Once perfusion has been quantified, the quantitative data must be displayed. In planar perfusion imaging, the myocardial samples were often displayed as a graph of relative counts versus angle (about the LV). SPECT perfusion data require more complex methods of display in order to present the larger amount of information clearly and logically. Polar maps were developed as a way to display the quantified perfusion data of the entire LV in a single picture. More recently, 3D displays have been adopted by many researchers, hospitals, and manufacturers as a more natural way to present the information.

Polar Maps

Polar maps, or bull's-eye displays, are the standard for viewing circumferential profiles. They allow a quick and comprehensive overview of the circumferential samples from all slices by combining these into a color-coded image. The points of each circumferential profile are assigned a color based on normalized count values, and the colored profiles are shaped into concentric rings. The most apical slice processed with circumferential profiles forms the center of the polar map, and each successive profile from each successive short-axis slice is displayed as a new ring surrounding the previous. The most basal slice of the LV makes up the outermost ring of the polar map. Figure 4-3 shows polar maps created from applying the CEqual quantification method to a perfusion study.

The use of color can help identify abnormal areas at a glance as well. Abnormal regions from the stress study can be assigned a black color, thus creating a blackout map. Blacked-out areas that normalize at rest are color-coded white, thus creating a whiteout reversibility map.[19] This can also be seen in Figure 4-3. Additional maps—for example, a standard deviation map that shows the number of standard deviations below normal of each point in each circumferential profile—can aid in evaluation of the study by indicating the severity of any abnormality.

Polar maps, while offering a comprehensive view of the quantitation results, distort the size and shape of the myocardium and any defects. There have been numerous improvements in the basic polar map display to help overcome some of these problems.[15] For instance, "distance-weighted" maps are created so that each ring is the same thickness. These maps have been shown to be useful for accurate localization of abnormalities. "Volume-weighted" maps are constructed such that the area of each ring is proportional to the volume of the corresponding slice. This type of map has been shown to be best for estimating defect size. However, more realistic displays have been introduced that do not suffer from the distortions of polar maps.

Three-Dimensional Displays

Three-dimensional graphics techniques can be used to overlay results of perfusion quantification onto a representation of a specific patient's LV. Figure 4-6 displays the same information seen in the polar maps of Figure 4-3, using a 3D representation. In its most basic form, the pixel locations of the maximal-count myocardial points sampled during quantitation are used to estimate the myocardial surface. More sophisticated methods may detect the epicardial surface boundaries of the perfusion scan.[16,24,34] These points can be connected into triangles, which are then color-coded similarly to the polar map; details of how such displays can be created may be found in the book by Watt, for example.[35] Such displays can routinely be rotated in real time and viewed from any angle with current computer power. They have the advantage of showing the actual size and shape of the LV and the extent and location of any defect in a very realistic manner. Some studies have shown that the 3D models are more accurate for evaluating the size and location of perfusion defects than polar maps[36] or slice-by-slice displays.[37]

A second approach to creating 3D displays from cardiac images generates the myocardial boundaries directly from image voxels without explicit boundary detection. These techniques are more helpful when used with computed tomography (CT) data; however, given the current interest in CT coronary angiography (CTCA), it is useful to understand the methods. Volume rendering is a 3D graphics technique that provides very realistic-appearing visualizations. For a volume of data, such as a stack of 2D tomographic slices, one assigns to every pixel a transparency, a color, and a reflectivity. The visual process is then simulated by recreating the physical process of light traveling

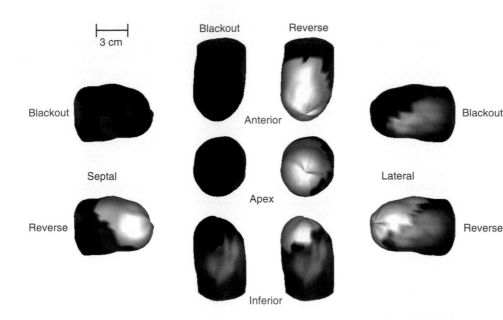

Figure 4-6 Three-dimensional surface-rendered displays of stress blackout and reversibility whiteout information from the same patient as in Figure 4-3. *From the top, clockwise,* are shown an anterior, lateral, inferior, and septal view. An apical view is shown in the *middle* of the display.

through or bouncing off the pixels that it encounters as it travels through the volume. More details of this process may also be found in the textbook by Watt.[35] For any given volume of data, the main problems involve the correct assignation of the pixel properties. Selecting a gray level threshold above which everything is opaque and below which everything is transparent, for example, will provide a 3D image with hard surfaces at that threshold. Unfortunately, very few medical images are accurately segmented with such simplistic threshold techniques. CT images are in fact probably the best adapted to this simple method of assigning pixel properties, since Hounsfield units are related to the electron density of particular tissues, and thus, bone can be made opaque and white, while muscle tissue can be made translucent and red, for example. Nonetheless, most 3D displays of the heart generated from CTCA require large amounts of preprocessing to remove extracardiac structures. The accuracy of this preprocessing is generally related to the quality of the images, and user intervention may be required to produce a useable 3D display. In addition, large amounts of memory and processing power are required for volume rendering of large data sets, although specialized algorithms that take advantage of specific data properties may be used to speed up the process.[38] Nevertheless, the realism, high resolution, and flexibility of volume renderings give them an advantage over surface renderings in many cases; this can be appreciated in Figure 4-7.

ARTIFICIAL INTELLIGENCE TECHNIQUES APPLIED TO SPECT

Interpretation of medical images by decision-support systems has made significant progress in recent years, mostly due to the implementation of artificial intelligence (AI) techniques. There are several major application areas associated with AI[39,40]: natural language

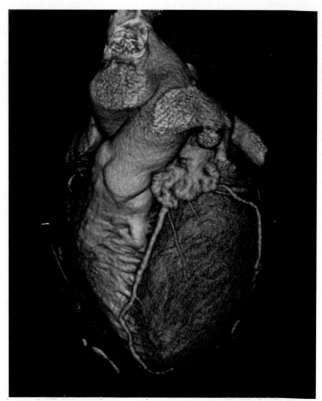

Figure 4-7 Volume-rendered display of a computed tomography coronary angiogram. Higher-intensity contrast in the coronary arteries has been assigned a white, opaque property; Hounsfield units associated with soft tissue have been assigned reddish, more translucent properties. Evidence of poor segmentation and user interaction is visible toward the apex on both sides of the left ventricle but particularly toward the right ventricle.

processing, problem solving and planning, computer vision, expert systems, and neural computing (neural networks). Expert systems and neural networks are two AI techniques that are currently being applied to nuclear medicine.

Expert System Analysis of Perfusion Tomograms

Expert systems are becoming commercially popular because they are designed to circumvent the problem of having few experts in areas where many are needed. Thus, expert systems attempt to capture the knowledge or expertise of the human domain expert and provide it to a large number of nonexperts. An example of the power of expert systems is found in PERFEX (PERFusion EXpert), a system that was originally developed to assist in diagnosing CAD from ^{201}Tl-myocardial distributions.[41,42] This type of approach has the potential for standardizing the image interpretation process. After reviewing 291 studies from patients with angiographically documented coronary artery disease, heuristic rules were derived that best correlated the presence and location of perfusion defects on ^{201}Tl-SPECT studies with coronary lesions. These rules operate on data that are input to the expert system from the CEqual SPECT quantification process, which identifies (1) *defects* as portions of the myocardium where normalized perfusion falls below a predetermined number of standard deviations when compared to a gender-matched normal file and (2) *reversibility* as defects at stress that improve at rest. An automatic feature extraction program then describes the location and severity of each defect or reversibility. The location is expressed in the form of 32 possible descriptors and is defined as coordinates of both depth (basal, medial, distal-apical, and proximal-apical) and angular location (eight subsets of the septal, inferior, lateral, and anterior myocardial walls). The severity is expressed in terms of certainty factors that range from -1 to $+1$ (-1 means there is definitely no disease, $+1$ means there is definitely disease, and the range from -0.2 to $+0.2$ means equivocal or indeterminable). Using the above features, the expert system automatically determines the location, size, and shape of each defect/reversibility. This information is used to "fire" or execute the 253 heuristic rules in order to produce new facts or draw new inferences. For each input parameter and for each rule, a certainty factor is assigned and is used to determine the certainty of the identification and location of a coronary lesion.

PERFEX has undergone extensive validation. Sixty prospective ^{99m}Tc-sestamibi patients (30 with angiographic correlation and 30 without, including 40 patients with CAD and 20 normals) were first used to validate the clinical efficacy of the CEqual/PERFEX program for detecting and localizing CAD.[43] The results showed excellent agreement between PERFEX and the human expert for detecting the presence (95%) and localizing CAD to the LAD (92%), LCx (100%), and RCA (96%) vascular territories. The results were good but less impressive for detecting the absence of CAD (50%) overall or in the vascular territories: LAD (46%), LCx (71%), and RCA (76%). These disagreements were concluded to be due mostly to the inherent limitation of not taking into account all of the clinical variables as is done by experts.

The purpose of a second study[44] was to validate PERFEX using a large prospective validation consisting of 376 stress/delayed ^{201}Tl-, 138 rest/stress ^{99m}Tc-sestamibi myocardial perfusion studies, and 141 rest ^{201}Tl-/stress ^{99m}Tc-sestamibi patients who also underwent coronary angiography. The visual interpretations of slices and maps, vessel stenosis from coronary angiography, and PERFEX interpretations were all accessed automatically from databases and used to automatically generate intercomparisons. This study showed that PERFEX demonstrated a higher sensitivity and correspondingly a lower specificity than visual interpretation by human experts for identifying the presence and location of CAD. It also showed that the agreement between PERFEX and the human expert was better than compared to coronary angiography.

Neural Networks

Neural networks have been developed as an attempt to simulate the highly connected biological system found in the brain through the use of computer hardware and/or software. In the brain, a neuron receives input from many different sources. It integrates all of these inputs and "fires" (sending a pulse down the nerve to other connected neurons) if the result is greater than a set threshold. In the same way, a neural network has nodes (the equivalent of a neuron) that are interconnected and receive input from other nodes. Each node sums or integrates its inputs and then uses a linear or nonlinear transfer function to determine if the node should "fire." A neural network can be arranged in many different ways; for example, it can have one or more layers of nodes, it can be fully connected (where every node is connected to every other node), or it can be partially connected. Also, it can have feed-forward processing (where processing only travels one direction), or it can have feedback processing (where processing travels both ways).

Another important aspect of neural networks is their ability to "learn" based on input patterns. A neural network can be trained in either a supervised or unsupervised mode. In the supervised mode, the net is trained by presenting it with an input and giving it the desired output. The error between the output of the net and the desired output is then propagated backward through the net, adjusting the weights of the inputs of all the nodes in such a way that the desired output is achieved. This is repeated for many input sets of training data and for multiple cycles per training set. Once the net has converged (i.e., the weights change very little for additional training sets or cycles), it can be tested with prospective data. This kind of training paradigm is very useful for finding patterns out of a known collection of patterns. Unsupervised training is similar to supervised training, but instead of providing the net with the desired output, it is free to find its own output. This type of training can be very useful for finding patterns in data where there is no known set of existing patterns. The main advantage of a neural network is the ability to solve a problem that can be represented by some sort of training data without needing an expert. However, if the training data are not complete, or if a problem is presented to the network that it has not been trained to solve, it may not give reliable answers.

With careful training, neural networks can provide a unique approach to solving problems. For example use neural networks have already been used by three different groups in nuclear cardiology to identify which coronaries are expected to have stenotic lesions for a specific hypoperfused distribution.[45–47] These methods vary on the number of input and output nodes used. The more training data available, the better the possibility for more nodes. The output of these systems can be as simple as a single node signifying that there is a lesion present in the myocardium.

WeAidU is one example of an automatic interpretation neural network for interpretation of myocardial perfusion scans.[48] In a European multicenter trial of this approach, perfusion studies from different hospitals along with the physicians' interpretations were transmitted to the neural network site where the images were processed and the interpretations compared. Agreement between hospitals varied between 74% and 92%.[49]

Data Mining

Data mining is a technique for discovering patterns in large data sets. These methods are generally statistical in nature and/or taken from pattern recognition approaches. Like neural nets, they require a training set for which the truth is known. However, instead of creating a neural network that may be able to process images for diagnostic purposes, the output of a data mining approach is associations between patterns in the data set. These associations may be used to help create an expert system or simply to investigate the data set more closely. Usually, the data input into a data mining algorithm is highly processed; for example, the scores from a typical 17-segment model may be used as the input. A data mining algorithm provided with this information for a large number of patients, along with each patient's actual diagnosis, may be able to predict the value of a score in each region that would indicate a fixed defect and statistics about its likelihood of being abnormal. Some examples of data mining applied to cardiac SPECT perfusion images can be read in research by Kurgan et al.[50] and Sacha et al.[51]

Commercial Implications

The PERFEX expert system approach described earlier has been integrated as part of the ECTb.[25] In this integrated view box display, all of the myocardial perfusion and function visual and quantitative data are available for the physician's review, as is a button that when depressed provides the expert system decision support. An example PERFEX processing within ECTb is shown in Figure 4-8.

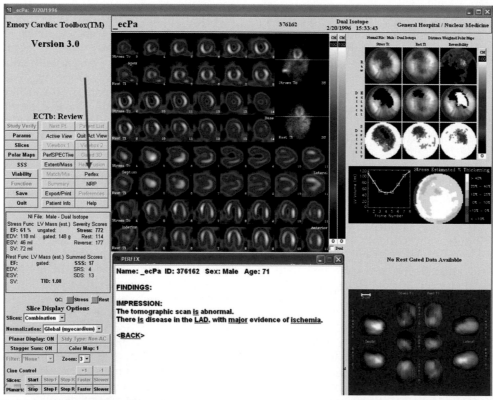

Figure 4-8 ECTb display of a patient with a reversible anterior wall stress-induced perfusion defect. Active comprehensive display that integrates: *(top-middle panel)* planar projections and oblique slices; *(top right)* polar maps, including normal database comparison; *(bottom right)* 3D displays; *(middle right)* LV volume/time curve and regional thickening map. *(Bottom middle)* Output of PERFEX expert system. PERFEX provides decision support by suggesting the study findings and impression. Each conclusion is underlined in the dialogue. By clicking on each underlined word, PERFEX provides justification for that conclusion reached. Note the quantitative measurements reported in the *middle left panel*. Also note the *blue arrow* pointing to the integrated PERFEX button in the *top-left panel* showing the available tools.

The WeAidU NEURAL NETWORK decision support approach has also been integrated into a cardiac software product called Care Heart and is now part of Exini Diagnostics (www.exini.com) under the name Exini Heart.

ASSESSMENT OF SERIAL STUDIES

In many cases, physicians are asked to evaluate changes in the heart, to evaluate the effects of therapy, or simply to follow a patient whose cardiac health may be improving or declining. Myocardial perfusion imaging is most often the method by which these changes are evaluated. Two processing steps may be applied to improve the assessment of changes in serial studies.

First, to optimally compare the images visually or quantitatively, they should be aligned with each other. MacDonald et al., for example, have demonstrated variabilities resulting from processing differences in serial SPECT studies,[52] and Faber et al.[53] demonstrated that explicit alignment of perfusion studies was necessary to allow accurate detection of even 10% changes in perfusion. The problem of matching one cardiac SPECT perfusion image to another has been investigated in the realm of aligning stress and rest images of the same patient or matching PET and SPECT images to each other. Historically, the images have been aligned to each other using only translation and rotation. In the simplest case, this alignment is achieved by finding and aligning the LV long axes in both images.[2,3] More complicated template matching that aligns over translation and rotation of two different images has also been described by Slomka et al.,[4] Turkington,[54] Peace,[55] and Faber,[53] for example. Some of these approaches were originally developed to align stress images to rest images,[3] to correct dynamic images for motion,[56] and to align a patient's image to a single standard for finding perfusion abnormalities,[57] but each of these applications is essentially similar to the problem of matching serial SPECT studies.

Others have matched extracted boundaries of the LV to align the images. Gilardi et al.[56] matched the extracted LV surfaces of PET and SPECT images of the same patient to find the rigid transform that best aligns the studies. Declerck et al.[57] used the iterative closest point approach to find the best rigid transform to align rest and stress surfaces to each other and to determine the best spline transform to align a specific SPECT study to a template image for diagnosing abnormalities. Thirion[58] used an elastic deformable model approach for intramodality registration of SPECT images. Use of this approach to align serial SPECT studies of patients acquired only days apart showed that it could improve reproducibility in quantitative perfusion measurements.[59]

Once the images are aligned, explicit statistical comparison between the perfusion distributions may help the physician determine if differences in perfusion are significant. This is because the use of standard measures of perfusion may not be sufficient to detect small changes. Faber et al. investigated using standard perfusion quantification measures, such as the summed stress score and summed total severity score, to analyze changes in perfusion.[60] In a set of simulations in which defect size and severity were varied, they showed that changes in summed stress scores did not correlate well with changes in severity ($r = 0.56$); summed stress scores correlated somewhat better ($r = 0.77$). This is unsurprising, since summed stress scores have a rather small range and may not be able to capture small changes. In general, scores such as the STSS and the total perfusion deficit (TPD),[61] which evaluate each pixel of the polar map and have a wide range of possible values, should be able to capture more of the variabilities of perfusion changes in serial studies. In fact, TPD has been used in large-scale clinical trials with success to analyze whether changes can be seen in groups of patients.[62] More recently, Berman et al. have shown that of TPD to assess serial studies is more reproducible than visual assessment.[13] In a set of patients whose condition was not expected to change, serial imaging performed within 22 months was analyzed by both visual analysis and quantitative TPD, and correlations of quantitative parameters between the serial studies were higher than correlations of visual indices.

However, use of a single global measure of perfusion will not give a complete picture of clinical changes when evaluating single patients. Instead, more information may be obtained by evaluating regional or even pixel-level changes in polar maps or the images themselves. Faber et al. investigated using a statistical comparison of the perfusion values within each segment of a 20-segment division of the polar maps.[60] While useful for detecting large perfusion changes, the approach failed entirely when changes were less than or equal to 5%. The method could only detect 10% changes when the size of the defect was greater than 1/8 of the LV. A more accurate approach looked at changes of pixel values within perfusion defects (determined by comparison of the perfusion values to a normal database). Perfusion values from the blacked-out area of one study were compared to those from the same region in the other study. This approach allowed high accuracy detection of both 10% and 15% differences in perfusion severity.[53] One of the few clinical studies performed to evaluate the efficacy of alignment and statistical comparison approaches for analysis of serial studies was carried out by Itti et al.[63] These investigators used the methods of Declerck et al.[57] to align both of the serial studies to a normal template and determine regions of abnormality in both. Changes within this abnormal region were computed and compared statistically. The method was applied in 49 patients to compare perfusion before and after PTCA, using QCA as a gold standard. They were able to show significant differences in perfusion changes between patients that did and did not reocclude 3 months after revascularization. Figure 4-9 shows an example from this work.

FUSION OF MULTIMODALITY CARDIAC IMAGERY

Frequently, patients being evaluated for cardiac disease have more than one imaging procedure. Depending upon the questions being asked, a patient may have

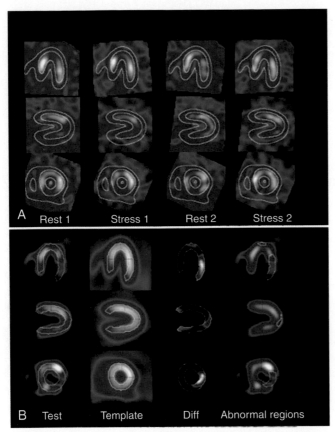

Figure 4-9 Use of image alignment and statistical comparison to find changes in serial perfusion images. (**A**) Example of image display allowing visual quality control of automated registration of serial image volumes. After each image has been fitted to a standard model of the ventricles, the boundaries of the model are overlaid on the perfusion images. These aligned images can then be statistically compared. (**B**) Representation of the key steps needed for calculation of differences. Patient's image volume (Test) is matched to reference template *(white overlay)*. All voxels with an intensity less than 1.8 standard deviations of the corresponding value from the normal population model (Template) are considered hypoperfused, as seen in the "Diff" column. These regions can be used as a mask (Abnormal regions) for the aligned test images, within which all further calculations will be performed. *(Adapted from Itti E, Klein G, Rosso, et al: Assessment of myocardial reperfusion after myocardial infarction using automatic 3D quantification and template matching, J Nucl Med 45:1981–1988, 2004.)*

coronary angiography to diagnose coronary artery stenosis, magnetic resonance imaging (MRI) to determine gross anatomy, and SPECT to evaluate myocardial perfusion. More recently, CT of the heart, with or without CTCA, is being utilized for calcium scoring and noninvasive analysis of coronary arteries. In the past, whenever more than one image of the same patient was used for evaluation, the physician mentally integrated the information in the two. However, it is now possible to align the two images so that they are in the same position and orientation as each other. This process is termed *registration, fusion,* or *unification.* Once this fusion is performed, each pixel, feature, or anatomic reference on one image can be immediately located on the other. Fused images can improve anatomical localization,

interpretation, and comprehension, as well as enhance confidence in observations.

Most manufacturers now supply interactive software so that the user can manipulate one image with 3D rotations and translations until it matches a second. However, these procedures are difficult and time-consuming, as well as subjective and irreproducible. To eliminate these drawbacks, automated methods are being developed. An excellent overview of cardiac image registration is given by Makela et al.[64] In the following sections, three applications of automatic integration of cardiac nuclear medicine with other modalities are described.

Registration of Myocardial Perfusion and Magnetic Resonance Images

Cardiac MRI is the gold standard for investigating cardiac anatomy and function. Its high resolution in space and time provides exquisite pictures of the moving heart, and in addition, delayed enhancement images using gadolinium may be used to visualize myocardial infarcts, including even small subendocardial infarcts that are impossible to analyze with nuclear medicine. Early imaging with gadolinium may provide some measure of perfusion with MRI, but nuclear medicine is still the gold standard for this. Therefore, the registration of MRI with myocardial perfusion imaging (MPI) should allow better integration of these three pieces of information: function, infarction, and perfusion.

Registration of SPECT perfusion images with cardiac MRI of the same patient is desirable because nuclear measurements of perfusion can be compared with the superior anatomical and functional information seen in MRI. In most cases, a boundary detection to isolate the ventricles is performed first, then the boundaries of these chambers are aligned to each other.

Various groups have published reports regarding surface-based registration of cardiac MRI and PET images.[65–69] In the work of Sinha et al.[65] the LV boundaries were detected interactively using morphologic and linear filtering tools. By combining this transform with the known pixel sizes and temporal resolution, either of the four-dimensional image sets could be transformed into the spatial and temporal coordinates of the other. This method was validated by calculating the difference between user-identified landmarks in the two images after transformation, using 6 MRI/PET image pairs and an average of 14 landmarks per pair. The accuracy was determined to be 1.3 + 1.1 mm for the end-diastolic images and 1.95 + 1.6 for end-systolic images.

Makela et al.[66] segment the MRI and PET data sets using deformable models fitted to edges in the MRI image and the PET transmission images. This gives 3D models of the important structures in the thorax, specifically, lungs, mediastinum, and body surface. The models are aligned rigidly using an optimization algorithm. The same group[67] extended this work by including an additional segmentation of the left and right ventricles from the MRI using a more sophisticated deformable model; since this step was done after registration, the model could be superimposed over the PET image and used to evaluate left and right ventricular perfusion.

More recently, volumetric approaches, which do not require explicit boundary detection as a first step, have been explored. These methods are commonplace in brain images, where even images from different modalities are very similar, and a good measure of similarity between the two images can be easily found. In cardiac applications, however, nuclear images of the thorax seldom look much like those from MRI. However, if the heart can be isolated from both MRI and nuclear images, then it is possible to align them using a cost function that operates on the original myocardial pixel values and attempts to reduce the differences between them. This is the approach taken by Aladl et al.[68] When they compared the automatic approach to an interactive one performed by an expert, they found differences in translation and orientation to average approximately 1 pixel and 4(o), respectively, based on 20 patients. Results from this method can be seen in Figure 4-10.

Misko et al[69] described the use and value of registered SPECT and cardiac MRI. They used manual alignment tools to reorient the ED frame of the SPECT study with the ED frame of the MRI. Perfusion data were obtained from this ED SPECT slice, whereas function was obtained from the MRI. They used delayed enhancement MRI techniques to define viability. The registered data sets were not displayed in 3D; instead, they were divided into 6 segments per short-axis slice, and the perfusion, motion, and viability information was combined in 18 patients. They computed a statistic called *MIBI uptake per volume* (MIV), which is made up of counts from the perfusion image normalized by the volume determined by the MRI LV boundaries. They were able to show strong relationships between reduced perfusion, delayed enhancement, and hypokinesis. Although this work is a preliminary example of how clinical fusion of SPECT and MRI might work, it does not address whether explicit alignment of these modalities aids diagnosis compared to mental integration which is typically performed by the clinician.

Registration of Myocardial Perfusion Images and Coronary Artery Data from Angiography

Often in current clinical practice, accurate assessment of the extent and severity of CAD requires the integration of physiologic information derived from SPECT perfusion images and anatomic information derived from coronary angiography. In most cases, the cardiologist mentally combines information about coronary artery blockages from the angiograms with that of cardiac perfusion from SPECT. However, the 2D nature of coronary angiography, which actually produces projection images, combined with the slice-by-slice display of cardiac perfusion studies makes subjective integration difficult. The location of a stenosis with respect to the LV epicardial surface can only be judged approximately, and thus, its physiologic effects may be difficult to determine. The existence of more than one blocked artery exacerbates this problem, especially if the degree of stenosis is near 50%, since such stenoses may or may not cause perfusion abnormalities. If the angiograms could be fused to the perfusion images, many of these difficulties would be alleviated.

Most approaches that attempt to combine nuclear with angiographic data perform the alignment by registering a 3D LV model representing myocardial perfusion with the patient's own 3D coronary artery tree and present both in a single unified display. One method creates a patient-specific coronary arterial tree from a 3D geometric reconstruction performed on simultaneously acquired, from digital biplane angiographic projections, or from two single-plane projections acquired at different angles. The 3D reconstructed arterial tree is approximated by successive conical segments and scaled and rotated to fit onto the myocardial surface. The left and/or right coronary arteries are registered with the myocardial perfusion surface model by automatically minimizing a cost function that describes the relationships of the coronary artery tree with the interventricular and atrioventricular groove and the surface of the myocardium.[70] A recent publication has described clinical validations of this technique.[71] Figure 4-11 shows an example of fusion on three different patient examples.

Similar work has been reported by Schindler et al.[72] Three-dimensional models of the LV epicardium were generated from SPECT and aligned with 3D models of the left coronary artery tree created from angiograms. In this work, however, the alignment was performed by using acquisition parameters for SPECT and angiography to determine "patient coordinates" of the two models. Once these coordinates were known, the models could be easily aligned, and a simple translation between the two models was applied if necessary to refine the match. A display was generated by reprojecting both 3D models into the desired view angle.

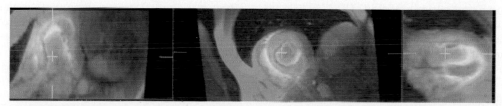

Figure 4-10 Three orthogonal slices obtained from a SPECT study registered and fused with the corresponding MRI. Automatic image registration of gated cardiac SPECT and magnetic resonance imaging. *(From Aladl UE, Hurwitz GA, Dey D, et al: Automatic image registration of gated cardiac single-photon emission computed tomography and magnetic resonance imaging, J Magn Reson Imaging 19:283–290, 2004.)*

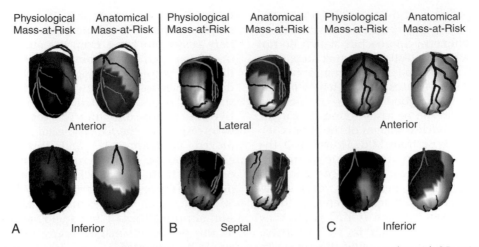

Figure 4-11 Validation of the fusion method for aligning 3D coronary trees from angiography with 3D epicardial surfaces from perfusion SPECT. Anatomic mass at risk *(purple areas)* computed from the coronary artery anatomy versus physiologic mass at risk *(black areas)* computed from perfusion quantitation. Vessels distal to the anatomic lesions are highlighted in *green*. Overlap of the purple and black areas is a measure of fusion accuracy, because in these patients, the perfusion abnormality was caused by the arterial blockage during balloon inflation for PTCA. **A**, Example of an LAD lesion. **B**, Example of an LCx lesion. **C**, Example of an RCA lesion. *(Reproduced with permission from Faber TL, Santana CA, Garcia EV, et al: 3D fusion of coronary arteries with myocardial perfusion distributions: Clinical validation. J Nucl Med 45:745–753, 2004.)*

A completely different approach was taken by Nishimura et al.[73] They used the original angiograms but superimposed these on top of a 3D model of perfusion obtained from SPECT quantification. The 3D LV was oriented to match the known angles of the angiogram and then automatically translated so that the endocardial surface in the 3D SPECT display matched the LV contour seen in a contrast left ventriculogram taken at the same angle as the arteriogram. A scaling factor was applied to the surface based on a previously calculated value determined using phantom studies.

Fusion of Myocardial Perfusion Images and CT Angiography (See Chapter 8)

More recently, the advent of combined PET/CT machines utilizing high-speed multislice CT has allowed the sequential acquisition of PET perfusion and CTCA. The images are in close alignment so that coronary artery anatomy can be visualized with the PET perfusion information. A visualization technique that displays volume-rendered CT surfaces with PET perfusion color-coding has been described by Namdar et al.[74]; in this case, the heart can be visualized in high resolution but with perfusion information overlaid on top. However, it is well understood that even in combined PET/CT scanners, the hearts are not perfectly aligned, owing to cardiac, breathing, and patient motion. Thus, additional alignment may need to be performed prior to display and analysis. Nakauro et al.[75] use an approach similar to that of Namdar et al.[74] for displaying SPECT and computed tomographic angiography (CTA) from a combined SPECT/CT scanner; however, this group does an explicit registration and volumetric display.

Faber et al.[76] take a surface-based approach in which coronary arteries segmented from the CT studies are explicitly aligned to and displayed on top of 3D models created from the PET perfusion data. The 3D LV epicardium is extracted from the PET image, and coronary arteries are extracted from the CT coronary angiogram. The left tree is aligned to the LV such that the LAD follows the anterior interventricular groove, and the LCx follows the left atrioventricular groove. The right tree is aligned so that the PDA follows the inferior interventricular groove. A final warping operation is performed so that the arteries are forced to lie on the epicardial surface.

Given that additional alignment is needed even from combined scanners and that high-resolution multislice CT scanners exist in radiology departments separate from any nuclear perfusion scanners, it is quite desirable to be able to align retrospectively CTA and SPECT or PET studies from different scanners. A study by Nakajo et al.[77] described using processed SPECT and CTA to create a combined surface display. They used manual identification of the coronary arteries in the CTA to define the trees and a threshold-based, semiautomatic algorithm to define the LV epicardium and endocardium. The CTA and SPECT images were aligned manually and also automatically using linear and nonrigid registration methods. For the automatic methods, a binary image of the LV was created from the CTA using the semiautomatically detected endocardial and epicardial surfaces. A linear transformation was computed that maximized the overlap between the SPECT and binary CT images. Then a second degree polynomial transformation was computed to maximize the same cost function. Three-dimensional polygonal surfaces were created from the aligned SPECT images and color-coded for perfusion, and then the manually detected coronary arteries were displayed on top of this surface.

Another group has taken a similar approach but with a volume-rendering type of display based on the CTA. Gaemperli et al.[78] describe an approach where the SPECT and CTA images are manually aligned. The LV epicardium is semiautomatically segmented from the CTA, and the SPECT intensity information is projected onto this epicardial surface. The coronary artery tree is segmented using an automated vessel-tracking technique. The results are displayed using a volume rendering technique. This group determined that fusion process was highly reproducible and accurate. They also published results of using this approach clinically.[79] One example of the results of this approach is shown in Figure 4-12.

Finally, it is also possible to use the methods of Faber et al. for aligning CTA with SPECT or PET images obtained from separate scanners. Since this method was developed to handle misalignment between the two studies, it is easily applied to scans that are not already in registration. This surface-based technique aligns the 3D coronary artery tree from CTA with the LV epicardial surface from MPI, which is automatically generated during standard perfusion quantification. Clinical assessment of this approach was described by both Rispler et al.[80] and Santana et al.[81] An example of the method applied to a CTA and SPECT study obtained from two separate scanners is shown in Figure 4-13.

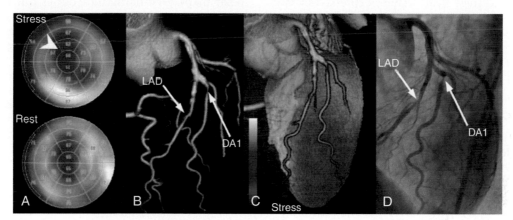

Figure 4-12 Utility of fused SPECT and computed tomography coronary angiography (CTCA), aligned and displayed using volumetric methods. (**A**) Stress and rest polar maps show a largely reversible anteroapical perfusion defect (*arrowhead*). (**B**) 3D volume-rendered CTCA images show the coronary vessel tree with mid-LAD and proximal first diagonal (DA1) branch stenoses. (**C**) Fused SPECT/CT images are able to identify DA1 stenosis as a functionally relevant lesion. (**D**) Findings were confirmed by invasive coronary angiography. (*Reproduced with permission from Gaemperli O, Schepis T, Valenta I, et al: Cardiac image fusion from stand-alone SPECT and CT: Clinical experience, J Nucl Med 48:696–703, 2007.*)

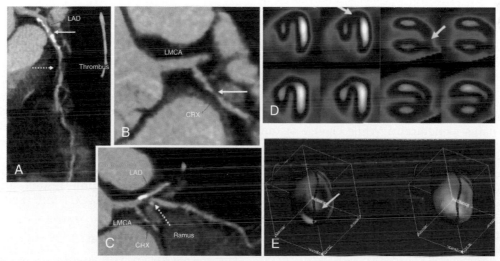

Figure 4-13 Utility of fused SPECT and computed tomography coronary angiography (CTCA) aligned and displayed using surface methods. (**A**) CTCA curved multilinear reformat of the LAD shows an irregular, mostly calcified plaque causing > 50% diameter stenosis (*arrow*). LCx (**B**) and RCA (**C**) multiplanar reformats show significant stenosis in the proximal portions of both arteries (*arrows*). (**D**) Perfusion SPECT at stress (*top*) and rest (*bottom*) shows a reversible defect in the apex and antero apical region (*arrows*). (**E**) Fused display shows overlap of arteries segmented from the CTCA and the epicardium detected from the perfusion SPECT. This display graphically demonstrates that the reversible antero apical defect is in fact a result of the LAD stenosis, and interventional therapy should be directed to the LAD lesion. (*Adapted with permission from Rispler S, Keidar Z, Ghersin E, et al: Integrated single photon emission computed tomography and computed tomography coronary angiography for the assessment of hemodynamically significant coronary artery lesions. J Am Coll Cardiol 49:1059–1067, 2007.*)

PHASE ANALYSIS OF GATED MYOCARDIAL PERFUSION SPECT IMAGES

It has been shown that phase analysis measured from gated myocardial perfusion SPECT images can differentiate patient cohorts who were expected to have different degrees of LV dyssynchrony.[82] LV dyssynchrony measured by phase analysis has been shown to correlate with that measured by 2D tissue Doppler imaging (TDI)[83] and 3D TDI,[84] and to predict patient response to cardiac resynchronization therapy (CRT),[85] in patients with end-stage heart failure, depressed LV ejection fraction, and prolonged QRS duration on surface electrocardiography. Phase analysis software packages have been recently developed and validated to quantitatively measure LV mechanical dyssynchrony from gated myocardial perfusion SPECT images.

Mathematical Principles in Phase Analysis

Jean-Baptiste Joseph Fourier (1768–1830) developed the mathematical technique of harmonic function decomposition. Fourier's theorem states that any physical function that varies periodically with time with a frequency f can be expressed as a superposition of sinusoidal components of frequencies: f, $2f$, $3f$, and so on. A quantitative statement of this theorem is usually given as if a periodic function F of t, with frequency of f, can be expressed as the following summation:

$$F(t) = \sum_{n=0}^{\infty} A_n \cos(2\pi nft + P_n)$$

Each term in the equation is called a *harmonic*. For example, A_0 is called the *zero harmonic*, $A_1\cos(2\pi ft + P_1)$ is called the *first harmonic*, and $A_2\cos(4\pi ft + P_2)$c is called the *second harmonic*, etc. For each harmonic, A represents its amplitude and P represents its phase.

Gated SPECT MPI produces a number of 3D LV images (frames) corresponding to different time points during the cardiac cycle. As these frames progress from the R-wave, both location and intensity of each myocardial segment change periodically. While change of the location of each myocardial segment allows assessment of regional wall motion, change of the intensity indicates regional wall thickening due to the partial volume effect.[86] It has been shown that the change in myocardial wall thickness is approximately linear to the change in maximum counts extracted from the same myocardial segment.[87,88] The phase analysis technique measures the first-harmonic phase of regional LV count changes throughout the cardiac cycle. This phase information is related to the time interval when a region in the 3D LV myocardial wall starts to contract (presumably, onset of mechanical contraction [OMC]). It provides information as to how uniform or inhomogeneous the distribution of these time intervals is for the entire LV (i.e., a measure of LV synchrony/dyssynchrony).

Processing and Quantification of Dyssynchrony

The basics of phase analysis are generally similar in most quantitative software packages, but implementations and processing details may vary significantly. For example, in the Emory Synctool, the input is a gated SPECT MPI short-axis image, which is reconstructed from a conventional gated SPECT MPI study using a conventional reconstruction algorithm. The short-axis image is then searched in 3D to obtain regional maximal counts using a 3D sampling algorithm previously implemented in the ECTb.[25] These samples can be displayed as gated polar maps. First-harmonic Fourier function is used to approximate the regional wall thickening curve and to calculate regional phase for each myocardial sample— that is, each pixel of the gated polar maps. This results in an OMC phase distribution, which is then quantitatively assessed for uniformity or heterogeneity. An example of this processing stream is shown in Figure 4-14. Five indices related to this distribution, including mean and standard deviation, for example, have been used to assess LV dyssynchrony. Normal limits for these indices were generated from gated SPECT MPI studies of 45 male and 45 female normal subjects.[89] Clinical validations of the phase analysis technique showed that phase standard deviation and histogram bandwidth had better clinical usefulness than the other derived quantitative indices.

Reproducibility

Phase analysis is largely automatic. Intra-observer and inter-observer reproducibility of this technique has been evaluated in a recent study using 10 consecutive subjects with LV dysfunction (LVEF $\leq$ 35%) and 10 normal controls.[90] For phase standard deviation and histogram bandwidth, intra-observer correlation coefficients were 1.00 and 1.00, and mean absolute differences between two reads by the same observer at different occasions were 0.8° and 1.4°, respectively. Inter-observer correlation coefficients were 0.99 and 0.99, and the mean absolute differences between two reads by two independent observers were 2.0° and 5.4°, respectively, for phase standard deviation and histogram bandwidth. The superior reproducibility of phase analysis over echocardiography is a promising advantage that may improve prediction of response to CRT, since 20% to 40% of the poor CRT outcome is based on echocardiographic results, and in none of these studies was gated SPECT MPI used.

Temporal Resolution

Since gated SPECT MPI studies are usually acquired as 8 or 16 frames/cardiac cycle, these data are perceived to have low temporal resolution. It is important to note that phase analysis uses continuous Fourier harmonic functions to approximate the discrete wall-thickening samples. Use of Fourier processing reduces the differences between phases measured from fewer gates. In the example in Figure 4-14, the phase difference

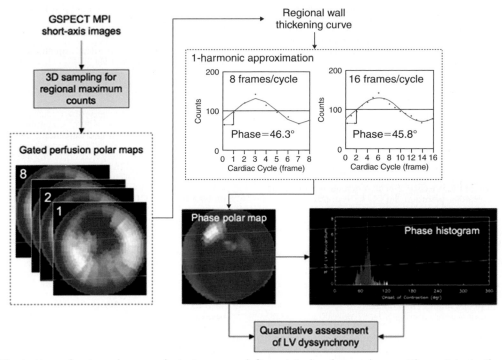

Figure 4-14 Illustration of using phase analysis to assess left ventricular dyssynchrony. The points in the graphs are the regional wall-thickening data. The first harmonic approximation for 8 or 16 frames/cycle is shown as *solid lines*. The phase difference between 8- versus 16-frames/cycle is very small—0.5 degrees (360 degrees corresponding to one cardiac cycle)—demonstrating that Fourier harmonic approximation improves the temporal resolution of the phase measurement. The phase polar map shows a significant phase delay *(bright region)* at the anterior and apical wall. The location of the phase delay matches well with the perfusion defect shown in the perfusion polar map.

between 8 versus 16 frames/cycle is very small: 0.5° (360° corresponds to one cardiac cycle), demonstrating that Fourier harmonic approximation improves the temporal resolution of the phase measurement. A recent simulation study based on digital phantoms has shown that in common clinical settings (≥ 10 counts per myocardial pixel) phase analysis can detect phase delays using gated SPECT MPI data acquired with 8 or 16 frames/cycle with the same accuracy as if they had been acquired using 64 frames/cycle but processed without Fourier analysis, indicating that the temporal resolution of phase analysis is equivalent to 1/64 cardiac cycle.[91]

CONCLUSION

Perfusion quantification methods will continue to evolve with and adapt to nuclear cardiology and the changing needs of physicians in particular, and to nuclear medicine technology and the health care system in general. The high level of automation already achieved in myocardial perfusion imaging is unmatched by any other cardiac imaging modality and continues to be its major strength. In addition, strong statistical evaluations of the accuracy and validity of the various techniques have been made possible simply because of the large amount of objectivity and standardization in the automated processes. These strengths should be built upon and enhanced to demonstrate the value of nuclear cardiology in patient management and, most important,

to maintain the highest quality of clinical care. Moreover, the superior reproducibility of quantitative techniques over visual analysis promotes the need for the use of quantification in randomized clinical trials and in monitoring the effects of therapy in an individual patient.

REFERENCES

1. Knollmann D, Winz OH, Meyer PT, et al: Gated myocardial perfusion SPECT: algorithm-specific influence of reorientation on calculation of left ventricular volumes and ejection fraction, *J Nucl Med* 49:1636–1642, 2008.
2. Germano G, Kavanagh PB, Su HT, et al: Automatic reorientation of 3-dimensional transaxial myocardial perfusion SPECT images, *J Nucl Med* 36:1107–1114, 1995.
3. Faber TL, Folks RD, Garcia EV: Development and analysis of an automatic reorientation program [abstract], *J Nucl Cardiol* 14:S99, 2007.
4. Slomka PJ, Hurwitz GA, Stephenson J, Cradduck T: Automated alignment and sizing of myocardial stress and rest scans to three-dimensional normal templates using an image registration algorithm, *J Nucl Med* 36:1115–1122, 1995.
5. Fitzgerald J, Danias TG: Effect of motion on cardiac SPECT imaging: recognition and motion correction, *J Nucl Cardiol* 8:701–706, 2001.
6. Cooper JA, Neumann PH, McCandless BK: Detection of patient movement during myocardial perfusion imaging, *J Nucl Med* 35:1341–1348, 1993.
7. O'Conner MK, Kanal KM, Gebhard MW, Rossman PJ: Comparison of four motion correction techniques in SPECT imaging of the heart: A cardiac phantom study, *J Nucl Med* 39:2027–2034, 1998.
8. Lee KJ, Barber DC: Use of forward projection to correct patient motion during SPECT imaging, *Phys Med Biol* 43:171–187, 1998.
9. Matsumoto N, Berman DS, Kavanagh PB, et al: Quantitative assessment of motion artifacts and validation of a new motion-correction program for myocardial perfusion SPECT, *J Nucl Med* 42:687–694, 2001.
10. Garcia EV, Van Train K, Maddahi J, et al: Quantification of rotational thallium-201 myocardial tomography, *J Nucl Med* 26:17–26, 1985.

11. DePasquale E, Nody A, DePuey G, et al: Quantitative rotational thallium-201 tomography for identifying and localizing coronary artery disease, *Circulation* 77:316–327, 1988.
12. Wackers FJT: Science, art, and artifacts: How important is quantification for the practicing physician interpreting myocardial perfusion studies? *J Nucl Cardiol* 1:S109–S117, 1994.
13. Berman DS, Kang X, Gransar H, et al: Quantitative assessment of myocardial perfusion abnormality on SPECT myocardial perfusion imaging is more reproducible than expert visual analysis, *J Nucl Cardiol* 16:45–53, 2009.
14. Ezekiel A, Van Train KF, Berman DS, et al: Automatic determination of quantitation parameters from Tc-sestamibi myocardial tomograms. In *Computers in Cardiology*, Los Alamitos, California, 1991, IEEE Computer Society, pp 237–240.
15. Garcia EV, Cooke CD, Van Train KF, et al: Technical aspects of myocardial perfusion SPECT imaging with Tc-99m sestamibi, *Am J Cardiol* 66:23–31E, 1990.
16. Germano G, Kavanaugh PB, Waechter P, et al: A new algorithm for the quantitation of myocardial perfusion SPECT. I: Technical principles and reproducibility, *J Nucl Med* 41:712–719, 2000.
17. Liu YH, Sinusa AJ, DeMan P, et al: Quantification of SPECT myocardial perfusion images: Methodology and validation of the Yale-CQ method, *J Nucl Cardiol* 6:190–203, 1999.
18. Watson DD: Quantitative SPECT techniques, *Semin Nucl Med* 29:192–203, 1999.
19. Klein JL, Garcia EV, DePuey EG, et al: Reversibility bullseye: A new polar bull's-eye map to quantify reversibility of stress-induced SPECT Tl-201 myocardial perfusion defects, *J Nucl Med* 31:1240–1246, 1990.
20. Diamond GA, Forrester JS: Analysis of probability as an aid in the clinical diagnosis of coronary artery disease, *N Engl J Med* 300:1350–1358, 1979.
21. Van Train KF, Areeda J, Garcia EV, et al: Quantitative same-day rest-stress technetium-99m-sestamibi SPECT: Definition and validation of stress normal limits and criteria for abnormality, *J Nucl Med* 34:1494–1502, 1993.
22. DePuey EG, Roubin GS, DePasquale EE, et al: Sequential multivessel coronary angioplasty assessed by thallium-201 tomography, *Cathet Cardiovasc Diagn* 18:213–221, 1989.
23. Berman DS, Hachamovitch R, Kiat H, et al: Incremental value of prognostic testing in patients with known or suspected ischemic heart disease: A basis for optimal utilization of exercise technetium-99m sestamibi myocardial perfusion single-photon emission computed tomography, *J Am Coll Cardiol* 26:639–647, 1995.
24. Faber TL, Cooke CD, Folks RD, et al: Left ventricular function and perfusion from gated SPECT perfusion images: An integrated method, *J Nucl Med* 40:650–659, 1999.
25. Garcia EV, Faber TL, Cooke CD, Folks RD, Chen J, Santana C: The increasing role of quantification in nuclear cardiology: The Emory approach, *J Nucl Cardiol* 14:420–432, 2007.
26. Ficaro EP, Kritzman JN, Corbett JR: Development and clinical validation of normal Tc-99m sestamibi database: comparison of 3D-MSPECT to CEqual [abstract], *J Nucl Med* 5:125P, 1999.
27. Ficaro EP, Lee BC, Kritzman JN, Corbett JR: Corridor 4DM: The Michigan method for quantitative nuclear cardiology, *J Nucl Cardiol* 14:455–465, 2007.
28. Germano G, Kavanagh PB, SLomka PJ, et al: Quantitation in gated perfusion SPECT imaging: The Cedars-Sinai approach, *J Nucl Cardiol* 14:433–454, 2007.
29. Liu YH: Quantification of nuclear cardiac images: The Yale approach, *J Nucl Cardiol* 14:483–491, 2007.
30. Sharir T, Germano G, Waechter PB, et al: A new algorithm for the quantitation of myocardial perfusion SPECT. II: Validation and diagnostic yield, *J Nucl Med* 41:720–727, 2000.
31. Van Train KF, Garcia EV, Maddahi J, et al: Multicenter trial validation for quantitative analysis of same-day rest-stress technetium-99m-sestamibi myocardial tomograms, *J Nucl Med* 35:609–1168, 1994.
32. Folks R, Garcia E, Van Train K, et al: Quantitative two-day Tc-99m sestamibi myocardial SPECT: Multicenter trial validation of normal limits, *J Med Tech* 24:158, 1996.
33. DePuey EG, Krawcynska EG, D'Amato PH, Patterson RE: Thallium-201 single-photon emission computed tomography with intravenous dipyridamole to diagnose coronary artery disease, *Coron Artery Dis* 1:75–82, 1990.
34. Ella A, Champier J, Bontemps L, Itti R: Three-dimensional automatic warping in cardiac SPECT, *Nucl Med Commun* 21:1135–1146, 2000.
35. Watt A: *3D Computer Graphics*, London, 1999, Addison Wesley.
36. Cooke CD, Vansant JP, Krawczynska E, et al: Clinical validation of 3-d color-modulated displays of myocardial perfusion, *J Nuclear Cardiol* 4:108–1106, 1997.
37. Santana CA, Garcia EV, Vansant JP, et al: Three-dimensional color-modulated display of myocardial SPECT perfusion distributions accurately assesses coronary artery disease, *J Nucl Med* 41:1941–1946, 2000.
38. Levin D, Aladl U, Germano G, Slomka P: Techniques for efficient, real-time 3D visualization of multi-modality cardiac data using consumer graphics hardware, *Comput Med Imaging Graph* 29:463–475, 2005.
39. Anderson JA, Rosenfeld E, editors: *Neurocomputing: Foundations of Research*, Cambridge, MA, 1988, MIT Press.
40. Nilsson N: *Principles of Artificial Intelligence*, Wellsboro, PA, 1980, Tioga Publishing.
41. Ezquerra NF, Garcia EV: Artificial intelligence in nuclear medicine imaging, *Am J Cardiac Imaging* 3:130–141, 1989.
42. Garcia EV, Herbst MD, Cooke CD, et al: Knowledge-based visualization of myocardial perfusion tomographic images. In *Proceedings of the First Conference on Visualization in Biomedical Computing*, Atlanta, GA, 1990, IEEE Press, pp 157–161.
43. Garcia EV, Cooke CD, Krawczynska E, Folks R, et al: Expert system interpretation of technetium-99m sestamibi myocardial perfusion tomograms: Enhancements and validation, *Circulation* 92:1–10, 1995.
44. Garcia EV, Cooke CD, Folks RD, et al: Diagnostic performance of an expert system for the interpretation of myocardial perfusion SPECT studies, *J Nucl Med* 42:1185–1191, 2001.
45. Fujita H, Katafuchi T, Uehara T, Nishimura T: Application of artificial neural network to computer-aided diagnosis of coronary artery disease in myocardial SPECT bull's-eye images, *J Nucl Med* 33:272–276, 1992.
46. Hamilton D, Riley PJ, Miola UJ, Amro AA: A feed forward neural network for classification of bull's-eye myocardial perfusion images, *Eur J Nucl Med* 22:108–115, 1995.
47. Porenta G, Dorffner G, Kundrat S, et al: Automated pnterpretation of Planar thallium-201-dipyridamole stress-redistribution scintigrams using artificial neural networks, *J Nucl Med* 35:2041–2047, 1994.
48. Lindahl D, Palmer J, Ohlsson M, et al: Automated interpretation of myocardial SPECT perfusion images using artificial neural networks, *J Nucl Med* 38:1870–1875, 1997.
49. Tagil K, Andersson L-G, Balogh I, et al: Evaluation of a new internet based system for interpretation of myocardial perfusion images, *J Nucl Cardiol* 8:S16, 1991 (abstr.)
50. Kurgan LA, Cios KJ, Tadeusiewicz R, et al: Knowledge discovery approach to automated cardiac SPECT diagnosis, *Artif Intell Med* 23:149–169, 2001.
51. Sacha JP, Goodenday L, Cios KJ: Bayesian learning for cardiac SPECT image interpretation, *Artif Intell Med* 26:109–143, 2002.
52. MacDonald LA, Elliott MD, Leonard SM, et al: Variability of myocardial perfusion SPECT: Contribution of repetitive processing, acquisition and testing [abstract], *J Nucl Med* 40:126P, 1999.
53. Faber TL, Modersitzki J, Folks RD, Garcia EV: Detecting changes in serial myocardial perfusion SPECT: A simulation study, *J Nucl Cardiol* 12:302–310, 2005.
54. Turkington TG, DeGrado TR, Hanson MW, Coleman RE: Alignment of dynamic cardiac PET images for correction of motion, *IEEE Trans Nucl Sci* 44:235–242, 1997.
55. Peace RA, Staff RT, Gemmell HG, et al: Automatic detection of coronary artery disease in myocardial perfusion SPECT using image registration and voxel to voxel statistical comparisons, *Nucl Med Commun* 23:785–794, 2002.
56. Gilardi MC, Rizzo G, Savi A, et al: Correlation of SPECT and PET cardiac images by a surface matching registration technique, *Comp Med Imaging Graph* 22:391–398, 1998.
57. Declerck J, Feldmar J, Goris ML, Betting F: Automatic registration and alignment on a template of cardiac stress and rest reoriented SPECT images, *IEEE Trans Med Imaging* 16:727–737, 1997.
58. Thirion JP: Image matching as a diffusion process: An analogy to Maxwell's demons, *Med Image Anal* 2:243–260, 1998.
59. Hendel RC, Thirion JP, Leonard SM: The impact of geometric and intensity normalization on the reproducibility of myocardial perfusion SPECT imaging [abstract], *J Nucl Med* 41:46P, 2000.
60. Faber TL, Galt JR, Chen J, et al: Detecting changes in myocardial perfusion. In Lemke HU, Vannier MW, Inamura K, et al: *Computer-Assisted Radiology and Surgery*, Berlin, 2002, Springer-Verlag, pp 879–883.
61. Slomka PJ, Nishina H, Berman DS, et al: Automated quantification of myocardial perfusion SPECT using simplified normal limits, *J Nucl Cardiol* 12:66–77, 2005.
62. Shaw LJ, Berman DS, Maron DJ, et al: Optimal medical therapy with or without percutaneous coronary intervention to reduce ischemic burden: Results from the Clinical Outcomes Utilizing Revascularization and Aggressive Drug Evaluation (COURAGE) trial nuclear substudy, *Circulation* 117:1283–1291, 2008.
63. Itti E, Klein G, Rosso J, Evangelista E, et al: Assessment of myocardial reperfusion after myocardial infarction using automatic 3D quantification and template matching, *J Nucl Med* 45:1981–1988, 2004.
64. Makela T, Clarysse P, Sipila O, et al: A review of cardiac image registration methods, *IEEE Trans Med Imaging* 21:1011–1021, 2002.
65. Sinha S, Sinha U, Czernin J, et al: Noninvasive assessment of myocardial perfusion and metabolism: feasibility of registering gated MR and PET images, *AJR Am J Roentgenol* 164:301–307, 1995.
66. Makela TJ, Clarysse P, Lotjonen J, et al: A new method for the registration of cardiac PET and MR images using deformable model-based segmentation of the main thorax structures. In Niessen WJ, Viergever MA, editors: *Lecture Notes in Computer Science, vol 2208: Medical Image Computing and Computer-Assisted Intervention*, Berlin, 2001, Springer-Verlag, pp 557–564.

67. Makela T, Pham QC, Clarysse P, et al: A 3D model-based registration approach for the PET, MR and MCG cardiac data fusion, *Med Image Anal* 7:377–389, 2003.
68. Aladl UE, Hurwitz GA, Dey D, et al: Automatic image registration of gated cardiac single photon emission computed tomography and magnetic resonance imaging, *J Magn Reson Imaging* 19:283–290, 2004.
69. Misko J, Dzluk M, Skrobowska E, et al: Co-registration of cardiac MRI and rest gated SPECT in the assessment of myocardial perfusion, function, and viability, *J Cardiovasc Magn Reson* 8:389–397, 2006.
70. Faber TL, Chiron F, Ezquerra NF, Rossignac J, et al: Registration of multimodal 3D cardiac information using the iterative closest point approach. In Wilson DC, et al: editor: *Mathematical Modeling, Estimation, and Imaging*, Bellingham, WA, 2000, SPIE, pp 233–241.
71. Faber TL, Santana CA, Garcia EV, et al: 3D fusion of coronary arteries with myocardial perfusion distributions: Clinical validation, *J Nucl Med* 45:745–753, 2004.
72. Schindler TH, Magosaki N, Jeserich M, et al: Fusion imaging: Combined visualization of 3D reconstructed coronary artery tree and 3D myocardial scintigraphic image in coronary artery disease, *Int J Card Imaging* 15:357–368, 1999.
73. Nishimura Y, Fukuchi K, Kataufchi T, et al: Superimposed display of coronary artery on gated myocardial perfusion scintigraphy, *J Nucl Med* 45:1444–1449, 2004.
74. Namdar M, Hany TF, Koepfli P, et al: Integrated PET/CT for the assessment of coronary artery disease: a feasibility study, *J Nucl Med* 46:930–935, 2005.
75. Nakauro T, Utsunomiya U, Shiraishi S, et al: Fusion imaging between myocardial perfusion single photon computed tomography and cardiac computed tomography, *Circulation* 112:e47–e48, 2005.
76. Faber TL, Garcia EV, Hertel S, et al: Evaluation of automatic fusion of coronary arteries onto left ventricular surfaces from PET/CT [abstract], *J Nucl Med* 45:399P, 2004.
77. Nakajo H, Kumita S, Cho K, Kumazaki T: Three-dimensional registration of myocardial perfusion SPECT and CT angiography, *Ann Nucl Med* 19:207–215, 2005.
78. Gaemperli O, Schepis T, Kalff V, et al: Validation of a new cardiac image fusion software for three-dimensional integration of myocardial perfusion SPECT and standalone 64-slice CT angiography, *Eur J Nucl Med Mol Imaging* 34:1097–1106, 2007.
79. Gaemperli O, Schepis T, Valenta I, et al: Cardiac image fusion from stand-alone SPECT and CT: Clinical experience, *J Nucl Med* 48:696–703, 2007.
80. Rispler S, Keidar Z, Ghersin E, et al: Integrated single photon emission computed tomography and computed tomography coronary angiography for the assessment of hemodynamically significant coronary artery lesions, *J Am Coll Cardiol* 49:1059–1067, 2007.
81. Santana CA, Garcia EV, Faber TL, et al: Diagnostic performance of fusion of myocardial perfusion imaging (MPI) and computed tomography coronary angiography, *J Nucl Cardiol* 16:201–211, 2009.
82. Trimble MA, Smalheiser S, Borges-Neto S, et al: Evaluation of left ventricular mechanical dyssynchrony as determined by phase analysis of ECG-gated myocardial perfusion SPECT imaging in patients with left ventricular dysfunction and conduction disturbances, *J Nucl Cardiol* 14:298–307, 2007.
83. Henneman MM, Chen J, Ypenburg C, Dibbets, et al: Phase analysis of gated myocardial perfusion SPECT compared to tissue Doppler imaging for the assessment of left ventricular dyssynchrony, *J Am Coll Cardiol* 49:1708–1714, 2007.
84. Ajmone Marsan N, Henneman MM, Chen J, et al: Left ventricular dyssynchrony assessed by two 3-dimensional imaging modalities: phase analysis of gated myocardial perfusion SPECT and tri-plane tissue Doppler imaging, *Eur J Nucl Med Mol Imaging* 35:166–173, 2008.
85. Henneman MM, Chen J, Dibbets P, et al: Can LV dyssynchrony as assessed with phase analysis on gated myocardial perfusion SPECT predict response to CRT? *J Nucl Med* 48:1104–1111, 2007.
86. Hoffman EJ, Huang SC, Phelps ME: Quantitation in positron emission computed tomography: 1. Effect of object size, *Comput Assist Tomogr* 3:299–308, 1979.
87. Galt JR, Garcia EV, Robbins WL: Effects of myocardial wall thickness on SPECT quantification, *IEEE Trans Med Imaging* 9:144–150, 1990.
88. Cooke CD, Garcia EV, Cullom SJ, et al: Determining the accuracy of calculating systolic wall thickening using a Fast Fourier Transform approximation: A simulation study based on canine and patient data, *J Nucl Med* 35:1185–1192, 1994.
89. Chen J, Garcia EV, Folks RD, et al: Onset of left ventricular mechanical contraction as determined by phase analysis of ECG-gated myocardial perfusion SPECT imaging: Development of a diagnostic tool for assessment of cardiac mechanical dyssynchrony, *J Nucl Cardiol* 12:687–695, 2005.
90. Trimble MA, Velazquez EJ, Adams GL, et al: Repeatability and reproducibility of phase analysis of gated SPECT myocardial perfusion imaging used to quantify cardiac dyssynchrony, *Nucl Med Commun* 29:374–381, 2008.
91. Chen J, Faber TL, Cooke CD, Garcia EV: Temporal resolution of multiharmonic phase analysis of ECG-gated myocardial perfusion SPECT studies, *J Nucl Cardiol* 15:383–391, 2008.

Chapter 5

Single-Photon Emission Computed Tomography Artifacts

E. GORDON DEPUEY

INTRODUCTION

Single-photon emission computed tomographic (SPECT) imaging of myocardial perfusion provides a sensitive means of detecting and localizing coronary artery disease (CAD) and assessing left ventricular (LV) function. However, the method suffers from the potential for poor specificity due to image artifacts related to both patient and technical factors. By recognizing the sources of such artifacts and understanding the means available to avoid them, the technologist and interpreting physician can substantially improve the specificity of SPECT studies and more meaningfully contribute to appropriate patient treatment.

TECHNICAL ARTIFACTS

Flood Field Nonuniformity

Flood field nonuniformity will result in "ring" artifacts in reconstructed SPECT images. These relatively photon-deficient rings may be apparent in tomographic slices and in severe cases may also appear in polar coordinate maps (Fig. 5-1). Because patients are frequently positioned differently within the camera field for rest and stress scans, flood field artifacts may occur in differents of the myocardium, mimicking reversible or partially reversible defects. Therefore, routine acquisition and inspection of intrinsic and extrinsic flood fields acquired according to vendor recommendations are absolutely critical to avoid such artifacts. Flood fields are routinely acquired the first thing in the morning each working day. However, if ring artifacts appear in clinical SPECT images, it may be necessary to reacquire flood field images in the middle of the day.

Center of Rotation and Camera-Held Alignment Errors

If the camera center of rotation (COR) is incorrect, filtered backprojection during SPECT reconstruction will result in image misregistration and apparent misalignment of the myocardial walls (Fig. 5-2). Technically, this is similar to the error created by cardiac motion. However, unlike motion artifacts, those due to COR error are usually more systematic and predictable. The severity of the apparent defect is directly proportional to the magnitude of the COR error. An error similar to that produced by the wrong center of rotation is produced when the detector is not aligned perpendicular to the radius of rotation.

To avoid these artifacts, camera COR checks should be performed according to the camera manufacturer's guidelines. The resultant plots should be inspected regularly by a knowledgeable technologist and physician before the camera is used for patient studies. With the observation of a myocardial defect suspected of representing such an artifact, the COR determination should be repeated immediately. Likewise for variable-angle multiheaded detector systems, camera head alignment should be assessed periodically, particularly after camera repair and whenever the detectors are impacted by objects such as stretchers.

Errors in Selecting Oblique Cardiac Axes and Subsequent Polar Map Reconstruction

If the long axis of the left ventricle (LV) is defined incorrectly on either the transaxial or midventricular vertical long-axis slice, the geometry of the heart in subsequently reconstructed orthogonal tomographic slices can be distorted. Consequently, the apparent regional

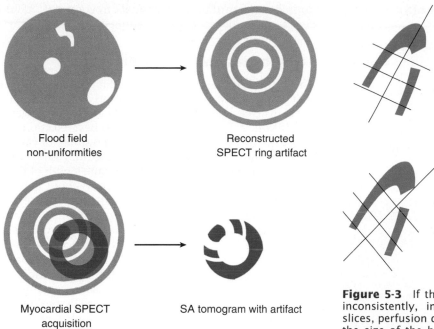

Flood field
non-uniformities

Reconstructed
SPECT ring artifact

Myocardial SPECT
acquisition

SA tomogram with artifact

Figure 5-1 Flood field nonuniformity resulting in ring artifacts and artifactual myocardial perfusion defects. *(Reproduced with permission from Iskandrian AE, Verani MS [eds]: Nuclear Cardiac Imaging: Principles and Applications, 3rd ed. New York: Oxford University Press, 2003.)*

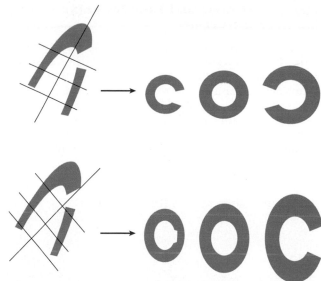

Figure 5-3 If the long axis of the left ventricle is selected inconsistently, in stress and rest transaxial tomographic slices, perfusion defect localization, cavity configuration, and the size of the basal septal defect due to the membranous septum will be represented inconsistently in reconstructed short-axis tomograms. *(Reproduced with permission from Iskandrian AE, Verani MS [eds]: Nuclear Cardiac Imaging: Principles and Applications, 3rd ed. New York: Oxford University Press, 2003.)*

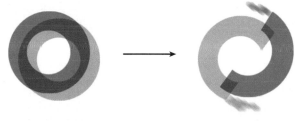

Misregistration by
filtered backprojection

Resulting SPECT
artifacts

Figure 5-2 Schematic representation of camera center of rotation error and resultant artifactual myocardial perfusion defects. Defects are in opposite sides of the "heart," and "tails" of activity are present extending from the edges of the defects. *(Reproduced with permission from Iskandrian AE, Verani MS [eds]: Nuclear Cardiac Imaging: Principles and Applications, 3rd ed. New York: Oxford University Press, 2003.)*

count density can be altered in polar maps, resulting in apparent perfusion defects. These may be accentuated by quantitative analyses in which patient data are compared to normal files (Fig. 5-3). In polar map reconstruction, such errors most often occur in basal myocardial regions at the periphery of the bull's-eye plot, owing to foreshortening of one of the myocardial walls (Fig. 5-4). Also, the apex, which often demonstrates physiologic thinning and decreased count density, is displaced from the exact center of the polar plot. The displaced apex may also consequently result in an artifact. Misregistration of perfusion defects in short-axis slices and polar maps is not infrequently encountered in patients with sizable severe infarcts

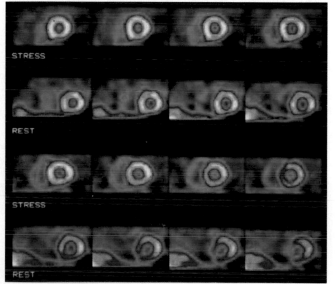

Figure 5-4 Stress tomograms *(top row)* were reconstructed correctly in this normal patient, whereas the long axis of the left ventricle was selected incorrectly for the resting tomograms. As a result, the ventricular cavity in the resting short-axis slices appears elliptical, and there is an artifactual perfusion defect in the basal inferoseptal region. *(Reproduced with permission from DePuey EG, Garcia EG, Berman DS [eds]: Cardiac SPECT Imaging, 2nd ed. New York: Raven, 2001, p 195.)*

Selection of Apex and Base for Polar Map Reconstruction

Accurate and reproducible selection of the apex and base of the LV myocardium is necessary in stress and rest images. Positioning limits for slice selection that lie too far apically or basally will result in apparent perfusion defects (Fig. 5-5). In contrast, positioning slice limits too tightly, so that they do not encompass the entire heart, will potentially result in underestimation of the size and extent of a defect. Likewise, in regions of

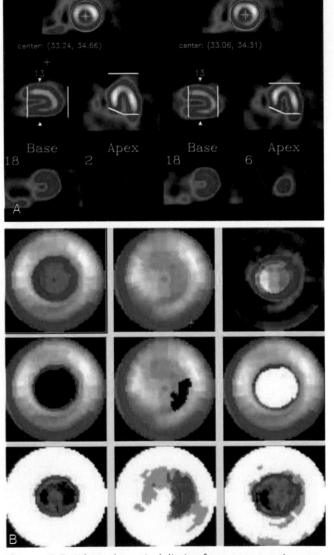

Figure 5-5 When the apical limits for reconstruction are defined distal to the left ventricular myocardium in stress images (**A**), an artifactual extensive and severe apical ischemic defect is produced in the polar plots (**B**). (**A**, *Reproduced with permission from DePuey EG, Garcia EG, Berman DS [eds]: Cardiac SPECT Imaging, 2nd ed. New York: Raven, 2001, p 98.* **B**, *Reproduced with permission from Iskandrian AE, Verani MS [eds]: Nuclear Cardiac Imaging: Principles and Applications, 3rd ed. New York: Oxford University Press, 2003.*)

normal myocardium, maximal myocardial count density may not be correctly sampled.

Arrhythmias and Gating Errors

If arrhythmia is present or if the heart rate changes during SPECT acquisition, inordinately short or long cardiac cycles will be rejected during an 8- or 16-frame/gated acquisition. If the degree of the regular beat rejection varies during the SPECT acquisition, the number of cardiac cycles acquired for each projection image may vary if each projection image is acquired for the same length of time. Therefore, projection images will vary in count density. When viewed in endless loop cinematic format, the projection images will appear to "flash." The most serious effect of arrhythmia is a decrease in image count density due to these "discarded" cardiac cycles. However, only with severe arrhythmias associated with atrial fibrillation and frequent premature ventricular contractions are clinically significant perfusion artifacts encountered. Although this problem may be overcome by prolonging SPECT acquisition until a prescribed number of regular cardiac cycles have been acquired, such longer acquisition times increase the probability of patient motion due to discomfort or anxiety. Recently, some manufacturers have established a "9th bin" wherein rejected cardiac cycles are stored temporarily and excluded from reconstruction of the gated tomograms, but added back into the summed, nongated images. Alternately, other manufacturers allow simultaneous acquisition of gated and nongated images so that arrhythmic beat rejection will not result in low count-density ungated images.

If the accepted cardiac cycles vary in length, and because each cycle begins at the R-wave used for gating, relative shorter beats will not fill the entire 8 or 16 "bins" of the cardiac cycle. When all of the acquired cardiac cycles are summed to create an 8- or 16-frame gated image, this will result in data "dropout" in the last few "bins" of the cardiac cycle.

Displays of cardiac image count density from individual planar projection images is now possible using some commercially available software programs (Fig. 5-6). Errors in LV volume and ejection fraction may result from gating errors, but these are beyond the scope of this chapter.[1]

PATIENT-RELATED ARTIFACTS

Soft-Tissue Attenuation (See Chapters 6 and 7)

The location of the attenuation artifact depends on the position of the soft-tissue attenuator in relation to the left ventricle. The severity of the artifact depends on the size and density of the attenuator in relation to adjacent tissue. Within the resultant SPECT image, the artifact may appear as a fixed or reversible defect or may mimic "reverse redistribution," depending on whether the attenuator is in a constant or variable position in stress and delayed image acquisitions. The severity of the attenuation artifact also depends on the energy of

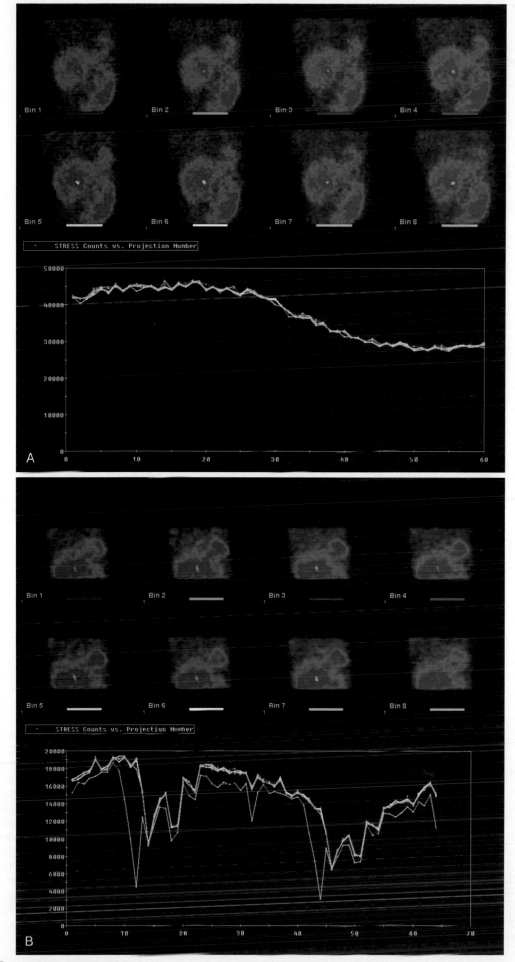

Figure 5-6 For Legend see Page 76

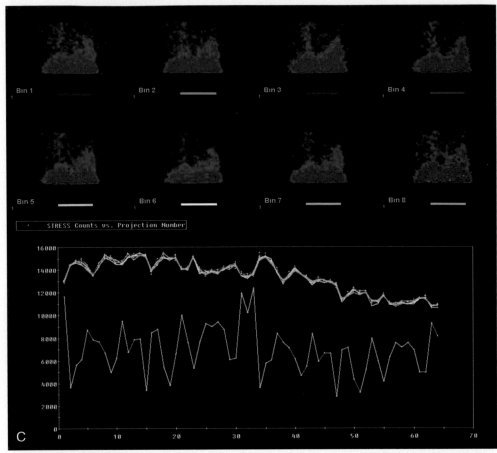

Figure 5-6—cont'd **A**, Count density is plotted on the y axis for each of the eight "bins" of an 8-frame per cardiac cycle gated post-stress myocardial perfusion scan for the 64 camera stops in the 180-degree SPECT imaging arc of a 90-degree-angled, two-detector scintillation camera. In this patient with no arrhythmia and a very regular R-R interval, the curves are superimposed for each of the eight gated "bins." **B**, In this arrhythmic patient, cardiac cycles are rejected during camera stops ~8 to 24 and simultaneously during stops ~40 to 56 for the other scintillation detector. This is manifested as a decrease in counts acquired/accepted at those stops. **C**, In this patient, all cardiac cycles were accepted during the SPECT acquisition. However, owing to variation of the R-R interval of the accepted beats, there is a decrease in count density in the eighth gated "bin."

the incident photon. Attenuation artifacts for technetium (^{99m}Tc)-labeled myocardial perfusion agents will be somewhat less marked than for thallium (^{201}Tl).[3] However, for either isotope, evaluation of regional wall motion is helpful in differentiating attenuation artifacts from myocardial scarring as a source of fixed perfusion defects.[4–6]

Breast Attenuation

Because breasts vary in size, position, configuration, and density, breast attenuation artifacts are extremely variable in appearance. In addressing the characteristics of breast attenuation, it is always necessary to consider the position and configuration of the breasts with the patient in the supine position, because patients are imaged in this position with most commercially available SPECT systems. In women of average body habitus, the left breast overlies the anterolateral wall of the heart. In women with large, pendulous breasts, the breasts lie adjacent to the lateral chest wall and more often

result in a lateral attenuation artifact. In some women with very large, pendulous breasts, the attenuation artifact may create apparent inferior or inferolateral perfusion defects. In women with very large breasts, the breast tissue may overlie the entire LV. In this instance, the resulting attenuation artifact may be diffuse and less discrete or may primarily involve the apex. In addition to breast position, the caudal angulation of the heart within the thorax will affect the appearance of the attenuation artifact.[2–3] Thus, in summary, the severity of breast attenuation artifacts is not necessarily directly proportional to breast size or chest circumference but may vary considerably according to the position, configuration, and density of the breast, body habitus of the patient, and orientation of the heart within the thorax. Additionally, when women are imaged upright or in a semi-upright, "reclining" position, the breasts are usually more pendulous than in the supine position. Therefore, apical and inferior breast attenuation artifacts are more frequent when women are imaged in these positions.

In some laboratories, a binder is used to flatten the breasts against the chest wall. Although this technique can be quite useful to decrease the thickness of the breast, there is often a degree of uncertainty about the exact position of the breast beneath the binder. Moreover, precise repositioning of the breast beneath the binder in stress and rest studies is difficult. Therefore, in most laboratories, breast binders are not used. For similar reasons, taping the breast upward in an attempt to avoid its overlying the heart is associated with uncertainty in reproducing the breast position for stress and rest SPECT acquisitions.

The interpreting physician must also be cognizant of factors that may further alter the position, configuration, and density of the breast. A bra positions the breast anteriorly and increases the amount of soft-tissue attenuation by thickening the breast. For this reason, it is recommended that SPECT imaging be performed with the bra off. Breast implants may be denser than normal breast tissue and may accentuate attenuation artifacts. Therefore, women who are candidates for SPECT should always be questioned about a history of breast implants or augmentation. Patients with previous left mastectomies may wear a breast prosthesis. Such prostheses may be quite dense, and women who have them must always be instructed to remove them before myocardial perfusion imaging.

Quantitative analysis of SPECT myocardial perfusion imaging is helpful, particularly to the novice, in differentiating normal, physiologic variations in radiotracer distribution from true perfusion defects. However, gender-matched normal files are derived from an average population, and normal limits are established on the basis of variations in regional count density within this population. However, this type of analysis does not take into account the marked variability in body habitus observed in the patient population referred for myocardial perfusion imaging. Therefore, quantitative analysis, instead of aiding the physician in identifying soft-tissue attenuation artifacts, may actually decrease the specificity of SPECT testing by incorrectly identifying such artifacts as abnormalities.

Attenuation correction for SPECT is now commercially available but is still a topic of intense interest and research. The methods for accomplishing it have used either scatter correction or attenuation correction using a separate radionuclide or x-ray transmission image. This approach has been demonstrated to significantly reduce breast and other attenuation artifacts in phantom and patient studies.[7–18] However, whereas attenuation correction may minimize attenuation artifacts created by overlying breast tissue, breast artifacts are frequently not totally eliminated.

Certain breast attenuation artifacts are unique to quantitative analysis in cardiac SPECT. The most common is an apparent inferior perfusion defect incorrectly identified by quantitative analysis in women who have had a left mastectomy. After removal of the breast, there is little or no anterior soft-tissue attenuation. In such cases, the anterior and inferior myocardial count densities are nearly the same as they are for males. Since the normal female file anticipates that the inferior wall will

be more intense than the anterior wall, and in the patient study the inferior wall has an identical or lower intensity than the anterior wall, the inferior wall will be identified as abnormal (Fig. 5-7). This quantitative error can be circumvented by comparison of the patient's data to the normal male file instead. Similar inferior artifacts have been observed in quantitative plots in women with very small breasts, and it might be argued that data from such patients should be compared to normal male limits. However, small breasts may be quite dense, and the assumption that they do not produce photon attenuation may be incorrect. Therefore, in most laboratories, the normal male file is used routinely only for women who have undergone left mastectomy.

The position of the breast may vary from stress to rest if a woman wears different clothing at the time of the two SPECT acquisitions. Breast position varies considerably with a bra on and off. The position of the breast may also vary depending upon the degree of elevation of the left arm, which is preferably positioned above the head for a SPECT acquisition. A shifting breast attenuation artifact can mimic a reversible perfusion defect (i.e., ischemia). For example, if during stress SPECT acquisition, the breast lies high over the anterior chest wall, an anterior attenuation artifact may result. However, if during the resting acquisition, the breast lies more laterally and inferiorly, the artifact will involve the inferolateral wall of the LV. The resulting attenuation artifacts are therefore different in the stress and rest images, so artifactual defect reversibility as well as artifactual "reverse distribution" may result. In this example, the anterior defect will appear to be reversible, whereas there will appear to be "reverse distribution" in the inferolateral wall (Fig. 5-8).

The astute physician and technologist can recognize breast attenuation artifacts by several means. From the following list, the observer should learn to anticipate artifacts:

1. The patient should always be instructed to remove her bra before every image acquisition. It is useful for the technologist to document that the bra has been removed.
2. A history of mastectomy should be documented, and breast prostheses must be removed if possible. Any history of breast augmentation should be noted.
3. Positioning of the patient on the SPECT imaging table should be reproduced as closely as possible for stress and rest images. Because the position of the elevated left arm greatly influences the position of the left breast, the imaging table's position should be identical for stress and rest image acquisitions, and the left arm should be positioned identically for each image acquisition. An arm holder is particularly useful to ensure reproducible arm positioning.
4. The planar images from which SPECT data are reconstructed should be viewed in rotating cinematic format. The position of the breast "shadow" should be observed with regard to the portion of

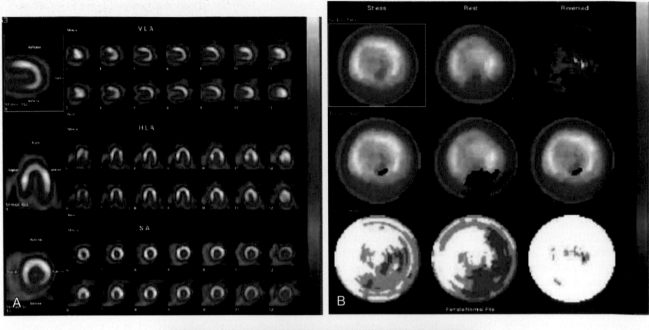

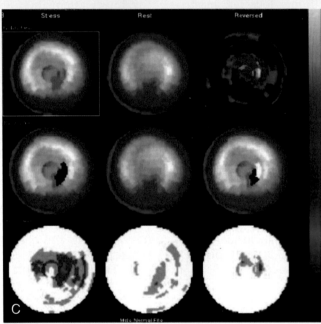

Figure 5-7 Technetium-99m-sestamibi stress and rest tomograms (**A**) and quantitative polar plots (**B**) in a patient with a left mastectomy. Patient data are compared to a normal female file, and quantitatively an inferior defect is identified artifactually. However, when patient data are compared to a normal male file (**C**), which anticipates no breast attenuation, quantitative analysis demonstrates no blackened pixels in the inferior wall. *(Reproduced with permission from Iskandrian AE, Verani MS [eds]: Nuclear Cardiac Imaging: Principles and Applications, 3rd ed. New York: Oxford University Press, 2003.)*

the LV myocardium that is eclipsed. Such a shadow is usually noted to extend beyond the heart to overlie the adjacent left hemithorax and can thereby be differentiated from a true myocardial perfusion defect in these rotating planar images. Moreover, the density of the breast can be estimated from the degree of attenuation of photons emanating from structures within the thorax, including the myocardium and lungs. The constancy (or inconstancy) of the position of the left breast in stress and rest images should be ascertained.

5. In reconstructed SPECT images, an area of markedly decreased photon density may be observed anterior or lateral to the heart in patients with very large or dense breasts. Adjacent to this photopenic defect are frequently observed accentuated streak artifacts due to nonisotropic attenuation.[3] The position of the breast is best evaluated from transaxial or horizontal long-axis slices. When such a large area of markedly decreased count density is noted, an attenuation artifact that may mimic a myocardial perfusion defect often occurs in the adjacent myocardium.

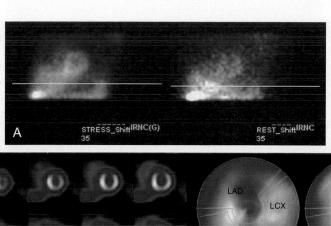

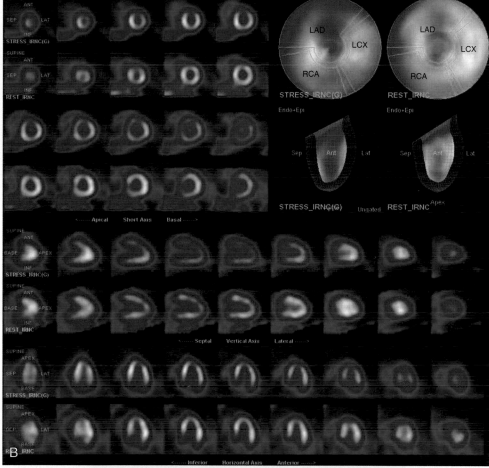

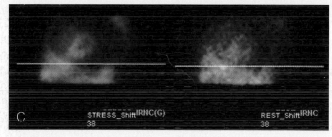

Figure 5-8　A, Left lateral planar projection images at stress *(left)* demonstrate a discrete breast shadow "eclipsing" the upper half to two-thirds of the left ventricle (LV). However, in the resting projection images *(right)*, the breast shadow covers the entire LV, indicating a more inferior position of the breast at the time of resting SPECT acquisition. **B,** Short-axis tomograms, polar plots, and 3D surface images demonstrate an anterior defect in stress images, not apparent at rest. Differentiation of a shifting breast attenuation artifact from anterior ischemia (and lateral "reverse distribution") is problematical. **C,** The stress SPECT acquisition was repeated with the patient's left arm lowered somewhat, not as fully extended above the head. In the repeat study, the breast "shadow" is comparable in the stress *(left)* and rest *(right)* planar projection images.

Continued

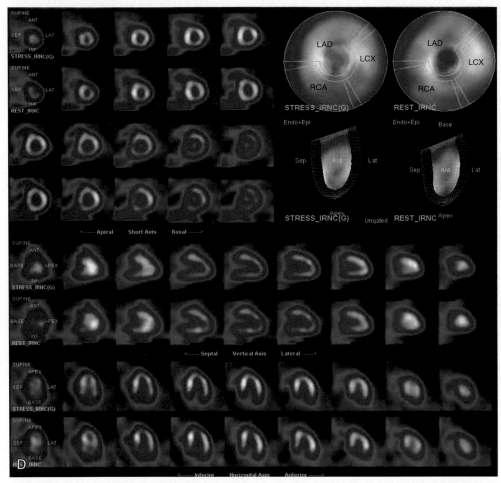

Figure 5-8—cont'd   **D**, With the breast repositioned, now eclipsing the entire left ventricle, stress and rest tomograms are both normal.

Gated myocardial perfusion SPECT is helpful in differentiating breast attenuation artifacts from scar, since artifacts will demonstrate normal wall motion and wall thickening, whereas infarcts, if they are transmural and sizable, will be hypokinetic with decreased wall thickening (Fig. 5-9).[4,5] However, patients with nontransmural myocardial infarctions might have normal wall motion, depending on the thickness of the infarct zone. For artifacts created by a breast that shifts in position from stress to rest, gating is less helpful to differentiate artifact from ischemia as a cause of the reversible or partially reversible defect.

Lateral Chest-Wall Fat Attenuation

In obese patients, there may be a considerable accumulation of fat in the lateral chest wall. When such a patient lies supine on the imaging palette, the thickness of soft tissue in the lateral chest wall is further accentuated. Although this tissue thickness may be the same as or greater than that of the breast, chest-wall fat is usually more uniformly distributed. Therefore, the resultant attenuation artifact is usually more diffuse, often involving the entire lateral wall of the LV.

Like breast attenuation artifacts, apparent perfusion defects due to lateral chest-wall fat should be anticipated before the actual inspection of tomographic slices, through awareness of the following points:

1. Height, weight, and chest-wall circumference should be recorded for all patients. In obese men and women, lateral chest-wall attenuation artifacts occur frequently, and in general their severity is directly proportional to the chest circumference.
2. In the planar images displayed in rotating cinematic format, the LV will exhibit a markedly decreased count density in lateral and left posterior oblique (LPO) views in patients with excessive lateral chest-wall fat. Although patients with true lateral perfusion defects in the distribution of the circumflex coronary artery may exhibit similar findings in the rotating planar images, a perfusion abnormality in the lateral wall is sometimes more often identifiable in the left anterior oblique (LAO) view in these patients, since lateral chest-wall fat usually lies more posterior when the patient lies supine.
3. As for breast attenuation artifacts, gated SPECT and attenuation correction are useful in differentiating

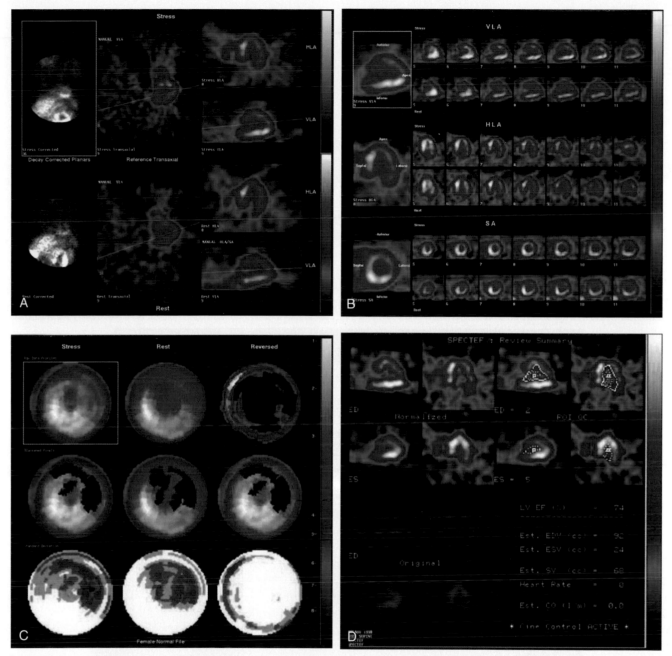

Figure 5-9 In planar projection images (**A**) a photopenic, curvilinear, photon-deficient area secondary to breast attenuation, "eclipsing" the superior portion of the left ventricle, is noted to extend to regions adjacent to the thorax. An anterior breast artifact is present in stress and rest ^{99m}Tc-sestamibi SPECT images. The artifact appears essentially fixed in tomographic slices (**B**) and polar coordinate plots (**C**). However, by careful inspection, the anterior/anterolateral defect appears somewhat more marked at rest. Gated end-diastolic and end-systolic midventricular short-axis *(top)* and vertical long-axis *(bottom)* slices (**D**) demonstrate normal anterior-wall motion and thickening, thus favoring an attenuation artifact rather than anterior infarction as a cause of the fixed defect.

lateral chest-wall attenuation artifacts from true perfusion defects. Normal lateral wall motion and wall thickening strongly favor the former.

Diffuse Depth-Dependent Soft-Tissue Attenuation

In some obese patients, soft-tissue attenuation may be diffuse. Under these circumstances, the entire myocardium may be attenuated. Because attenuation within soft tissue is distance dependent, the more basal portions of the LV myocardium will be attenuated to the greatest degree. Therefore, in obese patients, an apparent circumferential decrease in trace concentration may be present at the base. The artifact may be most pronounced at the base of the inferior and posterolateral walls, which, considering the normal anatomic position of the heart within the thorax, are furthest from the detector (Fig. 5-10). As for other attenuation artifacts, gating may be helpful to differentiate soft-tissue

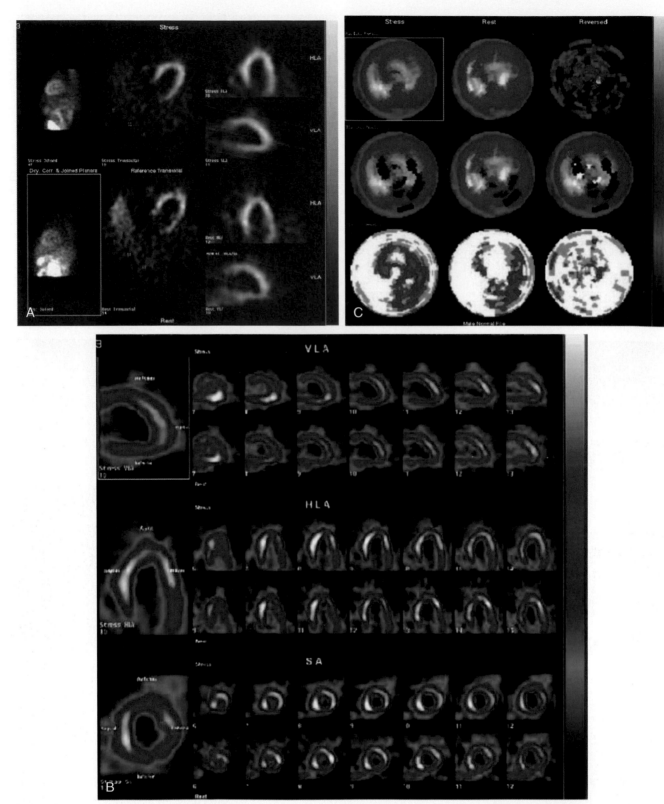

Figure 5-10 This study was performed on a 320-pound woman with a low clinical likelihood of coronary artery disease. **A,** A transaxial midventricular tomogram demonstrates apparently decreased technetium (^{99m}Tc)-sestamibi concentration in the base of the inferoposterior wall, which is the region of the left ventricle (LV) most distant from the detector and most attenuated by soft tissue. **B,** In ^{99m}Tc-sestamibi stress and rest tomograms, tracer concentration appears to be decreased at the base of the LV, particularly the base of the lateral wall. **C,** Polar plots similarly demonstrate an apparent circumferential decrease in activity at the base.

attenuation from scar. Normal wall motion and thickening of fixed basal perfusion defects in an obese patient favor the presence of attenuation artifacts rather than scar. Resolution recovery with or without attenuation correction likewise is helpful in circumventing this artifact.

Diaphragmatic Attenuation

The inferior wall of the LV of both men and women normally exhibits a decreased count density. This is most likely due to the attenuation of photons from the inferior wall of the LV by both the left hemidiaphragm and to a lesser degree the overlying right ventricle and right ventricular blood pool. In normal men, the anterior-to-inferior count-density ratio with ^{201}Tl SPECT is 1.2:1.[6] For ^{99m}Tc, the ratio is approximately 1:1.[1] In women, the ratio is approximately unity with both ^{201}Tl and [99m]Tc. This has been postulated to be due to the counterbalancing of inferior wall attenuation caused by the left hemidiaphragm in women by breast attenuation. However, it is doubtful whether that alone explains the difference, since the inferior-to-lateral wall ratio is also higher in women.

Left hemidiaphragmatic elevation can result in accentuated attenuation and inferior myocardial perfusion artifacts. Diaphragmatic elevation is common in obese patients. In patients with LV dilation, diaphragmatic attenuation may be accentuated. This may be because the dilated heart "sinks" down below the diaphragm, or possibly because the dilated ventricular blood pool results in enhanced attenuation of photons from the inferoposterior wall, which must pass through the ventricular cavity to reach the scintillation detector.

Attenuation artifacts due to left hemidiaphragmatic elevation are usually constant (fixed) in stress and rest images. However, the interpreting physician must anticipate unusual clinical circumstances in which the degree of diaphragmatic elevation is inconstant. A change in the position of the left hemidiaphragm may occur, for instance, in a patient who is anxious and swallows air during exercise but expels the air prior to subsequent resting images. This will result in more marked diaphragmatic attenuation in the stress images, mimicking a reversible ischemic perfusion defect in the inferior wall.

Infrequently, densities above or below the diaphragm may overlie the LV in planar projections used for SPECT reconstruction and result in attenuation artifacts. A left pleural effusion may attenuate the inferior and lateral walls of the LV. In patients with ascites, such as those with liver disease and those undergoing peritoneal dialysis, ascites fluid may accumulate below the left hemidiaphragm, elevating it and resulting in attenuation of photons from the inferior wall of the LV.[19] Patients with chest pain often undergo a battery of diagnostic tests that may include an upper gastrointestinal series with barium contrast. Occasionally, a loop of bowel containing barium may be superimposed on a portion of the left ventricle in the planar images used for SPECT reconstruction. Although very uncommon, such attenuation artifacts may be localized and mimic inferior wall perfusion defects.

To anticipate and recognize attenuation artifacts caused by the left hemidiaphragm and subdiaphragmatic contents and structures, the following factors should be considered before interpreting SPECT images:

1. The degree of abdominal protuberance should be noted as the patient is lying supine.
2. The hospital chart should be perused, or the patient should be questioned about having conditions predisposing to pleural effusion or free peritoneal fluid (e.g., liver disease, peritoneal dialysis).
3. The patient should be questioned about barium contrast studies within the preceding week. If there is a suspicion of barium contrast creating an attenuation artifact, an abdominal x-ray may help to confirm the presence and location of barium in the bowel.
4. The planar images used for SPECT reconstruction should be reviewed in a rotating cinematic format. The position of the left hemidiaphragm is usually identifiable in the left lateral or LPO views as a curvilinear region of tracer concentration representing the diaphragm itself or as a photopenic defect due to the stomach, which lies immediately below the diaphragm (Fig. 5-11). Attenuation of the inferior or inferoposterior wall of the LV is often evident from these views. To better define the position of the left hemidiaphragm and the associated potential for an attenuation artifact, some laboratories have obtained a separate left lateral planar view (preferably obtained with the patient

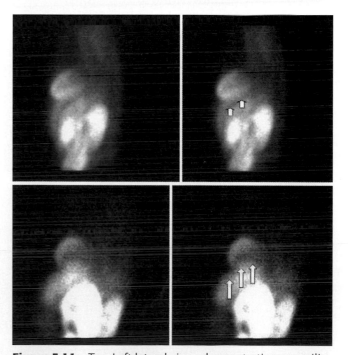

Figure 5-11 *Top,* Left lateral views demonstrating a curvilinear photopenic "shadow," indicating the position of the left hemidiaphragm. The *arrows* in the duplicate images *(right)* indicate the position of the diaphragm. In this case, the position of the diaphragm is normal, just below the inferior wall of the left ventricle. *Bottom,* Left hemidiaphragm elevation is indicated by tracer concentration in subdiaphragmatic structures "overlapping" the inferior wall.

in the right lateral decubitus position) with a higher count density.[20]

5. Gated ^{99m}Tc perfusion SPECT is very useful in differentiating diaphragmatic attenuation artifacts from inferior or inferoposterior myocardial infarction. Defects due to attenuation will move and thicken normally, whereas infarcts will exhibit decreased wall motion and wall thickening (Fig. 5-12).[4] As noted previously, however, some caution in this regard is appropriate; defects related to small subendocardial myocardial infarctions might move and thicken normally, thus mimicking attenuation, whereas some regions of hibernating myocardium that are viable may not move, simulating infarction.

SPECT image acquisitions in which the patient's position is altered to shift the level of the diaphragm and thereby minimize diaphragmatic attenuation have helped to increase diagnostic specificity. Upright imaging will cause the diaphragm to shift downward. Imaging in the prone

position is generally well tolerated by patients.[21] In the prone position, the heart shifts anteriorly to a slight degree, and the diaphragm and subdiaphragmatic contents are pushed down. There is also generally less motion of the anterior portion of the chest in the prone position and less upward creep.[21] Furthermore, the depth of respiration decreases, minimizing respiratory motion of the heart. Inferior myocardial perfusion defects noted with the patient supine but that are absent from prone images most likely represent diaphragmatic attenuation artifacts (Fig. 5-13).

Tracer washout and redistribution occur rapidly in stress ^{201}Tl SPECT, making it infeasible to repeat stress images in the prone position. Delayed redistribution images can be repeated with the patient in the prone position without appreciable tracer washout. However, this does not permit the differentiation of an attenuation artifact from a reversible ischemic abnormality. For that reason, some investigators have advocated prone imaging as an alternative to supine imaging in selected patients in whom diaphragmatic attenuation is

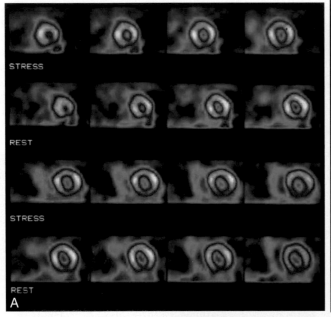

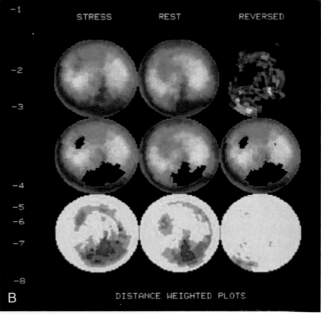

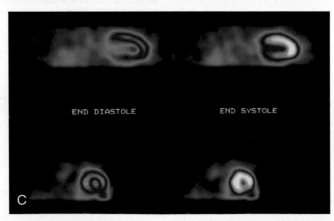

Figure 5-12 Technetium-99m-sestamibi stress and rest single-photon emission computed tomography (SPECT) tomographic slices (**A**) and polar coordinate plots (**B**) demonstrate an apparent mild relative decrease in tracer concentration in the inferior wall. Gated end-diastolic and end-systolic midventricular short-axis and vertical long-axis tomograms (**C**) demonstrate normal inferior-wall motion and wall thickening, thus favoring an attenuation artifact rather than inferior infarction as a cause of the fixed defect.

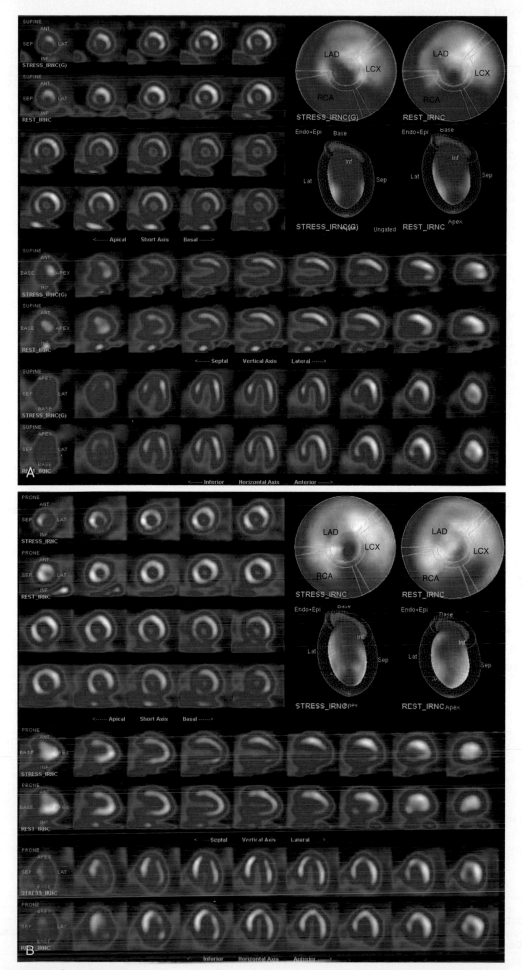

Figure 5-13 For Legend see Page 86

anticipated.[21,22] However, the physician must be cautious in interpreting routine prone SPECT myocardial perfusion images, because in the prone position, the heart lies more anteriorly than in the supine position, and there may be alterations in the geometric relationships between the detector and the heart. With the more anterior position of the heart, the anterior wall and septum may lie closer to the detector, thereby increasing the apparent anterior and septal count density. Because of this, supine SPECT studies should not be compared to a normal supine SPECT database for purposes of quantitative analysis. Also, artifactual perfusion decrease in the anteroseptal wall, probably secondary to increased sternal attenuation, has been reported.[22]

APPARENT WORSENING OF ATTENUATION ARTIFACTS IN LOW-DOSE REST IMAGES

Apart from the systematic approach of inspecting rotating projection images, viewing tomographic slices and polar plots or three-dimensional reconstructions, and observing wall motion and wall thickening in gated tomograms, another clue to a defect being attributable to soft-tissue attenuation is "pseudo–reverse distribution" in low-dose resting images (see Fig. 5-9).[23] The cause of this apparent worsening of attenuation artifacts in lower-dose resting images is most likely attributable to the filters routinely used to process data using filtered backprojection. In obese patients with low count-density images, it has been demonstrated that both breast and diaphragmatic attenuation artifacts may appear more marked in the lower count-density resting images acquired using a rest/stress 1-day protocol employing ^{99m}Tc-myocardial perfusion radiopharmaceuticals.

ADVANTAGES AND POTENTIAL DISADVANTAGES OF ATTENUATION CORRECTION IN RESOLVING ATTENUATION ARTIFACTS (See Chapters 6 and 7)

Attenuation correction using Gd-153 line sources or x-ray transmission sources are beneficial in differentiating attenuation artifacts from true perfusion defects. Currently, however, attenuation correction is in limited use because of the cost of the transmission sources or additional equipment and the fact that the method is presently not reimbursed by third-party payers. Also, there are artifacts unique to attenuation correction. If the emission and transmission scans are misregistered, significant myocardial perfusion artifacts may occur that mimic CAD[24,25] (Fig 5-14). This is particularly

problematical for x-ray attenuation methods where the transmission and emission scans are acquired sequentially as opposed to scanning line sources where the scans are "interleaved." Therefore, careful quality control of image registration is essential. In addition, scatter from subdiaphragmatic structures (see later) may be accentuated with attenuation correction, further confounding evaluation of the inferior wall of the LV.

SCATTERED ABDOMINAL VISCERAL ACTIVITY

Tracer uptake by the liver or reflux of tracer excreted by the liver into the stomach may degrade SPECT myocardial perfusion images through scatter of photons from the liver or stomach into the inferior wall of the LV. Thereby true inferior perfusion defects may be obscured. If scatter into the inferior wall is more marked at rest than with stress, the relative increase in inferior count density from rest to stress can easily mimic inferior reversibility (i.e., ischemia). Because the gallbladder is spatially separated from the heart, it seldom if ever creates such image artifacts.

To minimize scatter for SPECT with ^{99m}Tc-labeled tracers, a 15% to 20% window over the ^{99m}Tc photopeak is used. This finite window accepts photons scattered through as much as a 40-degree angle directly perpendicular to the detector, passing through the collimator holes. Such Compton scatter degrades ^{201}Tl images to an even greater degree because of the wider energy window used to encompass the emitted mercury x-rays.

In polar maps and some visual displays, as well as with quantitative analysis, SPECT images are normalized to the region of the myocardium having the greatest count density. If liver, stomach, or other abdominal visceral activity is superimposed upon the inferior wall, images will be incorrectly normalized to this area, making other areas of the heart appear count deficient. Therefore, visual or quantitative analysis may incorrectly identify defects in areas remote from the superimposed abdominal visceral activity (Fig. 5-15).

Recognition of the presence and location of abdominal visceral concentrations of tracer is essential to the accurate interpretation of myocardial perfusion SPECT studies and the avoidance of artifacts. Although abdominal visceral activity can usually be identified on tomographic slices, undeniably the best method to assess abdominal visceral activity is to inspect the multiple planar images used for SPECT reconstruction in a rotating cinematic format at the computer console. To optimize image reconstruction in the presence of abdominal visceral activity, or to determine the need to reimage selected patients, as described later, it is essential that the technologist or physician view these images before the patient leaves the laboratory.

Figure 5-13—cont'd **A,** In stress and rest technetium-99m-sestamibi single-photon emission computed tomography (SPECT) tomograms, polar plots, and 3D surface-rendered images, a decreased inferior count density secondary to diaphragmatic attenuation is present when the patient is imaged supinely. **B,** With repeat prone imaging for both stress and rest acquisitions, the diaphragmatic attenuation artifact is no longer present.

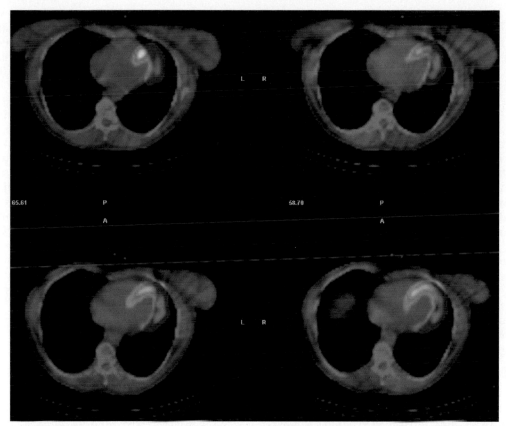

Figure 5-14 Severe misregistration of a fused transaxial single-photon emission computed tomography/computed tomography (SPECT/CT) image. *(Reproduced with permission from Goetze S, Wahl WL: Prevalence of misregistration between SPECT and CT for attenuation-corrected myocardial perfusion SPECT. J Nucl Cardiol 14:200–206, 2007.)*

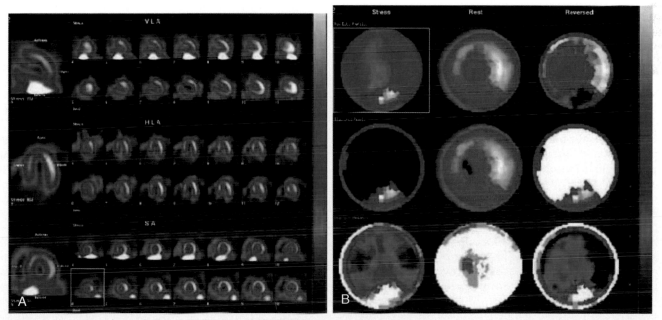

Figure 5-15 Dipyridamole stress and rest technetium-99m-sestamibi tomograms (**A**) and quantitative polar maps (**B**) in a patient with excessive subdiaphragmatic tracer concentration increasing left ventricular inferior-wall count density by means of Compton scatter. In reconstructing the stress polar map, abdominal visceral activity was included in the radius of search used for circumferential count-rate analysis, thus artifactually augmenting inferior-wall count density. By normalization to the inferior region, artifacts remote from the inferior wall were created in quantitative plots. *(Reproduced with permission from Iskandrian AF, Verani MS [eds]: Nuclear Cardiac Imaging: Principles and Applications, 3rd ed. New York: Oxford University Press, 2003, p 98.)*

For exercise images, abdominal tracer concentration can be minimized by ensuring that patients perform maximal exercise, resulting in the shunting of blood from the liver to the working skeletal musculature. For adenosine or dipyridamole, the added performance of dynamic, submaximal exercise (walking, pedaling, etc.) has been shown to significantly decrease tracer concentration in the liver in immediate images.[26] Exercise is performed during adenosine infusion or immediately after the infusion of dipyridamole, and the radiotracer is injected during exercise, at least 1 minute before its cessation. For ^{99m}Tc-sestamibi imaging, concentration in the liver decreases progressively after tracer injection, and injection-to-imaging times of 40 to 45 minutes for rest studies are recommended with this agent. For exercise ^{99m}Tc-tetrofosmin studies, the liver uptake is less problematic, and imaging at 20 to 30 minutes after injection is possible.

For pharmacologic stress studies with ^{99m}Tc-sestamibi, in which liver uptake of the agent is more marked, an interval of at least 45 minutes may be preferable. An 8-oz glass of milk or a light fatty meal may augment hepatic clearance of ^{99m}Tc-sestamibi and is offered to patients 15 minutes before both stress and rest SPECT imaging. However, this intervention may be counterproductive; tracer from the gallbladder will enter the small bowel and frequently the stomach, which may lie immediately adjacent to the inferior wall of the LV. For ^{99m}Tc-tetrofosmin imaging, injection-to-imaging times may be shortened because of more rapid liver clearance of tracer.

For ^{99m}Tc-sestamibi and ^{99m}Tc-tetrofosmin studies, additional maneuvers are available to decrease or eliminate tracer concentration in the stomach or bowel, after which repeat SPECT imaging can be performed. A large (at least 16-oz) glass of water can be given to clear activity from the stomach and promote bowel motility. If the patient ambulates after drinking water, gastric emptying may be further enhanced. Because the oral administration of water has been demonstrated to be so effective in minimizing gastric tracer concentration, most laboratories now routinely give patients water to drink 10 to 15 minutes before both stress and rest acquisitions using either ^{99m}Tc-sestamibi or tetrofosmin.

In tomographic sections, abdominal visceral activity is usually adequately distinguished from the left ventricular myocardium. However, artifacts are more common in reconstructed polar maps, because the radius of search used for the circumferential profile count-rate analysis of slices commonly extends to include abdominal visceral activity. The technologist must therefore be careful to exclude as much abdominal visceral activity as possible from regions used for reconstructing polar maps. However, care must be taken to be sure that the myocardial limiting region of interest (ROI) encompasses the entire left ventricular myocardium, particularly in basal slices where the epicardial dimensions are the greatest. If a portion of the myocardium is not encompassed, the maximal regional myocardial count density may not be detected in the bull's-eye radius of search, thereby resulting in an artifactually low regional count density in the polar plot. A deceptively attractive means for

eliminating abdominal visceral activity is to place a lead shield or apron over the areas of abdominal uptake. However, because abdominal visceral uptake can closely approximate that in the heart, and an apron may shift during SPECT image acquisition, there is the potential for attenuating the inferior myocardial wall as well.

Compton scatter of photons by overlying soft tissue significantly degrades cardiac image resolution, decreases image contrast, and decreases spatial resolution, thereby potentially decreasing test sensitivity in detecting CAD. Software methods are under development that estimate and correct for the distribution of scatter from the energy spectrum of detected photons. A "triple energy window" is used, selecting not only the ^{99m}Tc photopeak but also two narrow windows above and below that photopeak. This scatter correction method has been demonstrated to improve myocardial perfusion contrast in SPECT scans acquired with and without attenuation correction and processed with either filtered backprojection or maximum-likelihood expectation maximum (MLEM).[27-30]

THE RAMP FILTER ARTIFACT

As an inherent component of filtered backprojection, the Ramp filter is used to eliminate the "star artifact" associated with reconstruction of a finite number of projection images. This filtering process minimizes count density adjacent to an intense object, thereby better delineating its borders and increasing its contrast. However, when the Ramp filter is applied to intense tracer concentration adjacent to the heart—frequently present in the liver, stomach, or bowel—there may be an artifactual decrease in count density in the inferior wall of the LV (Fig. 5-16). Because the distribution and intensity of subdiaphragmatic activity often varies between stress and resting images (like the artifact due to scattered activity), the Ramp filter artifact is likewise variable. Therefore, both scatter of subdiaphragmatic activity and the Ramp filter may produce fixed, reversible, or reverse-distribution inferior artifacts.

Because iterative reconstruction does not incorporate the Ramp filter, it has been proposed as a means to avoid the Ramp filter artifact. Preliminary results have demonstrated, for instance, that ^{99m}Tc-sestamibi images may be acquired early (15 minutes) after resting tracer injection and processed with iterative reconstruction without artifactual inferior-wall defects, despite considerable liver radiotracer concentration.[31] However, not all nuclear medicine computer systems, particularly older models, are equipped with iterative reconstruction, so at the present time this alternative processing algorithm is not widely available.

MOTION ARTIFACTS (See Chapter 4)

Because of the process of filtered backprojection used for reconstructing SPECT images, cardiac motion relative to the detector can create image misregistration and

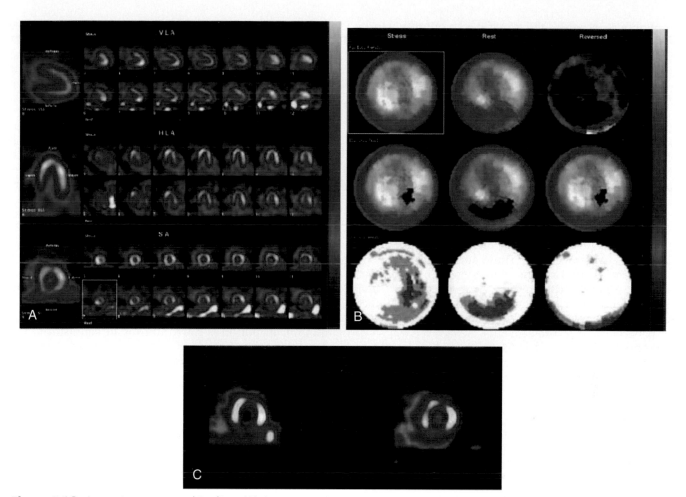

Figure 5-16 In resting tomographic slices (**A**), intense tracer concentration is present in the fundus of the stomach, localized adjacent to the inferior wall of the left ventricle (LV) in the *x* plane. By means of the Ramp filter in the resting scan, counts are subtracted from the adjacent inferior wall of the LV, creating an artifactual resting inferior perfusion defect and creating the impression of "reverse distribution" in both the tomographic slices and the polar plots (**B**). Oral administration of fluid usually "flushes out" tracer from the stomach. In **C**, stomach activity produces an inferior artifactual defect due to the Ramp filter *(left)*, which is eliminated after the patient drinks 16 oz of water *(right)*.

artifact. Cardiac motion has several sources. As it contracts, the heart rotates physiologically on its axis. It is unlikely that such motion creates artifacts large enough to be recognized or misconstrued as perfusion abnormalities. A reversible ^{201}Tl SPECT artifact may result from "upward creep" of the heart.[32] A patient's rate and depth of respiration increase markedly during dynamic exercise, resulting in more marked diaphragmatic excursion, increased lung volume, and a lower position of the diaphragm. If SPECT image acquisition is begun while the rate and depth of respiration are still increased, the position of the diaphragm and thus of the heart will be low. During the acquisition, as the depth of respiration decreases, the height of the diaphragm will progressively rise, with a gradual upward shift of the heart. Such cardiac motion will not be present in delayed resting images, when the rate of respiration is slower and more regular. Diaphragmatic creep artifacts are common with exercise ^{201}Tl, in which exercise SPECT images are acquired immediately after dynamic exercise. A 15-minute delay between exercise and ^{201}Tl image acquisition helps to allow for the respiratory rate to return to baseline.

Diaphragmatic creep artifacts are avoided with pharmacologic stress, which does not significantly increase respiration, and with ^{99m}Tc-sestamibi or tetrofosmin SPECT, for which there is a delay between exercise and stress image acquisition.

The most common source of motion artifact during SPECT image acquisition is patient movement. Such motion is unpredictable and thus most problematic. Patients may move at any time during the acquisition. The motion may be gradual or abrupt, may be vertical (axial), horizontal (sideways), or rotational, and may occur once or multiple times. With newer cameras that allow for upright patient positioning, additional patient motion in the "z-direction" is also possible if the patient slumps or leans forward in the imaging chair.

Artifact location, configuration, and severity will depend on all of these factors.[33-36] Cooper and colleagues evaluated the effect of patient motion in creating ^{201}Tl SPECT image artifacts.[34] The visual detectability of artifacts by experienced observers was directly proportional to the magnitude of motion. One-half pixel (3.25 mm) of motion was not visually detectable, 1 pixel of motion was recognized but judged to be clinically insignificant, and 2 pixels of motion resulted in artifacts potentially misconstrued as true perfusion defects. By quantitative analysis, 2 pixels of motion in the axial direction resulted in clinically significant artifacts in 5% of interpretations.

Patient motion is particularly problematic, because the location and severity of the resultant artifact depend not only on the magnitude of motion but also on its direction and the location within the 180-degree imaging arc. Cooper and coworkers observed that motion artifacts are more noticeable when axial motion occurs at the midpoint of the 180-degree acquisition.[34] They postulated that this was because the backprojected images were more evenly split between projections of two different distributions of radioactivity, one before and one after movement. These authors also observed that sideways motion results in more marked artifacts when it occurs in the anterior view, when the heart is parallel to the camera, and results in the least artifacts in the lateral projection, when the heart is more oblique or perpendicular to the camera.

The most reliable method for detecting the degree, direction, and frequency of cardiac motion is to inspect the rotating planar images at the computer console. An alternate, somewhat less reliable method is to add the individual planar frames to produce a summed image in which the heart forms a horizontal "stripe" as it moves left (45-degree right anterior oblique [RAO] projection) to right (45-degree LPO projection) across the field of view. Although abrupt downward or upward motion and diaphragmatic creep are reliably detected by this technique, it is difficult to detect sideways motion, z-direction motion, "cardiac bounce," or erratic up-and-down motion throughout the acquisition. A third method for detecting cardiac motion is by inspection of the cardiac sinogram (Fig. 5-17). The sinogram can be thought of as a "stack" of planar views in which

the y axis has been compressed. In the initial 45-degree RAO projection, the vertically compressed cardiac activity is therefore positioned in the lower left corner of the image. As the heart moves rightward across the field of view, subsequent compressed cardiac images are "stacked" in a sinusoidal configuration (reflecting a one-dimensional projection of an object rotating in a circular or elliptical orbit). Discontinuity of the sinogram indicates abrupt patient motion. However, gradual continuous motion is usually not apparent on the sinogram.

When cardiac motion occurs, misalignment of data by filtered backprojection often results in telltale artifacts in tomographic slices. The anterior and posterior walls of the LV may appear to be misaligned, with curvilinear tails of activity extending from the myocardium into adjacent background regions (Fig. 5-18).

It is essential that the physician interpreting a cardiac SPECT scan evaluate the study for motion and potential associated artifacts. It is equally or more important for the technologist to assess cardiac motion. If motion is noted during an acquisition, the acquisition may be terminated and restarted. Although this may be impractical for ^{201}Tl stress studies, reimaging is feasible for delayed ^{201}Tl studies and with ^{99m}Tc-sestamibi and ^{99m}Tc-tetrofosmin. Likewise, if motion is detected using the quality-control methods described previously, these studies may be reacquired. Therefore, it is important that rotating planar images be viewed before the patient leaves the laboratory to avoid a repeat visit and reinjection.

Motion artifacts can be avoided or minimized by an alert technologist. The patient should be positioned as comfortably as possible on the imaging table and should be observed during the entire SPECT acquisition. Stress on the low back should be minimized by supporting the lumbar spine and the knees. An arm rest is very helpful for maximizing patient comfort and thus minimizing motion. Nevertheless, patients often cannot hold their arms above their heads for the entire acquisition. Since arm movement often results in motion of the torso, the technologist should carefully reposition the patient's arm(s), avoiding any motion of the chest. The technologist should also encourage the patient to maintain a slow, steady rate of respiration. Similarly, coughing should be prevented if possible. SPECT imaging may be performed with the left arm by the side, providing it is posterior to the heart and does not attenuate the heart in any of the planar projection images, with the possible exception of the very last LPO views. A significant drawback of image acquisition with the left arm down is increased detector-to-heart distance, in turn resulting in significantly degraded tomographic spatial resolution.

One method of correcting studies for motion is to manually shift individual image frames, so that the heart remains within a constant, horizontal plane. However, this technique is relatively tedious and time-consuming and not available on all computer workstations. Automated computer methods to correct cardiac motion are now commercially available.[37–41] Their applicability may be limited if there is considerable

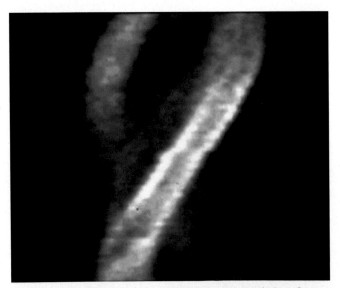

Figure 5-17 Sinogram of a 180-degree myocardial perfusion single-photon emission computed tomography (SPECT) acquisition. Discontinuity of the sinogram is indicative of patient motion.

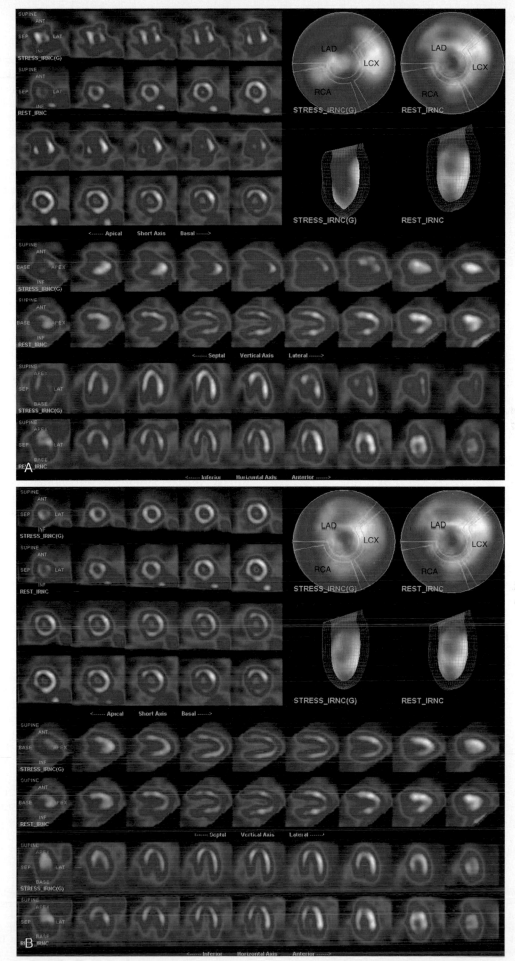

Figure 5-18 For Legend see Page 92

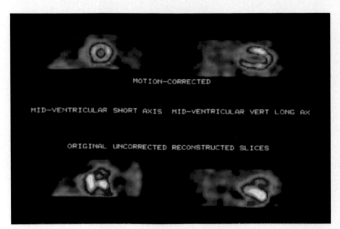

MOTION-CORRECTED

MID-VENTRICULAR SHORT AXIS   MID-VENTRICULAR VERT LONG AX

ORIGINAL UNCORRECTED RECONSTRUCTED SLICES

Figure 5-19 Tomograms acquired with greater than 3 pixels of vertical motion without *(bottom)* and with *(top)* motion correction applied.

concentration of tracer in the liver, which confounds the detection of myocardial borders.[37,38] In addition, whereas motion in the vertical direction is reliably corrected either by manual or computer methods, horizontal, rotational, and z-direction motion are not reliably corrected. Importantly, studies can often be salvaged with motion correction, obviating the need for repeat acquisition, and in some cases, reinjection (Fig. 5-19). Nevertheless, despite the development of these methods, to date, visual inspection of the rotating planar images remains the most important physician- and technologist-dependent method of quality control in cardiac SPECT.

ARTIFACTS RELATED TO NONCORONARY HEART DISEASE

Myocardial Hypertrophy

Diffuse myocardial hypertrophy often results from systemic hypertension or the increased volume or pressure overload associated with valvular heart disease. Such hypertrophy results in a generalized increase in uptake of the radiopharmaceuticals used for studying myocardial perfusion. Regional myocardial hypertrophy will appear as a localized increase in image count density.[42] If the tomographic slice or polar map is normalized to this region of increased count density, regions adjacent to and distant from the "hot spot" will appear to have relatively decreased count densities. Papillary muscle hypertrophy may occur in patients with LV hypertrophy, creating localized hot spots in the anterolateral and inferolateral wall. Occasionally there may be

localized apical hypertrophy, in which case there may be an apical hot spot with a consequent relative decrease in count density in the more basal aspects of the LV (Fig. 5-20). Additionally, a relative increase in septal-wall count density is common in hypertensive patients.[43] It is not clear whether this relative increase in septal count density is due to some degree of selective septal hypertrophy or to alterations in regional blood flow or metabolism in hypertensive patients. In patients with longstanding hypertension, a significant decrease in the lateral-to–septal wall count-density ratio as compared to that in normotensive controls has been reported.[43] Thus, in tomographic slices, raw polar maps, and quantitative plots, the lateral wall often displays a relative decrease in count density, simulating CAD in the territory of the circumflex coronary artery (Fig. 5-21). This defect is usually "fixed" in stress and rest images obtained with either ^{201}Tl or ^{99m}Tc-labeled agents, mimicking myocardial infarction. However, occasionally the septum may appear slightly less intense in resting images, rendering the defect partly reversible and raising a clinical suspicion of ischemia.

The physician interpreting the scan should anticipate this artifact in patients with hypertension. Therefore, it is important to obtain appropriate historical information. Similarly, the medical record should be examined for historical or echocardiographic evidence of idiopathic hypertrophic subaortic stenosis (IHSS) or asymmetric septal hypertrophy (ASH), which may produce a similar artifact. Moreover, inspection of the electrocardiograph (ECG) for evidence of LV hypertrophy is worthwhile. However, the standard voltage criteria are relatively insensitive to hypertrophy.[44] In gated SPECT studies in hypertensive patients without CAD, areas of relatively decreased count density, usually involving the lateral wall, will move and thicken vigorously.

Left Bundle Branch Block (See Chapter 16)

In exercise myocardial perfusion studies, reversible septal perfusion defects occur in patients with left bundle branch block (LBBB), mimicking exercise-induced septal ischemia. Such artifacts have been reported to occur in 30% to 90% of cases of LBBB, depending on whether visual or quantitative analysis was applied.[45,46] Hirzel and associates demonstrated in dog experiments that increased heart rates associated with right ventricular pacing, thus mimicking LBBB, result in a relative decrease in blood flow to the septum.[47] This decrease was not seen in experiments using atrial pacing, which mimics the sinus tachycardia of exercise. These investigators postulated that the decrease in septal blood flow is due to asynchronous relaxation of the septum, which is out of phase with diastolic filling of the remainder of the ventricle, during which coronary perfusion is

Figure 5-18—cont'd **A,** In a patient with marked downward motion during the 180-degree technetium-99m-sestamibi single-photon emission computed tomography (SPECT) post stress acquisition, reconstructed short-axis tomograms reveal apparent misalignment of the septal and lateral walls of the left ventricle, contralateral anterior and inferior defects, and "rabbit ears" or "tails" of activity streaming from the defects. In the stress vertical and horizontal long-axis tomograms, there appears to be discontinuity of the epicardial border. **B,** The stress SPECT acquisition was repeated, ensuring that the patient did not move. The resulting stress SPECT images are entirely normal.

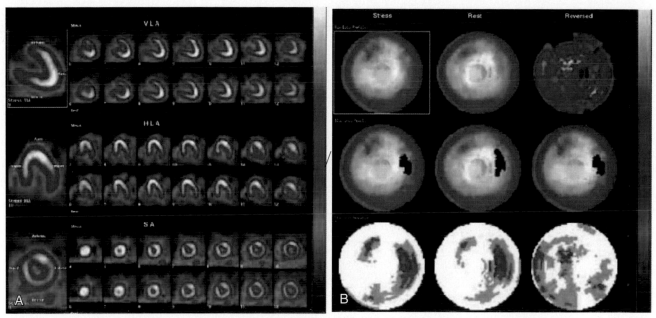

Figure 5-20 In this patient with hypertrophic cardiomyopathy with marked involvement of the apex, there is an increase in apical count density noted in tomographic slices (**A**). Polar plots, which are normalized to the apex in this particular case, demonstrate a relative decrease in count density in the more peripheral aspects of the left ventricle (**B**). *(Reproduced with permission from Iskandrian AE, Verani MS [eds]: Nuclear Cardiac Imaging: Principles and Applications, 3rd ed. New York: Oxford University Press, 2003, p 103.)*

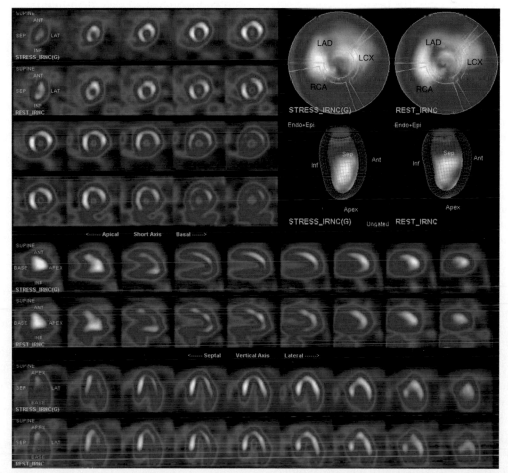

Figure 5-21 In this patient with longstanding systemic hypertension, there is a relative increase in count density in the septum in technetium-99m-sestamibi stress and rest tomograms, polar maps, and 3D surface-rendered images (viewing the septum of the left ventricle). Because images are normalized to the region of greatest count density (the septum), the remainder of the ventricle, particularly the lateral wall, appears abnormal.

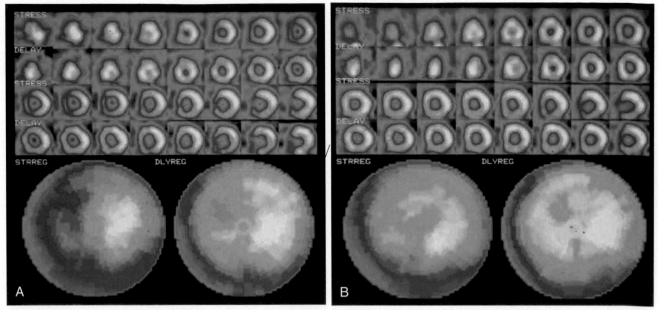

Figure 5-22 In this patient with left bundle branch block (LBBB) and no coronary artery disease, technetium-99m sestamibi short-axis tomograms and polar plots (**A**) were acquired after tracer injections at rest and during peak treadmill exercise. A reversible septal perfusion defect is present. The study was repeated, substituting dipyridamole pharmacologic stress for exercise (**B**). The reversible septal defect is no longer present. *(Courtesy of Alan Rozanski MD, St. Luke's-Roosevelt Hospital, New York.)*

maximal. At higher heart rates, the degree of septal asynchrony relative to the ECG R-R interval is greater than at rest, making septal perfusion defects appear reversible (Fig. 5-22). It has been reported that the severity of reversible perfusion defects is most marked in LBBB patients who achieve very high heart rates (>170 beats/min).[45]

It has been observed that perfusion defects associated with LBBB in patients without CAD spare the apex.[48] Thus, if an apical defect is present in a patient with LBBB, disease of the left anterior descending (LAD) coronary artery should be suspected. Also, quantitative techniques that analyze relative count density in only the more basal aspect of the septum have been reported to increase the specificity of detection of LAD CAD.[49] Perfusion abnormalities in the territories of the right and circumflex arteries carry a high sensitivity for the presence of CAD, despite the presence of LBBB.[45] Similar artifacts have not been reported for right bundle branch block (RBBB) or left anterior hemiblock. Thus, to anticipate reversible septal perfusion artifacts, it is imperative that the interpreting physician inspect the ECG tracing or report for the presence of LBBB.

It has been reported that septal artifacts associated with LBBB can be minimized by substituting pharmacologic stress with intravenous dipyridamole for exercise.[50,51] Because dipyridamole and adenosine have only a slight positive chronotropic effect, increasing the heart rate by only approximately 10 beats/min in most patients, there is little increase in septal asynchrony relative to the R-R interval. Thus, septal perfusion is kept relatively constant with dipyridamole and adenosine stress, and septal artifacts are avoided. In contrast, dobutamine has a positive inotropic effect,

so this pharmacologic agent should be avoided in LBBB patients. However, it should be cautioned that patients undergoing dipyridamole occasionally have high resting heart rates due to underlying medical conditions, and that in other individuals there may be a marked increase in heart rate associated with the infusion of pharmaceuticals. Therefore, septal artifacts may nonetheless be expected to occur if such patients also have LBBB. In most patients, it is advisable to perform low-level exercise in conjunction with dipyridamole and adenosine pharmacologic stress to minimize side effects and shunt blood away from the abdominal viscera to the working musculature. However, because of the associated increase in heart rate effected by low-level exercise, it should be avoided in LBBB patients.

SUMMARY

The list of technical and clinical circumstances that can result in SPECT image artifacts is considerable.[52] To avoid artifacts and optimize test specificity, both the technologist and interpreting physician must be aware of factors potentially contributing to the creation of artifacts.

REFERENCES

1. Nichols K, Yao SS, Kamran M, et al: Clinical impact of arrhythmias on gated SPECT cardiac myocardial perfusion and function assessment, *J Nucl Cardiol* 37:458, 2001.
2. Maddahi J, Kiat H, Van Train K, et al: Myocardial perfusion imaging with technetium-99m sestamibi SPECT in the evaluation of coronary artery disease, *Am J Cardiol* 66:55E–62E, 1990.

3. Manglos SH, Thomas FD, Gagne GM, et al: Phantom study of breast tissue attenuation in myocardial imaging, *J Nucl Med* 34:992–996, 1993.

4. DePuey EG, Rozanski A: Using gated technetium-99m sestamibi SPECT to characterize fixed myocardial defects as infarct or artifact, *J Nucl Med* 36.952–955, 1995.

5. Smanio PE, Watson DD, Segalla DL, et al: Value of gating of technetium-99m sestamibi single-photon emission computed tomographic imaging, *J Am Coll Cardiol* 29:69–77, 1997.

6. DePasquale EE, Nody AC, DePuey EG, et al: Quantitative rotational thallium-201 tomography for identifying and localizing coronary artery disease, *Circulation* 77:316–327, 1988.

7. Malko JA, Van Heertum RL, Gullberg GT, et al: SPECT liver imaging using an iterative attenuation correction algorithm and an external flood source, *J Nucl Med* 27:701–705, 1986.

8. Bailey DL, Hutton BF, Walter PJ: Improved SPECT using simultaneous emission and transmission tomography, *J Nucl Med* 28:844–851, 1987.

9. Galt JR, Cullum SJ, Garcia EV: SPECT quantification: A simplified method of attenuation and scatter correction for cardiac imaging, *J Nucl Med* 33:2232–2237, 1992.

10. Manglos SH, Bassano DA, Thomas FD: Cone-beam transmission CT for nonuniform attenuation compensation of SPECT images, *J Nucl Med* 32:1813–1820, 1991.

11. Tung C-H, Gullberg GT, Zeng GL, et al: Nonuniform attenuation correction using simultaneous transmission and emission converging tomography, *IEEE Trans Nucl Sci* 39:1134–1143, 1992.

12. Manglos SH, Bassano DA, Thomas FD: Imaging of the human torso using cone beam transmission CT implementation on a rotating gamma camera, *J Nucl Med* 33:150–156, 1992.

13. Corbett JR, Ficaro EP: Clinical review of attenuation-corrected cardiac SPECT, *J Nucl Cardiol* 6:54–68, 1999.

14. Kluge R, Seese A, Sattler B, Knapp WH: Non-uniform attenuation correction for myocardial SPECT using two Gd-153 line sources, *Nuklearmedizin* 35:205–211, 1996.

15. Kluge R, Sattler B, Seese A, et al: Attenuation correction by simultaneous emission-transmission myocardial single-photon emission tomography using a technetium-99m-labelled radiotracer: Impact on diagnostic accuracy, *Eur J Nucl Med* 24:1107–1114, 1997.

16. He ZX, Lakkis NM, America Y, et al: Qualitative and quantitative comparison of sestamibi SPECT without and with attenuation correction for detection of coronary artery disease in patients with large body habitus [abstract], *J Am Coll Cardiol* 29:302A, 1997.

17. Hendel RC, Berman DS, Cullom SJ, et al: Multicenter trial to evaluate the efficacy of correction for photon attenuation and scatter in SPECT myocardial perfusion imaging, *Circulation* 99:2742–2749, 1999.

18. Links JM, DePuey EG, Taillefer R, et al: Attenuation correction and gating synergistically improve the diagnostic accuracy of myocardial perfusion SPECT, *J Nucl Cardiol* 8:G1–G58, 2001.

19. Rab ST, Alazraki NP, Guertler-Krawczynska E: Peritoneal fluid causing inferior attenuation on SPECT thallium-201 myocardial imaging in women, *J Nucl Med* 29:1860–1864, 1988.

20. Johnstone D, Wakers F, Berger H, et al: Effect of patient positioning on left lateral thallium-201 myocardial images, *J Nucl Med* 20:183–188, 1979.

21. Machac J, George T: Effect of 360 SPECT prone imaging on Tl-201 myocardial perfusion studies, *J Nucl Med* 31:812, 1990.

22. Kiat H, Van Train KF, Friedman JD, et al: Quantitative stress-redistribution thallium-201 SPECT using prone imaging: Methodologic development and validation, *J Nucl Med* 33:1509–1515, 1992.

23. Araujo W, DePuey EG, Kamran M, et al: Artifactual reverse distribution pattern in myocardial perfusion SPECT with Tc-99m sestamibi, *J Nucl Cardiol* 7:633–638, 2000.

24. Goetze S, Wahl WL: Prevalence of misregistration between SPECT and CT for attenuation-corrected myocardial perfusion SPECT, *J Nucl Cardiol* 14:200–206, 2007.

25. Goetz S, Brown TL, Lavely WC, et al: Attenuation correction in myocardial perfusion SPECT/CT: Effects of misregistration and value of reregistration, *J Nucl Med* 48:1090–1095, 2007.

26. Stern S, Greenberg D, Corne R: Effect of exercise supplementation on dipyridamole thallium 201 image quality, *J Nucl Med* 33(Suppl):1559, 1992.

27. Zaidi H, Koral KF: *Quantitative Analysis in Nuclear Medicine Imaging*, New York, 2005, Springer-Verlag.

28. Kojima A, Matsumoto M, Tomiguchi S, et al: Accurate scatter correction for transmission computed tomography using an uncollimated line array source, *Ann Nucl Med* 18:45–50, 2004.

29. Changizi V, Takavar A, Babakhani A, Sohrabi M: Scatter correction for heart SPECT images using TEW method, *J Appl Clin Med Phys* 9:136–140, 2008.

30. Khalil M, Brown E, Heller E: Does scatter correction of cardiac SPECT improve image quality in the presence of high extracardiac activity? *J Nucl Cardiol* 11:424–434, 2004.

31. Lewin HC, Hyun ME, DePuey EG, et al: Validation of a very rapid rest/stress 1 day Tc-99m sestamibi stress protocol. *J Nucl Cardiol* 10:24S, 2003.

32. Friedman J, Van Train K, Maddahi J, et al: "Upward creep" of the heart: A frequent source of false-positive reversible defects during thallium-201 stress-redistribution SPECT, *J Nucl Med* 30:1718–1722, 1989.

33. Friedman J, Berman DS, Van Train K, et al: Patient motion in thallium-201 myocardial SPECT imaging. An easily identified frequent source of artifactual defect, *Clin Nucl Med* 13:321–324, 1988.

34. Cooper JA, Neumann PH, McCandless BK: Effect of patient motion on tomographic myocardial perfusion imaging, *J Nucl Med* 13:1566–1571, 1992.

35. Botvinick EH, Zhu YY, O'Connell WJ, et al: A quantitative assessment of patient motion and its effect on myocardial perfusion SPECT images, *J Nucl Med* 34:303–310, 1993.

36. Prigent FM, Hyun M, Berman DS, et al: Effect of motion on thallium-201 SPECT studies: A simulation and clinical study, *J Nucl Med* 34:1845–1850, 1993.

37. Eisner RL, Churchwell A, Noever T, et al: Quantitative analysis of the tomographic thallium-201 myocardial bullseye display: Critical role of correcting for patient motion, *J Nucl Med* 29:91–97, 1988.

38. Geckle WJ, Frank TL, Links JM, et al: Correction for patient and organ movement in SPECT: Application to exercise thallium-201 cardiac imaging, *J Nucl Med* 27:899, 1986.

39. Eisner RL, Noever T, Nowak D, et al: Use of cross-correlation function to detect patient motion during SPECT imaging, *J Nucl Med* 28:97–101, 1987.

40. Cooper JA, Neumann PH, McCandless BK: Detection of patient motion during tomographic myocardial perfusion imaging, *J Nucl Med* 34:1341–1348, 1993.

41. Germano G, Chua T, Kavanagh PB, et al: Detection and correction of patient motion in dynamic and static myocardial SPECT using a multi-detector camera, *J Nucl Med* 34:1349–1355, 1993.

42. Galt JR, Robbins WL, Eisner RL, et al: Thallium-201 myocardial SPECT quantitation: Effect of wall thickness, *J Nucl Med* 27:577, 1987.

43. DePuey EG, Guertler-Krawczynska E, Perkins JV, et al: Alterations in myocardial thallium-201 distribution in patients with chronic systemic hypertension undergoing single-photon emission computed tomography, *Am J Cardiol* 62:234–238, 1988.

44. Devereux RB, Alonso DR, Lutas EM, et al: Echocardiographic assessment of left ventricular hypertrophy: Comparison of necropsy findings, *Am J Cardiol* 57:450–458, 1986.

45. DePuey EG, Krawczynska EG, Robbins WL: Thallium-201 SPECT in coronary artery disease patients with left bundle branch block, *J Nucl Med* 29:1479–1485, 1988.

46. Burns RJ, Galligan L, Wright LM, et al: Improved specificity of myocardial thallium-201 single-photon emission computed tomography in patients with left bundle branch block by dipyridamole, *Am J Cardiol* 68:504–508, 1991.

47. Hirzel HO, Senn M, Nuesch K, et al: Thallium-201 scintigraphy in complete left bundle branch block, *Am J Cardiol* 53:764–769, 1984.

48. Matzer LA, Kiat H, Friedman JD, et al: A new approach to the assessment of tomographic thallium-201 scintigraphy in patients with left bundle branch block, *J Am Coll Cardiol* 17:1309–1317, 1991.

49. Civelek AC, Gozukara I, Durski K, et al: Detection of left anterior descending coronary artery disease in patients with left bundle branch block, *Am J Cardiol* 70:1565–1570, 1992.

50. Rockett JF, Chadwick M, Moinuddin M, et al: Intravenous dipyridamole thallium-201 SPECT imaging in patients with left bundle branch block, *Clin Nucl Med* 6:401–407, 1990.

51. Larcos G, Brown ML, Gibbons RJ: Role of dipyridamole thallium-201 imaging in left bundle branch block, *Am J Cardiol* 68:1097–1098, 1991.

52. DePuey EG, Garcia EV: Optimal specificity of thallium-201 SPECT through recognition of imaging artifacts, *J Nucl Med* 30:441–449, 1989.

Chapter 6

Attenuation/Scatter/ Resolution Correction: Physics Aspects

MICHAEL A. KING, TINSU PAN AND P. HENDRIK PRETORIUS

INTRODUCTION

A number of factors can cause artifacts in cardiac single-photon emission computed tomography (SPECT) imaging.[1] Among these are the attenuation and scattering of the photons in the patient's tissues and the finite and distance-dependent spatial resolution SPECT systems. A significant amount of research and development has gone into perfecting clinically robust compensation strategies for these. The present status of clinical trials has led the American Society of Nuclear Cardiology and the Society of Nuclear Medicine to jointly develop and publish a position statement on attenuation correction (AC), which concluded "that the adjunctive technique of attenuation correction has become a method for which the weight of evidence and opinion is in favor of its usefulness."[2] To achieve an improvement in diagnostic accuracy with AC, it is required for physicians to modify their "approach to image interpretation accounting for the effects of these methods on the resultant images,"[2] and "use hardware and software that have undergone clinical validation and include appropriate quality-control tools (see Chapter 7)."[2]

It is our belief this recognition of the utility of AC will be followed by that of the need for also correcting for scatter and distance-dependent spatial resolution. Our position is that the more completely the physics of imaging is correctly included in reconstruction, the more accurate will be the diagnosis from the reconstructed slices. Thus, the goals of this chapter are to (1) provide an introduction to the physics of imaging and how this can be incorporated into reconstruction and (2) illustrate that when this is done, diagnostic accuracy can be improved. Other related reviews on this have been published by Bacharach and Buvat,[3] King and colleagues,[4,5] Bailey,[6] and Zaidi and Hasegawa.[7]

IMPACT OF ATTENUATION, SCATTER, AND RESOLUTION ON CARDIAC SINGLE-PHOTON EMISSION COMPUTED TOMOGRAPHY (See Chapter 7)

Interactions and Exponential Attenuation

For a photon—whether gamma ray from technetium (^{99m}Tc) or x-ray subsequent to the decay of thallium (^{201}Tl)—to become part of a cardiac image, it must first escape the body (see photon A in Fig. 6-1). The chances of this occurring are reduced in proportion to the likelihood that it will interact in the patient's body before it can escape. At the photon energies of interest in nuclear cardiology, the major interactions in tissues are Compton scattering and photoelectric absorption.[8,9] In Compton scattering, a photon interacts with an electron that is loosely bound compared to the photon's energy. The result of this interaction is the ejection of the electron from the atom and the creation of a new photon having a lower energy and different direction (see photons B and C in Fig. 6-1). The probability of interaction per unit path length (characterized by the linear attenuation coefficient for Compton scattering) depends on the tissue density and number of electrons per gram and decreases slowly with increasing photon energy. In photoelectric absorption, the photon imparts all of its energy to an electron, which is then ejected from the atom. The ejected photoelectron carries a kinetic energy that is equal to the energy of the incident photon minus the binding energy with which it was held to the atom. No scattered photon is emitted in the photoelectric interaction (see photon D in Fig. 6-1). However, characteristic radiation will likely be emitted when the

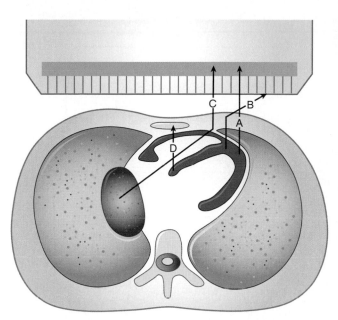

Figure 6-1 Illustration of photon interactions of interest in patient for cardiac imaging. **A,** Transmitted photon originating in myocardium. **B,** Compton scattered photon originating in myocardium that collimator stops from striking crystal. **C,** Compton scattered photon originating in the liver that collimator allows to pass and results in the detection of an event that apparently originated in the myocardium. **D,** Photoelectrically absorbed in bone, which originated in myocardium.

electrons of the atom rearrange to fill the vacancy left by the photoelectron. The linear attenuation coefficient for photoelectric absorption increases as the cube of the atomic number of the atom, depends on tissue density, and decreases as the inverse cube of the photon energy.

Mathematically, the fraction of photons that will be transmitted through an attenuator or the transmitted fraction (TF) is given by:

$$TF = e^{-\mu x} \qquad (1)$$

where μ is the linear attenuation coefficient (sum of all the coefficients for individual interactions) and x is the thickness of the attenuator the photons pass through. If the attenuator is made up of a number of materials of various compositions, then the product μx in Eq. 1 is replaced by a sum of the attenuation coefficient for each material times the thickness of the material the transmitted photons pass through (path length the photons travel in the material). As a result of the differences in attenuation coefficient with type of tissue, the TF will vary with the materials traversed, even if the total patient thickness between the site of the emission and the camera is the same. Thus, one needs to have patient-specific information on the spatial distribution of attenuation coefficients (an attenuation map) to calculate the attenuation, which decreases the probability of photon detection.

Attenuation Artifacts (See Chapter 6)

The change in TF with direction of the photons and between different locations in the patient results in a variation in attenuation. This can be visualized in planar images as, for example, breast shadows and decreased counts in the presence of an elevated diaphragm. In SPECT slices, these artificial shadows are difficult to recognize; however, there is a pattern of altered relative counts consistent with the influence of attenuation in the mean bull's eye polar maps of patients with a low likelihood of CAD. Eisner and colleagues reported decreased relative counts in the anterior wall of ^{201}Tl polar maps for females due to breast attenuation, and a relative decrease in the inferior wall of males, which may be due to diaphragmatic attenuation.[10] The problem is that the location, extent, and severity of these reduced-count regions vary from patient to patient as a function of their anatomy. Thus, the variation in the pattern of apparent localization in disease-free patients is increased, resulting in more false-positive results (lower specificity) at any given level of true-positive results (sensitivity).

The types of changes in the reconstructed activity distributions when attenuation is present are illustrated in Figure 6-2. The *top row* of this figure shows what can be expected in the simple case of an elliptically shaped uniform-activity distribution without and with the presence of attenuation caused by a uniform attenuation distribution within the object. Note that attenuation causes a scaling of the reconstructed activity distribution such that there is a decrease by more than a factor of 2 at the outside, and a further decrease as one moves toward the center or most attenuated portion of the distribution. Hence an extended object that has a uniform distribution to begin with would have a loss in uniformity dependent on the relative depths of locations within it. The *middle row* of the figure shows the more complex case of a uniform source distribution that is attenuated by a non-uniform attenuation distribution simulating that of a cross-section through a female patient. This attenuation distribution and subsequent source and attenuator distributions the employed in the figures of this chapter were obtained from the mathematic cardiac-torso (MCAT) digital anthropomorphic phantom.[11] Notice that because the lungs have an attenuation coefficient approximately one-third that of soft tissue, there is now less attenuation within them than would have occurred had the entire cross-section consisted of soft tissues. Thus with attenuation, there appears to be a higher concentration of activity within them than the surrounding soft tissue, when actually the concentration was uniform. Notice also the sharp transition in apparent concentration of activity between the medial boundary of the lung and the heart region. The heart lateral wall is attenuated significantly more than the lung next to it. This explains why AC correction is very sensitive to having the correct registration between emission imaging and attenuation maps. A small movement can cause a big difference in the correction applied. The *bottom row* shows the even more complex case of both non-uniform source and attenuation distributions from the MCAT phantom simulating that of ^{99m}Tc-sestamibi imaging. At the *far left*, in the absence of attenuation, the distribution of activity within the heart wall is uniform; however, when attenuation is included, a non-uniform

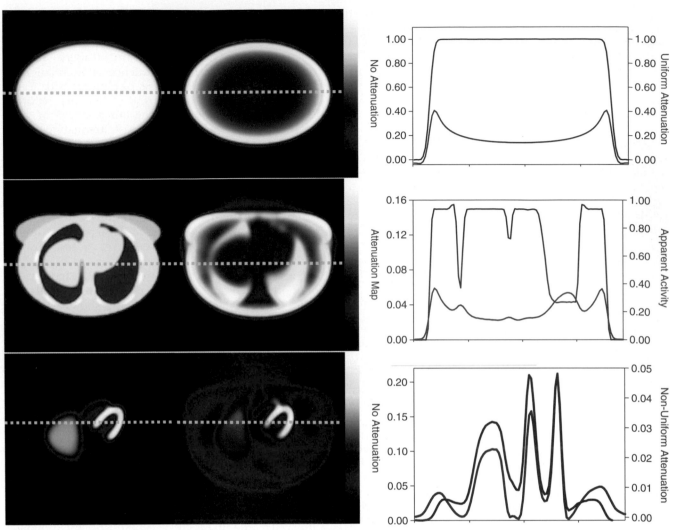

Figure 6-2   Transverse slices showing examples of the distortion in apparent activity distribution caused by attenuation for *(top)* uniform activity and attenuation distributions, *(middle)* non-uniform attenuation and a uniform attenuation distribution, and *(bottom)* non-uniform attenuation and activity distributions. *Top left* shows a comparison of a slice through an elliptically shaped uniform-activity distribution and its reconstruction when attenuation is included in the creation of the SPECT data used in reconstruction. The attenuation distribution used to simulate attenuation during acquisition was also assumed to be uniform, with an attenuation coefficient equal to that of water for (99mTc) photons. Notice that there is a significant decrease in the apparent activity in the reconstructed slice as one goes from the outside toward the center. The plots at the *upper right* are count profiles at the level indicated by the superimposed horizontal lines to the left for the original activity distribution *(red)* and the apparent distribution post reconstruction *(blue)*. These graphically illustrate the impact of attenuation on the originally uniform activity distribution. Note that the scaling of the two count profiles is different, and that attenuation decreases the counts, even at the edge of the original distribution. *Middle left* shows a non-uniform attenuation distribution from the mathematic cardiac-torso phantom simulating that of a cross-section through a female patient, and the resulting apparent activity distribution when a uniform activity distribution is simulated as having been present in the patient. The outermost portion of the apparent distribution is again hotter, but now the lungs—which have a significantly lower attenuation coefficient than soft tissues—are also hotter. Note also the false presence of activity beyond the anterior surface of the body. *Middle right* shows overlaid plots of a horizontal profile through the attenuation map *(red)* and through the apparent activity distribution *(blue)*, which clearly illustrate the impact of the less attenuating lungs. *Bottom left* shows 180-degree filtered backprojection reconstructed activity distribution that simulated that of 99mTc-sestamibi imaging for the cases of first, no attenuation and then, use of the attenuation distribution of the attenuation map, shown in the *middle row*. Notice the loss of uniformity of activity distribution within the walls of the heart, the presence of activity outside the body, and the significant distortion of the liver, with the inclusion of attenuation when simulating the SPECT data. *Bottom right* shows count profiles at the level indicated by the horizontal lines of the slices, showing the increased non-uniformity in wall apparent uptake when attenuation is included during simulation of the SPECT data.

distribution results, with the apex and lateral wall being brighter than the deeper lateral wall. Notice also that with attenuation present, there is now a mild change in the size and shape of the heart, as well as a significant distortion of the liver. With attenuation, there now is activity reconstructed as being outside the body. Such geometric distortion is greater for 180-degree reconstruction (as performed for these slices) than 360-degree reconstruction, owing to the greater inconsistencies in the emission profiles in the absence of their averaging by combining conjugate views.[12] The positive and negative tails from hot sources, which result from the incomplete cancellation of the inconsistent data in the emission profiles, can also lead to significant distortions in cardiac wall counts when there is significant extracardiac localization, such as with hepatic uptake. Germano and colleagues showed in phantom studies that an apparent reduction in counts occurs with the presence of a "hot" liver in the slices with the heart.[13] Nuyts and colleagues[14] observed that use of 360 degrees as opposed to 180 degrees with filtered backprojection (FBP) reconstruction reduced the magnitude of the artifact. The artifact was further reduced by use of attenuation compensation with maximum-likelihood expectation-maximization (MLEM) reconstruction.

The artifactual decrease in apparent activity within the heart walls due to nearby extracardiac activity is further illustrated in the short-axis slices and circumferential count profiles at the top of Figure 6-3 for 180-degree reconstruction of Monte Carlo simulations[15] of the MCAT phantom.[11] The *top set of slices* are with the liver uptake simulated as the same as that of the background. The *next lower set of three slices* shows the artifactual decrease in the inferior wall caused by the alteration of the liver activity to be the same as that of the heart. This alteration is illustrated graphically in the plots of the maximum count circumferential count to the *right*. There, one sees the typical pattern of a decrease in activity in the inferior versus the anterior wall due to the greater depth of the inferior wall, but this difference is dramatically accentuated by the increase in liver activity. This alteration in the apparent distribution of activity within the slices can be understood by the theory of the impact of attenuation on positron emission tomography (PET) and SPECT slices developed by Nuyts et al.,[16] Bai et al.,[17] and Bai and Shao.[18] By this theory, attenuation causes a scaling of the counts at a given position, as illustrated in Figure 6-2, and a shifting of the local counts due to the attenuation of the other activity within the slice. It is this shifting that creates a negative bias that is the cause of the artifactual decrease in the inferior wall of the heart.

That AC, when included within iterative reconstruction, can correct this artifactual decrease as illustrated in the *middle set* of three short-axis slices at the *left* in Figure 6-3, and in the corresponding circumferential profile at the *right*. Notice that with AC, the wall now becomes fairly uniform in uptake. Notice also that the liver now becomes more intense than the heart, even though they were simulated as having the same concentration of activity. The reason for the apparent difference is the partial volume effect (PVE),[9] which causes structures smaller in any dimension than two to three times the full-width-at-half-maximum (FWHM) measure of the system spatial resolution to be blurred such that their apparent activity is less than the actual value.

Broad Beam Attenuation and Scatter

Equation 1 is accurate only (1) for a beam of photons with the same energy and (2) under the "good geometry condition" that, as soon as a photon undergoes any

interaction, is no longer counted as a member of the beam.[8,9] Attenuation coefficients measured subject to these conditions are the "good-geometry" attenuation coefficients. Compton scattered photons, even though they are reduced in energy, are not necessarily excluded from being counted, owing to the finite width of the energy windows used because of the limited ability to distinguish different energy photons (finite energy resolution) of the cameras (Fig. 6-4). In fact, the ratio of scattered photons included in the energy window to primary photons in the energy window (scatter fraction) is typically 0.34 for ^{99m}Tc[19] and 0.95 for ^{201}Tl[20] for cardiac SPECT. Thus, Eq. 1 has to be modified to match the "broad beam" attenuation, which actually occurs in emission imaging by the inclusion of the buildup factor B, which is dependent on both μ and x. The result is[8,9]:

$$TF = B(\mu, x)e^{-\mu x} \qquad (2)$$

Numerically, the buildup factor is the ratio between the sum of primary and scatter counts over the primary counts only, or the relative increase in counts due to the inclusion of scattered photons. It thus depends on variables such as location in the attenuator, geometry and composition of the attenuator, energy of the photon, energy resolution of the camera, and energy window used in imaging.

When scatter is not removed from the emission profiles before reconstruction, or its presence is incorporated into the reconstruction process itself, an overcorrection will occur. This is illustrated by the three sets of short-axis slices and the circumferential profiles at the *bottom* of Figure 6-3. As discussed previously, the top row of these slices illustrates how successful AC included within MLEM reconstruction can be at correcting the artifactual change in apparent uptake of the inferior wall of the row of slices just above it. However, the success of AC returning this slice to an apparent uniform concentration of activity within the walls is due in part to just primary photons being present. When the scattered photons acquired within the photopeak of the simulated acquisition are included, the short-axis slices *next to the bottom* are obtained. Notice how scatter has caused the inferior wall to now appear brighter than the anterior wall, which is the opposite of the effect of attenuation. The presence of scatter has also decreased wall contrast compared to the heart chamber region and visually decreased the separation of the heart from the liver. The *bottom row* of short-axis slices shows this is due to the non-uniform presence of scatter being concentrated closer to the liver. The circumferential profiles at the *bottom right* in the figure show that quantitatively, scatter has added approximately 30% more counts to the heart wall and that the inferior wall was increased the most.

Finite and Distance-Dependent Spatial Resolution

The third source of degradation discussed in this chapter is the finite, distance-dependent spatial resolution of the

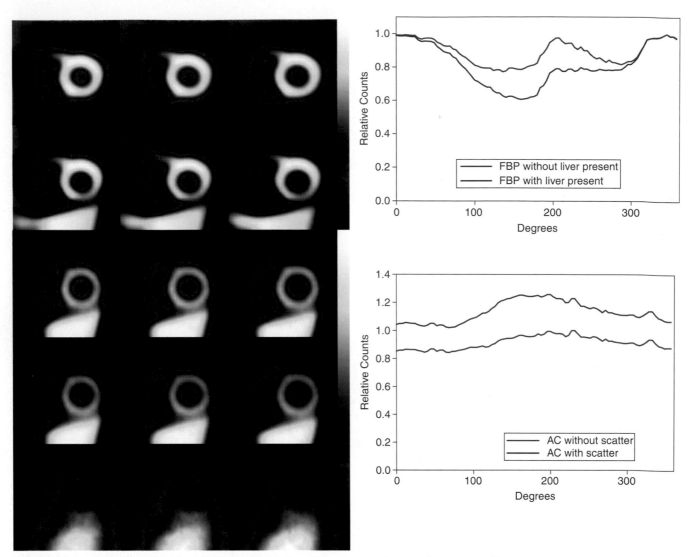

Figure 6-3 Comparison of Monte Carlo–simulated short-axis slices and circumferential profiles illustrating the impact of atten-uation, attenuation correction (AC), and the inclusion of scatter. The two sets of three short-axis slices at the *upper left* show the uniformity of the activity within the LV wall when reconstructing 180 degrees of data using filtered back projection (FBP) without AC. The simulated acquisitions included the presence of non-uniform attenuation and camera distance-dependent spatial resolu-tion but do not include scattered photons. In the first of these two sets, the concentration of activity within the liver was set to that of the background. In the second, it was set to be equal to that of the heart. Notice that the presence of a significant concen-tration of activity within the liver causes a significant apparent decrease in the inferior wall of the LV. This change is further demonstrated in the plots at the *upper right*, which show the maximum-count circumferential profiles from these short-axis slices. The *middle* of the five sets of short-axis slices shows the impact of using AC as part of maximum-likelihood expectation maximization reconstruction on the uniformity of the counts in the heart wall for acquisitions, with the liver activity concentra-tion equaling that of the heart. The dramatic improvement in wall uniformity seen in the slices can be seen graphically by com-paring the maximum-count circumferential profile plot for these slices at the *lower right* with those at the *upper right* for reconstruction without AC. The fourth set of three short-axis slices at the *lower left* illustrates the impact of the inclusion of scat-tered photons in imaging when the liver activity concentration is the same as in the heart. Notice that the apparent inferior-wall decrease seen without AC is now turned into an elevation in apparent inferior-wall counts with AC but no correction for scatter. This elevation is quantitatively demonstrated in the maximum-count circumferential profiles at the *lower right*. The bottom set of three short-axis slices is the reconstruction of solely the scatter contribution in the fourth set. Notice that scatter contributes to all regions of the slices, reducing wall contrast and apparent separation between the inferior heart wall and the liver.

imaging system. When imaging in air, the system spatial resolution consists of two independent sources of blur-ring.[9] The first is the intrinsic resolution of the detector and electronic components of the camera head. The sec-ond is the spatially varying geometric acceptance of the photons through the holes of the collimator. The colli-mator is the "lens" of the gamma camera; however, unlike optical lenses that form images by bending the

light photons, collimators work by stopping all but the few photons that can pass through their holes without being absorbed by the septa of the collimator (absorp-tive collimation). This is illustrated in Figure 6-5, which shows two images of a very small point source of ^{99m}Tc at the same location 10 cm from the detector face, first with no collimator and then with a low-energy high-resolution (LEHR) parallel-hole collimator on the

Tc-99m Energy Spectrum

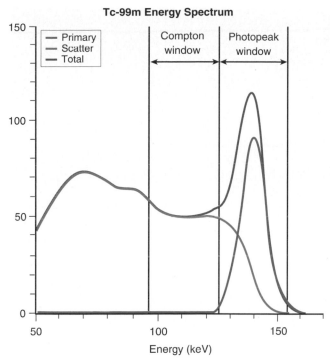

Figure 6-4 Illustration of the energy distribution of primary and scattered photons for a technetium (^{99m}Tc) point source in an attenuating medium. Shown also are the locations of the photopeak and Compton scatter windows.

camera head. The obvious need for the collimator is made clear by this figure, and so is the price paid for the use of the collimator in terms of loss in detection efficiency. Without the collimator, 7.2 million counts were collected in 1 minute. With the collimator, only 18,000 counts were collected in 1 minute, or 0.25% of that when the collimator was not on the system. The actual difference is greater because when the collimator was off, the count rate was near the maximum count rate of the system, so the recorded number of counts was depressed by resolving time count losses.[9]

As good as the image of the point source looks in Figure 6-5B compared to 6-5A, the ideal response would have been significantly better, since the point source

was approximately only 1 mm in any dimension, and its bright representation in Figure 6-5B is larger than 10 mm across. The image resulting from imaging a point source of activity such as illustrated in Figure 6-5B is called a *point spread function* (PSF),[9] and it portrays how a very small source of activity is blurred out during the course of imaging. Figure 6-6A illustrates plots through the center of Monte Carlo–simulated PSFs for an increasing distance of the point source in air from the face of a LEHR parallel-hole collimator. Notice how the PSF changes significantly in width and height as a function of distance. However, the area under the curves stays constant, consistent with no change in sensitivity with distance in air from the face of a parallel-hole collimator.

Figure 6-6B illustrates the impact of distance-dependent spatial resolution on one coronal slice through the MCAT phantom. As illustrated at the *upper left* in this figure, the concentrations of activity in the wall of the left ventricle (LV) and liver were the same, and that of the general tissue background was set to one-tenth that of the heart. All other organs had a concentration of activity of zero, as illustrated by the lungs, blood pool, and bones showing up as *black*. The slice at the *upper right* is that of the upper left blurred as if it were 10 cm from the face of a camera, as imaged with a LEHR collimator. The *lower left* slice is blurred as if acquired at 20 cm from the face of the collimator, and the *lower right* is 30 cm from the face. The FWHMs of the PSFs at these distances were 0.8 cm, 1.34 cm, and 1.88 cm. Notice how with increasing distance, the heart wall appears to become thicker and of apparently lower concentration relative to the liver. The apparent change in concentration is an illustration of the PVE or dependence of the apparent concentration of a structure on its size relative to the extent of blurring (FWHM).[9] Note that the thickness of the wall in the slice varies due to the angulation of the heart relative to the coronal plane. Thus, the PVE causes the heart wall to appear as though it does not have a uniform concentration, when it actually had to begin with. Notice also that with increased distance, the liver and heart blur together to an increasing extent.

Figure 6-5 Images of a (^{99m}Tc) point source 10 cm in air from the face of the camera detector. **A,** No collimator on the camera head. **B,** Low-energy high resolution collimator on the camera head.

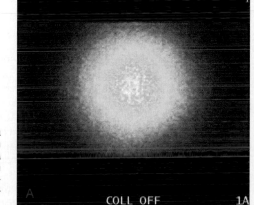
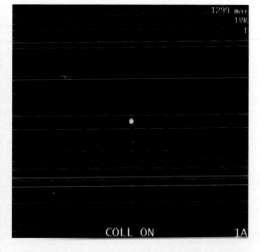

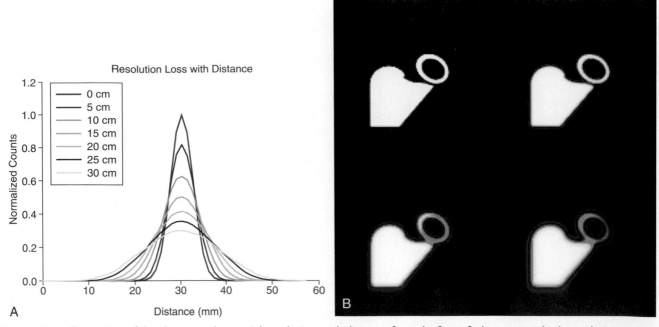

Figure 6-6 Illustration of the change in the spatial resolution with distance from the face of a low-energy high-resolution parallel-hole collimator for a (^{99m}Tc) point source as depicted by the system point spread function (PSF), and the impact of this change in spatial resolution on one coronal slice through the heart and liver of the mathematic cardiac-torso (MCAT) phantom. **A,** Variation in Monte Carlo–simulated PSFs with distance for a point source in air (no contribution of scatter is included). Since sensitivity does not change with distance for a parallel-hole collimator, the area under all of the PSFs is the same. Thus, as the blurring becomes greater (the PSF wider), the maximum of the PSF decreases. This illustrates that increasingly lower fractions of the counts are left in place (not blurred) as one moves farther from the collimator. **B,** Coronal slices of the MCAT phantom. From *upper left,* the source distribution, *upper right* imaged as 10 cm distant in air from the face of the collimator, *lower left* imaged as 20 cm distant, and *lower right* imaged as 30 cm distant. Notice that as the distance away from the camera increases, the activity distribution is increasingly blurred, as exemplified by the heart and liver becoming increasingly smoothed together.

ESTIMATION OF PATIENT-SPECIFIC ATTENUATION MAPS

As illustrated in Figure 6-2, to accurately correct a given patient for the decrease in counts resulting from attenuation, it is necessary to know how the photons were attenuated when imaging that patient. That is, a patient-specific map of attenuation coefficients (μ), or attenuation map, is required. A number of methods exist for estimating such maps.[3,4,6,7] In this chapter, we will discuss just those based on the idea of determining the attenuation of a beam of x-rays or gamma rays passing through the patient, which we will call *transmission imaging*. Transmission imaging consists of positioning a source of radiation (radionuclide or x-ray tube) on one side of the patient and a detector on the other side to measure the transmitted intensity. By taking the ratio of the transmitted intensity to the intensity without the patient present, the TF of Eq. 1 is determined. Because it is μ that we wish to estimate, Eq. 1 can be rearranged to solve for μ as follows:

$$\mu = [\ln(1/TF)]/x \qquad (3)$$

where x is the distance traveled by the photon through the medium. In actuality, what one obtains on the right side of Eq. 3 is the sum of the attenuation coefficients

that the photons travel through in going from the source to the detector, with each attenuation coefficient multiplied before summing by the length in pixels of that attenuation coefficient through which the beam passed. This is identical to the ideal case in emission imaging, where the counts one obtains in a pixel of an acquisition image are the result of the sum of the counts per pixel detected. Thus, just as the rows from the same level in emission images acquired around the patient can be used to reconstruct the emission image, rows from transmission images altered as per Eq. 3 can be used to reconstruct attenuation maps using FBP or some iterative algorithm. The question now is how one acquires the transmission information.

Basic Transmission Configurations

The basic transmission source and camera collimator configurations currently offered commercially are illustrated in Figure 6-7 for a 40-cm field of view (FOV) SPECT system imaging a 50-cm diameter patient. The first configuration illustrated in Figure 6-7*A* is that of a scanning line source.[21] The camera head opposed to the line source is electronically windowed to store only the events detected in a narrow region opposed to the line source in the transmission image. This results in significant reduction in the amount of scattered transmission radiation from the source itself, imaged compared

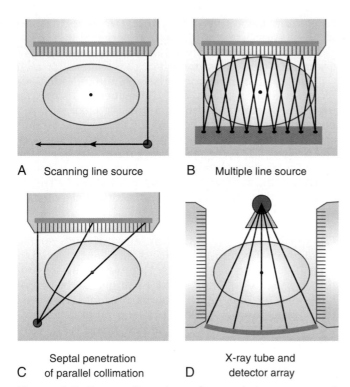

A   Scanning line source

B   Multiple line source

C   Septal penetration of parallel collimation

D   X-ray tube and detector array

Figure 6-7 Four configurations of transmission sources and collimators for use in transmission imaging. In each case, a 40-cm camera field of view (FOV) is shown imaging a patient with a 50-cm major axis. Truncation will vary with camera FOV, patient size, and focal distance for converging collimation.

to having a stationary planar source opposite the camera. It also decreases (but does not eliminate) the cross-contamination from emission photons, because only the portion of the camera face where there is a high likelihood of a transmission photon being detected is used to form the transmission image. The emission images can also be electronically windowed to store counts only when the transmission source is not opposed to the location of the detected event. This simplifies the correction for down-scatter from a higher-energy transmission source to a lower-energy emission source window if different radionuclides are used or for self-correction if the same radionuclide is used for both emission and transmission imaging. This type of system is susceptible to problems in the mechanical motion of the line source and coordination of mechanical scanning with electronic scanning. Therefore, as part of one's quality-control plan for attenuation compensation with such units, checks of the proper operation of the source scanning mechanism should be made frequently (daily) by performing a "blank" scan, which is a transmission scan with nothing, including the table, between the line source and camera head. One should also check individual patient transmission scans for signs of non-uniform motion in the axial (scanning) direction, truncation of the patient's body within the FOV of the system, significant crosstalk from the emission-to-transmission source, and excessive attenuation of the transmission source by extra-large patients or weak sources.[22] The merits of this configuration have made it the most widely available configuration for transmission imaging.

The second configuration, which is shown in Figure 6-7B, is that of the multiple line-source array.[23] With this configuration, the transmission flux comes from a series of collimated line sources aligned parallel to the axis of rotation of the camera. The spacing and activity of the line sources are tailored to provide a greater flux near the center of the FOV, where the attenuation from the patient is greater. As the line sources decay, new line sources are inserted into the center of the array. The rest of the lines are moved outward and the weakest is removed. The transmission profiles result from the overlapping irradiation of the individual lines, which varies with the distance of the source from the detector. The multiple line-source array provides full irradiation across the FOV of the parallel-hole collimator employed for emission imaging, without the need for translation of the source. An advantage of the configuration is that no scanning motion of the sources is required. A disadvantage of this system is the amount of crosstalk between the emission and transmission photons. Thus, attenuation maps formed with this system when imaging ^{99m}Tc-labeled agents should be checked for apparent decreases in the attenuation coefficients (display intensity) in regions of significant ^{99m}Tc accumulation, such as the heart and liver. Also, the down-scatter of the transmission source to the [201]Tl x-ray window makes the use of sequential or interleaved emission and transmission imaging favors. Another disadvantage is the high cost of replacing the line sources at short time intervals.

The first commercial transmission imaging system employed a line source at the focal distance of a fan-beam collimator.[24] The major problem with using fan-beam collimation for estimation of attenuation maps is that of truncation. Truncation of attenuation profiles results in the estimated attenuation maps exhibiting the "cupping artifact," or pile-up of information in the truncated region near its edge when the reconstruction is limited to reconstructing only the region within the FOV at every angle, or fully sampled region (FSR). If the reconstruction is not limited to the FSR, the area outside the FSR is distorted, and the inside is slightly reduced in value. Truncation can be eliminated, or at least dramatically reduced, by imaging with an asymmetric as opposed to a symmetric fan-beam collimator.[25–28] The use of asymmetric collimation results in one side of the patient being truncated instead of both. By rotating the collimator and source 360 degrees around the patient, conjugate views will fill in the region truncated. If a point source with electronic collimator is employed instead of a line source, then a significant improvement in crosstalk can be obtained.[29] The problem, however, is that fan-beam collimators acquire the emission profiles, which makes it difficult for physicians to use in cine-mode to check for attenuation artifacts when reading the patient studies. This difficulty is overcome by the third commercial method of transmission imaging currently being marketed, as illustrated in Figure 6-7C, by using photons from a medium-energy scanning point source to create an asymmetric fan-beam transmission projection through a parallel-hole collimator by penetrating the septa of the collimator.[30]

With this strategy, transmission imaging is performed sequentially after emission imaging to prevent transmission photons from contaminating the emission data. This lengthens the time the patient must remain motionless on the imaging table, thereby decreasing patient throughput and increasing the potential for patient motion. In particular, there is a change in motion of the heads between emission and subsequent transmission imaging, which can lead patients to momentarily relax, thinking the study is over, and thereby cause a misalignment between the emission data and attenuation map. Use of dual display in which the reconstructed emission slices are displayed in color "on top of" the reconstructed attenuation map displayed in grayscale, is recommended with this system to check for a possible misalignment.

High-resolution images from another modality can be imported and registered with the patient's SPECT data.[31,32] Of course, the task is made a lot simpler by acquiring the high-resolution slices while the patient is on the same imaging table.[33] The inclusion of a computed tomography (CT) system on the SPECT gantry is the fourth transmission imaging option currently being offered commercially[34] and is illustrated in Figure 6-7D. The use of a CT to estimate attenuation maps and provide anatomic correlation has essentially replaced the use of radionuclide-based transmission imaging in PET.[35] CT overcomes the noise limitations of radionuclide transmission imaging through use of the x-ray tube and a separate block of detectors for x-ray imaging. However, the x-ray beam is made up of photons of many different energies. Thus appropriate care must be taken in scaling the attenuation map measured with this polychromatic photon beam to that of the energy of the emission radionuclide.[36] Besides their use for attenuation maps, these images can also provide anatomic contexts for the emission distributions and compensation for the PVE.[37] Because different detectors are employed, the CT and SPECT acquisitions are performed sequentially. Thus, as with the scanning medium-energy point source, care must be taken to assess the possibility of patient motion between the two, and imaging time is protracted.

There are two types of CT scanners in hybrid SPECT/CT. The first type is with a low-output x-ray tube and a slow gantry rotation cycle.[34,38,39] A typical CT scan is taken with the x-ray tube current of 2.5 mA and the gantry rotation cycle of 23 seconds. It can be a single- or multiple-detector row CT scanner. It uses 13.6 seconds of data (little over half of a gantry rotation, due to fan-beam detector geometry) for reconstruction of a CT image. The CT image is not for diagnosis; rather, it is intended for attenuation correction of the SPECT data. The radiation dose of the slow CT is about 5 mGy, which is significantly less than that of CT when used for diagnostic imaging.[39] Studies have demonstrated its effectiveness for this purpose.[40] However, a recent study suggested caution when performing AC with this technology for evaluation of perfusion defects; the SPECT slices after AC might be compromised by misregistration between the attenuation map derived from the CT slices and the SPECT data.[38] In this study, motion resulted in 42% of the 60 patients having moderate to severe misregistration of the heart between the CT and the SPECT data. Since most respiratory cycles are in the range of 4 to 6 seconds,[41] the scan duration of 13.6 seconds for each CT image slice may not be slow enough to reduce reconstruction artifacts and subsequent misregistration. This is compounded by a possible change in respiration between emission and CT imaging, as well as a shifting in position of the patient. A recent study of using slow CT for respiratory gating suggested the gantry rotation cycle might have to be over 3 minutes to reduce the artifact caused by respiration.[42] This is to ensure that there is one respiratory cycle of data taken at each CT projection angle.

The second type of CT scanner is diagnostic-quality CT, capable of producing thin slices of high spatial and temporal resolutions with a fast gantry rotation cycle of less than 0.6 seconds. The number of detector rows is 2, 6, 16, 40, or 64. The CT scanner can be potentially used for imaging the coronary arteries. However, the 64-detector row CT with 0.35 second or faster gantry rotation cycle produces the best image quality for the coronary artery, owing to its larger coverage and higher temporal resolution. The combination of CT for imaging coronary arteries and SPECT for evaluation of myocardial perfusion provides a noninvasive evaluation of the heart in both anatomy and function. Calcium scoring can also be obtained from this type of CT scanner to provide long-term risk assessment.[43,44] Although the quality of CT is very good, it still poses problems in registration of the heart between CT and SPECT, because the CT image is taken in less than 1 second. Misregistration normally occurs when the CT image is taken at the end-inspiration phase, which is very different from the average respiration SPECT data of over several minutes. Recent development of "average CT" by averaging the CT images taken over one respiratory cycle may provide a solution.[41,45] Average CT is promising in cardiac PET/CT[46] and potentially useful for cardiac SPECT/CT. This approach uses a fast gantry rotation of less than 0.5 second to acquire CT images that are almost motion free in respiration, and averaging brings temporal resolution of the CT images to that of SPECT images. Acquisition of average CT data should be at least one respiratory cycle and can be carried out at a low tube current such as 10 mA and fast gantry rotation cycle of 0.5 seconds. The radiation dose of average CT is also about 5 mGy.[41] Since the patient is scanned sequentially, re-registration of the CT and SPECT data manually is necessary if the patient moves between the CT and SPECT scans.[46,47]

ATTENUATION CORRECTION METHODS

Not only has the ability to estimate attenuation maps improved greatly, but so has the ability to perform correction of attenuation once the attenuation maps are estimated. In part, this is due to the tremendous changes in computing power available, with computers in the clinic now making computations practical that could only be performed as research exercises 10 years ago. It is also due to an improvement in the algorithms used for correction and the efficiency of their implementations. An example of this is the development of ordered subset or block iterative algorithms for use with the statistically based reconstruction methods discussed elsewhere.[48-50] A number of algorithms have been developed for compensation of attenuation. The reader is referred to other reviews for more details and other algorithms.[3,5-7,51] In this review, we will focus on the group of methods that are replacing FBP.

In the following, we will use the term *projection* to mean the emission data acquired at one angle during SPECT acquisition. It is one row out of one of the set of images acquired as the camera rotates around the patient (or the patient rotates in front of the camera). The set of projections necessary to reconstruct a slice is thus the set consisting of the corresponding row taken out of each of the images acquired of the patient. Please note that the word *projection* can also be used to name the operation of creating acquisition data from an existing estimate of the source activity distribution. In this sense, it is the counterpart to the *backprojection* operation used in FBP to create an estimate of the source activity distribution from acquisition data. In iterative reconstruction, projection and backprojection are used alternately to obtain the final estimate of the source activity distribution.

Statistically Based Reconstruction Methods

The statistically based reconstruction algorithms start with a model for the noise in the emission data and then derive an estimate of the source distribution based on some statistical criterion. Many times they are named so that the first part of their name tells the statistical criterion that is to be optimized, and the second part of the name tells the mathematical algorithm employed to achieve optimization. For example, in MLEM,[52,53] the statistical criterion is to determine the source distribution in the slices with the maximum likelihood (ML) of having resulted in the measured SPECT projection data, given that the noise fluctuations in the acquisitions follow the Poisson distribution. The expectation maximization algorithm is employed for finding this ML solution. The success of this method of reconstruction is reflected by its becoming the standard for comparison against other reconstruction methods.

Conceptually, the MLEM algorithm works by iteratively refining an initial guess as to the distribution of the counts in the slices until the distribution is found that has the greatest likelihood of having resulted in the measured SPECT acquisitions. The rule or algorithm followed can be summarized as[51]:

$$\textbf{Slices}^{new} = \textbf{Slices}^{old} \times \textbf{Normalized Backprojection of}$$
$$\left(\frac{\textbf{Measured Projection Data}}{\textbf{Projection of Slices}^{old}} \right)$$

$$(4)$$

where $Slices^{new}$ is the resulting estimate of the counts in the voxels after the completion of one iteration during which the estimate of every voxel is updated, and $Slices^{old}$ is the current guess going into the iteration as to the counts in the slices. The initial guess is typically a uniform count in each voxel of the slice.

The algorithm starts on the bottom right hand side of Eq. 4 by mathematically emulating SPECT imaging of the current estimate (making projections from $Slices^{old}$). This is where the physics of imaging can come into play and is one of the major advantages of iterative methods over FBP reconstruction. One can include as much information as to how the estimated counts contribute to the acquired projections as one has the ability to mathematically model (and is willing to spend the computer time so doing) during each iteration. For example, given an aligned attenuation map for a slice, one could include attenuation by starting with the voxel on the side opposite the projection being created, and multiplying its value by the TF for passing through one-half the voxel distance of an attenuator of the given attenuation coeficient in the attenuation map. The value of half the pixel dimension is usually used as an approximation for the self-attenuation of the activity in the voxel. One would then move to the next voxel along the direction of projection, and add its value after correction for self-attenuation to the current projection sum attenuated by passing through the entire thickness of the voxel. One would then continue this process until having passed through all voxels along the path of projection. The result would be the discrete approximation to the calculation of the line integral through the emission estimate, with each voxel location corrected for attenuation. Similarly, one can include modeling of scatter-dependent and distance-dependent spatial resolution. It is our experience that the better one does at accurately mathematically modeling the imaging of the patient, the better the resulting image quality will be. Of course, without clever approximations, such modeling can be quite time-consuming, even with today's computers. Thus implementations of MLEM will vary, depending on the extent to which the physics is modeled and the approximations are employed in implementation.

The second step in the MLEM algorithm, as shown by the division on the right side of Eq. 4, is to divide the estimated projection values into the values actually measured. The ratio of the two indicates whether the voxel values along the given path of projection are too large (ratio less than 1), just right (ratio of 1), or too small (ratio larger than 1). These ratios are then backprojected as indicated in Eq. 4 to create an update matrix. That is, the ratios are combined for each slice voxel according to the probability they contributed to the projections from which the ratios were formed. This update matrix is then normalized by dividing by the backprojection of 1.0s to account for some ratios contributing more than others to the update matrix, based on the physics of imaging. The normalized update matrix is then multiplied voxel-by-voxel times the old estimate of the slice values to create the new estimate. This step is typically repeated until a set number of iterations has been performed. Ordered subset expectation

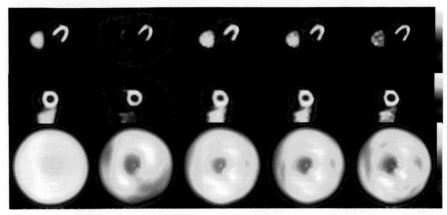

Figure 6-8 Comparison of transverse slices (*top row*), short-axis slices (*middle row*), and maximum count polar maps (*bottom row*) of mathematical cardiac-torso (MCAT) phantom simulations. *First column from the left* shows slices and polar map for OSEM reconstruction without attenuation, scatter, or noise included when creating the projections. Instead solely the influence of distance-dependent spatial resolution of a LEHR parallel-hole collimator is present. Shown are slices reconstructed by FBP with no post-reconstruction smoothing included in reconstruction because of no noise having been included in the simulated projections. This thus represents the ideal case of attenuation and scatter compensation. *Second column* shows slices and polar map for FBP reconstruction without attenuation correction when simulation included the influence of distance-dependent resolution, attenuation, and scatter with clinically equivalent noise. It represents how reconstruction is typically performed presently. *Third column* shows slices and polar map for OSEM reconstruction, which included modeling of attenuation in projection and back projection. *Fourth column* shows slices and polar map obtained with OSEM reconstruction which included attenuation and scatter correction. *Final column* shows slices and polar map for OSEM reconstruction which includes correction for attenuation, scatter, and distance-dependent spatial resolution.

maximization (OSEM)[48,49] and block iterative methods[50] accelerate reconstruction by forming and applying the update matrix from subsets of the projection set that are selected in an ordered fashion. The result is a reduction in the number of iterations by a factor approximately equal to the number of subsets used.[54] If fewer than four angles spaced as far apart as possible are used in forming subsets, then a loss in image quality with OSEM can result.[55]

Figure 6-8 shows a comparison of the transverse slices, short-axis slices, and polar maps for reconstructions of simulations of the MCAT phantom.[11] In the *first column on the right* are image slices and the polar map for the case FBP reconstruction over 360 degrees of Monte Carlo–simulated acquisition images created as imaged by a LEHR collimator but without inclusion of attenuation, scatter, or additional noise. Because no noise was added to the high-count Monte Carlo simulation, no low-pass smoothing was included with reconstruction. These images thus represent the case of ideal attenuation and scatter correction. Notice that the counts at the apex of the LV in the transverse slice and in the apical region of the polar map are not uniform. The non-uniformity reflects the impact of the PVE on wall counts due to the inclusion of apical thinning in the MCAT source distribution. This shows that even with ideal attenuation and scatter correction, one should not expect to obtain uniform counts in the polar maps. The *following columns* show what happens when attenuation and scatter in addition to distance-dependent spatial resolution are included in the Monte Carlo–simulated projections. Additionally, a noise level equivalent to that seen clinically is simulated, thus requiring low-pass filtering of the reconstructed slices. In the first column of these (*second column of images*

from the left) are shown the results for FBP reconstruction of projection data that include attenuation acquired over the 180 degrees centered on the heart. A two-dimensional pre-reconstruction Butterworth filter with an order of 5 and a cutoff frequency of 0.25 cycle/cm was used to suppress noise. Notice the significant count fall off as one moves basally (deeper into the patient) along the myocardial walls, especially for the inferior wall. Also notice the distortion in shape of the walls, especially near the base. The *center column* of images shows the result of one iteration of OSEM reconstruction that employed 15 subsets of 4 angles each and included AC as described in the proceeding paragraphs. Additionally, three-dimensional (3D) post-reconstruction Gaussian filtering was applied to reduce noise. Notice that the shape of the LV walls is improved with AC, and the decrease in counts inferiorly is replaced with an increase septally and inferiorly. This overcorrection is due to the presence of scattered photons in the projections, which add counts to the projection data such that the decrease due to attenuation is moderated. The correction of attenuation is usually based on correcting the losses of primary counts. When these losses are corrected and scatter has not been removed, an apparent overcorrection by attenuation correction occurs.

SCATTER CORRECTION METHODS

The best way to reduce the effect of scatter would be to improve the energy resolution of the imaging systems by using an alternative to NaI(T1) scintillation detection.[9] For such a system, the Gaussian function representing the distribution of primary photons with energy in Figure 6-4 would shrink to a single vertical line, with the result that very few scattered photons would be included in the energy window.

Currently, most SPECT systems use NaI(Tl) to detect the x-rays and gamma rays from patients. The scatter compensation methods employed with NaI(Tl) systems can be divided into two different categories. The first category, which we will call *scatter estimation*, consists of those methods that estimate the scatter contributions to the projections based on the acquired emission data. The data used may be information from the energy spectrum or a combination of the photopeak data and an approximation of scatter PSFs. The scatter PSF gives the spatial distribution of the relative probabilities of detecting scattered photons at each location in the projection for a given location in the source distribution. The scatter estimate can be used before, during, or after reconstruction. The second category consists of those methods that model the scatter PSFs during the reconstruction process. This second approach will be called *reconstruction-based scatter compensation* (RBSC) herein.

The Compton window subtraction (CWS) method of Jaszczak and colleagues represents a classic example of an energy domain scatter-estimation method that is still in clinical use.[56] In the CWS method, a second energy window placed below the photopeak window (see Fig. 6-4) is used to record an image that consists of scattered photons. This image is multiplied by a scaling factor, *k*, and then subtracted from the acquired image to yield a scatter-corrected image. This method assumes that (1) the spatial distribution of the scatter within the Compton scatter window is the same as that within the photopeak window, and (2) once determined from a calibration study, a single scaling factor (*k*) holds for all applications on a given system. That the distribution of scatter between the two windows is different can be seen by noting that the average angle of scattering, and hence degree of blurring, changes with energy. The difference in the distribution of scatter with energy can be minimized by making the scatter window smaller and placing it just below the photopeak window. With this arrangement, one obtains the two energy window (TEW) variant of the triple energy window (also TEW) scatter-correction method of Ogawa and colleagues[57] as applied to ^{99m}Tc. When down-scatter (scattered photons from a higher-energy emission) is present, a third small window is added above the photopeak, and scatter is estimated as the area under the trapezoid between the two narrow windows on either side of the photopeak.[58] In this way, TEW can be used with radionuclides such as ^{201}Tl, which emit photons of multiple energies, or for scatter correction when imaging multiple radionuclides.

In RBSC, a unique scatter PSF is estimated for each location in the patient, using a patient-specific attenuation map and the underlying principles of scattering interactions. This scatter PSF is then included in the projection and backprojection operations of iterative reconstruction. With RBSC methods, compensation is achieved in effect by mapping scattered photons back to their point of origin instead of trying to determine a separate estimate of the scatter contribution to the projections.[59] All of the photons are used in RBSC, and it has been argued that there should be less noise increase than with the other category of compensations.[59,60] The first RBSC method for SPECT was the inverse Monte Carlo method.[61] This algorithm provided compensation for scatter, attenuation, and system resolution by using a Monte Carlo simulation to estimate the PSFs. Because obtaining a "noise-free" estimate of the PSFs with Monte Carlo methods is extremely time-consuming, a number of approximate methods have been investigated, which provide excellent compensation in computationally acceptable reconstruction times.[59,60] More recently, methods of vastly speeding up Monte Carlo simulation have been developed such that for ^{99m}Tc, fully 3D reconstruction can be obtained in approximately 30 minutes on a personal computer.[62]

Comparison of the images of the *center* and *second from the right columns* in Figure 6-8 shows an example of the application of one of the RBSC methods to correct the simulated projection images from the MCAT phantom. OSEM reconstruction with the same reconstruction and smoothing parameters was used for both the images seen in both columns. Notice that with the addition of scatter correction, the cardiac blood-pool region is seen with higher contrast with respect to the walls, and the overcorrection in the septal and inferior walls is moderated somewhat. Also, there is slightly better separation between the liver and inferior wall. However, further separation between the two requires an improvement in reconstructed spatial resolution.

SPATIAL RESOLUTION COMPENSATION METHODS

If the PSF is the same for every point in the patient, then knowledge of it can be used to calculate restoration filters or mathematic filters that attempt to balance deblurring the slices with controlling noise.[63] However, the in-air PSF for nuclear medicine cameras increases in width with distance away from the face of collimators, as illustrated in Figure 6-6. Therefore, the accuracy of correction methods that assume it is unchanging is limited. The frequency-distance relationship (FDR) can be used to separate out the signal in sinograms (matrix containing all the projections to be used in reconstructing a slice arranged according to the angle they were acquired at) according to the distance at which the signal originated relative to the collimator face.[64] Once the distance is known, then a model for how spatial resolution changes as a function of distance from the face can be used to create restoration filters that account for the distance dependence of the PSF.[65,66] Application of the FDR to restoration filtering SPECT acquisitions has advantages in terms of computational load and being linear. It also has several disadvantages.[67] For example, it is limited as to how much resolution recovery can be obtained without excessive amplification of noise; modeling the distance-dependent spatial resolution directly in the projection and backprojection steps of iterative reconstruction has been determined to significantly improve the detection accuracy of tumors over use of it in observer studies using simulated images.[68]

Another method to correct for the distance-dependent camera response is the incorporation of a blurring model into iterative reconstruction.[69–71] Returning to Eq. 4, the idea is as follows: When creating the estimate of projection data acquired from the current estimate of the source activity distribution, the values in that distribution are smoothed equivalent to how the camera blurs counts at that given distance before they are combined to form the projection. This is illustrated in Figure 6-6B, where the coronal plane is smoothed various amounts as a function of the distance to the collimator face. You can envision this happening in reconstruction by dividing the current 3D estimate of the source into a set of oblique planes perpendicular to the rays making it through the parallel-hole collimator. Each plane is then smoothed an increasing amount as the distance between them and the collimator face increases. Combining the smoothed planes with accounting for attenuation and scatter results in the estimated projection values, which are then compared to the actual acquired values by being divided into them. The question then arises as to how smoothing can lead to an improvement in resolution. The answer is that the actual source distribution was smoothed during the process of acquisition, just as we are now smoothing our estimate of the source distribution. When our estimated projections, with smoothing included, match the actual projection data we acquire, the estimated source distribution should match the actual source distribution imaged. Thus as we iterate, we sharpen our estimate of the source distribution until the smoothed version of its projections matches the data we acquired.

The problem with this method has been the immense increase in computational burden imposed when an iterative reconstruction algorithm includes such modeling in its transition matrix. Combined with OSEM, blurring incrementally with distance, using the method of Gaussian diffusion[72] during projection and backprojection, can dramatically reduce the computational burden per iteration. With this method, correction for the system spatial resolution is incrementally changed with distance during projection and backprojection so that only a few voxels need to be combined at each distance from the face of the collimator. The increase in computational speed using this and similar algorithms is now such that reconstruction can be easily accomplished in clinically feasible times.

An illustration of the impact of including modeling of system spatial resolution in reconstruction is provided by a comparison of the images in the *last two columns* of Figure 6-8. The *last column* adds resolution compensation to compensation of attenuation and scatter, as illustrated in the *next to last column*. Notice the dramatic change in size of the blood-pool cavity, the thinning of the LV walls, and the improved separation from the liver. There is, however, a trade-off between gains in apparent image spatial resolution and increasing the noise content of the image. Thus

by increasing the number of iterations and/or decreasing extent of post-reconstruction filtering, a further increase in apparent resolution at the expense of a further increase in the noise content of the images can be obtained.

EXAMPLE OBSERVER STUDIES ILLUSTRATING THE UTILITY OF COMPENSATION

The following results from observer studies with simulated and clinical images are included in this chapter in support of our position that the more completely the physics of imaging is correctly included in the reconstruction algorithm, the more accurate will be the diagnosis from the reconstructed slices.

Using the channelized-Hotelling numeric observer, Frey and colleagues showed with simulated cardiac studies that the best coronary artery disease (CAD) detection accuracy results when attenuation, scatter, and spatial resolution are included in iterative reconstruction.[73] They determined an area under the receiver operating characteristic (ROC) curve, or AUC, of 0.90 for iterative reconstruction with solely AC, an AUC of 0.93 for iterative reconstruction with AC and spatial resolution compensation (RC), an AUC of 0.93 for AC and scatter correction (SC), and an AUC of 0.94 for combined AC, SC, and RC.

In a recent ROC comparison of detection accuracy for CAD of four different reconstruction strategies, using images from 100 patient studies read independently by seven physicians, Narayanan and colleagues determined that there was an additive improvement in detection accuracy as one progresses from FBP without additional compensation, to OSEM with AC, to OSEM with AC and SC, to OSEM with AC, SC, and Gaussian diffusion–based RC (Fig. 6-9).[74] OSEM with AC, SC, and RC was determined to have a statistically larger AUC compared with FBP, or OSEM with solely correction for AC, hence improved diagnostic accuracy.

In the previous study, as is standard for comparisons of FBP and iterative reconstruction, only the stress slices were viewed by the physicians. When interpreting studies, clinically significant additional information is available to the physician. Pretorius and colleagues performed an ROC comparison of FBP and OSEM with AC, SC, and RC in which present when viewing the FBP studies were the short- and long-axis slices for both stress and rest, cines of the acquisition data for both stress and rest, a cine of selected gated cardiac slices, polar maps, and indication of whether the patient was male or female.[75] Solely the stress short- and long-axis slices were made available to the observers for OSEM with combined correction. The inclusion of this additional information normally available clinically did increase the AUC for FBP from 0.81 for the previous study to 0.87 for this study. However, OSEM with combined correction still resulted in a statistically significant improvement in the detection accuracy of CAD, with an AUC of 0.90.

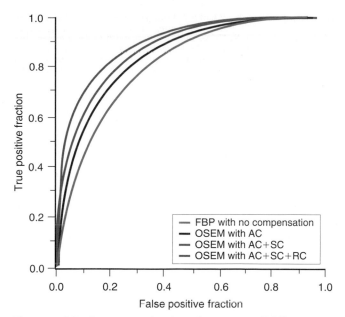

Figure 6-9 Reconstruction-based scatter (ROC) curves illustrating the progressive improvement in detection accuracy of CAD in patient studies as one progressively includes attenuation compensation (AC), scatter compensation (SC), and spatial resolution compensation (RC) in the reconstruction strategy.

CONCLUSIONS

When carefully implemented and validated hardware and software are used to perform attenuation compensation, an improvement in the detection accuracy can be achieved clinically. When attenuation compensation is combined with compensation for scatter and distance-dependent spatial resolution, an ever greater improvement in detection accuracy can be expected to occur. To achieve these increases, it is necessary that the physician take time to become familiar with the appearance of these corrected images.[76] Also, just as SPECT increased diagnostic accuracy over planar scintigraphy at the cost of increased demands on the performance of the imaging systems, so too the addition of attenuation compensation does increase diagnostic accuracy but at the price of needing to take more care with quality control. Finally, even though the degradation of SPECT images by attenuation, scatter, and the finite distance-dependent spatial resolution of the cameras employed in imaging is not debated, the extent to which these degradations can currently be routinely and robustly overcome in practice is still the subject of debate, exemplified in a pair of recent manuscripts.[77,78]

ACKNOWLEDGMENTS

This work was supported in part by U.S. Public Health grant HL50349 of the National Heart, Lung, and Blood Institute. Its contents are solely the responsibility of the authors and do not necessarily represent the official views of the National Heart, Lung, and Blood Institute. This work is based on a series of two review papers previously published in the *Journal of Nuclear Cardiology*. The authors thank the editor of that journal for permission to republish, in part, those reviews, including several of the figures.

REFERENCES

1. DuPuey DJ, Garcia EV: Optimal specificity of thallium-201 SPECT through recognition of imaging artifacts, *J Nucl Med* 30:441, 1989.
2. Hendel RC, Corbett JR, Cullom SJ, et al: The value and practice of attenuation correction for myocardial perfusion SPECT imaging: A joint position statement from the American Society of Nuclear Cardiology and the Society of Nuclear Medicine, *J Nucl Cardiol* 9:135, 2002.
3. Bacharach SL, Buvat I: Attenuation correction in cardiac positron emission tomography and single-photon emission computed tomography, *J Nucl Cardiol* 2:246, 1995.
4. King MA, Tsui BMW, Pan TS: Attenuation compensation for cardiac single-photon emission computed tomographic imaging: Part 1. Impact of attenuation and methods of estimating attenuation maps, *J Nucl Cardiol* 2:513, 1995.
5. King MA, Tsui BMW, Pan TS, et al: Attenuation compensation for cardiac single-photon emission computed tomographic imaging: Part 2. Attenuation compensation algorithms, *J Nucl Cardiol* 3:55, 1996.
6. Bailey DL: Transmission scanning in emission tomography, *Eur J Nucl Med* 25:774, 1998.
7. Zaidi H, Hasegawa BH: Determination of the attenuation map in emission tomography, *J Nucl Med* 44:291, 2003.
8. Attix FH: *Introduction to Radiological Physics and Radiation Dosimetry*, New York, 1983, John Wiley & Sons.
9. Cherry SA, Sorenson JA, Phelps ME: *Physics in Nuclear Medicine*, ed 3, Philadelphia, 2003, Saunders.
10. Eisner RL, Tamas M, Cloninger K, et al: Normal SPECT thallium-201 bull's-eye display: Gender differences, *J Nucl Med* 29:1901, 1988.
11. Pretorius PH, King M, Tsui BM, et al: A mathematical model of motion of the heart for use in generating source and attenuation maps for simulating emission imaging, *Med Phys* 26.2323, 1999.
12. Knesaurek K, King MA, Glick SJ, et al: Investigation of causes of geometric distortion in 180 degrees and 360 degrees angular sampling in SPECT, *J Nucl Med* 30:1666, 1989.
13. Germano G, Chua T, Kiat H, et al: A quantitative phantom analysis of artifacts due to hepatic activity in technetium-99m myocardial perfusion SPECT studies, *J Nucl Med* 35:356, 1994.
14. Nuyts J, Dupont P, Van DM, et al: A study of the liver-heart artifact in emission tomography, *J Nucl Med* 36:133, 1995.
15. Ljungberg M, Strand SE: A Monte Carlo program for the simulation of scintillation camera characteristics, *Comput Methods Programs Biomed* 29:257, 1989.
16. Nuyts J, Stroobants S, DuPuey DJ, et al: Reducing loss of image quality because of the attenuation artifact in uncorrected PET whole-body images, *J Nucl Med* 43:1054, 2002.
17. Bai C, Kinahan PE, Brasse D, et al: An analytic study of the effects of attenuation on tumor detection in whole-body PET oncology imaging, *J Nucl Med* 44:1855, 2003.
18. Bai C, Shao L: A study of the effects of attenuation correction on tumor detection in SPECT oncology, *IEEE Nucl Sci Symp Conf Rec (2004)* 5:3113–3117, 2004.
19. de Vries DJ, King MA: Window selection for dual photopeak window scatter correction in Tc-99m imaging, *IEEE Trans Nucl Sci* 41:2771, 1994.
20. Hademenos GJ, King MA, Ljungberg MH, et al: A scatter correction method for Tl-201 images: A Monte Carlo investigation, *IEEE Trans Nucl Sci* 40:1179, 1993.
21. Tan P, Bailey DL, Meikle SR, et al: A scanning line source for simultaneous emission and transmission measurements in SPECT, *J Nucl Med* 34:1752, 1993.
22. DePuey EG, Garcia EV, Borges-Neto S, et al: Imaging guidelines for transmission-emission tomographic systems to be used for attenuation correction, *J Nucl Cardiol* 8:G51, 2001.
23. Celler A, Sitek A, Stoub E, et al: Multiple line source array for SPECT transmission scans: Simulation, phantom and patient studies, *J Nucl Med* 39:2183, 1998.
24. Tung CH, Gullberg GT, Zeng GL, et al: Nonuniform attenuation correction using simultaneous transmission and emission converging tomography, *IEEE Trans Nucl Sci* 39:1134, 1991.
25. Chang W, Loncaric S, Huang G, et al: Asymmetric fan transmission CT on SPECT systems, *Phys Med Biol* 40:913, 1995.
26. Gilland DR, Jaszczak RJ, Greer KL, et al: Transmission imaging for nonuniform attenuation correction using a three-headed SPECT camera, *J Nucl Med* 39:1105, 1998.
27. Hollinger EF, Loncaric S, Yu DC, et al: Using fast sequential asymmetric fanbeam transmission CT for attenuation correction of cardiac SPECT imaging, *J Nucl Med* 39:1335, 1998.

28. LaCroix KJ, Tsui BMW: Investigation of 90 degree dual-camera half-fanbeam collimation for myocardial SPECT imaging, *IEEE Trans Nucl Sci* 46:2085, 1999.
29. Beekman FJ, Kamphuis C, Hutton BF, et al: Half-fanbeam collimators combined with scanning point sources for simultaneous emission-transmission imaging, *J Nucl Med* 39:1996, 1998.
30. Gagnon D, Tung CH, Zeng L, Hawkins WG: Design and early testing of a new medium-energy transmission device for attenuation correction in SPECT and PET, *IEEE Nucl Sci Symp Conf Rec (1998)* 3:1349–1353, 1999.
31. Fleming JS: A technique for using CT images in attenuation correction and quantification in SPECT, *Nucl Med Commun* 10:83, 1989.
32. Meyer CR, Boes JL, Kim B, et al: Demonstration of accuracy and clinical versatility of mutual information for automatic multimodality image fusion using affine and thin-plate spline warped geometric deformations, *Med Image Anal* 1:195, 1997.
33. Blankespoor SC, Xu X, Kaiki K, et al: Attenuation correction of SPECT using x-ray CT on an emission-transmission CT system: myocardial perfusion assessment, *IEEE Trans Nucl Sci* 43:2263, 1996.
34. Bocher M, Balan A, Krausz Y, et al: Gamma camera-mounted anatomical x-ray tomography: Technology, system characteristics and first images, *Eur J Nucl Med* 27:619, 2000.
35. Kinahan PE, Hasegawa BH, Beyer T: X-ray-based attenuation correction for positron emission tomography/computed tomography scanners, *Sem Nucl Med* 33:166, 2003.
36. LaCroix KJ, Tsui BMW, Hasegawa BH, et al: Investigation of the use of x-ray CT images for attenuation compensation in SPECT, *IEEE Trans Nucl Sci* 41:2793, 1994.
37. Da Silva AJ, Tang HR, Wong KH, et al: Absolute quantification of regional myocardial uptake of 99mTc-sestamibi with SPECT: Experimental validation in a porcine model, *J Nucl Med* 42:772, 2001.
38. Goetze S, Wahl RL: Prevalence of misregistration between SPECT and CT for attenuation-corrected myocardial perfusion SPECT, *J Nucl Cardiol* 14:200, 2007.
39. Patton JA, Turkington TG: SPECT/CT Physical Principles and Attenuation Correction, *J Nucl Med Technol* 36:1, 2008.
40. Masood Y, Liu YH, Depuey G, Taillefer R, Araujo LI, Allen S, Delbeke D, Anstett A, Peretz A, Zito MJ, et al: Clinical validation of SPECT attenuation correction using x-ray computed tomography-derived attenuation maps: multicenter clinical trial with angiographic correlation, *J Nucl Cardiol* 12:676, 2005.
41. Pan T, Mawlawi O, Luo D, Liu HH, Chi PC, Mar MV, Gladish G, Truong J, Erasmus J Jr, Liao Z, Macapinlac HA: Attenuation correction of PET cardiac data with low-dose average CT in PET/CT, *Med Phys* 33:3931, 2006.
42. Lu J, Guerrero TM, Munro P, Jeung A, Chi PC, Balter P, Zhu XR, Mohan T, Pan T: Four-dimensional cone beam CT with adaptive gantry rotation and adaptive data sampling, *Med Phys* 34:3520, 2007.
43. Berman DS, Hachamovitch R, Shaw LJ, Friedman JD, Hayes SW, Thomson DS, Fieno DS, Germano G, Wong ND, Kang X, Rozanski A: Roles of nuclear cardiology, cardiac computed tomography, and cardiac magnetic resonance: Noninvasive risk stratification and a conceptual framework for the selection of noninvasive imaging tests in patients with known or suspected coronary artery disease, *J Nucl Med* 47:1107, 2006.
44. Hecht HS, Budoff MJ, Berman DS, Ehrlich J, Rumberger JA: Coronary artery calcium scanning: Clinical paradigms for cardiac risk assessment and treatment, *Am Heart J* 151:1139, 2006.
45. Pan T, Mawlawi O, Nehmeh SA, Erdi YE, Luo D, Liu HH, Castillo R, Mohan Z, Liao Z, Macapinlac HA: Attenuation correction of PET images with respiration-averaged CT images in PET/CT, *J Nucl Med* 46:1481, 2005.
46. Gould KL, Pan T, Loghin C, Johnson NP, Guha A, Sdringola S: Frequent diagnostic errors in cardiac PET/CT due to misregistration of CT attenuation and emission PET images: a definitive analysis of causes, consequences, and corrections, *J Nucl Med* 48:1112, 2007.
47. Goetze S, Brown TL, Lavely WC, Zhang Z, Bengel FM: Attenuation correction in myocardial perfusion SPECT/CT: effects of misregistration and value of reregistration, *J Nucl Med* 48:1090, 2007.
48. Hudson HM, Larkin RS: Accelerated image reconstruction using ordered subsets of projection data, *IEEE Trans Med Imaging* 13:601, 1994.
49. Hutton BF, Hudson HM, Beekman FJ: A clinical perspective of accelerated statistical reconstruction, *Eur J Nucl Med* 24:797, 1997.
50. Byrne CL: Block iterative methods for image reconstruction from projections, *IEEE Trans Image Process* 5:792, 1996.
51. Bruyant PP: Analytic and iterative reconstruction algorithms in SPECT, *J Nucl Med* 43:1343, 2002.
52. Shepp LA, Vardi Y: Maximum likelihood reconstruction for emission tomography, *IEEE Trans Med Imaging* 1:113, 1982.
53. Lange K, Carson R: EM reconstruction algorithms for emission and transmission tomography, *J Comput Assist Tomogr* 8:306, 1984.
54. Meikle SR, Hutton BF, Bailey DL, et al: Accelerated EM reconstruction in total-body PET: Potential for improving tumour detectability, *Phys Med Biol* 39:1689, 1994.
55. Gifford HC, King MA, Narayanan MV, et al: Effect of block iterative acceleration on Ga-67 tumor detection in thoracic SPECT, *IEEE Trans Nucl Sci* 49:50, 2002.
56. Jaszczak RJ, Greer KL, Floyd CE Jr, et al: Improved SPECT quantification using compensation for scattered photons, *J Nucl Med* 25:893, 1984.
57. Ogawa K, Ichihara T, Kubo A: Accurate scatter correction in single photon emission CT, *Ann Nucl Med Sci* 7:145, 1994.
58. Ogawa K, Harata Y, Ichihara T, et al: A practical method for position-dependent Compton-scatter correction in single photon emission CT, *IEEE Trans Med Imaging* 10:408, 1991.
59. Kadrmas DJ, Frey EC, Tsui BMW: Application of reconstruction-based scatter compensation to thallium-201 SPECT: Implementations for reduced reconstructed image noise, *IEEE Trans Med Imaging* 17:325, 1998.
60. Beekman FJ, Kamphuis C, Frey EC: Scatter compensation methods in 3D iterative SPECT reconstruction: A simulation study, *Phys Med Biol* 42:1619, 1997.
61. Floyd CE, Jaszczak RJ, Coleman RE: Inverse Monte Carlo: A unified reconstruction algorithm, *IEEE Trans Nucl Sci* 32:785, 1985.
62. Beekman FJ, de Jong HWAM, van Geloven S: Efficient fully 3-D iterative SPECT reconstruction with Monte Carlo-based scatter compensation, *IEEE Trans Med Imaging* 21:867, 2002.
63. King MA, Schwinger RB, Doherty PW, et al: Two-dimensional filtering of SPECT images using the Metz and Wiener filters, *J Nucl Med* 25:1234, 1984.
64. Edholm PR, Lewitt RM, Lindholm B: Novel properties of the Fourier decomposition of the sinogram, *Proc Soc Photo Opt Instrum Eng* 671:8, 1986.
65. Lewitt RM, Edholm PR, Xia W: Fourier method of correction of depth-dependent collimator blurring, *Proc Soc Photo Opt Instrum Eng* 1092:232, 1989.
66. Glick SJ, Penney BC, King MA, et al: Noniterative compensation for the distance-dependent detector response and photon attenuation in SPECT imaging, *IEEE Trans Med Imaging* 13:363, 1994.
67. Kohli V, King MA, Glick SJ, et al: Comparison of frequency-distance relationship and Gaussian-diffusion-based methods of compensation for distance-dependent spatial resolution in SPECT imaging, *Phys Med Biol* 43:1025, 1998.
68. Gifford HC, King MA, Wells RG, et al: LROC analysis of detector-response compensation in SPECT, *IEEE Trans Med Imaging* 19:463, 2000.
69. Floyd CE Jr, Jaszczak RJ, Manglos SH, et al: Compensation for collimator divergence in SPECT using inverse Monte Carlo reconstruction, *IEEE Trans Med Imaging* 35:784, 1987.
70. Tsui BMW, Hu HB, Gilland DR, et al: Implementation of simultaneous attenuation and detector response correction in SPECT, *IEEE Trans Nucl Sci* 35:778, 1987.
71. Zeng GL, Gullberg GT, Tsui BMW, et al: Three-dimensional iterative reconstruction algorithms with attenuation and geometric point response correction, *IEEE Trans Med Imaging* 38:693, 1990.
72. McCarthy AW, Miller MI: Maximum likelihood SPECT in clinical computation times using mesh-connected parallel computers, *IEEE Trans Med Imaging* 10:426, 1991.
73. Frey EC, Gilland KL, Tsui BMW: Application of task-based measures of image quality to optimization and evaluation of three-dimensional reconstruction-based compensation methods in myocardial perfusion SPECT, *IEEE Trans Med Imaging* 21:1040, 2002.
74. Narayanan MV, King MA, Pretorius PH, et al: Human-observer ROC evaluation of attenuation, scatter, and resolution compensation strategies for Tc-99m myocardial perfusion imaging, *J Nucl Med* 44:1725, 2003.
75. Pretorius PH, King MA, Dahlberg ST, et al: Detection accuracy of coronary artery disease of FBP with all the clinically available imaging information compared to iterative reconstruction with combined compensation for imaging degradations, *J Nucl Cardiol* 12:284, 2005.
76. Corbett JR, Ficaro EP: Attenuation corrected cardiac perfusion SPECT, *Curr Opin Cardiol* 15:330, 2000.
77. Garcia EV: SPECT attenuation correction: an essential tool to realize nuclear cardiology's manifest destiny, *J Nucl Cardiol* 14:16, 2007.
78. Germano G, Slomka PJ, Berman DS: Attenuation correction in cardiac SPECT: the boy who cried wolf? *J Nucl Cardiol* 14:25, 2007.

Chapter 7

Attenuation Correction and Scatter Correction of Myocardial Perfusion SPECT Images

JAMES A. CASE

INTRODUCTION

Myocardial perfusion single-photon emission computed tomography (SPECT) has in large part been successful despite significant imaging limitations. Soft-tissue attenuation, photon scatter, distance dependent collimator blur, and partial volume artifacts are present in every single SPECT procedure performed in the world today. It is a testament to the robustness, utility, and clinical needs that SPECT continues to be such a dominant procedure for the management of patients with coronary artery disease, even with these limitations.

The field of medicine is changing dramatically, and the demands that will be placed on nuclear cardiology practitioners are increasing. Society is demanding greater accuracy, improved outcomes, and increased cost-effectiveness of procedures. To achieve these goals, attenuation correction will be a critical bridge that must be crossed if we are to achieve the gains society desires.

HISTORICAL PERSPECTIVE

The field of SPECT imaging was born out of pioneering work done at Duke University in the late 1970s under Ronald Jaszczak[1] and John Keyes.[2] It was demonstrated that three-dimensional radionuclide imaging could be obtained using an Anger camera rotating around a patient. As early as 1977, it was recognized that attenuation would be one of the major limitations of the new imaging modality.

The effort to solve the problem of attenuation artifacts in nuclear cardiology was carried forward by several groups around the world. Moore et al. demonstrated the feasibility of performing attenuation correction using x-ray computed tomography (CT),[3] and Greer KL et al.[4] demonstrated the feasibility of acquiring transmission data with a gamma camera system. A complete history of the development of attenuation correction can be found in King et al., 1995.[5]

The impact of attenuation was first quantitated in the work of Eisner et al. in 1988.[6] In this work, differences between males and females were correctly identified as arising from differences in anatomy. This led to significant differences in the mean normal distribution patterns in the left anterior descending (10% to 15% higher in males than females) and right coronary artery (8% to 10% higher in females than males). Later work by Galt et al. demonstrated that with the application of attenuation correction methods, these normal distributions were similar.[7] Depuey et al. developed techniques for identifying attenuation and presented algorithms for improving interpretive accuracy using deductive techniques.[8]

The first attempts at commercialization of attenuation correction were introduced by Picker with its STEP system (Fig. 7-1). This technique was based on the geometry proposed by Tung[9] and Jaszczak.[10] The system employed a fanning collimator design to collect photons from a fixed line source opposite the detector head on a triple-headed detector system. Early work using this system demonstrated that significant improvements in uniformity could be obtained using the fanbeam collimation system with attenuation correction.[11,12] This system failed to received widespread acceptance, because it employed a triple-detector SPECT system and fanbeam collimation. The use of fanbeam collimation led to very extreme truncation artifacts, owing to the small field of view of the fanbeam geometry (~30 cm). Furthermore, the added cost of a third detector system and loss of clinical efficiency from the

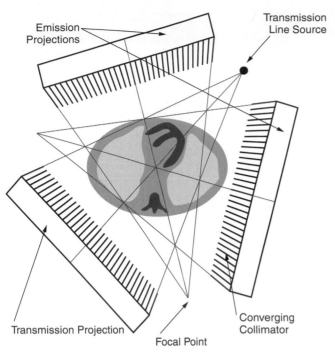

Figure 7-1 The Picker PRISM 3000 STEP system was the first commercially available attenuation correction system. It used a system of three fanbeam collimators and a stationary line source.

120-degree angles of the triple-head systems made this system cost prohibitive.

Other vendors introduced parallel-geometry scanning line source systems. The Vantage/ExSPECT system, introduced by ADAC laboratories, used a 90-degree parallel-hole geometry system for simultaneously acquiring emission and transmission data (Fig. 7-2).[13] Using this

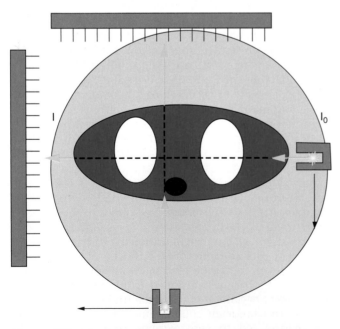

Figure 7-2 The scanning line source geometry employs a system of two radioactive sources, typically positioned opposite the detector face. A system of gears moves the arms across the field of view of the detector.

approach, one of the few multicenter trials of attenuation correction was conducted, demonstrating significant improvement in specificity and normalcy. These results were also duplicated in several single and multicenter imaging trials using various vendor approaches.[14–21]

One of the major limitations of the first-generation systems was that though they work reasonably well in clinical trials, they did not always perform well in the clinical setting.[22] Quality control (QC) of the attenuations correction systems was not well understood, and systematic QC procedures were not in place in most nuclear laboratories attempting to use attenuation correction. The result of this was a very uneven application of QC standards in the field and an eventual low rate of adoption by practitioners.

To address these limitations, ADAC laboratories introduced a second-generation processing suite for its Vantage scanning line source systems, the VantagePRO (Philips Medical, Milpitas, CA). This package used a combination of pre- and post-acquisition QC tools combined with a Bayesian iterative reconstruction algorithm to improve the consistency of the resulting images.[23] Clinical trials using this approach demonstrated significant improvement in normalcy and specificity; however, because of the retrospective nature of the study, sensitivity did not show improvement over conventional non-attenuation-corrected imaging.

Another approach that was investigated was the use of x-ray computed tomography to derive the patient-specific attenuation map. Because of the high count flux, very high-quality transmission maps can be obtained. Clinical results from these systems have been reported, and they have been shown to produce significant improvement in interpreter accuracy over non-attenuation-corrected image approaches.[24,25]

The limitation of x-ray-based approaches is that they are inherently sequential acquisition protocols. Transmission/emission image registration issues, as well as clinical efficiency concerns, have limited the acceptance of these systems. The Hawkeye System, introduced by General Electric, was a departure from the conventional line source attenuation correction, insofar as it employed a low-dose x-ray tube (140 kVp, 2.5 mAs) to generate a patient-specific x-ray-based CT attenuation map referred to as *hybrid imaging SPECT/CT*. This technique was capable of producing transmission maps and attenuation-corrected images of higher quality (Fig. 7-3). As the need for diagnostic-quality transmission maps has arisen, vendors have introduced SPECT/CT hybrid systems capable of detecting and measuring coronary calcium and performing vascular and coronary CT angiography (Siemens [Symbia], Philips [Precedence]).

Pressure for SPECT to evolve is mounting as payer and patient expectations rise. Positron emission tomography (PET) and CT are setting new standards for early detection of disease and in the management of complex patients. The expectations of a perfusion test are changing, and SPECT must improve the information content of its product or face obsolescence. Attenuation and scatter correction are likely to play a critical role in allowing SPECT to survive in this increasingly competitive medical environment.

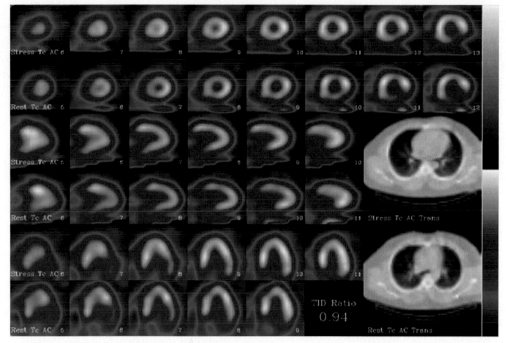

Figure 7-3 The Hawkeye SPECT/CT system employs a low-dosage CT system to produce x-rays for measuring the patient's anatomy. Though the CT images are not of diagnostic quality, they are of very high quality for the purpose of attenuation correction.

SCIENTIFIC FOUNDATION OF ATTENUATION: COMPTON SCATTERING AND THE PHOTOELECTRIC EFFECT (See Chapter 6)

Photon attenuation is a natural process of electromagnetic radiation with matter. For optical light, this process is easily recognized as the natural opacity of solid objects. Some materials—colored glass, polarizing sunglasses, and so forth—are translucent, allowing some of the photon beam to pass through the object. Logically, the thicker the translucent object, the fewer photons can survive the trip through the material.

This process is played out in a similar way in the high-energy regimen, albeit with different physical processes in play. Nuclear cardiology (and x-ray imaging as well) exists because of a very peculiar fact of nature: At these energies, the seemingly solid object of the human body is not nearly as solid as it appears. To understand this, we have to introduce an interesting concept, *the wave-particle duality of photons.*[1] At higher and higher energies, photons act as if they have smaller and smaller sizes. In the gamma ray and x-ray ranges, photons could pass through a solid object with little effort. To a high-energy gamma ray, the body looks less like a solid object and more like a cloud of electrons.[1]

To be precise, *attenuation* is a misnomer. Most of what is referred to as "attenuation" in nuclear cardiology is in reality photon scatter. The dominant process for "attenuating" photon signal in the energy range used in nuclear cardiology is known as *Compton scattering.*

This process, discovered by Arthur H. Compton in 1923 (resulting in Compton and his graduate student being awarded the Nobel Prize in physics[26]), is the quantum scatter of light off of matter and the transfer of significant amounts of energy from the photon to the electron.

The photon in a Compton scattering event can be thought of as a billiard ball striking the electron. The electron then absorbs some of the energy from the photon, lowering the energy of the photon (Fig. 7-4). The key parameters of a Compton scattering event are the incident energy of the photon (E_0) and the scattering angle of the photon relative to its incident and (θ). The higher the incident energy, the more relative energy can be delivered to the electron. (Imagine a compact car–against-truck head-on collision versus a truck-against-truck collision: The second truck will fare worse

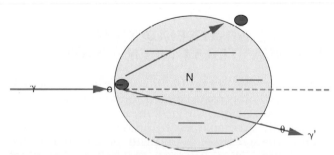

Figure 7-4 Compton scatter occurs when a high-energy photon collides with an electron in the media. The photon energy is changed by delivering energy to the electron, which is then ejected into the medium.

in the latter scenario.) Furthermore, the larger the scattering angle, the more energy that can be delivered to the electron. Compton demonstrated that the exact energy of the scattered photon can be calculated from the following formula:

$$E = \frac{E_0}{1 + \frac{E_0}{m_e c^2}(1 - \cos\theta)}$$

This is very important: Compton scattering does not destroy the incident photon. Each "attenuation" event is truly a scattering event. In other words, as we remove "good photons" from our signal, we add "bad photons" to the signal.

In the energy regimen of ^{99m}Tc (140 keV), Compton scattering dominates all scattering processes in human tissue. For lower-energy photons (^{201}Tl, ~72 keV), the photoelectric effect also plays a role. In photoelectric-effect absorption, the photon interacts with the atomic structure of the material. In these interactions, a significant fraction of the energy of the incident photons is used in ionizing the atom. For atoms such as oxygen and hydrogen, the k-shell binding energies are very low relative to the energies of the photons used in nuclear cardiology. Because of the energy difference between the binding energy and the incident photon, the likelihood of photoelectric effect ionization is low.

Example problem 1:

A 140-keV photon is completely backscattered by an electron. What is the resulting energy of the scattered photon?

Answer:

Using the Compton formula:

$$E = \frac{E_0}{1 + \frac{E_0}{m_e c^2}(1 - \cos\theta)}$$

where E_0 is the energy of the incident photon, $m_e c^2$ is the resting energy of an electron (511 keV), and θ is the angle of the scattered photon relative to the incident photon. For a backscattered photon: $\theta = 180$ degrees. Solving the Compton equation:

$$E = \frac{140\ keV}{1 + \frac{140\ keV}{511\ keV}(1 - (-1))} = \frac{140\ keV}{1 + 2*\frac{140\ keV}{511\ keV}} \approx 90\ keV$$

PHYSICS OF ATTENUATION AND SCATTER COMPENSATION

Attenuation and scatter of photons in nuclear cardiology can be compensated during the reconstruction process by knowing how the medium absorbs photons. This is typically accomplished by using a patient-specific map of the soft tissue to calculate the degree to which the photon signal has been reduced as a result of attenuation.

The degree to which photons are attenuated by the medium is calculated from this simple differential equation:

$$\frac{dI}{dl} = \mu * I$$

where I is the flux, μ is the linear attenuation coefficient, and $\frac{dI}{dl}$ is the change in I over a small distance. In other words, the change in the number of photons over a small distance of material is proportional to the single physical parameter, μ. Solving this equation yields:

$$I = I_0 \exp(-d * \mu)$$

The value of μ is dependent on the characteristics of the material in question and the energy of the incident photons. Examples of linear attenuation coefficients are given in Table 7-1.

To compensate for the impact of attenuation on the photo peak images, a model for the patient-specific attenuation is applied during the reconstruction. Conventional filtered backprojection reconstruction is not well suited for attenuation compensation; the attenuation profile cannot be easily expressed as a Fourier filter that can be applied to the projection data. To incorporate the attenuation profile data into the reconstruction, an iterative algorithm must be applied.

Iterative reconstruction algorithms can be broken down into three key components: the data, the estimate (or reconstruction), and the projection matrix (the model for how photons are moved out of the patient and into the camera). Ideally, a perfect model and perfect data will result in a perfect reconstruction. However, the reality is that perfect data and perfect models do not exist.

The most common iterative reconstruction algorithm is the maximum-likelihood expectation maximization (MLEM) algorithm.[27,28] This model employs an iterative approach for searching for the most likely source of the projection data, based on a physical model of how photons get from the patient to the camera. As one might expect, if the data are bad and the model is wrong, MLEM will not converge to the correct solution. The main strength of MLEM is the ease of which physics of attenuation can be modeled into the reconstruction. An example of the convergence of MLEM is given in Figure 7-5.

There are other iterative algorithms in addition to MLEM. Ordered subset expectation maximization (OSEM) is also commonly used. While its origins are similar to those of MLEM, OSEM has much more rapid convergence properties. OSEM uses pieces of the data to create each update of the data (subset). Each iteration of OSEM can result in several updates of the reconstruction map. This has the effect of greatly increasing the convergence time of the algorithm.[29]

Table 7-1 Examples of Linear Attenuation Coefficients for Water, Bone, and Air (in cm^{-1})

	70 keV	100 keV	150 keV
Water	0.195	0.171	0.151
Bone	0.516	0.362	0.284
Air	0.000213	0.000186	0.000163

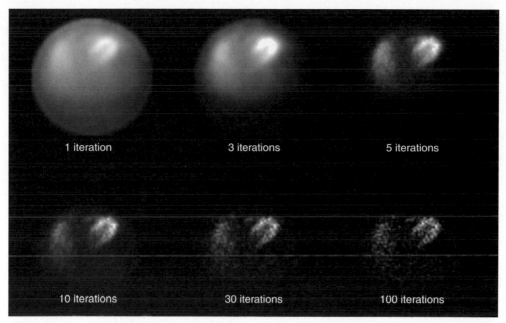

Figure 7-5 Iterative reconstruction successively improves the image fidelity by updating the image in small amounts at each iteration. Because the input data are not perfect, these algorithms can overfit the noise and produce a noisy reconstruction at high iteration numbers.

Example problem 2:

A beam of 140-keV photons penetrate a 10-cm slab of water. The attenuation coefficient for 140-keV photons is $\mu = 0.15$/cm.

Answer:

$$I = I_0 \exp(-d * \mu)$$

$$\frac{I}{I_0} = \exp(-d * \mu) = \exp(-10 * 0.14) \approx 0.25$$

where d is the thickness of the slab, I_0 is the flux of the incident beam, and I is the resulting flux.

Similar to attenuation correction, scatter correction relies on acquiring a patient-specific estimate of photon scatter. The most common technique for scatter estimation is the acquisition of adjacent energy windows to subtract the scatter component from the photo peak component (Fig. 7-6). These techniques typically use a secondary energy window placed at a lower energy from the primary photo peak to measure the distribution of Compton scatter photons.[30] These techniques can be effective in removing the scatter from ^{99m}Tc, but they have been less successful in correcting Tl-201 images. Furthermore, these techniques have been unable to demonstrate measurable improvements in sensitivity.

One possibility for the failure to observe improvement in sensitivity is that scatter window subtraction techniques do not model the smaller-angle scatter events responsible for defect fill-in (Fig. 7-7).[31] Several techniques have been described for more accurately modeling photon scatter. These techniques rely upon acquiring several energy windows and using multispectral techniques for modeling the large- and small-angle scattering events.[32]

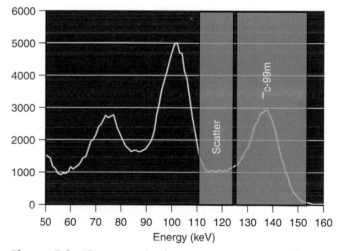

Figure 7-6 The most simple scatter correction technique uses a neighboring energy window to acquire a measurement of the down-scatter. This measurement is then subtracted from the primary peak data to produce a scatter-corrected projection data set.

TECHNIQUES OF ACQUIRING THE PATIENT-SPECIFIC ATTENUATION MAP

To perform attenuation correction, an estimate of the anatomy is required. This estimate of anatomy is typically obtained through the direct measurement of the patient using an external radiation source.

Line Source Attenuation Correction

One of the most common approaches to acquiring the transmission map is to use an external source of

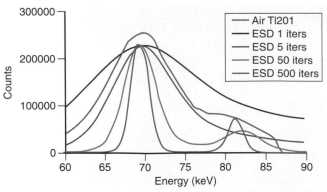

Figure 7-7 More sophisticated techniques use a model of the energy response of the detector system to "reconstruct" the energy spectrum at each pixel to achieve better energy discimination.

radioactivity to transmit gamma rays though the patient. This technique has several advantages:

1. The system design is relatively inexpensive to add onto a conventional SPECT system.
2. These systems produce a transmission map that is well matched to the patient in terms of breathing, photon energy, and resolution.
3. These systems can often acquire the transmission data simultaneous to the emission data, thereby having a minimal impact on laboratory efficiency.
4. These systems can use the same collimators and detectors that are used for emission imaging.
5. These transmission systems typically have very little additional radiation exposure.

Tung et al. and Jaszczak et al. proposed one of the first line source systems using a converging fanbeam collimation system.[9,10] This system used a triple-detector system with one of the heads dedicated to acquiring the transmission data. This system did not reach widespread acceptance, owing to the added expense of the third detector head and the need for having a second set of collimators.

Another approach was advanced by Tan et al., using a system of scanning line sources.[11] This system utilized a set of moving line sources to "scan" the patient. Though this system did require the purchase of robotic housings to contain the line sources, it was more widely accepted because it was more easily retrofitted to the 90-degree detector configuration used in cardiology.

Computed Tomography–Based Attenuation Correction

Another approach for acquiring the transmission map is to use an x-ray tube–based transmission system to acquire the transmission data. This system has an advantage in that the count flux from a conventional x-ray tube is very high relative to radionuclide-based approaches. X-ray-based CT images are typically characterized by their high spatial resolution and high signal to noise.

One of the earliest applications of CT-based attenuation correction for SPECT was the Hawkeye System from General Electric. This system used a small x-ray tube (140

kVp, 2.5 mAs) to create the attenuation map. Subsequent systems have been employed that use more advanced CT scanners capable of acquiring diagnostic-quality CT images (Symbia [Siemens], Precedence [Philips]).

Quality-Control Issues

Regardless of the techniques used for acquiring the transmission map, all attenuation correction systems require a high-quality transmission map to perform attenuation correction. A high-quality transmission map is defined as:

1. Near-uniform attenuation coefficients across the mediastinal area
2. Free of truncation artifacts
3. Well-defined lung boundaries
4. Registered with the emission data
5. Breathing cycle equivalent to a free breathing state averaged over several respiratory cycles

Examples of attenuation maps that do not meet these criteria are displayed in Figure 7-8.

Prior to interpretation, all transmission data sets should be routinely inspected for image quality. Data that do not meet these criteria should be suspect.

APPLICATIONS FOR ATTENUATION CORRECTION

The American Society of Nuclear Cardiology and the Society of Nuclear Medicine recommend the routine use of attenuation correction as an important adjunct to traditional filtered backprojection images.[33] These recommendations are based on the preponderance of evidence that demonstrates that superior specificity can be achieved using attenuation correction. Though anecdotal evidence exists for the improvement of sensitivity, study selection bias and suboptimal scatter correction techniques have been unable to demonstrate improvements in sensitivity.

Applications for attenuation correction fall into two broad categories: techniques that improve conventional perfusion imaging and techniques for which routine rest/stress perfusion imaging is not possible.

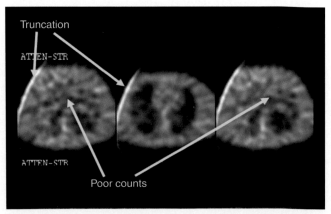

Figure 7-8 Low-quality transmission scans often have low counts, truncation, or both.

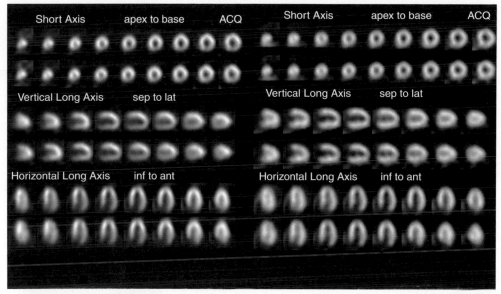

Figure 7-9 On the *left* is a filtered backprojection recontruction of a low-likelihood male patient. On the *right* is a reconstruction of the same patient, using attenuation correction. Note the change in the perfusion distribution after attenuation correction.

The most common application of attenuation correction is as supplementary data for rest/stress ^{99m}Tc- imaging. In these studies, a transmission data set is acquired in conjunction with the emission data set. The data are then reconstructed using a filtered backprojection algorithm for the non-attenuation-corrected data set and an iterative reconstruction for the attenuation-corrected data set. The filtered backprojection images can then be compared to the attenuation-corrected data sets to assess the significance of attenuation on the filtered backprojection images (Fig. 7-9).

Stress Only

Another application that has been promoted is the use of attenuation correction for assessing myocardial perfusion images in the absence of a resting study. In this application, patients presenting with a relatively low pretest likelihood for disease are tested with a stress-first myocardial perfusion test. The physician then will make a determination of the normalcy of the study based on the stress perfusion. If the stress images are normal, the patient is not brought back for rest testing (Fig. 7-10).[34]

One of the most significant challenges of stress-only imaging is the necessity of triaging patients to a stress-first protocol, which could require the patient to return for further testing on the second day.

Heller et al.[35,36] demonstrated that reader confidence was greatly improved when attenuation correction was applied. Other studies have demonstrated comparable accuracy in the normalcy rate when compared to full-rest stress studies.

Acute Imaging

There has also been considerable work on attenuation correction in the acute setting (during a chest pain episode). In this application, upon admission to the chest

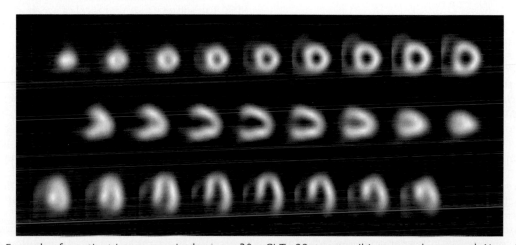

Figure 7-10 Example of a patient image acquired using a 30-mCi Tc-99m sestamibi stress-only protocol. Note: Because of the uniformity of this image, the patient would not be required to return for rest imaging.

pain center or emergency department, the patient is immediately injected with the radiotracer. Studies have demonstrated a high degree of positive predictive value for acute resting imaging if the patient can be injected before the chest pain resolves.[37] These studies are almost always performed as a single study (no true rest imaging). Because of the confounding problem of attenuation and the lack of a resting control study, attenuation can render non-attenuation-corrected images of little value.

The challenges for acute myocardial perfusion imaging are not the diagnostic strength of the test; rather it is the difficulty of managing the myocardial perfusion testing within the context of a busy chest pain center or emergency department. Iodine-based tracers such as Iodine-123 BMIPP, currently in Phase II clinical trial in the United States and in routine use in Japan, could resolve these crucial workflow issues in the acute setting.

Quantitative Single-Photon Emission Computed Tomography

As pressure builds for more and more accurate tests for myocardial perfusion imaging, the assessment of large epicardial disease may no longer be sufficient. Myocardial perfusion PET has already seen widespread interest in assessing true myocardial blood flow in terms of mL/g/min. These measurements, in principle, would be independent of the resting perfusion pattern, more sensitive to triple-vessel disease, and capable of measuring serial changes in perfusion.[38]

To obtain a quantitative measurement of myocardial perfusion, it is necessary to obtain a measurement in mCi/cc, the dynamic arterial tracer concentration, and the dynamic uptake of the tracer within the myocardium. To achieve this, it is necessary to acquire serial images of the input bolus in SPECT mode with attenuation. These rapid tomographic images must be acquired at such speed as to allow quantification of the input bolus to time less than 6 seconds (Fig. 7-11).

CHALLENGES FOR ATTENUATION CORRECTION

The story of attenuation correction in SPECT is best looked at as both a glass half empty and a glass half full. Most treatments of attenuation and scatter correction focus on either one or the other of these paradigms, best illustrated by the publications of dueling opinions in the *Journal of Nuclear Cardiology*, 2005.[22,39] Though there is little argument that specificity is improved with attenuation correction as is, there is also little argument that attenuation correction has not seen widespread adoption. A more appropriate question is "Why isn't the glass completely full?"—that is, what is missing to make attenuation correction an unquestionable necessity for SPECT? In fact, the "recommendation" for attenuation correction presented by the American Society of Nuclear Cardiology and the Society of Nuclear Medicine is qualified so as to relegate the attenuation-corrected images to adjunctive information to the patently incorrect

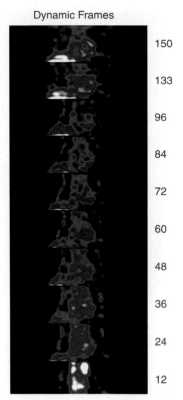

Dynamic Frames

150

133

96

84

72

60

48

36

24

12

Figure 7-11 Example of an attenuation-corrected "stress input function" sequence acquired using a Siemens (Symbia) system. Despite the high noise and low image fidelity in this image, counts are sufficient for measuring the integrated blood-pool concentration of tracer.

noncorrected images.[33] This is hardly a ringing endorsement.

In cardiac PET imaging, attenuation correction is always applied; in fact, non-attenuation-corrected images are never produced. Because of the unique geometry of PET (two photons produced simultaneously, traveling in opposite directions), attenuation and scatter correction are robust and very accurate. There is no added reimbursement for attenuation correction for PET; it is simply recognized as the correct way to process these images. For attenuation and scatter correction for SPECT to achieve a similar level of acceptance, it must produce a substantially better image than non-attenuation-corrected SPECT.

The most commonly cited limitation of attenuation-corrected SPECT is the lack of uniformity in some studies. This lack of uniformity is often referred to as *overcorrection* or *undercorrection* of the emission data.[22] The mathematics of attenuation correction is straightforward,[27–29] and its implementation within computer programs is straightforward. Attenuation correction is "working" when a high-quality transmission map is available. However, this may not be all that is going on. Poor scatter correction, partial volume effects, and distance-dependent blur all produce artifacts that are patient and protocol specific.

In a sense, the world without attenuation and scatter correction is a simpler world. Attenuation artifact plays such a dominant role that other effects pale in

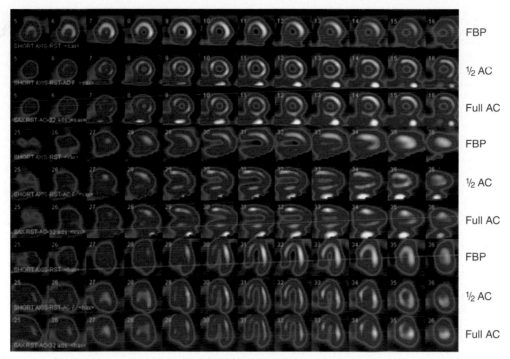

Figure 7-12 Example of attenuation correction combined with Astonish resolution recovery and scatter correction (Philips Medical Systems, Milipitas, CA). This study was performed using both full time (25/sec/stop) and half time (12.5 sec/stop). Note the clearly delineated papillary muscles in the Astonish images using both full- and half-time imaging.

comparison. When attenuation correction is applied, the myriad of other confounding artifacts become visible and can make the images more challenging to interpret, despite the fact they are more accurate.

Significant advances have been made in the implementation of resolution recovery and advanced scatter correction. Flash3D (Siemens, Hoffman Estates, IL), Astonish (Philips, Milpitas, CA) and Wide Beam Reconstruction (UltraSPECT, Haifa, Israel) all use a model for the blurring of the collimator. The results are higher-resolution images with fewer partial-volume artifacts (Fig. 7-12). Improvements in scatter correction will also be necessary for improving the sensitivity of myocardial perfusion SPECT images to smaller defects.[31]

CONCLUSION

It would be easy to recommend that attenuation and scatter correction should be applied in all cases; however, things are not that simple. Attenuation correction has been very well established as a technique that can yield significant and impressive improvements in specificity, and it can be useful in situations where two-stage rest/stress imaging is impossible. QC must be maintained, and protocols must be implemented to ensure accurate acquisition and reconstruction of the attenuation map, as well as the reconstruction of the emission data.

The future of attenuation correction mirrors the future of myocardial perfusion SPECT: Without a demonstrable change in the information that can be extracted from the data, SPECT will continue to lose out to other more sophisticated techniques such as CT, magnetic resonance imaging, and PET.

The next stage in the development of attenuation correction for SPECT is to create obsolescence for non-attenuation-corrected studies. This can be achieved through the further penetration of robust scatter correction and resolution recovery methodology. Many of these techniques are being brought to the commercial realm, and it is likely that attenuation, scatter, and resolution recovery methods will eclipse the techniques of today.

REFERENCES

1. Jaszczak RJ, Murphy PH, Huard D, Burdine JA: Radionuclide emission computed tomography of the head with Tc-99m and a scintillation camera, *J Nucl Med Inst Phys* 18(4):373–380, 1977.
2. Keyes WI: The fan-beam gamma camera, *Phys Med Biol* 20:489–491, 1975.
3. Moore SC, Ell PJ, Holman BL: *Attenuation Compensation in Computed Emission tomography*, New York, 1982, Oxford University Press.
4. Greer KL, Harris CC, Jaszczak, et al: Transmission computed tomography data acquisition with a SPECT system, *J Nucl Med Tech* 15:53–56, 1987.
5. King MA, Tsui BMW, Pan TS: Attenuation compensation for cardiac SPECT imaging, *J Nucl Cardiol* 2(6):513–523, 1995.
6. Eisner RL, Tamas MJ, Cloninger K, et al: Normal SPECT Thallium-201 bull's eye display: Gender differences, *J Nucl Med* 29(12):1901–1909, 1988.
7. Galt JR, Arram SM, Case JA, Cullom SJ, Habboush I, Shao L, Hines H, Bateman EV, Garcia EV: and the multicenter trial investigators. Multicenter evaluation of automated quality control of transmission scans for attenuation correction in myocardial perfusion SPECT, *J Am Coll Card* 37(2):425A, 2001.
8. Depuey GE, Garcia EV, Berman DS, "Cardiac SPECT Imaging", 2nd edition, Lippincott, Williams, and Wilkins, 2001.
9. Tung CH, Gullberg GT, Zeng GL, Christian PE, Datz FL, Morgan HT: Non-uniform attenuation correction using simultaneous transmission and emission converging tomography, *IEEE Trans. Nucl Sci* 39(4):1134–1143, 1992.
10. Jaszczak RJ, Gilliand DR, Hanson MW, Jang S, Greer KL, Coleman RE: Fast transmission CT for determining attenuation maps using a collimated line source, rotatable air-copper-lead attenuators and fanbeam collimation, *J Nucl Med* 34:1577–1586, 1993.

11. Ficaro EP, Fessler JA, Shreve PD, et al: Simultaneous transmission in emission myocardial perfusion imaging, *Circulation* 93(3):463–473, 1996.

12. Case JA: *A clinical Protocol for attenuation and scatter correction of Tl-201 and Tc-99m Sestamibi myocardial perfusion SPECT images [PhD dissertation]*, Amherst, 1998, University of Massachusetts.

13. Tan P, Bailey DL, Meikle SR, Eberl S, Fulton RR, Hutton BF: A scanning line source for simultaneous emission and transmission measurements in SPECT, *J Nucl Med* 34:1752–1760, 1993.

14. Ficaro EP, Fessler JA, Shreve PD, Kritzman JN, Rose PA, Corbett JR: Simultaneous transmission/emission myocardial perfusion tomography. Diagnostic accuracy of attenuation-corrected 99mTc-sestamibi single-photon emission computed tomography, *Circulation* 93(3):463–473, 1996.

15. Kluge R, Sattler B, Seese A, Knapp WH: Attenuation correction by simultaneous emission-transmission myocardial single-photon emission tomography using a technetium-99m-labelled radiotracer: impact on diagnostic accuracy, *Eur J Nucl Med* 24(9):1107–1114, 1997.

16. Gallowitsch HJ, Sykora J, Mikosch P, et al: Attenuation-corrected thallium-201 single-photon emission tomography using a gadolinium-153 moving line source: clinical value and the impact of attenuation correction on the extent and severity of perfusion abnormalities, *Eur J Nucl Med* 25(3):220–228, 1998.

17. Hendel RC, Berman DS, Cullom SJ, et al: Multicenter clinical trial to evaluate the efficacy of correction for photon attenuation and scatter in SPECT myocardial perfusion imaging, *Circulation* 99(21):2742–2749, 1999.

18. Links JM, DePuey EG, Taillefer R, Becker LC: Attenuation correction and gating synergistically improve the diagnostic accuracy of myocardial perfusion SPECT, *J Nucl Cardiol* 9(2):183–187, 2002.

19. Hendel RC, Corbett JR, Cullom SJ, DePuey EG, Garcia EV, Bateman TM: The value and practice of attenuation correction for myocardial perfusion SPECT imaging: a joint position statement from the American Society of Nuclear Cardiology and the Society of Nuclear Medicine, *J Nucl Cardiol* 9(1):135–143, 2002.

20. Thompson RC, Heller GV, Johnson LL, et al: Value of attenuation correction on ECG-gated SPECT myocardial perfusion imaging related to body mass index, *J Nucl Cardiol* 12(2):195–202, 2005.

21. Grossman GB, Garcia EV, Bateman TM, et al: Quantitative Tc-99m sestamibi attenuation-corrected SPECT: development and multicenter trial validation of myocardial perfusion stress gender-independent normal database in an obese population, *J Nucl Cardiol* 11(3):263–272, 2004.

22. Germano G, Slomka PJ, Berman DS: Attenuation correction in cardiac SPECT: the boy who cried wolf? *J Nucl Cardiol* 14:25–35, 2006.

23. Case JA, Hsu BL, Bateman TM, Cullom SJ: A Bayesian iterative transmission gradient reconstruction algorithm for cardiac SPECT attenuation correction, *J Nucl Cardiol* 14(3):324–333, 2007.

24. Masood Y, Liu YH, Depuey G, et al: Clinical validation of SPECT attenuation correction using x-ray computed tomography-derived attenuation maps: multicenter clinical trial with angiographic correlation, *J Nucl Cardiol* 12(6):676–686, 2005.

25. Fricke E, Fricke H, Weise R, et al: Attenuation correction of myocardial SPECT perfusion images with low-dose CT: evaluation of the method by comparison with perfusion PET, *J Nucl Med* 46(5):736–744, 2005.

26. Nobel Lectures: *Physics 1922–1941*, Amsterdam, 1965, Elsevier.

27. Shepp LA, Vardi Y: Maximum likelihood reconstruction for emission tomography, *IEEE Trans Med Imaging* MI-1(2):113–122, 1982.

28. Lange K, Carson R: EM reconstruction algorithms for emission and transmission tomography, *J Comput Assist Tomogr* 8:306–316, 1984.

29. Hudson MH, Larkin RS: Accelerated image reconstruction using ordered subsets of projection data, *IEEE Trans Med Imaging* 13(4):601–609, 1994.

30. Ogawa K, Harata Y, Ichihara T, Kubo A, Hashimoto S: A practical method for position-dependent Compton scatter correction in single photon emission CT, *IEEE Trans Med Imaging* 10:408–412, 1991.

31. Case JA, Hsu BL, Cullom SJ, Bateman TM: Importance of Tl-201 scatter compensation for resolution and contrast matching in rest Tl-201/stress Tc-99m myocardial perfusion SPECT imaging, *J Nucl Med* 46:173P, 2005.

32. Gagnon D, Todd-Pokropek A, Arsenault A, Dupras G: Introduction to holospectral imaging in nuclear medicine for scatter subtraction, *IEEE Trans Med Imaging* 8:245–250, 1989.

33. Hendel RC, Corbett JR, Cullom SJ, DePuey EG, Garcia EV, Bateman TM: The value and practice of attenuation correction for myocardial perfusion SPECT imaging: a joint position statement from the American Society of Nuclear Cardiology and the Society of Nuclear Medicine, *J Nucl Cardiol* 9(1):135–143, 2002.

34. Gibson PB, Demus D, Noto R, Hudson W, Johnson LL: Low event rate for stress-only perfusion imaging in patients evaluated for chest pain, *J Am Coll Cardiol* 39(6):999–1004, 2002.

35. Heller GV, Bateman TM, Johnson L, et al: Clinical value of attenuation correction in stress-only Tc-99m sestamibi SPECT imaging, *J Nucl Cardiol* 11(3):273–281, 2004.

36. Heller GV, Links J, Bateman TM, et al: American Society of Nuclear Cardiology and Society of Nuclear Medicine joint position statement: attenuation correction of myocardial perfusion SPECT scintigraphy, *J Nucl Cardiol* 11(2):229, 2004.

37. Holly TA, Toth BM, Leonard SM, et al: Incremental value of attenuation correction in SPECT myocardial perfusion imaging for patients with acute chest pain, *Circulation* 96:1735, 1997.

38. deKemp RA, Yoshinaga K, Beanlands RSB: Will 3-dimensional PET-CT enable the routine quantification of myocardial blood flow? *J Nucl Cardiol* 14:380–397, 2007.

39. Garcia E: SPECT Attenuation correction: An essential tool to realize nuclear cardiology's manifest destiny, *J Nucl Cardiol* 14:16–24, 2006.

Chapter 8

Hybrid Cardiac Imaging

PHILIPP A. KAUFMANN AND OLIVER GAEMPERLI

INTRODUCTION (See Chapter 22)

The constant technological developments of noninvasive imaging over the past decades have contributed to the enhancement of our pathophysiologic understanding of many cardiac conditions. Particularly in coronary artery disease (CAD), management is based upon assessment of both the presence of coronary stenoses and their hemodynamic consequences.[1,2] Hence, noninvasive imaging helps to guide therapeutic decisions by providing complementary information on coronary morphology and on myocardial perfusion and metabolism using different imaging tools,[3,4] including nuclear techniques such as single-photon emission computed tomography (SPECT) or positron emission tomography (PET), computed tomography (CT) techniques such as electron beam CT (EBCT) and multislice CT (MSCT), or cardiac magnetic resonance (CMR).

Advances in image processing software and the advent of hybrid scanners have paved the way for fusion of image data sets from different modalities, giving rise to multimodality or hybrid imaging. This technology avoids mental integration of functional and morphologic images and facilitates a comprehensive interpretation of the combined data sets. Integrating CT with SPECT or PET has different aims in cardiac imaging than body imaging. In body PET/CT, CT is merely used to localize the tracer accumulation seen on PET and for attenuation correction. Cardiac coronary anatomy is simpler but more difficult to image with CT because the speed and spatial resolution requirements are harder to meet. This has long been an unsuccessful quest, but with the latest advances in MSCT technology, noninvasive visualization of coronary artery anatomy has become reality.

Thus, the interest in hybrid imaging has rapidly spread onto cardiac applications and has changed the landscape of noninvasive cardiac imaging by bringing the different clinical specialties (i.e., cardiology, radiology, nuclear medicine) closer together.[5] Additionally, it has driven the development and production of dedicated hybrid scanners in an effort to simplify image coregistration and improve patient throughput for specialized cardiac imaging centers. For the evaluation of a patient with heart disease, hybrid imaging introduces a multifaceted approach to cardiovascular assessment. This approach facilitates the detection and quantification of coronary atherosclerosis through the use of coronary artery calcium scores (CACS) and coronary angiography, the quantification of vascular reactivity and endothelial integrity, the identification of flow-limiting coronary stenoses, and the assessment of myocardial viability and metabolism by means of PET. Thus, by revealing the burden of anatomic CAD and its physiologic relevance, hybrid imaging can provide noninvasively unique information that may help to improve diagnosis and risk stratification and guide management decisions in CAD patients.

TECHNICAL CONSIDERATIONS OF HYBRID IMAGING

Several pioneering attempts of software-based image fusion from conventional coronary angiography (CA) and SPECT paved the way for hybrid imaging but were not implemented into clinical practice because their invasiveness precluded use for noninvasive preinterventional decision making.[6–9] Fusion of CT and nuclear techniques for three-dimensional hybrid imaging was initially cumbersome, and the quality of the images suffered from several limitations (Fig. 8-1). The temporal and spatial resolution required for consistently good delineation of the coronary tree was not met by early 4- or 16-slice CT devices. Furthermore, the lack of dedicated cardiac fusion software rendered image processing tedious and time-consuming. Many new developments in hardware (e.g., 64-detector CT devices) and software (dedicated cardiac fusion software, high-powered postprocessing workstations) have helped to improve image quality and promote clinical availability of hybrid imaging (Fig. 8-2).

For cardiac applications, a three-dimensional display of the fused images (generated by volume-rendering

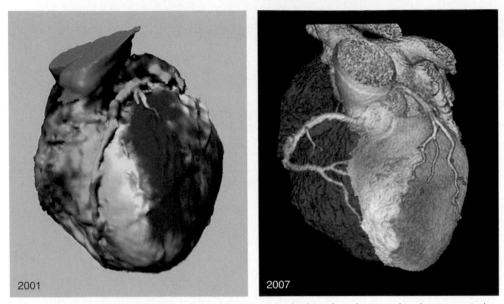

Figure 8-1 Advances in three-dimensional cardiac hybrid imaging. In the last decade, new developments in hardware (64-detector CT devices) and software (dedicated cardiac fusion software, high-powered postprocessing workstations) have helped to improve image quality and facilitate quick and reproducible image generation.

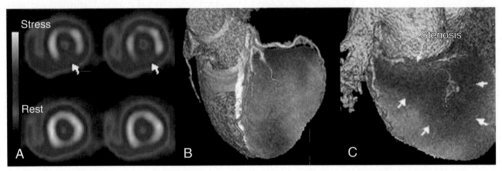

Figure 8-2 Image of the Year at the 2006 annual meeting of the Society of Nuclear Medicine, San Diego, CA, USA. The image shows a posterolateral ischemia *(arrows)* corresponding to a mid–left circumflex artery stenosis. *(Reprinted with permission of the Society of Nuclear Medicine.)*

technique)[10] is preferable compared to oncologic or neurologic applications, because it allows the best evaluation of myocardial territories and their respective tributaries. Thus, an important prerequisite of hybrid imaging is accurate image coregistration. Misalignment may result in erroneous allocation of perfusion defects and coronary artery territories. From a computational perspective, image coregistration can be achieved by a software-based or hardware-based approach.[11] Hardware-based image coregistration permits the acquisition of coregistered anatomic and functional images using hybrid scanners (such as PET/CT or SPECT/CT devices) with the capability to perform nuclear and CT image acquisition almost simultaneously, with the patient's position fixed. Inherently, image fusion is performed fully or semiautomatically by superposition of image data sets. With software-based coregistration, image data sets can be obtained on standalone scanners and fused manually through the use of landmark-based coregistration techniques (Fig. 8-3). Intuitively, the hardware-based approach appears preferable, since manual coregistration may be hampered

by issues of accuracy and user interaction. This is why, to date, hybrid PET/CT devices are widely used for whole-body PET/CT imaging, predominantly in oncology.

However, in contrast to whole-body PET/CT, the routine use of fully automated hardware-based image coregistration for cardiac hybrid applications is limited by organ-specific characteristics. Despite fixation of the patient's position and orientation, minor beat-to-beat variations in the heart's position may interfere with accurate image coregistration. Furthermore, CT image acquisition and analysis requires electrocardiographic gating, and images are generally reconstructed in mid-diastolic phases for obtaining optimal image quality.[12] By contrast, for sufficient quality of the SPECT images, the nongated data set is used, resulting in a slight mismatch of ventricular size between CT and SPECT images. Finally, the position of the heart is highly susceptible to respiratory motion. The CT scan is performed during a single inspiratory breath hold, but SPECT images are acquired during normal breathing, without accounting for respiratory motion unless respiratory gating is used.

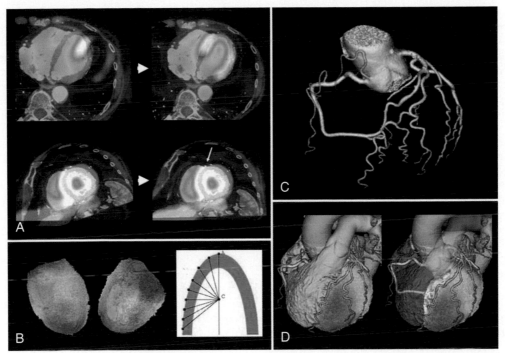

Figure 8-3 Illustration of the main protocols in the Cardiac Fusion software. **A,** Image co-registration. This first step is crucial and allows the user to align the images on axial, sagittal, and coronal image planes to obtain optimal matching of structural and functional information. In addition to translational alignment, this protocol allows for manual correction of the left ventricular (LV) rotation along its long axis, using the transition of right to left ventricle as a hinge point *(arrow).* **B,** Definition of left ventricular epicardium. This protocol displays a view containing the segmented computed tomography (CT) LV epicardium, using conventional volume-rendering technique, allowing addition or removal of structures from the LV epicardium if needed. Every voxel of the volume has an opacity value and a color. The opacity ramp is based on the Hounsfield units of the CT data. The color of the surface is generated based on the perfusion information. In each point of the surface of the volume-rendered image, the color is computed as being the maximum perfusion intensity on a ray going from the particular point to the center of the heart on CT. **C,** Coronary tree segmentation. This protocol allows the user to grow the coronary arteries from the ascending aorta, using automatic vessel tracking or manual segmentation. The algorithms used for adding or removing coronary arteries are based on morphologic techniques for segmentation, using the density value of the pixels and local shape parameters (tube likeliness for vessels). The protocol further extracts the ascending aorta and the coronary arteries from surrounding tissue, allowing them to be viewed in isolation. **D,** Three-dimensional volume-rendered fusion images. As the final step, the Hybrid Display protocol displays a volume rendering containing the LV epicardial volume, the volume-rendered coronary tree, and the left and right heart chambers acquired by an automatic segmentation algorithm. Implementation of a cardiac transparency tool enables the user to fade away any of these structures—for example, the right ventricle—allowing for better visualization of the septal wall. *(From Gaemperli O, Schepis T, Kalff V, et al: Validation of a new cardiac image fusion software for three-dimensional integration of myocardial perfusion SPECT and stand-alone 64-slice CT angiography, Eur J Nucl Med Mol Imaging 34:1097-1106, 2007. Reprinted with permission of the European Society of Nuclear Medicine.)*

In fact, whole-body PET/CT studies have shown significant misalignment of the heart between superimposed PET and CT acquired during inspiration.[13,14]

These factors contribute to the notion that despite the integration of high-end CT devices (with the capability to perform state-of-the-art coronary CT angiography) with nuclear scanners to form dedicated cardiac hybrid scanners, manual image coregistration may remain indispensable.[15] Published reports with x-ray-based attenuation correction have taught us that automated coregistration of CT and SPECT images is often unreliable, and manual correction for misalignment is needed in the vast majority of cases.[16,17] Dedicated cardiac fusion software packages are now commercially available, allowing software-based hybrid imaging with an excellent interobserver reproducibility and short processing durations (see Fig. 8-3). In a validation study using software-based SPECT/CT fusion from standalone scanners, reproducibility and feasibility of this method

were evaluated by assessing cardiac surface landmarks in 15 patients with a single coronary stenosis and a single perfusion defect.[18] The authors reported an excellent interobserver variability ($r = 0.99$; $P < 0.0001$) for landmark detection and reasonably short processing times of less than 15 minutes per patient. The full integration of these fusion software packages into the regular postprocessing applications for CT angiography will further minimize time expenditure and improve workflow for hybrid imaging (by avoiding repeat actions such as coronary artery tracking from CT angiography images).

HYBRID IMAGING: COMPREHENSIVE "ONE-STOP SHOP"

Atherosclerotic disease accounts for the majority of fatalities reported in industrialized countries. The diagnostic gold standard for establishing the presence of CAD is still x-ray coronary angiography, with all its drawbacks. A major limitation of this technique is its invasive nature, with considerable procedure-related morbidity (1.5%) and mortality (0.15%). In addition, the physiologic significance of any lesion is frequently difficult to assess from angiographic information alone. Furthermore, up to 75% of all invasive angiograms in the United States remain purely diagnostic, and between 20% and 40% of all diagnostic invasive coronary angiograms reveal no clinically significant disease,[19] so noninvasive procedures have the potential to play an important role in the future by eliminating a substantial fraction of these invasive angiograms (e.g., in cases of atypical chest pain, equivocal stress test results, and low to intermediate clinical probability of coronary disease).

Multislice CT angiography has rapidly evolved from an experimental technique to the most promising imaging modality for the noninvasive visualization of coronary arteries. Using the latest generation of CT scanners (dual-source CT, 256 detectors and more), excellent image quality can be achieved in the vast majority of patients, with values for sensitivity, specificity, and positive and negative predictive values averaging 92%, 96%, 79%, and 99%, respectively.[20] With its high negative predictive value, noninvasive angiography may play an important role when the clinical goal is to rule out CAD in patient populations with low clinical probability for CAD. Nonetheless, a minor drawback of CT angiography remains the moderate positive predictive value, insofar as stenoses tend to be overestimated owing to partial volume effects from coronary artery–wall calcifications and other image artifacts.

The value of hybrid imaging originates from the spatial correlation of structural and functional information on the fused images, which facilitates a comprehensive interpretation of coronary lesions and their pathophysiologic relevance. Although this can be achieved by mental integration, coronary artery anatomy may vary considerably, therefore standard myocardial distribution territories correspond in only 50% to 60% with the real anatomic coronary tree.[7] First clinical results with noninvasive hybrid imaging were presented by Namdar and coworkers using fusion of myocardial perfusion PET with ^{13}N-ammonia and 4-slice CT angiography in 25 patients with CAD. Sensitivity, specificity, and positive and negative predictive value of hybrid PET/CT for the detection of flow-limiting stenoses in the main coronary vessels were 90%, 98%, 82%, and 99%, respectively, compared to the clinical gold standard of PET and conventional coronary angiography. These encouraging results were confirmed by a similar study by Rispler and coworkers.[21] The authors compared the diagnostic accuracy of hybrid SPECT/CT imaging for the detection of flow-limiting coronary artery stenoses with CT angiography alone in 56 patients with angina pectoris. Hybrid SPECT/CT resulted in a significant improvement in specificity (from 63% to 95%) and positive predictive value (from 31% to 77%) compared to CT alone, without any change in sensitivity and negative predictive value. A similar study by Santana and colleagues showed an improved diagnostic accuracy of hybrid SPECT/CT imaging compared to SPECT alone ($P < 0.001$) and to the side-by-side analysis of SPECT and CT ($P = 0.007$) for diagnosis of obstructive CAD on conventional coronary angiography.[22] These data show that hybrid SPECT/CT imaging may play an important role in the noninvasive diagnosis of CAD as a decision-making tool for assessing the need for revascularization in coronary artery stenoses.

A recent publication focused on the role of hybrid SPECT/CT imaging for assessing the hemodynamic relevance of coronary artery stenoses and its potential added clinical value over side-by-side analysis in 38 high-risk patients with abnormal perfusion on SPECT (Fig. 8-4).[3] The main clinical benefit of hybrid SPECT/CT imaging was a significant reduction in the number of coronary lesions with equivocal hemodynamic significance (from $n = 40$ to $n = 16$; $P < 0.001$) (Fig. 8-5). Added diagnostic

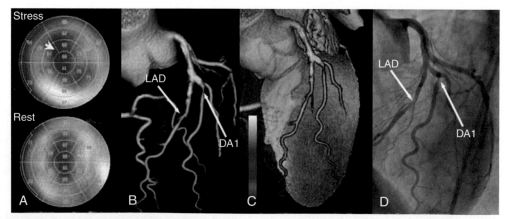

Figure 8-4 **A,** Perfusion polar maps of SPECT-MPI at stress and rest show a largely reversible anteroapical perfusion defect *(arrowhead).* **B,** Three-dimensional (3D) volume-rendered computed tomography angiography (CTA) images show the coronary vessel tree with a stenosis of the mid–left anterior descending (LAD) and a proximal stenosis of the first diagonal branch (DA1). **C,** Fused 3D SPECT/CT images are able to identify the DA1 stenosis as the functionally relevant lesion. **D,** Findings were confirmed by invasive coronary angiography. *(From Gaemperli O, Schepis T, Valenta I, et al: Cardiac image fusion from stand-alone SPECT and CT: Clinical experience. J Nucl Med 48:696-703, 2007. Reprinted with permission of the Society of Nuclear Medicine.)*

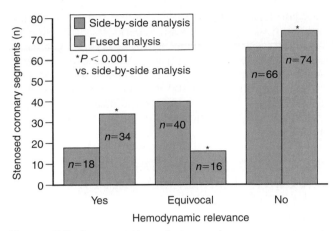

Figure 8-5 Interpretation of stenosed coronary segments with regard to their hemodynamic significance on side-by-side *(white columns)* or fused *(black columns)* analysis. *$P = 0.001$ for comparison of fused versus side-by-side analysis (chi-squared test). *(From Gaemperli O, Schepis T, Valenta I, et al: Cardiac image fusion from stand-alone SPECT and CT: Clinical experience. J Nucl Med 48:696-703, 2007. Reprinted with permission of the Society of Nuclear Medicine.)*

information of SPECT/CT fusion was more commonly found in patients with stenoses of small vessels such as diagonal or posterolateral branches. Hence, the hybrid approach allows reliable allocation of perfusion defects to its subtending coronary artery, compared to the side-by-side analysis—a finding that might be particularly useful to guide revascularization strategies in symptomatic patients with multivessel disease and/or intermediate-degree stenoses.

The role of elective PCI in patients with stable CAD is a matter of ongoing debate.[23,24] Guidelines recommend proof of ischemia prior to elective revascularization of coronary stenoses,[23,25,26] and several reports have demonstrated that PCI fails to improve prognosis in patients with stable CAD compared to conservative treatment.[24,27] These limitations have prompted the need for a comprehensive noninvasive CAD assessment prior to coronary revascularization. Hybrid cardiac imaging has the potential to fill this gap and become the long-awaited "One-Stop Shop," helping clinicians to more fully incorporate clinical evidence into their decision-making process in patients with CAD. Elective interventional therapy can be planned carefully, helping to avoid overuse of angioplasty and stent placement. This is extremely relevant because overuse of expensive intravascular stents is a key cost driver in invasive cardiology practice.[28] When lesion anatomy appears unsuitable for angioplasty, bypass grafting may be considered directly, without the need for further preoperative diagnostic coronary angiography, provided the noninvasive CT angiography images are of diagnostic quality.

VALUE OF HYBRID IMAGING FOR ATTENUATION CORRECTION

Strictly speaking, the term *hybrid imaging* refers to the combined or fused imaging of two data sets where both modalities equally contribute to image information. In a

wider sense, however, the use of low-dose CT information[29] for x-ray-based attenuation correction of myocardial perfusion images may also be considered "hybrid imaging." In this setting, the CT images do not provide added anatomic or functional information but are used to improve image quality of the other modality (i.e., PET or SPECT).

The sensitivity and specificity of cardiac SPECT or PET are commonly affected by image artifacts caused by photon attenuation. "Characteristic patterns" of attenuation in female and male patients are rendered unpredictable by the non-uniform attenuation characteristics of the human body, particularly in the chest area, and by the widely variable body habitus of individual patients. Breast and diaphragmatic attenuation are among the most common causes of these artifacts, but lateral wall artifacts due to obesity also occur.

Whereas the accuracy of cardiac PET imaging has long benefited from correction methods for tissue attenuation, in SPECT imaging, commercial methods have only recently been made available. Various techniques with different line sources, such as 241-americium (^{241}Am), 153-gadolinium (^{153}Gd), and 99m-technetium (^{99m}Tc) have been proposed. Initial reports indicate that some of these methods have achieved significant improvements, but that others have created more artifacts than they have remedied and have varied greatly in their clinical success.[30]

Certainly the use of CT for attenuation correction could well be an important step forward in solving some of the major attenuation-correction problems of the SPECT technique, allowing consistent image reading in male and female patients. Because of the recent introduction of this technique, only limited data are available. Although initial experiences seem promising,[31,32] there are some drawbacks that need to be overcome. For example, misalignment between SPECT and the attenuation map can lead to artifacts in the apical, septal, and anterior walls that will appear as defects. It also can cause overcorrection in the basal inferior and lateral segments. There is evidence that mismatches along the other directions may have a similar effect. The coregistration of SPECT and the attenuation map need to be verified for every patient, even when using integrated dual-modality imaging devices.[17]

In PET, the major advantage of using CT for attenuation correction is the short time duration (less than 5 seconds) compared with conventional correction with germanium sources (10 to 20 minutes). This allows the separation of the acquisitions of perfusion and viability PET scans, since the time loss for an additional transmission scan is minimal. Koepfli and coworkers reported a good feasibility and repeatability of this method for quantitative PET myocardial perfusion measurements. The results show that myocardial blood flow quantification is largely independent of CT tube current and document that electrocardiogram (ECG) gating of the CT beam seems not to be necessary.[29] Attenuation correction with CT provided results highly comparable to those obtained using germanium attenuation correction.

Although in SPECT, photon energies are lower (70 keV with 201-thallium [^{201}Tl], 140 keV with ^{99m}Tc

versus 511 keV with positron-emitting radionuclides) and thus more susceptible to photon attenuation, the use of x-ray-based attenuation correction is less well established compared to PET, because in general, attenuation correction for SPECT is more complex. Therefore, the latest developments in SPECT technology have aimed in a different direction: at reducing acquisition times and/or lowering radiation exposures, rather than addressing the issue of attenuation correction. Thus no attenuation correction is available in most dedicated cardiac SPECT scanners.[33] The lack of an inherent attenuation correction facility can be overcome by using low-dose native coronary artery CACs scans performed on a standalone high-end CT device for attenuation correction of the SPECT images. In contrast to present low-dose CT facilities of hybrid SPECT/CT scanners, CACS scans are ECG-triggered and acquired during a single breath hold. Furthermore, this approach requires the use of interface software for manual coregistration of SPECT and CT information to avoid misalignment between both images (Fig. 8-6). The feasibility and reproducibility of this method have been demonstrated in a recent publication by Schepis and coworkers using CACS scans during full inspiratory and expiratory breath hold.[16] Parametric attenuation maps from CACS scans provided accurate and reliable attenuation correction of SPECT images, resulting in a very good correlation compared to the established attenuation correction with the low-dose low-resolution CT facility included in

the hybrid SPECT/CT scanner. Interestingly, the expiratory CACS scan proved slightly superior to the inspiratory scan, particularly for regional tracer uptake values in apical and inferior segments, notably those segments most affected by attenuation artifacts (Fig. 8-7). This finding suggests that in hybrid scans, CACS scan may be performed during normal expiration to allow its additional use for attenuation correction of SPECT images.

PROGNOSTIC AND DIAGNOSTIC VALUE OF CORONARY ARTERY CALCIUM SCORES (See Chapter 20)

CACS provides an estimate of coronary atherosclerotic plaque burden and correlates strongly with the overall amount of coronary plaque (calcified and noncalcified) as determined at postmortem examination.[34] Assessment of the presence of subclinical coronary atherosclerosis with CACS provides an opportunity to identify asymptomatic patients who are at risk of developing clinical coronary artery disease (CAD) over the long term. Several studies in asymptomatic subjects have consistently shown that CACS provides accurate risk estimates for cardiac death and ischemic events beyond the risk calculations derived from clinical parameters.[35] These observations have led to the implementation of

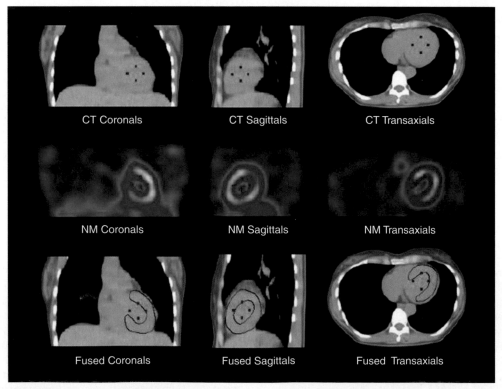

Figure 8-6 Coronal, sagittal, and transaxial computed tomography (CT) images are fused with the non-corrected SPECT images to verify the alignment of the coregistration. When necessary, misalignment may be corrected by manually adjusting CT images to obtain optimal alignment with the SPECT images. *(From Schepis T, Gaemperli O, Koepfli P, et al: Use of coronary calcium score scans from stand-alone multislice computed tomography for attenuation correction of myocardial perfusion SPECT. Eur J Nucl Med Mol Imaging 34:11-19, 2007. Reprinted with permission of the European Society of Nuclear Medicine.)*

APEX

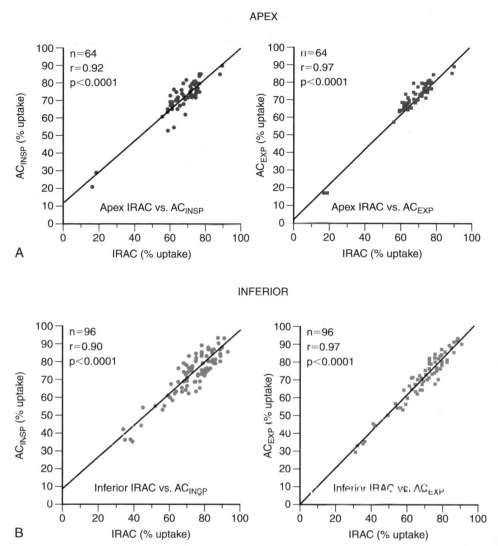

Figure 8-7 Linear regression analysis for percent radiotracer uptake between hybrid SPECT/CT scanner (with low-dose low-resolution CT facility incorporated for attenuation correction [AC]) and SPECT images reconstructed with coronary calcium scans obtained from standalone high-end CT scanner at inspiration (AC_{INSP}) and expiration (AC_{EXP}) in the (A) apical and (B) inferior myocardial regions. IRAC, Iterative reconstruction with AC. *(From Schepis T, Gaemperli O, Koepfli P, et al: Use of coronary calcium score scans from stand-alone multislice computed tomography for attenuation correction of myocardial perfusion SPECT. Eur J Nucl Med Mol Imaging 34:11-19, 2007. Reprinted with permission of the European Society of Nuclear Medicine.)*

CACS in current recommendations for coronary risk assessment.[35,36] Particularly in patients at intermediate clinical risk, CACS may prove helpful in further stratifying those patients into low-, intermediate-, and high-risk categories.[37]

In addition to its prognostic value, CACS may also offer diagnostic information. Coronary artery calcifications are almost always extant in the presence of angiographically significant CAD, so a CACS of 0 virtually excludes any significant angiographic CAD. In the largest study to date comparing CACS with conventional coronary angiography, sensitivity and negative predictive values of CACS for detecting angiographically significant CAD were 99% and 97%, respectively, indicating an excellent ability of CACS to rule out

obstructive CAD.[38] However, specificity and positive predictive value (23% and 62%) were low and increased only moderately when shifting the CACS cutoff from 0 to higher values. These limitations are the reason why CACS is not recommended as a single first-line imaging tool for the evaluation of symptomatic patients with suspected CAD.

An alternative approach, however, is using CACS in combination with myocardial perfusion imaging for the diagnosis of CAD, inasmuch as CACS is being made increasingly available with the introduction of hybrid scanners. In a recent study by Schepis and colleagues, the combination of SPECT and CACS resulted in a significant improvement in sensitivity and specificity for the diagnosis of angiographically significant CAD compared

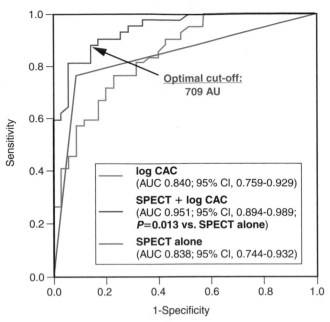

Figure 8-8 Receiver operating characteristic (ROC) curve for detection of significant coronary artery disease (≥ 50% stenosis on coronary angiography) by SPECT, coronary artery calcium score (CACS), and the combination of both. Combining SPECT and CACS results in a significant improvement in diagnostic accuracy. AU, Agatson units. AUC, area under the curve. *(Modified from Schepis T, Gaemperli O, Koepfli P, et al: Added value of coronary artery calcium score as an adjunct to gated SPECT for the evaluation of coronary artery disease in an intermediate-risk population. J Nucl Med 48:1424-1430, 2007.)*

to SPECT alone (Fig. 8-8). These findings suggest a potential role of CACS as an adjunct to SPECT for the noninvasive evaluation of CAD. It seems reasonable to elaborate algorithms where the combination of CACS with myocardial perfusion studies may help refine the interpretation of the latter. On the one hand, the presence of high atherosclerotic burden in a symptomatic patient with a normal perfusion scan may suggest significant multivessel disease with balanced ischemia. On the other hand, an equivocal perfusion result in the presence of very low CACS may raise the suspicion of an attenuation or respiratory artifact, justifying further CAD rule-out with CT angiography. However, despite encouraging results, the real role of the calcium score in the cascade of noninvasive investigations of CAD remains to be determined.

HYBRID SCANNERS VERSUS HYBRID IMAGING

Despite the widespread use of coronary CT angiography and myocardial perfusion imaging (MPI) with SPECT or PET, both techniques vary considerably in their image acquisition times. Whereas coronary CT angiography with the newest generation 64-slice or dual-source CT devices is performed in less than 12 seconds,[12] emission scans for stress and rest gated SPECT with 99mTc-based radiotracers at standard doses take at least 45 minutes.[39] This discrepancy between emission and transmission scan times determines that high-end CT facilities constituting the CT component of hybrid cardiac scanners will be blocked by long emission scan times and therefore operate at low capacity. Many advances in nuclear medicine, such as newly developed dedicated cardiac detector systems[33] and novel image reconstruction algorithms,[40] may contribute to reducing emission scan times considerably. However, to date, in hybrid scanners with high-end CT facilities, the rather long emission scan times preclude operating the high-end CT device at full capacity. Additionally, despite the promise of hybrid cardiac imaging, first clinical experiences with hybrid SPECT/CT imaging have shown that in an usual population referred for noninvasive workup of CAD, only a minority benefit from hybrid imaging, compared to side-by-side interpretation of MPI and CT.[3] Thus at present, it appears that seen from the standpoint of patient throughput, a dedicated cardiac hybrid scanner is less profitable than two standalone devices for normal-volume nuclear diagnostic centers. Nonetheless, it will depend on the individual setting of each institution to determine the type of approach—that is, software-based fusion or hybrid scanner—that is best tailored for its particular purpose, and highly specialized cardiac centers may prefer hybrid scanners for integrative cardiac imaging.

PERSPECTIVES OF HYBRID IMAGING

Hybrid imaging is a new and highly dynamic field of continuing research driven by constant advances in technology, innovations in noninvasive imaging, and increasing clinical interest in this promising tool. Efforts to improve techniques and implement hybrid imaging in daily clinical routine are ongoing. The advent of ultrafast dedicated cardiac SPECT scanners with short acquisition times[33] and their incorporation with multislice CT devices into hybrid scanners will reduce dead-time issues and allow for higher patient throughput and improvement of scanner efficiency. Furthermore, the increasing use of prospective ECG-gating protocols for coronary CT angiography will help to reduce radiation burden to approximately 2.0 to 2.5 mSv,[41] a dose that allows hybrid scanning at a reasonable radiation exposure (Fig. 8-9). First trials using hybrid imaging with PET/CT reported a reduction of 60% to 73% in radiation exposure using a prospective ECG-triggered protocol compared to retrospectively triggered spiral acquisition, without any loss in image quality.[42,43] In a recent SPECT/CT trial, a comparable reduction of 78% was reported for hybrid stress-only SPECT/CT in a low-pretest probability population. The resulting total effective dose was 5.4 mSv for hybrid imaging with prospective ECG-triggering for CT angiography.[44]

Myocardial perfusion imaging is by far the most important application of nuclear studies in cardiology.

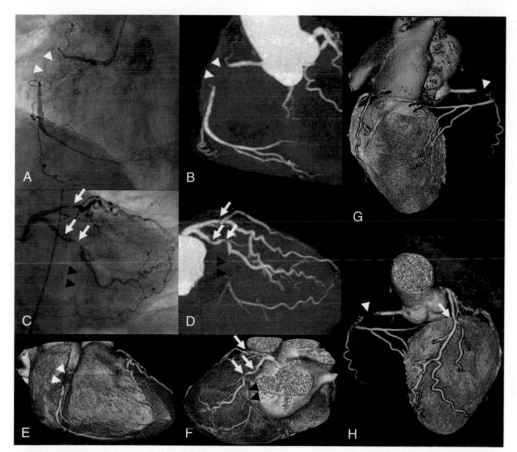

Figure 8-9 In a 66-year-old patient with prolonged episodes of chest pain, images **A-H** reveal total occlusions of the right coronary artery (RCA) *(white arrowheads)* and the distal left circumflex artery (LCX) *(black arrowheads)*, with retrograde filling of the vessels (**A** and **C,** catheter angiography; **B** and **D,** computed tomography angiography (CTA) maximum intensity projections; **E** and **F,** volume rendered CTA; **G** and **H,** fused PET/CTA images. Additionally, two sequential significant stenoses are demonstrated proximal to the total occlusion in the LCX and one in the proximal left anterior descending artery (LAD) *(white arrows)*. Noninvasive assessment of viability was performed by [18-F] fluorodeoxyglucose PET and fused with CTA to identify culprit lesions with their respective territory. CTA was performed using prospective gating; the applied radiation dose of CTA was 1.2 mSv. Fused PET/CTA images (**G** and **H**) demonstrated a large scar in the inferior myocardium, corresponding to the total occlusion of the RCA, and infarcted scar tissue with partially preserved viability in the anterior myocardium, corresponding to the presumably recanalized lesion in the LAD. The lateral myocardium was viable, despite the total occlusion in the distal LCX, most probably due to collaterals, which lead to retrograde filling of the vessel. *(From Husmann L, Valenta I, Weber K, et al: Cardiac fusion imaging with low-dose computed tomography using prospective electrocardiogram gating. Clin Nucl Med 33:490-491, 2008. Reprinted with permission from Clinical Nuclear Medicine.)*

However, software-based hybrid imaging allows free combination of morphologic images with any nuclear study. This widens the potential use of hybrid imaging by including studies for cardiac innervation, metabolism, gene expression and stem cell imaging, and plaque imaging, and by combining different modalities such as CT, nuclear techniques, or cardiac magnetic resonance (Fig. 8-10).[45,46] Nevertheless, atherosclerotic disease is responsible for high morbidity and mortality in industrialized countries. Despite major advances in treatment of CAD patients, a large number of victims of the disease who are apparently healthy die suddenly without prior symptoms. The recognition of the role of the vulnerable plaque has opened new avenues of opportunity in the field of cardiovascular medicine.[47] The hybrid technology has the unique potential to enable detection and quantification of the burden of calcified and noncalcified plaques, quantification of vascular reactivity and endothelial health, identification of flow-limiting coronary stenoses, and (potentially) identification of high-risk plaques using fusion of morphology and biology with molecularly targeted PET imaging.[48] By this means, in the future, hybrid imaging may allow easy and comprehensive noninvasive assessment of coronary plaque burden, its pathophysiologic relevance, and biological plaque activity, providing accurate individual risk estimates upon which further management decisions can be based.

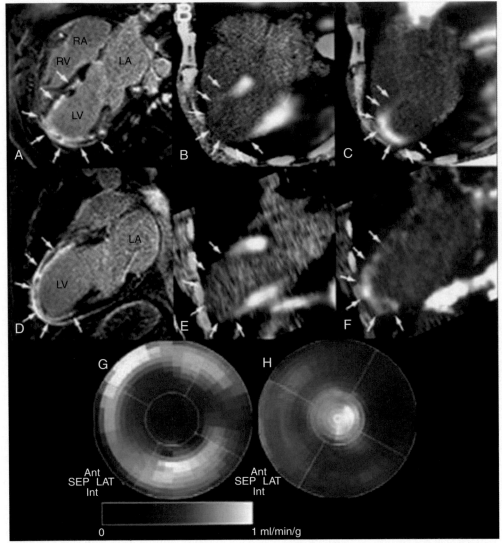

Figure 8-10 Multimodality imaging with cardiac magnetic resonance (CMR) and PET. **A** and **D** show horizontal and vertical long-axis slices of CMR. Late gadolinium hyperenhancement in the apex demonstrates a nearly transmural myocardial scar. **B** and **E** reveal diminished perfusion assessed with ^{13}N-ammonia PET in the apical, apicoanterior, and inferoseptal regions. In images **C** and **F,** PET with ^{18}F-RGD (a novel PET agent targeting $\alpha_v\beta_3$ integrin, a key mediator of angiogenesis) demonstrates focal tracer uptake in the infarcted area. This signal co-localizes to the regions of delayed hyperenhancement on CMR and indicates the presence of myocardial repair processes after ischemic injury. The complementary representation of perfusion with ^{13}N-ammonia (**G**) and angiogenesis in the infarcted apical myocardium (**H**) is visualized with polar maps. *(From Mankowski RM, Ebersberger U, Nekolla S, Schwaiger M: In vivo molecular imaging of angiogenesis, targeting alpha$_v$ beta$_3$ integrin expression in a patient after acute myocardial infarction. Eur Heart J 29:2201, 2008. Reprinted with permission of Oxford University Press.)*

REFERENCES

1. Topol EJ, Nissen SE: Our preoccupation with coronary luminology. The dissociation between clinical and angiographic findings in ischemic heart disease, *Circulation* 92(8):2333–2342, 1995.
2. Silber S, Albertsson P, Aviles FF, Camici PG, Colombo A, Hamm C, et al: Guidelines for percutaneous coronary interventions. The Task Force for Percutaneous Coronary Interventions of the European Society of Cardiology, *Eur Heart J* 26(8):804–847, 2005.
3. Gaemperli O, Schepis T, Valenta I, Husmann L, Scheffel H, Duerst V, et al: Cardiac image fusion from stand-alone SPECT and CT: clinical experience, *J Nucl Med* 48(5):696–703, 2007.
4. Namdar M, Hany TF, Koepfli P, Siegrist PT, Burger C, Wyss CA, et al: Integrated PET/CT for the assessment of coronary artery disease: a feasibility study, *J Nucl Med* 46(6):930–935, 2005.
5. Gourtsoyiannis N, McCall I, Reiser M, Silberman B, Bischof Delaloye A, Carrio I, et al: White paper of the European Society of Radiology (ESR) and the European Association of Nuclear Medicine (EANM) on multimodality imaging, *Eur Radiol* 17(8):1926–1930, 2007.
6. Faber TL, Santana CA, Garcia EV, Candell-Riera J, Folks RD, Peifer JW, et al: Three-dimensional fusion of coronary arteries with myocardial perfusion distributions: clinical validation, *J Nucl Med* 45(5):745–753, 2004.
7. Schindler TH, Magosaki N, Jeserich M, Oser U, Krause T, Fischer R, et al: Fusion imaging: combined visualization of 3D reconstructed coronary artery tree and 3D myocardial scintigraphic image in coronary artery disease, *Int J Card Imaging* 15(5):357–368, 1999 discussion 369–70.
8. Peifer JW, Ezquerra NF, Cooke CD, Mullick R, Klein L, Hyche ME, et al: Visualization of multimodality cardiac imagery, *IEEE Trans Biomed Eng* 37(8):744–756, 1990.
9. Nishimura Y, Fukuchi K, Katafuchi T, Sagou M, Oka H, Ishida Y, et al: Superimposed display of coronary artery on gated myocardial perfusion scintigraphy, *J Nucl Med* 45(9):1444–1449, 2004.
10. Fishman EK, Ney DR, Heath DG, Corl FM, Horton KM, Johnson PT: Volume rendering versus maximum intensity projection in CT angiography: what works best, when, and why, *Radiographics* 26(3):905–922, 2006.

11. Bax JJ, Beanlands RS, Klocke FJ, Knuuti J, Lammertsma AA, Schaefers MA, et al: Diagnostic and clinical perspectives of fusion imaging in cardiology: is the total greater than the sum of its parts? *Heart* 93(1):16–22, 2007.

12. Leschka S, Scheffel H, Desbiolles L, Plass A, Gaemperli O, Valenta I, et al: Image quality and reconstruction intervals of dual-source CT coronary angiography: recommendations for ECG-pulsing windowing, *Invest Radiol* 42(8):543–549, 2007.

13. Gilman MD, Fischman AJ, Krishnasetty V, Halpern EF, Aquino SL: Hybrid PET/CT of the thorax: when is computer registration necessary? *J Comput Assist Tomogr* 31(3):395–401, 2007.

14. Gould KL, Pan T, Loghin C, Johnson NP, Guha A, Sdringola S: Frequent diagnostic errors in cardiac PET/CT due to misregistration of CT attenuation and emission PET images: a definitive analysis of causes, consequences, and corrections, *J Nucl Med* 48(7):1112–1121, 2007.

15. Gaemperli O, Kaufmann PA: Hybrid cardiac imaging: more than the sum of its parts? *J Nucl Cardiol* 15(1):123–126, 2008.

16. Schepis T, Gaemperli O, Koepfli P, Ruegg C, Burger C, Leschka S, et al: Use of coronary calcium score scans from stand-alone multislice computed tomography for attenuation correction of myocardial perfusion SPECT, *Eur J Nucl Med Mol Imaging* 34(1):11–19, 2007.

17. Goetze S, Wahl RL: Prevalence of misregistration between SPECT and CT for attenuation-corrected myocardial perfusion SPECT, *J Nucl Cardiol* 14(2):200–206, 2007.

18. Gaemperli O, Schepis T, Kalff V, Namdar M, Valenta I, Stefani L, et al: Validation of a new cardiac image fusion software for three-dimensional integration of myocardial perfusion SPECT and stand-alone 64-slice CT angiography, *Eur J Nucl Med Mol Imaging* 34(7): 1097–1106, 2007.

19. Achenbach S, Daniel WG: Noninvasive coronary angiography—an acceptable alternative? *N Engl J Med* 345(26):1909–1910, 2001.

20. Schuijf JD, Jukema JW, van der Wall EE, Bax JJ: The current status of multislice computed tomography in the diagnosis and prognosis of coronary artery disease, *J Nucl Cardiol* 14(4):604–612, 2007.

21. Rispler S, Keidar Z, Ghersin E, Roguin A, Soil A, Dragu R, et al: Integrated single-photon emission computed tomography and computed tomography coronary angiography for the assessment of hemodynamically significant coronary artery lesions, *J Am Coll Cardiol* 49(10):1059–1067, 2007.

22. Santana CA, Garcia EV, Faber TL, Sinusas GK, Esteves FP, Sanyal R, et al: Diagnostic performance of fusion of myocardial perfusion imaging (MPI) and computed tomography coronary angiography, *J Nucl Cardiol* 16:201–211, 2009.

23. Fox K, Garcia MA, Ardissino D, Buszman P, Camici PG, Crea F, et al: Guidelines on the management of stable angina pectoris: executive summary: the Task Force on the Management of Stable Angina Pectoris of the European Society of Cardiology, *Eur Heart J* 27 (11):1341–1381, 2006.

24. Boden WE, O'Rourke RA, Teo KK, Hartigan PM, Maron DJ, Kostuk WJ, et al: Optimal medical therapy with or without PCI for stable disease, *N Engl J Med* 356(15):1503–1516, 2007.

25. Smith SC Jr, Feldman TE, Hirshfeld JW Jr, Jacobs AK, Kern MJ, King SB 3rd, et al: ACC/AHA/SCAI 2005 guideline update for percutaneous coronary intervention: a report of the American College of Cardiology/ American Heart Association Task Force on Practice Guidelines (ACC/ AHA/SCAI Writing Committee to Update the 2001 Guidelines for Percutaneous Coronary Intervention), *J Am Coll Cardiol* 47(1):e1–121, 2006.

26. Gibbons RJ, Abrams J, Chatterjee K, Daley J, Deedwania PC, Douglas JS, et al: ACC/AHA 2002 guideline update for the management of patients with chronic stable angina—summary article: a report of the American College of Cardiology/American Heart Association Task Force on practice guidelines (Committee on the Management of Patients With Chronic Stable Angina), *J Am Coll Cardiol* 41 (1):159–168, 2003.

27. Bucher HC, Hengstler P, Schindler C, Guyatt GH: Percutaneous transluminal coronary angioplasty versus medical treatment for non-acute coronary heart disease: meta-analysis of randomised controlled trials, *BMJ* 321(7253):73–77, 2000.

28. Kaiser C, Brunner-La Rocca HP, Buser PT, Bonetti PO, Osswald S, Linka A, et al: Incremental cost-effectiveness of drug-eluting stents compared with a third-generation bare-metal stent in a real-world setting: randomised Basel Stent Kosten Effektivitats Trial (BASKET), *Lancet* 366(9489):921–929, 2005.

29. Koepfli P, Hany TF, Wyss CA, Namdar M, Burger C, Konstantinidis AV, et al: CT attenuation correction for myocardial perfusion quantification using a PET/CT hybrid scanner, *J Nucl Med* 45(4):537–542, 2004.

30. Corbett JR, Ficaro EP: Attenuation corrected cardiac perfusion SPECT, *Curr Opin Cardiol* 15(5):330–336, 2000.

31. Utsunomiya D, Tomiguchi S, Shiraishi S, Yamada K, Honda T, Kawanaka K, et al: Initial experience with x-ray CT based attenuation correction in myocardial perfusion SPECT imaging using a combined SPECT/CT system, *Ann Nucl Med* 19(6):485–489, 2005.

32. Fricke E, Fricke H, Weise R, Kammeier A, Hagedorn R, Lotz N, et al: Attenuation correction of myocardial SPECT perfusion images with low-dose CT: evaluation of the method by comparison with perfusion PET, *J Nucl Med* 46(5):736–744, 2005.

33. Patton JA, Slomka PJ, Germano G, Berman DS: Recent technologic advances in nuclear cardiology, *J Nucl Cardiol* 14(4):501–513, 2007.

34. Rumberger JA, Simons DB, Fitzpatrick LA, Sheedy PF, Schwartz RS: Coronary artery calcium area by electron-beam computed tomography and coronary atherosclerotic plaque area. A histopathologic correlative study, *Circulation* 92(8):2157–2162, 1995.

35. Berman DS, Hachamovitch R, Shaw LJ, Friedman JD, Hayes SW, Thomson LE, et al: Roles of nuclear cardiology, cardiac computed tomography, and cardiac magnetic resonance: Noninvasive risk stratification and a conceptual framework for the selection of noninvasive imaging tests in patients with known or suspected coronary artery disease, *J Nucl Med* 47(7):1107–1118, 2006.

36. Grundy SM, Cleeman JI, Merz CN, Brewer HB Jr, Clark LT, Hunninghake DB, et al: Implications of recent clinical trials for the National Cholesterol Education Program Adult Treatment Panel III guidelines, *Circulation* 110(2):227–239, 2004.

37. Greenland P, Bonow RO, Brundage BH, Budoff MJ, Eisenberg MJ, Grundy SM, et al: ACCF/AHA 2007 clinical expert consensus document on coronary artery calcium scoring by computed tomography in global cardiovascular risk assessment and in evaluation of patients with chest pain: a report of the American College of Cardiology Foundation Clinical Expert Consensus Task Force (ACCF/AHA Writing Committee to Update the 2000 Expert Consensus Document on Electron Beam Computed Tomography) developed in collaboration with the Society of Atherosclerosis Imaging and Prevention and the Society of Cardiovascular Computed Tomography, *J Am Coll Cardiol* 49(3): 378–402, 2007.

38. Haberl R, Becker A, Leber A, Knez A, Becker C, Lang C, et al: Correlation of coronary calcification and angiographically documented stenoses in patients with suspected coronary artery disease: results of 1,764 patients, *J Am Coll Cardiol* 37(2):451–457, 2001.

39. Hansen CL, Goldstein RA, Berman DS, Churchwell KB, Cooke CD, Corbett JR, et al: Myocardial perfusion and function single photon emission computed tomography, *J Nucl Cardiol* 13(6):e97–e120, 2006.

40. Borges-Neto S, Pagnanelli RA, Shaw LK, Honeycutt E, Shwartz SC, Adams GL, et al: Clinical results of a novel wide beam reconstruction method for shortening scan time of Tc-99m cardiac SPECT perfusion studies, *J Nucl Cardiol* 14(4):555–565, 2007.

41. Husmann L, Valenta I, Gaemperli O, Adda O, Treyer V, Wyss CA, et al: Feasibility of low-dose coronary CT angiography: first experience with prospective ECG-gating, *Eur Heart J* 29(2):191–197, 2008.

42. Kajander S, Ukkonen H, Sipila H, Teras M, Knuuti J: Low radiation dose imaging of myocardial perfusion and coronary angiography with a hybrid PET/CT scanner, *Clin Physiol Funct Imaging* 29(1):81–88, 2009.

43. Javadi M, Mahesh M, McBride G, Voicu C, Epley W, Merrill J, et al: Lowering radiation dose for integrated assessment of coronary morphology and physiology: first experience with step-and-shoot CT angiography in a rubidium 82 PET-CT protocol, *J Nucl Cardiol* 15(6): 783–790, 2008.

44. Husmann L, Herzog BA, Gaemperli O, Tatsugami F, Burkhard N, Valenta I, et al: Diagnostic accuracy of computed tomography coronary angiography and evaluation of stress-only single-photon emission computed tomography/computed tomography hybrid imaging: comparison of prospective electrocardiogram-triggering vs. retrospective gating, *Eur Heart J* 2008.

45. Nekolla SG, Martinez-Moeller A, Saraste A: PET and MRI in cardiac imaging: from validation studies to integrated applications, *Eur J Nucl Med Mol Imaging* 2008.

46. Makowski MR, Ebersberger U, Nekolla S, Schwaiger M: In vivo molecular imaging of angiogenesis, targeting alphavbeta3 integrin expression, in a patient after acute myocardial infarction, *Eur Heart J* 29 (18):2201, 2008.

47. Naghavi M, Libby P, Falk E, Casscells SW, Litovsky S, Rumberger J, et al: From vulnerable plaque to vulnerable patient: a call for new definitions and risk assessment strategies: Part I, *Circulation* 108 (14):1664–1672, 2003.

48. Di Carli MF, Hachamovitch R: New technology for noninvasive evaluation of coronary artery disease, *Circulation* 115(11):1464–1480, 2007.

Chapter 9

Digital/Fast SPECT: Systems and Software

PIOTR SLOMKA, JAMES A. PATTON, DANIEL S. BERMAN
AND GUIDO GERMANO

"Dr. Berman has indicated that he has relationship with Spectrum Dynamics that, in the context of their participation in the writing of a chapter for the fourth edition of Clinical Nuclear Cardiology, could be perceived by some people as a real or apparent conflict of interest, but do not consider that it has influenced the writing of their chapter."

INTRODUCTION

Single-photon emission computed tomography (SPECT) myocardial perfusion imaging (MPI) has become a widely used and well-established medical imaging test. However, it suffers from some fundamental limitations that include long image acquisition, low image resolution, and patient radiation dose. Scan time is generally on the order of 15 to 20 minutes for each stress and rest acquisition, resulting in long overall test times and frequent artifacts from patient motion during the scan. Reduction of imaging times has been long recognized as an important factor in reducing patient motion artifacts and increasing throughput. Various efforts have been taken to reduce this time with standard equipment and cameras.[1–3] Furthermore, the recent increase in the use of coronary computed tomography angiography (CCTA) in patients who also have SPECT MPI studies has intensified the concern about the levels of radiation associated with SPECT.[4] Some of these limitations are intrinsically linked to each other; longer acquisition times could be used with lower injected doses, and higher doses could be used to shorten acquisition times.

The key performance parameter controlling these limitations is the scanner/camera photon sensitivity, which is primarily controlled by the type of collimator and imaging geometry used in the imaging system. Typically, obtaining higher resolution images requires lowering image sensitivity. For over 2 decades, dual-head scintillation cameras with parallel-hole collimators, typically configured in a 90-degree detector geometry, have been the workhorses of SPECT MPI. Image reconstruction for SPECT MPI has been performed with standard filtered backprojection (FBP) algorithms. Recently, however, there have been several efforts by industry and academic researchers to develop new imaging systems and new methods of image reconstruction that will simultaneously allow higher photon sensitivity and improve both image quality and resolution.

The initial clinical results that are being reported demonstrate potential for equivalent diagnostic performance by MPI scans obtained with much lower doses or in much shorter time periods. These efforts address the main limitations of SPECT MPI by multiple approaches such as changing the detector geometry and optimizing tomographic sampling of the field of view for myocardial imaging, improving the detector material and collimator design, and optimizing the image reconstruction algorithms. In this chapter, we summarize these recent developments by various groups and companies in the field.

DEDICATED CARDIAC IMAGING SYSTEMS

Several new dedicated hardware camera systems that have been introduced by various vendors for cardiac imaging attempt to improve imaging parameters primarily by optimizing acquisition geometry, collimator design, and reconstruction software.[5] Innovative designs of the gantry and detectors have been introduced that allow increased sampling of the myocardial region and thus allow better local sensitivity for MPI imaging. The primary goals for the development of these systems are twofold: (1) to achieve improved spatial resolution and sensitivity and therefore allow for faster imaging times and (2) to improve patient comfort by permitting imaging in an upright or reclining position, eliminating the need to position the patient's arms above the head. Furthermore, claustrophobic effects have been reduced or eliminated by technologies that reduce the size of the detector geometries and the associated mechanical structures. Overall sizes of the systems have also been reduced so they can be placed in locations with minimal available floor space. As a consequence of faster imaging times and more comfortable patient positioning, these systems have the additional benefit of reducing patient motion during a scan. In this section, we describe various available hardware designs and related reconstruction techniques.

Digirad Cardius 3 XPO

The first of these systems to be introduced was the Cardius XPO line manufactured by Digirad Corporation (Poway, CA). Although the initial design of a similar Digirad system was described in 1998 with the use of cadmium zinc telluride (CdZnTe, or CZT),[6] all manufactured systems use solid-state cesium iodide (CsI)-photodiode detectors. This system can be configured in 1-, 2-, or 3-detector configurations.[7] The Cardius 3 XPO is shown in Figure 9-1. Current models make use of pixilated CsI(Tl) detectors and photodiodes to configure detector heads that are more compact than conventional cameras equipped with photomultipliers. Each detector head is 21.2 × 15.8 cm and contains an array of 768 6.1 × 6.1 × 5 mm-thick CsI(Tl) crystals coupled to individual silicon photodiodes that are used to convert the light output of the crystals to electrical pulses. Digital software logic is used to process the signals and create images instead of analog Anger positional circuits. In the three-detector system, the detector heads are positioned at 67.5 degrees between heads, as shown in Figure 9-2. Heads are allowed to be moved in and out (closer to or farther away from the patient). For imaging, the patient sits on a chair with his arms placed on an armrest above the detectors. Data acquisition is typically accomplished in 7.5 minutes by rotating the patient chair by 67.5 degrees, producing a total acquisition arc of 202.5 degrees. With this system, the

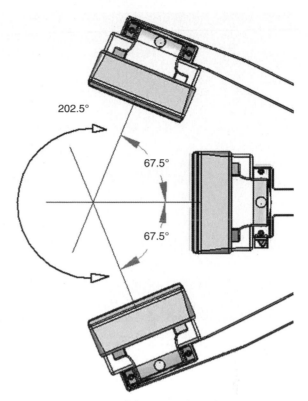

Figure 9-2 Geometry of the Digirad Cardius 3 XPO camera. Detectors remain fixed while patient is rotated through 202.5 degrees in a rotating chair. *(Images courtesy of Digirad Corp., San Diego, CA.)*

manufacturer reports a reconstructed spatial resolution of 8.95 mm (at a 20-cm orbit radius) and a sensitivity of 234 cpm/μCi, using the system's cardiac collimator and a three-dimensional (3D) version of the ordered subset expectation maximization (OSEM) approach for reconstruction. Images of a patient with an inferior-wall defect acquired with this system are shown in Figure 9-3. These systems are now used clinically in several sites, and preliminary reports have been published comparing

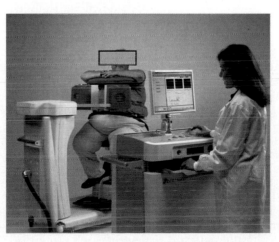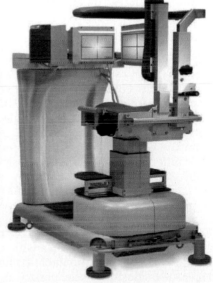

Figure 9-1 Upright patient position on the Digirad Cardius 3 XPO triple-head, pixilated detector camera *(left)* and photograph of the camera *(right)*. *(Images courtesy of Digirad Corp., San Diego, CA.)*

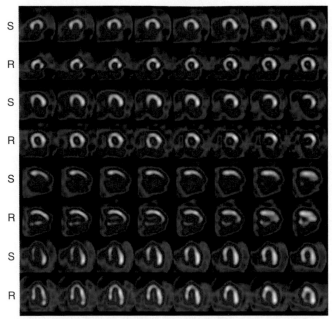

Figure 9-3 Typical SPECT scans obtained with Cardius 3 (C 3) XPO. A technetium-99m-sestamibi study of a patient with an inferior wall defect imaged with the C 3 XPO camera. Sex: male, Height: 5 feet 11 inches. Weight: 240 pounds. Age: 73. Stress: adenosine. Acquisition time: rest, 8.6 minutes; stress, 6.9 minutes. Dose: rest, 10.2 mCi (sestamibi); stress, 32.3 mCi (sestamibi). *(Images courtesy of Digirad Corp., San Diego, CA.)*

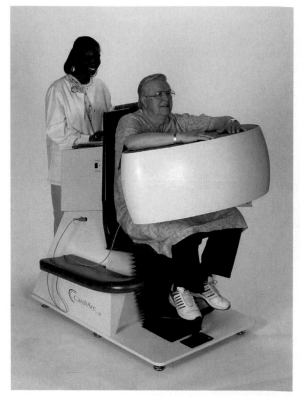

Figure 9-4 Photograph of the CardiArc SPECT-HD demonstrating patient positioning for optimal cardiac imaging and the technologist in the operating position, taking advantage of the built-in radiation shielding. *(Figure from CardiArc Ltd., with permission.)*

their performance to that of a standard dual-headed camera when it was found that similar quality could be obtained with a 38% reduction in acquisition time.[8]

Preliminary data have recently shown that the acquisition time can be further reduced with this scanner by the application of optimized image reconstruction protocols developed by Digirad. The nSPEED reconstruction[9] models the depth-dependent detector spatial response of the SPECT systems with a 3D version of the OSEM reconstruction method. In preliminary reports,[10] the image quality improvement with nSPEED, compared to a conventional two-dimensional OSEM technique,[11] enables the reduction of acquisition time by 50% while maintaining image quality and information.

CardiArc

CardiArc Limited (Canton, MI) has developed a dedicated nuclear cardiology SPECT camera in which the detector and collimator are redesigned and optimized specifically for cardiac imaging.[12] This device has no visibly moving parts but has a single internally moving part, which is hidden from the patient.[13] Therefore, from the outside, the detector appears motionless, and for comfort the patient can be positioned upright. Scan times reported by the company are as short as 2 minutes.[12] The camera system and a typical patient position are shown in Figure 9-4. This system was originally designed to use arrays of CZT crystals as detectors. However, owing to the high cost of CZT material and potential long-term stability issues with CZT,[14] the detector design was changed to enable commercial production. Figure 9-5 illustrates the design and the principle of

operation of the current model. The system incorporates a high-resolution detector with three curved sodium iodide–thallium (NaI[Tl]) crystals with graduated grooving technology and an array of 60 photomultiplier tubes arranged in three rows (see Fig. 9-5A). The gantry uses a proprietary digital process developed by CardiArc that replaces the conventional Anger logic. Horizontal photon collimation in each slice is accomplished using a thin, curved lead sheet with six narrow vertical slots (aperture arc; see Fig. 9-5A). Vertical slice collimation is accomplished using a series of stationary lead vanes that are stacked vertically between the aperture arc and the NaI(Tl) crystals (see Fig. 9-5B). In this way, data are collected as multiple 1 mm–thick slices using the six vertical apertures to collimate photons so they are detected continuously across the detector surface, with no overlap of data from different apertures. During acquisition, the aperture arc rotates to acquire data from multiple projections, providing 1280 angular samples in 0.14-degree increments over 180 degrees, which is an order of magnitude greater than the conventional camera angular sampling (typically 3 degrees). All detector pixels are active simultaneously, and photons can be detected from multiple angles (see Fig. 9-5C). The movement of the aperture arc is synchronized electronically with the areas of the NaI(Tl) crystals that are imaging the photons passing through the individual slots. The aperture arc's weight of 35 pounds is lighter than traditional moving gantries, which facilities motion control. The aperture arc movement ranges 9 inches to cover

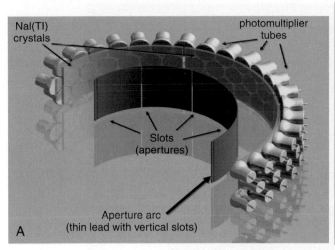

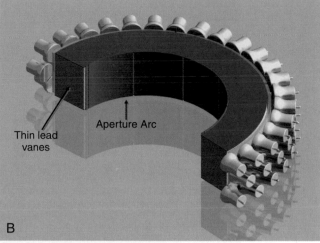

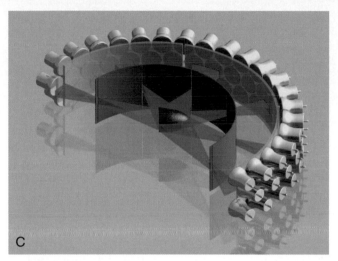

Figure 9-5 Design and principle of operation of CardiArc camera. The camera uses three stationary sodium iodide–thallium crystals and corresponding photomultiplier tubes for photon detection (**A**). The aperture arc has six slots (apertures) for horizontal collimation and continuously rotates while imaging. Vertical collimation is achieved by a stack of stationary thin lead vanes, individually separated by foam, that are set between the aperture arc and the detector crystals (**B**). All detector pixels are utilized simultaneously, allowing imaging of multiple angles (**C**). *(Figure from CardiArc Ltd., with permission.)*

the entire cardiac field of view, and each traverse of the arc takes 10 seconds.

SPECT reconstructed spatial resolution values (full-width half-maximum) quoted by CardiArc range from 3.6 mm (at 82 mm source-to-aperture arc distance) to 7.8 mm (at 337 mm source-to-aperture arc distance). An independent evaluation concluded that the CardiArc system appears to gain image quality by a factor of 5 to 10 when compared to the conventional dual-head camera.[15] A comparison of patient imaging capabilities is shown in Figure 9-6.

Spectrum Dynamics

Spectrum Dynamics (Haifa, Israel) has manufactured a system called *D-SPECT*. The design and principle of its operation are shown in Figure 9-7. The patient is imaged in either a semireclining position with the left arm placed on top of the camera (see Fig. 9-7A) or in the supine position. Acquisition time as short as 2 minutes has been reported.[16] This system uses pixilated CZT detector arrays (see Fig. 9-7B) mounted in nine vertical

columns and placed in a 90-degree gantry geometry (see Fig. 9-7C). While CZT detectors are higher in cost, they have advantages of superior energy resolution (by a factor of approximately 1.7 at 140 keV) and compact size compared to the combination of NaI(Tl) with photomultiplier tubes of the conventional Anger camera. With D-SPECT, each detector column is fixed in a mechanical mounting, and the data acquisition is performed by rotating these multiple columns in synchrony. The photons from a given location are detected at multiple angles by multiple columns as the fields of view of the detectors are swept through the region of interest. Each column (see Fig. 9-7B) consists of an array of 1024 CZT elements (2.46 × 2.46 × 5 mm thick) arranged in a 16 × 64 element array with an approximate size of 40 × 160 mm. Each column is fitted with square parallel-hole high-sensitivity collimators, such that the dimensions of each hole are matched to the size of a single detector element. The collimators are fabricated from tungsten to eliminate the production of lead x-rays that might interfere with technetium-201 (^{201}Tl) imaging. The collimators have a larger effective

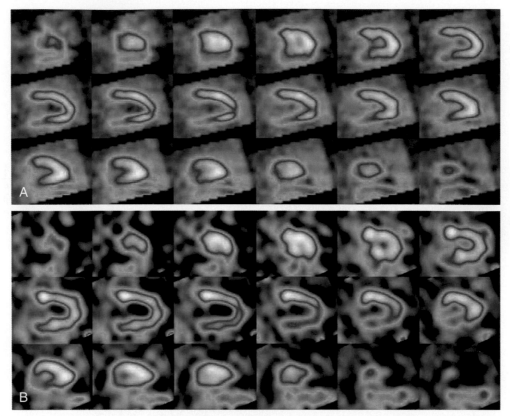

Figure 9-6 Stress images of a 55-year-old male, 6 feet 5 inches tall, 235 pounds, with substernal chest pain and shortness of breath. Father had CABG at the same age. Cholesterol = 240. Developed 1.5 to 2.0 mm ST depression in inferior leads at stress, injected with 31.2 mCi technetium-99m-sestamibi at peak stress. Image set (**A**) was acquired with a conventional dual-head scintillation camera using low-energy high-resolution collimators for 10.6 minutes, and demonstrated an inferobasal defect. Image set (**B**) was acquired with the CardiArc SPECT-HD for 4.7 minutes and correctly demonstrated a more severe and more extensive defect in the inferior wall to the apex. Angiography revealed high-grade, proximal PDA stenosis. *(Figure from CardiArc Ltd., with permission.)*

diameter than conventional low-energy high-resolution collimators used with scintillation cameras, yielding a significant gain in their geometric efficiency. The collimator has a hole length of 24.5 mm, with a 2.46-mm pitch and 2.26-mm hole diameter. The compensation for the loss in geometric spatial resolution that results from this design is accomplished by the software compensation methods. All data are collected in list mode. A proprietary Broadview iterative reconstruction algorithm based on the maximum-likelihood expectation

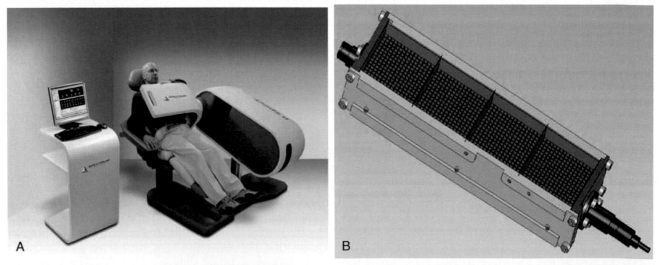

Figure 9-7 D-SPECT camera. Photograph of the D-SPECT camera showing patient position (**A**). A diagram of a single detector column from the D-SPECT camera (**B**), and a photograph of 9-detector columns configuration (**C**). *(Photograph courtesy of Spectrum Dynamics, Haifa, Israel.)*

Continued

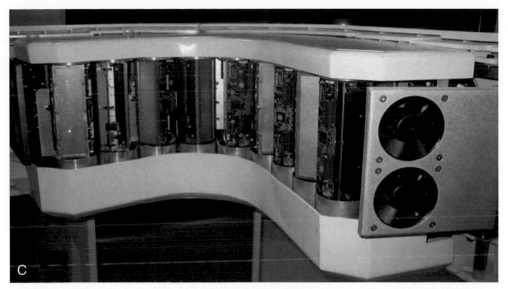

Figure 9-7—cont'd

maximization (MLEM) approach, with resolution recovery and use of the cardiac shape priors, has been developed and patented by the manufacturer.[17] It allows the recovery of image resolution to 5 mm in line source experiments.

Data acquisition is accomplished in a two-step process. First, a 1-minute pre-scan is performed to identify the location of the region of interest. Scan limits and timings are then set for each detector column, and the final scan is performed with each detector column rotating within the limits set from the pre-scan data. This process is shown diagrammatically in Figure 9-8. This process is termed *region-of-interest-centric scanning* by the manufacturer, because the scan field is limited to only the myocardial region. It has not been possible to measure an absolute value of sensitivity for this system as prescribed by the National Electrical Manufacturers Association quality-control standards,[18] because the sensitivity is significantly dependent on the field of view, defined individually for each patient by the pre-scan process. However, the most centrally located point has been reported to demonstrate a sensitivity of 1407 counts/μCi/min compared to the 160 to 240 counts/ μCi/min range generally observed with standard cameras.[19] A case example showing image quality on both D-SPECT and A-SPECT, obtained with the same isotope injection, is shown in Figure 9-9. In a recently published study, when D-SPECT was compared to A-SPECT, the myocardial count rate (with the same injection of the isotope) was 7 to 8 times higher for D-SPECT (Fig. 9-10).[16] Preliminary work has shown that simultaneous dual-isotope SPECT MPI with this camera is feasible using ^{201}Tl and technetium-99m, taking advantage of the improved energy resolution of CZT.[20]

The higher sensitivity of this system has been exploited to develop new clinical protocols. Cedars-Sinai Medical Center has reported the routine clinical use of this scanner in more than 400 patients using a stress [201]Tl (2 mCi)/rest tetrofosmin or sestamibi (8 to 10 mCi)

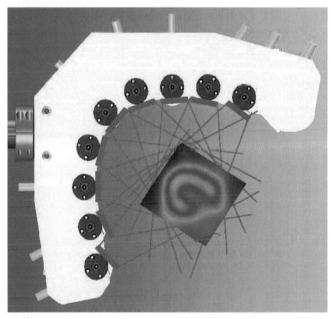

Figure 9-8 The ROI-centric technique utilized by the D-SPECT camera to optimize data collection from the myocardium.

protocol. Using half of the radioactivity associated with standard dual-isotope procedures, this protocol includes upright and supine immediate poststress images of 6 minutes each followed by rest injection and immediate 4-minute rest imaging. The total imaging time of this protocol is 19 minutes. Good to excellent image quality without significant extracardiac interference was observed in over 96% of the cases.[21]

Multipinhole Systems

An alternative approach to standard parallel-hole collimation is multipinhole tomography. Previously, promising results with the multipinhole SPECT systems have been

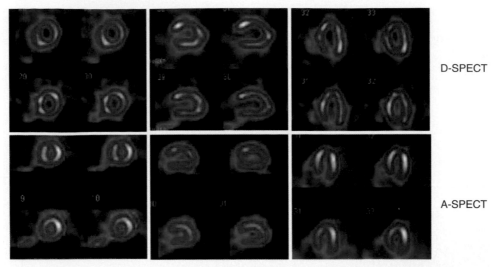

D-SPECT

A-SPECT

Figure 9-9 A study with standard dual-head SPECT camera (A-SPECT) and D-SPECT. Gender: Male, Age: 61 years, Weight: 200 lbs. Patient had history of coronary disease LAD stent, atypical angina, shortness of breath, diabetes, hypertension, or current smoking. The rest/stress MIBI protocol was performed with rest 8.2 mCi, and stress 37 mCi dose. X-ray angiography found proximal to mid-LAD 70% long lesion correlation. Both A-SPECT and D-SPECT correlate to coronary angiography, but D-SPECT shows more ischemia correlating better to coronary angiography. The acquisition times for both stress and rest were: ASPECT: rest 17 minutes, and stress 15 minutes; D-SPECT: rest 4 minutes, stress 2 minutes. *(Images courtesy of Dalia Dickman, Spectrum Dynamics, Haifa, Israel.)*

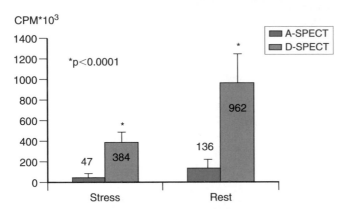

Figure 9-10 The higher system sensitivity of the D-SPECT system is demonstrated by a significantly higher myocardial count rate (7 to 8 times), compared with conventional SPECT at stress and rest images. CPM, Counts/min. *(From Sharir T, Ben-Haim S, Merzon K, et al: High-speed myocardial perfusion imaging: Initial clinical comparison with conventional dual-detector Anger camera imaging. JACC Cardiovasc Imaging 1:156–163, 2008. Reproduced with permission.)*

presented by several groups in small-animal imaging, surpassing the spatial resolution and detection efficiency of parallel-hole collimation.[22–24] Because all views are active throughout the entire image acquisition period, SPECT imaging in this technique is accomplished without the need for motion of the detector, collimator, or patient. Since image acquisition is accomplished without any electromechanical motion, the manufacturing and servicing costs could potentially be significantly reduced.

The design of the cardiac system for human imaging was reported by Funk et al., with two 9-pinhole collimators attached to the standard dual-headed gamma camera,[25] forming, in effect, an 18-pinhole imaging system. This cardiac imaging technology utilizes pinhole collimation to project a simultaneous set of images onto one or more large-area detectors. The principle of operation and a photograph of the actual prototype systems are shown in Figure 9-11. In experiments with the first prototype system, the authors found that spatial resolution of the 9-pinhole collimator with 8-mm diameter pinholes was 30% poorer than that for the parallel-hole collimator. However, the detection efficiency was increased by more than ten-fold. These data allowed them to predict that in comparison to a standard gamma camera, a five-fold increase in sensitivity could be achieved with this technology without degradation of image resolution. Similar increase in sensitivity has been demonstrated by the same group in the small-animal full-ring multipinhole SPECT system.[26]

With the use of a stationary detector, patient motion–induced inconsistencies between views are eliminated because all views are acquired simultaneously, and multiple isotopes can be imaged simultaneously. All views are active over the entire image acquisition period, leading to a consistent data set for the reconstruction by iterative reconstruction techniques, similar to the acquisition obtained in the full-ring positron emission tomography (PET) system. Correction for patient respiratory motion could also be potentially more reliable compared to standard systems, since all the data acquisition is performed simultaneously from multiple angles.

Multipinhole design potentially suffers from some limitations that will need to be addressed. The approach may be prone to greater formation of artifacts, because it inherently produces an incomplete tomographic data set, and it acquires images from only limited views.[25] Background activity from other organs may not be seen in all of the views, which could lead to inconsistencies in the reconstructed data. It is also known that the resolution and sensitivity of pinhole collimators decrease with the distance from the collimator[27]; however,

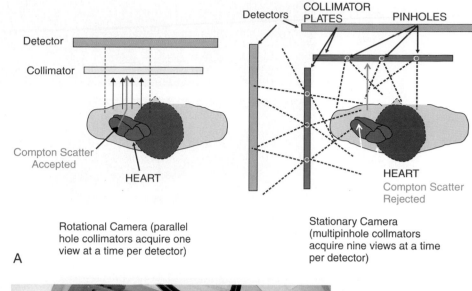

Rotational Camera (parallel hole collimators acquire one view at a time per detector)

Stationary Camera (multipinhole collmators acquire nine views at a time per detector)

A

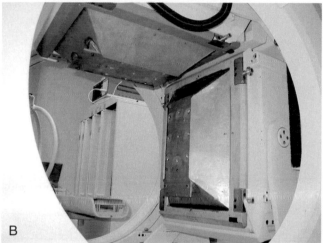

Figure 9-11 Principle of operation (**A**) and photograph of the prototype multipinhole collimator (**B**) mounted on standard SPECT camera. *(Images courtesy of Dennis Kirch, Nuclear Cardiology Research, Denver, CO.)*

B

resolution recovery can be applied during the reconstruction to compensate for this spatial variation. Nuclear Cardiology Research (NCR), located in Denver, Colorado, is currently commercializing this design.

Original acquisition images are shown in Figure 9-12, and the reconstructed views are shown in Figure 9-13. The result of breath-by-breath motion correction is shown in Figure 9-14.

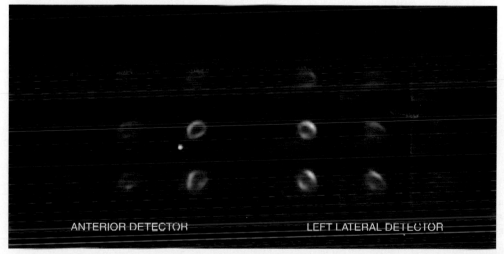

Figure 9-12 Original ungated raw views of myocardial perfusion obtained on a 9-pinhole system. *(Images courtesy of Dennis Kirch, Nuclear Cardiology Research, Denver, CO.)*

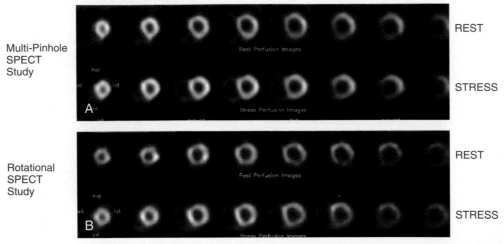

Figure 9-13 Tomographic slices are reconstructed from pinhole views using iterative reconstruction techniques (**A**) resulting in comparable image quality to the standard MPI reconstruction (**B**). *(Images courtesy of Dennis Kirch, Nuclear Cardiology Research, Denver, CO.)*

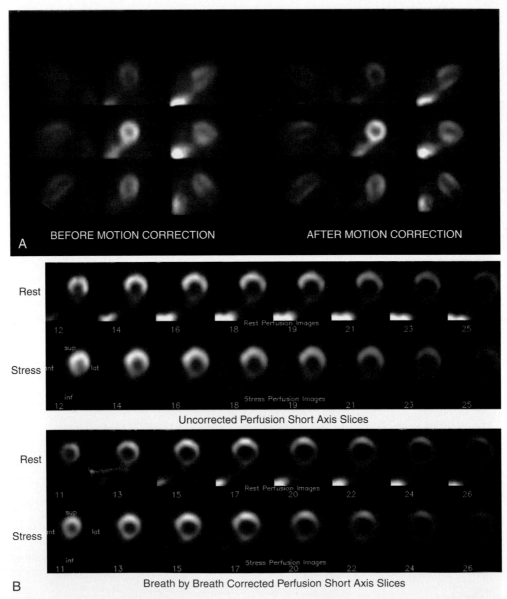

Figure 9-14 Multipinhole SPECT images shown before and after motion correction prior to (**A**) and after (**B**) reconstruction. Note that the myocardial outline appears slightly smaller, and the interior of the cardiac chamber is better defined. *(Images courtesy of Dennis Kirch, Nuclear Cardiology Research, Denver, CO.)*

FAST MYOCARDIAL PERFUSION IMAGING SOFTWARE WITH STANDARD SYSTEMS

Software improvements of image reconstruction have centered on the development of new proprietary algorithms that have evolved from the early work in iterative reconstruction techniques, MLEM,[28,29] and later the accelerated method of OSEM.[11] These techniques were developed to improve image contrast and reduce noise levels inherent in images with low counts reconstructed with FBP.

For purposes of comparison to the iterative methods, standard FBP reconstruction assumes that the object is detected equally in all of the angular projections. This leads to various artifacts caused by variations in attenuation, scatter, resolution, and count density. Iterative reconstruction methods based on MLEM and OSEM allow the geometry of the acquisition to vary for each projection, greatly enhancing the flexibility in modeling the physical parameters. SPECT imaging is greatly affected by Poisson noise, scatter, attenuation correction, and variable image resolution.[30] The iterative methods make it possible to incorporate projection-specific corrections for these image-degrading factors into the reconstruction process so that the reconstructed image is a better representation of the object being imaged.

Currently, the most widely used iterative technique is based on the OSEM approach, which is an accelerated version of the MLEM algorithm and allows efficient computer processing. This technique groups projection data into an ordered sequence of subsets. *One iteration* of the OSEM algorithm is defined as a single pass through all of the subsets.[11] Typically, 2 to 4 projections per subset are used with 4 to 12 iterations, which is computationally less demanding than 1 iteration of the standard MLEM algorithm (assuming 64 projections). Even with 1 iteration of OSEM and 32 subsets, it is possible to obtain a reasonable initial reconstruction. Typically, OSEM results in a degree of magnitude decrease of computing time without measurable loss of image quality, as demonstrated by Hudson and Larkin.[11]

OSEM techniques incorporate both backprojection and forward projection. *Backprojection* is the process of filling in a matrix by projecting back the data contained in the projection images. In this process, individual pixels in the reconstruction matrix are filled in along a ray corresponding to the direction from the projection data (Fig. 9-15). *Forward projection* is the reverse process: The data from the image reconstruction matrix are projected (summed) data from the image display matrix with movement out of the image matrix to form estimated projection data. Note also that MPI spatial resolution is a function of distance from the collimator, and that this can be modeled in the iterative reconstruction process (see Fig. 9-15).

In OSEM, reconstruction image data are updated during each iteration and for each subset. Therefore the number of updates is the product of iterations and projections subsets. As the number of updates increases, the spatial resolution increases, but the noise increases at the same time. This is demonstrated in Figure 9-16. This increase necessitates an optimization process where the noise-smoothing filter, the number of iterations, and the number of subsets are properly balanced to obtain optimal image quality—that is, spatial resolution and uniformity.

These iterative algorithms were extended to include depth-dependent and resolution recovery techniques, developed to correct for losses in spatial resolution due to the line response function of the collimator.[31] Other physical effects that can be corrected are scatter and attenuation compensation. The algorithms currently available simultaneously address these problems by modeling the instrumentation and imaging parameters used for a specific application to eliminate the degrading effects of the line spread function (LSF) and to suppress noise in the image reconstruction process. The resolution recovery aspects of these algorithms can be emphasized to provide significant improvements in spatial resolution and image quality of SPECT sets, and the noise suppression aspects can be emphasized to permit decreased imaging times for SPECT acquisitions.

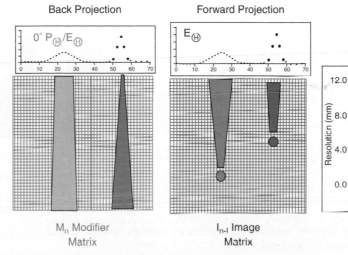

Figure 9-15 An overview of the iterative reconstruction technique. In the backprojection process, the modifier matrix is filled in by apportioning "counts" into pixels along the respective light and dark green rays. This is repeated for each of the ordered subset angles. In the forward projection process, the data from the image matrix is summed along the ray path to produce an estimated projection (EΘ). Images obtained with Astonish reconstruction. *(Courtesy of Horace Hines, Philips, Milpitas, CA).*

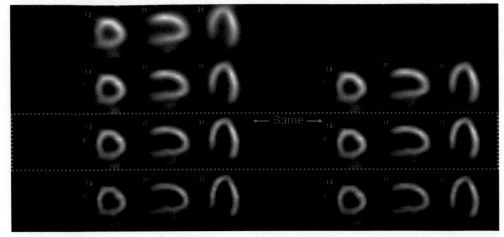

Figure 9-16 Improved spatial resolution as the number of updates increases in the iterative process. Note that with more updates, the noise level increases. This decreases the uniformity in normal myocardial regions. *(Courtesy of Horace Hines, Philips, Milpitas, CA).*

Astonish

Philips (Milpitas, CA) has developed a fast SPECT reconstruction algorithm (Astonish) that includes corrections for the major factors degrading SPECT image quality. It is based on the OSEM reconstruction method, with built-in noise reduction methods during the iterative process and incorporating corrections for photon scatter, photon attenuation, and variations in spatial resolution. Correction for Compton scattering in the patient improves lesion contrast and is required for accurate attenuation correction. Correction for photon attenuation provides a more accurate representation of the counts from lesions that are at different depths inside the patient. Correction for variations in spatial resolution with depth allows the preservation of sharper details and small lesions with greater conspicuity. The company has developed this approach to shorten the MPI acquisition time without compromising the image quality.

The corrections for variations in spatial resolution use measurements of the changes in spatial resolution with distance from the collimator, as is shown in a general case in Figure 9-15. Calibrations for each of the collimators are measured initially by the manufacturer. Astonish software incorporates this collimator information into both the backprojection and the forward projection parts of the reconstruction. The resolution recover correction in Astonish can be performed with or without attenuation correction.

In Astonish, the corrections for the photon scatter are performed by the ESSE method described by Kadrmas et al.[32] The corrections for the photon scatter are performed prior to the attenuation correction in each iterative OSEM step. Corrections for attenuation are performed during the forward projection process. Attenuation correction requires knowledge of both the photon attenuation coefficient and the density of each pixel that the "counts" are forward projected through. The density information is accessed in an attenuation map, modified from a previously acquired density image, with either a scanning line source or from a CT scanner.

One problem that all iterative methods must address is amplification of statistical noise during the reconstruction process. Astonish uses a proprietary (patent pending) noise-reduction method of smoothing both the estimated projection data and the measured projection data internally during the reconstruction process.[33,34] This modification of OSEM allows for optimized control of Poisson image noise while maintaining higher image resolution. In addition, a Hanning prefilter (or optionally no filter) is used to smooth the projection images prior to starting reconstruction. The estimated projections are also smoothed with the same filter prior to the measured/estimated comparison being taken during each subset. This approach can be compared with other methods that smooth the image data after the reconstruction process.[35]

The clinical performance of Astonish has been tested in a multicenter trial consisting of 221 patients, and preliminary results have been reported.[36] Image quality, interpretative certainty, and diagnostic accuracy were evaluated by three "blinded" readers for standard reconstruction for full-time FBP, full-time Astonish (FTA)

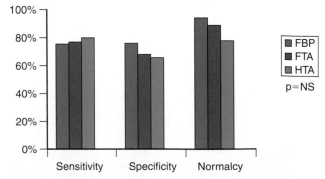

Figure 9-17 The sensitivity, specificity, and normalcy were determined for filtered backprojection (FBP), full-time Astonish (FTA), and half-time Astonish (HTA). *(From Van Laere K, Koole M, Lemahieu I, Dierckx R: Image filtering in single-photon emission computed tomography: Principles and applications. Comput Med Imaging Graph 25:127–133, 2001. Reproduced with permission.)*

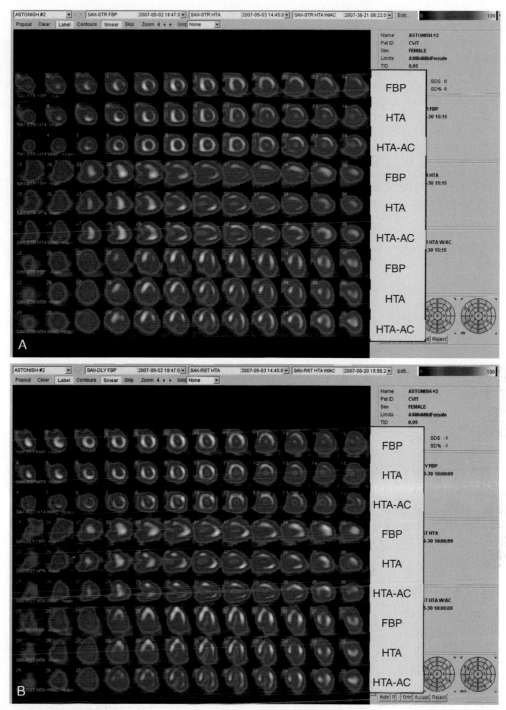

Figure 9-18 Example of image quality with Astonish. Stress (**A**) and rest (**B**) images are reconstructed with standard filtered backprojection (FBP) image reconstruction, half-time Astonish reconstruction (HTA), and half-time Astonish reconstruction with attenuation correction (HTA-AC). Images of a 209-pound male were acquired with a technetium/technetium protocol with 64 projections and 25 seconds per view full-time and with 32 projections and 25 seconds per view half-time, acquired on CardioMD Philips camera. *(Images courtesy of Philips Healthcare.)*

(64 projections, 20 to 25 sec/projection), and half-time Astonish (HTA) (32 projections, 20 to 25 sec/projection). The HTA data were obtained from the full-time data by using half of the original projections. Stress and rest perfusion image qualities (excellent/good) were 87.8%/83.3% (FBP), 97.7%/95.9% (FTA), and 96.8%/95.5% (IITA), respectively ($P < 0.001$). Interpretive certainty and diagnostic accuracy (Fig. 9-17) were the same for

all these techniques. An example of MPI image quality achievable with Astonish is shown in Figure 9-18.

GE Healthcare's Evolution Software

GE Healthcare (Waukesha, WI) has also developed a modification of the OSEM algorithm that incorporates resolution recovery named "Evolution for Cardiac" or

OSEM-RR. Their approach includes modeling of the integrated collimator and detector response function (CDR) in an iterative reconstruction algorithm, and performs image resolution recovery[37] based on these parameters. This technique has been described in detail in a recent publication by DePuey et al.[38] The OSEM-RR modeling includes basic collimator geometric response function for round-hole-shaped collimators[31,39] that can be applied with good approximation to hexagonal holes.

The CDR compensation technique utilized in OSEM-RR was developed at the University of North Carolina, Chapel Hill, and Johns Hopkins University by Tsui et al.[37,39,40] It is accomplished by convolving the projected photon ray with the corresponding LSF during iterative projection and backprojection. The following parameters are accounted for and compensated: collimator hole and septa dimensions, intrinsic detector resolution, crystal thickness, collimator-to-detector gap, and projection-angle-specific center of rotation–to–collimator face distances. These collimator-specific data are embedded in the software in the form of lookup tables. Some of the relevant acquisition parameters (such as object-to-collimator distance) are obtained directly from the raw projection data.

Additionally, similar to other optimized reconstruction methods, OSEM-RR incorporates noise suppression, which is required since the resolution recovery during the iterative reconstruction process amplifies noise, which can lead to the formation of hot spots in the final image. A maximum a posteriori technique[41] is incorporated to control image noise in the OSEM-RR design. A modified one-step-late algorithm with a Green prior[42] is utilized. The specific parameters in these reconstructions are optimized separately for each clinical protocol and separately for gated and attenuation-corrected images. The last iteration is performed using a median root prior.[43]

Siemens Medical Solutions

Siemens has recently released its software (Flash3D) incorporating iterative fast OSEM reconstruction with 3D resolution recovery, 3D collimator and detector response correction, and attenuation and scatter compensation.[44] SPECT cardiac acquisition protocols (Cardio-Flash) have been developed utilizing Flash3D, where the acquisition time can be reduced to between 33% and 50%, compared to the standard acquisition protocols with FBP reconstruction. An example of the image quality obtained with CardioFlash is shown in phantoms (Fig. 9-19) and in clinical images (Fig. 9-20). To date, it has been shown in phantom data in combination with a few clinical scans that Flash3D allows faster acquisition protocols but still provides sufficient myocardial uniformity and lesion detectability.[44] Prospective clinical studies are currently being conducted to assess the performance of this technique with a protocol using 6-degree angular sampling, thus reducing acquisition time by 50%.

The computer reconstruction times of the 2007 release of Flash3D (Siemens OSEM reconstruction with

Torso Phantom, normal (33kcts/view; 64^2, 4.8 mm)

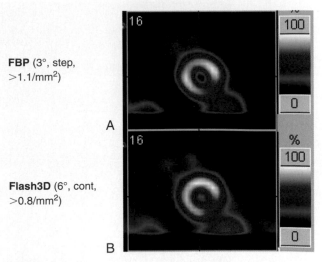

FBP (3°, step, >1.1/mm²)

Flash3D (6°, cont, >0.8/mm²)

Figure 9-19 Example images comparing a standard protocol and a protocol using Flash3D in 36% of the acquisition time. The inferolateral artifact due to lack of attenuation correction is well visible in phantoms. *(From Alenius S, Ruotsalainen U: Bayesian image reconstruction for emission tomography based on median root prior. Eur J Nucl Med Mol Imaging 24:258–265, 1997. Reproduced with permission.)*

Example Patient data (rest; 64^2, 6.6 mm)

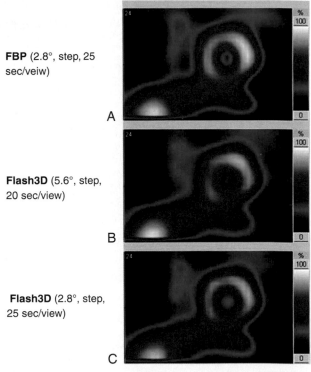

FBP (2.8°, step, 25 sec/veiw)

Flash3D (5.6°, step, 20 sec/view)

Flash3D (2.8°, step, 25 sec/view)

Figure 9-20 Example patient data acquired with Cardio-Flash. For images (**A**) and (**C**), the original projection data are used but reconstructed with filtered backprojection and Flash3D. The projection data in (**B**) are extracted from the original data and represent a "what-if" protocol data set with twice the angular step size and 80% dwell time reduction, and reconstructed with Flash3D. *(From Alenius S, Ruotsalainen U: Bayesian image reconstruction for emission tomography based on median root prior. Eur J Nucl Med Mol Imaging 24:258–265, 1997. Reproduced with permission.)*

3D distance-dependent resolution recovery and optional scatter and attenuation corrections) were improved, and it is now possible to process an entire clinical gated cardiac data set in less then 1 minute on a standard workstation. High correlation ($r^2 > 0.97$) has been shown between the ejection fractions obtained from conventional FBP-based protocol and the CardioFlash reconstructions in a preliminary study.[45]

UltraSPECT Wide Beam Reconstruction

UltraSPECT Limited (Haifa, Israel) has developed a standalone workstation (Xpress.cardiac) that utilizes the patented wide beam reconstruction (WBR) algorithm.[46] The WBR reconstruction technique, phantom validation, and its clinical application have been recently described by Borges-Neto et al.[47] This solution is available as an additional workstation and can reconstruct data from most existing gamma cameras with standard collimator design. Similar to other methods, WBR models the physics and geometry of the emission and detection processes and attempts resolution recovery. During the iterative reconstruction, it corrects reconstructed voxels, given the information regarding the collimator's geometry (such as the dimensions and shape of holes or the septa thickness). Furthermore, the detector's distance from the patient is considered. New gamma cameras provide this information automatically for each angular position from their body contour tracking systems used for orbit prescription. However, this distance can also be obtained by image-processing techniques and definition of the 3D patient body contour, from which the distance of the detector to the body at a given location can be calculated.[47] In addition, this technique applies statistical modeling of the expected photon emission in order to suppress Poisson noise. The standard approach to overcome noise is the application of Fourier domain post filtering; however, Fourier filtering does not distinguish between the actual signal and noise at a given frequency. WBR instead regularizes the likelihood objective function with a combination of the Poisson and Gaussian distributions. This is accomplished by Fourier analysis of a projection to determine the approximate signal-to-noise ratio that is present in the acquired data and the selection of an optimal noise model to yield the appropriate balance between resolution and noise. An example of WBR image quality is shown in Figure 9-21.

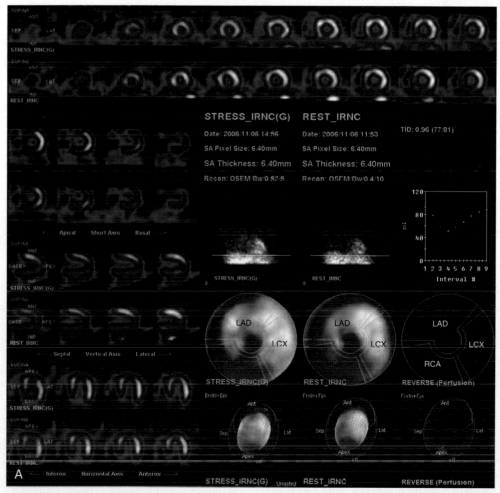

Figure 9-21 For Legend see Page 146

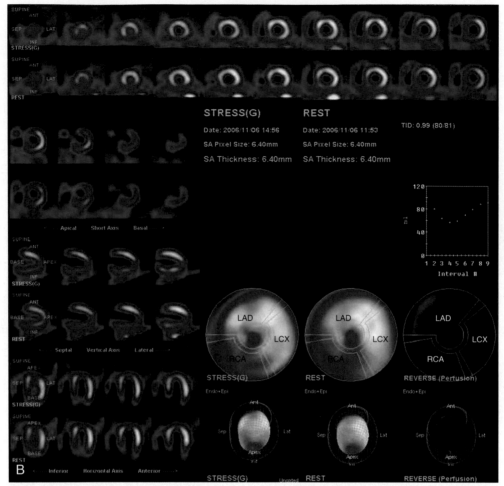

Figure 9-21—cont'd SPECT scans of a 56-year-old male hypertensive smoker with no prior history of coronary disease. Images obtained with technetium-99m-sestamibi (dose: 8 mCi at rest and 32 mCi at stress) protocol and acquired with dual-head scintillation camera without attenuation correction. Images were reconstructed with full-time ordered subset expectation maximization (OSEM) (15 minutes rest, 12 minutes stress) (**A**) and with separate wide beam reconstruction (WBR) (9 minutes rest, 7 minutes stress) acquisitions (**B**) following the rest and stress OSEM acquisitions, respectively. The actual acquisition time for "half-time" WBR is slightly longer than half as a result of the dead time associated with gantry rotation. However, the WBR acquisition time per camera stop is one-half that for OSEM. Both WBR and OSEM images show the same small apical defect, which is likely physiologic apical thinning. *(Images courtesy Dr. Gordon DePuey, Columbia University, New York, NY.)*

Motion-Frozen Reconstruction

Another development related to the quality and therefore potential time reduction in image reconstruction is the "motion-frozen" processing of gated cardiac images, which eliminates blurring of perfusion images due to cardiac motion.[48] This technique applies a nonlinear, thin-plate-spline warping algorithm and shifts counts from the whole cardiac cycle into the end-diastolic (ED) position. The "motion-frozen" images have the appearance of ED frames but are significantly less noisy, since the counts from the entire cardiac cycle are used. The spatial resolution of such images is higher than that of summed gated images. This technique has been successfully applied to SPECT and PET images. Figure 9-22 shows an example of a SPECT image reconstructed with motion-frozen technique. A significant improvement in image resolution can be observed when compared to standard summed images. The combination of such advanced approaches dedicated to cardiac

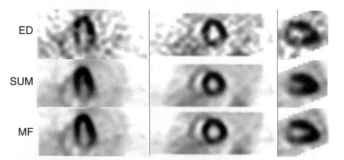

Figure 9-22 Short-axis and vertical long-axis of motion-frozen (MF) reconstruction and standard summed reconstruction (SUM) of gated SPECT images. Motion-frozen perfusion images compared to the summed perfusion images in the case of double-vessel disease confirmed by angiography (100% LAD occlusion and 80% LCx occlusion). Both standard quantification technique and visual analysis of summed data identified only the LAD lesion; the additional LCX lesion was identified only by the motion-frozen quantification. *(From Slomka PJ, Nishina H, Berman DS, et al: "Motion-frozen" display and quantification of myocardial perfusion. J Nucl Med 45:1128–1134, 2004. Reproduced with permission.)*

imaging and the general advances in image reconstruction described could result in further gains in image quality.

CONCLUSIONS

In summary, a variety of new approaches have been introduced that may substantially reduce both the time of acquisition and the radiation doses associated with SPECT MPI. In general, software methods can facilitate the acceleration of image acquisition on standard gamma cameras by a factor of approximately 2 without significant degradation of image quality. When these new software reconstruction techniques are coupled with the use of novel dedicated detectors and collimators optimized specifically for SPECT MPI imaging, a further significant reduction of acquisition time is possible, achieving scan times as short as 2 minutes. These new approaches will likely result in innovative imaging protocols that improve patient comfort, improve throughput, and reduce radiation dose associated with SPECT MPI.

ACKNOWLEDGMENTS

Daniel Berman has equity position in Spectrum Dynamics Ltd. We would like to acknowledge help from the following individuals who have sent material, data, and images relating to specific technologies: Gordon DePuey, Columbia University, New York, NY; Gary Heller, University of Connecticut School of Medicine; Hans Vija, Siemens Medical, Hoffman Estates, IL; Horace Hines and Angela Da Silva of Philips, Milpitas, CA; Dennis Kirch, Nuclear Cardiology Research, Denver, CO; Dalia Sherry, Spectrum Dynamics, Haifa, Israel; Terri Garner, CardiArc, Lubbock, TX); Richard Conwell, Digirad Corporation, San Diego, CA; and Frank Ansett of GE Healthcare.

In addition, we would like to thank Joyoni Dey, University of Massachusetts, Worcester, and Gillian Haemer, University of Southern California, Los Angeles, for comments and proofreading the text.

REFERENCES

1. DePuey EG, Nichols KJ, Slowikowski JS, Scarpa WJ, Smith C, Melancon S: Fast stress (8 minute) and rest (10 minute) acquisitions for Tc-99m sestamibi separate day SPECT, *J Nucl Med* 36(1):569–574, 1995.
2. Mazzanti M, Germano G, Kiat H, Friedman J, Berman DS: Fast technetium 99m-labeled sestamibi gated single-photon emission computed tomography for evaluation of myocardial function, *J Nucl Cardiol* 3(2):143–149, 1996.
3. Germano G, Kavanagh PB, Berman DS: Effect of the number of projections collected on quantitative perfusion and left ventricular ejection fraction measurements from gated myocardial perfusion single-photon emission computed tomographic images, *J Nucl Cardiol* 3(5): 395–402, 1996.
4. Einstein AJ, Henzlova MJ, Rajagopalan S: Estimating risk of cancer associated with radiation exposure from 64-slice computed tomography coronary angiography, *JAMA* 298(3):317–323, 2007.
5. Patton JA, Slomka PJ, Germano G, Berman DS: Recent technologic advances in nuclear cardiology, *J Nucl Cardiol* 14(4):501–513, 2007.
6. Butler JF, Lingren CL, Friesenhahn SJ, et al: CdZnTe solid-state gamma camera, *IEEE Trans Nucl Sci* 45(3 Part 1):359–363, 1998.
7. Babla H, Bai C, Conwell R: A triple-head solid state camera for cardiac single photon emission tomography (SPECT), *Proc Soc Phot Opt Instrum Eng* 6319:63190M, 2006.
8. Lewin HC, Hyun MC: [Abstract] A clinical comparison of an upright triple-head digital detector system to a standard supine dual-head gamma camera, *J Nucl Cardiol* 12(4):113, 2005.
9. Bai C, Conwell R, Babla H, et al: *Improving Image Quality and Imaging Efficiency Using nSPEED*, 2008. http://www.digirad.com/downloads_2007/nSPEED_white_paper.pdf Accessed 05/30/2008.
10. Maddahi J, Mendez R, Chuanyong B, et al: [Abstract] Validation of a method for fast myocardial perfusion gated SPECT imaging, *J Nucl Cardiol* 14:16, 2007.
11. Hudson HM, Larkin RS: Accelerated image reconstruction using ordered subsets of projection data, *IEEE Trans Med Imaging* 13(4): 601–609, 1994.
12. www.CardiArc.com. 2008. Accessed 05/30/2008.
13. Madsen MT: Recent Advances in SPECT Imaging, *J Nucl Med* 48(4): 661–673, 2007.
14. Arlt R, Rundquist DE: Room temperature semiconductor detectors for safeguards measurements, *Nucl Instrum Methods Phys Res A* 380(1): 455–461, 1996.
15. O'Connor M: *Evaluation of the CardiArc dedicated cardiac system [unpublished independent evaluation]*, Rochester, MN, 2005, Mayo Clinic.
16. Sharir T, Ben-Haim S, Merzon K, et al: High-speed myocardial perfusion imaging: Initial clinical comparison with conventional dual detector anger camera imaging, *JACC Cardiovasc Imaging* 1:156–163, 2008.
17. Rousso B, Nagler M, Rousso B, Nagler MRousso B, Nagler Ms: Spectrum Dynamics LLC, assignee: *Multi-dimensional image reconstruction*, 2007. US patent 7176466. Feb 13, 2007.
18. Hines H, Kayayan R, Colsher J, et al: Recommendations for implementing SPECT instrumentation quality control, *Eur J Nucl Med Mol Imaging* 26(5):527–532, 1999.
19. Patton J, Sandler M, Berman D, et al: D-SPECT: [Abstract] A new solid state camera for high speed molecular imaging abstract, *J Nucl Med* 47:189, 2006.
20. Ben-Haim S, Hutton B, Van Gramberg D, et al: Simultaneous dual isotope myocardial perfusion scintigraphy (DI MPS): Initial experience with fast D-SPECT [Abstract], *J Nucl Med* 49(Suppl 1):72P, 2008.
21. Berman DS, Kang X, Tamarappoo B, et al: Stress thallium-201/rest technetium-99m sequential dual isotope high-speed myocardial perfusion imaging, *JACC Cardiovasc Imaging* 2:273–282, 2009.
22. Jaszczak RJ, Li J, Wang H, Zalutsky MR, Coleman RE: Pinhole collimation for ultra-high-resolution, small-field-of-view SPECT, *Phys Med Biol* 39:425–437, 1994.
23. Schramm NU, Ebel G, Engeland U, Schurrat T, Behe M, Behr TM: High-resolution SPECT using multipinhole collimation, *IEEE Trans Nucl Sci* 50(3):315–320, 2003.
24. Beekman FJ, Vastenhouw B: Design and simulation of a high-resolution stationary SPECT system for small animals, *Phys Med Biol* 49(19):4579–4592, 2004.
25. Funk T, Kirch DL, Koss JE, Botvinick E, Hasegawa BH: A Novel Approach to Multipinhole SPECT for Myocardial Perfusion Imaging, *J Nucl Med* 47(4):595–602, 2006.
26. Funk T, Després P, Barber WC, Shah KS, Hasegawa BH: A multipinhole small animal SPECT system with submillimeter spatial resolution, *Med Phys* 33:1259–1268, 2006.
27. Metzler SD, Bowsher JE, Smith MF, Jaszczak RJ: Analytic determination of pinhole collimator sensitivity with penetration, *IEEE Trans Med Imaging* 20(8):730–741, 2001.
28. Shepp LA, Vardi Y: Maximum likelihood reconstruction for emission tomography, *IEEE Trans Med Imaging* 1:113–122, 1982.
29. Lange K, Carson R: EM reconstruction algorithms for emission and transmission tomography, *J Comput Assist Tomogr* 8(2):306–316, 1984.
30. El Fakhri G, Buvat I, Benali H, Todd-Pokropek A, Di Paola R: Relative Impact of Scatter, Collimator Response, Attenuation, and Finite Spatial Resolution Corrections in Cardiac SPECT, *J Nucl Med* 41(8):1400–1408, 2000.
31. Metz CE: The geometric transfer function component for scintillation camera collimators with straight parallel holes, *Phys Med Biol* 25(6):1059–1070, 1980.
32. Kadrmas DJ, Frey EC, Karimi SS, Tsui BMW: Fast implementation of reconstruction-based scatter compensation in fully 3D SPECT image reconstruction, *Phys Med Biol* 43(4):857–873, 1998.
33. Ye J, Song X, Zhao Z, Da Silva AJ, Wiener JS, Shao L: Iterative SPECT Reconstruction Using Matched Filtering for Improved Image Quality, *IEEE Nucl Sci Symp Conf Rec (2006)* 4:2285–2287, 2006.
34. Ye J, Shao L, Zhao Z, Durbin M: *Iterative Reconstruction with Enhanced Noise Control Filtering*, 2007. WO Patent WO/2007/034,342.
35. Van Laere K, Koole M, Lemahieu I, Dierckx R: Image filtering in single-photon emission computed tomography: principles and applications, *Comput Med Imaging Graph* 25(2):127–133, 2001.
36. Venero CV, Ahlberg AW, Bateman TM, et al: Enhancement of Nuclear Cardiac Laboratory Efficiency: Multicenter Evaluation of a New Post-Processing Method with Depth-Dependent Collimator Resolution Applied to Full and Half-Time Acquisitions, *J Nucl Cardiol* 2008;15:S4.

37. Tsui BMW, Hu HB, Gilland DR, Gullberg GT: Implementation of simultaneous attenuation and detector response correction in SPECT, *IEEE Trans Nucl Sci* 35(1):778–783, 1988.

38. DePuey E, Gadiraju R, Clark J, Thompson L, Anstett F, Shwartz S: Ordered subset expectation maximization and wide beam reconstruction "half-time" gated myocardial perfusion SPECT functional imaging: A comparison to "full-time" filtered backprojection, *J Nucl Cardiol* 15:547–563, 2008.

39. Tsui BMW, Gullberg GT: The Geometric Transfer-Function for Cone and Fan Beam Collimators, *Phys Med Biol* 35(1):81–93, 1990.

40. Tsui BMW, Frey EC, Zhao X, Lalush DS, Johnston RE, McCartney WH: The importance and implementation of accurate 3D compensation methods for quantitative SPECT, *Phys Med Biol* 39(3):509–530, 1994.

41. Bruyant PP: Analytic and iterative reconstruction algorithms in SPECT, *J Nucl Med* 43(10):1343–1358, 2002.

42. Green PJ: Bayesian reconstructions from emission tomography data using a modified EM algorithm, *IEEE Trans Med Imaging* 9(1):84–93, 1990.

43. Alenius S, Ruotsalainen U: Bayesian image reconstruction for emission tomography based on median root prior, *Eur J Nucl Med Mol Imaging* 24 (3):258–265, 1997.

44. Vija AH, Zeintl J, Chapman JT, Hawman EG, Hornegger J: Development of Rapid SPECT Acquisition Protocol for Myocardial Perfusion Imaging, *IEEE Nucl Sci Symp Conf Record* 3:1811–1816, 2006.

45. Zeintl J, Ding X, Vija AH, Hawman EG, Hornegger J, Kuwert T: Estimation accuracy of ejection fraction in gated cardiac SPECT/CT imaging using iterative reconstruction with 3D resolution recovery in rapid acquisition Protocols, *IEEE Nucl Sci Symp Conf Rec* 6:4491–4496, 2007.

46. UltraSPECT. www.UltraSPECT.com. Accessed 09/06, 2008.

47. Borges-Neto SPR, Shaw LK, et al: Clinical results of a novel wide beam reconstruction method for shortening scan time of Tc-99m cardiac SPECT perfusion studies, *J Nucl Cardiol* 14:555–565, 2007.

48. Slomka PJ, Nishina H, Berman DS, et al: Motion-frozen" display and quantification of myocardial perfusion, *J Nucl Med* 45(7):1128–1134, 2004.

Radiation Considerations for Cardiac Nuclear and Computed Tomography Imaging

S. JAMES CULLOM AND TIMOTHY M. BATEMAN

INTRODUCTION

The contribution of nuclear cardiology and computed tomography (CT) to the diagnosis and management of cardiovascular disease is undeniable. In contrast to other imaging modalities, they rely on the use of ionizing radiation, which has been associated with the risk of harmful effects. Of greatest concern is increasing the risk of cancer occurrence and mortality.[1-4] In recent years, the number of diagnostic imaging studies using "low-level" doses of ionizing radiation increased dramatically. Concern over the risk to the population grew accordingly.[2,3] Industry data show that cardiac imaging applications using single-photon emission computed tomography (SPECT), positron emission tomography (PET), and CT experienced greater relative increases compared with other imaging areas. Within these groups, there was an increase in the proportion of studies performed in women and pediatric populations, raising additional concern over exposure in these populations.[3,4] These developments have fueled the debate over the accuracy and appropriateness of the estimated rates of cancer predicted by current models and assumptions that have been at times highly disputed. While it is generally accepted that excessive exposure to ionizing radiation can cause certain types of malignancies and other diseases, this relationship is far less accepted for the amounts of radiation used in most diagnostic imaging tests. In clinical practice, the debate is largely centered on the uncertainty in risk estimates relative to the counterprevailing risk of misdiagnosed disease or underutilization of appropriate testing.[5] In parallel, advances in imaging technology have reduced radiation dose while preserving image quality, particularly for CT—and

cardiac CT specifically—and are rapidly being adopted into clinical application.[6] New SPECT reconstruction algorithms and detector configurations for myocardial perfusion imaging allow studies to be acquired in half the time or less[7-9] of conventional protocols and theoretically may allow tradeoff of acquisition time advantage for imaging with less injection activity.[7] Cardiac PET studies overall deliver favorable radiation dose compared with SPECT and are therefore an option for radiation dose reduction.

Cardiac imaging decisions at the patient and strategic laboratory level are increasingly influenced by perceptions about radiation dosimetry. This chapter presents an overview of current issues surrounding radiation dosimetry for nuclear cardiology and cardiac CT. Reference to resources with greater detailed discussion are included and recommended for further reading.

RADIATION DOSIMETRY

The science of radiation dosimetry focuses on characterizing the propagation and transfer of energy to tissues in the body, with the intent of estimating biological damage. Using these calculations, the risk of harmful effects or disease is estimated using complex models. Of particular concern is the risk of increasing the frequency of fatal cancer from additional ionizing radiation exposure. The debate for diagnostic imaging is whether the amount of ionizing radiation delivered from typical diagnostic imaging methods at one or more times over a lifetime can be associated with cause of disease. The physical quantities and related interactions measured in radiation dosimetry are well standardized, but the subsequent characterization of the risk of causing disease is far more complex and unresolved. Major factors cited include:

1. Passage of decades before exposure-induced malignancy appears
2. Dependency of disease presentation on age of the individual at time of exposure
3. Impact of multiple exposures over many years
4. Very low rate of confirmable radiation-induced cancer events
5. Reliability of data over the early years of ionization-based imaging
6. Lack of prospective evidence in humans
7. Difficulties differentiating among the various causes of cancers, including "natural" causes

For diagnostic imaging, radiation dosimetry is approached from two perspectives: *Internal radiation dosimetry* describes the deposition of energy and biological damage resulting from radiation sources located internal to the body, such as with radiopharmaceuticals or inhaled industrial radionuclides. *External radiation dosimetry* refers to characterization of biological damage from radiation sources external to the body, such as with conventional x-ray or CT imaging. They share common elements in their formalism and descriptors but have distinct differences. As will be described, radiation dosimetry strives toward a common framework for estimation of risk that is applicable to different types of radiation energy levels and exposure.

Fundamentals, Definitions, and Quantities

The amount of energy absorbed from incident radiation per unit mass of tissue is defined as the *absorbed dose*.[10] It is expressed in units of rads, where *1 rad* is defined as the absorption of 100 ergs per gram of tissue (or 1 joule per kilogram [J/kg]). The absorbed dose definition applies to most forms of radiation relevant to medical imaging, including photons, (x-rays, gamma) and particles with mass (e.g., electrons, positrons). The International System (SI) unit for absorbed dose is the gray (Gy); 1 gray is equal to 100 rads, or 1 rad = 10 mGy. Absorbed dose is also expressed in terms of the *roentgen* (R), a unit of radiation exposure defined as the amount of radiation producing 2.58×10^{-4} coulombs (C) of ionization charge per kilogram of air under standard conditions.[11] Because this is such a complex definition to relate to various materials, the rad or gray are most frequently utilized.

The deposition of energy in tissue occurs through a number of mechanisms that are dependent on the magnitude of energy and atomic properties of the tissue.[10,11] Since the same amount of energy deposited by different forms of radiation can produce different amounts of biological damage, a quantity called the *quality factor* is used to describe the difference.[12] The International Commission on Radiation Protection (ICRP), an important policy-setting body for radiation dosimetry, defines the quality factors as: 20 for alpha particles (helium nucleus), 10 for protons, and 1 for beta particles, gamma rays, and x-rays.[12] Quality factors are dimensionless quantities defined such that the product of the absorbed dose and quality factor give an estimate of the biological damage for the type and amount of radiation. The resulting quantity is called the *dose equivalent* and is expressed in units of rem (roentgen equivalent man) or the SI units of sieverts (Sv).[10] In principle, dose equivalent and absorbed dose have the same units, since the quality factors are dimensionless. However, to differentiate them, the units of dose equivalent are given the names *rems* or *sieverts*. The risk of cancer or harmful effects developing from the biological damage from ionizing radiation are derived from organ-specific dose equivalent values by use of a tissue weighting factor, w_T, reflecting the sensitivity to developing fatal cancer, or, in the latest 2007 revision, including lethality and loss of life quality (ICRP-103). Two quantities commonly used to quantify risk are the *effective dose* (ED)[12] and the *effective dose equivalent* (EDE).[13] The ED has generally replaced the older concept of EDE. Recent changes in the w_T values in 2007 are an increase for breast tissue (from 0.05 to 0.12), a decrease for gonads (from 0.2 to 0.08), and inclusion of more organs and tissues in the "remainder" component (from 0.05 to 0.12). Table 10-1 lists tissue weighting factors for representative organs from the ICRP-30, ICRP-60, and most recent ICRP-103 publications.[13,14] The basic equation relating ED to these quantities is given as:

$$\text{Effective dose} = E = \sum_{T} w_T H_T \qquad (1)$$

where H_T is the tissue-specific equivalent doses and w_T is the tissue-specific weighting factors. Complex mathematic simulation programs are used with standardized

Table 10-1 Tissue Radiation Sensitivity Factors (w_T) from the ICRP-36, ICRP-60, and the Recent ICRP-103 Reports*

	ICRP-26	ICRP-60	ICRP-103
Bladder	—	0.05	0.04
Bone	0.03	0.01	0.01
Brain	—	—	0.01
Breasts	0.15	0.05	0.12
Colon	—	—	0.12
Esophagus	—	0.05	0.04
Liver	—	0.05	0.04
Lower large intestine	—	0.12	—
Lungs	0.12	0.12	0.12
Ovaries/testes	0.25	0.20	0.08
Red marrow	0.12	0.12	0.12
Remainder tissues	0.30	0.05	0.12
Salivary glands	—	—	0.01
Skin	—	0.01	0.01
Stomach	—	0.12	0.12
Thyroid	0.03	0.05	0.04

*A larger value indicates greater risk for biological damage and cancer causation.
ICRP, International Commission on Radiation Protection.

anatomic models of the human body,[15,16] kinetic parameters, and voiding assumptions to estimate H_T. Initially in early ICRP models, organs were simulated as spheres containing uniform amounts of radioactivity, and only self-irradiation was included. Two systems exist for calculation of ED and EDE values: the Medical Internal Radiation Dose (MIRD) system,[16] developed by the Society of Nuclear Medicine specifically for calculating patient radiation doses, and the ICRP system, developed initially for studying and regulating the protection of nuclear industry workers.[13] The MIRD approach includes so-called S-factor's[17] which relate the cumulative activity[16] (integral number of decays in an organ) to the exposure of other organs in order to calculate the dose equivalent. A limiting assumption of the MIRD approach is that the radioactivity in each organ is uniformly distributed. Organs containing no activity may have a non-zero absorbed dose value resulting from the surrounding sources. A total body radiation dose is then calculated from the contributions of all organs and compartments (blood, other structures) of the body by a weighted summation of the values that include the "risk" from each organ's exposure resulting in an equivalent risk from a whole body uniform exposure. Note that the ED is not the same as a "total body dose" often reported on the package insert for many radiopharmaceuticals. The *total body dose* is the total energy deposited anywhere in the body divided by the total mass of the body. The intent is to provide ED and EDE values that quantify the risk in a single number so that exposures under different circumstances (internal, external, amount of radiation, type of radiation, rate and route of delivery, and other factors) can be compared as a common quantity. The values are intended to be independent of the number of exposures or whether a single or multiple organs were exposed.

Values reported for ED or EDE for a specific application and protocol often differ, leading to uncertainty in evaluating risk.[18] This is attributable to differences in assumptions and methodologies in the models and differences in the input data origin. It is important to note that ED and EDE represent expected or average values for a given population. Application to an individual is inappropriate. While radiation dose estimates are provided for an "individual" study by modern CT scanners, it has yet to be implemented for nuclear imaging procedures, as is done for radiation therapy protocols using internal sources.

The package insert (PI) for a radiopharmaceutical is the primary resource for radiation dosimetry values. The dose values are indication-specific and expressed in either rads (rem) or grays (Sv) for a total amount of injected radiopharmaceutical, or "per unit" of injected radiopharmaceutical. The values are typically obtained from studies on normal volunteers under resting conditions, but stress values are included for stress/rest imaging protocols such as myocardial perfusion. The standard stress modality for the PI is exercise stress when given. However, values for pharmacologic stress are often published but are not routine, probably given the many types of pharmacologic stress agents and protocols. The PI also contains relevant dosimetry and safety

information for both toxicity and radiation dose contributions from radionuclide contaminants resulting from the radioisotope or radiopharmaceutical manufacturing process.[19]

The use of ED and EDE as standards for risk is controversial but is the most accepted standard. Individual investigators and position statements reflecting the opinion of health-related professional societies[20-22] have questioned the use of this approach. Issues cited in the debate include the omission of molecular repair mechanisms for biological damage in the risk calculations, differences in the tissue radiosensitivity values across species, or differences in the model and specific assumptions in the methodology. Many of the complex factors affecting the development and response by the body to the many forms of cancer are not well understood nor included in the models. The risk values are thus theoretical calculations with limited outcome of data. Adaptation of the EDE and ED is not universal, and some countries have not accepted them as a standard.

Environmental Sources of Radiation Exposure

When comparing risk values for ionizing radiation exposure, it is useful to contrast them with risk values resulting from environmental sources alone. The risk to the general population from background radiation of all types (naturally occurring and man-made) in the United States is estimated at 3.0 to 3.6 mSv annually.[23,24] The worldwide annual mean value has been estimated at 2.4 mSv, considerably lower than the US value, although some regions are considerably higher, with a range of 1.5 to 10 mSv.[24] One-half to two-thirds of the background radiation dose in the United States is estimated to originate from the alpha particle emissions of radon absorbed by the lungs.[23] Individuals living at higher elevations, where shielding by the atmosphere from high-energy cosmic rays is reduced may receive greater exposure. The background values can be helpful when responding to radiation dose questions.

Radiation Dosimetry of Single-Photon Emission Computed Tomography Myocardial Perfusion Tracers

The technetium (Tc)-99m-labeled tracers ($T_{1/2}$ = 6.02 hours) for myocardial perfusion imaging are Tc-99m sestamibi,[25] Tc-99m tetrofosmin[26] and Tc-99m-teboroxime,[27] although the latter is not currently marketed. Thallium (Tl)-201 chloride ($T_{1/2}$ = 72 hours) is used for myocardial perfusion and viability assessment in single- and dual-isotope protocols.[28] Table 10-2 lists dosimetry values for these tracers from PIs and other sources. Tl-201 dosimetry has attracted particular interest recently because of its high ED and EDE values compared to the Tc-99m perfusion agents and the PET myocardial perfusion agents.[3,18] Shown in Table 10-3 are values for Tl-201 SPECT protocols that can be more than double the values for the Tc-99m agents. Using the PI values, Tc-99m tetrofosmin shows an EDE value

Table 10-2   ICRP and Manufacturers' Data on Effective Doses, Total Body Doses, and Absorbed Doses per Unit Activity for Technetium-99m-Tetrofosmin and Technetium-99m Sestamibi Single-Photon Emission Computed Tomography

Radiopharmaceutical	^{99m}Tc SESTAMIBI						^{99m}Tc TETROFOSMIN			
DATA SOURCE	ICRP-80		PRODUCT INSERT				ICRP-80		PI	
REST/STRESS (VOID TIME)	REST	STRESS	REST (2 H)	REST (4.8 H)	STRESS (2 H)	STRESS (4.8 H)	REST	STRESS	REST	STRESS
Effective dose (mSv/MBq)	9.0E-03	7.9E-03	—	—	3.8E-03	—	7.6E-03	7.0E-03	1.1E-02	8.6E-03
Total body dose (mGy/MBq)	—	—	4.3E-03	4.3E-03	3.8E-03	3.8E-03	—	—	—	—
Organ absorbed doses (mGy/MBq)										
Adrenals	7.5E-03	6.6E-03					3.4E-03	3.3E-03	4.1E-03	4.3E-03
Bladder	1.1E-02	9.8E-03	1.8E-02	3.7E-02	1.4E-02	2.7E-02	1.7E-02	2.6E-02	1.9E-02	1.6E-02
Bone	8.2E-03	7.8E-03	6.1E-03	5.8E-03	5.6E-03	5.4E-03	4.5E-03	4.8E-03	5.6E-03	6.2E-03
Bone marrow	5.5E-03	5.0E-03	4.6E-03	4.5E-03	4.1E-03	4.0E-03	2.9E-03	2.9E-03	4.0E-03	4.1E-03
Brain	5.2E-03	4.4E-03					3.9E-04	4.6E-04	2.2E-03	2.7E-03
Breasts	3.8E-03	3.4E-03	1.8E-03	1.7E-03	1.8E-03	1.6E-03	9.0E-04	1.0E-03	1.8E-03	2.2E-03
Colon	2.4E-02	1.9E-02					2.4E-02	1.8E-02		
Colon (lower large intestine)	1.9E-02	1.6E-02	3.6E-02	3.7E-02	2.9E-02	2.9E-02	2.0E-02	1.5E-02	2.2E-02	1.5E-02
Colon (upper large intestine)	2.7E-02	2.2E-02	5.0E-02	5.0E-02	4.0E-02	4.0E-02	2.7E-02	2.0E-02	3.0E-02	2.0E-02
Esophagus	4.1E-03	4.0E-03					2.1E-03	2.4E-03		
Gallbladder	3.9E-02	3.3E-02	1.8E-02	1.8E-02	2.6E-02	2.5E-02	3.6E-02	2.7E-02	4.9E-02	3.3E-02
Heart	6.3E-03	7.2E-03	4.6E-03	4.4E-03	5.0E-03	4.8E-03	4.4E-03	4.8E-03	3.9E-03	4.1E-03
Kidneys	3.6E-02	2.6E-02	1.8E-02	1.8E-02	1.5E-02	1.5E-02	1.4E-02	1.1E-02	1.3E-02	1.0E-02
Liver	1.1E-02	9.2E-03	5.2E-03	5.1E-03	3.8E-03	3.7E-03	4.0E-03	3.3E-03	4.2E-03	3.2E-03
Lungs	4.6E-03	4.4E-03	2.5E-03	2.4E-03	2.3E-03	2.2E-03	2.0E-03	2.2E-03	2.1E-03	2.3E-03
Muscles	2.9E-03	3.2E-03					3.7E-03	4.1E-03	3.3E-03	3.5E-03
Ovaries	9.1E-03	8.1E-03	1.4E-02	1.4E-02	1.1E-02	1.2E-02	8.4E-03	7.6E-03	9.6E-03	7.9E-03
Pancreas	7.7E-03	6.9E-03					4.1E-03	3.9E-03	5.0E-03	5.0E-03
Remaining organs	3.1E-03	3.3E-03					3.9E-03	4.1E-03		
Salivary glands	1.4E-02	9.2E-03					1.4E-02	9.3E-03	1.2E-02	8.0E-03
Skin	3.1E-03	2.9E-03					1.3E-03	1.4E-03	1.9E-03	2.2E-03
Small intestine	1.5E-02	1.2E-02	2.7E-02	2.7E-02	2.2E-02	2.2E-02	1.5E-02	1.1E-02	1.7E-02	1.2E-02
Spleen	6.5E-03	5.8E-03					3.0E-03	3.0E-03	3.8E-03	4.1E-03
Stomach	6.5E-03	5.9E-03	5.5E-03	5.2E-03	4.8E-03	4.7E-03	3.7E-03	3.5E-03	4.6E-03	4.6E-03
Testes	3.8E-03	3.7E-03	3.1E-03	3.5E-03	2.8E-03	3.1E-03	2.4E-03	2.9E-03	3.1E-03	3.4E-03
Thalamus										
Thymus	4.1E-03	4.0E-03					2.1E-03	2.4E-03	2.5E-03	3.1E-03
Thyroid	5.3E-03	4.4E-03	6.3E-03	6.3E-03	2.4E-03	2.2E-03	5.7E-03	4.8E-03	5.8E-03	4.3E-03
Uterus	7.8E-03	7.2E-03					7.2E-03	7.6E-03	8.4E-03	7.3E-03

ICRP, International Commission on Radiation Protection.
Andrew J. Einstein; Kevin W. Moser; Randall C. Thompson; Manuel D. Cerqueira; Milena J. Henzlova. Online-only Data Supplement to *Radiation Dose to Patients from Cardiac Diagnostic Imaging Circulation.* 2007;116:1290–1305.

Table 10-3 ICRP and Manufacturers' Data on Effective Doses, Total Body Doses, and Absorbed Doses per Unit Activity for PET Cardiac Imaging and Other Radiopharmaceuticals

Radiopharmaceutical	^{201}Tl				^{99m}Tc-LABELED ERYTHROCYTES		^{82}Rb		^{13}N-ammonia	^{15}O-water	^{18}F-FDG
DATA SOURCE	ICRP-53A5	PI 1	PI 2	PI 3	ICRP-80	PI	ICRP-80	PI	ICRP-80	ICRP-53A5	ICRP-80
EFFECTIVE DOSE (mSv/MBq)	1.7E-01	3.6E-01	5.9E-02	3.6E-01	7.0E-03	4.1E-03	3.4E-03	4.3E-04	2.0E-03	1.1E-03	1.9E-02
TOTAL BODY DOSE (mGy/MBq) — DATA SOURCE	ICRP-53A5	PI 1	PI 2	PI 3	ICRP-80	PI	ICRP-53	PI	ICRP-53	ICRP-53A5	ICRP-80
Organ absorbed doses (mGy/MBq)											
Adrenals	5.8E-02	6.2E-02		6.5E-02	9.9E-03		2.0E-02	9.7E-04	2.3E-03	1.4E-03	1.2E-02
Bladder	4.1E-02	5.2E-02	5.3E-02	5.3E-02	8.5E-03	6.5E-03	1.7E-04	1.7E-04	8.1E-03	2.6E-04	1.6E-01
Bone	3.8E-01	8.8E-02	8.5E-02	8.5E-02	7.4E-03	6.5E-03	6.7E-04	6.6E-06	1.6E-03	6.3E-04	1.1E-02
Bone marrow	1.1E-01	5.5E-02	5.6E-02	5.6E-02	6.1E-03	4.1E-03	9.9E-04	3.8E-04	1.7E-03	8.9E-04	1.1E-02
Brain	2.3E-02	5.9E-02	6.1E-02	6.1E-02	3.6E-03				4.2E-03	1.3E-03	2.8E-02
Breasts	2.5E-02	3.6E-02	3.6E-02	3.6E-02	3.5E-03		1.9E-04	1.9E-04	1.8E-03	2.8E-04	8.6E-03
Colon	2.5E-01				3.7E-03					1.6E-03	1.3E-02
Colon (lower large intestine)	3.4E-01	5.9E-02	5.9E-02	3.4E-01	3.4E-03		3.9E-03	8.6E-04	1.9E-03	1.6E-03	1.5E-02
Colon (upper large intestine)	1.8E-01	7.0E-02	7.0E-02	3.3E-01	4.0E-03		3.9E-03	8.6E-04	1.8E-03	1.6E-03	1.2E-02
Esophagus	3.6E-02				6.1E-03					3.3E-04	1.1E-02
Gall bladder	6.6E-02	8.3E-02		8.4E-02	6.5E-03					4.5E-04	1.2E-02
Heart	1.9E-01	2.8E-01	1.4E-01	2.8E-01	2.3E-02	2.7E-02	3.3E-03	1.9E-03	2.1E-03	1.9E-03	6.2E-02
Kidneys	4.8E-01	4.6E-01	3.2E-01	4.6E-01	1.8E-02		1.8E-02	8.7E-03	4.6E-03	1.7E-03	2.1E-02
Liver	1.5E-01	9.9E-02	1.6E-01	9.9E-02	1.3E-02	7.8E-03	9.7E-04	8.7E-04	4.0E-03	1.6E-03	1.1E-02
Lungs	1.1E-01	4.7E-02	4.8E-02	4.8E-02	1.8E-02		2.4E-03	1.7E-03	2.5E-03	1.6E-03	1.0E-02
Muscles	5.2E-02	4.6E-02	4.7E-02	4.7E-02	3.3E-03					2.9E-04	1.1E-02
Ovaries	1.2E-01	1.0E-01	1.3E-01	1.0E-01	3.7E-03	4.3E-03	2.4E-04	3.8E-04	1.7E-03	8.5E-04	1.5E-02
Pancreas	5.8E-02	7.4E-02		7.5E-02	6.6E-03		4.5E-03	6.3E-04	1.9E-03	1.4E-03	1.2E-02
Remaining organs	5.4E-02				3.5E-03	1.1E-02	2.3E-04	2.3E-04	1.6E-03	4.0E-04	1.1E-02
Salivary glands											
Skin	2.2E-02	3.3E-02		3.4E-02	2.0E-03		3.9E-03	1.4E-03	1.8E-03	2.5E-04	8.0E-03
Small intestine	1.4E-01	4.5E-01	1.1E-01	4.5E-01	3.9E-03		5.0E-03		1.7E-03	1.3E-03	1.3E-02
Spleen	1.2E-01	1.8E-01		1.8E-01	1.4E-02	3.0E-02	3.8E-03	8.6E-04	2.5E-03	1.6E-03	1.1E-02
Stomach	1.2E-01	1.9E-01		1.9E-01	4.6E-03		1.3E-04	3.0E-04	1.7E-03	1.7E-03	1.1E-02
Testes	4.5E-01	8.2E-01	1.5E-01	8.3E-01	2.3E-03	3.0E-03			1.8E-03	7.4E-04	1.2E-02
Thalamus				4.7E-02							
Thymus	3.6E-02	4.6E-02			6.1E-03				1.7E-03	3.3E-04	1.1E-02
Thyroid	2.2E-01	6.2E-01	1.3E-01	6.2E-01	5.7E-03		3.8E-03	3.8E-04	1.7E-03	1.5E-03	1.0E-02
Uterus	5.1E-02	8.5E-02	8.6E-02	8.6E-02	3.9E-03		2.1E-04	2.1E-04	1.9E-03	3.5E-04	2.1E-02

ICRP 53A5 denotes ICRP Publication 53 Addendum 5. Three manufacturers currently produce ^{201}Tl for medical use in the United States; Their package inserts are referred to as PI, PI 1, PI 2, and PI 3.
^{18}F-FDG, ^{18}F-fluorodeoxyglucose; ICRP, International Commission on Radiation Protection; ^{82}Rb, rubidium-82; ^{99m}Tc, technetium-99m; ^{201}Tl, thallium-201.
Adapted from Andrew J. Einstein; Kevin W. Moser; Randall C. Thompson; Manuel D. Cerqueira Milena J. Henzlova. Online-only Data Supplement to *Radiation Dose to Patients from Cardiac Diagnostic Imaging Circulation.* 2007;116:1290–1305 with permission.

of 8.61E-03 mSv/MBq for exercise stress and 1.12E-02 mSv/MBq for the resting dose.[18] Therefore, a conventional rest/stress SPECT imaging protocol using a 30 mCi (1110 MBq) stress injection and 10 mCi (370 MBq) rest injection yields a total EDE of approximately 14.0 mSv. A rest/stress protocol using Tc-99m sestamibi from the PI values for the same injected activity and protocol yields an absorbed radiation dose of 570 mrad.[25] Based on the PI for Tl-201, a stress-redistribution protocol utilizing 3.0 mCi of activity results has an EDE of 37 mSv.[18] A dual-isotope SPECT protocol using a 3.0 mCi dose of Tl-201 at rest and a 30 mCi dose of a Tc-99m agent at stress results in an EDE of approximately 41 mSv.[3,18] Thus, the inclusion of a Tl-201 injection results in a significant increase in radiation dose compared with the other protocols. Thomas et al. recently examined the dose from Tl-201 chloride to the testes in adults and children, important for fertility considerations. The study recommended a downward revision from the current ICRP values for testicular dose by a factor of almost 2.[29] The impact, however, on total ED or EDE values was not significant. For breastfeeding women who must have a nuclear medicine study, a temporary suspension of breastfeeding following the scans currently recommended. The delay (2 weeks) is somewhat unique for Tl-201 studies, given the longer physical half-life. The Nuclear Regulatory Commission (NRC)[30] provides specific guidance for the recommended suspension of breastfeeding following a nuclear study, based on the radiopharmaceutical and protocol. Data suggesting that some studies may not warrant suspension of breastfeeding are provided in Refs. 31 and 32. Lastly, radiation dose considerations specific to males and females may be important if the same injected activity is given to both genders, due to organ mass differences, biokinetics, and other factors.[32]

Radiation Dosimetry for Cardiac Positron Emission Tomography Tracers

Table 10-3 lists radiation dose values for the approved cardiac PET tracers and other cardiac imaging tracers. Rubidium-82 chloride (Rb-82) ($T_{1/2}$ = 75 sec) is a chemical analog of Tl-201 chloride used for the assessment of coronary artery disease with PET.[19,33] Rb-82 is produced as the daughter radionuclide of strontium-82 (Sr-82) eluted from a portable on-site generator renewed approximately monthly due to the physical half-life of Sr-82 ($T_{1/2}$ = 25 days).[19,34] Assay of the eluent for trace contaminants of Strontium (Sr-85) ($T_{1/2}$ = 64.8 days) and Sr-82 is required as part of daily quality control. SR-82 activity levels toward the end of the month result in a lower maximum available Rb-82 dose for injection, with a concordant reduced exposure.

The Rb-82 PI reports dosimetry values based on data from Kearfott et al.[35] in animals and Ryan et al.[36] in normal human volunteers. For an adult, an absorbed radiation dose of 0.95 mGy/2220 MBq or 0.096 rads for each 60 mCi injected is reported. Lodge et al.[37] computed effective dose equivalent values of 5.5 mSv for combined rest/stress doses of 60 mCi each. Effective dose equivalent values were reported in ICRP-80 of

15.8 mSv for combined rest/stress (60 mCi total) injections.[38] Recently, deKemp et al.[39] reexamined ED values for Rb-82 myocardial perfusion PET, specifically the role of conservative assumptions used in early dose studies. The authors suggest that the ICRP-80 values may overestimate ED by as much as fivefold, lending weight to the PI values.

Nitrogen-13 ammonia chloride (N-13; $T_{1/2}$ = 10 min) is used for PET imaging in the diagnosis of coronary artery disease[40] and for quantitative assessment of myocardial bloodflow.[41] N-13 production requires on-site cyclotron and radiochemistry facilities for rapid preparation and injection into the patient. By comparison, the positrons emitted from N-13 are significantly lower in energy (492 keV) compared to those from Rb-82 and contribute to less radiation dose from N-13 (Valentin et al.) in ICRP-80, reported values for N-13 ammonia chloride for rest/stress injections of 550 MBq (15 mCi) each, equal to 2.2 mSv.[41]

F-18-labeled fluorodeoxyglucose (F-18DG; $T_{1/2}$ = 110 min) is utilized with PET cardiac imaging for the assessment of myocardial viability, evaluating the extent of scar, hibernating myocardium, and stunned myocardium.[42] FDG provides complimentary information to poorly perfused or equivocal regions on rest/stress images. FDG cardiac imaging is performed conventionally at rest after metabolically preparing the myocardium for optimal FDG uptake. The FDG PI reports dose values for a single 10 mCi injection of FDG.[43] ICRP-80 reports that for this amount of activity, the effective dose is 7 mSv.[44] The Oak Ridge Associated Laboratories reported an effective dose equivalent 3.0E-02 mSv/MBq, which for a 10 mCi (370 MBq) injection yields 11.2 mSv.[44] FDG is provided in unit dose syringes, and thus as with N-13 ammonia, there are important radiation safety considerations for the technologist and clinical personnel involved with the study.[45,46] Shown for reference in Table 10-4 are representative values of doses from other common medical imaging procedures using ionizing radiation.

Table 10-4 Radiation Exposure Estimates from Common Medical Imaging Procedures

STUDY TYPE	RELEVANT ORGAN	RELEVANT ORGAN DOSE (mGy or mSv)
Dental radiography	Brain	0.005
Posterior-anterior chest radiography	Lung	0.01
Lateral chest radiography	Lung	0.15
Screening mammography	Breast	3
Adult abdominal CT	Stomach	10
Barium enema	Colon	15
Neonatal abdominal CT	Stomach	20

CT, Computed tomography.
Brenner DJ, Hall EJ. Computed tomography—an increasing source of radiation exposure. *N Engl J Med* 2007;357:2277-2284.

MODELS FOR RADIATION RISK

The Linear No-Threshold Model for Radiation Risk

The linear no-threshold (LNT) model[47,48] describes a relationship between risk of harmful effects and the amount of exposure to ionizing radiation (Fig. 10-1). The LNT model implies that there is no level of exposure to ionizing radiation below which there is zero risk of causing cancer. It also implies that risk will increase in direct linear proportion to the amount of radiation exposure, and typically refers to an "instantaneous" exposure and a lifetime risk of fatal cancer. The model stands in contrast to alternative proposed models suggesting that an exposure threshold exists below which the risk of cancer induction is negligible, nonexistent, or potentially beneficial. A key criticism of the LNT model centers on the extrapolation of data based primarily on observed health effects following the high-intensity exposures from the Hiroshima and Nagasaki events of World War II to the "low-level" ionizing radiation exposure values of diagnostic imaging. The appropriateness of the LNT model was reemphasized in the 2005 report by the Biological Effects of Ionizing Radiation (BEIR) Committee report number 7, following examination of the weight of current evidence.[48] Of particular interest in the report was the implication for so-called low-level (<100 mSv) exposures typical of diagnostic imaging procedures. The cancer risk coefficient predicted from the LNT model is 4.8×10^{-4} per rem. Or, an additional five cancers would be expected above a baseline rate of 3000 for an individual receiving a 1-rem exposure in their lifetime. This would be approximately the same exposure from a conventional CT angiography study or SPECT rest/stress myocardial perfusion imaging (MPI) study with Tc-99m agents.

As exposure levels become very high (>100 mSv), the risk of causing cancer becomes more predictable. Effects for an exposure that are certain to result are referred to as *deterministic* and are typically associated with values well above 100 mSv. When effects are not confidently predictable, they are referred to as *stochastic*, implying the intrinsic uncertainty in the frequency of occurrence. The LNT model is considered conservative and promotes that the only conclusively "safe" exposure level is zero. A balance of risk from exposure in diagnostic testing and the risk of fatal cardiovascular disease or associated comorbidity from inappropriate diagnosis in the population is a critical debate framed by the LNT model. The model stands as the primary reference for guiding imaging and radiation dosimetry exposure policies.

Attributable Lifetime Risk from Radiation Exposure

The theoretical risk of harmful effects from ionizing radiation exposure over a lifetime is dependent on the age of the individual at the time of exposure. Individual exposures at various times during a lifetime are combined through a weighting that takes into account the probabilistic nature of delay between exposure and development of cancer, which changes with age.[49] The cumulative effect has been described by the attributable lifetime risk (ALR).[49,50] The ALR differs from the simple additive approach of exposures occurring at times that are negligibly separated compared to the expected human lifetime. There are also differences in ALR for males and females.[49] The issue of repeated cardiac CT studies on ALR has been reported in several studies recently, based on the models and data described in the BEIR VII report. Einstein et al.[50] examined the ALR of fatal cancer from cardiac CT exposures using models and data from the BEIR VII report. Among their findings, the authors reported that ALR estimates for standard cardiac scans varied from 1 in 143 for a 20-year-old woman to 1 in approximately 3300 for an 80-year-old male. Sodicksin et al.[51] examined data retrospectively from more than 190,000 CT studies focusing on ALR of individuals having repeat CT examinations over the previous 22 years. 33% of patients had 5 or more lifetime CT examinations, 5% had more than 22 over their lifetime, and 15% received more than 100 mSv collectively over their lifetime. The resulting ALR values had mean and maximum values of 0.3% and 12% for cancer incidence and 0.2% and 6.8% for cancer mortality, respectively, showing that cumulative exposure from CT examinations had an incremental lifetime of cancer above baseline. Importantly, the subjects of this study did not have the advantages of modern CT dose-reduction techniques, which hypothetically would have reduced the increased incidence for this population.

In a similar study on whole-body PET/CT using 18-FDG and comparing U.S. and Hong Kong populations, Huang et al. also found an increase in the ALR for cancer, which interestingly was significantly greater for the Hong Kong population.[52] Quantitation of risk from "low-dose" ionizing radiation is controversial because of the lack of definitive outcome-based studies linking low levels of radiation exposure with health effects as acknowledged in the BEIR VII report. Approximately 2000 to 4000 of every 10,000 individuals will die of

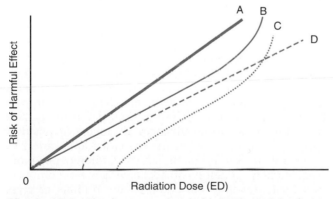

Figure 10-1 The linear no-threshold (LNT) model relating exposure to ionizing radiation and the incremental risk of developing cancer. **A,** LNT. **B,** LNT and nonlinear response above a threshold dose. **C,** Threshold at lower dose and nonlinear at higher doses. **D,** Threshold at a lower dose and linear at higher doses.

cancers of all origins.[53] It has been estimated that 1 rem (10 mSv) of exposure received annually, or approximately three times the expected annual value, from background radiation sources for the U.S. population received in "small doses" over an individual's lifetime will result in 5 to 6 additional fatal cancers per 10,000 individuals (1 in 2000 to 1 in 2500)[54,55]. It could therefore be concluded that up to 0.06% (6/10,000) additional deaths from cancer will result, or the 2000 possible deaths is increased to 2006 out of 10,000. If the average lifetime of an individual is 76 years, extrapolating this relationship to a 10-mSv exposure would increase the risk approximately threefold to 2018 out of 10,000 is implied.

Another important risk consideration is the so-called genetic effects that extend beyond an individual's risk to the progeny through passing of genetic mutation. The genetically significant dose (GSD)[56] represents the estimated dose to the population gene pool that can result in genetic effects in its offspring. *GSD* is defined as the dose that, if received by every member of the population, would produce the total genetic effect on the population as the sum of the individual doses actually received. It is a complex quantity related to age, number of expected children, gender, type of exposure and other factors. The GSD is currently estimated to be 20 mrad above the annual background radiation exposure levels. This dose is well below a detectable level and is well within radiation exposure tolerance for the population.

Occupational Radiation Exposure and Limitations

The NRC provides well-enforced legal limits for professional staff exposure to radiation in the provision of medical services.[57] The key sources of exposure for a nuclear cardiac imaging facility likely include the management of waste and preparation of patient doses in the hot laboratory, exposure to radiopharmaceuticals at the time of injection, and secondary radiation exposure from the patient post injection, during monitoring or image acquisition. The cumulative exposure values are dependent upon the number of studies performed annually, the role of the individual in relation to interaction with the radiopharmaceutical and patient, and the properties of the radionuclides and protocols used at the facility. For CT facilities, the exposure can be considerably less than nuclear laboratories because of the separation of patients and staff during x-ray exposure and the cessation of exposure at the end of the study, compared with the finite half-lives of radiopharmaceuticals. Exposure to staff from combined SPECT/CT or PET/CT includes the additive exposure from both modalities. Schleipman et al.[58] described the radiation exposure to staff in a nuclear medicine department performing Rb-82 rest/stress PET and Tc-99m sestamibi rest/stress myocardial perfusion studies. In particular, they examined the role of physical position of the technologist with respect to the patient. For this laboratory performing pharmacologic stress protocols, the dose to personnel was less than that for the Tc-99m studies. Additionally,

the exposure to the personnel for routine stress testing at variable distances from the patient was equivalent to background.

"As Low As Reasonably Achievable" Principle

The "as low as reasonably achievable" (ALARA) principle[59] applies to all aspects of radiation exposure, including diagnostic imaging. The principle is intended to promote a culture and mindset resulting in minimizing exposure to ionizing radiation at all reasonable costs. For patients, if no benefit is obtained, there is no justification for the medical radiation exposure. For laboratory personnel, there is no benefit receiving unnecessary radiation exposure, particularly if it is not essential to performing their duties. In general, perhaps with the exception of mammography, there are no federal regulations limiting the radiation dose to patients.[60] Beyond these considerations, adherence to the structure imposed by the ALARA concept supports an overall efficiency of laboratory operations for all imaging modalities, and limitation of patient radiation dose is largely entrusted to the physician and technologist. In 1994, the ALARA principle was adopted as part of Title 10 of the Code of Federal Regulations (10 CFR 35.20), which is binding on all institutions as an NRC regulation.

COMPUTED TOMOGRAPHY (See Chapter 21)

CT scanner technology has advanced at an unprecedented pace, including increases in the number of slices, temporal resolution, spiral resolution and electrocardiogram (ECG)-gating strategies, and dual-source dual-energy capabilities.[61] The temporal resolution and multislice capabilities are particularly important for improving imaging of the heart during the cardiac cycle by reducing image blurring. CT is also used routinely to obtain transmission scans for attenuation correction of PET images and calcium scoring studies. The growth in the number of CT studies has raised concern about the cumulative effect of radiation exposure and ALR for cancer. Brenner and Hall[2] examined CT utilization, reporting the number of scans performed in the United States increased from 3 million in 1980 to 62 million in 2006. The authors highlight that the greatest proportional increase in CT studies has occurred in the pediatric population, citing advances in image acquisition speed (<1 second) and in the increased application to screening of asymptomatic adults. Children are more susceptible to radiation damage, having greater numbers of actively dividing cells and a greater number of years in which a "lifetime cancer" can be realized. In response to these factors, medical imaging societies have produced position statements, guidelines, and other publications to advance education on the issues of radiation exposure in diagnostic imaging.[60,62,63]

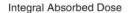

Integral Absorbed Dose

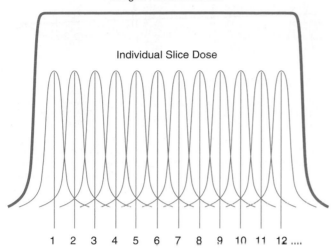

Individual Slice Dose

1 2 3 4 5 6 7 8 9 10 11 12 ....

Figure 10-2 Irradiation of tissues in adjacent regions to each transaxial slice with computed tomography (CT). Minimizing the amount of overlapping radiation is an important objective in system design and imaging protocol implementation. As overlap is reduced, integral dose—and therefore CT dose index and effective dose—are proportionally reduced.

CT Radiation Dosimetry: Fundamentals, Definitions, and Quantities

The approach to dosimetry for CT is similar in many ways to the internal dosimetry approach. Radiation risk calculations from x-ray CT exposure are based on the use of the CT dose index (CTDI).[64-66] The CTDI is calculated as the integral over the range of exposure along the z-axis (system or patient axis) of the radiation dose profile. It represents the average absorbed dose for the series of contiguous irradiated sections of tissue. It is calculated assuming that the "tails" of the exposure profiles are included, which is a theoretical approximation (Fig. 10-2). Common variants of the CTDI include $CTDI_{FDA}$, $CTDI_{100}$, $CTDI_{W}$, and $CTDI_{vol}$; the definitions and differences are discussed in detail elsewhere.[64-67] The differences are related to the multislice capabilities of the system, as expressed by pitch, calibration of the measurements against known geometries, and other factors. The $CTDI_{vol}$ is commonly implemented on modern CT scanners to provide individual patient dose estimates. The SI units of CTDI are the milligray (mGy). The American College of Radiology requires sites applying for accreditation to measure CTDI and ED values for a range of pediatric and adult imaging applications.

From the CTDI, the dose length product, which represents the overall energy absorbed for a CT scan, is obtained by integration of the CTDI over the z-axis length of the scan.[67] DLP represents the potential biological effect delivered by the absorbed energy of the scan but is not yet a measure of risk, which requires incorporation of the specific sensitivity of each tissue to the type and amount of radiation. The DLP is most commonly calculated using Monte Carlo calculations, which track the path of individual x-rays and their ionization products and the location of energy deposition in models of standard anatomic geometries much like the MIRD approach described earlier. ED values for various studies

and specific regions of the body (e.g., head, neck, abdomen, pelvis, thorax) can then be calculated as the product of the DLP and a factor, k, representing the proportion and sensitivity of tissues in the scan region.[67] The units of k are $mSv\text{-}mGy^{-1}\text{-}cm^{-1}$, so that the product is expressed in units of mSv. The values of k are dependent upon the parameters of the acquisition (mAs, kVp, pitch), but the calibration is typically performed automatically by the system. The appropriateness of these values in larger patients or specific populations is a concern, and deviations in the values may be significant. It is important to note that in all cases, the ED represents an "expected" dose and is not an exact dose for each patient, as with the internal dosimetry values. However, while certain values have become standard, these models have intrinsic variability,[67] as with other quantitative dose methods. It should be emphasized that at the time of this writing, CT system estimates for DLP are highly dependent upon specific 'default' study acquisition parameters defined by the manufacturer. Deviation from these default settings may result in erroneous DLP values, and therefore exposures that differ significantly from expected values. This would have the unintended consequence of potentially delivering a higher dose than suggested by the calculations. It is highly recommended that the DLP values be calibrated or confirmed to be accurate when acquisition parameters are manually adjusted. This is most effectively performed by a medical or health physicist with expertise in cardiac CT technologies and imaging protocols.

Dose Reduction Techniques for Cardiac Computed Tomography

The most important consideration in avoiding unnecessary radiation exposure is the appropriateness of the scan. There have been remarkable technical advances, resulting in a significant reduction in the radiation dose from CT studies, and they have been rapidly implemented in clinical practice. Details of specific technical approaches are described in the sections that follow. However, there are important practical considerations that should be applied regularly to help minimize excessive dose exposure:

1. Limiting the axial length of the scan to only those regions essential to the clinical question
2. Selecting appropriate beam collimation and filtration if available
3. Use of optimal mAs and kVp values, taking patient body habitus or other special considerations into consideration
4. Use of preferred angular projection ranges to minimize exposure of radiosensitive tissues
5. Shielding of organs not directly in the field of view

Scanners with fewer slices have been reported to provide lower radiation exposure than those with a higher number of slices.[68] However, this should now be considered on balance with radiation dose reduction methods; the generalization may not hold true. The application of highly standardized protocols emphasizing all aspects of dose limitation are important and needed. Hausleiter et al. recently[69] reported the wide variability in radiation dose associated with cardiac CT angiography. In their study, 94% of systems were 64 slice and the remainder 16 slice, and primarily single source. They reported that radiation dose estimates differed significantly, ranging from 5.7 mSv to 36.5 mSv, with a median of 15.4 mSv. Furthermore, they reported the widely variable application of standardized dose reduction strategies when available. Extended discussion of other important considerations and in-depth detail for a range of imaging circumstances are described elsewhere.[61]

Tube Current Modulation

Modulation of the tube current (mA) or effective tube current (mAs) based on the patient's anatomy, specific region of interest, or susceptibility to radiation exposure of certain organs is a highly effective method for optimizing radiation dose.[70,71] Modulation of the dose may be applied along the z-axis of the patient (longitudinal variation), angularly to respond to thicker regions of the body, or both (angular-longitudinal).[61] The current may be modulated to rise and fall with variable frequency and by various amounts, depending on the parameters of the acquisition. The principle is based on recognition that attenuations through different regions or at different angles through the body are quite different and can be exploited to reduce dose. In general, most methods utilize a "scout" or "topogram" image just prior to the study scan combined with a second lateral scan or an anteroposterior scan, with predictive algorithms to (1) estimate attenuation along projections through the body and (2) predict the expected image noise levels to avoid compromising image reconstruction accuracy at the expense of reduced dose. The small additional exposure from the scout scans is easily offset by the reduction in exposure of the modulated study scan. Body mass index (BMI) or other body habitus descriptors may be used in some systems. Based on the predicted optimal intensity required for each projection, the tube current is varied as the scanner translates through the acquisition. Additionally, tube current modulation may be used with automatic exposure-control algorithms that will assist in predicting overall noise or contrast-to-noise values requested by the operator.

ECG-Pulse Modulation

For cardiac imaging, minimizing the effects of heart motion during the cardiac cycle is critical to maximizing image quality. While tube current modulation can be applied to general radiologic CT studies, additional reduction in radiation dose for cardiac CT scans can be obtained from the use of ECG-pulse modulation techniques during image acquisition (Fig. 10-3).[72,73] With these methods, the tube current rapidly rises to a plateau, followed by a rapid descent to a baseline, resulting in a proportional change in x-ray beam exposure triggered at points in the R-R cycle by the ECG.[74] The technique may be applied in a retrospective or prospective mode, and the degree of dose reduction for each is very different. *Retrospective ECG-gated pulse-modulation* refers to the reconstruction of image data acquired as with a conventional acquisition, where projection data are

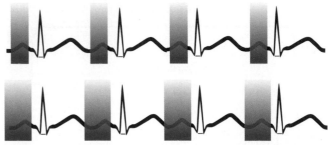

Figure 10-3 The principles of ECG-gating of cardiac computed tomography images by use of a window placed over a region of the cardiac cycle. Retrospective gating applies a windowing to the data after they are acquired over the full cardiac cycle. Prospective gating uses a predictive algorithm that samples the cardiac cycle prior to imaging and acquires the data over the windowed region only. Top and bottom show two possible windows based on ECG-patterns.

obtained over the full R-R cycle. The image data are stored such that the user may select a specific subset of data from the cardiac cycle. Image data weighted toward the ED phase is typically used, since the heart is most static at this phase. Prospective ECG-pulse modulation utilizes a prediction algorithm to estimate the time of subsequent phases of the cardiac cycle to predict a preset window for imaging, such that image data are acquired only for this region of the cardiac cycle.[73] By modulating the acquisition in this way, exposure during the other phases is avoided, with a proportional reduction in radiation dose.

Organ and Breast Shielding

A specific concern for CT radiation exposure has been related to the female population, where a higher effective dose to the breast results from elevated radiosensitivity of breast tissue[75,76] and direct positioning in the beam. Several groups have recently reported the utilization of breast shielding methods to minimize exposure to certain organs, applied in pediatric studies and to women. A primary concern with these approaches has been the effect on image noise, which may compromise image quality, and the introduction of image artifacts related to projection sampling. At this time, these methods have not been widely adopted, owing to concerns about image quality, but they continue to be investigated and have shown effectiveness for dose reduction.

Dosimetry Values for Cardiac CT Procedures

Table 10-5 lists radiation dose results from a large number of recent studies in the literature, conducted over various populations, methods, and CT systems.[77–96] As can be seen, the results are variable. Additionally, studies using a form of modulation, whether ECG or contrast (exposure control) based, tend to yield ED values approximately one-half or less the values without. Additional information on the differences is captured in the recent publication by Hausleiter et al.[69] concluding that dose reduction techniques, although available, are not routinely used and may reflect practical limitations that remain in their implementation.

Table 10-5 Cardiac Computed Tomography Angiography Radiation Dose Values Collated from a Number of Studies

STUDY	SLICES	VENDOR	METHOD	MEAN EFFECTIVE DOSE ESTIMATES, mSv					
				CTCA			CALCIUM SCORING		
				WITHOUT ECTCM	MIXED	WITH ECTCM	WITHOUT ECTCM	WITH ECTCM	PROSPECTIVE GATING
Hunold et al.[77]	4	Siemens	TLD-ARP (low)	6.7♂ 8.1♀	—	—	3.0♂ 3.6♀	—	1.5♂ 1.8♀
	4	Siemens	TLD-ARP (high)	10.9♂ 13.0♀	—	—	5.2♂ 6.2♀	—	—
McCollough[78]	4	– (1st)	Multiple	9.0	—	—	2.5	—	0.9
	4	– (2nd)	Multiple	12.0	—	—	4.5	—	1.1
Poll et al.[74]	4	Siemens	DLP	8.3♂ 11.0♀	—	4.0♂ 5.4♀	1.9♂ 2.5♀	1.2♂ 1.6♀	—
	4	Siemens	TLD-ARP	10.3♂ 12.7♀	—	4.6♂ 5.6♀	2.4♂ 2.9♀	1.5♂ 1.8♀	—
Hacker et al.[79]	12	Siemens	—	—	—	4.3	—	4.1	—
Coles et al.[80]	12	Siemens	CTDosimetry.xls	14.2	—	—	4.1	2.6	—
	16	Siemens	CTDosimetry.xls	15.3	—	—	—	—	—
Flohr et al.[81]	16	Siemens	WinDose	7.3♂ 10.5♀	—	4.3♂ 6.4♀	2.2♂ 3.1♀	—	0.45♂ 0.65♀
Garcia et al.[76]	16	Philips	DLP	—	8	—	—	—	—
Gerber et al.[83]	16	Siemens	Modified DLP	11.3	—	8.1	—	—	—
Hoffmann et al.[82]	16	Philips	Modified DLP	4.0	—	8.1	—	—	—
Nawfel and Yoshizumi[84]	16	GE	MOSFET-CIRS	20.6	—	—	—	—	—
	16	Siemens	MOSFET-CIRS	18.8	—	—	—	—	—
Sato et al.[85]	4	Siemens	—	4-5	—	—	—	—	—
	16	Toshiba	—	7-8	—	—	—	—	—
Trabold et al.[86]	16	Siemens	TLD-ARP	8.1♂ 10.9♀	—	4.3♂ 5.6♀	2.9♂ 3.6♀	1.6♂ 2.0♀	—
Gaspar et al.[87]	40	Philips	Modified DLP	9.9	—	—	—	—	—
Caussin et al.[88]	64	Siemens	—	—	8.4	—	—	—	—
Hausleiter et al.[89]	16	Siemens	DLP	10.5	—	6.4	—	—	—
	64	Siemens	DLP	14.3	—	9.4	—	—	—
Chostine et al.[90]	64	Siemens	DLP	—	—	7	—	—	—
Leber et al.[91]	64	Siemens	—	—	—	10-14	—	—	—
Mollet et al.[92]	64	Siemens	WinDose	15.2♂ 21.4♀	—	—	—	1.3♂ 1.7♀	—
Muhlenbruch et al.[93]	64	Siemens	—	13.6♂ 17.2♀	—	—	—	—	—
Nikolaou et al.[94]	64	Siemens	WinDose	8-10	—	—	—	—	—
Pugliese et al.[95]	64	Siemens	—	15♂ 20♀	—	—	—	—	—
Raff et al.[95]	64	Siemens	—	13♂ 18♀	—	—	—	—	—

Gender symbols refer to the number of subjects in each group.

Adapted from Andrew J. Einstein; Kevin W. Moser; Manuel D. Cerqueira; Milena J. Henzlova. *Radiation Dose to Patients from Cardiac Diagnostic Imaging Circulation.* 2007;116:1290-1305 with permission.

X-RAY AND RADIONUCLIDE SOURCE–BASED RADIATION EXPOSURE FOR PET AND SPECT ATTENUATION CORRECTION

PET imaging requires attenuation correction as a standard for effective image accuracy. Some dedicated PET systems utilize radionuclide sources (germanium-68 or cesium-137) for transmission attenuation correction.[97] Transmission imaging using radionuclide sources for SPECT remains an option,[98] as well as CT[99] using low-dose protocols. Absorbed dose values from transmission exposure for attenuation correction have been reported and show minimal additional dose is added compared with the internal radiation dose of most procedures: typically less than 1.0 mSv and often lower than 0.6 mSv. PET/CT and SPECT/CT hybrid systems, combined, therefore deliver greater radiation dose for attenuation correction compared with the radionuclide sources alone but the amount is minimal.

SUMMARY

The risk of inducing harmful effects from the levels of ionization radiation in diagnostic imaging is accepted as a real possibility that current management strategies must address. However, for appropriately applied studies, the risk-benefit relationship favors the risk of testing under these conditions. The options and range of values that technical variables can assume, and the influence on the delivery of radiation dose vary considerably by modality. Dose reduction methods are currently continuing a rapid evolution, which likely will yield new dose considerations in the near term. The resources on radiation dosimetry are highly technical and distributed broadly across the scientific and clinical literature; significant effort continues toward improving standardization. However, prospective outcomes-based evidence required for establishing broad consensus remains elusive, and thus a conservative approach to minimizing exposure is still the prudent approach.

REFERENCES

1. Mettler FA Jr, Thomadsen BR, Bhargavan M, et al: Medical radiation exposure in the U.S. in 2006: preliminary results, *Health Phys* 95:502–507, 2008.
2. Brenner DJ, Hall EJ: Computed tomography—an increasing source of radiation exposure, *N Engl J Med* 357:2277–2284, 2007.
3. Einstein AJ, Moser KW, Thompson RC, Cerqueira MD, Henzlova MJ: Radiation Dose to Patients from Cardiac Diagnostic Imaging, *Circulation* 116:1290–1305, 2007.
4. National Cancer Institute: *Radiation Risks and Pediatric Computed Tomography (CT): A Guide for Health Care Providers.* http://www. cancer. gov/cancertopics/causes/radiation-risks-pediatric-CT.
5. Zanzonico P, Rothenberg LN, Strauss HW: Radiation exposure of computed tomography and direct intracoronary angiography: risk has its reward, *J Am Coll Cardiol* 47:1846–1849, 2006.
6. McCollough CH, Primak AN, Braun N, Kofler J, Yu L, Christner J: Strategies for reducing radiation dose in CT, *Radiol Clin North Am* 47 (1):27–40, 2009.
7. Patton JA, Slomka PJ, Germano G, Berman DS: Recent technologic advances in nuclear cardiology, *J Nucl Cardiol* 14(4):501–513, 2007.
8. Heller GV, et al: A Multicenter Evaluation of a New Post-Processing Method with Depth-Dependent Collimator Resolution Applied to Full and Half-Time Acquisitions Without and With Simultaneously Acquired Attenuation, *J Nucl Cardiol* (in press).
9. DePuey EG, Gadiraju R, Clark J, Thompson L, Anstett F, Shwartz SC: Ordered subset expectation maximization and wide beam reconstruction "half-time" gated myocardial perfusion SPECT functional imaging: a comparison to "full-time" filtered backprojection, *J Nucl Cardiol* (in press).
10. Zanzonico PB: Internal radionuclide radiation dosimetry: a review of basic concepts and recent developments, *J Nucl Med* 41(2):297–308, 2000.
11. Bushberg JT, Siebert JA, Leidholdt EM, Boone JM: *The essential Physics of Medical Imaging*, ed 1, Philadelphia, 1994, Williams & Wilkins.
12. International Commission on Radiological Protection: *1990 Recommendations of the International Commission on Radiological Protection*, New York, 1991, Pergamon Press ICRP Publication 60.
13. International Commission on Radiological Protection: *Limits for Intakes of Radionuclides by Workers*, New York, 1979, Pergamon Press ICRP Publication 30.
14. 2007 Recommendations of the International Commission on Radiological Protection: *Annals of the ICRP*, New York, 2007, Elsevier ICRP Publication 103.
15. Cristy M: Development of mathematical pediatric phantoms for internal dose calculations: designs, limitations, and prospects. In Watson ATS, Stelson ATS, Coffey JL, Cloutier RJ, editors: *Proceedings of the Third International Radiopharmaceutical Dosimetry Symposium (FDA 81-8166)*, Oak Ridge, TN, 1981, Oak Ridge Associated Universities, pp 496–517.
16. Loevinger R, Budinger T, Watson E: *MIRD Primer for Absorbed Dose Calculations*, New York, 1991, Society of Nuclear Medicine.
17. Snyder W, Ford M, Warner G, Watson S: *"S," absorbed dose per unit cumulated activity for selected radionuclides and organs, MIRD Pamphlet No. 11*, New York, 1975, Society of Nuclear Medicine.
18. Thompson RC, Cullom SJ: Issues Regarding Radiation Dosage of Cardiac Nuclear and X-Ray Procedures, *J Nucl Cardiol* 13(1):19–23, 2006.
19. Cardiogen package insert. http://www.nuclearonline.org/PI/Cardiogen.pdf.
20. Mossman KL, Goldman M, Masse F, Mills WA, et al: *Radiation Risk in Perspective. Health Physics Society Position Statement*, McLean, VA, 2004, Health Physics Society.
21. Lazo T: The evolution of the international system of radiological protection: food for thought from the Nuclear Energy Agency Committee on Radiation Protection and Public Health, *J Radiol Prot* 23(3):241–246, 2003.
22. Mossman KL: The linear no-threshold debate: where do we go from here? *Med Phys* 25(3):279–284, 1998.
23. National Council on Radiation Protection and Measurements: *Exposure of the population in the United States and Canada from natural background radiation NCRP Report 94*, Bethesda, MD, 1988, National Council on Radiation Protection and Measurements.
24. United Nations Scientific Committee on the Effects of Atomic Radiation (UNSCEAR): *Epidemiological studies of radiation and cancer*, Paper presented at 54th Session of UNSCEAR; May 29-June 2, Vienna, Austria, 2006.
25. Wackers FJ, Berman DS, Maddahi J, et al: Technetium-99m hexakis 2-methoxyisobutyl isonitrile: human biodistribution, dosimetry, safety, and preliminary comparison to thallium-201 for myocardial perfusion imaging, *J Nucl Med* 30:301–311, 1989.
26. Tc-99m tetrofosmin package inserthttp://www.fda.gov/medwatch/SAFETY/2003/03NOV_PI/Myoview_PI.pdf.
27. Berman DS, Kiat H, Maddahi J: The new 99mTc myocardial perfusion imaging agents: 99mTc-sestamibi and 99mTc-teboroxime [review], *Circulation* 84(3 Suppl):I7–I21, 1991.
28. Thallium-201 Chloride package insert.
29. Thomas SR, Stabin MG, Castronovo FP: Radiation-Absorbed Dose from ^{201}Tl-Thallous Chloride. J Nucl Med 46:502–508.
30. Siegel JA: *Guide for Diagnostic Nuclear Medicine and Radiopharmaceutical Therapy*, Reston, VA, 2004, Society of Nuclear Medicine.
31. Stabin MG, Breitz HB: Breast milk excretion of radiopharmaceuticals: mechanisms, findings, and radiation dosimetry, *J Nucl Med* 41(5):863–873, 2000.
32. Stabin MG: Health concerns related to radiation exposure of the female nuclear medicine patient, *Environ Health Perspect* 105(Suppl 6):1403–1409, 1997.
33. Di Carli MF, Dorbala S, Meserve J, El Fakhri G, Sitek A, Moore SC: Clinical myocardial perfusion PET/CT [review], *J Nucl Med* 48(5):783–793, 2007.
34. Alvarez-Diez TM, deKemp R, Beanlands R, Vincent J: Manufacture of strontium-82/rubidium-82 generators and quality control of rubidium-82 chloride for myocardial perfusion imaging in patients using positron emission tomography, *Appl Radiat Isot* 50(6):1015–1023, 1999.
35. Kearfott KJ: Radiation absorbed dose estimates for positron emission tomography (PET): K-38, Rb-81, Rb-82, and Cs-130, *J Nucl Med* 23(12):1128–1132, 1982.

36. Ryan JW, Haiper PV, Stark Vi, Peterson EL, Lathrop KA: Radiation absorbed dose estimate for rubidium-82 determined from in vivo measurements in human subjects. In Schiafice-Stelson AT, Watson EE, eds. *Fourth international radiopharmaceutical dosimetry symposium*, Oak Ridge, TN: Oak Ridge Associated University Publishers; 1986:346–358.

37. Lodge MA, Braess H, Mahmoud F, et al: Developments in nuclear cardiology: transition from single photon emission computed tomography to positron emission tomography-computed tomography [review], *J Invasive Cardiol* 17(9):491–496, 2005.

38. Valentin J: Radiation dose to patients from radiopharmaceuticals (addendum 2 to ICRP publication 53): ICRP publication 80 approved by the Commission in September 1997, *Ann ICRP* 28:1–126, 1998.

39. deKemp RA, Beanlands RS: A revised effective dose estimate for the PET perfusion tracer Rb-82. [abstract], *J Nucl Med* 49(Suppl 1):183P, 2008.

40. Schelbert HR: Blood flow and metabolism by PET, *Cardiol Clin* 12 (2):303–315, 1994.

41. Hutchins GD, Schwaiger M, Rosenspire KC, Krivokapich J, Schelbert H, Kuhl DE: Noninvasive quantification of regional blood flow in the human heart using N-13 ammonia and dynamic positron emission tomographic imaging, *J Am Coll Cardiol* 15(5):1032–1042, 1990.

42. Beller GA: Assessment of myocardial perfusion and metabolism for assessment of myocardial viability, *Q J Nucl Med* 40(1):55–67, 1996.

43. Jones SC, Alavi A, Christman D, Montanez I, Wolf AP, Reivich M: The radiation dosimetry of 2-F-18 fluoro-2-deoxy-D-glucose in man, *J Nucl Med* 23:613–617, 1982.

44. Oak Ridge FDG data. *Radiation Dose to Patients from Radiopharmaceuticals*. Oxford, U.K.: Pergamon Press; 1999:76. ICRP Publication 80, Addendum 2 to ICRP Publication 53.

45. Bixler A, Springer G, Lovas R: Practical aspects of radiation safety for using fluorine-18, *J Nucl Med Technol* 27(1):14–16, 1999.

46. Zanzonico P, Dauer L, St Germain J: Operational radiation safety for PET-CT, SPECT-CT, and cyclotron facilities, *Health Phys* 95 (5):554–570, 2008.

47. Upton AC: National Council on Radiation Protection and Measurements Scientific Committee 1–6: The state of the art in the 1990's: NCRP Report No. 136 on the scientific bases for linearity in the dose-response relationship for ionizing radiation, *Health Phys* 85 (1):15–22, 2003.

48. Committee to Assess Health Risks from Exposure to Low Levels of Ionizing Radiation, National Research Council: *Health Risks from Exposure to Low Levels of Ionizing Radiation: BEIR VII Phase 2*, Washington, DC, 2005, National Academy Press.

49. Brenner D, Elliston C, Hall E, Berdon W: Estimated risks of radiation-induced fatal cancer from pediatric CT, *AJR Am J Roentgenol* 176 (2):289–296, 2001.

50. Einstein AJ, Henzlova MJ, Rajagopalan S: Estimating risk of cancer associated with radiation exposure from 64-slice computed tomography coronary angiography, *JAMA* 298(3):317–323, 2007.

51. Sodickson A, Baeyens PF, Andriole KP, et al: Recurrent CT, cumulative radiation exposure, and associated radiation-induced cancer risks from CT of adults, *Radiology* 251(1):175–184, 2009.

52. Huang B, Law MW, Khong PL: Whole-body PET/CT scanning: estimation of radiation dose and cancer risk, *Radiology* 251(1):166–174, 2009 Epub 2009 Feb 27.

53. United States Cancer Statistics: *Centers for Disease Control*, Atlanta, Georgia, 2000.

54. Instruction Concerning Risks from Occupational Radiation Exposure. US Nuclear Regulatory Commission Regulatory Guide 8.29, Revision 1, February 1996.

55. NCRP. National Council on Radiation Protection and Measurements. Statement No. 10. December 2004. *Recent Applications of the NCRP Public Dose Limit Recommendation for Ionizing Radiation*. http://www.ncrponline.org/NCRP%20Statement%20No.%2010.pdf.

56. Hall EJ, Brenner DJ, Worgul B, Smilenov L: Genetic susceptibility to radiation, *Adv Space Res* 35(2):249–253, 2005.

57. United States Nuclear Regulatory Commission: *Standards for Protection against radiation*, http://www.nrc.gov/reading-rm/doc-collections/cfr/part020/.

58. Schleipman AR, Castronovo FP Jr, Di Carli MF, Dorbala S: Occupational radiation dose associated with Rb-82 myocardial perfusion positron emission tomography imaging, *J Nucl Cardiol* 13(3):378–384, 2006.

59. Limacher, et al: Radiation safety in the practice of cardiology, *J Am Coll Cardiol* 31:892, 1998.

60. Gerber TC, Carr JJ, Arai AE, et al: Ionizing radiation in cardiac imaging. A science advisory from the American Heart Association Committee on Cardiac Imaging of the Council on Clinical Cardiology and Committee on Cardiovascular Imaging and Intervention of the Council on Cardiovascular Radiology and Intervention, *Circulation* 119: 1056–1065, 2009.

61. McCollough CH, Bruesewitz MR, Kofler JM Jr, : CT dose reduction and dose management tools: overview of available options, *Radiographics* 26(2):503–512, 2006.

62. Amis E, et al: American College of Radiology white paper on Radiation Dose in Medicine, *Radiat Prot Dosimetry* 114:11–25, 2005.

63. American Society of Nuclear Cardiology. *Information statement on variability in radiation dose estimates*. 2008 by the American Society of Nuclear Cardiology. doi:10.1007/s12350-008-9026-0.

64. Morin RL, Gerber TC, McCollough CH: Radiation dose in computed tomography of the heart, *Circulation* 107(6):917–922, 2003.

65. Flohr T: Radiation exposure estimation and reduction approaches. In Ohnesorge T, Becker T, Flohr T, Reiser T, editors: *Multi-Slice CT in Cardiac Imaging*, 2nd ed., 2006, Berlin, Springer Publishing.

66. McNitt-Gray MF: Radiation dose in CT. AAPM/RSNA Physics Tutorial for Residents: Topics in CT, *Radiographics* 22:1541–1553, 2002.

67. Huda W, Ogden KM, Khorasani MR: Converting dose-length product to effective dose at CT, *Radiology* 248(3):995–1003, 2008.

68. Mahesh M, Cody DD: Physics of cardiac imaging with multiple-row detector CT, *Radiographics [review]* 27(5):1495–1509, 2007.

69. Hausleiter J, Meyer T, Hermann F, et al: Estimated radiation dose associated with cardiac CT angiography, *JAMA* 301(5):500–507, 2009.

70. Kalra MK, Naz N, Rizzo SM, Blake MA: Computed tomography radiation dose optimization: scanning protocols and clinical applications of automatic exposure control, *Curr Probl Diagn Radiol* 34(5): 171–181, 2005.

71. Kalender WA, Wolf H, Suess C: Dose reduction in CT by anatomically adapted tube current modulation. II. Phantom measurements, *Med Phys* 26:2248–2253, 1999.

72. Shuman WP, Branch KR, May JM: et al: Prospective versus retrospective ECG gating for 64-detector CT of the coronary arteries: Comparison of image quality and patient radiation dose, *Radiology*. 248 (2):431–437, Aug 2008.

73. Ertel D, Pflederer T, Achenbach S, Kalender WA: Real-time determination of the optimal reconstruction phase to control ECG pulsing in spiral cardiac CT, *Phys Med* 25(3):122–127, Sep 2009.

74. Poll LW, Cohnen M, Brachten S, et al: Dose reduction in multi-slice CT of the heart by use of ECG-controlled tube current modulation ("ECG pulsing"): phantom measurements, *Rofo* 174:1500–1505, 2002.

75. Parker MS, Kelleher NM, Hoots JA, Chung JK, Fatouros PP, Benedict SH: Absorbed radiation dose of the female breast during diagnostic multidetector chest CT and dose reduction with a tungsten-antimony composite breast shield: preliminary results, *Clin Radiol* 63(3):278–288, 2008.

76. Garcia MJ, Lessick J, Hoffmann MH: CATSCAN Study Investigators: Accuracy of 16-row multidetector computed tomography for the assessment of coronary artery stenosis, *JAMA* 296(4):403–411, 2006.

77. Hunold P, Vogt FM, Schmermund A, et al: Radiation exposure during cardiac CT: effective doses at multi-detector row CT and electron-beam CT, *Radiology* 226:145–152, 2003.

78. McCollough CH: Patient dose in cardiac computed tomography, *Herz* 28:1–6, 2003.

79. Hacker M, Jakobs T, Matthiesen F, et al: Comparison of spiral multidetector CT angiography and myocardial perfusion imaging in the noninvasive detection of functionally relevant coronary artery lesions: first clinical experiences, *J Nucl Med* 46:1294–1300, 2005.

80. Coles DR, Smail MA, Negus IS, et al: Comparison of radiation doses from multislice computed tomography coronary angiography and conventional diagnostic angiography, *J Am Coll Cardiol* 47: 1840–1845, 2006.

81. Flohr TG, Schoepf UJ, Kuettner A, et al: Advances in cardiac imaging with 16-section CT systems, *Acad Radiol* 10:386–401, 2003.

82. Hoffmann MH, Shi H, Schmitz BL, et al: Noninvasive coronary angiography with multislice computed tomography, *JAMA* 293: 2471–2478, 2005.

83. Gerber TC, Stratmann BP, Kuzo RS, Kantor B, Morin RL: Effect of acquisition technique on radiation dose and image quality in multidetector row computed tomography coronary angiography with submillimeter collimation, *Invest Radiol* 40:556–563, 2005.

84. Nawfel R, Yoshizumi T: Update on radiation dose in CT, *Am Assoc Physicists Med Newsl* 30:12–13, 2005.

85. Sato Y, Matsumoto N, Ichikawa M, et al: Efficacy of multislice computed tomography for the detection of acute coronary syndrome in the emergency department, *Circ J* 69:1047–1051, 2005.

86. Trabold T, Buchgeister M, Kuttner A, et al: Estimation of radiation exposure in 16-detector row computed tomography of the heart with retrospective ECG-gating, *Rofo* 175:1051–1055, 2003.

87. Gaspar T, Halon DA, Lewis BS, et al: Diagnosis of coronary in-stent restenosis with multidetector row spiral computed tomography, *J Am Coll Cardiol* 46:1573–1579, 2005.

88. Caussin C, Larchez C, Ghostine S, et al: Comparison of coronary minimal lumen area quantification by sixty-four-slice computed tomography versus intravascular ultrasound for intermediate stenosis, *Am J Cardiol* 98:871–876, 2006.

89. Hausleiter J, Meyer T, Hadamitzky M, et al: Radiation dose estimates from cardiac multislice computed tomography in daily practice: impact of different scanning protocols on effective dose estimates, *Circulation* 113:1305–1310, 2006.

90. Ghostine S, Caussin C, Daoud B, et al: Non-invasive detection of coronary artery disease in patients with left bundle branch block using 64 slice computed tomography, *J Am Coll Cardiol* 48: 1929–1934, 2006.

91. Leber AW, Knez A, von Ziegler F, et al: Quantification of obstructive and nonobstructive coronary lesions by 64-slice computed tomography: a comparative study with quantitative coronary angiography and intravascular ultrasound, *J Am Coll Cardiol* 46:147–154, 2005.

92. Mollet NR, Cademartiri F, van Mieghem CA, et al: High-resolution spiral computed tomography coronary angiography in patients referred for diagnostic conventional coronary angiography, *Circulation* 112:2318–2323, 2005.

93. Muhlenbruch G, Seyfarth T, Soo CS, Pregalathan N, Mahnken AH: Diagnostic value of 64-slice multi-detector row cardiac CTA in symptomatic patients, *Eur Radiol* 17:603–609, 2007.

94. Nikolaou K, Knez A, Rist C, et al: Accuracy of 64-MDCT in the diagnosis of ischemic heart disease, *AJR Am J Roentgenol* 187:111–117, 2006.

95. Pugliese F, Mollet NR, Runza G, et al: Diagnostic accuracy of non-invasive 64-slice CT coronary angiography in patients with stable angina pectoris, *Eur Radiol* 16:575–582, 2006.

96. Raff GL, Gallagher MJ, O'Neill WW, Goldstein JA: Diagnostic accuracy of noninvasive coronary angiography using 64-slice spiral computed tomography, *J Am Coll Cardiol* 46:552–557, 2005.

97. Wu TH, Huang YH, Lee JJ, et al: Radiation exposure during transmission measurements: comparison between CT- and germanium-based techniques with a current PET scanner, *Eur J Nucl Med Mol Imaging* 31(1):38–43, 2004 Epub 2003 Oct 8.

98. Almeida P, Bendriem B, de Dreuille O, Peltier A, Perrot C, Brulon V: Dosimetry of transmission measurements in nuclear medicine: a study using anthropomorphic phantoms and thermoluminescent dosimeters, *Eur J Nucl Med* 25(10):1435–1441, 1998.

99. Fricke E, Fricke H, Weise R, et al: Attenuation correction of myocardial SPECT perfusion images with low-dose CT: evaluation of the method by comparison with perfusion PET, *J Nucl Med* 46(5):736–744, 2005.

State-of-the-Art Instrumentation for PET and SPECT Imaging in Small Animals

DAVID K. GLOVER, BIJOY KUNDU
AND HEINRICH R. SCHELBERT

INTRODUCTION

Cardiovascular molecular imaging is an emerging field that will have tremendous impact on the diagnosis and treatment of heart disease in the years ahead. While traditional cardiac imaging provides important information regarding myocardial perfusion, function, or heart structure and dimensions, cardiovascular molecular imaging utilizes tracers or contrast agents to measure physiologic and pathologic processes at the cellular and molecular level. These tracers are designed to target specific cell types, receptors or transporters, peptides, or even the expression of a particular gene product. Targeted tracers are currently being used or investigated for imaging cellular processes such as glucose transport or metabolism (i.e., FDG, BMIPP), apoptosis (annexin-V), sympathetic innervation (MIBG), as well as inflammation, hypoxia, angiogenesis, matrix metalloproteinase expression, and the transition of atherosclerotic plaques from the stable to the unstable state. In addition, cardiovascular molecular imaging approaches are being investigated as a tool for monitoring cell trafficking and tissue localization of injected therapeutic stem cells and the delivery and efficacy of targeted gene therapy.

Small animals such as mice, rats, and guinea pigs have long been utilized as models in most areas of molecular biology, toxicology, and drug discovery research, and well-characterized models of specific diseases have been developed using these animals. With the relatively recent development of transgenic mice, mouse models have gained even greater importance. The ability to manipulate the mouse genome to produce accurate models of many human diseases has resulted in significant progress in understanding these diseases. Historic methodologies for assessing molecular changes require euthanizing the animal and performing invasive and destructive assays such as autoradiography and in vitro histopathologic assays on specific tissue types. These techniques are not ideal, because they do not provide information in real time and in situ. As a result, large numbers of animals must often be euthanized to screen for the desired phenotypic changes, resulting in significantly higher cost as well as lost time. The full potential of these new transgenic mouse models can only be realized with the ready availability of accurate, noninvasive imaging methods to investigate disease progression and its response to therapeutic agents. For these reasons, there has been increasing interest in developing noninvasive imaging techniques that allow repeated in vivo imaging at the cellular and molecular level in small animals such as mice. Importantly, repeated imaging studies allow for the delineation of temporal changes of these functional processes.

While other imaging modalities like magnetic resonance imaging (MRI), myocardial contrast echocardiography (MCE), and the newer optical imaging modality are being utilized for small-animal imaging and have their particular strengths, imaging techniques based on radiolabeled probes and positron emission tomography (PET) and single-photon emission computed tomography (SPECT) instrumentation will remain at the forefront because of their unparalleled sensitivity. Unfortunately, however, the spatial resolution of commercially available SPECT and PET cameras designed for clinical imaging is on the order of 4 to 6 mm, which limits their usefulness in small animals such as mice in which the heart is typically 3 to

4 mm across the short axis and the left ventricular wall thickness is less than 1 mm (~0.8 to 0.9 mm). Accordingly, there has been a tremendous effort in recent years to develop high-resolution SPECT and PET cameras specifically designed for imaging small animals in biomedical research. At the present time, there are multiple commercial versions of both microSPECT and microPET cameras available, and intensive work is underway in both academic settings and industry to further develop and improve these cameras.

MICRO–POSITRON EMISSION TOMOGRAPHY

PET extends the investigative possibilities of radionuclide approaches that have historically focused mostly on the evaluation of myocardial blood flow. With PET tracers, it is now possible to explore and, more important, to noninvasively quantify functional processes such as substrate metabolism, oxygen consumption, receptor density and occupancy, and activation and expression of transfected genes. Because of PET's quantitative and high temporal resolution capability, it is possible to accurately measure regional activity concentrations in the myocardium and blood as well as their changes over time. As described later, the radiotracer input function and the tissue response can be determined from serially acquired PET images. When combined with appropriate tracer kinetic models, absolute estimates of rates of functional processes can be derived (e.g., mL blood or mol substrate per minute per gram myocardium).

Dedicated, high spatial resolution small-animal PET imaging devices have become available. Some are in-house-developed systems at several research institutions,[1-5] but more recently, dedicated small-animal systems have become available through several commercial suppliers. The spatial resolution of these imaging devices is typically in the range of 1.0 to 1.5 mm full-width at half-maximum (FWHM) and enables mapping of the distribution of positron-emitting radiotracer and its changes over time throughout the body of small animals. These imaging systems have been used quite extensively for measuring substrate metabolism and cell replication rates of tumors as indices of tumor growth rates and tumor aggressiveness, and for determining responses of tumor growth to investigational therapeutic agents.[6-10] Other research has utilized these small-animal imaging devices for the development and validation of novel noninvasive assays for identifying activation and expression of transgenes.[6,9-11]

POSITRON EMISSION TOMOGRAPHY IMAGING OF THE RODENT HEART

The small dimensions of the rodent heart pose formidable challenges for PET studies of the cardiovascular system in rodents. In general, dedicated small-animal PET systems employ two different technical concepts: (1) crystal detector–based and (2) multiwire proportional chamber–based systems.[12,13] As shown in Figure 11-1, multiwire proportional chamber–based systems may

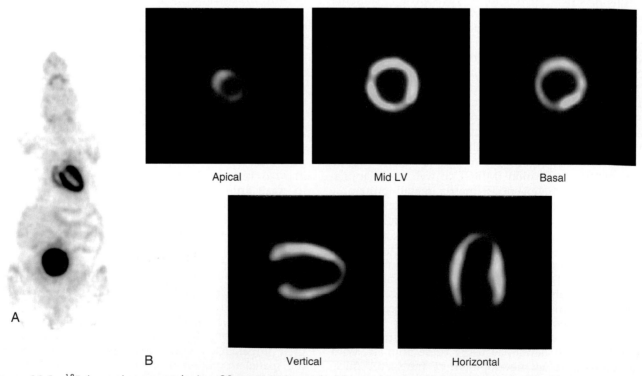

Apical   Mid LV   Basal

A   B   Vertical   Horizontal

Figure 11-1 ^{18}F-deoxyglucose uptake in a 29-g mouse imaged with a multiwire proportional chamber-based system (QuadHIDAC-PET, Oxford Positron Systems, Cambridge, England). The 15-minute whole body image was recorded 1 hour after injection of 10 MBq ^{18}F-deoxyglucose. **A,** Coronal whole body slice. **B,** Reoriented myocardial slices. *(Courtesy of K. Schäfers, University of Münster, Münster, Germany.)*

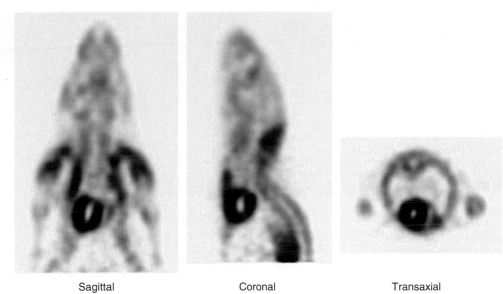

| Sagittal | Coronal | Transaxial |

Figure 11-2 Sagittal, coronal, and transaxial images slices of ^{18}F-deoxyglucose uptake in a mouse, obtained with a crystal-based, dedicated small-animal PET system (Concorde Microsystems, Knoxville, TN; Focus microPET system) and reconstructed using maximum a posteriori probability at 60 minutes after a tail-vein injection of ^{18}F-deoxyglucose. *(Courtesy of David Stout, University of California, Los Angeles.)*

offer superior spatial or volume resolution but generally are less sensitive and require longer image acquisition times. Conversely, crystal-based systems offer higher sensitivity (count rate per unit radioactivity) and offer superior temporal resolution but at the expense of somewhat lower spatial resolution (Fig. 11-2).

Several commercial small-animal scanners are now available since the first prototype scanner was built at University of California, Los Angeles. Figure 11-3 shows

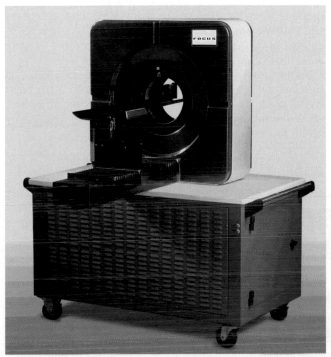

Figure 11-3 MicroPET Focus 120 scanner. *(Image courtesy of Siemens Medical Solutions USA, Inc.)*

one such small-animal PET scanner, the microPET Focus 120.[14] This system consists of 96 scintillation detectors arranged in four rings with a 14.7-cm diameter and 7.6-cm axial extent. Each detector consists of a 12 × 12 array of 1.52 × 1.52 × 10 mm lutetium oxyorthosilicate (LSO) crystals coupled to a position-sensitive photomultiplier tube (PS-PMT) via optical fiber bundles. Data are acquired in three-dimensional (3D) mode. With standard filtered backprojection reconstruction algorithms, the system achieves an isotropic (in all three directions) spatial resolution of 1.5 mm in the center of the field of view (FOV) and remains less than 2.0 mm within 5 cm of the center of the FOV. Imaging of the myocardium in mice and rats with the flow tracer ^{13}N-ammonia or the glucose analogue ^{18}F-deoxyglucose typically requires activity doses of 0.5 to 1.5 mCi.[15] Count rates at these radioactivity doses remain relatively low so that dead-time losses are small. Image reconstruction with the more recently developed maximum a posteriori probability (MAP) algorithm, now employed for cardiac studies in mice, provides images of myocardial perfusion and glucose uptake of good to excellent diagnostic quality (see Fig. 11-2).[16] The MAP reconstruction algorithm improves the spatial resolution in the center of the FOV to 1.2 mm FWHM so that a volumetric resolution of less than 5 microliters is now possible.

The emission data are reconstructed initially into a set of contiguous transaxial slices with a 0.75-mm interplane spacing (Fig. 11-4).[17] The transaxial images are typically reoriented into short-axis and vertical and horizontal long-axis cuts (Fig. 11-5)[17] that can be assembled into polar maps analogous to those of myocardial perfusion studies in humans (Fig. 11-6).[17] Images of glucose uptake obtained with ^{18}F-deoxyglucose are of greater contrast and higher quality than images of perfusion obtained with ^{13}N-ammonia. This is most likely because of the more complete clearance of ^{18}F-deoxyglucose

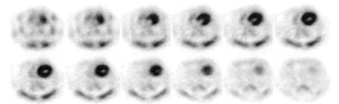

Figure 11-4 Contiguous transaxial images of the chest in a mouse (inferior to superior from *top left to bottom right*, interplane spacing 0.75 mm) obtained 30 minutes after intravenous ^{18}F-deoxyglucose. *(Reproduced with permission from Schelbert HR, Inubushi M, Ross RS: PET imaging in small animals, J Nucl Cardiol 10:513–520, 2003.)*

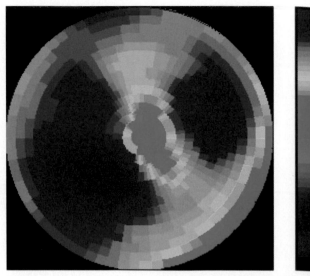

Figure 11-6 Polar map display of the ^{18}F-deoxyglucose uptake in the left ventricular myocardium in the mouse depicted in Figures 11-4 and 11-5. *(Reproduced with permission from Schelbert HR, Inubushi M, Ross RS: PET imaging in small animals. J Nucl Cardiol 10:513–520, 2003.)*

from blood and higher tracer activity concentrations in the myocardium. Another reason is the slower physical decay of ^{18}F-deoxyglucose so that over the total image acquisition time, more counts are recorded. On the other hand, the shorter physical half-life of ^{13}N-ammonia affords the ability to perform repeat examinations of myocardial blood flow during the same study session so that effects of interventions can be evaluated. ECG gated image acquisition is also possible with small PET systems so that left ventricular function can be assessed.[18] For example, in normal 300-g rats, the left ventricular ejection fraction was about 60% to 70%, and the stroke volume was about 300 μL.[18]

The image reconstruction algorithm corrects for radioactive decay and for dead-time losses. It also includes routines for photon attenuation correction. These routines utilize transmission images that are typically acquired prior to radiotracer administration and are performed using a Co57 point source or, for hybrid microPET/CT systems, an x-ray attenuation map. Despite the small body size of rats, photon attenuation causes about 30% systematic underestimation of the true myocardial radioactivity concentration.[19] Albeit somewhat less in mice, photon attenuation still amounts to about 17% underestimation of the true activity. Accordingly, even in small animals, proper attenuation correction is important for the measurement of the true absolute intensities in cardiac imaging. Chow et al.[19] have shown that CT-based attenuation correction methods result in less noise correction to

emission images compared to the transmission-based attenuation corrections.

The stationary imaging gantry of microPET permits rapid serial (or "dynamic") acquisition of images. Theoretically, images can be recorded at sampling rates of less than 1 second. For practical purposes, however, image acquisition rates depend on the number of counts required for statistically adequate image frames. Framing rates in the range of 2 to 10 seconds per image following an intravenous bolus of ^{13}N-ammonia, ^{18}F-deoxyglucose, or ^{11}C-palmitate produce statistically adequate images for generating tissue time-activity curves and thus are appropriate for radiotracer kinetic studies.[20] Figure 11-7 depicts selected frames acquired during and shortly after an intravenous bolus injection of ^{13}N-ammonia in a rat. High temporal-resolution tissue time-activity curves for the right and left ventricular blood pools and the left ventricular myocardium in a rat following an intravenous bolus of ^{18}F-deoxyglucose into a tail vein are shown in Figure 11-8.

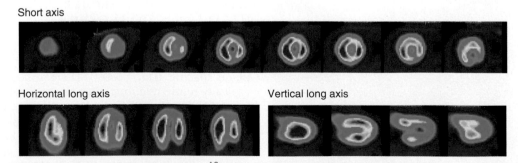

Short axis

Horizontal long axis

Vertical long axis

Figure 11-5 Reoriented images of the myocardial ^{18}F-deoxyglucose uptake in the same mouse as depicted in Figure 11-4. Selected short-axis *(upper row)* and vertical and horizontal long-axis cuts are shown. *(Reproduced with permission from Schelbert HR, Inubushi M, Ross RS: PET imaging in small animals. J Nucl Cardiol 10:513–520, 2003.)*

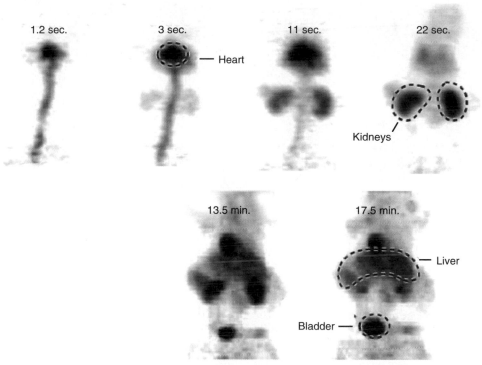

Figure 11-7 Selected serially acquired images during and following a bolus administration of ^{13}N-ammonia into the tail vein of a rat. The initial two images depict the tracer transit through the inferior vena cava through the right and then to the left ventricle, and the third image depicts the arrival and retention of tracer in both kidneys. Delayed (13.5 and 17.5 minutes) images demonstrate declining tracer activities in the kidneys and continued accumulation of tracer in the bladder. Tracer activity is also noted in the myocardium and throughout the liver. *(Reproduced with permission from Schelbert HR, Inubushi M, Ross RS: PET imaging in small animals, J Nucl Cardiol 10:513–520, 2003.)*

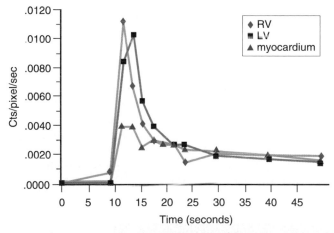

Figure 11-8 Time-activity curves derived from the right and the left ventricular (RV, LV) blood pool and the left ventricular myocardium in a mouse. Serial images were recorded beginning with a tail vein injection of ^{18}F-deoxyglucose. Note the high temporal resolution of the time-activity curves, with clearly separated activity peaks in the right and left ventricular blood pool. *(Courtesy of Michael Kreissl.)*

IMAGING THE CARDIOVASCULAR SYSTEM IN MICE AND RATS

Experimental Coronary Occlusions in the Rat

The extent and severity of regional myocardial perfusion defects that are experimentally induced by transient coronary occlusions in rats can be accurately determined with microPET.[15] In Figure 11-9, myocardial perfusion was imaged with intravenous ^{13}N-ammonia at baseline, 45 minutes later during a 20-minute coronary occlusion, and again 45 minutes following reperfusion. Figure 11-10 shows the corresponding polar map displays. The location and extent of the image perfusion defects corresponded well with the actual regions observed on postmortem stained tissue. Using a threshold of 50% of the maximum myocardial activity concentration as the lower limit of normal, the size of the flow defect derived from polar maps of myocardial perfusion correlated linearly with the defect sizes determined by postmortem examination (Fig. 11-11).

Studies in Genetically Modified Mice

Initial studies have demonstrated the possibility of phenotyping genetically modified mice. For example, cardiac myocyte-specific excision of the murine β-1 integrin gene results in extensive myocardial fibrosis.[21] In adulthood, the mice develop a form of dilated cardiomyopathy and symptoms of congestive heart failure. MicroPET imaging with ^{18}F-deoxyglucose in β-1-integrin knockout mice revealed heterogeneously distributed tracer uptake consistent with either replacement of myocytes by fibrotic tissue or as a consequence of regional alterations in substrate metabolism (Fig. 11-12). Assessment of myocardial perfusion with ^{13}N-ammonia in the β-1-integrin knockout mouse further revealed heterogeneously

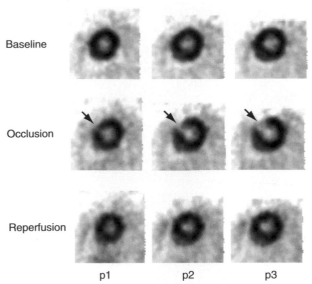

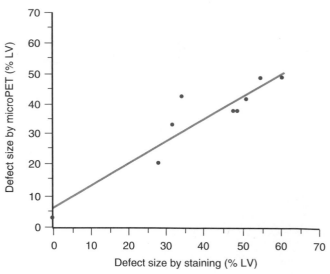

Figure 11-9 Serial images of the regional myocardial perfusion with intravenous ^{13}N-ammonia in a rat. Selected short axis slices through the left ventricular myocardium are shown. The initial image obtained at baseline depicts the homogenously distributed myocardial blood flow. The images in the center were recorded after a second ^{13}N-ammonia injection during a transient coronary occlusion. The severe perfusion defect is seen in the base portion of the anterior wall *(arrows)*. The defect has resolved completely at 45 minutes after release of the coronary occlusion, as seen on the third image set *(right panel)* obtained after another intravenous dose of ^{13}N-ammonia. *(Reproduced with permission from Kudo T, Fukuchi K, Annala AJ, et al: Noninvasive measurement of myocardial activity concentrations and perfusion defect sizes in rats with a new small-animal positron emission tomograph, Circulation 106:118–123, 2002.)*

Figure 11-11 Extent of perfusion defects induced by coronary occlusions in nine rats. Note the close linear correlation between the PET image–derived defect extents and the perfusion defect sizes determined following blue dye staining and postmortem measurements. *(Reproduced with permission from Kudo T, Fukuchi K, Annala AJ, et al: Noninvasive measurement of myocardial activity concentrations and perfusion defect sizes in rats with a new small-animal positron emission tomograph, Circulation 106:118–123, 2002.)*

distributed myocardial blood flow in addition to patchy regions of reduced tracer uptake.

Development of Novel Radiotracer Assay Approaches

Noninvasive, image-based probe systems for studying location, extent, magnitude, and duration of gene expression have also been explored and are now being used in small animals. One approach used in oncologic studies in mice has been the PET reporter gene/reporter probe system.[9–11,22] In one of these systems, a mutant herpes simplex virus thymidine kinase gene is delivered by an adenoviral vector and represents the PET reporter gene. If expressed in tissue, thymidine kinase phosphorylates the radiolabeled 9-(4-[^{18}F]-fluoro-3 hydroxymethylbutyl) (guanine) (^{18}FHBG) that serves as the PET reporter probe. Because the phosphorylated product of ^{18}FHBG is relatively impermeable to the cell membrane, it becomes effectively trapped in tissue and thus can be imaged with PET. Details on this in vivo assay approach and on other probe systems are described in several recent reviews.[6,9,10,23]

Pilot studies with in vitro imaging approaches had explored the feasibility of adapting these probe systems

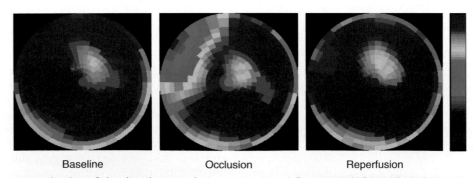

Figure 11-10 Polar map display of the distribution of myocardial blood flow recorded serially before, during, and following a transient coronary occlusion in the rat depicted in Figure 11-7. Note the perfusion defect on the polar map during the occlusion, as indicated in *blue*. *(Reproduced with permission from Kudo T, Fukuchi K, Annala AJ, et al: Noninvasive measurement of myocardial activity concentrations and perfusion defect sizes in rats with a new small-animal positron emission tomograph, Circulation 106:118–123, 2002.)*

Figure 11-12 Transaxial images of myocardial perfusion and of exogenous glucose utilization, obtained with intravenous ^{13}N-ammonia and ^{18}F-deoxyglucose in a β-1 integrin knockout mouse. Note the left ventricular enlargement and the heterogeneous tracer retentions. *(Reproduced with permission from Schelbert HR, Inubushi M, Ross RS: PET imaging in small animals, J Nucl Cardiol 10:513–520, 2003.)*

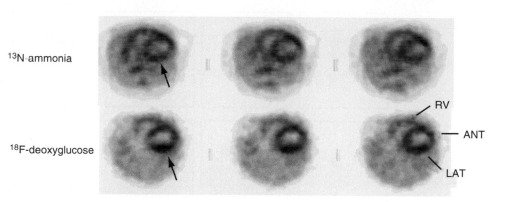

to the heart.[24] Optical and microPET imaging approaches have more recently been utilized to examine the feasibility of using these probe systems for in vivo studies of the heart. In these investigations, the PET reporter gene was introduced into the myocardium by direct needle injection during a thoracotomy. Images of the PET reporter probe were then obtained several days after transfection.[25,26] Another study in rats explored quantitative aspects of the probe system (Fig. 11-13).[27] The site of the reporter gene expression in the myocardium as identified by microPET correlated closely with that determined postmortem. In vivo measured activity concentrations of the PET reporter probe accurately represented those measured by in vitro tissue counting and, importantly, correlated with the tissue activity of the expressed thymidine kinase. Further, as shown in Figure 11-14, repeat imaging up to 17 days following transfection of the PET reporter gene defined the time course of the gene expression. The expression was highest on days 3 and 5, was still identifiable in some animals between days 10 and 14, but was no longer observed on day 17.

PET imaging studies with the reporter gene/reporter probe system in rats also appear promising for investigations on cardiac cell therapy.[28] Embryonic rat cardiomyoblasts were transfected with the PET reporter gene and were delivered by direct needle injection into the myocardium of rats. Engraftment and survival of the transplanted myoblasts were then demonstrated noninvasively and repeatedly by microPET imaging of the myocardial retention of the intravenously delivered PET reporter probe.

Quantification of Functional Processes

Adoption of PET's advantages and full quantitative capabilities to the cardiovascular system of mice and rats remains difficult and is still incomplete. The potential of PET for measuring rates of functional processes is based on the ability to accurately measure tracer activity concentrations in the myocardium and in arterial blood or left ventricular blood pool and to dynamically monitor their changes over time. Major limitations have been the small size of the left ventricular cavity, the thin left ventricular wall, and the rapid heart rates in rodents (~400 to 600 beats/min). Therefore, measurements of tracer activity concentrations in the less than 1-mm-thick myocardium require substantial corrections for partial

Figure 11-13 Retention of the PET reporter probe ^{18}FHBG in the myocardium of a rat 3 days following transfection of herpes simplex virus type into the myocardium. The *upper row* shows contiguous ^{13}N-ammonia images of the myocardium, the *middle row* depicts the retention of ^{18}FHBG in the myocardium, and the *bottom row*, the superimposed images. *(Reproduced with permission from Inubushi M, Wu JC, Gambhir SS, et al: Positron-emission tomography reporter gene expression imaging in rat myocardium, Circulation 107:326–332, 2003.)*

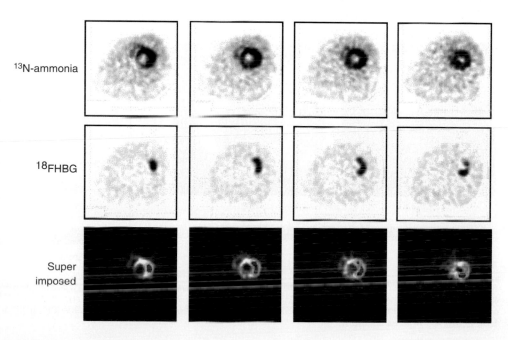

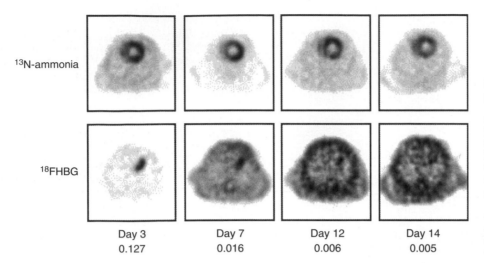

Figure 11-14 Repeat images of the myocardial retention of ^{18}FHBG and myocardial perfusion in a rat. The images show the ^{18}FHBG retention highest on day 3 of the transfection; the activity subsequently declines and is no longer seen on day 14. *(Reproduced with permission from Inubushi M, Wu JC, Gambhir SS, et al: Positron-emission tomography reporter gene expression imaging in rat myocardium, Circulation 107:326–332, 2003.)*

volume effects that might lead to considerable errors. The small inner diameter of the LV cavity together with the rapid heart rate causes considerable spillover of activity between myocardium and blood, and results in considerable contaminations of counts recovered from regions of interests assigned to the myocardium and the blood pool. Difficulties in serial sampling of arterial blood needed for validation of noninvasively derived radiotracer input functions, mostly due to the small blood volume in mice or rats, has further limited development and implementation of tracer kinetic approaches in small animals. Nevertheless, significant advances have been made over the last couple of years in obtaining accurate measurement of the blood input function, either by direct arterial blood sampling[29,30] or by derivation of the input function from PET images. A recent study by Fang et al.[31] validated a new method for deriving the arterial input function from dynamic PET image data that is less susceptible to spillover (SP) and partial volume (PV) effects. This method accounts for the SP and PV effects in a physiologic model to obtain

a model-corrected input function that compared well with the physically derived arterial blood samples. These investigators speculated that the addition of cardiac and respiratory gating, in combination with iterative algorithms such as MAP, would further reduce the SP and PV effects in the image-derived input function. This is supported by recent studies at the University of Virginia that demonstrated that high-resolution iterative reconstruction algorithms, combined with cardiac gating, minimized SP from the blood pool to the myocardium and vice versa.[32] Partial volume corrections for the blood pool were small because the dimensions were approximately two times the intrinsic spatial resolution of the Siemens Focus 120 scanner.[33] Performing PV corrections for the myocardium enabled accurate estimates of the kinetic rate constants and hence the rates of glucose uptake, K_i, and utilization, rMGU, using a three-compartment model approach in a mouse model of pressure-overload left ventricular hypertrophy produced by transverse aortic constriction (TAC) over 4 weeks (Fig. 11-15).

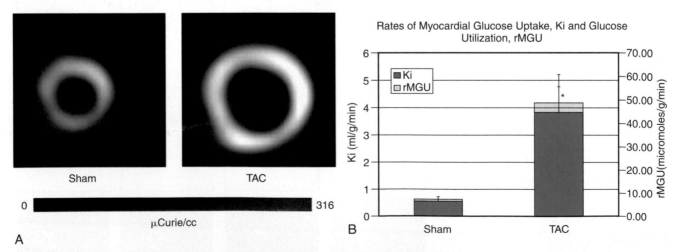

Figure 11-15 **A,** End-diastolic PET transverse slices from sham-operated and transverse aortic constricted (TAC) mice that developed left ventricular hypertrophy (LVH) over 4 weeks. **B,** Measured K_i (mL/g/min) and rMGU (micromoles/g/min) values obtained from PET images, showing increased rates of myocardial glucose uptake and utilization in the TAC mice with LVH. *$P < 0.001$ compared to sham.

Measurements of Myocardial Activity Concentrations

Regional radiotracer activity concentrations can be measured in absolute units in the myocardium of rats.[15] Following intravenous injection of ^{18}F-deoxyglucose and tracer accumulation in the myocardium, regions of interest were assigned to the left ventricular myocardium on the attenuation-corrected images. The PV-related underestimation of true tissue activity concentrations was corrected for with a recovery coefficient of 0.59, a value derived from postmortem measurements of the myocardial wall thickness and from the performance characteristics of the imaging system. Additional adjustments were needed for method-related differences in activity measurements between microPET and in vitro well counting of tissue samples. A calibration factor adjusted for differences in in vitro and in vivo measurements in tissue concentrations was obtained from images of a "rat phantom" that mimics the distribution of radioactivity in the body of the rat, and that contained in the region of the heart a solution of known radioactivity concentration.[15] Once corrected for PV effect and for differences in measurement sensitivities, values of tissue activity concentrations determined in vivo correlated closely and linearly with those obtained by postmortem well counting of myocardial tissue samples and ranging from 0.89 to 10.46 MBq/g. (Fig. 11-16).

Assays of Time-Dependent Changes in Tissue Activity Concentrations

Other studies have explored semiquantitative PET approaches for identifying alterations in the myocardium's substrate metabolism as phenotypic consequences

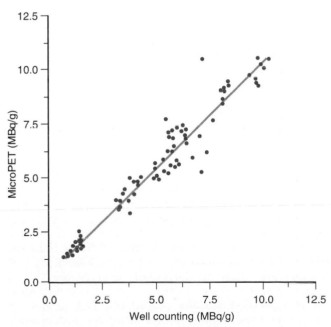

Figure 11-16 Comparison of ^{18}F-deoxyglucose concentrations in vivo and by well counting. *(Reproduced with permission from Kudo T, Fukuchi K, Annala AJ et al: Noninvasive measurement of myocardial activity concentrations and perfusion defect sizes in rats with a new small-animal positron emission tomograph, Circulation 106:118-123, 2002.)*

of gene alterations in mice. In addition to ^{18}F-deoxyglucose, these studies also employed ^{11}C-palmitate as a tracer of fatty acid metabolism in transgenic mice with cardiac-specific overexpression of peroxisome proliferator–activated receptor alpha (PPARα).[20] Beginning with the intravenous tracer administration, serial images were recorded for up to 40 minutes, and whole heart time-activity curves were generated. Consistent with the expression of PPARα target genes involved in free fatty acid and glucose metabolism, myocardial ^{18}F-deoxyglucose uptake in these transgenic mice was found to be diminished, whereas ^{11}C-palmitate uptake and clearance as indices of myocardial fatty acid uptake and oxidation were found to be increased. The images and derived time-activity curves in these mice clearly indicated trends of the alterations in substrate metabolism that were in agreement with findings by in vitro assays of the heart.

Measurements of Absolute Blood Flow in the Myocardium of Rats

The possibility to extract time-dependent activity concentrations from the serially acquired images in both arterial blood and myocardium has also been demonstrated in the somewhat larger heart of rats.[34] Time-activity curves for myocardium and left ventricular blood pool were derived in these studies with ^{13}N-ammonia and ^{11}C-acetate from regions of interest assigned to the serially acquired images. Model fitting of the time-activity curves yielded estimates of myocardial blood flow that averaged 4.56 mL/m/g, a value consistent with that reported for rat myocardium.[35] Further, the myocardial clearance rate of ^{11}C-acetate as an index of regional myocardial oxidative metabolism averaged 1.48 min^{-1} and thus was markedly higher than clearance rates of 0.48 ± 0.004 min^{-1} reported for human myocardium at baseline.[36] Although the noninvasively derived estimates of myocardial blood flow and oxidative metabolism lacked independent validation in this study in rats, and although heart rate and blood pressure were not reported, the high values of blood flow and oxidative metabolism, at least relative to those in humans, are consistent with the high heart rate and consequently high levels of cardiac work in the rodent heart. The findings of this study support the possibility of extracting quantitative information on functional processes of the myocardium in rodents. However, estimates of regional myocardial blood flow and oxidative metabolism varied considerably between myocardial regions, as for example the septum and the lateral wall, highlighting the difficulties and current limitations in extracting accurate and uncontaminated regional tracer activity concentrations from the serially acquired images.

Semiquantitative Estimates of Changes in Myocardial Blood Flow in Mice

Experimentally induced genetic alterations in mice may affect myocardial blood flow homogenously rather than regionally. Demonstration of phenotypic consequences of genetic alterations therefore requires estimates of myocardial blood flow in absolute units rather than identification of regional alterations in the relative flow

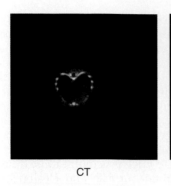
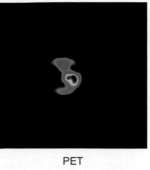
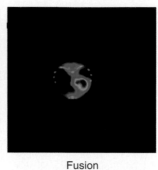

CT PET Fusion

Figure 11-17 Transaxial PET/CT images in a mouse in the prone position. The computed tomography (CT) image is shown on the *left*, the corresponding transaxial positron emission tomography (PET) image in the *middle*, and the PET/CT fusion image on the *right*. Note the ^{18}F-deoxyglucose uptake in the left ventricular myocardium.

distribution of blood flow. Additional factors complicating such measurements include the already high levels of myocardial blood flow at rest. Even though myocardial blood flow has not been measured in vivo in mice, values may be as high as 4 mL/m/g, judging from the high resting heart rates of 400 to 600 beats/min in mice and from estimates of 3.5 to 4.0 mL/min/g as observed in rat myocardium.[35] Consequently, the myocardial net retention of most tracers of myocardial blood flow resides in the plateau region of the nonlinear relationship between the tracer net retention and myocardial blood flow. Further increases in blood flow, as for example induced by pharmacologic vasodilatation, would be associated with only small increments in radiotracer uptake. Because of this, one microPET study in mice with ^{13}N-ammonia attempted to lower rather than increase myocardial blood flow, and examined whether associated decreases in flow could be demonstrated noninvasively with microPET imaging.[37] With an approximate 50% reduction in the heart rate after intraperitoneal administration of the α^2-adrenoreceptor agonist clonidine, the myocardial retention of ^{13}N-ammonia expressed as percent of the total injected dose declined significantly but by modest 14%. Even if the 50% reduction in heart rate produced more substantial decreases in myocardial blood flow, the observed modest decrease in tracer retention most likely was because of the nonlinear relationship between tracer net uptake and myocardial blood flow, at least in the hyperemic flow range.

Limitations and Challenges

With the recent development of high-resolution and high-sensitivity small-animal PET scanners, accurate imaging of the murine heart is now possible. Obtaining the arterial blood input function has been a challenge in dynamic PET imaging of the mouse heart in the past, but adoption of the factor analysis approach to serially acquired microPET images appears promising for determining accurate estimates of the arterial tracer input function and likely also of the myocardial tissue response.[38] The high-resolution iterative ordered subset expectation maximization (OSEM)-MAP reconstruction algorithms improve the reconstructed image resolution as compared to the conventional analytic filtered backprojection algorithm.[39] Nevertheless, even the relatively high spatial resolution of the dedicated microPET systems remains low relative to the myocardial wall thickness of about 0.9 mm in the mouse.

Accordingly, the necessary partial volume corrections have to be applied for accurate estimates of the myocardial tracer uptake. This along with cardiac and/or respiratory gating enables accurate estimates of the blood input function.[32]

Other refinements to existing methodologies include small-animal PET/CT and PET/MRI approaches and thus coregistration of functional with anatomic information (Fig. 11-17).[40,41] Besides offering improved accuracy in localizing regional functional processes, the addition of anatomic information may prove useful for more accurate determination of regional tracer activity concentrations. With these method- and instrumentation-related refinements, it will likely become possible to fully utilize the potential of PET in mice as a noninvasive probe of a broad range of tissue assays. Such assays include tracer kinetic approaches already fully validated and employed in large-animal studies and in humans for measurements of myocardial blood flow, oxidative metabolism and consumption, and myocardial substrate metabolism.

MICRO–SINGLE-PHOTON EMISSION COMPUTED TOMOGRAPHY

Imaging with microSPECT offers a number of advantages over microPET for cardiovascular molecular imaging using small-animal models. One advantage is the ready availability of isotopes with excellent properties for imaging. Commonly used isotopes for medical imaging such as ^{201}Tl, ^{99m}Tc, ^{111}In, and ^{123}I can be ordered from local radiopharmacies or commercial vendors and are fairly inexpensive. Furthermore, new single-photon, radiolabeled probes can usually be developed quite easily because the chemistry techniques for iodination (^{123}I) or for chelating metals such as ^{99m}Tc or ^{111}In and linking them to a specific protein or ligand are well established. Many of the radiolabeled probes can be prepared when needed in the research laboratory using simple kit-based labeling procedures. PET probes, on the other hand, require access to an on-site cyclotron for isotopes with short half-lives (i.e., ^{15}O, ^{13}N, ^{18}F). Although ^{18}F-FDG can also be ordered from regional suppliers, the synthesis of other PET probes on-site can be difficult or require expensive synthesis equipment. Another advantage of microSPECT is that the isotopes typically have longer half-lives (hours to days) that permit repeated monitoring of tracer activities over time. This is especially useful for longitudinal studies or for tracking the movement of specific cell types (e.g., inflammatory cells or stem cells). Another major advantage of microSPECT is the ability to discriminate between the energy photopeaks of different isotopes, allowing one to image multiple isotopes simultaneously in the same animal. For example, ^{99m}Tc-sestamibi perfusion could be imaged at the same time as an ^{111}In-labeled tracer of hypoxia. With PET, if multiple processes are to be measured in the same animal, imaging must be performed sequentially rather than simultaneously. Finally, another reason for the growing interest in SPECT-based imaging systems is the ability to achieve greater spatial resolution with SPECT. PET spatial resolution is ultimately limited by the diffusion of high-energy positrons emitted from the radioisotope before annihilation (i.e., generation of two 511-keV gamma rays). As mentioned earlier in this chapter, the spatial resolution of the current generation of microPET scanners is on the order of 1.2 to 1.5 mm FWHM; microSPECT systems do not suffer from this inherent limitation and ultimately can achieve even higher spatial resolution. Commercial microSPECT systems from several vendors are currently achieving submillimeter spatial resolution.

MicroSPECT Instrumentation

There have been tremendous advances made in small-animal SPECT instrumentation over the past several years in both hardware and software. As with clinical SPECT cameras, a typical microSPECT system often consists of a rotating gantry with one or more single-photon detectors. Hybrid systems are also available whereby the gantry is equipped with a microfocus x-ray source and detector that allow dual microSPECT/CT studies to be performed in the same animals. The single-photon detectors can be based on scintillation crystals (NaI) coupled with photomultiplier tubes, or they can be solid-state such as cadmium telluride detectors. Single-photon gamma cameras require some form of collimation for accurate localization of the position of origin of a gamma photon. The collimators are interchangeable, depending upon the resolution and FOV required, and can be either parallel-hole for whole body imaging or, to achieve high spatial resolution, pinhole collimators

with 0.5- to 2.0-mm apertures; the latter are most commonly employed. Because the photon detection efficiency is diminished with the use of a collimator, state-of-the-art high resolution microSPECT systems often employ multiple detectors, with each detector having more than one pinhole to improve sensitivity. Sensitivity and magnification are also enhanced by the use of a relatively tight radius of rotation whereby the animal is in close proximity to the pinhole apertures.

One drawback to gantry-based microSPECT systems is that they are not optimal for imaging rapid, dynamic processes, because there is a finite time required to rotate the detector head to the next position. The investigators from the Radiology Research Laboratory at the University of Arizona Health Sciences Center developed a unique "gantryless" stationary SPECT system called *FASTSPECT* for small-animal imaging. The system consists of 24 modular gamma cameras arranged in two circular arrays: one array of 11 cameras and a second array of 13 cameras. Each of the modular cameras consists of a 10 cm × 10 cm NaI(Tl) scintillation crystal coupled to a photomultiplier tube with an optical light guide. The collimator consists of 24 1-mm-diameter pinholes drilled into a cylindrical aperture in such a manner that an object placed in the center of the FOV is simultaneously projected onto the center of each of the 24 detectors. Compared with a single-pinhole aperture and detector system, having multiple pinholes and detectors markedly improves the overall system sensitivity. Importantly, because the detectors are placed in a circular pattern around the animal, there is no need to rotate a gantry. A full 3D dynamic image set can be acquired in only 5 to 10 minutes. Another unique stationary approach to rapid dynamic microSPECT imaging is a second-generation system called *U-SPECT-II* that was developed by Beekman and colleagues and is now available commercially (Fig. 11-18A).[42] The system consists of interchangeable tungsten ring collimators with 75 pinholes (see Fig. 11-18B) that yield non-overlapping projections of the imaging volume onto three 508 × 381 × 9.5 mm detectors. Using the mouse collimator with 0.35-mm pinhole apertures, a resolution of less than 0.35 mm was obtained using a rod phantom filled with [99m]Tc (see Fig. 11-18C). The U-SPECT-II system acquires the data set simultaneously in list mode, and both ECG and respiratory gating can be performed. Figure 11-19 is an example image of myocardial

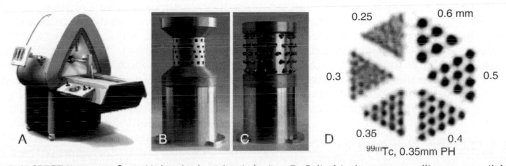

Figure 11-18 **A,** U-SPECT-II system from Molecular Imaging Labs Inc. **B,** Cylindrical tungsten collimators available in two different sizes for mice and rats, respectively. **C,** High-resolution technetium-99m hot rod phantom acquired using USPECT-II with a cylindrical collimator consisting of 75 0.35-mm pinholes. *(Image courtesy of MILabs Inc.)*

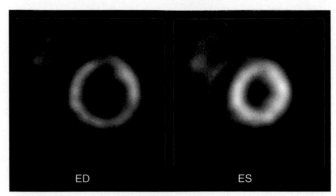

Figure 11-19 End-diastolic (ED) and end-systolic (ES) images of perfusion (technetium-99m-tetrofosmin) in a mouse heart obtained using the U-SPECT camera. The ED and ES frames were obtained from a gated SPECT study. *(Image courtesy of MILabs Inc.)*

perfusion (^{99m}Tc-tetrofosmin) in a mouse heart at end-diastole and end-systole that was obtained with U-SPECT. The ultra-high-resolution images clearly show both papillary muscle and the thin right ventricular wall of the mouse heart. With U-SPECT-II, CT imaging can also be performed using a separate CT module, and the reconstructed image data sets can be co-registered and fused with postacquisition software.

Uses of MicroSPECT Instrumentation for Cardiovascular Molecular Imaging

In the remainder of this chapter, we will give a few specific examples of how microSPECT imaging is playing an important role in cardiovascular research using rodent models.

Myocardial Perfusion and LV Function

State-of-the-art, standalone microSPECT systems have many attractive features, but for some applications, excellent results have been obtained using clinical SPECT cameras with pinhole collimators. In one study, Maskali et al. used such a system to image myocardial perfusion and LV function by gated SPECT in a rat model of postinfarction LV remodeling over 12 weeks.[43] The rats were serially imaged over 12 weeks using 400 to 700 MBq of ^{99m}Tc-sestamibi injected intravenously (300-500-μL volume) at each time point. The camera system consisted of a single-head clinical SPECT camera with a 3-mm diameter pinhole and a magnification factor of approximately 4.5 (195 mm focal length, 43 mm radius of rotation). Image reconstruction was performed using an OSEM iterative algorithm, and LV function was determined using clinical QGS software. The investigators demonstrated that in the post-MI setting, the initial (48-hour) infarct size measured by sestamibi SPECT predicts the extent of subsequent LV remodeling in rats (Fig. 11-20).[43]

Quantitative Assessment of Myocardial Viability Using Technetium-99m-Glucarate

In a recent study by Liu et al. at the University of Arizona,[44] the FASTSPECT camera (described earlier)

was used to image ^{99m}Tc-glucarate uptake in the hearts of rats as a measure of the extent of myocardial necrosis following experimental coronary occlusion (Fig. 11-21). The investigators demonstrated that administration of the α1 adenosine receptor agonist 2-chloro-N6-cyclopentyladenosine reduced infarct size to the same extent as that obtained with ischemic preconditioning (IPC), and that the degree of protection was lost in the presence of a nonselective adenosine receptor antagonist, SPT.[44] This study is an excellent example of how quantitative microSPECT imaging can be used as an endpoint when assessing the efficacy of new therapies in experimental models.

Dual-Isotope Imaging of Myocardial Perfusion and Inflammation

Sato et al. reported on the use of a radiolabeled anti-tenascin-C monoclonal antibody for imaging myocardial inflammation.[45] In a rat model of autoimmune myocarditis produced by immunization with porcine myosin twice over a 7-day interval, these investigators demonstrated high accumulation of ^{111}In-labeled anti-tenascin-C antibody in the inflamed myocardial region. Using a dual-isotope approach with ^{111}In-anti-tenascin-C and ^{99m}Tc-sestamibi (Fig. 11-22) and SPECT imaging, these investigators demonstrated that the focal uptake of ^{111}In-anti-tenascin-C antibody in the septal wall could easily be visualized in vivo. The camera system utilized for these experiments was a three-headed clinical SPECT camera with 1-mm pinholes on each detector. The fused image shown in *panel C* of Figure 11-22 highlights the multi-isotope advantage of SPECT instrumentation, whereby the sestamibi perfusion image can serve as an anatomic marker that is helpful for localizing the focal uptake of the "hot spot" tracer in the myocardium. Even with dual-modality hybrid microSPECT/CT systems where the CT image is extremely valuable as an anatomic reference point, the use of different isotopes to simultaneously image different aspects of cardiovascular system under study is advantageous.

Monocyte Trafficking in Atherosclerosis

In another recent study, Kircher et al. used a commercially available dual-modality microSPECT/CT (X-SPECT, Gamma Medica Ideas, Inc.) to follow monocyte trafficking in a murine model of atherosclerosis.[46] ApoE$^{-/-}$ subjects were fed for several weeks on the Western diet to produce atherosclerotic plaques. Monocytes were isolated from donor wild-type mice and labeled ex vivo with ^{111}In-oxine. Approximately 3×10^6 labeled cells were then injected into a tail vein, and serial microSPECT/CT imaging was performed over 5 days. Figure 11-23 depicts the CT *(row A)*, fused microSPECT/CT *(row B)*, and postmortem phosphor plate autoradiographs of the excised aortas *(row C)*. The panel on the left shows an ApoE$^{-/-}$ mouse that received the indium-labeled monocytes. As shown, the monocytes homed in on the atherosclerotic region of the ascending aorta, which was confirmed by immunohistochemistry. The binding specificity was demonstrated using a mouse that received a fraction of cells that had been depleted

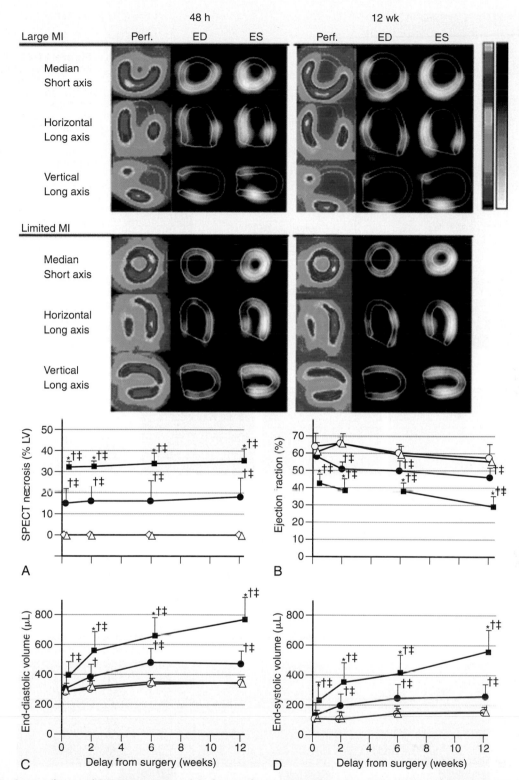

Figure 11-20 Sestamibi gated SPECT in a rat model of postinfarction LV remodeling. The *left panel* depicts perfusion at 48 hours and 12 weeks in rats with large or limited infarct size at 48 hours. The *right panel* depicts changes in LV volume and functional parameters in the same rats, as compared with sham-operated controls *(open triangles)*, as well as in rats with no detectable infarcts *(open circles)*. *(Reproduced with permission from Maskali F, Franken PR, Poussier S, et al: Initial infarct size predicts subsequent cardiac remodeling in the rat infarct model: An in vivo serial pinhole gated SPECT study, J Nucl Med 47:337–344, 2006.)*

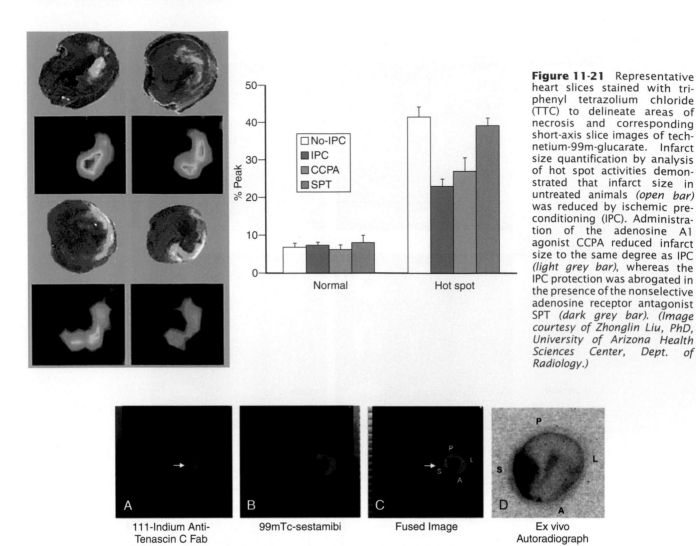

Figure 11-21 Representative heart slices stained with triphenyl tetrazolium chloride (TTC) to delineate areas of necrosis and corresponding short-axis slice images of technetium-99m-glucarate. Infarct size quantification by analysis of hot spot activities demonstrated that infarct size in untreated animals *(open bar)* was reduced by ischemic preconditioning (IPC). Administration of the adenosine A1 agonist CCPA reduced infarct size to the same degree as IPC *(light grey bar)*, whereas the IPC protection was abrogated in the presence of the nonselective adenosine receptor antagonist SPT *(dark grey bar)*. *(Image courtesy of Zhonglin Liu, PhD, University of Arizona Health Sciences Center, Dept. of Radiology.)*

| 111-Indium Anti-Tenascin C Fab | 99mTc-sestamibi | Fused Image | Ex vivo Autoradiograph |

Figure 11-22 Dual-isotope SPECT of inflammation (^{111}In-anti-tenascin C Fab), perfusion (^{99m}Tc-sestamibi), and fused images in a rat model of experimental myocarditis. The use of a myocardial perfusion agent provides anatomic localization for a "hot spot" tracer that is labeled with a second isotope. *(Figure adapted and reproduced with permission from Sato M, Toyozaki T, Odaka K, et al: Detection of experimental autoimmune myocarditis in rats by ^{111}In monoclonal antibody specific for tenascin-C. Circulation 106:1397–1402, 2002.)*

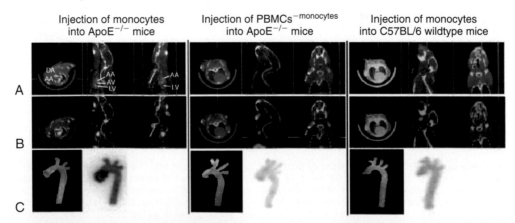

Injection of monocytes into ApoE$^{-/-}$ mice   Injection of PBMCs$^{-monocytes}$ into ApoE$^{-/-}$ mice   Injection of monocytes into C57BL/6 wildtype mice

Figure 11-23 Example of imaging monocyte cell trafficking in a murine model of atherosclerosis. Radiolabeled monocytes homed to the ascending aorta in ApoE$^{-/-}$ mice *(left column)*, but not in mice where the injected cell fraction had been depleted of monocytes or in wild-type mice with no atherosclerosis. Cells labeled with ^{111}In can be followed over several days with micro-SPECT imaging to monitor their fate and ultimate site of localization. *(Figure reproduced with permission from Kircher MF, Grimm J, Swirski FK, Libby P, et al: Noninvasive in vivo imaging of monocyte trafficking to atherosclerotic lesions, Circulation 117:388–395, 2008.)*

of monocytes *(middle panel)* and with a negative control wild-type mouse with no atherosclerosis *(right panel)*. In both of these negative controls, no uptake of the indium-labeled tracer was observed in the aortic arch. The longer half-life of the single photon isotope [111]In (2.7 days) allowed for the monitoring of the same population of labeled cells over time. As mentioned earlier, this ability to track cells over a period of days is one of the advantages of using microSPECT over microPET.

Imaging Matrix Metalloproteinase Expression in Vascular Remodeling

Zhang et al. utilized high-resolution microSPECT/CT to image activated matrix metalloproteinases (MMPs) using a novel ^{111}In-labeled tracer (RP782).[47] ApoE[−/−] mice that had been fed a high-cholesterol diet were subjected to left common carotid injury. RP782 was administered at 1, 2, 3, and 4 weeks after injury. The microSPECT camera utilized 1-mm-diameter pinhole collimators. To enhance CT contrast, an infusion of an iodinated contrast agent (iohexol, 100 μL/min) was given. As shown in Figure 11-24, at 3 weeks postinjury, an RP782 hotspot was observed in the injured left carotid artery but not in the uninjured right carotid artery. Importantly, image quantification *(panel D)* allowed for the determination of the time course of MMP activation. This study provides an excellent example of the importance of using a second modality, in this case CT, to help localize the uptake of the radiolabeled probe. It also demonstrates that the use of an iodinated CT contrast agent can greatly enhance the CT image for this purpose.

Limitations and Challenges

As mentioned previously, mainly because of the need for collimation, the sensitivity of microSPECT is roughly an order of magnitude less than microPET. Accordingly, to achieve reasonable count statistics and shorten image acquisition times, human-scale activities of between 5 and 20 mCi have been administered to mice and rats weighing only 20 or 300 g, respectively. Obviously, administering such high doses of radiation to small animals is not optimal because of the potential adverse effects of the radiation on the biological system under study. In the case of receptor-targeted tracers, there is also the danger of saturating the specific receptor sites with an excessive concentration of tracer, which may also affect the system under study. Furthermore, depending upon the labeling efficiency and specific activity of a particular radiotracer, it can be quite challenging to deliver a high dose of activity in a small volume. In the mouse, for example, injection volumes must be kept to less than 200 μL. Over the past several years, advances in microSPECT instrumentation, as well as improvements in software reconstruction techniques, have improved both the sensitivity and resolution of these new systems tremendously, and further advances are expected in the future.

In recent years, hybrid imaging systems have become more commonplace. All of the commercially available microSPECT systems provide some means of obtaining dual SPECT and CT images in the same animal, although with most of these systems, the SPECT and CT image data sets must be acquired sequentially. While the addition of CT provides an anatomic road map that can be extremely helpful in localizing "hot spot" radiotracers, one must also be careful to minimize the exposure of the animal to additional ionizing radiation. Exciting work is underway to develop SPECT (and PET) inserts for MRI systems that will allow simultaneous radionuclide and MRI.

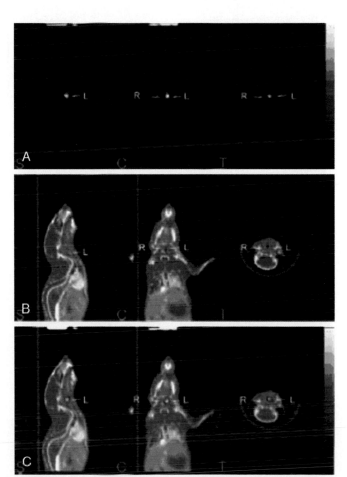

Figure 11-24 An example of (**A**) RP782 microSPECT, (**B**) CT angiography, and (**C**) fused microSPECT/CT in vivo imaging at 3 weeks after carotid injury. *Arrows* point to the injured left (L) and noninjured right (R) carotid arteries. The small hot spot in the abdomen is likely the upper pole of the kidney on the edge of the SPECT field of view and/or a pinhole imaging artifact. S indicates sagittal; C, coronal; and T, transverse slices.

Continued

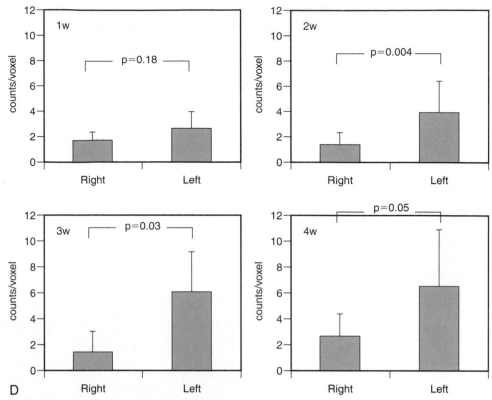

Figure 11-24—cont'd **D**, Image-derived quantitative analysis of background-corrected RP782 carotid uptake. N = 5 to 7 in each group. w, week. *(Figure reproduced with permission from Zhang J, Nie L, Razavian M, et al: Molecular imaging of activated matrix metalloproteinases in vascular remodeling. Circulation 118:1953–1960, 2008.)*

REFERENCES

1. Lecomte R, Cadorette J, Richard P, et al: Initial results from Sherbrooke avalanche photodiode positron tomograph, *IEEE Trans Nucl Sci* 41:1446–1452, 1996.
2. Cherry SR, Shao Y, S RW, et al: MicroPET: a high resolution PET scanner for imaging small animals, *IEEE Trans Nucl Sci* 44:1161–1166, 1997.
3. Chatziioannou AF, Cherry SR, Shao Y, et al: Performance evaluation of microPET: a high-resolution lutetium oxyorthosilicate PET scanner for animal imaging, *J Nucl Med* 40(7):1164–1175, 1999.
4. Chatziioannou A, Tai YC, Doshi N, Cherry SR: Detector development for microPET II: a 1 microl resolution PET scanner for small animal imaging, *Phys Med Biol* 46(11):2899–2910, 2001.
5. Ziegler SI, Pichler BJ, Boening G, et al: A prototype high-resolution animal positron tomograph with avalanche photodiode arrays and LSO crystals, *Eur J Nucl Med* 28(2):136–143, 2001.
6. Blasberg R: PET imaging of gene expression, *Eur J Cancer* 38(16): 2137–2146, 2002.
7. Cherry SR, Gambhir SS: Use of positron emission tomography in animal research, *ILAR J* 42(3):219–232, 2001.
8. Chatziioannou AF: Molecular imaging of small animals with dedicated PET tomographs, *Eur J Nucl Med* 29(1):98–114, 2002.
9. Herschman HR, MacLaren DC, Iyer M, et al: Seeing is believing: non-invasive, quantitative and repetitive imaging of reporter gene expression in living animals, using positron emission tomography, *J Neurosci Res* 59(6):699–705, 2000.
10. Gambhir SS: Molecular imaging of cancer with positron emission tomography, *Nat Rev Cancer* 2(9):683–693, 2002.
11. Gambhir SS, Herschman HR, Cherry SR, et al: Imaging transgene expression with radionuclide imaging technologies, *Neoplasia* 2(1–2): 118–138, 2000.
12. Schafers KP: Imaging small animals with positron emission tomography, *Nuklearmedizin* 42(3):86–89, 2003.
13. Rowland DJ, Lewis JS, Welch MJ: Molecular imaging: the application of small animal positron emission tomography, *J Cell Biochem Suppl* 39:110–115, 2002.
14. Laforest R, Longord D, Siegel S, Newport DF, Yap J: *Performance evaluation of the microPET-Focus-F120*, Paper presented at: IEEE Nuclear Science Symposium and Medical Imaging Conference, Rome, Italy 2004.
15. Kudo T, Fukuchi K, Annala AJ, et al: Noninvasive measurement of myocardial activity concentrations and perfusion defect sizes in rats with a new small-animal positron emission tomograph, *Circulation* 106(1):118–123, 2002.
16. Chatziioannou A, Qi J, Moore A, et al: Comparison of 3-D maximum a posteriori and filtered backprojection algorithms for high-resolution animal imaging with microPET, *IEEE Trans Med Imaging* 19(5): 507–512, 2000.
17. Schelbert HR, Inubushi M, Ross RS: PET imaging in small animals, *J Nucl Cardiol* 10(5):513–520, 2003.
18. Lecomte R, Croteau E, Gauthier M-E, et al: Cardiac PET imaging of blood flow, metabolism and function in normal and infarcted rats, *IEEE Trans Nucl Sci* 2003 (in press).
19. Chow PL, Rannou FR, Chatziioannou AF: Attenuation correction for small animal PET tomographs, *Phys Med Biol* 50(8):1837–1850, 2005.
20. Finck BN, Lehman JJ, Leone TC, et al: The cardiac phenotype induced by PPARalpha overexpression mimics that caused by diabetes mellitus, *J Clin Invest* 109(1):121–130, 2002.
21. Shai SY, Harpf AE, Babbitt CJ, et al: Cardiac myocyte-specific excision of the beta-1 integrin gene results in myocardial fibrosis and cardiac failure, *Circ Res* 90(4):458–464, 2002.
22. Blasberg R: Imaging gene expression and endogenous molecular processes: molecular imaging, *J Cereb Blood Flow Metab* 22(10): 1157–1164, 2002.
23. Min JJ, Gambhir SS: Gene therapy progress and prospects: noninvasive imaging of gene therapy in living subjects, *Gene Ther* 11(2):115–125, 2004.
24. Bengel FM, Anton M, Avril N, et al: Uptake of radiolabeled 2′-fluoro-2′-deoxy-5-iodo-1-beta-D-arabinofuranosyluracil in cardiac cells after adenoviral transfer of the herpesvirus thymidine kinase gene: the cellular basis for cardiac gene imaging, *Circulation* 102(9):948–950, 2000.
25. Wu JC, Inubushi M, Sundaresan G, Schelbert HR, Gambhir SS: Positron emission tomography imaging of cardiac reporter gene expression in living rats, *Circulation* 106(2):180–183, 2002.
26. Wu JC, Inubushi M, Sundaresan G, Schelbert HR, Gambhir SS: Optical imaging of cardiac reporter gene expression in living rats, *Circulation* 105(14):1631–1634, 2002.
27. Inubushi M, Wu JC, Gambhir SS, et al: Positron-emission tomography reporter gene expression imaging in rat myocardium, *Circulation* 107 (2):326–332, 2003.
28. Wu JC, Chen IY, Sundaresan G, et al: Molecular imaging of cardiac cell transplantation in living animals using optical bioluminescence and positron emission tomography, *Circulation* 108(11):1302–1305, 2003.

29. Pain F, Laniece P, Mastrippolito R, Gervais P, Hantraye P, Besret L: Arterial input function measurement without blood sampling using a beta-microprobe in rats, *J Nucl Med* 45(9):1577–1582, 2004.

30. Laforest R, Sharp TL, Engelbach JA, et al: Measurement of input functions in rodents: challenges and solutions, *Nucl Med Biol* 32 (7):679–685, 2005.

31. Fang YH, Muzic RF Jr, : Spillover and partial-volume correction for image-derived input functions for small-animal 18F-FDG PET studies, *J Nucl Med* 49(4):606–614, 2008.

32. Kundu BK, Locke L, Berr S, Matherne G, Lankford A: Dynamic FDG-PET imaging in-vivo to evaluate glucose metabolism in a mouse model of myocardial hypertrophy, *J Nucl Med* 49(Suppl 1):184P, 2008.

33. Phelps ME: *PET: Molecular Imaging and Its Biological Applications*, New York, NY, 2004, Springer-Verlag.

34. Bentourkia M, Croteau E, Aliaga A, et al: Cardiac studies in rats with ^{11}C-acetate and PET: A comparison with ^{13}N-ammonia, *IEEE Trans Nucl Sci* 49(5):2322–2327, 2002.

35. Waller C, Kahler E, Hiller KH, et al: Myocardial perfusion and intracapillary blood volume in rats at rest and with coronary dilatation: MR imaging in vivo with use of a spin-labeling technique, *Radiology* 215 (1):189–197, 2000.

36. Armbrecht JJ, Buxton DB, Brunken RC, Phelps ME, Schelbert HR: Regional myocardial oxygen consumption determined noninvasively in humans with [1-11C]acetate and dynamic positron tomography, *Circulation* 80(4):863–872, 1989.

37. Inubushi M, Jordan MC, Roos KP, et al: Nitrogen-13 ammonia cardiac positron emission tomography in mice: effects of clonidine-induced changes in cardiac work on myocardial perfusion, *Eur J Nucl Med Mol Imaging* 31(1):110–116, 2004.

38. Wu HM, Stout D, Shoghi-Jadid K, Schiepers C, Chatziioannou A, Huang SC: Derivation of input function from dynamic FDG-microPET images of mice (abstract), *Mol Imaging Biol* 4(Suppl 1):S43, 2002.

39. Qi J, Leahy RM, Cherry SR, Chatziioannou A, Farquhar TH: High-resolution 3D Bayesian image reconstruction using the microPET small-animal scanner, *Phys Med Biol* 43(4):1001–1013, 1998.

40. Goertzen AL, Meadors AK, Silverman RW, Cherry SR: Simultaneous molecular and anatomical imaging of the mouse in vivo, *Phys Med Biol* 47(24):4315–4328, 2002.

41. Judenhofer MS, Catana C, Swann BK, et al: PET/MR images acquired with a compact MR-compatible PET detector in a 7-T magnet, *Radiology* 244(3):807–814, 2007.

42. van der Have F, Vastenhouw B, Ramakers RM, et al: U-SPECT-II: An ultra-high-resolution device for molecular small-animal imaging, *J Nucl Med* 50:599–605, 2009.

43. Maskali F, Franken PR, Poussier S, et al: Initial infarct size predicts subsequent cardiac remodeling in the rat infarct model: an in vivo serial pinhole gated SPECT study, *J Nucl Med* 47(2):337–344, 2006.

44. Liu Z, Barrett HH, Stevenson GD, Furenlid LR, Pak KY, Woolfenden JM: Evaluating the protective role of ischaemic preconditioning in rat hearts using a stationary small-animal SPECT imager and 99mTc-glucarate, *Nucl Med Commun* 29(2):120–128, 2008.

45. Sato M, Toyozaki T, Odaka K, et al: Detection of experimental autoimmune myocarditis in rats by ^{111}In monoclonal antibody specific for tenascin-C, *Circulation* 106(11):1397–1402, 2002.

46. Kircher MF, Grimm J, Swirski FK, et al: Noninvasive in vivo imaging of monocyte trafficking to atherosclerotic lesions, *Circulation* 117(3):388–395, 2008.

47. Zhang J, Nie L, Razavian M, et al: Molecular imaging of activated matrix metalloproteinases in vascular remodeling, *Circulation* 118(19):1953–1960, 2008.

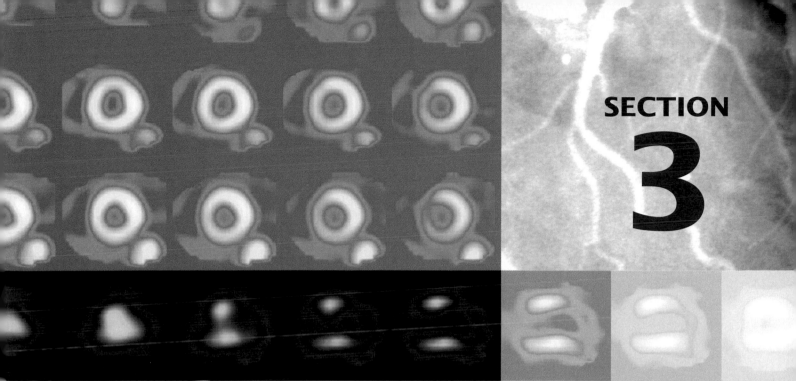

Ventricular Function

Chapter 12

Cardiac Performance

BARRY L. ZARET

INTRODUCTION

An assessment of cardiac performance constituted the first nuclear cardiology studies performed in man. As early as 1927, Blumgart and Weiss in a series of elegant papers identified characteristics of hemodynamic performance as measured by circulation times in normals and in patients with significant cardiovascular disease, utilizing injected radon followed by measurements obtained with a modified Wilson cloud chamber over the thorax and contralateral upper extremity.[1] These pioneering studies called attention to the potential of utilizing radioisotope technology for answering relevant clinical questions.

Presently, cardiac performance can be evaluated by nuclear cardiology in three general manners. Two involve measurement of radioactivity within the blood pool, while the third applies the principles of electrocardiography (ECG) gating to conventional myocardial perfusion single-photon emission computed tomography (SPECT) studies. This latter technique is discussed in detail in Chapter 13 and consequently will not be developed here. This chapter will concentrate on the initial techniques of equilibrium intravascular labeling, which allows repeated imaging over several hours (equilibrium radionuclide angiocardiography [ERNA]), and the first-pass technique during which analysis of the first transit of a radionuclide bolus through the central circulation is assessed (first-pass radionuclide angiocardiography [FPRNA]). Although the intravascular radionuclide approaches for the evaluation of ventricular function have been challenged by both echocardiography and gated perfusion SPECT, these specific techniques still play a role in the quantitative assessment of cardiac performance. These intravascular approaches and their clinical implications and applications are discussed subsequently.

EQUILIBRIUM RADIONUCLIDE ANGIOCARDIOGRAPHY

The basic concept of utilizing a physiologic input to "gate" or physiologically control radioisotope-labeled equilibrium cardiac blood pool data to measure left ventricular ejection fraction was first introduced in 1971.[2,3] The physiologic signal chosen was the electrocardiogram, and the blood pool was initially labeled with technetium [99mTc] human serum albumin. Left ventricular ejection fraction was measured and regional wall motion assessed visually from end-systolic and end-diastolic summed data.[2] This approach built on earlier studies whereby "gating" had been achieved with intravenous first-pass or intraventricular injections of radioisotope and left ventricular ejection fraction evaluated from respective maxima and minima of the generated curves.[4–7] ERNA uses the electrocardiographic signal to establish the temporal relationships between acquired nuclear data and volumetric events of the cardiac cycle. To accomplish this, sampling is performed during the time of radioisotopic equilibrium within the blood pool such that sequential data can be summed over several hundred cardiac cycles. These data are then segregated physiologically according to their time of occurrence within the cardiac cycle as determined by the simultaneously acquired electrocardiogram (Fig. 12-1). Data are accumulated until the radioactive count density over the cardiac region of interest is of sufficient magnitude for generation of statistically meaningful analysis. The data from the individual components of this temporal segregation of nuclear data are displayed in an endless-loop scintigraphy movie and as a ventricular volume curve for qualitative visual assessment as well as for quantification of global left ventricular function (Fig. 12-2).

Technical Issues

The duration of study necessitated by utilizing the equilibrium technique can be both an advantage and a disadvantage.[8] Because studies involve summation of several hundred cardiac cycles, a number of time-related specific issues must be considered. First, the patient must be able to remain relatively still beneath the detector during the period of acquisition. Second, most studies continue to be obtained with the planar technique.

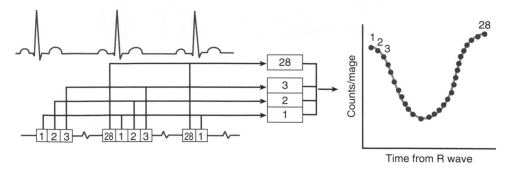

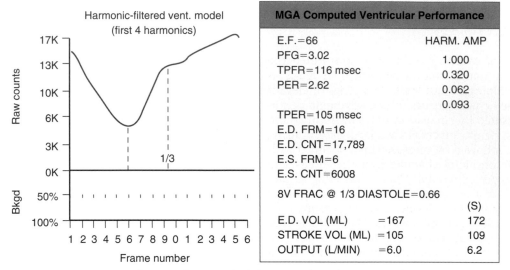

Figure 12-1 Diagrammatic representation of the ERNA technique. Each cardiac cycle is divided into 28 equal segments. For each heartbeat, data are accumulated then stored in a separate file. To the *right*, these data for the 28 portions of the cycle are displayed as a single summed ventricular volume curve. The numbers *1* to *28* refer to temporal sequence within the cardiac cycle. *(Reprinted from Wackers FJTh, Soufer R, Zaret BL: Nuclear cardiology. In Braunwald E, Zipes DP, Libby P [eds]: Heart Disease, 6th ed. Philadelphia: WB Saunders, 2001, p 273, with permission from the American College of Cardiology Foundation.)*

Figure 12-2 Computer screen capture of a normal ERNA. The left ventricular volume curve shows a normal appearance. There is some count dropoff in the last frame due to respiratory heart rate variability. On the *right* are quantitative results of analysis from the volume curve. LVEF is normal at 66%. End-diastolic (ED) counts (CNT) are excellent (17,789), ensuring good statistical reliability. Peak filling rate (PFR) is normal at 3.82 EDV/sec. The ED volume (VOL) is at the upper limit of normal at 167 mL. *(From Wackers FJTh, Bruni W, Zaret BL: Planar equilibrium radionuclide angiocardiography: Acquisition and processing protocols. In Nuclear Cardiology: The Basics. Totowa, NJ: Humana, 2003.)*

Consequently, data are acquired in multiple views in order for complete interpretation. Generally, this involves the anterior, left anterior oblique, and either left lateral or left posterior oblique views. The need for multiple views is inherent in the planar technique to account for superimposed radioactivity in multiple cardiac and noncardiac structures that can at times obscure analysis of a given region of interest. Such views are also important for defining specific regional left ventricular abnormalities such as ventricular aneurysm or severe akinesis. Third, intrinsic to this approach is the assumption that cardiac performance will remain relatively stable during the entire period of acquisition. Such stability is not present in instances of rapidly changing ventricular responses to atrial fibrillation or frequent premature beats of either ventricular or atrial origin. Fourth, the radionuclide label must remain stable during the period of analysis. (For conventional clinical imaging, this is usually not a problem). Fifth, the framing acquisition interval also must be of sufficient duration

to allow statistically meaningful data as well as adequate temporal resolution for definition of parameters of systolic and diastolic ventricular performance.

Gated Blood Pool Single-Photon Emission Computed Tomography

The equilibrium radionuclide technique can also be readily applied to SPECT rather than planar studies.[9-14] SPECT blood pool imaging would have some obvious advantages with respect to three-dimensional visualization and elimination of problems induced by overlapping structures (Fig. 12-3). Recently, new algorithms have been developed to improve calculations of both left ventricular ejection fraction and ventricular volumes from gated SPECT studies. It is likely that algorithms such as those recently proposed will enhance the ability to move gated SPECT technology from the research to the clinical environment for assessment of ventricular function.[14] However, at the present time, work has

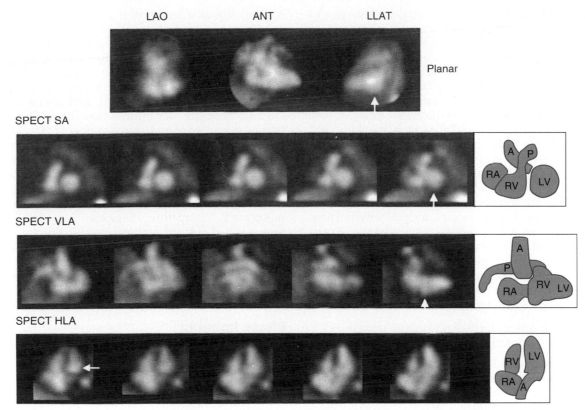

LAO   ANT   LLAT

Planar

SPECT SA

SPECT VLA

SPECT HLA

Figure 12-3 Planar and SPECT ERNA at rest in a patient with a basal inferior aneurysm. Planar images in the LAO, anterior (ANT), and left lateral (LLAT) views *(top)*. The basal inferior aneurysm is best appreciated in the LLAT *(arrow)*. SPECT images in the same patient *(bottom)*. Short axis (SA), vertical long-axis (VLA), and horizontal long-axis (HLA) slices are shown. The basal inferior aneurysm is appreciated on multiple reconstructive slices *(arrows)*. A schematic drawing of the anatomy is shown on the right. *(Reprinted from Wackers FJTh, Soufer R, Zaret BL: Nuclear cardiology. In Braunwald E, Zipes DP, Libby P [eds]: Heart Disease, 6th ed. Philadelphia: WB Saunders, 2001, p 273, with permission from the American College of Cardiology Foundation.)*

been primarily experimental, and advantages have not been of sufficient magnitude to replace the less time-consuming and complex planar approach.

A recent study by Nichols et al. analyzed automated quantitative analysis of gated blood pool SPECT for assessing regional and global wall motion using magnetic resonance imaging as a standard. They found good agreement with independent magnetic resonance imaging calculations and demonstrated that the automated technique was superior to visual analysis.[14]

Performance

Labeling of the blood pool at equilibrium is obtained using ^{99m}Tc fixed to the patient's own red blood cells.[16] This technique is standard and can be done using either an in vitro or modified in vivo technique employing unlabeled stannous pyrophosphate as a facilitator of the labeling process. The in vitro approach has a labeling efficiency of greater than 97% and is the current method of choice.[15] A single labeling procedure will involve sufficient radioactivity present in the blood pool to allow for serial studies over a period of 4 to 6 hours. A dose of 25 to 30 mCi is used.

Conventional Anger scintillation cameras are used for these studies. If planar imaging devices are not available, then the single head of a SPECT instrumentation camera can be employed. A 64 ∞ 64 matrix

should be used. Pixel size should be less than 4 mm/pixel. No zoom should be applied to a 10-inch field of view camera, and 1.5 to 22 zoom used in a large field of view camera.[16] Data are analyzed by computer, either totally automatically or with operator interaction. There must be sufficient radioactivity within the field to allow for quantitative analysis. Generally, studies are acquired over sufficient time to accumulate greater than 4 million counts. At the present time, most studies are performed in the resting state. This evaluation can be performed in multiple views within 15 minutes. Collimation generally involves low-energy high-resolution collimators. If exercise studies are used, high-sensitivity collimators or low-energy all-purpose or low-energy high-sensitivity collimators should be used. Background subtraction is necessary because there is activity throughout the intravascular space. In some programs, the background region is placed 4 pixels outside the lateral border of the left ventricular region of interest. In other programs, this may be done manually. In either case, it is key to be sure that background is not chosen over a very high count area such as the aorta or spleen, since this will lead to erroneous measurements.[16]

There are two general modes of data acquisition: frame mode or list mode. At the present time, frame mode is most widely used.[16–18] In this approach, a specified duration for each portion of the cardiac cycle is established. For resting studies this usually is between 10 and 40 msec or, generally, 16 frames/cycle, depending on the patient's intrinsic heart rate and the conditions of the study. This same frame duration will be utilized throughout the study, irrespective of any changes in the heart rate. Beat rejection programs are possible, which allow after the fact elimination of pre-specified duration premature and post-extrasystolic beats. A 10% to 15% window around the R-R peak is standard, and beats not falling within this window are rejected. This window will take into account normal physiologic variability. With list mode, analysis is made after acquisition and depends on cycle length. Consequently, with this technique a more accurate evaluation can be obtained in the presence of changes in cardiac cycle length. However, this approach is a bit more complicated and expensive and is for the most part limited to research studies.

Data are obtained in the left anterior oblique view for quantitative analysis of global left ventricular function. In this view, there is no overlap between the two ventricles. Ejection fraction is measured in a standard manner:

$$\frac{\text{End-diastolic counts } (bc) - \text{End-systolic counts } (bc)}{\text{End-diastolic counts } (bc)}$$

where bc = background corrected. With this technique, the lower count of normal is 0.50 (50%).[18] In addition to the conventional measurement of left ventricular ejection fraction, other indices of left ventricular ejection as well as ventricular filling can be made. These include ejection time, ejection rate, peak filling rate, and time to peak filling rate. Filling indices are measured in units of end-diastolic volumes per second (EDV/sec, normal < 2.5). To measure diastolic parameters, data must either be acquired at higher temporal resolution (i.e., 24 frames/R-R cycle) or have Fourier filtering applied to the standard 16 frame/cycle ERNA.[19] In the generated volume curve, a smooth diastolic upslope concludes with a visible "atrial kick" (see Fig. 12-2).

Ventricular volumes can also be determined by count-based methods. Because at equilibrium blood pool radioactivity is proportional to volume, by using an appropriate region of interest and accounting for attenuation, it is possible to measure chamber volume.[20–23] This may be accomplished by either acquisition and counting of a reference blood sample or by measuring pixel size for calibration. Volumes measured in this manner correlate well with other analyses. Because analysis is count-based, the data are free from errors associated with geometric analysis of volume. Ventricular volume measurements are increasingly important clinically with respect to serial monitoring and assessing ventricular remodeling.

Interpretation of ERNA studies requires both visual and quantitative analysis. Quantitative evaluation of right ventricular function is difficult with this technique because of contamination from anterior overlying right atrial activity. Consequently, right ventricular global function is best evaluated by concomitant first-pass techniques.[24,25] The degree of left anterior obliquity chosen for ERNA requires operator interaction to ensure optimal separation of right and left ventricles. This is generally achieved at a 45-degree angle but often

requires operator interaction to account for individual anatomic variation. From this view, measurement of global left ventricular function such as LV ejection fraction is obtained. Each of the three views employed provides qualitative information concerning regional contraction. The left anterior oblique view provides views of the septal, inferoapical, and lateral walls. The anterior view provides information concerning contraction of the anterior and apical segments. The left lateral or left posterior oblique views allow insight into contraction of the inferior wall and posterobasal segments. In addition, since the entire intravascular blood pool is labeled, information is derived concerning all cardiac and vascular structures such as the atria, aorta, and pulmonary vasculature. Regional function can also be quantified utilizing regional ejection fraction measurements with this approach; the left ventricular blood pool is divided into four to five segments, and ejection fraction is derived from each segment (Fig. 12-4).[26,27] This analysis is also done in the left anterior oblique view.

Phase Imaging

Parametric phase images are derived from the same radionuclide data utilized for standard ERNA measures of right and left ventricular function.[28,29] Commercially

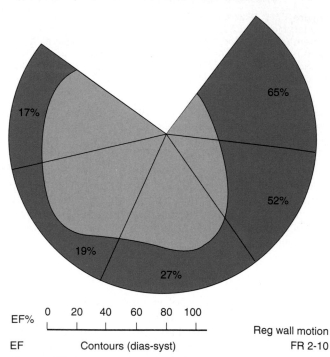

Figure 12-4 A typical regional ejection fraction display obtained from a left anterior oblique ERNA study. The left ventricle is divided into five sectors. An upper sector involving the valve planes is excluded. The sectors from *upper left to upper right, counterclockwise,* involve the upper septum, lower septum, and apex, and inferior lateral and posterolateral segments. In this particular study, regional ejection fraction is decreased in the upper and lower septum as well as the apex, with maintained contraction of the two lateral segments. *(Reprinted from Wackers FJTh, Soufer R, Zaret BL. Nuclear cardiology. In Braunwald E, Zipes DP, Libby P [eds]: Heart Disease, 6th ed. Philadelphia: WB Saunders, 2001, p 273, with permission from the American College of Cardiology Foundation.)*

available computer programs are utilized. A phase angle is assigned to each pixel of the phase image. This is derived from the first Fourier harmonic of time. The phase angle (ϕ) corresponds to the relative pattern and sequence of contraction in the cardiac chamber of interest throughout a single cardiac cycle. Generally, color coding is used and corresponding histograms are generated in each study. Dyssynchrony of cardiac contraction, whether intraventricular or interventricular, is evaluated from the difference in appropriate mean phase angles (Fig. 12-5). In the case of intraventricular dyssynchrony, right ventricle–left ventricle delays are evaluated. In the case of intraventricular dyssynchrony, this is measured by the standard deviation of the mean phase angle for the left ventricle. The technique has been used to identify sites of bypass tracks, sites of arrhythmogenesis, and altered contraction patterns in cardiomyopathy, and to assess the impact of biventricular pacer resynchronization therapy on the efficiency of cardiac contraction.[20],[34] The technique has also recently been employed to localize ventricular tachycardia exit sites as well as subsequent contraction sequence and functional effects of arrhythmia. In this very technically challenging study, a total of 26 patients with 32 episodes of ventricular tachycardia were studied. This occurred both in the electrophysiology laboratory and spontaneously. The phase analysis technique was quite accurate when compared to electrophysiologic study for defining exit site of the arrhythmia. In addition, there were good correlations between the imaging findings and the patient's ability to tolerate the specific arrhythmia.[34]

Ambulatory Monitoring

An additional application of the ERNA principle involves utilization of miniaturized portable equipment for monitoring patients during routine activities.[35] Instrumentation has been developed that allows for monitoring over several hours following equilibrium blood pool labeling. The device, called the *VEST*, is worn by patients such that they may be fully ambulatory. Radionuclide and electrocardiographic signals are stored on tapes comparable to Holter monitoring for analysis of arrhythmias. Off-line analysis allows trending of data concerning left ventricular ejection fraction and relative volumes (Fig. 12-6). This approach has been

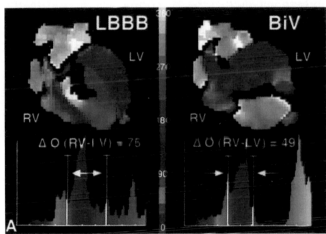

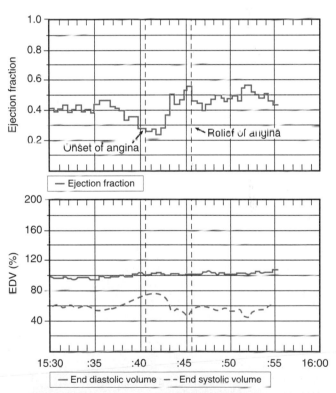

Figure 12-5 Phase images acquired in a patient with dilated cardiomyopathy and left bundle branch block (LBBB) before *(left)* and after *(right)* biventricular pacing. The contraction sequence, from early to late, is *green, azure, navy, violet, orange,* and *yellow.* Histograms illustrate dispersion of phase angles during ejection fraction plotted as phase angle (*x* axis) versus number of pixels (*y* axis). *Vertical bars* represent the arithmetic mean phase angle (ϕ) computed for RV and LV blood pools. On the *left*, an abnormal phase pattern in sinus rhythm with right-to-left ventricular contraction sequence is noted. The left ventricular apex and septum contract with extreme delay in phase with atrial systole *(orange segment at top of figure)*. The histogram illustrates abnormal dispersion of phase angles spanning the cardiac cycle with a $\Delta\phi$ of 75 degrees. At the right, a characteristic apex to base contraction sequence during biventricular pacing is noted. The phase pattern is more symmetric across the interventricular septum. Despite close proximity to pacing stimulus sites *(green)*, the LV apex *(yellow)* fails to contract in sequence. A decrease in phase angle occurs with pacing. *(Reprinted from Kerwin WF, Botvinick EH, O'Connell JW, et al: Ventricular contraction abnormalities in dilated cardiomyopathy: Effect of biventricular pacing to correct interventricular dyssynchrony, J Am Coll Cardiol 35:1221, 2000, with permission from the American College of Cardiology Foundation.)*

Figure 12-6 Trended data obtained with VEST in a patient in whom post–myocardial infarction ischemia is developing. Data for ejection fraction are shown in the *upper panel*, and data for relevant end-diastolic volume (EDV) and end-systolic volume are shown in the *lower panel*. Continuous data are shown for a 25-minute period. The times of onset and relief of angina are indicated. The decrease in ejection fraction precedes clinical occurrence of angina. This decrease is associated predominately with the increase in end-systolic volume and a minimal change in end-diastolic volume. *(Reprinted from Wackers FJTh, Soufer R, Zaret BL: Nuclear cardiology. In Braunwald E, Zipes DP, Libby P [eds]: Heart Disease, 6th ed. Philadelphia: WB Saunders, 2001, p 273, with permission from the American College of Cardiology Foundation.)*

standardized in several laboratories and has been utilized for the assessment of silent myocardial ischemia as well as pharmacologic intervention.[36-38] Newer-generation equipment has been developed for this assessment.

First-Pass Radionuclide Angiocardiography

The first-pass approach offers an alternative to ERNA.[8,39] However, because it is somewhat more technically demanding, it is performed less frequently. Nevertheless, it can be used routinely at the time of any ^{99m}Tc-labeled pharmaceutical injection such as myocardial perfusion agents.[40-44] This option presents a distinct advantage.

With the first-pass technique, sampling occurs only during the initial seconds of transit of the radioactivity bolus through the central circulation. Analysis is made of the high-frequency components of this signal. The basic assumption of this approach is that there has been sufficient admixture of radioactivity with circulating blood such that the count rate changes recorded represent a true proportionality to volumetric changes within the cardiac chamber of interest. The temporal segregation of the radioactivity bolus allows independent evaluation of right and left ventricular function (Fig. 12-7). Regional function can also be assessed.

Any technetium-labeled radiopharmaceutical can be used for a first-pass technique. For the most part, this had previously either been ^{99m}Tc-pertechnetate or ^{99m}Tc complexed to other carriers such as DTPA or sulfur colloid. In such a manner, multiple injections can be made for assessment of function at both rest and exercise.[39,45,46] Currently, first-pass studies are generally done at the time of tracer injection for either ERNA or perfusion SPECT. Other short-lived generator systems have been employed experimentally; these include

generators involving tungsten-178-tantalum-178,[47] osmium-191-iridium-191m,[48-51] and mercury-195m-gold-195m.[52-55] However, none have been used clinically to any substantial extent.

The scintillation camera used for first-pass studies is extremely important. To provide statistically meaningful high count rate data, cameras must be able to provide high sensitivity with system linearity and no major dead-time losses.[8,56] Initial approaches utilizing this technique involved multicrystal scintillation cameras. This instrumentation has since been replaced by second- and third-generation digital scintillation cameras suitable for rapid acquisition of high count rate data. Another experimental imaging system is the multiwire proportional chamber gamma camera.[57] However, this system provides optimal data only for low energies less than 100 keV, such as those provided by tantalum-178.

As with ERNA, a number of relevant technical issues must be considered for each study. The injection technique must provide delivery of a compact bolus without associated streaming of the radioactivity input function. To accomplish this, injections must be made from either the antecubital vein or a more central site. Since analysis occurs over a few cardiac cycles lasting only seconds, the presence of significant change in cardiac cycle length or arrhythmia during the procedure will invalidate the data. In addition, in stable arrhythmias such as atrial fibrillation, it is impossible to get a meaningful assessment, since only a few variable beats are available for analysis.

Studies are obtained in the anterior or right anterior oblique views. Data from FPRNA are computer processed in frame mode. Regions of interest are selected over the chamber of interest. Generally these are fixed regions. Activity is analyzed only as the initial bolus traverses the chamber of interest, the right or left ventricle. A background correction is necessary. A number of approaches to background have been described, but generally a fixed background is used.[16,24] The first-pass approach is the best technique for assessing global right ventricular function. This can also be used in the process of ERNA studies evaluating the left ventricle, with analysis performed at the time of initial radionuclide injection.

A variation called the *gated first-pass technique* can be used as well. With this technique, there is a merging of first-pass and equilibrium technology. First-pass data are acquired in concert with the ECG signal. These data are stored and summed, and several beats are used to form a representative cardiac cycle assessing the right heart phase of transit. Separate regions of interest are defined for end-systole and end-diastole. No background subtraction is necessary.[16] This provides higher count data than that obtainable with a simple bolus injection.

Shunt Detection

The first-pass study also may be utilized to detect and quantify intracardiac shunts.[58-63] A region of interest is selected over the lung field. The pulmonary time-activity curve from this region is then analyzed. Under normal circumstances there will be a sharp rise in the

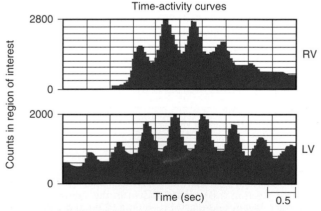

Figure 12-7 Radionuclide time-activity curves obtained from a right ventricular (RV) and left ventricular (LV) region of interest during first-pass radionuclide angiocardiography. Each peak and valley represents a single cardiac cycle. Data from this study are summed to provide RV and LV ejection fraction. *(Reprinted from Wackers FJTh, Soufer R, Zaret BL: Nuclear cardiology. In Braunwald E, Zipes DP, Libby P [eds]: Heart Disease, 6th ed. Philadelphia: WB Saunders, 2001, p 273, with permission from the American College of Cardiology Foundation.)*

time-activity curve as the bolus enters the pulmonary circulation, with a subsequent rapid falloff before recirculation. In the presence of a significant left-to-right shunt, activity will remain in the lung, and pulmonary washout will be relatively slow. The degree of shunting measured by this technique correlates well with other standard techniques. While this technique remains a viable option, it is clear that Doppler echocardiographic techniques are the method of choice and the most widely applied technology for assessing shunts.

Comparison of First-Pass and Equilibrium Techniques

There clearly are advantages and limitations to each approach. It is generally recommended that a particular laboratory use the technique with which it has greatest familiarity and experience and for which equipment is optimized. With respect to direct comparisons, several issues are relevant. ERNA allows multiple studies to be performed from a single injection. This simplifies performance of combined rest and exercise studies as well as same-day therapeutic intervention studies. Regional functional analysis can be done with much greater qualitative and quantitative accuracy using ERNA. The statistical reliability of the high count rate ERNA studies is superior to FPRNA techniques. The entire blood pool is visualized. Consequently, one may get insight into abnormalities in other cardiovascular structures. FPRNA is the best approach to evaluating right ventricular function. It can also be combined with perfusion analysis using technetium tracers. FPRNA can be done far more rapidly and consequently can improve patient throughput in the laboratory.

CLINICAL APPLICATIONS

Resting Ventricular Performance

Measurement of left and right ventricular performance in the resting state provides important insight with respect to a large number of cardiovascular conditions. This includes prognosis in both coronary and noncoronary cardiovascular disease.[8,56,64] Evaluation of global left ventricular function can assist in therapeutic decisions ranging from implantation of automatic internal defibrillators[64] to monitoring of cancer chemotherapy (see Chapter 24).[66,67] Distinction can be made between systolic and diastolic heart failure (see Chapter 23).[68–72] Assessment can be made of relative chamber sizes, thereby providing reasonable inferences concerning the hemodynamic relevance of valvular lesions. Distinction can be made between cardiac and pulmonary etiologies of symptoms.

Coronary Artery Disease

Perhaps the widest clinical application of resting radionuclide ventricular function studies has involved the assessment of patients with both acute and stable coronary artery disease. Numerous reports over several

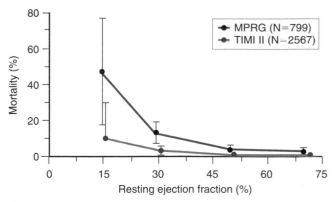

Figure 12-8 Relationship of ejection fraction at rest to cardiac mortality in the thrombolysis and myocardial infarction (TIMI) phase II study *(blue circles)* and the Multicenter Post Infarction Research Group Study (MPRG; *purple circles*). Note the comparable shape of both mortality curves and a significantly lower mortality associated with lower ejection fraction levels in the TIMI II study. *(Modified from Wackers FJTh, Soufer R, Zaret BL: Nuclear cardiology. In Braunwald E, Zipes DP, Libby P [eds]: Heart Disease, 6th ed. Philadelphia: WB Saunders, 2001, p 273, with permission of the American College of Cardiology Foundations.)*

decades have documented the importance of left ventricular function at rest as an important prognostic indicator in patients with coronary artery disease, with or without documented prior myocardial infarction.[69–77] This prognostic importance has transcended the therapeutic approaches available in any one clinical era (Fig. 12-8). This evaluation was first established over 3 decades ago in the coronary artery surgery study (CASS), where the importance of prognostic stratification based on ejection fraction in patients with multivessel disease was first noted.[78] In the present era, the relevance of ejection fraction in defining the need for placement of internal defibrillators following acute myocardial infarction has also been well established and has led to a major paradigm shift in how such patients are approached.[65]

Exercise Studies

A large volume of information has been generated concerning the value of exercise ventricular performance utilizing either ERNA or FPRNA techniques.[56,64] Exercise may be performed in supine, semisupine, or upright positions. In patients with coronary artery disease, measurements during exercise may be expressed either in absolute terms of the exercise ejection fraction or as the change in ejection fraction from rest to exercise (Δ LVEF). Specific prognostic levels vary among studies.[79–91] However, in general, risk of either death or myocardial infarction is at least 5% per year when (Δ) ejection fraction involves a decrease of 5% or more (in absolute numbers; Fig. 12-9).[92] Data are parallel using absolute LVEF during exercise, with a cut level being less than 30%.[93] However, despite these excellent results, exercise ventricular function studies are currently not widely performed and have been largely replaced by either exercise myocardial perfusion SPECT or stress echocardiography (see Chapters 13, 15, and 17).

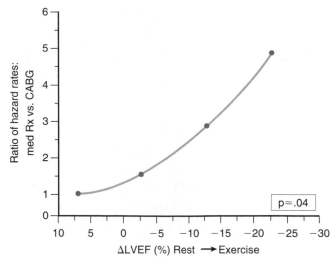

Figure 12-9 Relation of baseline ischemic severity to benefit coronary bypass surgery among 167 patients with three-vessel coronary disease. *P* value reflects differences among cardiac-event hazard ratios for death or myocardial infarction derived from non-bypass-treated versus bypass-treated patients, stratified according to sequential 10% increments of change in left ventricular ejection fraction (ΔLVEF) from rest to exercise at initial study. *(From Borer JS, Supino P: Equilibrium imaging. In Iskandrian AE, Verani MS [eds]: Nuclear Cardiac Imaging. Principles and Applications, 3rd ed. London: Oxford University Press, 2003, p 346.)*

Silent Myocardial Ischemia

Prognosis in ischemia appears to be comparable whether symptoms are present or not. This has been noted over decades with exercise studies.[94] Using ambulatory ventricular function, silent myocardial ischemia can be readily evaluated. This has been noted during routine activities as well as under conditions of mental stress (see Chapter 25).[35,95–98]

Valvular Heart Disease

It is recognized that both diagnosis and accurate assessment of hemodynamic severity in valvular heart disease are best accomplished by echocardiography and Doppler techniques. Nevertheless, important prognostic information can be obtained utilizing radionuclide approaches, particularly with exercise.[99] In aortic regurgitation, left ventricular ejection fraction at rest is a primary determinant of prognosis. Abnormal ejection fraction, even in the absence of symptoms, is considered an indication for valve surgery.[100] Changes in ejection fraction with exercise also have provided important information concerning prognosis in patients with asymptomatic aortic regurgitation and normal ventricular function at rest.[101] This parameter is even more accurate when combined with echocardiographically defined wall stress, in the form of a new myocardial contractility index (Fig. 12-10).[102] Borer and colleagues demonstrated that this particular measurement is more predictive with respect to outcomes than either radionuclide or echocardiographic measures alone.

In mitral regurgitation, measurement of right and left ventricular ejection fraction can also have important

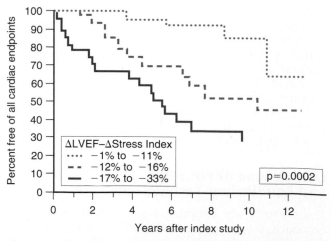

Figure 12-10 Relationship of myocardial contractility index to occurrence of any cardiac endpoint over follow-up. *(From Borer JS, Supino P: Equilibrium imaging. In Iskandrian AE, Verani MS [eds]: Nuclear Cardiac Imaging. Principles and Applications, 3rd ed. London: Oxford University Press, 2003, p 346.)*

applications with respect to assessing outcome. Because in mitral regurgitation there is unloading of the left ventricle by virtue of the pathophysiology of the specific valvular lesion, greater hemodynamic stress is placed on the right ventricle. Consequently, it has been suggested that right ventricular ejection fraction at rest and/or exercise is a more sensitive indicator of prognosis in this condition (Fig. 12-11).[103–105] It is also recognized that right ventricular ejection fraction is extremely sensitive to changes in the afterload conditions faced by this chamber.[25,106] The interaction of measures of both left and right ventricular ejection fraction can play an important role in assessing prognosis in patients with mitral regurgitation.

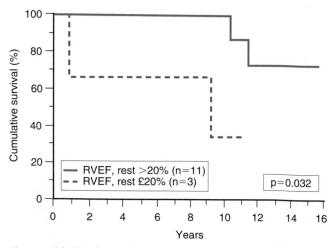

Figure 12-11 Survival in operated patients with mitral regurgitation and left ventricular ejection fraction less than or equal to 30% as a function of right ventricular ejection fraction. *(From Wencker D, Borer JS, Hochreiter C, et al: Preoperative predictors of late post-operative outcome among patients with nonischemic mitral regurgitation with "high risk" descriptors, and comparison with unoperated patients. Cardiology 93:37, 2000, with permission from S. Karger AG, Basel.)*

Congestive Heart Failure

Analysis of right and left ventricular ejection fraction plays an important role in the assessment of patients with known or presumed heart failure (see Chapter 23). Resting studies allow assessment of systolic versus diastolic dysfunction. Assessment of relative chamber sizes may provide additional insight into both the hemodynamic impact of silent valvular disease and the results of intervention. Serial measures at rest provide important insights into monitoring chemotherapeutic cardiotoxic effects (see Chapter 24). Assessment of global function can play an important role in patient selection for cardiac transplantation or ventricular assist device implantation.

Measurements of ejection fraction currently play a substantial role in defining suitability for implantation of cardioverter-defibrillators. Based on a number of major clinical trials, a clear-cut survival benefit has been demonstrated in individuals who have sustained a myocardial infarction or who have chronic congestive heart failure with substantial depressions in ejection fraction.[106] Clearly the ability of the nuclear procedure to define ejection fraction in most precise terms would make this the most suitable modality for evaluating such patients.

Phase analysis has been used in two studies to assess the impact of biventricular pacing on interventricular and intraventricular dyssynchrony in patients with cardiomyopathy. Kerwin and colleagues evaluated a small series of patients with dilated cardiomyopathy and intraventricular conduction delay before and after biventricular pacing.[33] The degree of interventricular dyssynchrony as measured by phase analysis present at baseline correlated with left ventricular ejection fraction. During biventricular pacing, interventricular dyssynchrony decreased. Left ventricular ejection fraction increased in all patients with biventricular pacing and the increment in ejection fraction correlated with improvement in interventricular dyssynchrony (Fig. 12-12).

Fauchier and colleagues evaluated 103 patients with idiopathic dilated cardiomyopathy.[34] Patients were studied with phase ERNA and followed up for a mean of 27 ± 23 months. Eighteen patients had a major cardiac event. The degree of left and right ventricular dyssynchrony and QRS duration were predictors of cardiac events. However, the degree of interventricular dyssynchrony was not. The degree of left ventricular intraventricular dyssynchrony was an independent predictor of future cardiac events.

Chronic Obstructive Pulmonary Disease

The use of first-pass technology for monitoring right ventricular function can play an important role in assessing the hemodynamic consequences of longstanding lung disease. Since right ventricular performance is extremely afterload dependent, these measurements can provide important insights into associated pulmonary hypertension and its concomitant effects in patients with pulmonary disease.[24,25]

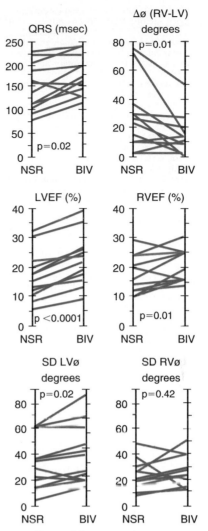

Figure 12-12 Effect of biventricular pacing on measured parameters. BiV, atrial sensed biventricular pacing; Δ ø (RV − LV), difference in RV and LV mean phase angles; LVEF, left ventricular ejection fraction; NSR, normal sinus rhythm; RVFF, right ventricular ejection fraction; SDLV ø, standard deviation of LV mean phase angle; SDRV ø, standard deviation of RV mean phase angle. *(From Kerwin WF, Botvinick EH, O'Connell JW, et al: Ventricular contraction abnormalities in dilated cardiomyopathy: Effect of biventricular pacing to correct interventricular dyssynchrony, J Am Coll Cardiol 35:1221, 2000.)*

REFERENCES

1. Blumgart HL, Weiss S: Studies on the velocity of blood flow. VII: The pulmonary circulation time in normal resting individuals, *J Clin Invest* 4:399, 1927.
2. Strauss WH, Zaret BL, Hurley PJ, et al: A scintigraphic method for measuring left ventricular ejection fraction in man without cardiac catheterization, *Am J Cardiol* 28:575, 1971.
3. Zaret BL, Strauss HW, Hurley PJ, et al: A noninvasive scintiphotographic method for detecting regional ventricular dysfunction in man, *N Engl J Med* 284:1165, 1971.
4. Folse R, Braunwald E: Determination of fraction of left ventricular volume ejected per beat and of ventricular end-diastolic and residual volumes, *Circulation* 25:674, 1962.
5. Hoffmann G, Kleine N: Die methode der radiokardiographischen funktions analyse, *Nuklearmedizin* 7:350, 1968.
6. Bacharach SL, Green MV, Borer JS, et al: ECG-gated scintillation probe measurement of left ventricular function, *J Nucl Med* 18:1176, 1977.
7. Van Dyke DC, Anger HO, Sullivan RW, et al: Cardiac evaluation for radioisotope dynamics, *J Nucl Med* 13:585, 1972.

8. Wackers FJTh, Soufer R, Zaret BL: Nuclear cardiology. In Braunwald E, Zipes DP, Libby P, editors: *Heart Disease*, 6th ed., Philadelphia, 2001, WB Saunders, p 273.

9. Corbett JR, Jansen DE, Lewis SE, et al: Tomographic gated blood pool radionuclide ventriculography: Analysis of wall motion and left ventricular volumes in patients with coronary artery disease, *J Am Coll Cardiol* 6:349, 1985.

10. Corbett JR: Tomographic radionuclide ventriculography: Opportunity ignored?*J Nucl Cardiol* 1:567, 1994.

11. Lu P, Liu X, Shi R, et al: Comparison of tomographic and planar radionuclide ventriculography in the assessment of regional left ventricular function in patients with left ventricular aneurysm before and after surgery, *J Nucl Cardiol* 1:537, 1994.

12. Groch MW, DePuey EG, Belzberg AC, et al: Planar imaging versus gated blood-pool SPECT for assessment of ventricular performance: a multicenter study, *J Nucl Med* 42:1773, 2001.

13. Harel F, Finnerty V, Nao Q, et al: *J Nucl Cardiol* 14:544, 2007.

14. Nichols KJ, Van Tosh A, Wang Y, et al: Validation of gated blood-pool SPECT regional left ventricular function measurements, *J Nucl Med* 50:53, 2009.

15. Callahan RJ, Froelich JW, McKusick KA, et al: A modified method for the in vivo labeling of red blood cells with Tc-99m: Concise communication, *J Nucl Med* 23:315, 1982.

16. Wackers FJTh, Bruni W, Zaret BL: Planar equilibrium radionuclide angiocardiography: Acquisition and processing protocols. In *Nuclear Cardiology: The Basics*, Totowa, NJ, 2003, Humana, p 81.

17. Bacharach SL, Green MV, Borer JS, et al: A real-time system for multi-image gated cardiac studies, *J Nucl Med* 18:79, 1977.

18. DePuey GE, Garcia EV: Updated imaging guidelines for nuclear cardiology procedures, part I, *J Nucl Cardiol* 8:G1, 2001.

19. Bacharach SL, Green MV, Borer JS, et al: Left ventricular peak ejection rate, filling rate and ejection fraction: Frame rate requirements at rest and exercise, *J Nucl Med* 20:189, 1979.

20. Starling MR, Dell'Italia LJ, Walsh RA, et al: Accurate estimates of absolute ventricular volumes from equilibrium radionuclide angiographic count data using a simple geometric attenuation correction, *J Am Coll Cardiol* 3:789, 1984.

21. Links JM, Becker LC, Shindledecker JG, et al: Measurement of absolute left ventricular volume from gated blood pool studies, *Circulation* 65:82, 1982.

22. Massardo T, Gal RA, Grenier RP, et al: Left ventricular volume calculation using a count-based ratio method applied to multigated radionuclide angiography, *J Nucl Med* 31:450, 1990.

23. Levy WC, Cerqueira MD, Matsuoka DT, et al: Four radionuclide methods for left ventricular volume determinations: Comparison of a manual and automated technique, *J Nucl Med* 33:763, 1992.

24. Zaret BL, Wackers FJTh: Measurement of right ventricular function. In Gerson MC, editor: *Cardiac Nuclear Medicine*, 3rd ed., New York, 1997, McGraw-Hill, p 387.

25. Shulman DS: Assessment of the right ventricle with radionuclide techniques, *J Nucl Cardiol* 3:253, 1996.

26. Maddox DE, Wynne J, Uren R, et al: Regional ejection fraction: a quantitative radionuclide index of regional left ventricular performance, *Circulation* 59:1001, 1979.

27. Zaret BL, Wackers FJ, Terin M, et al: Assessment of global and regional left ventricular performance at rest and during exercise after thrombolysis in Myocardial Infarction (TIMI II) study, *Am J Cardiol* 69:1, 1992.

28. Botvinick E, Dunn R, Frais M, et al: The phase image: Its relationship to patterns of contraction and conduction, *Circulation* 65:551, 1982.

29. Botvinick EH: Scintigraphic blood pool and phase image analysis: the optimal tool for the evaluation of resynchronization therapy, *J Nucl Cardiol* 10:424, 2003.

30. Botvinick E, Schechtmann N, Dae M, et al: Augmented pre-excitation assessed by scintigraphic phase analysis during atrial pacing, *Am Heart J* 114:738, 1987.

31. Munoz L, Chin M, Krishnan R, et al: Scintigraphic phase analysis in the study of ventricular tachycardia (abstract), *J Clin Res* 40:19A, 1992.

32. Botvinick E, Frais M, Shosa D, et al: An accurate means of detecting and characterizing abnormal patterns of ventricular activation by phase image analysis, *Am J Cardiol* 50:289, 1982.

33. Kerwin WF, Botvinick EH, O'Connell JW, et al: Ventricular contraction abnormalities in dilated cardiomyopathy, effect of biventricular pacing to correct interventricular dyssynchrony, *J Am Coll Cardiol* 35:1221, 2000.

34. Fauchier L, Marie O, Casset-Senon D, et al: Interventricular and intraventricular dyssynchrony in idiopathic dilated cardiomyopathy. A prognosis study with Fourier phase analysis of radionuclide angioscintigraphy, *J Am Coll Cardiol* 40:2022, 2002.

35. Zaret BL, Jain D: Monitoring of left ventricular function with miniaturized non-imaging detectors. In Zaret BL, Beller GA, editors: *Nuclear Cardiology: State-of-the-Art and Future Directions*, 2nd ed., St. Louis, 1999, Mosby, p 91.

36. Burg MM, Jain D, Soufer R, et al: Role of behavioral and psychological factors in mental stress induced silent left ventricular dysfunction in coronary artery disease, *J Am Coll Cardiol* 22:440, 1993.

37. Jain D, Burg M, Soufer R, et al: Prognostic implications of mental stress induced silent left ventricular dysfunction of patients with stable angina pectoris, *Am J Cardiol* 76:31, 1995.

38. Ciampi Q, Betocchi S, Violante A, et al: Hemodynamic effects of isometric exercise in hypertrophic cardiomyopathy: Comparison with normal subjects, *J Nucl Cardiol* 10:154, 2003.

39. Marshall RC, Berger HJ, Costin JC, et al: Assessment of cardiac performance with quantitative radionuclide angiocardiography: Sequential left ventricular ejection fraction, normalized left ventricular ejection rate, and regional wall motion, *Circulation* 56:820, 1977.

40. Baillet GY, Mena IG, Kuperus JH, et al: Simultaneous technetium-99m MIBI angiography and first-pass radionuclide angiography, *J Nucl Med* 30:38, 1989.

41. Williams KA, Taillon LA: Gated planar technetium-99m-sestamibi myocardial perfusion image inversion for quantitative scintigraphic assessment of left ventricular function, *J Nucl Cardiol* 2:285, 1995.

42. Elliott AT, McKillop JH, Pringle SD, et al: Simultaneous measurement of left ventricular function and perfusion, *Eur J Nucl Med* 17:310, 1990.

43. Boucher CA, Wackers FJ, Zaret BL, et al: Technetium-99m sestamibi myocardial imaging at rest for assessment of myocardial infarction and first-pass ejection fraction. Multicenter Cardiolite Study Group, *Am J Cardiol* 69:22, 1992.

44. Borges-Neto S, Curtis MA, Morris EI, et al: Combined Tc-99m sestamibi first-pass radionuclide angiography and cardiac SPECT imaging during arbutamine infusion delivered by a computerized closed-loop system, *Clin Nucl Med* 24:42, 1999.

45. Francis CK, Cleman M, Berger HJ, et al: Left ventricular systolic performance during upright bicycle exercise in patients with essential hypertension, *Am J Med* 75:40, 1983.

46. Williams KA, Taillon LA, Draho JM, et al: First-pass radionuclide angiographic studies of left ventricular function with Tc-99m-teboroxime, Tc-99m-sestamibi and Tc-99m-DTPA, *J Nucl Med* 34:394, 1993.

47. Lacy JL, Layne WW, Guidry GW, et al: Development and clinical performance of an automated, portable tungsten-178/tantalum-178 generator, *J Nucl Med* 32:2158, 1991.

48. Treves S, Cheng C, Samuel A, et al: Iridium-191 angiocardiography for the detection and quantitation of left-to-right shunting, *J Nucl Med* 21:1151, 1980.

49. Packard AB, Day PJ, Treves ST: An improved 1910s/191mIr generator using a hybrid anion exchanger, *Nucl Med Biol* 22:887, 1995.

50. Hellman C, Zafrir N, Shimoni A, et al: Evaluation of ventricular function with first-pass iridium-191m radionuclide angiocardiography, *J Nucl Med* 30:450, 1989.

51. Heller GV, Treves ST, Parker JA, et al: Comparison of ultra-short-lived iridium-191m with technetium-99m for first pass radionuclide angiocardiographic evaluation of right and left ventricular function in adults, *J Am Coll Cardiol* 7:1295, 1986.

52. Wackers FJ, Giles RW, Hoffer PB, et al: Gold-195m, a new generator-produced short-lived radionuclide for sequential assessment of ventricular performance by first pass radionuclide angiocardiography, *Am J Cardiol* 50:89, 1982.

53. Mena I, Narahara KA, de Jong R, et al: Gold-195m, an ultra-short-lived generator-produced radionuclide: Clinical application in sequential first pass ventriculography, *J Nucl Med* 24:139, 1983.

54. Elliott AT, Dymond DS, Stone DL, et al: A 195mHg-195mAu generator for use in first-pass nuclear angiocardiography, *Phys Med Biol* 28:139, 1983.

55. Fazio F, Gerundini P, Margonato A, et al: Quantitative radionuclide angiocardiography using gold-195m, *Am J Cardiol* 53:1442, 1984.

56. Williams KA, Borer JS, Supino P: Radionuclide angiography. In Iskandrian AE, Verani MS, editors: *Nuclear Cardiac Imaging, Principles and Applications*, 3rd ed., London, 2003, Oxford University Press, p 323.

57. Verani MS, Lacy JL, Guidry GW, et al: Quantification of left ventricular performance during transient coronary occlusion at various anatomic sites in humans: A study using tantalum-178 and a multiwire gamma camera, *J Am Coll Cardiol* 19:297, 1992.

58. Maltz DL, Treves S: Quantitative radionuclide angiocardiography: Determination of Qp:Qs in children, *Circulation* 47:1049, 1973.

59. Arheden H, Holqvist C, Thilen U, et al: Left-to-right cardiac shunts: comparison of measurements obtained with MR velocity mapping and with radionuclide angiography, *Radiology* 211:453, 1999.

60. Tian JH, Murray IP, Walker B, et al: First-pass radionuclide angiocardiography in the determination of left-to-right cardiac shunt site in children, *Cathet Cardiovasc Diagn* 8:459, 1982.

61. Baker EJ, Ellam SV, Lorber A, et al: Superiority of radionuclide over oximetric measurement of left to right shunts, *Br Heart J* 53:535, 1985.

62. Eterovic D, Dujic Z, Popovic S, et al: Gated versus first-pass radioangiography in the evaluation of left-to-right shunts, *Clin Nucl Med* 20:534, 1995.

63. Kelbaek H, Aldershvile J, Svendsen JH, et al: Evaluation of left-to-right shunts in adults with atrial septal defect using first-pass radionuclide cardiography, *Eur Heart J* 13:491, 1992.

64. Borer JS, Supino P: Equilibrium imaging. In Iskandrian AE, Verani MS, editors: *Nuclear Cardiac Imaging. Principles and Applications*, 3rd ed., London, 2003, Oxford University Press, p 346.

65. Moss AJ, Zareba W, Hall WJ, et al: Prophylactic implantation of a defibrillator in patients with myocardial infarction and reduced ejection fraction, *N Engl J Med* 346:877, 2002.

66. Schwartz RG, Zaret BL: The diagnosis and treatment of drug-induced myocardial disease. In Muggia FM, Green MD, Speyer JL, editors: *Cancer Treatment and the Heart*, Baltimore, 1992, Johns Hopkins University Press, p 173.

67. Jain D: Cardiotoxicity of doxorubicin and other anthracycline derivatives, *J Nucl Cardiol* 7:53, 2000.

68. Setaro JF, Zaret BL, Schulman DS, et al: Usefulness of verapamil for congestive heart failure, abnormal diastolic filling and normal left ventricular systolic performance, *Am J Cardiol* 66:981, 1990.

69. Bonow RO, Vitale DF, Bacharach SL, et al: Asynchronous left ventricular regional function and impaired global diastolic filling in patients with coronary artery disease: reversal after angioplasty, *Circulation* 71:297, 1985.

70. Bonow RO, Frederick TM, Bacharach SL, et al: Atrial systole and left ventricular filling in hypertrophic cardiomyopathy: Effect of verapamil, *Am J Cardiol* 51:1386, 1983.

71. Bonow RO: Radionuclide angiographic evaluation of left ventricular diastolic function, *Circulation* 84:1208, 1991.

72. Bonow RO, Bacharach SL, Green MV, et al: Impaired left ventricular diastolic filling in patients with coronary artery disease; assessment with radionuclide angiography, *Circulation* 64:315, 1981.

73. The Multicenter Post Infarction Research Group: Risk stratification and survival after myocardial infarction, *N Engl J Med* 309:331, 1983.

74. Rogers WJ, Papapietro SE, Wackers FJTh, et al: Variables predictive of good functional outcome following thrombolytic therapy in the Thrombolysis in Myocardial Infarction Phase II (TIMI II) Pilot Study, *Am J Cardiol* 63:503, 1989.

75. Cerqueira MD, Maynard C, Ritchie JL, et al: Long-term survival in 618 patients from the Western Washington Streptokinase in Myocardial Infarction Trials, *J Am Coll Cardiol* 20:1452, 1992.

76. Candell-Riera J, Permanyer-Miralda G, Castell J, et al: Uncomplicated first myocardial infarction: Strategy for comprehensive prognostic studies, *J Am Coll Cardiol* 18:1207, 1991.

77. Zaret BL, Wackers FJTh, Terrin ML, et al: Value of radionuclide rest and exercise left ventricular ejection fractions in assessing survival of patients after thrombolytic therapy for acute myocardial infarction: Results of Thrombolysis in Myocardial Infarction (TIMI) phase II study, *J Am Coll Cardiol* 26:73, 1995.

78. CASS principal Investigators: Coronary Artery Surgery Study (CASS): A randomized trial of coronary bypass surgery. Survival data, *Circulation* 68:939, 1983.

79. Bonow RO, Kent KM, Rosing DR, et al: Exercise-induced ischemia in mildly symptomatic patients with coronary artery disease and preserved left ventricular function, *N Engl J Med* 311:1339, 1984.

80. Clements IP, Brown ML, Zinsmeister AR, et al: Influence of left ventricular diastolic filling on symptoms and survival in patients with decreased left ventricular systolic function, *Am J Cardiol* 67:1245, 1991.

81. Mazotta G, Bonow RO, Pace L, et al: Relation between exertional ischemia and prognosis in mildly symptomatic patients with single- or double-vessel coronary artery disease and left ventricular function at rest, *J Am Coll Cardiol* 13:567, 1989.

82. Miller TD, Taliercio CP, Zinsmeister AR, et al: Risk stratification of single- or double-vessel coronary artery disease and impaired left ventricular function using exercise radionuclide angiography, *Am J Cardiol* 65:1317, 1990.

83. Supino PS, Wallis JB, Chlouoverakis G, et al: Risk Stratification in the elderly patient after coronary artery bypass grafting: The prognostic value of radionuclide cineangiography, *J Nucl Cardiol* 1:159, 1994.

84. Iqbal A, Gibbons RJ, Zinsmeister AR, et al: Prognostic value of exercise radionuclide angiography in a population-based cohort of patients with known or suspected coronary artery disease, *Am J Cardiol* 74:119, 1994.

85. Morlel M, Rozanski A, Klein J, et al: The differing prognostic utility of exercise radionuclide ventriculography in coronary artery disease patients with and without prior myocardial infarction, *Int J Card Imaging* 13:403, 1997.

86. Shapira I, Heller I, Isakov A, et al: Impact of early exercise radionuclide cineangiography on long-term prognosis after CABG, *Ann Thorac Surg* 64:473, 1997.

87. Griffin BP, Shah PK, Diamond GA, et al: Incremental prognostic accuracy of clinical, radionuclide and hemodynamic data in acute myocardial infarction, *Am J Cardiol* 68:707, 1991.

88. Abraham RD, Harris PJ, Roubin GS, et al: Usefulness of ejection fraction response to exercise one month after acute myocardial infarction in predicting coronary anatomy and prognosis, *Am J Cardiol* 60:225, 1987.

89. Zhu WX, Gibbons RJ, Bailey KR, et al: Predischarge exercise radionuclide angiography in predicting multivessel coronary artery disease and subsequent cardiac events after thrombolytic therapy for acute myocardial infarction, *Am J Cardiol* 74:554, 1994.

90. Roig E, Magrina J, Armengol X, et al: Prognostic value of exercise radionuclide angiography in low-risk acute myocardial infarction survivors, *Eur Heart J* 14:213, 1993.

91. Mazotta G, Camerini A, Scopinaro G, et al: Predicting severe ischemic events after uncomplicated myocardial infarction by exercise testing and rest and exercise radionuclide ventriculography, *J Nucl Cardiol* 1:246, 1994.

92. Supino PG, Borer JS, Herrold EM, et al: Prognostication in 3-vessel coronary artery disease based on left ventricular ejection fraction during exercise: Influence of coronary artery bypass grafting, *Circulation* 100:924, 1999.

93. Shaw LJ, Heinle SK, Borges-Neto S, et al: Prognosis by measurements of left ventricular function during exercise, *J Nucl Med* 39:140, 1998.

94. Bonow RO, Bacharach SL, Green MV, et al: Prognostic implications of symptomatic vs asymptomatic (silent) myocardial ischemia induced by exercise in mildly symptomatic and in asymptomatic patients with angiographically documented coronary artery disease, *Am J Cardiol* 60:778, 1987.

95. Burg MM, Jain D, Soufer R, et al: Role of behavioral and psychological factors in mental stress induced silent left ventricular dysfunction in coronary artery disease, *J Am Coll Cardiol* 22:440, 1993.

96. Jain D, Burg M, Soufer R, et al: Prognostic implications of mental stress induced silent left ventricular dysfunction of patients with stable angina pectoris, *Am J Cardiol* 76:31, 1995.

97. Kayden DS, Wackers FJ, Zaret BL: Silent left ventricular dysfunction during routine activity following thrombolytic therapy for acute myocardial infarction: A predictor of subsequent cardiac morbidity, *J Am Coll Cardiol* 15:1500, 1990.

98. Jain D, Joske T, Lee FA, et al: Day-to-day reproducibility of mental stress-induced left ventricular dysfunction in patients with coronary artery disease and its relationship to autonomic activation, *J Nucl Cardiol* 8:317, 2001.

99. Borer JS, Wencker D, Hochreiter C: Management decisions in valvular function and performance, *J Nucl Cardiol* 3:72, 1996.

100. Bonow RO, Picone AL, McIntosh CL, et al: Survival and functional results after valve replacement for aortic regurgitation from 1976 to 1983: Impact of preoperative left ventricular function, *Circulation* 72:1244, 1985.

101. Borer JS, Hochreiter C, Herrold EM, et al: Prediction of indications for valve replacement among asymptomatic or minimally symptomatic patients with chronic aortic regurgitation and normal left ventricular performance, *Circulation* 97:525, 1998.

102. Borer JS, Supino P: Equilibrium imaging. In Iskandrian AE, Verani MS, editors: *Nuclear Cardiac Imaging*, London, 2003, Oxford University Press, p 362 Fig. 17-22.

103. Niles N, Borer JS, Kamen M, et al: Pre-operative left and right ventricular performance in combined aortic and mitral regurgitation and comparison with isolated mitral or aortic regurgitation, *Am J Cardiol* 65:1372, 1990.

104. Wencker D, Borer JS, Hochreiter C, et al: Preoperative predictors of late post-operative outcome among patients with nonischemic mitral regurgitation with "high risk" descriptors, and comparison with unoperated patients, *Cardiology* 93:37, 2000.

105. Hochreiter C, Niles N, Devereux RB, et al: Mitral regurgitation: relationship of non-invasive descriptors of right and left ventricular performance to clinical and hemodynamic findings and to prognosis in medically and surgically treated patients, *Circulation* 73:900, 1986.

106. Brent BN, Mahler D, Matthay RA, et al: Noninvasive diagnosis of pulmonary hypertension in chronic obstructive pulmonary disease: Utility of resting right ventricular ejection fraction, *Am J Cardiol* 53:1349, 1984.

Chapter 13

Regional and Global Ventricular Function and Volumes from SPECT Perfusion Imaging

GUIDO GERMANO, SERGE D. VAN KRIEKINGE AND DANIEL S. BERMAN

The authors receive royalties from Cedars-Sinai Medical Center for algorithms incorporated in commercially distributed software that performs automatic quantification of perfusion, function and other cardiac parameters.

INTRODUCTION

Electrocardiographic (ECG)-gated myocardial perfusion single-photon emission computed tomography (SPECT) is one of the most frequently performed techniques in nuclear cardiology, and in 2007 it accounted for over 90% of all myocardial perfusion SPECT imaging in the U.S.A. Key to its diffusion has been the relative ease with which gated SPECT acquisitions can be accomplished, especially in conjunction with technetium-99m ^{99m}Tc-based radioisotopes, multidetector cameras, and fast processing computers. Gated myocardial perfusion SPECT (gated SPECT) permits the assessment and quantification of various parameters of global and regional function for the left ventricle (LV), which in turn translates into improved diagnostic capabilities and better prognostic power. This chapter will start by identifying and discussing a number of issues connected with the acquisition and processing of gated SPECT data sets, then quantification of global and regional LV function will be addressed in terms of different algorithmic approaches, validation, and practical limitations to quantitative accuracy. Finally, the incremental diagnostic value of gated SPECT parameters over myocardial

perfusion parameters will be described and evaluated. Their prognostic value will be addressed later in Chapter 16.

ACQUISITION

As Figure 13-1 shows, a gated SPECT acquisition is essentially equivalent to a standard SPECT acquisition, the only difference being that 8 to 16 projection images instead of one are acquired at each camera angle. Each of those 8 to 16 images is representative of a specific phase of the cardiac cycle, since count accumulation is triggered by the QRS complex of the patient's ECG wave. It is therefore possible to reconstruct three-dimensional (3D) tomographic representations of the LV's location and count distribution throughout the cardiac cycle and display them in rapid cinematic succession to achieve a realistic rendition of the four-dimensional (4D) LV motion (three dimensions plus time). Ideally it would be desirable that the number of gating intervals or "frames" employed be as high as possible so as to better follow changes in myocardial position and volumes; however, this consideration is balanced by the need for each projection image to contain adequate counts. Count statistics are influenced by numerous factors, including radioisotope used, injected dose, acquisition time, patient size, camera configuration and sensitivity, collimation, number of frames, and count acceptance criteria. For assessment of systolic ventricular function, gated myocardial perfusion SPECT has traditionally been performed using either 8-frame or 16-frame gating. We

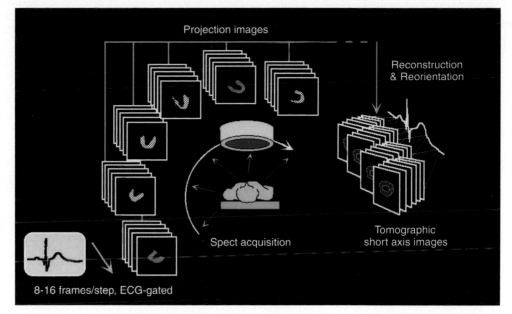

Figure 13-1 Schematic representation of ECG-gated perfusion SPECT acquisition and processing. *(Reproduced with permission from Germano G, Berman D: Acquisition and processing for gated perfusion SPECT: Technical aspects. In Germano G, Berman D [eds]: Clinical Gated Cardiac SPECT. Armonk, NY: Futura Publishing, 1999, pp 93-113.)*

prefer the latter, since it can more reliably than the 8-frame approach contain a frame that will correspond closely to true end-systole, important for assessment of systolic function, and because it has a greater number of diastolic frames, important for assessment of diastolic function.

Importance of "Bad Beat" Rejection

Since gated SPECT acquisitions involve the summation of ventricular function information from hundreds of cardiac cycles, the accuracy of the functional measurements derived from the method are dependent on the degree to which the successive cardiac cycles are of similar length. Arrhythmias—particularly when due to premature ventricular contractions (PVCs)—can be a significant source of error in function measurements with this method. PVCs often reduce ventricular function and affect the systolic and diastolic timing of the beat as well as that of the successive beat. Virtually all arrhythmias, atrial or ventricular, if not addressed by "bad beat" rejection, have a profound effect on diastolic function assessment, which is derived from measurements of the rate of filling of the LV. Frequent premature beats also lead to selective reduction of counts in the last frames of a gated acquisition, rendering those frames inaccurate for assessing diastolic filling. In atrial fibrillation, variable beat length severely impairs the assessment of diastolic function, since diastole is the portion of the cardiac cycle demonstrating the greatest variability. However, since systolic time intervals are relatively constant with atrial arrhythmias, ejection fraction measurements by gated SPECT are usually considered to represent a reasonable estimation of the true average ejection fraction and remain relatively accurate in atrial fibrillation. Additionally, an inaccuracy even for systolic function remains unless both the arrhythmic beat and the successive beat are eliminated from analysis, owing

to the increased systolic function associated with the post-extrasystolic beat.

Cardiac Beat Length Acceptance Window as a Tool for "Bad Beat" Rejection

As explained earlier, the peak or R point of each QRS complex in the ECG triggers the binning of counts into projection images. If a "fixed temporal resolution framing" approach is employed,[1] usually based on a sampling of the beats at the beginning of a gated SPECT acquisition, all gating intervals will be set to the same temporal length. For example, in 8-frame gating, the 8 intervals will span 125 milliseconds each if the *expected* heartbeat duration (R-R computer) is 1 second (Fig. 13-2). Because the actual time between successive R points (R-R patient) typically varies during the course of the acquisition, and particularly because of the impact of PVCs on systolic function and the systolic and diastolic timing noted, if there is no "bad beat" rejection, an error in the function measurements will be embedded in the data, with the magnitude of the error being proportional to the frequency of the premature beats. To circumvent this problem, most computers used in the acquisition process have beat length tolerances built into the count collection process. This is done by defining a beat length acceptance window, which essentially specifies how much shorter (or longer) than its 1-second expected duration a cardiac beat can be to not have its counts discarded for purposes of assessing ventricular function. As Figure 13-2 shows, a beat length acceptance window of 20% allows accumulation of data from cardiac beats of 900 to 1100 milliseconds' duration. An acceptance window of 100%, on the other hand, allows accumulation of data from beats with duration in the range of 500 to 1500 milliseconds. Note that this is *not* equivalent to accepting 100% of the beats, which is instead consistent with having a window of infinite width.

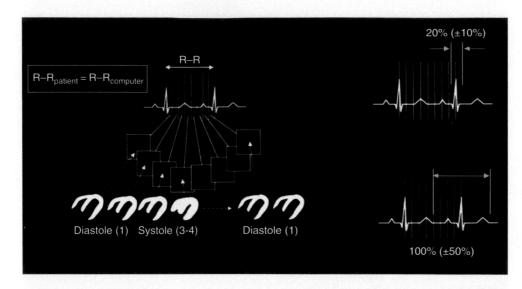

Figure 13-2 The cardiac beat length acceptance window. *(Adapted and reproduced with permission from Cullom SJ, et al: Electrocardiographically gated myocardial perfusion SPECT: Technical principles and quality control considerations. J Nucl Cardiol 5:418-425, 1998.)*

Figure 13-3 shows that a gated SPECT acquisition produces both gated SPECT images (through reconstruction and reorientation of the projection data sets corresponding to the individual gating intervals) and standard SPECT images (through reconstruction and reorientation of the sum of the projection sets across all intervals). Whereas cardiac function is assessed from the former, myocardial perfusion is derived from the latter. Since the primary purpose of gated SPECT is usually to assess myocardial perfusion, it is optimal to include all of the data in the perfusion assessment, not just data from the accepted beats. To this end, a useful option is an "extra frame" in which all counts "rejected" by being outside the acceptance window for purposes of gated ventricular function assessment are still accumulated and used for perfusion assessment, leading to optimal count statistics for perfusion assessment purposes and optimal beats for function assessment. Cameras with

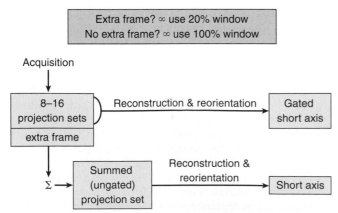

Figure 13-3 Setting the cardiac beat length acceptance window. *(Adapted and reproduced with permission from Germano G, Berman D: Gated single-photon emission computed tomography. In Iskandrian AS, Verani MS [eds]: Nuclear Cardiac Imaging: Principles and Applications, 3rd ed. New York: Oxford University Press, 2003, pp 121-136.)*

this feature allow the use of a narrow acceptance window, typically 20% to 30%. If, on the other hand, no "extra frame" exists, it may be advisable to open the acceptance window to 100% or infinity so as to maximize the quality of the images from which perfusion will be assessed. The downside of the wide acceptance window is that counts from arrhythmic beats are allowed into the gated SPECT images, decreasing the accuracy of cardiac function assessment. Most camera manufacturers today do provide the "extra frame" feature in conjunction with gated SPECT imaging, as currently recommended.[2] Another approach to the same end is to have simultaneous, independent acquisition of the gated and ungated data sets, a potentially optimal approach because it allows the use of a narrow window on the gated portion and no window at all on the ungated portion of the study.[3]

Gating Errors

If a wide cardiac beat length acceptance window is used in the presence of arrhythmias (e.g., the 100% window mentioned), some arrhythmic beats will not be rejected. A typical example of this problem is the "count dropoff" phenomenon, in which shorter cardiac beats, but not short enough to be rejected, do not contribute counts to the later gating intervals of a "fixed temporal resolution" acquisition; this in turn causes "flickering" of gated SPECT images displayed in cinematic mode (Fig. 13-4).

Excessive "bad beat" rejection can result in inadequate counting statistics for accurate function assessment from the remaining beats. In these circumstances, it is recommended that the ventricular function assessments not be considered valid. Examples of such arrhythmias are bigeminy, trigeminy, and frequent ventricular PVC couplets. In many laboratories, patients with more than 20% PVCs present are considered poor candidates for ventricular function measurements with gated SPECT.[4] To detect cases in which arrhythmias develop *during* a gated acquisition employing a wide window, however, additional quality-control

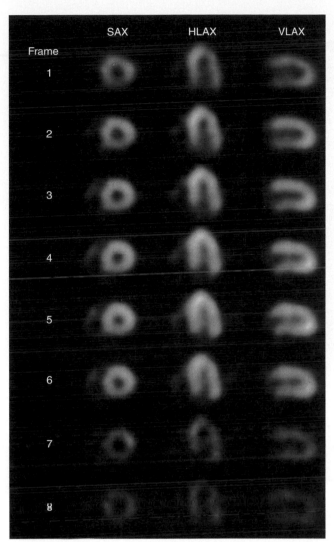

Figure 13-4 Example of the "count drop-off" phenomenon: Cardiac arrhythmias in combination with a wide cardiac beat length acceptance window cause fewer counts to be accumulated in frames 7 and 8 of this gated ^{99m}Tc-sestamibi SPECT acquisition, which in turn generates "flickering" when images are displayed in cinematic mode. HLAX, horizontal long axis; SAX, short axis; VLAX, vertical long axis.

strategies can be useful, including (1) the generation, from an independent heart monitor, of paper printouts of the patient's heart rate throughout the acquisition, (2) the use of software that aims at detecting gating errors from postacquisition analysis of the relative counts and count patterns in the various gated frames,[5] and (3) when provided by the camera manufacturer, the review of graphs of accepted counts or heart rate as a function of the projection angle, as well as beat length histograms (Fig. 13-5).

In addition to arrhythmia, gating errors can be caused by poor contact of ECG electrodes with the skin, resulting in noise, triggering off of a signal other than the R wave (e.g., an atrial pacing spike in patients with atrial pacemakers), and excessive patient motion, among other sources.

A simple yet effective quality-control tool that can easily be used postprocessing to identify gating errors is visual assessment of the time-volume curve generated by the quantification software available with most systems. A "canonical" curve would be expected to be approximately U-shaped, with the maximal volume (end-diastolic volume [EDV]) corresponding to the first gating interval, and the minimal volume (end-systolic volume [ESV]) slightly before the midpoint of the R-R interval (Fig. 13-6). If major deviations from this expected shape occur, the ECG gate has most likely sensed the R-R interval incorrectly or there have been excessive arrhythmic beats. As Figure 13-7 exemplifies, both arrhythmias and various gating errors are capable of causing severe deformations of the time-volume curve from which EDV, ESV, and left ventricular ejection fraction (LVEF) are calculated, naturally resulting in quantitative errors.

PROCESSING

As is the case with ungated acquisitions, projection images corresponding to the individual frames of a gated acquisition are tomographically reconstructed into transaxial images, which are in turn reoriented into short-axis images perpendicular to the long axis of the LV.[6] Projection images are typically smoothed before reconstruction to reduce statistical noise; this is most frequently accomplished using a Butterworth filter, which in the frequency (f) domain is described by the following equation:

$$B(f) = \frac{1}{1 + \left(\frac{f}{f_c}\right)^{2n}}$$

The degree of smoothing applied is proportional to f_c, the critical or "cutoff" frequency, and depends to a lesser degree on n, the order of the filter. The cutoff frequency can be expressed as a value either in the 0 to 1 range or in the 0 to 0.5 range, depending on the particular convention adopted[6]—in any event, it is generally agreed that gated images must be smoothed more heavily than ungated or summed images because they contain fewer counts. A summary of the filters settings used at the authors' institution can be found in Table 13-1.

Gated SPECT images are reconstructed using either the classic filtered backprojection approach, first described by Bracewell and Riddle for astronomical applications in 1967[7] and later extended to medical imaging by Shepp and Logan,[8] or iterative reconstruction techniques. The latter have the potential advantages of reducing reconstruction artifacts caused by hepatic or other extracardiac activity,[9] as well as the ease of incorporation of attenuation correction and other compensations into the reconstruction process. Iterative techniques are intrinsically slower than filtered backprojection; however, the speed of modern computers makes it both practical and advisable to reconstruct gated and ungated data sets using the same iterative reconstruction approach.

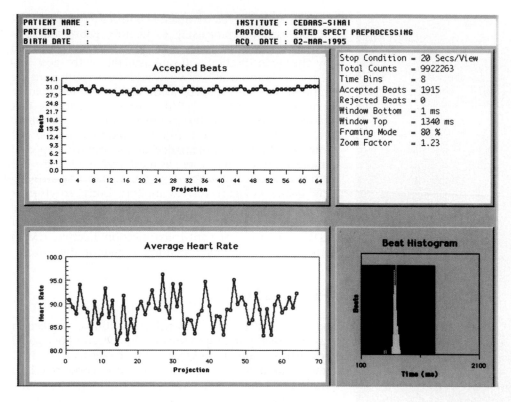

Figure 13-5 Graphs of accepted beats and heart rate as a function of the projection number. Together with the cardiac beat length histogram, these tools are useful to assess the reliability of the gated data sets. Gating errors are more likely to have occurred if the graphs do not show a uniform function, or if the histogram is wide or bimodal. *(Reproduced with permission from Germano G, Berman D: Acquisition and processing for gated perfusion SPECT: Technical aspects. In Germano G, Berman D [eds]: Clinical Gated Cardiac SPECT. Armonk, NY: Futura Publishing, 1999, pp 93-113.)*

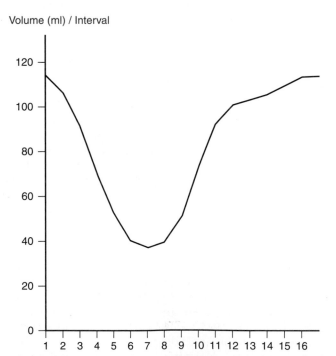

Figure 13-6 "Canonical" shape of the time-volume curve for a 16-frame gated SPECT study of a patient with normal LV function.

Automated algorithms to filter, reconstruct, and reorient gated SPECT images are widely available in modern nuclear cardiology[10–13] and can greatly improve the accuracy and reproducibility of processing. One particularly useful feature of these approaches is that even though different filter cutoffs are used (see Table 13-1 and Fig. 13-8), the same reconstruction limits (see Fig. 13-8) and reorientation angles (Fig. 13-9) can be applied in lockstep to the gated and ungated image data sets, improving consistency between the perfusion and the function assessment.

QUANTIFICATION

Gated perfusion SPECT images can be quantitatively analyzed with respect to a remarkable number of parameters of cardiac function, both global and regional, both systolic and diastolic. As Table 13-2 shows, global systolic function is typically characterized by measurement of the LVEF, EDV and ESV, whereas global diastolic function is similarly defined by assessment of the peak filling rate, time to PFR, peak ejection rate, time to PER, and mean filling fraction MFR/3. Regional parameters of LV function include myocardial wall motion and wall thickening. When these are semiquantitatively scored using a segmental model, the individual segment scores can be added to generate a global or summed wall motion score and a summed wall thickening score. Quantitative phase analysis can also be performed both in a global manner (synchrony of contraction of the LV as a whole) or regionally as the difference between the onset of contraction in different myocardial walls.

Gated SPECT imaging also offers interesting potential advantages, such as the ability to "freeze" LV motion so as to better identify mild perfusion defects,[14–16] as

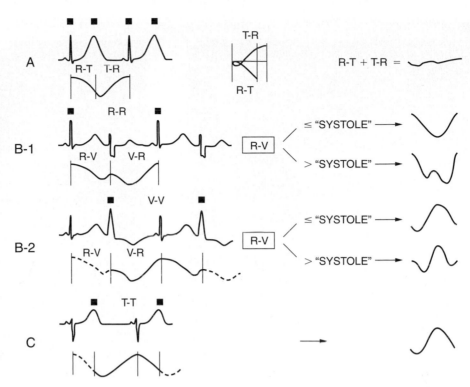

Figure 13-7 Potential errors in electrocardiographic (ECG) gating. If the ECG gate senses the R-R interval incorrectly, an erroneous time-volume curve will be produced. **A,** Both T and R waves trigger the ECG gate. **B,** The original R waves are sensed for B-1, and the ventricular premature beats are sensed for B-2. Two entire cardiac cycles are involved in the sensed R-R interval for B-1 and B-2. **C,** The T waves are sensed instead of R waves. R-T, T-R, R-R, R-V, V-R, and V-V each represent an interval, respectively. V, ventricular premature beat; square, trigger for gating. *(Reproduced with permission from Kasai T, DePuey EG, Shah AA, Merla VC: Impact of gating errors with electrocardiography gated myocardial perfusion SPECT, J Nucl Cardiol 10:709-711, 2003.)*

Table 13-1 Butterworth Filter Parameters

	⁹⁹ᴹTc-BASED AGENTS		²⁰¹Tl-BASED AGENTS	
	Ungated	**Gated**	**Ungated**	**Gated**
Order	2.5		5	
Cutoff	0.3	0.25	0.25	0.2

Butterworth filter parameters employed at the authors' institution using the 0-0.5 cutoff range, a pixel size of 0.53-0.64 cm, and the dual isotope doses and acquisition times described in Table 1.
⁹⁹ᵐTc, technetium-99m; ²⁰¹Tl, thallium-201.
Modified and reproduced with permission from Germano G, Berman D: Acquisition and processing for gated perfusion SPECT: Technical aspects. In Germano G, Berman D [eds]: Clinical Gated Cardiac SPECT. Armonk, NY: Futura Publishing, 1999, pp 93-113.

well as the ability to measure *gated* transient ischemic dilation of the LV,[17] which in its ungated form has proven a highly specific marker of severe and extensive coronary artery disease (CAD).[18]

Recent years have seen the development and validation of numerous algorithms aimed at quantifying parameters of cardiac function from gated SPECT images, and it is indeed estimated that the overwhelming majority of institutions and laboratories performing gated SPECT imaging today also employ quantification to some degree. Although many of those algorithms are important for historical reasons,[19–27] only the four commercially available algorithms will be discussed in detail within this chapter. The algorithms are usually referred to as: (1) Cedars-Sinai's software, or "Quantitative Gated SPECT" (QGS), also a component of AutoQUANT; (2) Emory University's software, a component of the

Emory Cardiac Toolbox (ECT); (3) the University of Michigan's software, or 4D-MSPECT; and (4) Yale University's CQ software.

The Cedars-Sinai Approach: Quantitative Gated SPECT

This approach is entirely automated and based in the 3D space. It starts with the segmentation of the LV myocardium using heuristic image thresholding, binarization, and clusterification, followed by iterative cluster refinement using pixel erosion and pixel growing. When a mask consistent with the expected size, shape, and location of the LV is obtained, ellipsoidal fitting is used to define a new sampling coordinate system, along which rays are drawn and count profiles measured normally to the myocardium. These count profiles are fitted to asymmetric Gaussian curves. The Gaussians' maxima represent the midmyocardial surface, while the endocardial and epicardial surfaces are determined based on a phantom-determined fraction of the Gaussians' standard deviations, and the valve plane is determined by fitting a plane to the most basal myocardial points. Surfaces can usually be accurately determined even in the apparent absence of perfusion, thanks to count gradient continuity constraints. LV cavity and myocardial volumes are calculated for each gating interval as the number of voxels bound by myocardial surfaces and the valve plane, and cavity volumes are displayed in the time-volume curve, from which diastolic function can be assessed, while the LVEF is derived from the EDV and ESV.[28]

Myocardial motion is computed as the excursion of the endocardial surface from end-diastole to end-systole, and myocardial thickening is based on both geometric and

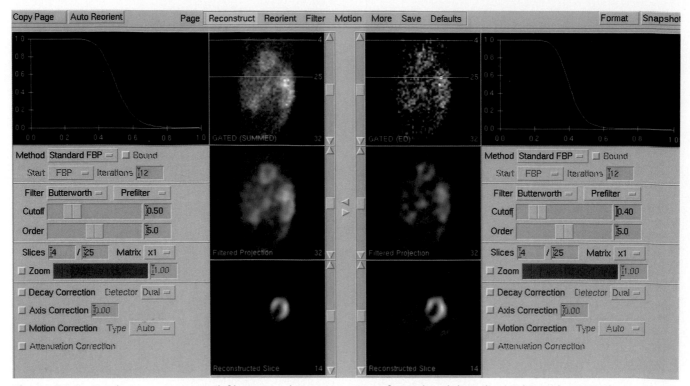

Figure 13-8 Simultaneous automated filtering and reconstruction of gated end-diastolic (*right*) and summed gated (*left*) projection images from a thallium-201 gated SPECT acquisition. Note that despite the difference in count statistics, the same reconstruction limits *(yellow lines)* are calculated for and applied to the two data sets. Cutoff frequencies are based on Table 13-1 but expressed using the 0 to 1 scale.

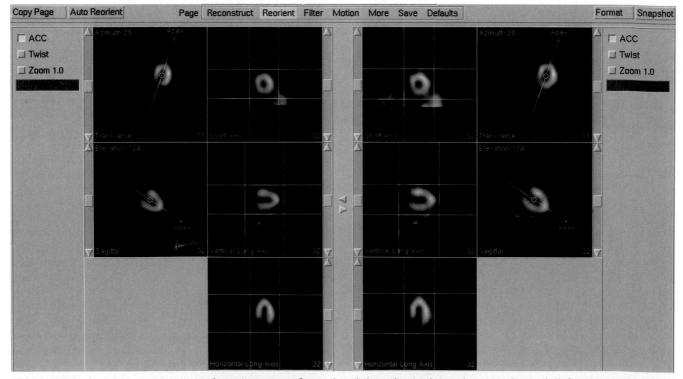

Figure 13-9 Simultaneous automated reorientation of gated end-diastolic *(right)* and summed gated *(left)* transaxial images from a thallium-201 gated SPECT acquisition. Note that despite the difference in count statistics, the same reorientation angles *(blue arrowed lines)* are calculated for and applied to the two data sets.

Table 13-2 Global and Regional Parameters of Systolic and Diastolic Left Ventricular Function Measured from Gated Myocardial Perfusion SPECT Images

Parameter	Systolic	Diastolic
Global	LVEF	PFR, TPFR
	EDV	PER, TPER
	ESV	MFR/3
	SWM	
	SWT	
	Phase	
Regional	WM	
	WT	
	Phase	

Global and regional parameters of systolic and diastolic LV function that can be effectively measured from gated myocardial perfusion SPECT images. EDV, end-diastolic volume; ESV, end-systolic volume; MFR/3, mean filling fraction; LVEF, left ventricular ejection fraction; PER, peak ejection rate; PFR, peak filling rate; SWM, summed wall motion score; SWT; summed wall thickening score; TPER, time to PER; TPFR, time to PFR; WM, myocardial wall motion; WT, myocardial wall thickening.

count considerations.[29] Synchrony of contraction can be measured for the LV as a whole, or as differences in the time of contraction of individual portions of the LV quantified.[30] Both myocardial motion and thickening can be visualized through various 2D and 3D cinematic displays, and motion and thickening scores are calculated automatically using normal databases.[31] A sample QGS display is presented in Figure 13-10, and a comprehensive description of the Cedars-Sinai approach can be found in Ref. 32.

The Emory University Approach: Emory Cardiac Toolbox

In this approach, maximal myocardial count samples are extracted at many locations about the LV during perfusion analysis for each gated frame of the study. Because of the SPECT point spread function, it is assumed that the maximum count value occurs in the middle of the myocardium at each sample. Therefore, these sample points define a midmyocardial surface at each frame. The frame where the volume of this midmyocardial surface is maximum is considered the probable end-diastolic frame, and the myocardium is assumed to be uniformly 1-cm thick at each sample of that frame.[33] Wall thickening through the cardiac cycle at each myocardial sample is determined by fitting the change in counts to a cosine function and computing its amplitude. The ED wall thickness value of 1 cm is modified according to the percent thickening curve to compute wall thickness for each sample in each additional frame. Finally, the endocardial or epicardial surfaces are estimated at each frame by subtracting or adding, respectively, half of the thickness to the midmyocardial surface at each sample. Using these surfaces, a final calculation of volume is made for the endocardial surface to determine end-diastole, end-systole, LV volumes, and LVEF. A phase histogram from which global dyssynchrony measures are derived is also generated from the phase angles of the fitted cosine curves for each sample point.[34] A sample ECT display is presented in Figure 13-11, and a comprehensive description of the Emory approach can be found in Ref. 35.

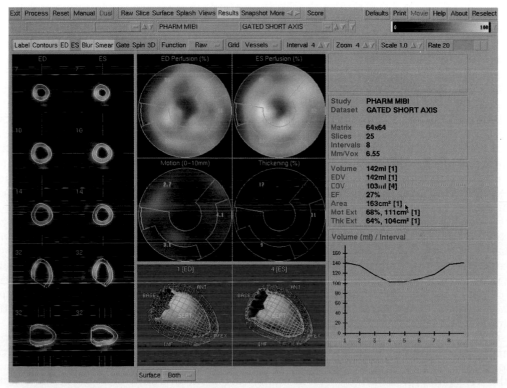

Figure 13-10 Representative display for Cedars-Sinai Medical Center's QGS software.

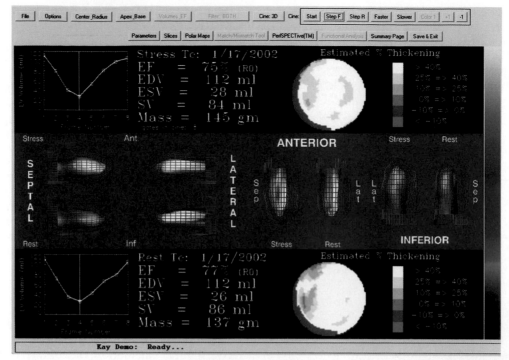

Figure 13-11 Representative display for Emory University's Cardiac Toolbox software.

The University of Michigan Approach: 4D-MSPECT

The surface estimation algorithm for 4D-MSPECT (4DM) utilizes a 2D gradient operator in conjunction with a segmented image and a contiguity constraint to provide initial surface estimates for the endocardial and epicardial surfaces. Weights are assigned based on measured intensity profiles within these initial surface boundaries. Using these weights and the estimated curvature of the heart, 2D and 1D weighted splines are utilized to "fill in" missing data (i.e., perfusion defects) while minimizing the inclusion of extracardiac activity.[36] Using the intensity profiles bounded by these new surfaces, a Gaussian fit is used to find the peak activity and an estimate of the myocardial thickness. To compensate for the limited resolution of emission tomography, the myocardial thickness at end-diastole (max endocardial volume) is scaled to provide an average thickness of 10 mm. This scale factor in conjunction with a myocardial mass constraint is used to adjust the myocardial thickness throughout the cardiac cycle. Using the endocardial surfaces, a volume curve is generated that spans the cardiac cycle. From the volume curve data, systolic (LVEF, volumes, cardiac output, myocardial mass) and diastolic (peak and time to peak filling, and ejection rates) parameters are calculated. For diastolic function, a minimum of 16 frames of data are required to provide adequate sampling or the harmonic fitting to compute to the diastolic parameters. Use of 4DM also provides 2D and 3D regional wall motion and wall thickening maps with database comparisons, wall motion and wall thickening segmented scoring maps,[37] and 2D and 3D cinematic displays for the visual interpretation of wall motion and wall thickening. To complement the functional

estimates, 2D and 3D analysis of the myocardial intensity information within the detected LV surfaces is compared with normal databases to quantify myocardial perfusion, thereby providing correlative information of perfusion with function for the improved diagnosis of CAD. A sample 4DM display is presented in Figure 13-12, and a comprehensive description of the University of Michigan approach can be found in Ref. 38.

The Yale University Approach

In this approach, gated SPECT images are preprocessed using a temporal filter. Then the "mid-wall" of the ungated LV is estimated according to cylindrical and semispherical models, using a maximal count search followed by a median search. The median count search is extended to all gated frames, with a basic thickness of 12 mm assumed for the gated myocardial sector in which the median count is detected, and homologous thicknesses in the other gated frames weighted by the ratio of the sector count to the median count. This calculation is implemented on all sectors. Endocardial and epicardial edges are determined for all gating frames by expanding a sector's mid-wall inward and outward, based upon the total counts within predefined endocardial and epicardial areas. End-diastolic and end-systolic volumes are computed from the total number of voxels enclosed in the endocardial edges, and the LVEF is derived accordingly.

Quantification of regional myocardial wall thickening is based on the generation of circumferential maximal count profiles for each gating frame, and measurement of count changes in each sector from end-diastole to end-systole.[39] End-diastole is defined as the

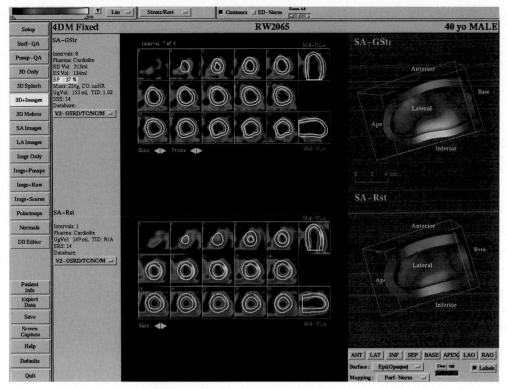

Figure 13-12 Representative display for the University of Michigan's 4D-MSPECT software.

first frame that corresponds to the R wave, and end-systole as the frame with maximal sectorial count density. The normalized maximal thickening profile is displayed in conjunction with the lower limit of normal wall thickening (mean thickening in normal subjects is 2SD). A sample Yale University display is presented in Figure 13-13, and a comprehensive description of the Yale approach can be found in Ref. 10.

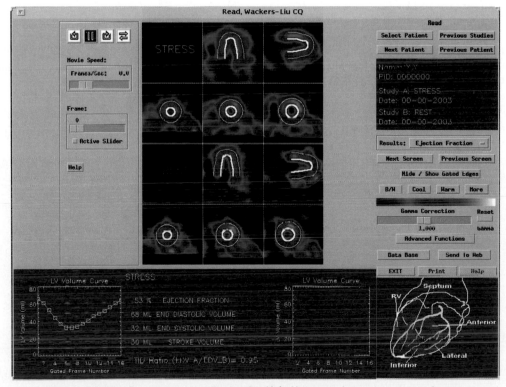

Figure 13-13 Representative display for Yale University's Wackers-Liu software.

EJECTION FRACTION

LVEF is typically measured using a volume-based rather than a count-based approach. In other words, the location of the LV endocardium is estimated in the 2D or 3D space, and the LV cavity volume is calculated as the territory bound by the endocardium and its valve plane. The process is repeated for every interval in the cardiac cycle, after which the EDV and ESV are identified as the largest and smallest LV cavity volume, respectively, and the LVEF derived as:

$$\% \, LVEF = (EDV - ESV)/EDV * 100$$

As Table 13-3 shows, the agreement between gated SPECT and reference standard measurements of quantitative LVEF is in the very good to excellent range and relatively independent of the isotope, protocol, standard, and algorithm used. Reproducibility (defined as the agreement between independent measurements of LVEF resulting from multiple applications of the same quantitative algorithm to *the same* gated SPECT study) is also excellent, being directly related to the degree of automation of the algorithm.[22,57,66,67]

Repeatability (defined as the agreement between independent measurements of LVEF resulting from separate applications of the same quantitative algorithm to different, but presumably equivalent, gated SPECT studies) is also extremely good, both for sequential studies[74-76] and for acquisition involving different isotopes,[50,52,58,76-79] injected dose and acquisition time,[80-82] acquisition orbit,[83] cameras,[84,85] number of gating intervals,[53] and patient position.[86,87] Moreover, the use of attenuation correction or resolution recovery in conjunction with gated SPECT imaging does not appear to greatly affect quantitative measurements of LVEF.[88,89]

Cross-algorithm reproducibility (defined as the agreement between LVEF values measured by different quantitative algorithms applied to *the same* gated SPECT study) has been reported to be in the very good to excellent range. However, it is also well established that systematic differences among algorithms do exist and effectively prevent the direct comparison (or pooling) of differently analyzed data.[55,59,90-95] Normal limits for LVEF are similarly algorithm dependent[55,73,96-100] and also gender specific,[98,100-108] as shown in Table 13-4 for the QGS software.

There are some limitations common to most algorithms connected with the quantification of LVEF from gated perfusion SPECT. For example, it is well known that the relatively low resolution of nuclear cardiology images may make it difficult to visualize small objects, such as the LV cavity of patients with small ventricles, particularly at end-systole (Fig. 13-14). This phenomenon, also referred to as *partial volume effect*,[26] will lead to the underestimation of LV cavity volumes (particularly the ESV), with consequent overestimation of the LVEF.[109-111] The problem can be alleviated through magnification of the LV either in acquisition (by employing a larger acquisition zoom) and/or in reconstruction (by employing zoomed centered or zoomed off-axis reconstruction),[111-114] or by applying numerical modeling and compensation of blurring.[115,116] However, a simpler solution is to discard the overestimated

Table 13-4 Normal Limits for Quantitative Measurements of Global Left Ventricular Function from 8-Frame Gated Perfusion SPECT Images, Using the QGS Algorithm

Gender	LVEF [%]	EDV [mL]	ESV [mL]	EDV [mL/m²]	ESV [mL/m²]
F	51	102	46	60	27
M	43	149	75	75	39

EDV, end-diastolic volume; ESV, end-systolic volume; LVEF, left ventricular ejection fraction.
From Sharir T, Kang XP, Germano G, et al: Prognostic value of post-stress left ventricular volume and ejection fraction by gated myocardial perfusion SPECT in women and men: Gender-related differences in normal limits and outcomes, J Nucl Cardiol 13:495-506, 2006.

Table 13-3 Clinical Validation of Quantitative Measurements of Left Ventricular Ejection Fraction Volume from Gated Perfusion SPECT

Algorithm	No. Reports	No. Patients	Gold Standard	Spearman's R	Isotope	References
Cedars	30 papers	1,846	First pass, MUGA, 2D echo, contrast ventricul., MRI	0.72-0.95	⁹⁹ᵐTc-sestamibi, ⁹⁹ᵐTc-tetrofosmin, ²⁰¹Tl, BMIPP	28,41-68
Emory	5 papers, 2 abstracts	238	First pass, MUGA, 2D echo, MRI	0.70-0.88	⁹⁹ᵐTc-sestamibi	33,49,57,59,67,68
Michigan	2 papers, 5 abstracts	347	MUGA, 2D echo, contrast ventricul., MRI	0.69-0.97	⁹⁹ᵐTc-sestamibi, ⁹⁹ᵐTc-tetrofosmin	36,55,57,67,69-71
Yale	1 paper, 1 abstract	171	First pass, MUGA	0.78-0.90	⁹⁹ᵐTc-sestamibi	72,73
TOTAL	**38 papers, 8 abstracts**	**2,602**		**0.69-0.97**		

BMIPP, [¹²³I]β-methyl-iodophenyl pentadecanoic acid; MRI, magnetic resonance imaging; MUGA, multigated acquisition scan; ⁹⁹ᵐTc, technetium-99m; ²⁰¹Tl, thallium-201.

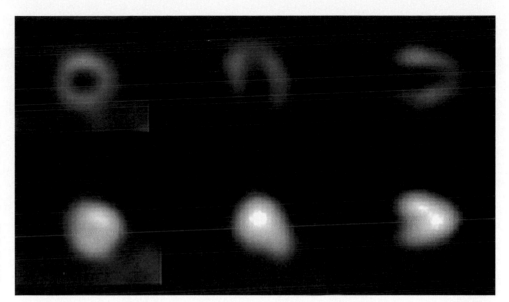

Figure 13-14 End-diastolic *(top)* and end-systolic *(bottom)* midventricular short-axis *(left)*, horizontal long-axis *(middle)* and vertical long-axis *(right)* images from a gated ^{99m}Tc-sestamibi SPECT study of a patient with a small left ventricle. *(Reproduced with permission from Germano G, Berman D: Quantitative gated perfusion SPECT: Technical aspects. In Germano G, Berman D [eds]: Clinical Gated Cardiac SPECT. Armonk, NY. Futura Publishing, 1999, pp 115-146.)*

value and report the LVEF as being "in the normal range."

Another limitation related to the partial volume effect is that nuclear cardiology techniques are incapable of measuring myocardial thickness with high accuracy. Most quantitative gated SPECT algorithms are either calibrated for the range of thicknesses most typically encountered in clinical practice[28] or assume a fixed myocardial thickness in the normal range[33]; consequently, gated SPECT LVEFs measured in patients with left ventricular hypertrophy are likely to be underestimated.[117]

Gated SPECT imaging traditionally has been performed with 8-frame gating, which undersamples the time-volume curve compared to 16-frame gating, and thus leads to mild underestimation of the LVEF. However, Figure 13-15 shows that the degree of underestimation is small (3 to 4 LVEF percentage points) and remarkably uniform over a wide range of ejection fractions, as also confirmed by other published reports.[28,53,54,56,118–120]

Finally, most quantitative gated SPECT algorithms tend to assume a regular or "smooth" LV shape in areas with severely reduced or absent perfusion,[28] and this would be expected to result in the "cutting off" of aneurysms, with consequent overestimation of the measured LVEF. Although a large number of published reports deny the presence of major discrepancies between true and quantitatively measured LVEF in patients with large perfusion defects and/or low LVEF,[42,13,45,46,48,50,56,121–125] the possibility of aneurysms should always be considered in the presence of perfusion defects.[69,126]

END-SYSTOLIC AND END-DIASTOLIC VOLUME

As Table 13-5 shows, the agreement between gated SPECT and reference standard measurements of quantitative end-diastolic and end-systolic volumes is in the very good to

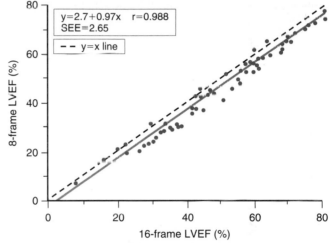

Figure 13-15 Left ventricular ejection fractions (LVEFs) measured by QGS on 65 patients, using 16-frame and 8-frame gated ^{99m}Tc-sestamibi SPECT, showing that the latter underestimates LVEF.[28] The correlation between the two measurements is excellent, and the standard error of the estimate (SEE) low, making their relationship quite predictable. *(Reproduced with permission from Germano G, Berman D: Quantitative gated perfusion SPECT: Technical aspects. In Germano G, Berman D [eds]: Clinical Gated Cardiac SPECT. Armonk, NY: Futura Publishing, 1999, pp 115-146.)*

excellent range and relatively independent of the isotope, protocol, standard, and algorithm used. These published findings are similar to those for LVEF (see Table 13-3), even though the LVEF can be considered relatively less vulnerable to errors in the EDV and ESV volume estimates (errors in the determination of EDV and ESV would be expected to occur in the same general direction and therefore would at least partially cancel out when the volumes are ratioed). As with LVEF, reproducibility is excellent,[28,46,66,67,74] and repeatability has also been reported to be extremely high, both for sequential studies[74] and for acquisition involving different isotopes,[58,76,79] injected dose and acquisition time,[80,81] number of gating intervals,[53] and patient

Table 13-5 Clinical Validation of Quantitative Measurements of Volumes from Gated Perfusion SPECT

Algorithm	No. Reports	No. Patients	Gold Standard	Spearman's R	Isotope	References
Cedars	20 papers	954	First pass, MUGA, 2D echo, contrast ventricul., thermodilution, MRI	0.67-0.94 (EDV), 0.75-0.97 (ESV)	^{99m}Tc-sestamibi, ^{99m}Tc-tetrofosmin, ^{201}Tl, BMIPP	41,44–47,49,55, 57–63,65,66, 127,128
Emory	4 papers, 2 abstracts	246	First pass, MUGA, 2D echo, MRI	0.85-0.97 (EDV), 0.91-0.99 (ESV)	^{99m}Tc-sestamibi	33,49,57,59,68,129
Michigan	2 papers, 1 abstract	105	MUGA, contrast ventricul., MRI	0.85-0.95 (EDV), 0.96-0.98 (ESV)	^{99m}Tc-sestamibi	57,69
Yale	1 abstract	Phantom				130
TOTAL	**27 papers, 4 abstracts**	**1,305**		**0.67-0.97 (EDV), 0.75-0.99 (ESV)**		

BMIPP, [^{123}I]β-methyl-iodophenyl pentadecanoic acid; MRI, magnetic resonance imaging; MUGA, multigated acquisition scan; ^{99m}Tc, technetium-99m; ^{201}Tl, thallium-201.

position.[86,87] Cross-algorithm reproducibility of LV volume measurements at ES and ED has also been reported to be very high,[57,94,95,99,129] although, as for LVEF, systematic differences among algorithms do exist and can be quite large.[59,90,92,94,95]

Limitations connected with the quantification of EDV and ESV are essentially the same as previously described for LVEF, with one additional caveat: Whenever the pixel size is set incorrectly in the image file header, volumes calculated by counting the number of pixels (voxels) corresponding to a given structure will also be incorrect, causing a more severe problem than with LVEF, where volumes are ratioed and errors tend to cancel out. A typical case in which this situation might occur is with hybrid camera-computer systems, where pixel size information is not properly transmitted from the acquisition computer to the processing workstation, and the latter sets it to a default value.

REGIONAL SYSTOLIC FUNCTION

The quantitative measurement of regional LV myocardial wall motion and wall thickening from gated SPECT images poses a unique problem. While it is certainly possible to measure (at many sampling locations) the absolute motion of the endocardial surface of the LV or the "brightening" of the LV myocardium from ED to ES,[29] these measurements are not as directly interpretable as regional measurements of myocardial perfusion. For example, neither myocardial wall motion nor thickening are uniform across the myocardium of a normal patient,[131] as shown in Figure 13-16, so dark areas in the motion or thickening polar maps cannot be considered a visual clue that myocardial function is abnormal in those areas. Indeed, it has been demonstrated that normal regional myocardial contraction by gated myocardial perfusion SPECT is characterized by a substantial apex-to-base decline in thickening and circumferential heterogeneity in endocardial motion (Fig. 13-17).[31]

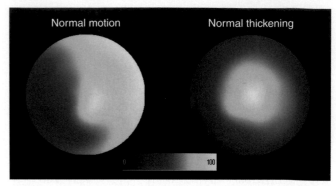

Figure 13-16 Polar maps showing average regional myocardial wall motion *(left)* and wall thickening *(right)* in 30 normal male patients undergoing post stress ^{99m}Tc-sestamibi gated SPECT. "Normal" motion is usually less (in absolute terms) at the septum compared to the lateral wall, whereas normal thickening is usually higher at the apex compared to the base. These patterns are independent of patient gender or radioisotope used. Unlike with regional perfusion, normal regional function does NOT result in uniform polar maps.

Validation of absolute quantitative measurements of regional myocardial function can be performed by comparing gated SPECT results to results from a high-resolution reference standard like MRI.[132] However, absolute measurements have greater clinical value if translated into an assessment of function abnormality through the development of region-specific normal limits[133–137] and criteria for abnormality.[31] Normal limits are usually developed based on an expert observer's classification of segmental motion and thickening using a semiquantitative or categorical scale and a multi-segment model of the myocardium. The standardized 17-segment model recommended by the American Heart Association[138] uses three short-axis slices (distal [apical], mid, and basal), with the apex represented by one segment visualized in a midvertical long-axis image,[139] and each segment is scored with a 6-point (motion) or 4-point (thickening) scale, as exemplified in Figure 13-18.

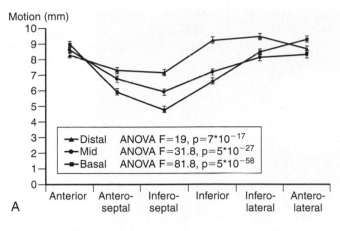

Motion (mm)

- Distal   ANOVA F=19, p=$7*10^{-17}$
- Mid   ANOVA F=31.8, p=$5*10^{-27}$
- Basal   ANOVA F=81.8, p=$5*10^{-58}$

A

Anterior / Antero-septal / Infero-septal / Inferior / Infero-lateral / Antero-lateral

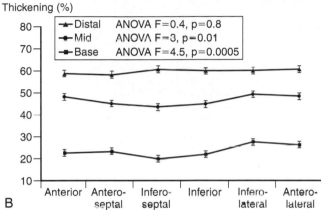

Thickening (%)

- Distal   ANOVA F=0.4, p=0.8
- Mid   ANOVA F=3, p=0.01
- Base   ANOVA F=4.5, p=0.0005

B

Anterior / Antero-septal / Infero-septal / Inferior / Infero-lateral / Antero-lateral

Figure 13-17 Circumferential variations in **A,** normal segmental motion and **B,** normal segmental thickening at distal ventricular, midventricular, and basal ventricular levels. *(Reproduced with permission from Sharir T, Berman DS, Waechter PD, et al. Quantitative analysis of regional motion and thickening by gated myocardial perfusion SPECT: Normal heterogeneity and criteria for abnormality, J Nucl Med 42:1630-1638, 2001.)*

Semiquantitative scoring of myocardial wall motion and thickening can now be generated automatically by computer algorithms based on normal limits and has been validated against reference semiquantitative visual assessment (Fig. 13-19).[31,37,139]

DIASTOLIC FUNCTION

While it is generally agreed that 8-frame gated SPECT imaging does not allow for meaningful measurement of LV diastolic function,[140] it has also been reported that 12-frame imaging may be somewhat adequate,[141] 16-frame imaging quite effective,[142] and 32-frame imaging feasible and resulting in excellent agreement with a MUGA standard.[51,53,54,143] As shown in Figure 13-20, parameters of LV diastolic function that can be quantitatively measured from gated myocardial perfusion SPECT images include the peak filling rate (PFR), the time at which the PFR occurs (TTPF), the peak ejection rate (PER), the time at which the PER occurs (TPER), and MFR/3. Normal limits for PFR and TTPF have been quantitatively determined by QGS from 16-frame gated SPECT images and proved very similar to those reported with gated blood pool studies.[144]

PHASE ANALYSIS

Phase analysis, initially described with nuclear cardiology methods in the 1970s, has reemerged as being of clinical interest in assessing the likelihood of benefit from and evaluation of the benefit from cardiac resynchronization therapy (CRT),[145,146] as well as for potentially evaluating and guiding internal cardiac defibrillators (ICDs). Phase analysis can be applied to gated myocardial perfusion SPECT or gated blood pool SPECT. In the former, when

REGIONAL WALL MOTION/THICKENING

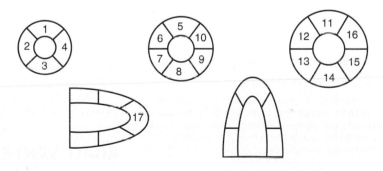

Figure 13-18 Illustration of the 17-segment model for semiquantitative visual assessment of gated myocardial perfusion SPECT. Scores are based on what is "normal" for a region.

WALL MOTION
0 = NORMAL
1 = MILD HYPOKINESIS
2 = MODERATE HYPOKINESIS
3 = SEVERE HYPOKINESIS
4 = AKINESIS
5 = DYSKINESIS

WALL THICKENING
0 = NORMAL
1 = MILD (EQUIVOCAL) REDUCTION
2 = MODERATE-SEVERE (DEFINITE) REDUCTION
3 = NO DETECTABLE THICKENING

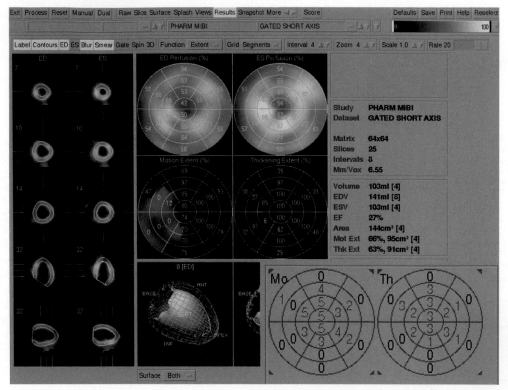

Figure 13-19 Quantitative gated SPECT automatic scoring of regional myocardial wall motion (Mo) and thickening (Th) based on the 20-segment, 6-point (motion) or 4-point scale (thickening) in a patient with severe cardiac disease.

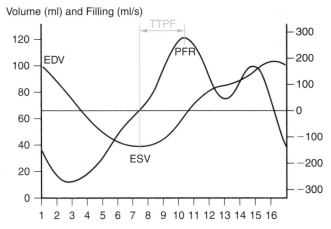

Volumes | **ED 103.5ml [16.2], ES 38.5ml [7.5]**

Rates | **PFR 2.66 EDV/s [10.4], BPM 69.2**

Misc | **MFR/3 1.36 EDV/s, TTPF 161ms**

Figure 13-20 Parameters of global diastolic left ventricular function can be readily quantified from the first derivative (*magenta curve*) of the time-volume curve (*in black*). (*Adapted and reproduced with permission from Germano G, Berman D: Quantification of ventricular function. In Germano G, Berman D [eds]: Clinical Gated Cardiac SPECT, 2nd ed. Oxford, UK: Blackwell Publishing, 2006, pp 93-137.*)

sampling the LV myocardium for the purpose of quantitative perfusion and function assessment, it is also straightforward to create two one-dimensional arrays for each LV myocardium sampling point, the first one containing the distance (amount of wall motion) between the mid-myocardial surface and a reference position for each gating interval, and the second one containing the myocardial thickness (distance between the endo- and epicardial surfaces normally to the mid-myocardial surface), also for each gating interval. Each array represents a time-varying, periodic function that can be reduced to its first fourier harmonic (FFH), in turn defined by its phase and amplitude.[147] Motion and thickening phase and amplitude for all the sampling points representative of the LV can be displayed in polar maps or global histograms, as shown in Figure 13-21, where thickening phase is compared between a low-likelihood patient and a patient with left bundle branch block. In addition, motion and thickening curves showing onset and peak of contraction can be derived and compared across different portions of the LV (segments, walls, coronary territories), which makes it easier to evaluate dyssynchrony between the lateral wall of the LV and the septum (Fig. 13-22). As previously mentioned, phase analysis calculations have been implemented in the ECT and the Cedars-Sinai software.

RIGHT VENTRICULAR FUNCTION

Quantitative assessment of right ventricular (RV) function is generally not performed with gated perfusion SPECT, because (a) the RV myocardium is thinner and on a per-gram basis has lower blood flow than the LV, so its perceived intensity of uptake is about 50% of that in the LV, and for that reason it is generally difficult to visualize, unless the patient has RV hypertrophy, and

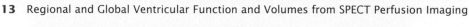

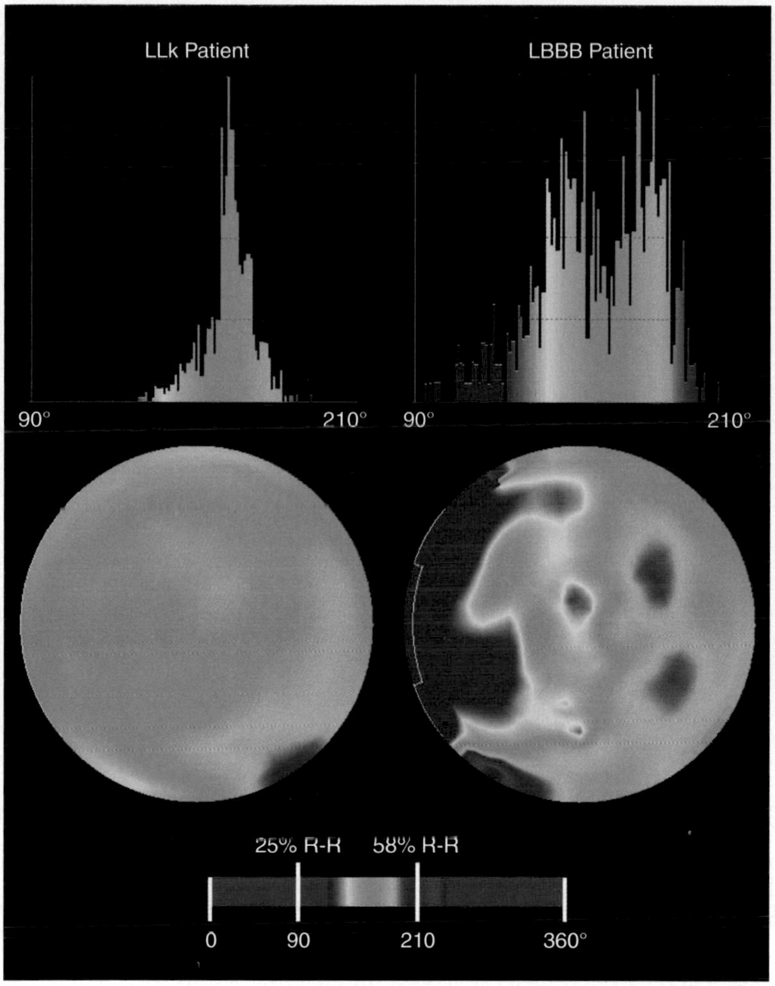

Figure 13-21 Comparison of global and regional thickening phase in a typical low-likelihood (LLk) and a left bundle branch block (LBBB) patient. The global histograms *(top row)* show overall increased dyssynchrony (histogram width or standard deviation) in the LBBB patient compared to the LLk patient. The polar maps *(middle)* demonstrate the differences in regional left ventricular contraction timing for each individual myocardial sampling point, with uniform contraction for the LLk patient and a clear septum-to-lateral wall delay for the LBBB patient, as evidenced by the red-to-green color shift. The color scale used for both patients *(bottom)* has been adjusted to emphasize contraction timing differences during a third of the cardiac cycle (25% to 50% R-R).

(b) the geometric shape of the RV is less straightforward to model than that of the LV.

Nevertheless, it is conceptually possible to apply to the RV algorithms similar to those used for LV function quantitation, determine RV myocardial contours even in non hypertrophic RVs (Fig. 13-23), and derive estimates of both RVEF and RV volumes. It is anticipated that RV quantitation will become an integral part of gated perfusion SPECT quantification, even though it is not currently widely available or fully validated.

BLOOD POOL SPECT

If tomographic assessment of both LV *and* RV function is required, the most widespread nuclear medicine technique available today for that purpose is gated blood pool SPECT using ^{99m}Tc-labeled red blood cells[148–151]; unlike with traditional gated blood pool planar imaging, no background subtraction is needed with the SPECT approach, since the LV and RV are well separated in the 3D space.

Most of the technical issues examined in this chapter with respect to the acquisition and processing of gated perfusion SPECT studies also apply to gated blood pool SPECT imaging. However, in blood pool imaging, no perfusion information is acquired, and therefore it is

advisable to always set the cardiac beat length acceptance window to 20% to 30% to minimize the effects of arrhythmia. With the use of 10% to 20% acceptance windows and 16-frame studies, assessment of diastolic function could be both feasible and accurate. Several quantitative algorithms have been recently introduced that aim at identifying the endocardial surfaces of the LV and (in a minority of cases) of the RV throughout the cardiac cycle (Fig. 13-24), so as to determine ventricular volumes and ejection fractions in a manner similar to gated perfusion SPECT. Although reported validations of these algorithm measurements are generally satisfactory,[132,152–179] the gold standards used are very often planar, and RV parameters are rarely validated. Still, the increase in computer speed, the greater diffusion of multidetector cameras, and the general acceptance of state-of-the-art 3D analysis and display techniques (Fig. 13-25) have already considerably strengthened the case for gated blood pool SPECT imaging. The clinical circumstances in which this procedure is likely to become effective are the same as those in which resting blood pool scintigraphy is currently applied. Chief among these is the assessment of Adriamycin cardiotoxicity. Blood pool scintigraphy is also commonly employed in serial assessment of patients with aortic insufficiency, congestive heart failure, and patients who have undergone cardiac transplantation.

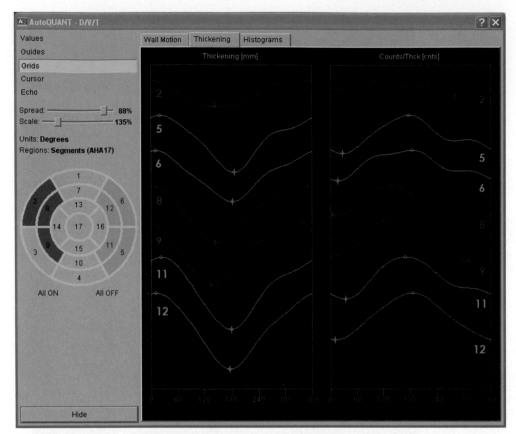

Figure 13-22 Comparison of segment-derived thickening *(left)* and counts *(right)* curves versus time in a typical patient with left bundle branch block. The vertical scales are omitted for clarity, and time is expressed in degrees from 0° to 360°. Curves that relate to the septal segments (2, 8, and 9) are drawn in *red*, and curves that relate to the lateral segments (5, 6, 11, and 12) are drawn in *green*. The polar map to the left of the graphs indicates the location of the selected segments. Peak contraction can clearly be seen to occur earlier in septal segments than in lateral segments, as demonstrated by the location of the minima for the thickening curves (which are flipped upside-down in this display to resemble time-volume curves) and the maxima of the counts curves (where counts are higher at peak contraction due to the partial volume effect).

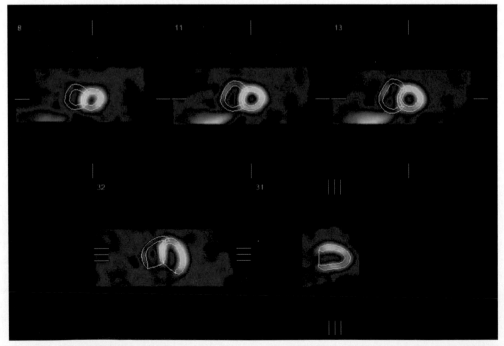

Figure 13-23 Left ventricular and right ventricular contours automatically determined for a gated myocardial perfusion SPECT study. *(Reproduced with permission from Germano G, Kavanagh PB, Slomka PJ, et al: Quantitation in gated perfusion SPECT imaging: The Cedars-Sinai approach. J Nucl Cardiol 14:433-454, 2007.)*

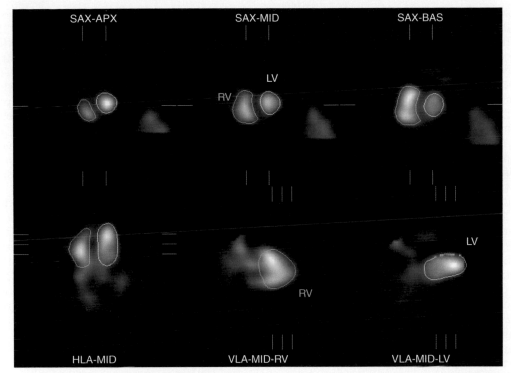

Figure 13-24 Reconstructed and reoriented short-axis (*top row; left to right, apex to base*), midventricular horizontal (*bottom left*) and vertical long-axis (*bottom center and right*, respectively, through the right ventricle [RV] and left ventricle [LV]) images for a gated blood pool SPECT study at end-diastole. Automatically determined and overlaid contours are displayed for both ventricles (*white*, LV; *yellow*, RV). *(Reprinted with permission from Van Kriekinge S, Berman D, Germano G: Quantitative gated blood pool SPECT. In Germano G, Berman D [eds]: Clinical Gated Cardiac SPECT, 2nd ed. Oxford, UK: Blackwell Publishing, 2006, pp 273-284.)*

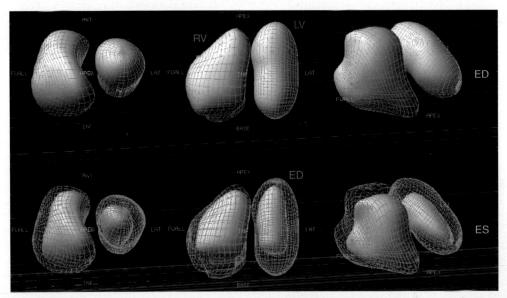

Figure 13-25 Three-dimensional representation of the left and right ventricles displayed in three standard orientations at end-diastole (*top row*) and end-systole (*bottom row*). *Shaded grey* surfaces indicate endocardia (*red grid*, LV; *blue grid*, RV), *green* grid indicates reference endocardial location at end-diastole. *(Reprinted with permission from Van Kriekinge S, Berman D, Germano G: Quantitative gated blood pool SPECT. In Germano G, Berman D [eds]: Clinical Gated Cardiac SPECT, 2nd ed. Oxford, UK: Blackwell Publishing, 2006, pp 273-284.)*

DIAGNOSTIC VALUE OF GATED SPECT

An important clinical role of myocardial perfusion SPECT stems from its ability to reduce the number of diagnoses deemed equivocal when based on perfusion assessment alone. The principal way in which this occurs is by defining the motion characteristics of segments with apparent nonreversible perfusion defects that are considered to possibly represent soft-tissue attenuation. The assumption is that regions with true perfusion defects that are nonreversible would contract abnormally, while those associated with attenuation artifacts would demonstrate normal motion and thickening. The incremental value of gated SPECT in this area was demonstrated by Smanio et al.,[180] who interpreted myocardial perfusion SPECT studies using (1) perfusion information and (2) both perfusion and regional function information in 285 consecutive patients undergoing same-day rest and gated post-stress ^{99m}Tc sestamibi SPECT. Based on a 4-point classification of perfusion (normal, borderline normal, borderline abnormal, and abnormal), 31% of the patients had a "borderline" interpretation using the perfusion images alone; when wall motion from the gated SPECT images was also considered, the number of borderline interpretations fell to 10% (Fig. 13-26). Of note, the increase in normal interpretations occurred mostly in the subsample of patients with a low (<10%) pretest likelihood of disease, whereas the increase in abnormal interpretations was associated with the subsample of patients with documented CAD, suggesting that the addition of regional myocardial function assessment to perfusion assessment was improving the diagnostic accuracy of SPECT imaging.

The differentiation of true perfusion defects from attenuation artifacts with gated SPECT has been shown to increase the specificity of myocardial perfusion assessment in a population of 115 women with known or suspected CAD (n = 85) or with a less than 5% likelihood of CAD (n = 30) undergoing nongated stress/rest ^{99m}Tc sestamibi plus post stress gated ^{99m}Tc sestamibi SPECT,[181] as well as in a mixed population of 91 patients (71 males) with equivocal fixed perfusion defects on stress/rest ^{99m}Tc tetrofosmin SPECT.[182] In the latter study, two independent observers classified the defects as true or artifactual in three separate steps, by visually assessing (1) the stress/rest perfusion images, (2) the stress/rest perfusion images plus the stress/rest rotating projection images, and (3) all of the above plus myocardial wall motion from the rest gated SPECT images. The main finding was that the diagnostic accuracy for each observer (measured by ROC curve analysis) increased at each step. Moreover, the κ coefficient of agreement between the two observers improved with each step, signifying an increase in interobserver reproducibility.

Since attenuation artifacts are relatively frequent in both women (mainly breast attenuation) and men (diaphragmatic attenuation), combining gated SPECT with attenuation correction might further improve the specificity of myocardial perfusion SPECT imaging. This has been suggested by preliminary studies,[183] although considerable concerns still exist concerning the cost, standardization, and validation of currently available attenuation-correction protocols.[184,185] If accurate and standardized attenuation correction could be achieved, however, its utilization in conjunction with gating could facilitate the diffusion of "stress-only" SPECT protocols in some types of patients.[186-190] In essence, if a perfusion defect is present and can be assumed to be real because of attenuation correction, and if the myocardial region corresponding to the defect contracts or thickens on gated SPECT,[191] the defect can be considered to be reversible and indicative of ischemia. As Figure 13-27 shows, in the gated SPECT with attenuation correction scenario, only patients with stress perfusion defects that do not contract or thicken would need to return for a resting perfusion study. This single-injection, single-acquisition protocol would offer advantages in regard to cost reduction and maximization of patient throughput, although it also would have the disadvantage of requiring a 2-day study in some patients, and possibly of decreasing the sensitivity associated with observing mild reversible perfusion defects, which might be interpreted as normal in stress-only protocols.

Myocardial wall motion abnormalities detected by postexercise gated SPECT may be a sign of prolonged postischemic stunning. Since exercise-induced stunning is considered to be a marker of severe ischemia and is usually related to a high-grade coronary stenosis, this finding can be of value in the attempts to use gated SPECT for risk stratification. Sharir et al. studied 98 patients who underwent nongated rest thallium-201/gated postexercise ^{99m}Tc sestamibi SPECT, with the latter acquisition commencing 15 to 30 minutes after exercise, and semiquantitatively scored both myocardial perfusion and function using a 20-segment model and a 5-point (perfusion) or 6-point (motion) scale.[192] These investigators found, and others[193] later confirmed, that in patients with normal resting myocardial perfusion, postexercise wall motion abnormalities are strongly associated with critical coronary stenoses. As a rule of thumb, approximately 90% of segments displaying this pattern are associated with a greater than or equal to 90% stenosis in the vessels supplying the segment. Sharir et al. also demonstrated that this "post stress stunning" had significantly higher sensitivity for the detection of severe CAD compared to severe perfusion defects. A mechanism by which to explain this finding is that perfusion SPECT images are normalized to the area of highest uptake within the myocardium, so that

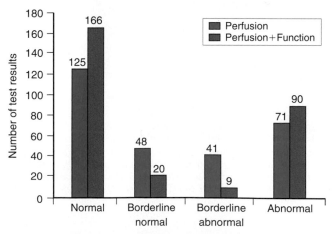

Figure 13-26 The incremental clinical value of gated SPECT relative to perfusion assessment alone is demonstrated by the reduction in equivocal diagnoses. *(Modified and reproduced with permission from Smanio PE, Watson DD, Segalla DL, et al: Value of gating of technetium-99m sestamibi single-photon emission computed tomographic imaging, J Am Coll Cardiol 30:1687-1692, 1997.)*

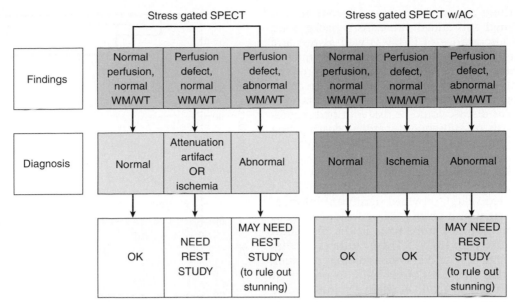

Figure 13-27 Role of attenuation correction in eliminating diagnostic ambiguity in stress-only gated SPECT protocols. AC, attenuation correction; WM, myocardial wall motion; WT, myocardial wall thickening.

in the setting of multivessel ischemia, only the most severely abnormal region shows a perfusion defect, because myocardial perfusion SPECT depends on a regional decrease in perfusion compared to the "normal zone" for perfusion defect detection. This phenomenon can lead to an interpretation of single-vessel rather than multivessel disease, even when the patient actually has multivessel ischemia. An extreme (albeit rare) generalization of this scenario pertains to patients with balanced reduction of flow due to triple-vessel disease (where image normalization might lead to apparent normal perfusion across the myocardium), with the clue to its presence being the finding of diffuse post stress stunning. Table 13-6 summarizes the ways in which gated SPECT improves diagnostic assessment.

Several studies have confirmed and added to these observations. Lima et al. demonstrated that the combination of perfusion and function (i.e., wall motion abnormalities) resulted in a significant increase in correct identification of multivessel CAD in patients with angiographically documented triple-vessel disease. The

addition of functional data from gated SPECT to clinical, stress, and perfusion information also yielded a significant increase in the prediction of triple-vessel disease.[194] Cullom et al. furthered this concept by showing added benefit of using gated acquisition during rest as well as post stress studies, demonstrating that a fall in ejection fraction on post stress is associated with higher risk. Following this work, it has become standard in our laboratories and many laboratories to use gated acquisitions as a routine for all gated SPECT acquisitions, even when the tracer employed is thallium-201 (rest or redistribution imaging), with its associated lower count rates.[4,195,196] Emmett et al. subsequently also demonstrated that combined rest and post stress regional wall motion abnormality added incremental value to perfusion defect analysis with gated SPECT for the assessment of the severity of angiographic CAD.[193] We have shown that gated SPECT wall motion assessment and EF assessment at the time of reporting adds to perfusion defect assessment in the correct classification of patients with left main CAD as being at high risk.[197]

Table 13-6 Role of Gated SPECT Imaging in the Assessment of Cardiac Disease

Detection of nonischemic cardiomyopathy
Identification of attenuation artifacts
  Increased specificity for coronary artery disease
Identification of post stress stunning
  Increased sensitivity in balanced ischemia
  Increased identification of multivessel disease
  Increased identification of severe stenosis
Detection of diastolic dysfunction

PROGNOSTIC VALUE OF GATED SPECT

Increasingly, the most useful application of myocardial perfusion SPECT is that of risk stratification and guiding management decisions, where the focus is not on predicting who has CAD but on identifying patients at risk for specific adverse events (cardiac death or non-fatal myocardial infarction) and guiding subsequent management to reducing the risk of those outcomes. Although there are fewer reports of the incremental value of function measurements from gated SPECT over perfusion in these assessments, several recent studies have documented this added value. As a background regarding the importance of LVEF, as well as rest and peak-stress end-systolic volumes measured by nuclear cardiology methods, a series of reports from the Duke databank using rest and exercise first-pass radionuclide angiography demonstrated that patients with suspected cardiac disease could be risk-stratified according to their risk of subsequent cardiac death using a diagnostic threshold of resting LVEF equal to 50%.[198–203]

Using the Cedars-Sinai database, Sharir et al.[204] demonstrated in 1680 patients that post stress LVEF, as measured by gated SPECT, provided significant information over the extent and severity of perfusion defect as measured by the summed stress score in the prediction of cardiac death (Fig. 13-28). These authors further demonstrated that LV end-systolic volume provided added information over post stress LVEF in prediction of cardiac death (Fig. 13-29). A relatively low cardiac death rate in patients with abnormal perfusion and normal LV function reported in this study is probably explained by a referral bias in which patients with greatest ischemia by summed stress score were preferentially sent for early revascularization and thus censored from assessment of the prognostic value of the test, whereas the referral bias was likely less prominent based on ventricular function. In a subsequent report in more than 2600 patients, Sharir et al. noted that while post stress EF provides incremental information over prescan and perfusion variables in prediction of cardiac death, the extent of ischemia was a stronger predictor of nonfatal

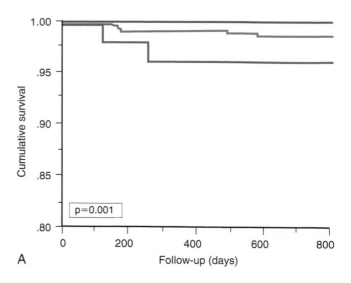

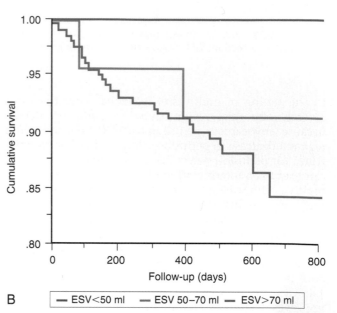

A

B — ESV<50 ml — ESV 50–70 ml — ESV>70 ml

Figure 13-29 Use of quantitative gated SPECT to measure cumulative survival of patients with post stress LVEF greater than or equal to 45% (**A**) and less than 45% (**B**) stratified by end-systolic volume (ESV), also measured by gated SPECT. *(Reproduced with permission from Sharir T, Germano G, Kavanagh PB, et al: Incremental prognostic value of post-stress left ventricular ejection fraction and volume by gated myocardial perfusion single photon emission computed tomography, Circulation 100:1035-1042, 1999.)*

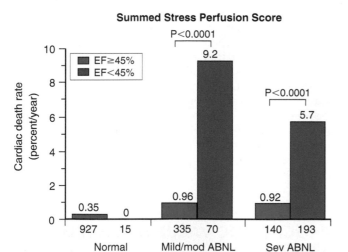

Figure 13-28 Cardiac death (percent per year) as a function of perfusion abnormality and post stress LVEF by gated SPECT. The number of patients within each category is indicated below each column. The categories for summed stress score are normal 0-3, mild/moderate 4-13, and severe >13. ABNL, abnormality; LVEF, left ventricular ejection fraction; MOD, moderate; Sev, severe. *(Adapted and reproduced with permission from Sharir T, Germano G, Kavanagh PB, et al: Incremental prognostic value of post-stress left ventricular ejection fraction and volume by gated myocardial perfusion single photon emission computed tomography, Circulation 100:1035-1042, 1999.)*

myocardial infarction. Once prescan and perfusion variables were known, post stress LVEF did not provide incremental information with respect to the risk of nonfatal MI.[205]

Sharir et al. further reported that the combination of the ejection fraction and reversible ischemia can be used in the prediction of cardiac events.[205] If post stress EF is less than 30%. Cardiac death or nonfatal MI rates appear to be high regardless of the amount of ischemia as assessed by the summed difference score. In patients with post stress EF of 30% to 50%, mild amounts of ischemia were associated with relatively high cardiac

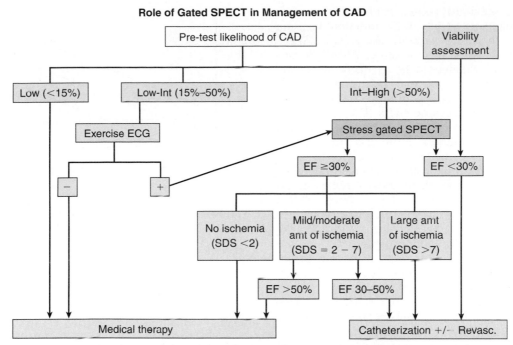

Figure 13-30 Schematic diagram showing role of gated SPECT in the management of coronary artery disease (CAD), based on pretest likelihood of CAD and the results of exercise ECG or stress gated SPECT. Patients with a low pretest likelihood of CAD do not generally require testing. Patients with a low intermediate (Int) likelihood generally only require stress gated SPECT when the exercise ECG is abnormal (or uninterruptible, or when the patient cannot exercise). Patients with a high intermediate to high likelihood of CAD (>50%) might be considered for direct referral to stress gated SPECT. The diagram illustrates how the combination of ventricular function and stress-induced ischemia (SDS) interact in judging the need for referral to catheterization (in patients without limiting angina). In patients with ejection fraction (EF) < 30%, catheterization is usually performed. Frequently, viability assessment with rest redistribution thallium or nitroglycerin augmented sestamibi or tetrofosmin, FDG PET, or low-dose dobutamine echo can be helpful in determining the likelihood of benefit from revascularization in these patients with severely reduced EF. *(Based on Refs. 205 and 207.)*

event rates. In patients with ejection fractions of greater than 50%, only patients with moderately extensive ischemia were at high risk of cardiac events. The work of Sharir et al. was based on the summed difference score as a measure of ischemia, but we have recently advocated the use of a ratio between this score and the maximal score as a more useful clinical measurement.[206] An algorithm incorporating myocardial perfusion scintigraphy and gated SPECT LVEF based on these findings is shown in Figure 13-30.

Similar findings were reported by Liao et al.,[208] who studied 997 patients (75% male; median age = 60 years) who underwent exercise treadmill testing with first-pass ejection fraction (RNA-EF)-measured and myocardial perfusion SPECT imaging as a single test. During a median follow-up of 4.1 years, 175 patients experienced outcome events. In clinically risk-adjusted models, RNA-EF was the most powerful predictor of cardiovascular death compared with the Duke Treadmill Score (DTS) and myocardial perfusion SPECT (X^2 = 40.5, 27.6, and 19.8, respectively). Conversely, exercise myocardial perfusion SPECT was a stronger predictor of nonfatal MI than the DTS or RNA-EF (X^2 = 26.7, 15.7, and 16.7, respectively).

A recent report by Thomas et al. illustrated the added value of the post stress EF from gated SPECT over myocardial perfusion measurements from a community-based nuclear cardiology laboratory that followed 1612 consecutive patients undergoing stress gated SPECT over a follow-up period of 24 ± 7 months.[209] These authors found that post stress EF added incremental prognostic value over pre-SPECT and perfusion data. Even after adjustment for these variables, each 1% change in LVEF was associated with a 3% increase in risk of adverse events. In this study, perfusion data also added incremental value over EF data in both patients with EF lower than 40% and those with EF of 40% or greater. Travin et al. subsequently reported a series of 3207 patients who underwent stress SPECT and were followed up for adverse events.[210] They found that both abnormal wall motion and abnormal EF were associated with increased risk; furthermore, they demonstrated that an abnormal gated SPECT wall motion score was also predictive of outcome. Similar to previous studies, myocardial infarction was predicted by the number of territories with a perfusion defect but not by EF. These authors also demonstrated that the results of gated SPECT added incremental value over both normal and abnormal SPECT perfusion. Similarly, Petix et al. studied 333 patients undergoing gated myocardial perfusion SPECT with both rest and post stress gating, demonstrating that addition of function data from gated SPECT provided a significant increase in the prediction of hard cardiac events.[211]

Most of the previously noted studies documenting the added prognostic value of LV function measurements over perfusion assessment using gated SPECT employed exercise as the form of stress. Although vasodilator stress is considered to be as likely as exercise stress to produce an abnormal perfusion study in patients with CAD, it less commonly produces true ischemia compared to exercise stress. Thus, vasodilator stress is expected to less commonly produce abnormalities of ventricular function. Little has been written regarding the added value of function measurements from gated SPECT for prognosis in patients undergoing vasodilator stress. Mast et al. reported findings in 240 patients undergoing pharmacologic gated SPECT, demonstrating that a significant minority of patients with CAD undergoing pharmacologic stress develop stress-induced wall motion abnormalities.[212]

A problem of particular interest with regard to outcome research dealing with the use of nuclear cardiology procedures in guiding patient management is the impact of including both patients treated medically and those treated with early revascularization on the results of survival analyses. In a landmark manuscript dealing with myocardial perfusion variables without gating, Hachamovitch et al. demonstrated that the amount of ischemia by myocardial perfusion SPECT was predictive of benefit from revascularization.[213] More recently, these investigators included the gated SPECT findings to examine the hypothesis that although EF predicts the risk of cardiac death, only measures of ischemia will identify which patients will accrue a survival benefit from revascularization compared with medical therapy after stress SPECT. In this study, 5366 consecutive patients without prior revascularization were followed up for 2.8 ± 1.2 years, during which 146 cardiac deaths occurred (2.7%, or 1% per year). After adjustment for pre-SPECT data and the use of a propensity score to adjust for nonrandomized treatment assignment, the authors found several interesting findings. First, as previously shown by Sharir et al., LVEF was the most powerful predictor of cardiac death. In addition, as shown before, stress perfusion results added incremental value over EF for prediction of cardiac death.[214] Most important, only the percent ischemic myocardium was able to predict which patients would accrue a survival benefit with revascularization over medical therapy. On the other hand, LVEF played a crucial role in identifying the absolute benefit (number of lives saved per 100 treated, number of years of life gained with treatment) for a given patient (Figs. 13-31 and 13-32).

As previously described, prediction of absolute benefit after gated SPECT is also a function of clinical risk factors such as patient age, sex, diabetes mellitus, and type of stress performed.[214] Optimal implementation of the results of gated SPECT for purposes of guiding patient management will require complex algorithms that incorporate all of the information from the perfusion and function variables derived from gated SPECT as well as the clinical response to stress and comprehensive assessment of variables that define the baseline risk of the patient.

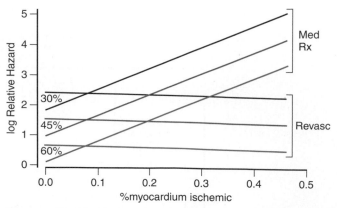

Figure 13-31 Predicted relationship based on Cox proportional hazards modeling between log hazard ratio versus percent ischemic myocardium in patients treated medically (Med Rx) or with early revascularization (Revasc) after stress SPECT. Three pairs of lines are shown for post-stress left ventricular ejection fractions (LVEFs) of 30%, 45%, and 60%. Within each pair, patient risk is unchanged across values of percent ischemic myocardium with early revascularization, and increases significantly in patients treated medically. With decreasing EF, risk in both patients who underwent early revascularization and those treated medically increases for any level of percent ischemic myocardium. This increase in risk demonstrates the incremental value of LVEF over other factors. Similarly, the increase in risk with increasing percent ischemic myocardium in the setting of medical therapy demonstrates the incremental value of SPECT measures of inducible ischemia. Finally, the differential risk with medical therapy versus revascularization identified by percent ischemic myocardium demonstrates its ability to identify treatment benefit. Model $P < 0.00001$. *(Reprinted with permission from Hachamovitch R: Clinical value of combined perfusion and function imaging in the diagnosis, prognosis, and management of patients with suspected or known coronary artery disease. In Germano G, Berman D [eds]: Clinical Gated Cardiac SPECT, 2nd ed. Oxford, UK: Blackwell Publishing, 2006, pp 189-215.)*

ASSESSING MYOCARDIAL VIABILITY

An underappreciated potential use of gated SPECT is in assessment of myocardial viability by examining the recruitment of contractile function in asynergic segments in response to inotropic stimulation. Low-dose dobutamine echocardiography has become a commonly employed, established method in this regard.[215] Gated SPECT can also be applied for this purpose. In this regard, Leoncini et al. documented the usefulness of dobutamine ^{99m}Tc sestamibi gated SPECT for prediction of improvement (or lack of improvement) of LVEF after coronary revascularization.[216] In 37 patients undergoing this procedure as well as revascularization with follow-up gated SPECT, an increase in LVEF of ≥ 5 units during dobutamine was the optimal cutoff value for predicting a significant post revascularization improvement in LVEF, with sensitivity and specificity of 79% and 78%, respectively.

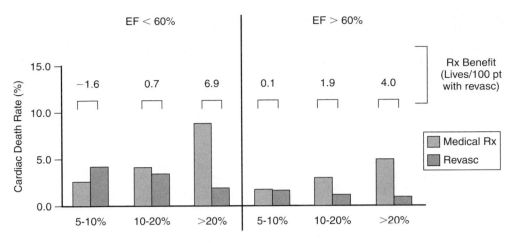

Figure 13-32 Predicted cardiac death rates based on final Cox proportional hazards model for patients with ejection fraction (EF) < 60% versus those with EF > 60%. Results were further stratified by percent ischemic myocardium (5-10%, 10-20%, and > 20%). Within each category of inducible ischemia, predicted cardiac death rates are shown separately for medical therapy (Rx) after stress SPECT *(black bars)* versus early revascularization (Revasc) *(white bars)*. In both low-EF and high-EF subgroups, the risk associated with revascularization is significantly lower in the setting of marked ischemia. The number of lives saved per 100 patients treated (difference between predicted survival with early revascularization versus medical therapy) is shown over the bars. The number of lives saved per 100 patients treated is significant in patients with 20% ischemic myocardium and is greater in those with low EF than in those with high EF. Model $P < 0.0001$. *(Reprinted with permission from Hachamovitch R: Clinical value of combined perfusion and function imaging in the diagnosis, prognosis, and management of patients with suspected or known coronary artery disease. In Germano G, Berman D [eds]: Clinical Gated Cardiac SPECT, 2nd ed. Oxford, UK: Blackwell Publishing, 2006, pp 189-215.)*

REFERENCES

1. Bacharach SL, Bonow RO, Green MV: Comparison of fixed and variable temporal resolution methods for creating gated cardiac blood-pool image sequences, *J Nucl Med* 31:38–42, 1990.
2. Bar Harbor Invitation Meeting 2000: *J Nucl Cardiol* 8:224–316, 2001.
3. Philips Medical Systems: Personal communication.
4. Cullom SJ, Case JA, Bateman TM: Electrocardiographically gated myocardial perfusion SPECT: technical principles and quality control considerations, *J Nucl Cardiol* 5:418–425, 1998.
5. Nichols K, Dorbala S, DePuey EG, et al: Influence of arrhythmias on gated SPECT myocardial perfusion and function quantification, *J Nucl Med* 40:924–934, 1999.
6. Germano G: Technical aspects of myocardial SPECT imaging, *J Nucl Med* 42:1499–1507, 2001.
7. Bracewell R, Riddle A: Inversion of fan-beam scans in radioastronomy, *Astrophys J* 150:427–434, 1967.
8. Shepp LA, Logan BF: The Fourier reconstruction of a head section, *IEEE Trans Nucl Sci* NS-21:21–43, 1974.
9. Germano G, Chua T, Kiat H, et al: A quantitative phantom analysis of artifacts due to hepatic activity in technetium-99m myocardial perfusion SPECT studies, *J Nucl Med* 35:356–359, 1994.
10. Cauvin JC, Boire JY, Maublant JC, et al: Automatic detection of the left ventricular myocardium long axis and center in thallium-201 single photon emission computed tomography, *Eur J Nucl Med* 19:1032–1037, 1992.
11. Cooke C, Folks R, Jones M, et al: Automatic program for determining the long axis of the left ventricular myocardium used for thallium-201 tomographic reconstruction, *J Nucl Med* 30:806, 1989. (abstract).
12. Germano G, Kavanagh PB, Chen J, et al: Operator-less processing of myocardial perfusion SPECT studies, *J Nucl Med* 36:2127–2132, 1995.
13. Germano G, Kavanagh PB, Su HT, et al: Automatic reorientation of three-dimensional, transaxial myocardial perfusion SPECT images [commentary], *J Nucl Med* 36:1107–1114, 1995.
14. Slomka PJ, Nishina H, Berman DS, et al: "Motion-Frozen" Display and quantification of myocardial perfusion, *J Nucl Med* 45:1128–1134, 2004.
15. Suzuki Y, Slomka P, Wolak A, et al: Motion-frozen myocardial perfusion SPECT improves detection of coronary artery disease in obese patients, *J Nucl Med* 49:1075–1079, 2008.
16. Taillefer R, DePuey EG, Udelson JE, et al: Comparison between the end-diastolic images and the summed images of gated 99mTc-sestamibi SPECT perfusion study in detection of coronary artery disease in women, *J Nucl Cardiol* 6:169–176, 1999.
17. Bestetti A, Di Leo C, Alessi A, et al: Transient left ventricular dilation during myocardial perfusion gated-SPECT in hypertensive patients, *Eur J Nucl Med* 28:OS239, 2001. (abstract).
18. Mazzanti M, Germano G, Kiat H, et al: Identification of severe and extensive coronary artery disease by automatic measurement of transient ischemic dilation of the left ventricle in dual-isotope myocardial perfusion SPECT, *J Am Coll Cardiol* 27:1612–1620, 1996.
19. Buvat I, Bartlett ML, Kitsiou AN, et al: A "hybrid" method for measuring myocardial wall thickening from gated PET/SPECT images, *J Nucl Med* 38:324–329, 1997.
20. DePuey EG, Nichols K, Dobrinsky C: Left ventricular ejection fraction assessed from gated technetium-99m-sestamibi SPECT, *J Nucl Med* 34:1871–1876, 1993.
21. Everaert H, Franken PR, Flamen P, et al: Left ventricular ejection fraction from gated SPET myocardial perfusion studies: a method based on the radial distribution of count rate density across the myocardial wall, *Eur J Nucl Med* 23:1628–1633, 1996.
22. Goris ML, Thompson C, Malone LJ, Franken PR: Modelling the integration of myocardial regional perfusion and function, *Nucl Med Commun* 15:9–20, 1994.
23. Marcassa C, Marzullo P, Parodi O, et al: A new method for noninvasive quantitation of segmental myocardial wall thickening using technetium-99m 2-methoxy-isobutyl-isonitrile scintigraphy: Results in normal subjects, *J Nucl Med* 31:173–177, 1990.
24. Mochizuki T, Murase K, Fujiwara Y, et al: Assessment of systolic thickening with thallium-201 ECG-gated single-photon emission computed tomography: a parameter for local left ventricular function, *J Nucl Med* 32:1496–1500, 1991.
25. Nichols K, DePuey EG, Rozanski A: Automation of gated tomographic left ventricular ejection fraction, *J Nucl Cardiol* 3:475–482, 1996.
26. Smith WH, Kastner RJ, Calnon DA, et al: Quantitative gated single photon emission computed tomography imaging: a counts-based method for display and measurement of regional and global ventricular systolic function, *J Nucl Cardiol* 4:451–463, 1997.
27. Williams KA, Taillon LA: Left ventricular function in patients with coronary artery disease assessed by gated tomographic myocardial perfusion images. Comparison with assessment by contrast ventriculography and first-pass radionuclide angiography, *J Am Coll Cardiol* 27:173–181, 1996.
28. Germano G, Kiat H, Kavanagh PB, et al: Automatic quantification of ejection fraction from gated myocardial perfusion SPECT, *J Nucl Med* 36:2138–2147, 1995.
29. Germano G, Erel J, Lewin H, et al: Automatic quantitation of regional myocardial wall motion and thickening from gated technetium-99m sestamibi myocardial perfusion single-photon emission computed tomography, *J Am Coll Cardiol* 30:1360–1367, 1997.
30. Van Kriekinge SD, Nishina H, Ohba M, et al: Automatic global and regional phase analysis from gated myocardial perfusion SPECT

imaging: application to the characterization of ventricular contraction in patients with left bundle branch block, *J Nucl Med* 49:1790–1797, 2008.

31. Sharir T, Berman DS, Waechter PB, et al: Quantitative analysis of regional motion and thickening by gated myocardial perfusion SPECT: Normal heterogeneity and criteria for abnormality, *J Nucl Med* 42:1630–1638, 2001.

32. Germano G, Kavanagh PB, Slomka PJ, et al: Quantitation in gated perfusion SPECT imaging: The Cedars-Sinai approach, *J Nucl Cardiol* 14:433–454, 2007.

33. Faber TL, Cooke CD, Folks RD, et al: Left ventricular function and perfusion from gated SPECT perfusion images: an integrated method, *J Nucl Med* 40:650–659, 1999.

34. Chen J, Garcia EV, Folks RD, et al: Onset of left ventricular mechanical contraction as determined by phase analysis of ECG-gated myocardial perfusion SPECT imaging: Development of a diagnostic tool for assessment of cardiac mechanical dyssynchrony, *J Nucl Cardiol* 12:687–695, 2005.

35. Garcia EV, Faber TL, Cooke CD, et al: The increasing role of quantification in clinical nuclear cardiology: The Emory approach, *J Nucl Cardiol* 14:420–432, 2007.

36. Chugh A, Ficaro EP, Moscucci M, et al: Quantification of left ventricular function by gated perfusion tomography: Testing of a new fully automatic algorithm, *J Am Coll Cardiol* 37:394A, 2001. (abstract).

37. Ficaro EP, Kritzman JN, Corbett JR: Automatic segmental scoring of myocardial wall thickening and motion: validation of a new semi-quantitative algorithm, *J Nucl Med* 42:171P, 2001. (abstract).

38. Ficaro EP, Lee BC, Kritzman JN, Corbett JR: Corridor4DM: The Michigan method for quantitative nuclear cardiology, *J Nucl Cardiol* 14:455–465, 2007.

39. Shen MY, Liu YH, Sinusas AJ, et al: Quantification of regional myocardial wall thickening on electrocardiogram-gated SPECT imaging, *J Nucl Cardiol* 6:583–595, 1999.

40. Liu YH: Quantification of nuclear cardiac images: The Yale approach, *J Nucl Cardiol* 14:483–491, 2007.

41. Abe M, Kazatani Y, Fukuda H, et al: Left ventricular volumes, ejection fraction, and regional wall motion calculated with gated technetium-99m tetrofosmin SPECT in reperfused acute myocardial infarction at super-acute phase: comparison with left ventriculography, *J Nucl Cardiol* 7:569–574, 2000.

42. Atsma DE, Bavelaar-Croon CDL, Germano G, et al: Good correlation between gated single photon emission computed myocardial tomography and contrast ventriculography in the assessment of global and regional left ventricular function, *Int J Card Imaging* 16:447–453, 2000.

43. Bacher-Stier C, Müller S, Pachinger O, et al: Thallium-201 gated single-photon emission tomography for the assessment of left ventricular ejection fraction and regional wall motion abnormalities in comparison with two-dimensional echocardiography, *Eur J Nucl Med* 26:1533–1540, 1999.

44. Bavelaar-Croon CD, Kayser HW, van der Wall EE, et al: Left ventricular function: correlation of quantitative gated SPECT and MR imaging over a wide range of values, *Radiology* 217:572–575, 2000.

45. Bax JJ, Lamb H, Dibbets P, et al: Comparison of gated single-photon emission computed tomography with magnetic resonance imaging for evaluation of left ventricular function in ischemic cardiomyopathy, *Am J Cardiol* 86:1299–1305, 2000.

46. Chua T, Yin LC, Thiang TH, et al: Accuracy of the automated assessment of left ventricular function with gated perfusion SPECT in the presence of perfusion defects and left ventricular dysfunction: correlation with equilibrium radionuclide ventriculography and echocardiography, *J Nucl Cardiol* 7:301–311, 2000.

47. Cwajg E, Cwajg J, He ZX, et al: Gated myocardial perfusion tomography for the assessment of left ventricular function and volumes: comparison with echocardiography, *J Nucl Med* 40:1857–1865, 1999.

48. Everaert H, Bossuyt A, Franken PR: Left ventricular ejection fraction and volumes from gated single photon emission tomographic myocardial perfusion images: comparison between two algorithms working in three-dimensional space, *J Nucl Cardiol* 4:472–476, 1997.

49. Faber TL, Vansant JP, Pettigrew RI, et al: Evaluation of left ventricular endocardial volumes and ejection fractions computed from gated perfusion SPECT with magnetic resonance imaging: Comparison of two methods, *J Nucl Cardiol* 8:645–651, 2001.

50. He ZX, Cwajg E, Preslar JS, et al: Accuracy of left ventricular ejection fraction determined by gated myocardial perfusion SPECT with Tl-201 and Tc-99m sestamibi: comparison with first-pass radionuclide angiography, *J Nucl Cardiol* 6:412–417, 1999.

51. Higuchi T, Nakajima K, Taki J, et al: Assessment of left ventricular systolic and diastolic function based on the edge detection method with myocardial ECG-gated SPET, *Eur J Nucl Med* 28:1512–1516, 2001.

52. Inubushi M, Tadamura E, Kudoh T, et al: Simultaneous assessment of myocardial free fatty acid utilization and left ventricular function using 123I-BMIPP-gated SPECT, *J Nucl Med* 40:1840–1847, 1999.

53. Kikkawa M, Nakamura T, Sakamoto K, et al: Assessment of left ventricular diastolic function from quantitative electrocardiographic-gated (99)mTc-tetrofosmin myocardial SPET (ERRATA in vol 28, pg 1579, 2001), *Eur J Nucl Med* 28:593–601, 2001.

54. Kumita S, Cho K, Nakajo H, et al: Assessment of left ventricular diastolic function with electrocardiography-gated myocardial perfusion SPECT: Comparison with multigated equilibrium radionuclide angiography, *J Nucl Cardiol* 8:568–574, 2001.

55. Lipke CSA, Kuhl HP, Nowak B, et al: Validation of 4D-MSPECT and QGS for quantification of left ventricular volumes and ejection fraction from gated Tc-99m-MIBI SPET: comparison with cardiac magnetic resonance imaging, *Eur J Nucl Med Mol Imaging* 31:482–490, 2004.

56. Manrique A, Koning R, Cribier A, Véra P: Effect of temporal sampling on evaluation of left ventricular ejection fraction by means of thallium-201 gated SPET: comparison of 16- and 8-interval gating, with reference to equilibrium radionuclide angiography, *Eur J Nucl Med* 27:694–699, 2000.

57. Nakajima K, Higuchi T, Taki J, et al: Accuracy of ventricular volume and ejection fraction measured by gated myocardial SPECT: Comparison of 4 software programs, *J Nucl Med* 42:1571–1578, 2001.

58. Nanasato M, Ando A, Isobe S, et al: Evaluation of left ventricular function using electrocardiographically gated myocardial SPECT with I-123- labeled fatty acid analog, *J Nucl Med* 42:1747–1756, 2001.

59. Nichols K, Lefkowitz D, Faber T, et al: Echocardiographic validation of gated SPECT ventricular function measurements, *J Nucl Med* 41:1308–1314, 2000.

60. Tadamura E, Kudoh T, Motooka M, et al: Use of technetium-99m sestamibi ECG-gated single-photon emission tomography for the evaluation of left ventricular function following coronary artery bypass graft: comparison with three-dimensional magnetic resonance imaging, *Eur J Nucl Med* 26:705–712, 1999.

61. Tadamura E, Kudoh T, Motooka M, et al: Assessment of regional and global left ventricular function by reinjection T1-201 and rest Tc-99m sestamibi ECG-gated SPECT: comparison with three-dimensional magnetic resonance imaging, *J Am Coll Cardiol* 33:991–997, 1999.

62. Thorley PJ, Plein S, Bloomer TN, et al: Comparison of Tc-99m tetrofosmin gated SPECT measurements of left ventricular volumes and ejection fraction with MRI over a wide range of values, *Nucl Med Commun* 24:763–769, 2003.

63. Vaduganathan P, He ZX, Vick GW 3rd, , et al: Evaluation of left ventricular wall motion, volumes, and ejection fraction by gated myocardial tomography with technetium 99m-labeled tetrofosmin: a comparison with cine magnetic resonance imaging, *J Nucl Cardiol* 6:3–10, 1999.

64. Vallejo E, Dione DP, Sinusas AJ, Wackers FJ: Assessment of left ventricular ejection fraction with quantitative gated SPECT: accuracy and correlation with first-pass radionuclide angiography, *J Nucl Cardiol* 7:461–470, 2000.

65. Vourvouri EC, Poldermans D, Bax JJ, et al: Evaluation of left ventricular function and volumes in patients with ischaemic cardiomyopathy: gated single-photon emission computed tomography versus two-dimensional echocardiography, *Eur J Nucl Med* 28:1610–1615, 2001.

66. Yoshioka J, Hasegawa S, Yamaguchi H, et al: Left ventricular volumes and ejection fraction calculated from quantitative electrocardiographic-gated 99mTc-tetrofosmin myocardial SPECT, *J Nucl Med* 40:1693–1698, 1999.

67. Higuchi T, Nakajima K, Taki J, et al: Accuracy and reproducibility of four softwares for the left-ventricular function with ECG-gated myocardial perfusion SPECT, *J Nucl Cardiol* 8:S64, 2001. (abstract).

68. Vansant J, Pettigrew R, Faber T, et al: Comparison and accuracy of two gated-SPECT techniques for assessing left ventricular function defined by cardiac MRI, *J Nucl Med* 40:166P, 1999. (abstract).

69. Cahill J, Chen M, Corbett J, Quaife R: Validation of three-dimensional analysis method for calculation of the LV mass and ejection fraction using Tc-99m sestamibi gated-SPECT perfusion imaging: Comparison between 4D-MSPECT and magnetic resonance imaging, *J Nucl Med* 44:197P, 2003. (abstract).

70. Ficaro E, Quaife R, Kritzman J, Corbett J: Accuracy and reproducibility of 3D-MSPECT for estimating left ventricular ejection fraction in patients with severe perfusion abnormalities, *Circulation* 100:I-26, 1999. (abstract).

71. Gayed IW, Cid E, Boccalandro F: Correlation of left ventricular ejection fraction using Gated SPECT automated programs with echocardiography, *J Nucl Med* 42:177P–178P, 2001. (abstract).

72. Lam PT, Wackers FJT, Liu YH: Validation of a new method for quantification of left ventricular function from ECG-gated SPECT, *J Nucl Med* 42:93P–94P, 2001. (abstract).

73. Liu YH, Sinusas AJ, Khaimov D, et al: New hybrid count- and geometry-based method for quantification of left ventricular volumes and ejection fraction from ECG-gated SPECT: Methodology and validation, *J Nucl Cardiol* 12:55–65, 2005.

74. Hyun IY, Kwan J, Park KS, Lee WH: Reproducibility of Tl-201 and Tc-99m sestamibi gated myocardial perfusion SPECT measurement of myocardial function, *J Nucl Cardiol* 8:182–187, 2001.

75. Johnson LL, Verdesca SA, Aude WY, et al: Postischemic stunning can affect left ventricular ejection fraction and regional wall motion on post-stress gated sestamibi tomograms [commentary], *J Am Coll Cardiol* 30:1641–1648, 1997.

76. Lee DS, Ahn JY, Kim SK, et al: Limited performance of quantitative assessment of myocardial function by thallium-201 gated myocardial single-photon emission tomography, *Eur J Nucl Med* 27:185–191, 2000.

77. Agostini D, Filmont J, Darlas Y, et al: LVEF and LV volumes determinations with gated 123I-MIBG SPECT in dystrophic myotony, *J Nucl Med* 41:49P, 2000. (abstract).

78. Germano G, Erel J, Kiat H, et al: Quantitative LVEF and qualitative regional function from gated thallium-201 perfusion SPECT, *J Nucl Med* 38:749–754, 1997.

79. Maunoury C, Chen CC, Chua KB, Thompson CJ: Quantification of left ventricular function with thallium-201 and technetium-99m-sestamibi myocardial gated SPECT, *J Nucl Med* 38:958–961, 1997.

80. Everaert H, Vanhove C, Franken PR: Gated SPET myocardial perfusion acquisition within 5 minutes using focusing collimators and a three-head gamma camera, *Eur J Nucl Med* 25:587–593, 1998.

81. Franken PR, Everaert H, Momen A, Vanhove C: Automatic left ventricular cavity volume and ejection fraction measurements from one-day rest/stress perfusion gated tomograms, *Eur J Nucl Med* 26:1079, 1999. (abstract).

82. Mazzanti M, Germano G, Kiat H, et al: Fast technetium 99m-labeled sestamibi gated single-photon emission computed tomography for evaluation of myocardial function, *J Nucl Cardiol* 3:143–149, 1996.

83. Vanhove C, Franken PR, Defrise M, Bossuyt A: Comparison of 180 degrees and 360 degrees data acquisition for determination of left ventricular function from gated myocardial perfusion tomography and gated blood pool tomography, *Eur J Nucl Med Mol Imaging* 30:1498–1504, 2003.

84. Kritzman J, Ficaro E, Corbett J: Reproducibility of 3-D MSPECT for quantitative gated SPECT sestamibi perfusion analysis, *J Nucl Med* 41:166P, 2000. (abstract).

85. Nakajima K, Nishimura T: Inter-institution preference-based variability of ejection fraction and volumes using quantitative gated SPECT with Tc-99m-tetrofosmin: a multicentre study involving 106 hospitals, *Eur J Nucl Med Mol Imaging* 33:127–133, 2006.

86. Berman D, Germano G, Lewin H, et al: Comparison of post-stress ejection fraction and relative left ventricular volumes by automatic analysis of gated myocardial perfusion single-photon emission computed tomography acquired in the supine and prone positions, *J Nucl Cardiol* 5:40–47, 1998.

87. Kubo N, Mabuchi M, Katoh C, et al: Validation of left ventricular function using gated SPECT with a scintillation crystal and semiconductor detectors camera system: A study of dynamic myocardial phantom, *J Nucl Med* 43:199P–200P, 2002. (abstract).

88. Daou D, Pointurier I, Coaguila C, et al: Performance of OSEM and depth-dependent resolution recovery algorithms for the evaluation of global left ventricular function in Tl-201 gated myocardial perfusion SPECT, *J Nucl Med* 44:155–162, 2003.

89. Ficaro E, Kritzman J, Hamilton J, et al: Effect of attenuation corrected myocardial perfusion SPECT on left ventricular ejection fraction estimates, *J Nucl Med* 41:166P–167P, 2000. (abstract).

90. Boussaha MR, Storto G, Antonescu C, Delaloye AB: Ejection fraction evaluation by gated myocardial perfusion SPECT: Comparison between gated SPECT quantification (GSQ) and Emory Cardiac Tool Box (ECTB), *Eur J Nucl Med* 28:OS240, 2001. (abstract).

91. Dede F, Narin Y: Can different software programs give the same functional measurements in ECG gated SPECT: Comparison of two software programs, *Eur J Nucl Med* 29:S209, 2002. (abstract).

92. Franken PR, Everaert H, Momen A, Vanhove C: Comparison of three automatic software to measure left ventricular cavity volume and ejection fraction from perfusion gated tomograms, *Eur J Nucl Med* 26:1076, 1999. (abstract).

93. Hambye AS, Vervaet A, Dobbeleir A: Variability of left ventricular ejection fraction and volumes with quantitative gated SPECT: influence of algorithm, pixel size and reconstruction parameters in small and normal-sized hearts, *Eur J Nucl Med Mol Imaging* 31:1606–1613, 2004.

94. Lewis T, Grewal K, Calnon D: Discrepancies in estimating left-ventricular volumes and ejection fraction by two commercially available gated SPECT algorithms: comparison to echocardiography, *J Nucl Cardiol* 8:S18, 2001. (abstract).

95. Nichols K, Folks R, Cooke D, et al: Comparisons between "ECTb" and "QGS" software to compute left ventricular function from myocardial perfusion gated SPECT, *J Nucl Cardiol* 7:S20, 2000. (abstract).

96. Kang D, Kim M, Kim Y: Functional data of gated myocardial perfusion SPECT by QGS and 4D-MSPECT program cannot exchanged each other (sic), *J Nucl Med* 45:225P, 2004. (abstract).

97. Krasnow J, Trask I, Dahlberg S, et al: Automatic determination of left ventricular function (LVEF) by gated SPECT; comparison of four quantitative software programs, *J Nucl Cardiol* 8:S138, 2001. (abstract).

98. Rozanski A, Nichols K, Yao SS, et al: Development and application of normal limits for left ventricular ejection fraction and volume measurements from 99mTc-sestamibi myocardial perfusion gates SPECT, *J Nucl Med* 41:1445–1450, 2000.

99. Santana CA, Garcia EV, Folks R, et al: Comparison of normal values of left ventricular function between two programs: QGS and emory cardiac toolbox (ECTB), *J Nucl Med* 42:166P, 2001. (abstract).

100. Sharir T, Germano G, Friedman J, et al: Prognostic value of gated myocardial perfusion single photon emission computed tomography in women versus men, *Circulation* 102:II–544, 2000. (abstract).

101. Ababneh A, Sciacca R, Bergmann S: Normal limits for left ventricular ejection fraction, end-diastolic, and end-systolic volume as estimated with gated perfusion imaging, *Circulation* 102:II–724, 2000. (abstract).

102. Ababneh AA, Sciacca RR, Kim B, Bergmann SR: Normal limits for left ventricular ejection fraction and volumes estimated with gated myocardial perfusion imaging in patients with normal exercise test results: influence of tracer, gender, and acquisition camera, *J Nucl Cardiol* 7:661–668, 2000.

103. De Bondt P, De Sutter J, De Winter F, et al: Normal values of left ventricular ejection fraction (LVEF) and left ventricular volumes (LVV) measured by gated myocardial SPECT in women and men at rest and after bicycle or dipyridamole (DIP) stress testing, *J Nucl Med* 41:159P, 2000. (abstract).

104. De Bondt P, Van de Wiele C, De Sutter J, et al: Age- and gender-specific differences in left ventricular cardiac function and volumes determined by gated SPET, *Eur J Nucl Med* 28:620–624, 2001.

105. Ficaro F, Kritzman J, Stephens G, Corbett J: Gender specific differences in normal ranges of cardiac functional parameters from gated SPECT, *J Nucl Med* 44:205P–206P, 2003. (abstract).

106. Hyun I, Kim D, Seo J, et al: Normal parameters of left ventricular volume and ejection fraction measured by gated myocardial perfusion SPECT: comparison of Tc99m MIBI and Tl-201, *Eur J Nucl Med* 29:S205, 2002. (abstract).

107. Kim J, Kim N: Normal LVEF measurements are significantly higher in females assessed by 99m Tc-MIBI and Tetrofosmin quantitative gated myocardial perfusion SPECT: age and gender matched statistical analysis, *J Nucl Med* 44:106P, 2003. (abstract).

108. Sharir T, Germano G, Kang XP, et al: Prognostic value of post-stress left ventricular volume and ejection fraction by gated myocardial perfusion single photon emission computed tomography in women: Gender related differences in normal limits and outcome, *Circulation* 106:II–523, 2002. (abstract).

109. Case J, Cullom S, Bateman T, et al: Overestimation of LVEF by gated MIBI myocardial perfusion SPECT in patients with small hearts, *J Am Coll Cardiol* 31:43A, 1998. (abstract).

110. Ford PV, Chatziioannou SN, Moore WH, Dhekne RD: Overestimation of the LVEF by quantitative gated SPECT in simulated left ventricles, *J Nucl Med* 42:454–459, 2001.

111. Nakajima K, Taki J, Higuchi T, et al: Gated SPET quantification of small hearts: mathematical simulation and clinical application, *Eur J Nucl Med* 27:1372–1379, 2000.

112. Fzuddin S, Sfakianakis G, Pay L, Sanchez P: Comparative study to determine the effect of different zoom factors on the calculation of LVEF from gated myocardial perfusion SPECT with Tl-201 and Tc-99m-sestamibi in patients with small hearts, *J Nucl Med* 40:169P, 1999. (abstract).

113. Manrique A, Gardin I, Brasse D, et al: Effect of reconstruction parameters on LV volume measurements from Tl-201 SPECT: a phantom study, *J Nucl Cardiol* 8:S71, 2001. (abstract).

114. Schwartz R, Mixon L, Germano G, et al: Gated SPECT reconstruction with zoom and depth dependent filter improves accuracy of volume and LVEF in small hearts, *J Nucl Cardiol* 6:S17, 1999. (abstract).

115. Case J, Bateman T, Cullom S, et al: Improved accuracy of SPECT LVEF using numerical modeling of ventricular image blurring for patients with small hearts, *J Am Coll Cardiol* 33:436A, 1999. (abstract).

116. Faber T, Cooke C, Folks R, et al: Correction of artifactually high EF from gated perfusion SPECT in small ventricles, *J Nucl Cardiol* 7:S20, 2000. (abstract).

117. Santos M, Lewin H, Hayes S, et al: A potential cause for underestimation of LVEF by QGS, *J Nucl Cardiol* 8:S130, 2001. (abstract).

118. Cohade C, Taillefer R, Gagnon A, et al: Effect of the number of frames per cardiac cycle and the amount of injected dose of radionuclide on the determination of left ventricular ejection fraction (LVEF) with gated SPECT myocardial perfusion imaging (GS), *J Nucl Med* 41:154P, 2000. (abstract).

119. Imal K, Azuma Y, Nakajima S, et al: Frames a cardiac cycle in quantitative gated SPECT (QGS) for clinical use: 8 versus 16, *J Nucl Cardiol* 6:S17, 1999. (abstract).

120. Manrique A, Vera P, Hitzel A, et al: 16-interval gating improves thallium-201 gated SPECT LVEF measurement in patients with large

myocardial infarction, *J Am Coll Cardiol* 33:436A–437A, 1999. (abstract).

121. Everaert H, Vanhove C, Franken PR: Low-dose dobutamine gated single-photon emission tomography: comparison with stress echocardiography, *Eur J Nucl Med* 27:413–418, 2000.
122. Itti E, Rosso J, Damien P, et al: Assessment of ejection fraction with Tl-201 gated SPECT in myocardial infarction: Precision in a rest-redistribution study and accuracy versus planar angiography, *J Nucl Cardiol* 8:31–39, 2001.
123. Nichols K, Tamis J, DePuey EG, et al: Relationship of gated SPECT ventricular function parameters to angiographic measurements, *J Nucl Cardiol* 5:295–303, 1998.
124. Stollfuss JC, Haas F, Matsunari I, et al: Regional myocardial wall thickening and global ejection fraction in patients with low angiographic left ventricular ejection fraction assessed by visual and quantitative resting ECG-gated 99mTc-tetrofosmin single-photon emission tomography and magnetic resonance imaging, *Eur J Nucl Med* 25:522–530, 1998.
125. Stollfuss JC, Haas F, Matsunari I, et al: 99mTc-tetrofosmin SPECT for prediction of functional recovery defined by MRI in patients with severe left ventricular dysfunction: additional value of gated SPECT, *J Nucl Med* 40:1824–1831, 1999.
126. Canbaz F, Basoglu1 T, Durna K, et al: Left ventricular aneurysm in the scope of gated perfusion SPECT: accuracy of detection and ejection fraction calculation, *Int J Cardiovasc Imaging* 24: 585–596, 2008.
127. Iskandrian AE, Germano G, VanDecker W, et al: Validation of left ventricular volume measurements by gated SPECT 99mTc-labeled sestamibi imaging, *J Nucl Cardiol* 5:574–578, 1998.
128. Zuber E, Rosfors S: Effect of reversible hypoperfusion on left ventricular volumes measured with gated SPECT at rest and after adenosine infusion, *J Nucl Cardiol* 7:655–660, 2000.
129. Nichols K, Lefkovitz D, Faber T, et al: Ventricular volumes compared among three gated SPECT methods and echocardiography, *J Am Coll Cardiol* 33:409A, 1999. (abstract).
130. Liu Y: A new approach of quantification of left-ventricular volume for gated SPECT imaging: preliminary validation using a phantom, *J Nucl Cardiol* 8:S61, 2001. (abstract).
131. Adachi I, Morita K, Imran MB, et al: Heterogeneity of myocardial wall motion and thickening in the left ventricle evaluated with quantitative gated SPECT, *J Nucl Cardiol* 7:296–300, 2000.
132. Faber TL, Stokely EM, Peshock RM, Corbett JR: A model-based four-dimensional left ventricular surface detector, *IEEE Trans Med Imaging* 10:321–329, 1991.
133. Cooke C, Garcia E, Folks R, Ziffer J: Myocardial thickening and phase analysis from Tc-99m sestamibi multiple gated SPECT: development of normal limits, *J Nucl Med* 33:926–927, 1992. (abstract).
134. Everaert H, Vanhove C, Franken PR: Effects of low-dose dobutamine on left ventricular function in normal subjects as assessed by gated single-photon emission tomography myocardial perfusion studies, *Eur J Nucl Med* 26:1298–1303, 1999.
135. Fujino S, Masuyama K, Kanayama S, et al: Early and delayed technetium-99m labeled sestamibi myocardial ECG-gated SPECT by QGS program in normal volunteers, *J Nucl Med* 40:180P, 1999. (abstract).
136. Itoh Y, Adachi I, Kohya T, et al: Heterogeneity in myocardial perfusion, wall motion and wall thickening with Tc-99m-sestamibi quantitative gated SPECT in normal subjects, *J Nucl Med* 40:165P, 1999. (abstract).
137. Shirakawa S, Hattori N, Tamaki N, et al: [Assessment of left ventricular wall thickening with gated 99mTc-MIBI SPECT—value of normal file], *Kaku Igaku* 32:643–650, 1995.
138. Cerqueira MD, Weissman NJ, Dilsizian V, et al: Standardized myocardial segmentation and nomenclature for tomographic imaging of the heart: A statement for healthcare professionals from the Cardiac Imaging Committee of the Council on Clinical Cardiology of the American Heart Association, *J Nucl Cardiol* 9:240–245, 2002.
139. Berman D, Germano G: An approach to the interpretation and reporting of gated myocardial perfusion SPECT. In Germano G, Berman D, editors: *Clinical Gated Cardiac SPECT*, Armonk, NY, 1999, Futura Publishing Company, pp 147–182.
140. Damrongpipatkij Y, Mohammed F, Brown E, et al: Quantitative cardiac SPECT: measuring diastolic function, *J Nucl Med* 41:154P, 2000. (abstract).
141. Higuchi T, Taki J, Yoneyama T, et al: Diastolic and systolic parameters obtained by myocardial ECG-gated perfusion study, *J Nucl Med* 41:160P, 2000. (abstract).
142. Nakajima K, Taki J, Kawano M, et al: Diastolic dysfunction in patients with systemic sclerosis detected by gated myocardial perfusion SPECT: an early sign of cardiac involvement, *J Nucl Med* 42:183–188, 2001.
143. Higuchi T, Nakajima K, Taki J, et al: The accuracy of left-ventricular time volume curve derived from ECG-gated myocardial perfusion SPECT, *J Nucl Cardiol* 8:S18, 2001. (abstract).
144. Akincioglu C, Berman DS, Nishina H, et al: Assessment of diastolic function using 16-frame Tc-99m-sestamibi gated myocardial perfusion SPECT: Normal values, *J Nucl Med* 46:1102–1108, 2005.
145. Boogers MM, Van Kriekinge SD, Henneman MM, et al: QGS derived phase analysis on gated myocardial perfusion SPECT detects LV dyssynchrony and predicts response to CRT, *J Nucl Med* 2009 (in press).
146. Henneman MM, Chen J, Dibbets-Schneider P, et al: Can LV Dyssynchrony as Assessed with Phase Analysis on Gated Myocardial Perfusion SPECT Predict Response to CRT, *J Nucl Med* 48:1104–1111, 2007.
147. Chen J, Henneman MM, Trimble MA, et al: Assessment of left ventricular mechanical dyssynchrony by phase analysis of ECG-gated SPECT myocardial perfusion imaging, *J Nucl Cardiol* 15:127–136, 2008.
148. Berman DS, Salel AF, DeNardo GL, et al: Clinical assessment of left ventricular regional contraction patterns and ejection fraction by high-resolution gated scintigraphy, *J Nucl Med* 16:865–874, 1975.
149. Maublant J, Bailly P, Mestas D, et al: Feasibility of gated single-photon emission transaxial tomography of the cardiac blood pool, *Radiology* 146:837–839, 1983.
150. Moore ML, Murphy PH, Burdine JA: ECG-gated emission computed tomography of the cardiac blood pool, *Radiology* 134:233–235, 1980.
151. Tamaki N, Mukai T, Ishii Y, et al: Multiaxial tomography of heart chambers by gated blood-pool emission computed tomography using a rotating gamma camera, *Radiology* 147:547–554, 1983.
152. Alexanderson E, Espinola N, Meavel A, Victoria D: Assessment of ventricular perfusion and function with nuclear scan and echocardiography in patients with corrected transposition of great arteries, *J Nucl Cardiol* 10:S66, 2003. (abstract).
153. Barat JL, Brendel AJ, Colle JP, et al: Quantitative analysis of left-ventricular function using gated single photon emission tomography, *J Nucl Med* 25:1167–1174, 1984.
154. Bartlett ML, Srinivasan G, Barker WC, et al: Left ventricular ejection fraction: comparison of results from planar and SPECT gated blood-pool studies, *J Nucl Med* 37:1795–1799, 1996.
155. Bunker SR, Hartshorne MF, Schmidt WP, et al: Left ventricular volume determination from single-photon emission computed tomography, *Am J Roentgenol* 144:295–298, 1985.
156. Chin BB, Bloomgarden DC, Xia W, et al: Right and left ventricular volume and ejection fraction by tomographic gated blood-pool scintigraphy, *J Nucl Med* 38:942–948, 1997.
157. Corbett JR, Jansen DE, Lewis SE, et al: Tomographic gated blood pool radionuclide ventriculography: analysis of wall motion and left ventricular volumes in patients with coronary artery disease, *J Am Coll Cardiol* 6:349–358, 1985.
158. Daou D, Harel F, Mariano-Goulart D, et al: Left ventricular function estimated with ECG-gated blood pool SPECT: Comparison of two different processing softwares, *J Nucl Med* 42:137P, 2001. (abstract).
159. Daou D, Van Kriekinge SD, Coaguila C, et al: Automatic quantification of right ventricular function with gated blood pool SPECT, 11: 293–304, 2004.
160. Druz RS, Akinboboye OA, Grimson R, et al: Postischemic stunning after adenosine vasodilator stress, *J Nucl Cardiol* 11:534–541, 2004.
161. Ficaro EP, Kritzman' JN, Corbett JR: Normal LV ejection fraction limits using 4D MSPECT: Comparisons of gated perfusion and gated blood pool SPECT data with planar blood pool imaging, *J Nucl Cardiol* 10:S9, 2003. (abstract).
162. Ficaro EP, Quaife RF, Kritzman JN, Corbett JR: Validation of a new fully automatic algorithm for quantification of gated blood pool SPECT: Correlations with planar gated blood pool and perfusion SPECT, *J Nucl Med* 43:97P, 2002. (abstract).
163. Gill JB, Moore RH, Tamaki N, et al: Multigated blood-pool tomography: new method for the assessment of left ventricular function, *J Nucl Med* 27:1916–1924, 1986.
164. Groch M, Belzberg A, DePuey E, et al: Evaluation of ventricular performance using gated blood pool SPECT: a multicenter study, *J Nucl Med* 41:5P, 2000. (abstract).
165. Groch M, Marshall R, Erwin W, et al: Left ventricular ejection fraction computed from gated SPECT blood pool imaging correlates with conventional planar imaging, *J Nucl Med* 41:98P, 2000. (abstract).
166. Groch MW, Erwin WD, DePuey EG, et al: Multicenter clinical evaluation of gated blood pool SPECT for the assessment of ventricular function, *Eur J Nucl Med* 28:PS85, 2001. (abstract).
167. Keng F, Chua T, Koh T: Quantitative blood pool single-photon emission computed tomography (QBS) program: comparison with conventional planar equilibrium blood pool imaging (MUGA), *J Nucl Cardiol* 10:S25, 2003. (abstract).
168. Keng F, Tan H, Chua T: Gated SPECT blood pool imaging: a comparison with equilibrium blood pool imaging, *J Nucl Cardiol* 7:S3, 2000. (abstract).
169. Nakajima K, Higuchi T, Taki J, et al: Quantitative gated SPECT with myocardial perfusion and blood-pool studies to determine ventricular volumes and stroke volume ratio in congenital heart diseases, *J Nucl Cardiol* 10:S11, 2003. (abstract).

170. Nichols K, Saouaf R, Ababneh AA, et al: Validation of SPECT equilibrium radionuclide angiographic right ventricular parameters by cardiac magnetic resonance imaging, *J Nucl Cardiol* 9:153–160, 2002.

171. Rouzet F, Ederhy S, Daou D, et al: Respective role of inter and intraventricular delays in patients candidates to biventricular pacing evaluated by multiharmonic analysis of radionuclide angiography, *J Nucl Med* 45:242P, 2004. (abstract).

172. Schwartz R, Le Guludec D, Holder L, et al: Blood pool gated SPECT: validation of left ventricular volumes and ejection fraction with planar radionuclide angiography, *J Nucl Cardiol* 7:S2, 2000. (abstract).

173. Stadius ML, Williams DL, Harp G, et al: Left ventricular volume determination using single-photon emission computed tomography, *Am J Cardiol* 55:1185–1191, 1985.

174. Underwood SR, Walton S, Ell PJ, et al: Gated blood-pool emission tomography: a new technique for the investigation of cardiac structure and function, *Eur J Nucl Med* 10:332–337, 1985.

175. Van Kriekinge S, Berman D, Germano G: Automatic quantification of left and right ventricular ejection fractions from gated blood pool SPECT, *Circulation* 100:I–26, 1999. (abstract).

176. Van Kriekinge S, Paul AK, Hasegawa S, et al: Validation of quantitative left-ventricular end-diastolic and end-systolic volumes from gated blood pool SPECT, *J Am Coll Cardiol* 37:500A, 2001. (abstract).

177. Van Kriekinge SD, Berman DS, Germano G: Automatic quantification of left ventricular ejection fraction from gated blood pool SPECT, *J Nucl Cardiol* 6:498–506, 1999.

178. Vanhove C, Everaert H, Bossuyt A, Franken P: Automatic determination of LV ejection fraction and volumes by gated blood pool SPECT, *J Nucl Med* 41:187P, 2000. (abstract).

179. Vanhove C, Franken PR: Left ventricular ejection fraction and volumes from gated blood pool tomography: Comparison between two automatic algorithms that work in three-dimensional space, *J Nucl Cardiol* 8:466–471, 2001.

180. Smanio PE, Watson DD, Segalla DL, et al: Value of gating of technetium-99m sestamibi single-photon emission computed tomographic imaging, *J Am Coll Cardiol* 30:1687–1692, 1997.

181. Taillefer R, DePuey EG, Udelson JE, et al: Comparative diagnostic accuracy of Tl-201 and Tc-99m sestamibi SPECT imaging (perfusion and ECG-gated SPECT) in detecting coronary artery disease in women, *J Am Coll Cardiol* 29:69–77, 1997.

182. Choi JY, Lee KH, Kim SJ, et al: Gating provides improved accuracy for differentiating artifacts from true lesions in equivocal fixed defects on technetium 99m tetrofosmin perfusion SPECT, *J Nucl Cardiol* 5:395–401, 1998.

183. Links JM, DePuey EG, Taillefer R, Becker LC: Attenuation correction and gating synergistically improve the diagnostic accuracy of myocardial perfusion SPECT, *J Nucl Cardiol* 9:183–187, 2002.

184. Hendel RC, Corbett JR, Cullom SJ, et al: The value and practice of attenuation correction for myocardial perfusion SPECT imaging: A joint position statement from the American Society of Nuclear Cardiology and the Society of Nuclear Medicine, *J Nucl Med* 43:273–280, 2002.

185. O'Connor MK, Kemp B, Anstett F, et al: A multicenter evaluation of commercial attenuation compensation techniques in cardiac SPECT using phantom models, *J Nucl Cardiol* 9:361–376, 2002.

186. Bateman TM, Kolobrodov VV, Vasin AP, O'Keefe JH Jr: Extended acquisition for minimizing attenuation artifact in SPECT cardiac perfusion imaging, *J Nucl Med* 35:625–627, 1994.

187. Gibson PB, Demus D, Noto R, et al: Low event rate for stress-only perfusion imaging in patients evaluated for chest pain, *J Am Coll Cardiol* 39:999–1004, 2002.

188. Heller GV, Bateman TM, Botvinick EH, et al: Value of attenuation correction in interpretation of stress only exercise Tc-99m sestamibi SPECT imaging: Results of a multicenter trial, *J Am Coll Cardiol* 39:343A, 2002. (abstract).

189. Santana CA, Garcia EV, Vansant JP, et al: Gated stress-only Tc-99m myocardial perfusion SPECT imaging accurately assesses coronary artery disease, *Nucl Med Commun* 24:241–249, 2003.

190. Thompson RC, Heller GV, Johnson LL, et al: Value of attenuation correction on ECG-gated SPECT myocardial perfusion imaging related to body mass index, *J Nucl Cardiol* 12:195–202, 2005.

191. Chua T, Kiat H, Germano G, et al: Gated technetium-99m sestamibi for simultaneous assessment of stress myocardial perfusion, postexercise regional ventricular function and myocardial viability. Correlation with echocardiography and rest thallium-201 scintigraphy, *J Am Coll Cardiol* 23:1107–1114, 1994.

192. Sharir T, Bacher-Stier C, Dhar S, et al: Identification of severe and extensive coronary artery disease by postexercise regional wall motion abnormalities in Tc-99m sestamibi gated single-photon emission computed tomography, *Am J Cardiol* 86:1171–1175, 2000.

193. Emmett L, Iwanochko RM, Freeman MR, et al: Reversible regional wall motion abnormalities on exercise technetium-99m-gated cardiac single photon emission computed tomography

194. Lima RSL, Watson DD, Goode AR, et al: Incremental value of combined perfusion and function over perfusion alone by gated SPECT myocardial perfusion imaging for detection of severe three-vessel coronary artery disease, *J Am Coll Cardiol* 42:64–70, 2003.

195. Abidov A, Bax JJ, Hayes SW, et al: Transient ischemic dilation ratio of the left ventricle is a significant predictor of future cardiac events in patients with otherwise normal myocardial perfusion SPECT, *J Am Coll Cardiol* 42:1818–1825, 2003.

196. Hachamovitch R, Rozanski A, Hayes SW, et al: Predicting therapeutic benefit from myocardial revascularization procedures: Are measurements of both resting left ventricular ejection fraction and stress-induced myocardial ischemia necessary, *J Nucl Cardiol* 13:768–778, 2006.

197. Berman DS, Kang X, Slomka PJ, et al: Underestimation of extent of ischemia by gated SPECT myocardial perfusion imaging in patients with left main coronary artery disease, *J Nucl Cardiol* 14:521–528, 2007.

198. Johnson SH, Bigelow C, Lee KL, et al: Prediction of death and myocardial infarction by radionuclide angiocardiography in patients with suspected coronary artery disease, *Am J Cardiol* 67:919–926, 1991.

199. Jones RH, Johnson SH, Bigelow C, et al: Exercise radionuclide angiocardiography predicts cardiac death in patients with coronary artery disease, *Circulation* 84:I52–I58, 1991.

200. Lee KL, Pryor DB, Pieper KS, et al: Prognostic value of radionuclide angiography in medically treated patients with coronary artery disease. A comparison with clinical and catheterization variables, *Circulation* 82:1705–1717, 1990.

201. Morris KG, Palmeri ST, Califf RM, et al: Value of radionuclide angiography for predicting specific cardiac events after acute myocardial infarction, *Am J Cardiol* 55:318–324, 1985.

202. Pryor DB, Harrell FE Jr, Lee KL, et al: Prognostic indicators from radionuclide angiography in medically treated patients with coronary artery disease, *Am J Cardiol* 53:18–22, 1984.

203. Upton MT, Palmeri ST, Jones RH, et al: Assessment of left ventricular function by resting and exercise radionuclide angiocardiography following acute myocardial infarction, *Am Heart J* 104:1232–1243, 1982.

204. Sharir T, Germano G, Kavanagh PB, et al: Incremental prognostic value of post-stress left ventricular ejection fraction and volume by gated myocardial perfusion single photon emission computed tomography, *Circulation* 100:1035–1042, 1999.

205. Sharir T, Germano G, Kang XP, et al: Prediction of myocardial infarction versus cardiac death by gated myocardial perfusion SPECT: Risk stratification by the amount of stress-induced ischemia and the poststress ejection fraction, *J Nucl Med* 42:831–837, 2001.

206. Hachamovitch R: Personal communication, 2006.

207. Klocke FJ, Baird MG, Lorell BH, et al: ACC/AHA/ASNC guidelines for the clinical use of cardiac radionuclide imaging—Executive summary—A report of the American College of Cardiology/American Heart Association Task Force on Practice Guidelines (ACC/AHA/ASNC Committee to revise the 1995 guidelines for the clinical use of cardiac radionuclide imaging), *J Am Coll Cardiol* 42:1318–1333, 2003.

208. Liao L, Smith WT, Tuttle RH, et al: Prediction of death and nonfatal myocardial infarction in high-risk patients: A comparison between the Duke treadmill score, peak exercise radionuclide angiography, and SPECT perfusion imaging, *J Nucl Med* 46:5–11, 2005.

209. Thomas GS, Miyamoto MI, Morello AP, et al: Technetium(99m) sestamibi myocardial perfusion imaging predicts clinical outcome in the community outpatient setting—The Nuclear Utility in the Community (NUC) Study, *J Am Coll Cardiol* 43:213–223, 2004.

210. Travin MI, Heller GV, Johnson LL, et al: The prognostic value of ECG-gated SPECT imaging in patients undergoing stress Tc-99m sestamibi myocardial perfusion imaging, *J Nucl Cardiol* 11:253–262, 2004.

211. Petix NR, Sestini S, Coppola A, et al: Prognostic value of combined perfusion and function by stress technetium-99m Sestamibi gated SPECT myocardial perfusion imaging in patients with suspected or known coronary artery disease, *Am J Cardiol* 95:1351–1357, 2005.

212. Mast ST, Shaw LK, Ravizzini GC, et al: Incremental prognostic value of RNA ejection fraction measurements during pharmacologic stress testing: A comparison with clinical and perfusion variables, *J Nucl Med* 42:871–877, 2001.

213. Hachamovitch R, Hayes SW, Friedman JD, et al: Comparison of the short-term survival benefit associated with revascularization compared with medical therapy in patients with no prior coronary artery disease undergoing stress myocardial perfusion single photon emission computed tomography, *Circulation* 107:2900–2907, 2003.

214. Abidov A, Germano G, Hachamovitch R, Berman DS: Gated SPECT in assessment of regional and global left ventricular function: Major tool of modern nuclear imaging, *J Nucl Cardiol* 13:261–279, 2006.

215. Cheitlin MD, Armstrong WF, Aurigemma GP, et al: ACC/AHA/ASE 2003 guideline update for the clinical application of echocardiography: Summary article: A report of the American College of Cardiology/American Heart Association Task Force on Practice Guidelines (ACC/AHA/ASE Committee to update the 1997 guidelines for the clinical application of echocardiography), *Circulation* 108: 1146–1162, 2003.

216. Leoncini M, Marcucci G, Sciagrà R, et al: Nitrate-enhanced gated technetium 99m sestamibi SPECT for evaluating regional wall motion at baseline and during low-dose dobutamine infusion in patients with chronic coronary artery disease and left ventricular dysfunction: comparison with two-dimensional echocardiography, *J Nucl Cardiol* 7:426–431, 2000.

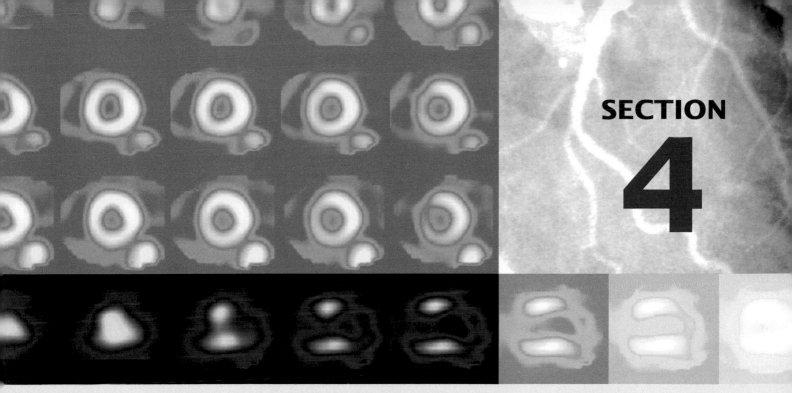

Perfusion Imaging

Chapter 14

Coronary Artery Disease Detection: Exercise Stress SPECT

RAYMOND R. RUSSELL AND FRANS J. TH. WACKERS

INTRODUCTION

In the United States alone, more than 7.7 million patients are referred yearly for diagnostic cardiac stress testing with radionuclide imaging. Although patients may require pharmacologic stress testing because they are unable to perform adequate physical exercise, dynamic exercise on treadmill or bicycle remains the preferred stress modality. In our nuclear stress laboratory, the percentage of myocardial perfusion studies performed with exercise has remained approximately 50% since 2004. Exercise variables, including maximal workload, duration, hemodynamic response, exercise-induced symptoms, and electrocardiographic (ECG) changes provide invaluable additional information for assessing a patient's prognosis that are not available with pharmacologic stress. The Duke exercise treadmill score incorporates some of these important exercise variables and allows for risk stratification.[1] However, because of the inherent diagnostic limitations of the exercise ECG and subjective symptoms, patients stratified by the Duke Treadmill Score can be further stratified on the basis of (semi)quantitative stress radionuclide myocardial perfusion imaging (MPI).[2]

PHYSIOLOGY OF EXERCISE STRESS TESTING

Dynamic exercise increases the metabolic demand of the exercising skeletal muscle which can be met only by increasing the blood flow to the exercising muscle. Under conditions of maximal exertion, the cardiac output may increase more than fourfold to meet this need.[3] As shown in Figure 14-1, at low levels of exercise, the increase in cardiac output is due to an increase in both stroke volume and heart rate. However, as the intensity of exercise increases, the contribution of the stroke volume to cardiac output reaches a plateau, and the augmentation of cardiac output becomes primarily dependent on the ability to increase the heart rate further. Of note, the inability to appropriately increase the heart rate in response to exercise predicts severity of coronary artery disease (CAD) and mortality.[4,5] The increase in cardiac output results in a greater myocardial metabolic demand, inducing coronary vasodilation. A recent positron emission tomography (PET) study in human subjects quantifying the change in myocardial perfusion with exercise demonstrated that myocardial blood flow can increase more than fourfold to meet the metabolic demands of the heart during exercise.[6]

The above-mentioned hemodynamic changes occur through both neurohormonal and metabolic mechanisms. With the onset of exercise, heart rate and stroke volume both increase through sympathetic activation and parasympathetic withdrawal. During exercise there are several peripheral effects that augment the effects provided by the central sympathetic activation. These include α-adrenergic stimulation of the venous capacitance vessels, resulting in venoconstriction and enhanced venous return, which will increase preload and cardiac inotropy. In addition, skeletal muscle production of lactic acid and adenosine during exercise causes dilation of the arteriolar resistance vessels, reducing the systemic vascular resistance and thereby increasing cardiac output and blood flow to the exercising skeletal muscle.

Metabolic changes occur in association with these hemodynamic adaptations. Specifically, in exercising skeletal muscles, there is a decreasing dependence on fatty acid oxidation and an increasing dependence on glucose oxidation to meet the energy needs until maximum oxygen consumption is achieved. At that point, glucose is the exclusive oxidative substrate. Further

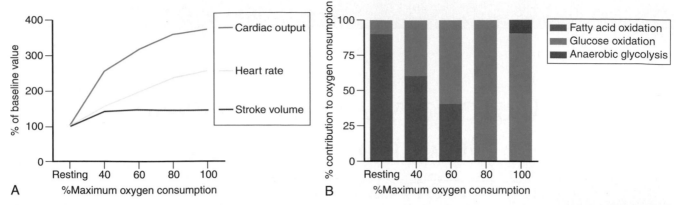

Figure 14-1 Hemodynamic and metabolic responses to exercise. **A,** During low levels of exercise, the increase in cardiac output is due to increases in both heart rate and stroke volume. However, as the exercise increases, stroke volume cannot increase further, and the augmentation of cardiac output is due to continued increases in heart rate. These changes are related to increased sympathetic drive as well as withdrawal of parasympathetic stimulation to the heart. **B,** Under resting, fasted conditions, fatty acid oxidation is the predominant fuel source for the body. However, with increasing levels of exercise, glucose oxidation plays an increasingly important role in meeting the energy demands of the exercising skeletal muscle. At the point of exhaustion, anaerobic glycolysis and glucose oxidation are required to meet the energy demands.

increases in the level of exercise above the anaerobic threshold cause the release of lactate from exercising skeletal muscle. Interestingly and in contrast, with increasing exercise, the myocardium continues to oxidize both fatty acids and glucose and also increases the utilization of lactate produced by the exercising skeletal muscle for energy (see Fig. 14-1).

The intensity of exercise can continue to increase until the point at which the heart cannot meet the metabolic demands of the exercising muscles (i.e., blood flow to muscles can no longer provide adequate amounts of substrate or remove metabolic byproducts). In the case of a healthy individual, this is generally at the level of the exercising skeletal muscle. However, in the case of an individual with critical coronary artery stenoses, the inability to exercise can be due to the limited ability to provide adequate blood flow to the heart muscle. It is in this latter scenario that myocardial ischemia is manifested and provides the rationale for exercise stress testing.

Table 14-1 Contraindications to Exercise Stress Testing

Absolute Contraindications	Relative Contraindications
Acute myocardial infarction	Aortic stenosis
Unstable angina	Suspected left main equivalent
Acute myocarditis or pericarditis	Severe hypertension (>240/130)
Ongoing ventricular or atrial tachyarrhythmias	Severe outflow tract obstruction
Second- or third-degree heart block	Left bundle branch block
Known severe left main disease	
Decompensated heart failure	
Acutely ill patients	
Patients unable to exercise due to neurologic or musculoskeletal limitations	

EXERCISE PROTOCOLS

In the United States, most exercise tests are performed using a motorized treadmill and graded Bruce, modified Bruce, or Naughton protocols. In many other countries, the upright bicycle is the preferred exercise equipment. An important aspect of diagnostic exercise protocols is the gradual, linear increase in workload from a very low level to the maximally tolerated workload. This gradual increase in workload is of importance, since the purpose of physical exercise testing is to reproduce symptoms, and one can generally not predict at which workload symptoms will occur. It is therefore important to also evaluate the patient carefully prior to starting a stress test to determine if the patient is appropriate for exercise stress testing (Table 14-1). Exercise protocols are generally terminated because of the onset of symptoms or fatigue, but they may also be

terminated because of the development of significant ECG changes or because the patient becomes hypotensive or develops pulmonary edema. Termination of exercise solely because the predicted target heart rate (85% of age-predicted max) was achieved is a commonly made mistake. Many elderly patients, for example, are capable of achieving a considerably higher heart rate and workload at which symptoms may be unmasked.

PREPARATION FOR EXERCISE

As mentioned, the purpose of exercise testing is to provoke and to reproduce ischemic symptoms during maximal physical effort. The patient should be well informed about the details of the procedure and be motivated to give his/her best effort. Cardioactive medications, such as β-blockers, calcium blockers, or nitrates, may diminish the sensitivity of testing. Therefore, if the exercise test is performed specifically to diagnose CAD in a patient with no prior cardiac history, such medications should be stopped for at least 24 hours and in the case of long-acting medications, 48 hours before the day of testing. On the other hand, in patients with known CAD, a physician may be more interested in the results of testing with the patient on his/her routine medication, which will provide insight into the effectiveness of treatment.

Patients should be instructed to wear comfortable clothing and shoes and be in a fasted state on the morning of the exercise test. Moreover, it is prudent to instruct all patients scheduled for stress testing not to consume any caffeine-containing beverages or food on the morning of testing. The reason for this is that it is not uncommon that a patient is not able to perform adequate exercise. If the patient has not consumed caffeine-containing items, it is easy to switch to pharmacologic stress and ensure a diagnostic test result without having to reschedule the patient. On the other hand, a recent study suggested that a small amount of caffeine does not significantly affect the presence and magnitude of perfusion abnormalities. Although it appears prudent to continue to recommend that patients abstain from caffeine usage prior to the test, consumption of a single cup of coffee may not be a valid reason for cancellation of a vasodilator stress test.[7]

BASIS OF STRESS IMAGING

The conceptual underpinning of radionuclide imaging is the visualization of heterogeneity of regional myocardial blood flow secondary to impaired regional coronary flow reserve downstream of coronary arteries with significant obstructive disease (Fig. 14-2).

In order to visualize such heterogeneity of blood flow reliably, a linear relationship must exist between regional myocardial blood flow and regional myocardial uptake of a radiotracer.[8] Although in general this is true for relatively low flow ranges (up to 1 mL/min/g), as is present under resting conditions and resting myocardial ischemia, at the higher flow ranges (>2 mL/min/g) achieved during stress, especially during vasodilator stress, regional myocardial radiotracer uptake may no longer be linear. At higher rates of blood flow, the uptake of many radiotracers presently used in clinical imaging demonstrates a plateau (Fig. 14-3) known as the *roll-off phenomenon*.

The suboptimal linearity at higher flow ranges is caused by the limited first-pass extraction fraction of many single-photon radiopharmaceuticals used for MPI. Table 14-2 shows the myocardial extraction fractions of commonly used radiotracers. In addition to myocardial extraction fraction, mechanisms involved in the transmembrane transport and myocardial washout and wash-in affect net myocardial uptake of radiopharmaceuticals. Fortunately this roll-off phenomenon does not significantly affect the ability to identify

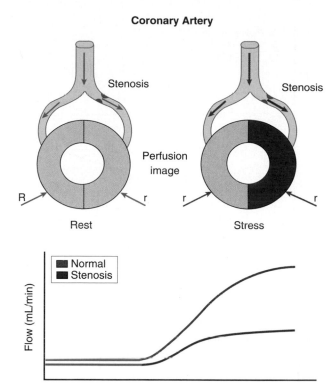

Coronary Artery

Figure 14-2 Schematic representation of the principle of rest/stress myocardial perfusion imaging. *Top*: Two branches of a coronary artery are schematically shown; the left branch is normal, and the right branch has a significant stenosis. *Middle*: Rest and stress myocardial perfusion images of the territories supplied by the two branches. *Bottom*: Schematic representation of coronary blood flow in the coronary branches at rest and during stress. At rest, myocardial blood flow is similar in both coronary artery branches. Coronary blood flow in the abnormal vascular bed was maintained through autoregulatory mechanisms that lower vascular resistance (r) distal of a significant stenosis. When a myocardial perfusion imaging agent is injected at rest, myocardial uptake therefore will be homogenous *(normal image on the left)*. During stress, peripheral vascular resistance (R) decreases in the normal bed (r), resulting in a 2 to 2.5-fold increase of blood flow over baseline. In the abnormal bed, distal from the stenosis, peripheral vascular resistance (r) cannot decrease much further. This creates heterogeneity of regional myocardial blood flow that can be visualized with thallium-201- or technetium-99m-labeled agents as an area with relatively decreased radiotracer uptake *(darker left area on stress image)*. *(Modified from Wackers FJ: Exercise myocardial perfusion imaging, J Nucl Med 35:726–729, 1994.)*

patients with high-degree (>70%) coronary stenoses. However, in patients with relatively mild CAD, the roll-off phenomenon may potentially result in falsely normal images (Fig. 14-4).

Thallium (^{201}Tl), a potassium analog, has a relatively high initial extraction fraction and good linearity to flow. After intravenous administration, continuous washout and wash-in occurs in the myocardium, resulting in Tl-201 myocardial redistribution. Technetium (^{99m}Tc)-labeled agents, such as sestamibi and tetrofosmin, are lipophilic compounds that have lower first-pass extraction fractions than ^{201}Tl and bind to mitochondrial membranes in a stable manner based on the mitochondrial membrane potential, and demonstrate

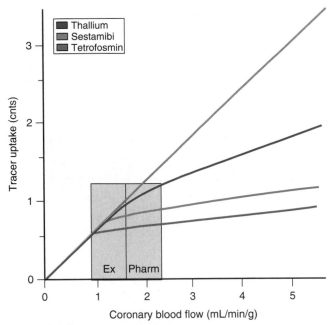

Figure 14-3 Relationship between coronary blood flow and radiotracer uptake. An ideal flow imaging agent would be plotted on the line of identity. All commonly used radiotracers deviate below the line of identity and show a plateau ("roll-off") at higher blood flow levels. Typical ranges of coronary blood flow during physical exercise (EX) and pharmacologic vasodilation (Pharm) are shown. As shown on the graph, the roll-off is the least for thallium-201 and more for technetium-99m sestamibi and ^{99m}Tc tetrofosmin.

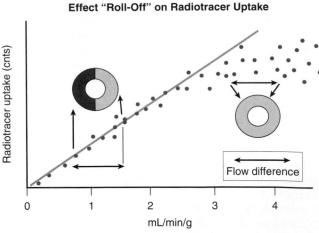

Figure 14-4 Effect of radiotracer "roll-off" on myocardial perfusion images. In the graph, regional myocardial uptake of a radiotracer is plotted against regional coronary blood flow. The radiotracer shows significant roll-off at flows exceeding 2.5 mL/min/g. In the relative low flow range, because of good linearity of uptake, a myocardial region with 0.75 mL/min/g has significantly less radiotracer uptake than a region with1.5 mL/min/g, resulting in an abnormal image with defect *(left image)*. However, at higher flow ranges, a similar 0.75 mL/min/g flow difference may result in no significant difference in myocardial radiotracer uptake and in a normal image without perfusion defect *(right image)*.

Table 14-2 First-Pass Myocardial Extraction Fraction of Various Radiopharmaceuticals

Thallium-201	82%–88%
Technetium (^{99m}Tc) sestamibi	55%–68%
^{99m}Tc tetrofosmin	54%
^{99m}Tc teboroxime	>90%
^{99m}Tc NOET	75%–85%

minimal washout. Consequently the ultimate net retention of ^{201}Tl-labeled and ^{99m}Tc-labeled agents in the myocardium is similar.[9]

INJECTION OF RADIOTRACER

The timing of injection of radiotracer relative to peak exercise and termination of exercise is an important and often not well-appreciated aspect of stress testing. Because the first-pass extraction of the radiotracers is not 100%, myocardial uptake of a radiotracer is not instantaneous at the moment of injection. After injection during stress, the injected bolus reaches the central circulation in about 10 to 15 seconds, and first-pass myocardial extraction takes place. After the initial first transit, recirculation occurs with a rapidly decreasing blood concentration of radiotracer. On average, it takes about 1.5 to 2 minutes for blood radioactivity to decrease to 50% of maximum (Fig. 14-5).

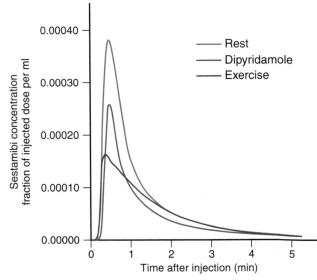

Figure 14-5 Blood clearance of radiotracer. Arterial blood disappearance curve of technetium-99m-sestamibi after injection at peak exercise or pharmacologic vasodilation with dipyridamole. Peak blood pool activity occurs at 0.5 minute for both exercise and pharmacologic testing. At 1.5 minutes after injection, the blood pool activity is 50% of maximum for exercise stress testing. The decrease in blood pool activity is relatively quicker for pharmacologic stress testing. *(From Sand NP, Juelsgaard P, Rasmussen K, et al.: Arterial concentration of ^{99m}Tc-sestamibi at rest, during peak exercise and after dipyridamole infusion. Clin Physiol Funct Imaging 24:394–397, 2004.)*

This may differ among patients, depending on the level of exercise effort. Furthermore, blood clearance curves are different for various radiotracers (e.g., slightly faster for ^{99m}Tc-labeled agents than for ^{201}Tl). The timing of radioisotope injection is based on the fact that it is important to have most of the dose accumulate in the myocardium under conditions in which the heterogeneity of blood flow is maximal, that is, at peak exercise. Termination of exercise at about 1 minute after injection, as is frequently done in clinical practice, may be too early. A substantial amount of radiotracer may still be recirculating at that time. Therefore, it is advisable to encourage patients to continue exercising for at least 2 minutes after injection of radiotracer.

IMAGING PROTOCOLS

Reliable interpretation of stress myocardial perfusion images depends for a large part on optimal quality images. Consistently good quality can be ensured by following image acquisition guidelines published by the American Society of Nuclear Cardiology.[10]

Two important variables affect quality of images: the amount of radiotracer injected and imaging time. The injected dose can be adjusted to a patient's weight, keeping in mind the balance between the image quality and radiation exposure. Imaging time, or time per stop per projection, can also be adjusted to the dose and the patient's weight. One way to anticipate suboptimal image quality is to record the count rate emanating from a patient's chest before setting image acquisition parameters. If the count rate is less than that usually recorded for good-quality studies, the time per stop should be lengthened.

At present, four image-acquisition protocols are most commonly used: the 1-day or 2-day rest-exercise ^{99m}Tc-agent imaging protocol, the exercise-redistribution Tl-201 imaging protocol, and the rest/exercise dual-isotope imaging protocol. Numerous studies have shown that each of these protocols yields equivalent clinical results for detection of CAD and for risk stratification. If many patients referred to an imaging facility are overweight (body mass index > 30 kg/m^2), ^{99m}Tc-labeled agents and 2-day imaging protocols may be preferred. The most frequently used imaging protocols for ^{201}Tl and ^{99m}Tc-labeled agents are schematically shown in Figure 14-6A-D. Technical details of imaging are tabulated in Table 14-3.

Increasing attention is being paid to the radiation exposure associated with imaging procedures, including myocardial perfusion studies. The exposure and the biological effect of radiation, generally assessed in terms of the effective dose, is dependent not only on the absolute amount of radioactivity that is injected but also the quality of the radiation that is emitted, which is the same for the gamma-photon emitting radionuclides used in single-photon emission computed tomography (SPECT) MPI, the half-life of the agent, and the sensitivities of specific organs to the radiation. Based on these factors, the lowest effective dose is

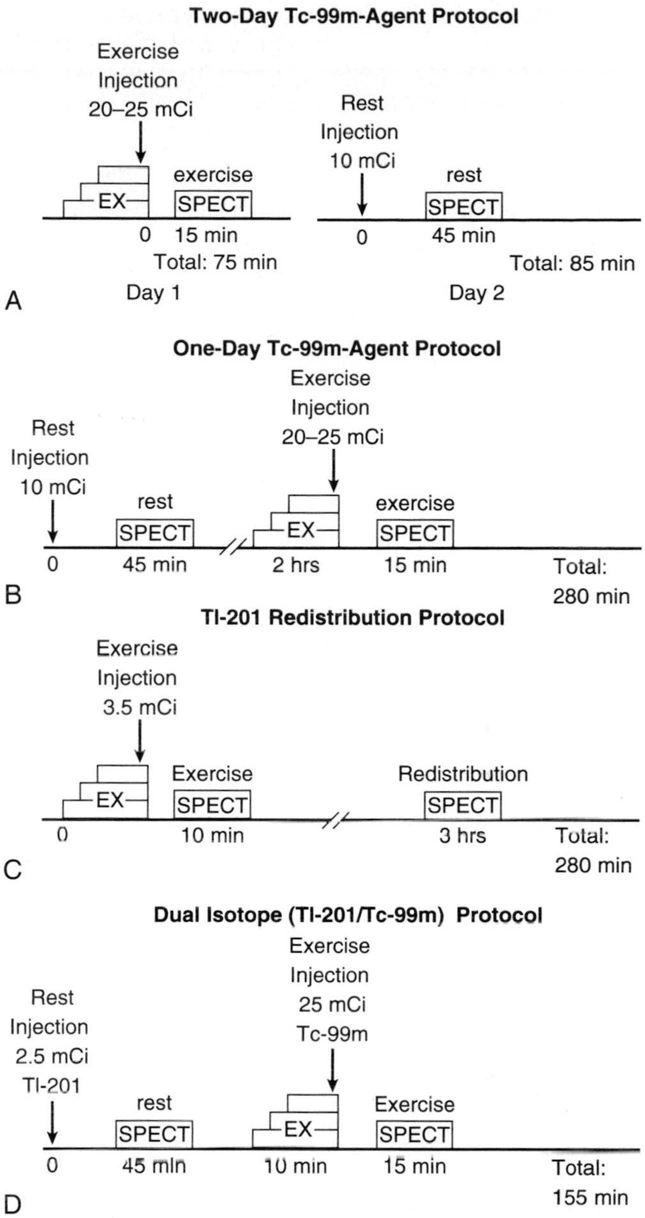

Figure 14-6 Commonly used rest/exercise (EX) SPECT imaging protocols. **A,** Two-day imaging protocol used for ^{99m}Tc-based radiotracer stress/rest imaging, typically used in obese patients. **B,** One-day imaging used for Tc-99m-based radiotracer stress/rest imaging, typically used in nonobese patients. **C,** One-day, stress-redistribution imaging protocol used for thallium-201 imaging. **D,** One-day, dual-isotope imaging protocol. Time intervals and total protocol times are shown.

achieved with ^{99m}Tc-labeled agents used in a 1-day stress/rest protocol, whereas the highest effective dose is achieved with a dual-isotope protocol (Table 14-4).[11] In patients with low to intermediate pretest likelihood of CAD, normal exercise parameters, and normal MPI, it may be possible to perform only stress imaging, thereby reducing the radiation exposure.

Table 14-3 Summary of Typical Acquisition Parameters for SPECT Myocardial Perfusion Imaging with ^{201}Tl and ^{99m}Tc-Labeled Imaging Agents

	^{201}Tl	^{99m}Tc Agents	^{99m}Tc Agents
Dose	3.5–4 mCi	Low: 10–15 mCi	High: 20–30 mCi
Start Imaging After Injection:			
During exercise	10–15 min	15–30 min	15–30 min
During pharmacologic	5–10 min	45–60 min	45–60 min
At rest	45 min	45–60 min	45–60 min
Imaging interval:			
Redistribution Stress/rest, rest/stress	2–4 hr	1–4 hr	1–4 hr
Imaging position	Supine or prone	Supine or prone	Supine or prone
Collimator	Low-energy, all-purpose	Low-energy, high-resolution	Low-energy, high-resolution
Orbit	Circular 180°	Circular, 360° or 180°	Circular, 360° or 180°
Energy peak	70 keV 167 keV	140 keV	140 keV
Energy window	20% and 30% symmetric	20% symmetric	20% symmetric
Matrix	64 × 64	64 × 64	64 × 64
Pixel size	6.4. ± 0.2 mm	6.4. ± 0.2 mm	6.4.± 0.2 mm
Acquisition type	Step-and-shoot	Step-and-shoot	Step-and-shoot
No. of projections	32	64	64
Time/projection	40 sec	25 sec	20 sec
Total imaging time	22 min	27 min	22 min

Table 14-4 Estimated Effective Doses for Various Myocardial Perfusion Imaging Protocols

Protocol	Effective Dose (mSv)
Thallium stress/redistribution	22.0
One-day stress/rest ^{99m}Tc sestamibi	11.3
Two-day stress/rest ^{99m}Tc sestamibi	15.7
One-day stress/rest ^{99m}Tc tetrofosmin	9.3
Two-day stress/rest ^{99m}Tc tetrofosmin	12.8

Based on data from Einstein AJ, Moser KW, Thompson RC, et al: Radiation dose to patients from cardiac diagnostic imaging. Circulation 116:1290–1305, 2007.

DIAGNOSTIC VALUE OF EXERCISE SPECT IMAGING

Since the introduction of stress radionuclide MPI in the mid-1970s, numerous clinical studies have demonstrated the clinical usefulness for detection of CAD. The main objective of exercise SPECT imaging in present-day clinical practice is still predominantly to elucidate whether symptoms suggestive of CAD, such as chest discomfort or dyspnea on exertion, are caused by CAD or whether other etiologies should be pursued. Management decisions may then be guided by extensive published evidence that certain image patterns have important prognostic significance.

Because of the proven prognostic value of stress MPI, it is unlikely that angiographic correlation and sensitivity and specificity will continue to be assessed in large numbers of patients using state-of-the-art technology, other than for local quality assurance purposes or to evaluate new technical advances such as attenuation-correction devices. The sensitivity, specificity, and normalcy values for exercise SPECT MPI have been evaluated in multiple studies and confirm the diagnostic power of this modality.[12–24] Based on a meta-analysis of 79 studies that included a total of 8964 patients, the sensitivity, specificity, and normalcy rate of SPECT MPI are 86%, 74%, and 89%, respectively.[25,26] Figure 14-7 shows representative data for the diagnostic yield for identifying disease in individual coronary arteries.[27] Sensitivity for recognizing disease in the left anterior descending coronary artery is higher than that for disease in the right coronary artery or left circumflex coronary artery, with no significant difference in accuracy. The relatively low specificity of SPECT imaging suggests that artifacts due to attenuation and motion are not always recognized. Referral bias has been proposed as another potential explanation for the limited specificity of SPECT imaging.

Through the years, it has also become clear that complete agreement with coronary angiography is an elusive goal, because stress perfusion imaging and coronary angiography evaluate two different aspects of CAD. Whereas contrast coronary angiography visualizes coronary anatomy and the presence or absence of regional coronary luminal narrowings, radionuclide stress MPI provides noninvasive information about the pathophysiologic consequences of coronary atherosclerosis. Specifically, patients with apparently significant angiographic

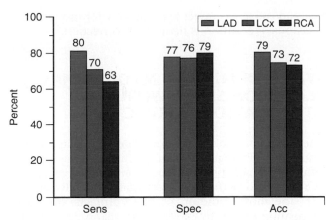

Figure 14-7 Detection of coronary artery disease in individual coronary arteries. The sensitivity (Sens), specificity (Spec), and accuracy (Acc) for detecting $\geq 50\%$ stenosis in the left anterior descending coronary artery (LAD), right coronary artery (RCA), and left circumflex coronary artery (LCx) are shown. *(Reproduced with permission from Elhendy A, Sozzi FB, van Domburg RT, et al: Accuracy of exercise stress technetium-99m sestamibi SPECT imaging in the evaluation of the extent and location of coronary artery disease in patients with an earlier myocardial infarction, J Nucl Cardiol 7:432–438, 2000.)*

CAD but normal exercise myocardial perfusion images nevertheless have a favorable prognosis.[28] In contrast, patients with relatively mild angiographic CAD but markedly abnormal SPECT images have a less favorable outcome. One study[29] demonstrated that in patients with apparently "false-positive" [201]Tl images and "normal" epicardial coronary arteries, coronary blood flow response to acetylcholine infusion was blunted, indicating endothelial dysfunction (Fig. 14-8). This suggests

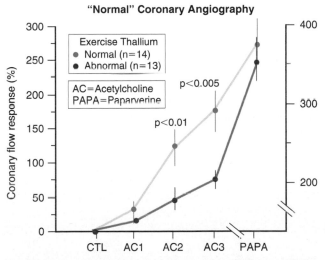

Figure 14-8 Impaired endothelium-dependent vasodilation in abnormal exercise SPECT. Coronary blood flow response to increasing doses of acetylcholine (AC) and to papaverine (PAPA) in patients with normal or minimally diseased (<30% luminal narrowing) epicardial coronary arteries and abnormal (n = 13) or normal (n = 14) exercise SPECT thallium-201 (^{201}Tl) imaging. Patients with abnormal ^{201}Tl SPECT showed blunted response to endothelial-dependent vasodilation with AC compared to those with normal ^{201}Tl SPECT. *(Modified from Zeiher AM, Krause T, Schachinger V, et al: Impaired endothelium-dependent vasodilation of coronary resistance vessels is associated with exercise-induced myocardial ischemia. Circulation 91:2345–2352, 1995.)*

that "false-positive" images probably were true positives. A better measure of the true specificity of stress MPI is the assessment of normalcy rate in subjects with low (<3%) likelihood of CAD. In our own laboratory, the normalcy rate of ^{99m}Tc sestamibi SPECT was 99% using quantitative analysis of exercise myocardial perfusion SPECT images acquired in 40 normal subjects.

ECG-GATED SPECT

Evaluating the left ventricular ejection fraction (LVEF) is important in any cardiac patient. Currently, more than 80% of all SPECT studies are acquired with ECG gating. Gated SPECT provides a means of assessing postexercise resting LVEF, as well as regional wall motion and wall thickening. The routine assessment of LVEF by ECG-gated SPECT has added an important dimension to the overall assessment of patients referred for exercise testing and MPI.[30] Although the appearance of motion and the change in count density on cine display of ECG-gated SPECT myocardial perfusion studies is in fact artifactual and caused by improved count recovery during the cardiac cycle due to diminishing partial volume effect, a linear relationship exists with myocardial thickening.[31]

Assessment of LVEF, either normal or abnormal, in a patient with exercise-induced ischemia has important clinical and management consequences.[32,33] Furthermore, it is not rare that a patient is diagnosed as having a previously unknown cardiomyopathy on the basis of the information from a gated SPECT. In some patients, postexercise LVEF may be significantly lower than LVEF on rest SPECT imaging.[34] This may indicate postexercise ischemic stunning, which is a marker signifying severe CAD, although the specificity of this finding reflecting stunning may be limited in the setting of a large reversible defect.[35]

Visual assessment of regional myocardial thickening on gated SPECT has also improved the diagnostic yield of exercise MPI by improving identification of attenuation artifacts and thereby increasing the certainty of the image interpretation. Specifically, the inspection of gated SPECT images has been shown to decrease the number of "borderline" interpretations by 68%, increasing the number of normal studies in patients with a low likelihood of CAD and increasing the detection of abnormal perfusion in patients with a known history of CAD.[36]

When nongated exercise thallium SPECT was compared to ECG-gated exercise sestamibi SPECT images in women, specificity improved from 67% to 92%, mainly because of better identification of breast attenuation.[37] A fixed defect that shows normal wall thickening is most likely due to attenuation. Unfortunately, attenuation artifacts, either caused by breast or diaphragm, may be at times more severe on stress images than on rest images, mimicking myocardial ischemia. In this scenario, normal wall thickening is unhelpful in differentiating between the two possibilities. It is then necessary to consider other available clinical and exercise information to solve this conundrum. However, when a rest defect is more severe than a stress defect and regional wall thickening is normal, the defect in question is very likely artifactual.

It has been shown that the quality and accuracy of LVEF derived from ECG-gated SPECT studies are dependent on the amount of injected dose, stable heart rhythm, size of left ventricle, and the amount of gastrointestinal activity adjacent to the heart.[38] Sixteen frames per R-R interval acquisition provide more accurate (~5% higher) LVEF than the traditionally used 8-frame acquisition.[39] Although in many laboratories, both the rest and exercise studies are acquired in ECG-gated mode, gated SPECT acquisition is preferably applied to the higher dose study. Provided that a SPECT study has adequate count density, no gating problems due to arrhythmias, no intense adjacent gastrointestinal activity, and normal left ventricular size, LVEF quantification by gated SPECT is highly reproducible and accurate in most patients.[40] Most software packages also provide end-diastolic and end-systolic volumes.[41] These volume measurements generally demonstrate greater variation than that of LVEF. Normal values for gated SPECT LVEF are significantly lower in men than in women (median LVEF: 52% versus 56%), whereas normal end-diastolic volumes are larger in men than in women (median volume: 109 mL versus 79 mL). In addition to the assessment of global left ventricular function, which is an important diagnostic and prognostic variable in cardiac patients, evaluation of regional wall motion has become an extremely useful aid for identifying attenuation artifacts and thus has helped to improve specificity.[37]

MOTION CORRECTION

Technologists use a number of ways to ensure that patients remain immobile during image acquisition. Velcro straps are commonly used to immobilize a patient's arms and body. Furthermore, technologists emphasize to patients the importance of lying still during image acquisition. Nevertheless, a substantial number of patients show motion during the acquisition. All vendors provide motion correction software. However, it is not always possible to correct appropriately for motion in all directions. Prevention is better than correction.[42]

STATE-OF-THE-ART MYOCARDIAL PERFUSION SPECT WITH ATTENUATION CORRECTION

One of the main obstacles encountered in the interpretation of SPECT myocardial perfusion images is the influence of soft-tissue attenuation on the generation of a perceived perfusion defect that is actually an artifact. The most common of these artifacts arise from attenuation caused by breast tissue, diaphragm, or obesity. Although the artifacts can be evaluated to a certain extent through the use of prone imaging to identify diaphragmatic attenuation or gating of the SPECT images to evaluate regional wall motion, attenuation correction is the optimum method of dealing with these artifacts.

Many gamma cameras are presently equipped with non-uniform attenuation correction devices as an option. Each vendor has championed different approaches consisting of scanning external line sources in varying configurations or x-ray CT for generating transmission attenuation maps. No one approach has yet been identified as clearly superior over the others, but the increasing interest in hybrid imaging will likely result in a greater reliance on x-ray CT for attenuation correction.

Recent clinical studies using non-uniform attenuation-correction devices (Table 14-5) show improved specificity and normalcy rate with preserved sensitivity compared to uncorrected studies.[43-47] In one study, it was suggested that attenuation correction not only improves specificity but also enhances the identification of multivessel disease.[48] In clinical practice, experienced interpreters are well capable of recognizing attenuation artifacts from indirect evidence and thus avoiding false-positive interpretations. However, it is of interest to note that the application of attenuation correction has been shown to improve the overall diagnostic performance of individual readers with different interpretive attitudes.[47,49]

Table 14-5 Comparative Diagnostic Results of Non-Attenuation-Corrected (NC) and Attenuation-Corrected (AC) SPECT Myocardial Perfusion Imaging

Authors	No. Patients	Sensitivity %		Specificity %		Normalcy %	
		NC	AC	NC	AC	NC	AC
Ficaro et al.[91]	119	78	84	48	82	88	98
Gallowitsch et al.[46]	49	89	94	69	84	NA	NA
Hendel et al.[44]	200	76	78	44	50	86	96
Links et al.[45]	112	84	88	69	92	69	92
Lenzo et al.[92]	171	93	93	84	88	78	85
Shotwell et al.[93]	118	NA	NA	NA	NA	74	88
Links et al.[94]	66	78	96	NA	NA	62	85
Grossman et al.[95]	95	90	97	29	57	52	90
Thompson et al.[96]	116	88	86	50	79	NA	NA
Utsunomiya et al.[97]	30	67	76	86	93	NA	NA
Masood et al.[47]	156	79	81	60	64	90	90

In clinical practice, the performance of attenuation correction devices has not been consistently successful, in part due to the accentuation of scatter from adjacent bowel activity or improper registration of CT and SPECT images.[50] Although significant progress has been made, further development of scatter correction algorithms is necessary. It is important that rigorous and practical criteria for quality assurance of attenuation maps and their registration with the SPECT images be developed to improve the reliability of attenuation correction in every patient.

DISPLAY OF EXERCISE SPECT IMAGES

Tomographic reconstruction of the heart generates a multitude of images. To simplify image interpretation, the display of SPECT images has been standardized (Fig. 14-9).[51] This is also important for communication and exchange of images between imaging facilities. Three sets of reconstructed tomographic slices are usually displayed for interpretation: short-axis slices, horizontal long-axis slices, and vertical long-axis slices (Fig. 14-10). Stress and rest (or delayed) images are displayed in two rows (stress on top and rest below) to facilitate comparison. The short-axis slices are displayed from apex (upper left) to base (lower right), the vertical long-axis slices are displayed from septum (left) to lateral wall (right), and the horizontal long-axis slices are displayed from inferior wall (left) to anterior wall (right).

Images are preferably displayed on a monitor using a linear grayscale, a monochromatic color scale, or a multicolor scale. It is important for the interpreter to routinely use one standard display mode and not change frequently to different color scales. Certain color scales have a tendency to exaggerate subtle differences in myocardial radiotracer uptake, whereas other color scales may have the opposite effect.

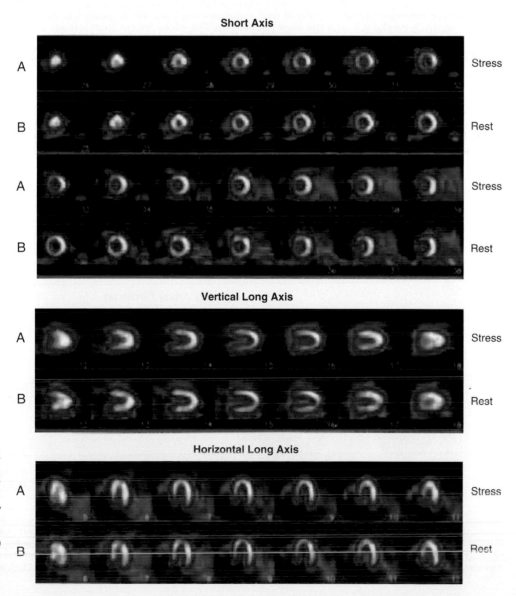

Figure 14-9 Standardized display of stress/rest SPECT images. Representative normal exercise stress and rest SPECT images. The reconstructed short axis slices *(top four rows)*, vertical long-axis slices *(rows 5 and 6)*, horizontal long-axis slices *(rows 7 and 8)* shown are displayed according to the format explained in Figure 14-7.

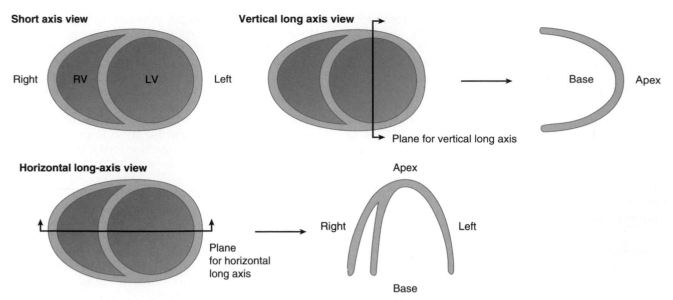

Figure 14-10 Standardized display of reconstructed SPECT slices. Stress and rest slices are displayed in alternating rows with the stress slices on top. Short-axis slices are displayed with the right ventricle at the left on the image. The slices are cut from apex to base and displayed from left to right. Vertical long-axis slices are displayed with the apex pointing towards, the right. The slices are cut from septum to lateral wall and displayed from left to right. Horizontal long-axis slices are displayed with the right ventricle on the left with the apex pointing up. The slices are cut from inferior wall to anterior wall and displayed from left to right. *(Reproduced with permission from Standardization of cardiac tomographic imaging. From the Committee on Advanced Cardiac Imaging and Technology, Council on Clinical Cardiology, American Heart Association; Cardiovascular Imaging Committee, American College of Cardiology; and Board of Directors, Cardiovascular Council, Society of Nuclear Medicine, Circulation 86:338–339, 1992.)*

To simplify and standardize interpretation further, myocardial slices are divided into segments.[51] The American Heart Association, the American College of Cardiology, and the American Society of Nuclear Cardiology adopted a 17-segment model for interpretation of nuclear, echocardiographic, and magnetic resonance images (Fig. 14-11).[51,52] Each segment can be assigned to one of three coronary artery perfusion territories, as shown in the diagram in Figure 14-11. A detailed three-dimensional atlas of coronary anatomy territories for MPI has been developed based on extensive angiographic correlation (Fig. 14-12).[53] Last, the nomenclature for each segment has been standardized as well (Fig. 14-13). The most important difference with the older nomenclature is that the term *posterior* is no longer used.

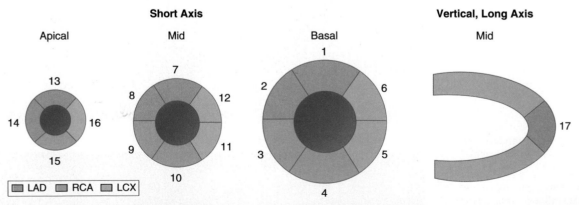

Coronary Artery Territories

Figure 14-11 Coronary artery territories on SPECT reconstructed slices. The standard 17-segment model is shown with assignment of segments to the territories of the left anterior descending coronary artery (LAD), right coronary artery (RCA), and left circumflex coronary artery (LCX). *(Reproduced with permission from Cerqueira MD, Weissman NJ, Dilsizian V, et al: Standardized myocardial segmentation and nomenclature for tomographic imaging of the heart: A statement for healthcare professionals from the Cardiac Imaging Committee of the Council on Clinical Cardiology of the American Heart Association, J Nucl Cardiol 9:240–245, 2002.)*

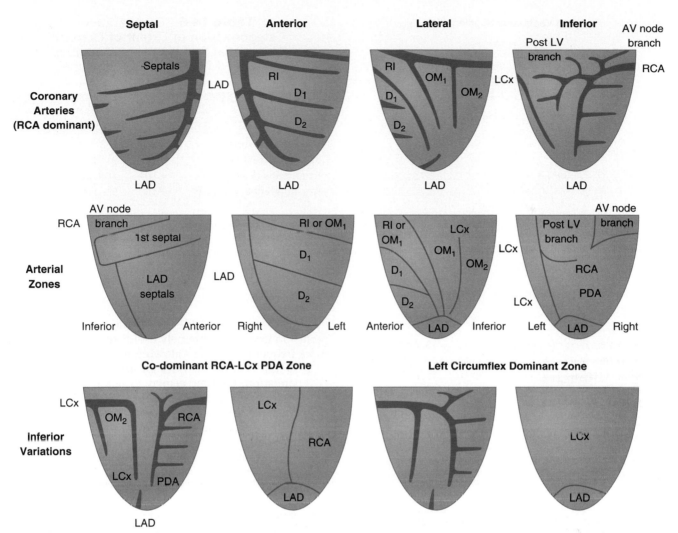

Figure 14-12 SPECT myocardial perfusion zones and atlas of coronary arteries. AV, atrioventricular; D1, first diagonal branch; D2, second diagonal branch, RI, ramus intermedius. *(Reproduced with permission from Nakagawa Y, Nakagawa K, Sdringola S, et al: A precise, three-dimensional atlas of myocardial perfusion correlated with coronary arteriographic anatomy, J Nucl Cardiol 8:580–590, 2001.)*

SEMIQUANTITATIVE VISUAL ANALYSIS AND QUANTITATIVE ANALYSIS OF MYOCARDIAL PERFUSION IMAGES

Myocardial perfusion images should not be interpreted simply in a binary fashion as either "normal" or "abnormal." Myocardial perfusion abnormalities should be characterized according to the degree of decreased radiotracer uptake. A commonly employed scoring system uses a 4-point scale: 0 = normal; 1 = mildly reduced; 2 = moderately reduced; 3 = severely reduced; 4 = absent uptake.[54] By applying this scoring system to each segment of the 17-segment model, to both the rest and stress images, a summed stress score, a summed rest score, and a summed difference score can be derived. These semiquantitative visual scores have been shown to provide important prognostic information.[2] A normal image thus has a score of 0, whereas the maximal abnormal score is 68 (no heart visualized). A summed score of less than 8 is considered a small perfusion abnormality, 9 to 13 a moderate abnormality, and over 13 a large perfusion abnormality.

A purely visual assessment of SPECT images is subjective and may result in suboptimal reproducibility of the results. Therefore, an important complement to visual inspection of images is the quantitative evaluation of perceived perfusion defects, which is based on the inherently quantifiable nature of nuclear images. A number of validated software packages based on the concept of count profiles extracted from the emission tomographic images have been developed, and most are commercially available for quantification of myocardial perfusion and function (QPS-QGS; Emory Toolbox; 4D-MSPECT, and WLCQ). While evaluation of SPECT images using a quantitative program provides greater reproducibility than visual assessment,[55] a recent comparative study showed that the performance of currently available software packages for quantification of myocardial perfusion differs significantly in their diagnostic performance and therefore cannot be used interchangeably.[56]

Left Ventricular Segmentation

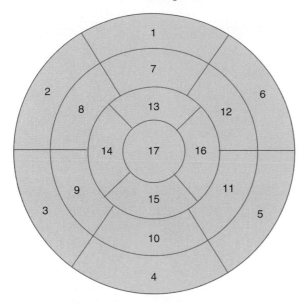

1. Basal anterior
2. Basal anteroseptal
3. Basal inferoseptal
4. Basal inferior
5. Basal inferolateral
6. Basal anterolateral

7. Mid anterior
8. Mid anteroseptal
9. Mid inferoseptal
10. Mid inferior
11. Mid inferolateral
12. Mid anterolateral

13. Apical anterior
14. Apical septal
15. Apical inferior
16. Apical lateral
17. Apex

Figure 14-13 Standardized nomenclature of 17 segments. The display is the bull's eye plot. The segmentation and numbers are the same as in Figure 14-8. *(Reproduced with permission from Cerqueira MD, Weissman NJ, Dilsizian V, et al: Standardized myocardial segmentation and nomenclature for tomographic imaging of the heart: A statement for healthcare professionals from the Cardiac Imaging Committee of the Council on Clinical Cardiology of the American Heart Association, J Nucl Cardiol 9:240–245, 2002.)*

The basic quantitative approaches are similar for each of the programs: regional radiotracer uptake is quantitatively compared to normal databases, although each of the programs is based on slightly different models that are used to generate the quantitative profiles. Specific information about the various quantitative programs has been published in a recent review that will provide the reader with a greater understanding of the assumptions and modeling upon which the programs are based.[57–61] The difference is largely in the display of data. Four of the programs display relative radiotracer uptake on SPECT images as polar plots or bull's eyes. The fourth package, WLCQ, used routinely in our laboratory, involves the generation of circumferential count distribution profiles.[62] Circumferential count profiles are generated for each of the short-axis slices and displayed with a curve representing the lower limit of normal myocardial count distribution. This provides a readily appreciable quantitative measure of the degree of abnormality of the patient's image compared to normal image files. Table 14-6 compares various ways to categorize the extent of myocardial perfusion abnormalities.[63]

Table 14-6 Comparative Categorization of Extent of Exercise Myocardial Perfusion Abnormalities (Modified from Wintergreen Panel Summaries)

	DEFECT EXTENT		
	Small	Moderate	Large
Vascular territories	≤1	1–2	2 or 3
Summed stress score	4–8	9–13	>13
Polar maps (% of LV)	<10%	10%–20%	>20%
Circumferential profile (% of LV)	<5%	5%–10%	>10%

Modified from Iskandrian A: Risk assessment of stable patients (panel III, Wintergreen Panel Summaries). *J Nucl Cardiol* 6(1 Pt 1):93–155, 1999.

We believe that reliable quantification of myocardial perfusion images is extremely useful and should be used more frequently for the following reasons:

1. Quantification provides *greater confidence* in interpretation. Graphic display of relative count distribution serves as an objective and consistent "second observer." The normal database serves as a fixed benchmark against which images are compared.
2. Quantification provides *enhanced intra-* and *interobserver reproducibility.*[64]
3. Quantification provides a reproducible measure for the *degree of abnormality.* This is important, since it is well established that the more abnormal a myocardial perfusion image, the poorer the patient's outcome.[2]

However, quantitative analysis should always be viewed as *complementary* to visual analysis. Image interpretation should always start with visual inspection of images. Quantitative display then serves *to confirm* the visual impression.

INTERPRETATION OF EXERCISE SPECT STUDIES

It is recommended that clinical interpretation of exercise SPECT images should follow a systematic approach to extract the maximal amount of information. The following routine is used in our laboratory:

1. Inspection of cine display of rotating planar projection images. This should always be the first step before interpretation of SPECT images. The rotating images allow assessment of overall study quality: (a) Is the left ventricle well visualized? (b) Is there excessive intestinal activity? Is there extracardiac activity immediately adjacent to the heart? (c) Is there patient motion or upward creep of the heart? (d) Is there a breast shadow obscuring the heart in certain projections? (e) Is there abnormal extracardiac activity in the lungs, mediastinum,

breast, or axilla? This must be mentioned in the final report, in that it could signify malignancy, and further clinical evaluation may be justified.

2. The interpreter should have access to the technologists' acquisition work sheets to address the following questions: (a) Was an appropriate dose of the radiopharmaceutical administered? (b) What was the count density within the left ventricle? Software used in our laboratory displays automatically the maximal number of counts in the "hottest" pixel in the heart in one of the anterior projection images. This information combined with the rotating planar projection images may alert the reader to potential problems with inadequate dose administration, dose infiltration, or inefficient tagging of the tracer with radionuclide. (c) Did the patient continue to exercise after injection of the radiotracer for 1 to 2 minutes? (d) Was timing of imaging appropriate after injection of radiotracer?

3. Are displayed reconstructed tomographic slices appropriately chosen? Are stress and rest slices paired and aligned correctly? Incorrect pairing of slices may result in errors in judging the presence of transient ischemic dilation, discussed later. Furthermore, incorrect alignment of the tomographic slices may result in artifactual perfusion abnormalities.

4. Are there artifacts possibly due to patient motion, breast, or diaphragmatic attenuation? If needed, one should inspect the cine of the rotating planar images again. Inspection of cine display of ECG-gated slices may be helpful for identifying attenuation artifacts.

5. Quantification of SPECT by either polar map or circumferential profiles should be compared with visual analysis, and the reader should feel confident that any discrepancies can be explained.

6. Was ECG-gating optimal? "Blinking" or a decrease in image intensity in one or more of the frames on cine display of the left ventricle indicates that there was a problem due to arrhythmia and that the LVEF may be overestimated. Is the shape of the LVEF volume curve appropriate (Fig. 14-14)? Specifically, is diastolic volume at the beginning and end of the volume curve similar?

IMAGE INTERPRETATION

It is helpful to divide the numerous reconstructed short-axis slices into three groups: apical slices, midventricular slices, and basal slices. After interpretation of the myocardial free walls on short-axis slices, the apex and base of the left ventricle are reviewed on the long-axis slices. The following define the various image patterns and abnormalities that can be seen in myocardial perfusion images:

Normal. The uptake of radiopharmaceutical is homogeneous throughout the left ventricular myocardium. However, in studies that are not attenuation corrected, normal regional variation in uptake can occur in specific areas. Specifically, the lateral wall is usually hotter than other walls because of its closer proximity to the gamma camera head. Quantitatively normal images show regional radiotracer uptake that is above lower limits of normal distribution.

Care should always be taken in interpreting SPECT images as showing no perfusion abnormalities. SPECT imaging only reflects relative flow heterogeneity but offers no information about absolute flow. As a result, multivessel disease causing balanced ischemia may not be appreciated. It is therefore critical to evaluate all of the imaging and exercise data to identify any findings that might suggest the presence of diffuse ischemia.[65] For example, the evaluation of function by gated SPECT can increase the identification of abnormal segments in patients with three-vessel disease by almost 50% compared to perfusion imaging alone.[66] Furthermore, identification of transient ischemic dilation will increase the identification of high-risk patients with left main disease from 56% to 83%.[67]

Defect. A defect represents a localized myocardial area with a relative decrease in radiotracer uptake exceeding normal variation. Quantitatively abnormal regional radiotracer uptake is below lower limits of normal. Defects may vary in intensity from slightly reduced activity to almost total absence of activity. Using the earlier-mentioned semiquantitative scoring system, mildly reduced uptake = 1; moderately reduced uptake = 2; severely reduced uptake = 3; and absent uptake = 4.[54] The degree of abnormality can be quantified in terms of the extent and severity of abnormal uptake. A defect can be further quantified as "percent of total

Figure 14-14 Evidence of poor gating of SPECT images. In the volume curve for the optimally gated study (left panel), the end-diastolic volumes in the first and last frame bin are the same. In contrast, in the study with poor gating due to the presence of frequent premature ventricular contractions (right panel), the end-diastolic volume in the last frame bin is 50% greater than the end-diastolic volume in the first frame bin.

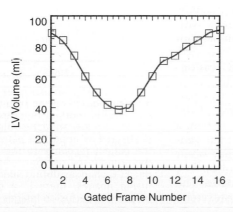
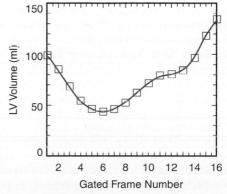

left ventricle." Severe breast or diaphragmatic attenuation may occasionally create a quantitative defect, but it is vital that the reader exclude the possibility that a true perfusion abnormality is contributing to the defect before interpreting the defect as being artifact.

Reversible Defect. A *reversible defect* is defined as a defect that is present on the initial stress images and no longer present, or present to a lesser degree, on resting or delayed images. This pattern usually indicates myocardial ischemia. Visually discerniable reversibility corresponds quantitatively to at least a 25% improvement of defect.

Fixed Defect. A *fixed defect* is defined as a defect that is unchanged and present on both exercise and rest (delayed) images. This pattern generally indicates infarction and the presence of scar tissue. However, in some patients with fixed ^{201}Tl defects on redistribution imaging, improved uptake can be noted after a new resting injection of ^{201}Tl or on 24-hour redistribution imaging. Similarly resting reinjection of ^{99m}Tc-labeled agents after administration of oral nitrates may reveal defect reversibility. These additional imaging maneuvers can help to identify viable myocardium with severely decreased resting blood flow.

Reverse Defect. The initial images are either normal or show a defect, whereas the delayed or rest images show a more severe defect. This pattern is frequently observed in patients who had thrombolytic therapy or percutaneous coronary intervention for acute coronary syndrome. This pattern may persist for years, and the phenomenon is thought to be caused by initial excess radiotracer uptake in a reperfused myocardial area consisting of a mixture of scar tissue and viable myocytes. Initial excess accumulation is subsequently followed by rapid clearance from scar tissue. Although the clinical significance of this finding is controversial, it does not represent evidence of exercise-induced ischemia.[68]

Lung Uptake. Normally no, or very little, radiotracer is noted in the lung fields on postexercise images. Increased lung uptake on planar images can be quantified as the lung-to-heart ratio (normal < 0.5 for ^{201}Tl and < 0.4 for ^{99m}Tc-labeled agents).[69-71] Increased lung uptake of radiotracer represents an important abnormal image pattern, which is associated with an elevated left ventricular end-diastolic pressure,[72] and indicates exercise-induced ischemic left ventricular dysfunction and severe multivessel CAD. Occasionally, increased lung uptake is also observed after pharmacologic stress and has a similar unfavorable significance. Not surprisingly, increased lung uptake occurs also in patients with severely decreased resting LVEF, with or without demonstrable exercise-induced ischemia.

Transient Left Ventricular Dilation. Occasionally, the left ventricle is noted to be larger following exercise than on the rest or delayed image.[73] This pattern is more likely caused by apparent thinning of the myocardium by circumferential endocardial ischemia rather than true and persistent dilation of the left ventricular cavity.[74] At times this image pattern may occur without apparent regional perfusion abnormalities.[75]

Transient Right Ventricular Visualization. The right ventricle is more clearly visualized on postexercise

images than on rest images. This pattern indicates ischemic left ventricular dysfunction during exercise.[76] The mechanism responsible for this finding remains unknown but may involve either increased right ventricular strain or a relative decrease in count intensity in the left ventricle due to diffuse hypoperfusion.

LOW-RISK AND HIGH-RISK IMAGE PATTERNS

Interpretation of myocardial perfusion images must take into account all of the above factors, because certain image patterns have important diagnostic and prognostic significance. It is important to consider both ends of the diagnostic spectrum of SPECT imaging. Categorization of outcome based on these various imaging parameters has been stratified into low, intermediate, and high risk, which are associated with a $< 1\%$, 1% to 5%, and $> 5\%$ annual risk of cardiac death or nonfatal myocardial infarction, respectively.

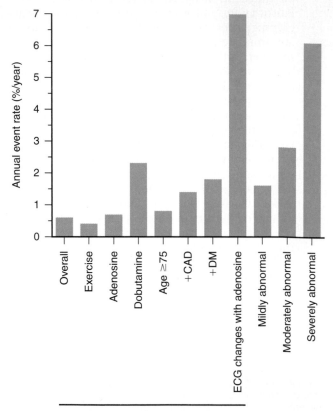

Normal perfusion images

Figure 14-15 Annual rates of cardiac death or myocardial infarction based on the results of myocardial perfusion imaging. Overall, normal myocardial perfusion images are associated with low annual cardiac event rates, although the risk is affected by important patient factors and factors related to the patient response to the stressor. With the exception of the pronounced risk of cardiac events in patients with ischemic ECG changes during adenosine infusion with normal perfusion images, there is a graded increase in risk as the myocardial perfusion images become more abnormal.

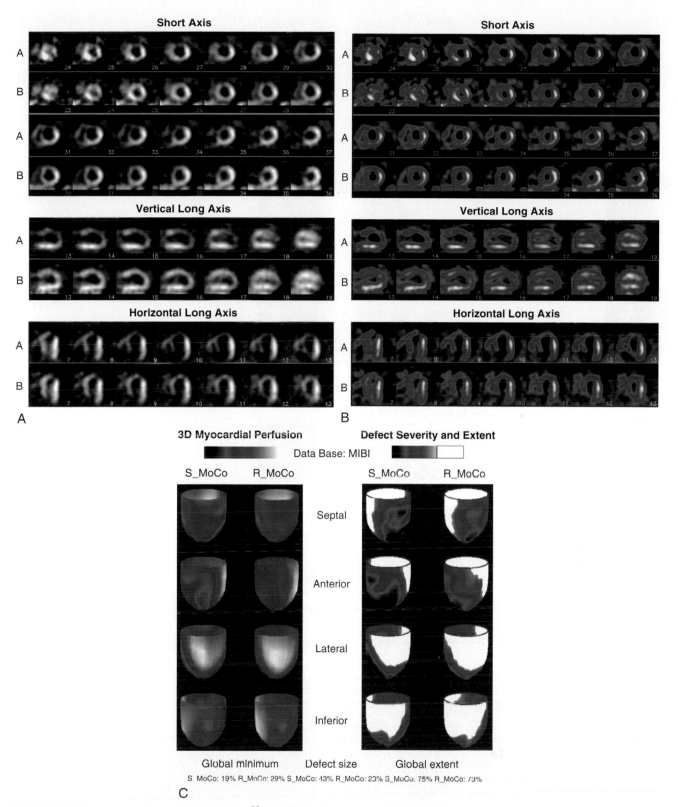

Figure 14-16 **A-D**, Abnormal and high-risk ^{99m}Tc sestamibi exercise/rest SPECT images of a 63-yr-old male with diabetes and atypical chest discomfort. **A and B**, The reconstructed exercise SPECT slices show an enlarged left ventricle with a large antero-septal and apical myocardial perfusion defect that shows partial reversibility. Transient ischemic dilation and transiently enhanced visualization of the right ventricle can be noted. These three image features indicate a high-risk study. **C**, Three-dimensional repre-sentation of the slices shown in *A* and *B*. On the *left*, surface rendering of four myocardial walls: septal, anterior, lateral, and inferior. Relative radiotracer uptake is shown normalized to the area with maximal uptake (i.e., lateral wall). The large perfusion defect involving all walls except the lateral wall can be appreciated. Although partial defect reversibility is present in the anteroapical wall, a large rest defect in the same area is present. On the *right*, comparison to normal data files. Abnormal areas are indicated in color and normal areas in white.

Continued

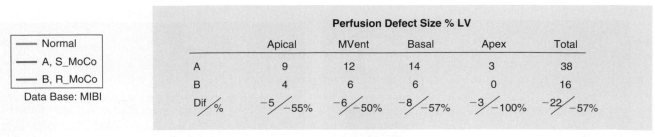

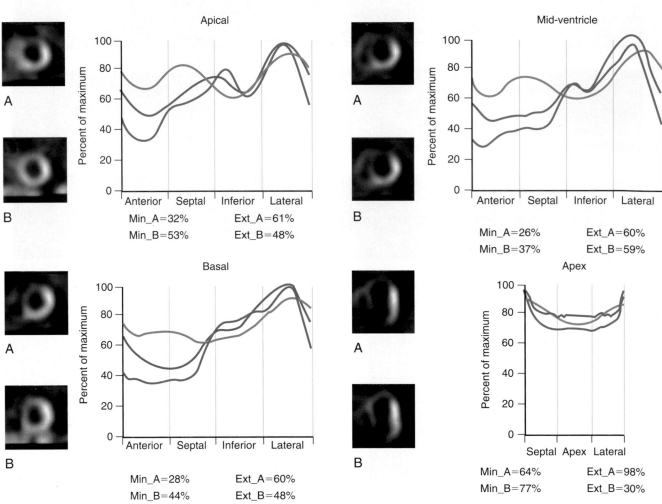

Figure 14-16—cont D, Quantification of relative radiotracer uptake by circumferential profile analysis in comparison to a normal database. Blue, stress count distribution profiles; red, rest count distribution profiles; green, lower limit of normal count distribution. Representative apical, midventricular, and basal and apex profiles are shown. The blue exercise curves are below the lower limit of normal in the anteroseptal region from apex to base. The red rest curves show improvement—that is, closer to the lower limit of normal—from apex to base. The overall exercise defect is large (38% of the left ventricle), the rest defect is also large (16% of the left ventricle), and the ischemic burden is large as well, involving 22% of the left ventricle.

Low-Risk Patterns

Patients with entirely normal or near-normal exercise myocardial perfusion images, even in the presence of known angiographic CAD, have a very low (<1%) yearly cardiac event rate.[28,54,77–84] This was already demonstrated in the early 1980s for planar exercise ^{201}Tl and sestamibi images, and was subsequently confirmed in the 1990s in large numbers of patients with SPECT imaging. In recent years, it has been recognized that although this notion is generally correct, there are small but important subgroups of patients with a less favorable outcome (Fig. 14-15).[84] These subgroups are elderly patients, patients (especially women) with diabetes,[85] African-Americans,[86] and patients with known CAD. In addition, patients who require pharmacologic testing with either adenosine or dobutamine[87] have a relatively poorer outcome despite normal myocardial perfusion images. Obviously, patients who require pharmacologic stress testing often have additional significant comorbidity. Furthermore, patients who exercise less than 7 METs, patients who have ischemic ECG changes during adenosine infusion,[88] or patients who have transient ischemic dilation of the left ventricle[75] may have a higher cardiac event rate even though myocardial perfusion images appear normal. It was assumed previously that the "warranty period" of normal stress myocardial perfusion images was about 2 years. In view of the data, it seems reasonable that patients in the higher-risk categories should undergo repeat stress imaging after 1 year.[84]

High-Risk Patterns

When assessing the overall results of an exercise SPECT study, exercise variables should be taken into consideration as well. The Duke Treadmill Score provides a simple first estimate of risk that can be refined subsequently by considering additional information derived from SPECT imaging.[1] The Duke Treadmill Score is calculated as follows: exercise time (minutes) *minus* 5 times maximal exercise ST segment deviation (mm) *minus* 4 times angina index (0 = no angina, 1 = angina occurs; 2 = exercise-limiting angina) or can be assessed from a simple nomogram.[1] In addition to low exercise tolerance (<7 METs), exercise-limiting angina, and marked ST depression, exercise-induced hypotension, or exercise-induced ventricular arrhythmias indicate also poor outcome.

High-risk SPECT myocardial perfusion images (Fig. 14-16) are characterized by any one or more of the following image patterns:

- A large exercise-induced myocardial perfusion defect (see Table 14-2)
- Multiple myocardial perfusion defects in more than one coronary artery territory (see Table 14-6)
- Extensive reversibility of an exercise-induced defect
- Abnormal postexercise LVEF, normal rest LVEF
- Increased postexercise lung uptake
- Transient (postexercise) ischemic left ventricular dilation
- Transient (postexercise) right ventricular visualization
- Abnormal rest LVEF

When one or more of these exercise/image patterns are present, the patient should be considered to be at high risk for future cardiac events.

REPORTING SPECT IMAGING RESULTS

The results of exercise SPECT may have an important impact on decision making and management of cardiac patients. If communication with referring physicians is ineffective, patients may not fully benefit from nuclear cardiology procedures. In recent years it has become clear that in many imaging facilities, the quality of reporting was inadequate.[89] Reports should be concise and clear. In most circumstances, it is possible to decide if a study is normal or abnormal. If a study is abnormal, the degree of abnormality should be defined (i.e., small, moderate, or large) as well as the type of abnormality, fixed or reversible. The anatomic location of a perfusion defect, the possible coronary territory involved, and presence of high-risk features should be stated. Interpretation should also be formulated with consideration of exercise parameters: one should never interpret images alone. A relatively small exercise-induced myocardial perfusion abnormality has markedly different clinical significance in a patient who achieved only a low workload as compared to a patient who exercised for 15 minutes. Reasons for suboptimal quality of images that affect the confidence of interpretation (attenuation artifacts, intense gastrointestinal uptake, motion) should be mentioned as well. Examples of optimized reports have been published.[89,90]

Exercise radionuclide MPI is a mature, powerful, and well-validated clinical tool. Optimal results are obtained when careful attention is paid to many details of the entire process, from performing the exercise stress, to optimized image acquisition, thoughtful image interpretation, and formulating a meaningful report.

REFERENCES

1. Mark DB, Shaw L, Harrell FE Jr, et al: Prognostic value of a treadmill exercise score in outpatients with suspected coronary artery disease, *N Engl J Med* 325(12):849–853, 1991.
2. Hachamovitch R, Berman DS, Kiat H, et al: Exercise myocardial perfusion SPECT in patients without known coronary artery disease: incremental prognostic value and use in risk stratification, *Circulation* 93 (5):905–914, 1996.
3. Christie J, Sheldahl LM, Tristani FE, et al: Determination of stroke volume and cardiac output during exercise: comparison of two-dimensional and Doppler echocardiography, Fick oximetry, and thermodilution, *Circulation* 76(3):539–547, 1987.
4. Hammond HK, Kelly TL, Froelicher V: Radionuclide imaging correlatives of heart rate impairment during maximal exercise testing, *J Am Coll Cardiol* 2(5):826–833, 1983.
5. Lauer MS, Okin PM, Larson MG, et al: Impaired heart rate response to graded exercise. Prognostic implications of chronotropic incompetence in the Framingham Heart Study, *Circulation* 93(8):1520–1526, 1996.
6. Laaksonen MS, Kalliokoski KK, Luotolahti M, et al: Myocardial perfusion during exercise in endurance-trained and untrained humans, *Am J Physiol Regul Integr Comp Physiol* 293(2):R837–R843, 2007.
7. Zoghbi GJ, Htay T, Aqel R, et al: Effect of caffeine on ischemia detection by adenosine single-photon emission computed tomography perfusion imaging, *J Am Coll Cardiol* 47(11):2296–2302, 2006.
8. Kailasnath P, Sinusas AJ: Comparison of Tl-201 with Tc-99m-labeled myocardial perfusion agents: technical, physiologic, and clinical issues, *J Nucl Cardiol* 8(4):482–498, 2001.
9. Marshall RC, Leidholdt EM Jr., Zhang DY, Barnett CA: Technetium-99m hexakis 2-methoxy-2-isobutyl isonitrile and thallium-201 extraction, washout, and retention at varying coronary flow rates in rabbit heart, *Circulation* 82(3):998–1007, 1990.
10. DePuey E, Garcia E: Updated imaging guidelines for nuclear cardiology procedures, part 1, *J Nucl Cardiol* 8(1):G5–G58, 2001.
11. Einstein AJ, Moser KW, Thompson RC, et al: Radiation dose to patients from cardiac diagnostic imaging, *Circulation* 116(11):1290–1305, 2007.
12. Wackers FJ, Bodenheimer M, Fleiss JL, Brown M: Factors affecting uniformity in interpretation of planar thallium-201 imaging in a multicenter trial. The Multicenter Study on Silent Myocardial Ischemia (MSSMI) Thallium 201 Investigators, *J Am Coll Cardiol* 21(5): 1064–1074, 1993.
13. Kiat H, Maddahi J, Roy LT, et al: Comparison of technetium 99m methoxy isobutyl isonitrile and thallium 201 for evaluation of coronary artery disease by planar and tomographic methods, *Am Heart J* 117(1):1–11, 1989.
14. Iskandrian AS, Heo J, Kong B, et al: Use of technetium-99m isonitrile (RP-30A) in assessing left ventricular perfusion and function at rest and during exercise in coronary artery disease, and comparison with

coronary arteriography and exercise thallium-201 SPECT imaging, *Am J Cardiol* 64(5):270–275, 1989.

15. Kahn JK, McGhie I, Akers MS, et al: Quantitative rotational tomography with 201Tl and 99mTc 2-methoxy-isobutyl-isonitrile. A direct comparison in normal individuals and patients with coronary artery disease, *Circulation* 79(6):1282–1293, 1989.

16. Solot G, Hermans J, Merlo P, et al: Correlation of 99Tcm-sestamibi SPECT with coronary angiography in general hospital practice, *Nucl Med Commun* 14(1):23–29, 1993.

17. Chae SC, Heo J, Iskandrian AS, et al: Identification of extensive coronary artery disease in women by exercise single-photon emission computed tomographic (SPECT) thallium imaging, *J Am Coll Cardiol* 21 (6):1305–1311, 1993.

18. Van Train KF, Garcia EV, Maddahi J, et al: Multicenter trial validation for quantitative analysis of same-day rest-stress technetium-99m-sestamibi myocardial tomograms, *J Nucl Med* 35(4):609–618, 1994.

19. Rubello D, Zanco P, Candelpergher G, et al: Usefulness of 99mTc-MIBI stress myocardial SPECT bull's-eye quantification in coronary artery disease, *Q J Nucl Med* 39(2):111–115, 1995.

20. Hambye AS, Vervaet A, Lieber S, Ranquin R: Diagnostic value and incremental contribution of bicycle exercise, first-pass radionuclide angiography, and 99mTc-labeled sestamibi single-photon emission computed tomography in the identification of coronary artery disease in patients without infarction, *J Nucl Cardiol* 3(6 Pt 1):464–474, 1996.

21. Iskandrian AE, Heo J, Nallamothu N: Detection of coronary artery disease in women with use of stress single-photon emission computed tomography myocardial perfusion imaging, *J Nucl Cardiol* 4(4): 329–335, 1997.

22. Santana-Boado C, Candell-Riera J, Castell-Conesa J, et al: Diagnostic accuracy of technetium-99m-MIBI myocardial SPECT in women and men, *J Nucl Med* 39(5):751–755, 1998.

23. Azzarelli S, Galassi AR, Foti R, et al: Accuracy of 99mTc-tetrofosmin myocardial tomography in the evaluation of coronary artery disease, *J Nucl Cardiol* 6(2):183–189, 1999.

24. Elhendy A, van Domburg RT, Sozzi FB, et al: Impact of hypertension on the accuracy of exercise stress myocardial perfusion imaging for the diagnosis of coronary artery disease, *Heart* 85(6):655–661, 2001.

25. Schuijf JD, Poldermans D, Shaw LJ, et al: Diagnostic and prognostic value of non-invasive imaging in known or suspected coronary artery disease, *Eur J Nucl Med Mol Imaging* 33(1):93–104, 2006.

26. Underwood SR, Anagnostopoulos C, Cerqueira M, et al: Myocardial perfusion scintigraphy: the evidence, *Eur J Nucl Med Mol Imaging* 31(2):261–291, 2004.

27. Elhendy A, Sozzi FB, van Domburg RT, et al: Accuracy of exercise stress technetium 99m sestamibi SPECT imaging in the evaluation of the extent and location of coronary artery disease in patients with an earlier myocardial infarction, *J Nucl Cardiol* 7(5):432–438, 2000.

28. Brown KA, Rowen M: Prognostic value of a normal exercise myocardial perfusion imaging study in patients with angiographically significant coronary artery disease, *Am J Cardiol* 71(10):865–867, 1993.

29. Zeiher AM, Krause T, Schachinger V, et al: Impaired endothelium-dependent vasodilation of coronary resistance vessels is associated with exercise-induced myocardial ischemia, *Circulation* 91(9): 2345–2352, 1995.

30. Sharir T, Germano G, Kavanagh PB, et al: Incremental prognostic value of post-stress left ventricular ejection fraction and volume by gated myocardial perfusion single photon emission computed tomography, *Circulation* 100(10):1035–1042, 1999.

31. Shen MY, Liu YH, Sinusas AJ, et al: Quantification of regional myocardial wall thickening on electrocardiogram-gated SPECT imaging, *J Nucl Cardiol* 6(6):583–595, 1999.

32. Sharir T, Germano G, Kang X, et al: Prediction of myocardial infarction versus cardiac death by gated myocardial perfusion SPECT: risk stratification by the amount of stress-induced ischemia and the post-stress ejection fraction, *J Nucl Med* 42(6):831–837, 2001.

33. Spinelli L, Petretta M, Acampa W, et al: Prognostic value of combined assessment of regional left ventricular function and myocardial perfusion by dobutamine and rest gated SPECT in patients with uncomplicated acute myocardial infarction, *J Nucl Med* 44(7):1023–1029, 2003.

34. Johnson LL, Verdesca SA, Aude WY, et al: Postischemic stunning can affect left ventricular ejection fraction and regional wall motion on post-stress gated sestamibi tomograms, *J Am Coll Cardiol* 30(7): 1641–1648, 1997.

35. Ward RP, Gundeck EL, Lang RM, et al: Overestimation of postischemic myocardial stunning on gated SPECT imaging: correlation with echocardiography, *J Nucl Cardiol* 13(4):514–520, 2006.

36. Smanio PE, Watson DD, Segalla DL, et al: Value of gating of technetium-99m sestamibi single-photon emission computed tomographic imaging, *J Am Coll Cardiol* 30(7):1687–1692, 1997.

37. Taillefer R, DePuey EG, Udelson JE, et al: Comparative diagnostic accuracy of Tl-201 and Tc-99m sestamibi SPECT imaging (perfusion and ECG-gated SPECT) in detecting coronary artery disease in women, *J Am Coll Cardiol* 29(1):69–77, 1997.

38. Vallejo E, Dione DP, Sinusas AJ, Wackers FJ: Assessment of left ventricular ejection fraction with quantitative gated SPECT: accuracy and correlation with first-pass radionuclide angiography, *J Nucl Cardiol* 7 (5):461–470, 2000.

39. Navare SM, Wackers FJ, Liu YH: Comparison of 16-frame and 8-frame gated SPET imaging for determination of left ventricular volumes and ejection fraction, *Eur J Nucl Med Mol Imaging* 30(10):1330–1337, 2003.

40. Germano G, Kiat H, Kavanagh PB, et al: Automatic quantification of ejection fraction from gated myocardial perfusion SPECT, *J Nucl Med* 36:2138–2147, 1995.

41. Iskandrian AE, Germano G, VanDecker W, et al: Validation of left ventricular volume measurements by gated SPECT 99mTc-labeled sestamibi imaging, *J Nucl Cardiol* 5(6):574–578, 1998.

42. Fitzgerald J, Danias PG: Effect of motion on cardiac SPECT imaging: recognition and motion correction, *J Nucl Cardiol* 8:701–706, 2001.

43. Ficaro EP, Fessler JA, Shreve PD, et al: Simultaneous transmission/emission myocardial perfusion tomography. Diagnostic accuracy of attenuation-corrected 99mTc-sestamibi single-photon emission computed tomography, *Circulation* 93(3):463–473, 1996.

44. Hendel RC, Berman DS, Cullom SJ, et al: Multicenter clinical trial to evaluate the efficacy of correction for photon attenuation and scatter in SPECT myocardial perfusion imaging, *Circulation* 99(21): 2742–2749, 1999.

45. Links JM, Becker LC, Rigo P, et al: Combined corrections for attenuation, depth-dependent blur, and motion in cardiac SPECT: a multicenter trial, *J Nucl Cardiol* 7(5):414–425, 2000.

46. Gallowitsch HJ, Sykora J, Mikosch P, et al: Attenuation-corrected thallium-201 single-photon emission tomography using a gadolinium-153 moving line source: clinical value and the impact of attenuation correction on the extent and severity of perfusion abnormalities, *Eur J Nucl Med* 25(3):220–228, 1998.

47. Masood Y, Liu YH, Depuey G, et al: Clinical validation of SPECT attenuation correction using x-ray computed tomography-derived attenuation maps: multicenter clinical trial with angiographic correlation, *J Nucl Cardiol* 12(6):676–686, 2005.

48. Duvernoy CS, Ficaro EP, Karabajakian MZ, et al: Improved detection of left main coronary artery disease with attenuation-corrected SPECT, *J Nucl Cardiol* 7(6):639–648, 2000.

49. O'Connor MK, Kemp B, Anstett F, et al: A multicenter evaluation of commercial attenuation compensation techniques in cardiac SPECT using phantom models, *J Nucl Cardiol* 9(4):361–376, 2002.

50. Goetze S, Wahl RL: Prevalence of misregistration between SPECT and CT for attenuation-corrected myocardial perfusion SPECT, *J Nucl Cardiol* 14(2):200–206, 2007.

51. Standardization of cardiac tomographic imaging: From the Committee on Advanced Cardiac Imaging and Technology, Council on Clinical Cardiology, American Heart Association; Cardiovascular Imaging Committee, American College of Cardiology; and Board of Directors, Cardiovascular Council, Society of Nuclear Medicine, *Circulation* 86 (1):338–339, 1992.

52. Cerqueira MD, Weissman NJ, Dilsizian V, et al: Standardized myocardial segmentation and nomenclature for tomographic imaging of the heart: a statement for healthcare professionals from the Cardiac Imaging Committee of the Council on Clinical Cardiology of the American Heart Association, *J Nucl Cardiol* 9(2):240–245, 2002.

53. Nakagawa Y, Nakagawa K, Sdringola S, et al: A precise, three-dimensional atlas of myocardial perfusion correlated with coronary arteriographic anatomy, *J Nucl Cardiol* 8(5):580–590, 2001.

54. Hachamovitch R, Berman DS, Shaw LJ, et al: Incremental prognostic value of myocardial perfusion single photon emission computed tomography for the prediction of cardiac death: differential stratification for risk of cardiac death and myocardial infarction, *Circulation* 97(6):535–543, 1998.

55. Berman DS, Kang X, Gransar H, et al: Quantitative assessment of myocardial perfusion abnormality on SPECT myocardial perfusion imaging is more reproducible than expert visual analysis, *J Nucl Cardiol* 16 (1):45–53, 2009.

56. Wolak A, Slomka PJ, Fish MB, et al: Quantitative myocardial-perfusion SPECT: comparison of three state-of-the-art software packages, *J Nucl Cardiol* 15(1):27–34, 2008.

57. Garcia EV, Faber TL, Cooke CD, et al: The increasing role of quantification in clinical nuclear cardiology: The Emory approach, *J Nucl Cardiol* 14(4):420–432, 2007.

58. Germano G, Kavanagh PB, Slomka PJ, et al: Quantitation in gated perfusion SPECT imaging: The Cedars-Sinai approach, *J Nucl Cardiol* 14 (4):433–454, 2007.

59. Ficaro EP, Lee BC, Kritzman JN, Corbett JR: Corridor4DM: The Michigan method for quantitative nuclear cardiology, *J Nucl Cardiol* 14(4):455–465, 2007.

60. Watson DD, Smith Ii WH: The role of quantitation in clinical nuclear cardiology: The University of Virginia approach, *J Nucl Cardiol* 14(4):466–482, 2007.

61. Liu Y-H: Quantification of nuclear cardiac images: The Yale approach, *J Nucl Cardiol* 14(4):483–491, 2007.

62. Liu YH, Sinusas AJ, DeMan P, et al: Quantification of SPECT myocardial perfusion images: methodology and validation of the Yale-CQ method, *J Nucl Cardiol* 6(2):190–204, 1999.

63. Iskandrian A: Risk assessment of stable patients (panel III Wintergreen Panel Summaries), *J Nucl Cardiol* 6(1 Pt 1):93–155, 1999.
64. Wackers FJ: Science, art, and artifacts: how important is quantification for the practicing physician interpreting myocardial perfusion studies? *J Nucl Cardiol* 1(5 Pt 2):S109–S117, 1994.
65. Higgins JP, Higgins JA, Williams G: Stress-induced abnormalities in myocardial perfusion imaging that are not related to perfusion but are of diagnostic and prognostic importance, *Eur J Nucl Med Mol Imaging* 34(4):584–595, 2007.
66. Lima RSL, Watson DD, Goode AR, et al: Incremental value of combined perfusion and function over perfusion alone by gated SPECT myocardial perfusion imaging for detection of severe three-vessel coronary artery disease, *J Am Coll Cardiol* 42(1):64–70, 2003.
67. Berman DS, Kang X, Slomka PJ, et al: Underestimation of extent of ischemia by gated SPECT myocardial perfusion imaging in patients with left main coronary artery disease, *J Nucl Cardiol* 14(4):521–528, 2007.
68. Smith EJ, Hussain A, Manoharan M, et al: A reverse perfusion pattern during Technetium-99m stress myocardial perfusion imaging does not predict flow limiting coronary artery disease, *Int J Cardiovasc Imaging* 20(4):321–326, 2004.
69. Gill JB, Ruddy TD, Newell JB, et al: Prognostic importance of thallium uptake by the lungs during exercise in coronary artery disease, *N Engl J Med* 317(24):1486–1489, 1987.
70. Choy JB, Leslie WD: Clinical correlates of Tc-99m sestamibi lung uptake, *J Nucl Cardiol* 8(6):639–644, 2001.
71. Bacher-Stier C, Sharir T, Kavanagh PB, et al: Postexercise lung uptake of 99mTc-sestamibi determined by a new automatic technique: validation and application in detection of severe and extensive coronary artery disease and reduced left ventricular function, *J Nucl Med* 41(7):1190–1197, 2000.
72. Patel GM, Hauser TH, Parker JA, et al: Quantitative relationship of stress Tc-99m sestamibi lung uptake with resting Tl-201 lung uptake and with indices of left ventricular dysfunction and coronary artery disease, *J Nucl Cardiol* 11(4):408–413, 2004.
73. Weiss AT, Berman DS, Lew AS, et al: Transient ischemic dilation of the left ventricle on stress thallium-201 scintigraphy: a marker of severe and extensive coronary artery disease, *J Am Coll Cardiol* 9(4):752–759, 1987.
74. McLaughlin MG, Danias PG: Transient ischemic dilation: a powerful diagnostic and prognostic finding of stress myocardial perfusion imaging, *J Nucl Cardiol* 9(6):663–667, 2002.
75. Abidov A, Bax JJ, Hayes SW, et al: Transient ischemic dilation ratio of the left ventricle is a significant predictor of future cardiac events in patients with otherwise normal myocardial perfusion SPECT, *J Am Coll Cardiol* 42(10):1818–1825, 2003.
76. Williams KA, Schneider CM: Increased stress right ventricular activity on dual isotope perfusion SPECT: a sign of multivessel and/or left main coronary artery disease, *J Am Coll Cardiol* 34(2):420–427, 1999.
77. Wackers FJ, Russo DJ, Russo D, Clements JP: Prognostic significance of normal quantitative planar thallium-201 stress scintigraphy in patients with chest pain, *J Am Coll Cardiol* 6(1):27–30, 1985.
78. Raiker K, Sinusas AJ, Wackers FJ, Zaret BL: One-year prognosis of patients with normal planar or single-photon emission computed tomographic technetium 99m-labeled sestamibi exercise imaging, *J Nucl Cardiol* 1(5 Pt 1):449–456, 1994.
79. Soman P, Parsons A, Lahiri N, Lahiri A: The prognostic value of a normal Tc-99m sestamibi SPECT study in suspected coronary artery disease, *J Nucl Cardiol* 6(3):252–256, 1999.
80. Gibbons RJ, Hodge DO, Berman DS, et al: Long-term outcome of patients with intermediate-risk exercise electrocardiograms who do not have myocardial perfusion defects on radionuclide imaging, *Circulation* 100(21):2140–2145, 1999.
81. Vanzetto G, Ormezzano O, Fagret D, et al: Long-term additive prognostic value of thallium-201 myocardial perfusion imaging over clinical and exercise stress test in low to intermediate risk patients : study in 1137 patients with 6-year follow-up, *Circulation* 100(14):1521–1527, 1999.
82. Groutars RG, Verzijlbergen JF, Muller AJ, et al: Prognostic value and quality of life in patients with normal rest thallium-201/stress technetium 99m-tetrofosmin dual-isotope myocardial SPECT, *J Nucl Cardiol* 7(4):333–341, 2000.
83. Galassi AR, Azzarelli S, Tomaselli A, et al: Incremental prognostic value of technetium-99m-tetrofosmin exercise myocardial perfusion imaging for predicting outcomes in patients with suspected or known coronary artery disease, *Am J Cardiol* 88(2):101–106, 2001.
84. Hachamovitch R, Hayes S, Friedman JD, et al: Determinants of risk and its temporal variation in patients with normal stress myocardial perfusion scans: what is the warranty period of a normal scan? *J Am Coll Cardiol* 41(8):1329–1340, 2003.
85. Giri S, Shaw LJ, Murthy DR, et al: Impact of diabetes on the risk stratification using stress single-photon emission computed tomography myocardial perfusion imaging in patients with symptoms suggestive of coronary artery disease, *Circulation* 105(1):32–40, 2002.
86. Akinboboye OO, Idris O, Onwuanyi A, et al: Incidence of major cardiovascular events in black patients with normal myocardial stress perfusion study results, *J Nucl Cardiol* 8(5):541–547, 2001.
87. Calnon DA, McGrath PD, Doss AL, et al: Prognostic value of dobutamine stress technetium-99m-sestamibi single-photon emission computed tomography myocardial perfusion imaging: stratification of a high-risk population, *J Am Coll Cardiol* 38(5):1511–1517, 2001.
88. Abbott BG, Afshar M, Berger AK, Wackers FJ: Prognostic significance of ischemic electrocardiographic changes during adenosine infusion in patients with normal myocardial perfusion imaging, *J Nucl Cardiol* 10(1):9–16, 2003.
89. Wackers FJ: Intersocietal Commission for the Accreditation of Nuclear Medicine Laboratories (ICANL) position statement on standardization and optimization of nuclear cardiology reports, *J Nucl Cardiol* 7(4):397–400, 2000.
90. Hendel RC, Wackers FJ, Berman DS, et al: American Society of Nuclear Cardiology consensus statement: Reporting of radionuclide myocardial perfusion imaging studies, *J Nucl Cardiol* 13(6):e152–e156, 2006.
91. Ficaro EP, Fessler JA, Ackermann RJ, et al: Simultaneous transmission-emission thallium-201 cardiac SPECT: effect of attenuation correction on myocardial tracer distribution, *J Nucl Med* 36(6):921–931, 1995.
92. Lenzo N, Ficaro E, Kritzman JN, Corbett JR: Clinical comparison of Profile attenuation correction and the Michigan modified STEP method, *J Nucl Cardiol* 8:S19, 2001.
93. Shotwell M, Singh BM, Fortman C, et al: Improved coronary disease detection with quantitative attenuation-corrected Tl-201 images, *J Nucl Cardiol* 9(1):52–62, 2002.
94. Links JM, DePuey EG, Taillefer R, Becker LC: Attenuation correction and gating synergistically improve the diagnostic accuracy of myocardial perfusion SPECT, *J Nucl Cardiol* 9:183–187, 2002.
95. Grossman GB, Garcia EV, Bateman TM, et al: Quantitative Tc-99m sestamibi attenuation-corrected SPECT: development and multicenter trial validation of myocardial perfusion stress gender-independent normal database in an obese population, *J Nucl Cardiol* 11(3):263–272, 2004.
96. Thompson RC, Heller GV, Johnson LL, et al: Value of attenuation correction on ECG-gated SPECT myocardial perfusion imaging related to body mass index, *J Nucl Cardiol* 12(2):195–202, 2005.
97. Utsunomiya D, Tomiguchi S, Shiraishi S, et al: Initial experience with X-ray CT based attenuation correction in myocardial perfusion SPECT imaging using a combined SPECT/CT system, *Ann Nucl Med* 19(6):485–489, 2005.

Coronary Artery Disease Detection: Pharmacologic Stress SPECT

GILBERT J. ZOGHBI AND AMI E. ISKANDRIAN

INTRODUCTION

Pharmacologic stress is used in approximately 40% of the stress myocardial perfusion imaging (MPI) studies performed for the detection of coronary artery disease (CAD) in the United States.[1] Approximately 75% of inpatients, 40% of outpatients, 30% of patients younger than 75 years, and 50% of patients older than 75 years cannot perform maximal exercise.[2] Submaximal exercise lowers the sensitivity of exercise MPI and underestimates the degree and extent of ischemia.[3] Exercise is the preferred stress modality for patients who can exercise and achieve adequate exercise endpoints, whereas pharmacologic stress is reserved for patients who have left bundle branch block (LBBB) electronically paced rhythms, or are unable to exercise or achieve adequate exercise endpoints (Table 15-1).[3–5] Pharmacologic stress agents include vasodilators such as adenosine, dipyridamole, adenosine triphosphate (ATP), or the newer selective adenosine A2A receptor agonists and inotropic and chronotropic agents such as dobutamine and arbutamine. Adenosine triphosphate and arbutamine are not used in the United States and thus will not be discussed in this chapter.

PHARMACOLOGY

Adenosine

Adenosine, a small heterocyclic compound made of a purine base and a sugar ribose, is produced endogenously by endothelial and vascular smooth muscle cells in small amounts during normal cellular conditions and in larger amounts under ischemic conditions.[6] The intracellular adenosine production involves two different pathways. In the S-adenosyl pathway, S-adenosyl methionine is converted to adenosine and homocysteine via the intermediary of S-adenosyl homocysteine.[1,3,6] In the ATP pathway that predominates during episodes of ischemia, ATP is dephosphorylated sequentially to adenosine diphosphate (ADP), adenosine monophosphate (AMP), and finally to adenosine and phosphate by the catalytic action of a 5′nucleotidase.[1,3,6] A carrier-mediated transporter transports the produced adenosine into the extracellular space, where it interacts with its cell membrane receptors on endothelial and smooth muscle cells.[1,3,6] It subsequently reenters the intracellular space of endothelial cells, smooth muscle cells, or red blood cells via facilitated transport, where it gets degraded to xanthine and uric acid in a pathway that involves adenosine deaminase, nucleoside phosphorylase, and xanthine oxidase or to AMP via an adenosine kinase pathway.[1,3,6] Adenosine can also be produced extracellularly from the dephosphorylation of ATP and ADP that are released from mast cells, nerve endings, or platelets.[1]

Adenosine receptors are divided into at least four types: A1, A2A, A2B, and A3.[1,3,6,7] The different adenosine receptor subtypes, their location, and action are listed in Table 15-2.[1,7,8] Activation of the A2A receptor causes coronary vasodilatation, and activation of the other receptors is responsible for undesirable effects.[8] Adenosine binding to the A2 receptor activates adenylate cyclase and increases intracellular cyclic AMP production via G_s protein activation.[8] This causes opening of potassium channels, inhibition of voltage-gated calcium channels, and hyperpolarization of smooth muscle cells, with resultant decrease in calcium uptake and intracellular calcium release that lead to smooth muscle relaxation and arteriolar dilation.[3,8] Adenosine binding to A1 receptors inhibits norepinephrine release, stimulates endothelial-derived relaxing factor production, and activates G_i proteins that inhibit adenylate cyclase, decrease intracellular cyclic AMP, and increase potassium channel conductance—all of which result in smooth muscle contraction.[1,3,8] Adenosine also

Table 15-1 Factors That Favor Pharmacologic Myocardial Perfusion Imaging

Neurologic disorders

Muscular disorders

Skeletal disorders

Peripheral vascular disease

Limited exercise capacity
  o Chronic obstructive lung disease
  o Diabetes mellitus
  o Poor physical conditioning
  o Poor motivation
  o Morbid obesity

Chronotropic incompetence

Inability to achieve maximal exercise

Left bundle branch block (vasodilators are the preferred agents)

Electronically paced rhythms (vasodilators are the preferred agents)

From Zoghbi G, Iskandrian AE: Pharmacologic stress testing. In Garcia EV, Iskandrian AE (eds): *Nuclear Cardiac Imaging: Principles and Applications*. New York: Oxford University Press, 2008, pp 293-315, with permission.

has direct effects on sympathetic nerve endings, resulting in the increase in heart rate (HR) and the rise in blood pressure (BP) seen occasionally.[1] Xanthine-containing compounds, such as theophylline and caffeine, competitively inhibit the action of adenosine on these receptors.[4]

Adenosine has a very short half-life of less than 2 seconds and a rapid onset of action.[4,9] Its peak hyperemic effect is reached within 2 minutes after beginning its infusion and returns to baseline within 2 minutes after termination of its infusion.[4,9]

Dipyridamole

Dipyridamole, a pyrimidine base, increases interstitial adenosine level by inhibiting adenosine-facilitated reuptake across vascular, endothelial, and red blood cell membranes that are responsible for its degradation.[3,4] Thus, dipyridamole indirectly increases endogenous adenosine production at its receptor sites, mediating its various effects.[3,4] Its peak vasodilatory effect occurs within 3 to 7 minutes from beginning of infusion, and its half-life lasts around 30 to 45 minutes.[3,4]

Dobutamine

Dobutamine is a synthetic sympathomimetic amine that has a direct weak β_2 and α_1 receptor agonist activity and a strong β_1 agonist activity with dose-dependent inotropic and chronotropic effects.[3,10] Dobutamine doses less than 10 µg/kg/min cause cardiac β_1 and peripheral α_1 receptor stimulation resulting in augmentation of stroke volume and cardiac output and minimal changes in HR and BP.[3,10] Dobutamine doses over 10 µg/kg/min cause predominant cardiac β_1 receptor stimulation resulting in significant dose-dependent increases in HR, contractility, and cardiac output, with minimal increase in systemic BP.[3,10] The systemic BP occasionally decreases due to peripheral vasodilatation caused by more effects on the peripheral β_2 receptor.[3,10,11] Myocardial blood flow (MBF) increases, predominantly due to the increase in myocardial oxygen demand and a minimal direct vasodilatory effect on the coronary bed.[3,10,11]

Dobutamine's onset of action is within 2 minutes of its infusion and reaches steady state after several minutes.[3,10,11] Dobutamine has a 2-minute half-life and is metabolized in the liver through methylation and conjugation.[11] The cardiovascular effects of the various pharmacologic stressors are summarized in Table 15-3.

MYOCARDIAL BLOOD FLOW

The hemodynamic significance of coronary lesions can be evaluated invasively with Doppler catheters that measure flow velocities (coronary flow reserve [CFR]), with

Table 15-2 Adenosine Receptor Types, Location, and Action

Receptor Type	Location	Action
A1	• Sinoatrial node	• Negative dromotropic, inotropic and chronotropic effects
	• Atrioventricular node	• Preconditioning
	• Atrial myocytes	• Chest pain production
	• Ventricular myocytes	• Tachypnea production
A2A	• Smooth muscle cells	• Coronary vasodilatation (predominant)
		• Peripheral vasodilatation (partial)
		• Antiinflammatory effect
		• Sympathetic stimulation
A2B	• Smooth muscle cells	• Vasodilatation in most vascular beds
		• Vasoconstriction in renal afferent arterioles and hepatic veins
		• Bronchiolar constriction
		• Mast cell degranulation
A3	• Ventricular myocytes	• Preconditioning
		• Bronchospasm

From Zoghbi G, Iskandrian AE: Pharmacologic stress testing. In Garcia EV, Iskandrian AE (eds): *Nuclear Cardiac Imaging: Principles and Applications*. New York: Oxford University Press, 2008, pp 293-315, with permission.

Table 15-3   The Cardiovascular Effects of the Various Pharmacologic Stressors

	Adenosine	Dipyridamole	Regadenoson	Binodenoson	Dobutamine
Coronary vasodilatation	+++	++	+++	+++	+
Heart rate	+	+	++	++	+++
Blood pressure	−	−	−	−	++
Inotropy	↔	↔	↔	↔	++
Chronotropy	↔	↔	↔	↔	+++
Ischemic response	+	+	+	+	+++
Side effects	+++	++	++	++	++

+ increase; − decrease; ↔ no change.
Modified from Refs. 2 and 5.

pressure catheters that measure pressure gradients (fractional flow reserve [FFR]), or with both to measure stenosis resistance (resistance index).[12,13] Coronary flow can be measured noninvasively using positron emission tomography (PET). Resting and hyperemic MBF are mainly dependent on myocardial oxygen demand expressed by the double-product of BP × HR, as well as other factors such as contractility, coronary driving pressure, left ventricular (LV) hypertrophy, blood viscosity, anemia, and microvascular disease (Table 15-4).[5,14–17]

Myocardial Blood Flow in Normal Patients

Wilson and associates first compared the effect of intravenous adenosine to intracoronary papaverine using a Doppler wire.[18] In patients with normal CFR by papaverine, intravenous adenosine caused a dose-dependent increase in CFR up to a dose of 140 μg/kg/min.[18] Most patients (92%) achieved near-maximal hyperemia comparable to papaverine. This compares to 50% of patients who achieved maximal vasodilatation with 0.56 mg/kg of dipyridamole infused over 4 minutes and to 84% of the subjects who received adenosine doses of 70 μg/kg/min.[18] CFR was submaximal with adenosine doses of 35 and 70 μg/kg/min compared to papaverine and the 100 and 140 μg/kg/min adenosine doses (Fig. 15-1). The maximum CFR achieved with adenosine (3.4 ± 1.2) or with dipyridamole (3.1 ± 1.2) was lower than that achieved with papaverine (3.9 ± 1.1).[19] The coronary vascular resistance by adenosine and papaverine was significantly lower than by dipyridamole.[19] The peak flow velocity was achieved quicker with adenosine (within 55 ± 34 seconds) compared to dipyridamole (within 287 ± 101 seconds).[19] In a PET study, the CFR was 4.0 ± 1.3 with dipyridamole and 4.3 ± 1.6 with adenosine, with considerable interindividual variation (range of 1.5 to 5.8 with dipyridamole; 2.0 to 8.4 with adenosine).[20] The peak MBF was similar between a standard dipyridamole dose of 0.56 mg/kg (2.13 ± 0.28 mL/min/g) compared to a higher dipyridamole dose of 0.8 mg/kg (2.08 ± 0.20 mL/min/g).[21]

The effect of dobutamine on MBF was studied in the normal coronary arteries of 15 patients with CAD, using ^{13}N-ammonia PET.[22] The CFR increased 2.4-fold in the normal coronary arteries, corresponding to a 2.2-fold increase in the double-product.[22] Dobutamine produced a lower peak MBF (2.16 ± 0.99 mL/min/g) than adenosine (3.10 ± 0.90 mL/min/g).[23] Dobutamine-atropine infusion caused a greater increase in peak MBF (5.89 ± 1.58 mL/mg/min) than dipyridamole (4.33 ± 1.23 mL/mg/min), though with no difference in coronary vascular resistance.[24] The 8.8-fold increase in peak MBF with dobutamine-atropine was out of proportion to the 4-fold increase in the double-product, possibly because of the atropine-mediated increase in HR.

Table 15-4   Factors Affecting Myocardial Blood Flow in Patients Without CAD as Measured by PET

	MYOCARDIAL BLOOD FLOW		
	Rest	Hyperemia	CFR
Ant + lat versus inf areas	Higher	Higher	Same
Women versus men	Higher	Same	Lower
Older versus younger	Higher	Lower	Lower
Acute versus nonsmoker	Higher	Lower	Lower
Acute versus long-term smoker	Higher	Lower	Lower
Diabetics versus nondiabetics	Same	Lower	Lower
↑ Low-density lipoprotein			Decrease
↑ High-density lipoprotein			±Increase

Ant, anterior; CAD, coronary artery disease; CFR, coronary flow reserve; PET, positron emission tomography; inf, inferior; lat, lateral; ↑, increase; ±, slight increase. From Zoghbi G, Iskandrian AE: Pharmacologic stress testing. In Garcia EV, Iskandrian AE (eds): *Nuclear Cardiac Imaging: Principles and Applications.* New York: Oxford University Press, 2008, pp 293–315, with permission.

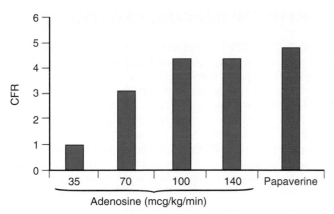

Figure 15-1 Dose-response effect of intravenous adenosine on coronary flow reserve (CFR) compared to intracoronary papaverine. Modified from Zoghbi G, Iskandrian AE: *Coronary artery disease detection: pharmacologic stress.* Zaret BL, Beller GA, eds. *Clinical Nuclear Cardiology: State of the Art and Future Directions, 3rd ed.* Philadelphia: Elsevier Mosby, 2005, pp 233–253 with permission from Elsevier.

Myocardial Blood Flow with Modified Pharmacologic Stress Protocols

The effect of 140 µg/kg/min intravenous adenosine was studied alone or in combination with supine bicycle exercise in 11 healthy volunteers using ^{13}N-ammonia PET.[25] Compared to adenosine stress alone, adenosine combined with exercise resulted in significantly higher systolic and mean BP, HR, and double-product. Adenosine combined with exercise resulted in significantly lower peak MBF (2.2 ± 0.4 mL/min/g) compared to adenosine alone (2.6 + 0.4 mL/min/g).[25] The CFR and coronary vascular resistance were also lower with the combined protocol.[25] Similarly, the addition of isometric handgrip to dipyridamole caused a significant decrease rather than an increase in MBF.[21]

In summary, adenosine and dipyridamole cause a threefold to fivefold increase in MBF in normal coronary arteries, independent of myocardial oxygen demand (unlike dobutamine and exercise). Adenosine and dipyridamole cause a higher CFR than exercise and dobutamine.[22] The hyperemic response is more predictable with adenosine than with dipyridamole and is much shorter lived.[26] Addition of exercise to either adenosine or dipyridamole decreases the peak MBF compared to either alone.[25]

Myocardial Blood Flow in Patients with CAD

The landmark study of Gould showed that the resting MBF in dogs remained normal up to a diameter stenosis of 90%, while the CFR progressively decreased starting at 45% to 50% diameter stenosis (≈75% area stenosis).[27] These results were later confirmed using PET in patients with single-vessel CAD and normal LV function.[28] The resting MBF was not affected by stenosis severity, but the hyperemic MBF after intravenous adenosine progressively decreased with increasing percent diameter stenosis and decreasing minimal luminal diameter.[28] The CFR started to decline at 40% diameter stenosis

(≈60% area stenosis) and reached 1 at 80% diameter stenosis (≈90% area stenosis).[28] Wilson et al. studied 50 patients with limited and discrete one- or two-vessel CAD using papaverine with Doppler and pressure wires.[29] The CFR significantly correlated with percent area stenosis, minimal cross-sectional area, and translesional pressure gradient.[29] Lesions with less than 70% area stenosis (<50% diameter stenosis) or more than 2.5 mm^2 cross-sectional area had a CFR greater than 3.[29]

Dobutamine-induced CFR was significantly lower in regions supplied by vessels with more than 50% diameter stenoses compared to less than 50% (1.7 versus 2.3).[30] A maximally tolerated dobutamine dose was compared to a standard dose of adenosine in 13 patients with CAD using PET.[23] In normal segments, dobutamine caused a peak MBF of 2.16 ± 0.99 mL/min/g, which was 25% less than that achieved with adenosine ($P < 0.001$). In abnormal segments, dobutamine caused an MBF of 0.83 ± 0.43 mL/min/g compared to 0.90 ± 0.49 mL/min/g with adenosine ($P = NS$). The hyperemic response to dobutamine was in excess of that expected by the double-product and was attributed to the inotropic, oxygen-wasting, and β$_2$ agonist effects of dobutamine. The effects of dobutamine and adenosine on MBF and CFR were compared in patients with 50% to 75% and greater than 75% diameter stenosis severity using PET.[31] CFR was significantly greater with adenosine than with dobutamine stress in control subjects and remote territories not subtended by significant CAD.[31] Flow heterogeneity was achieved across all coronary stenoses greater than 50% with adenosine but only in the presence of greater than 75% coronary stenoses with dobutamine.[31]

MYOCARDIAL BLOOD FLOW AND PERFUSION IMAGING

The conduit epicardial coronary arteries provide little resistance to flow under physiologic conditions.[27] The MBF is primarily autoregulated by the arteriolar bed.[27] In the presence of a stenosis in the epicardial artery, the translesional pressure drops, and the arteriolar bed progressively dilates proportional to the stenosis severity, maintaining normal flow to the myocardium.[29] However, the arteriolar autoregulation and the vasodilatory reserve reach a maximum when the diameter stenosis approaches 85% to 90%, after which the coronary perfusion pressure drops to less than 45 mm Hg, along with a drop in the resting MBF.[29] The ability of a stenosed artery to further augment the MBF during hyperemic conditions becomes limited because of the limited vasodilatory reserve of the arteriolar bed. The capillaries are important for exchange at the cellular level and contain 90% of the blood volume in the myocardium.[32] A constant capillary pressure of 30 mm Hg is required to maintain hemostasis.[32] During hyperemia of a stenosed vessel, the capillary resistance increases (derecruitment) to maintain a constant hydrostatic pressure in the face of dropping perfusion pressure and limited vasodilatory reserve.[32] The hyperemic capillary resistance is directly proportional to the stenosis severity.[32]

The radiotracer uptake is dependent on its concentration, the MBF, and the capillary surface area for exchange.[32] Thus the capillary surface area becomes an important limiting factor to radiotracer uptake. The more the derecruitment, the less the surface area available for radiotracer extraction, leading to a perfusion defect in the area supplied by a stenosed artery.[32]

Perfusion defects during stress MPI are generated from the disparity in MBF (or myocardial blood volume) and the differential radiotracer uptake between regions supplied by diseased compared to normal coronary arteries (Fig. 15-2).[5] The regional tracer concentration also depends on the roll-off phenomenon in extraction at high rates of MBF.[33] The first-pass extraction fraction of most radiotracers decreases when the flow rate reaches 2.5× the baseline value and leads to underestimation of the flow in relation to the myocardial tracer concentration.[33] This roll-off effect is thought to be related to a disproportional increase in blood flow velocity compared to the increase in myocardial oxygen demand and may limit the ability of vasodilator MPI to detect mild to moderate coronary artery stenoses.[5,33] The effect of the roll-off phenomenon is greater with technetium-99m tracers than thallium-201.[33]

The comparison of the results of Doppler flow wires to MPI has provided further insight into the generation of perfusion defects. Using dual Doppler flow wires to measure dipyridamole-induced relative CFR in normal (2.6) and diseased (1.1) coronary arteries, Voudris et al. showed a strong correlation ($r = 0.90$, $P < 0.001$) between CFR and the relative tracer uptake ratio on single-photon emission tomography (SPECT).[34] In another study, a CFR less than 1.8 predicted the presence of a reversible perfusion defect on MPI with a 96% concordance rate.[35] Other theories have been postulated as mechanisms for perfusion abnormalities during vasodilator stress such as decrease in distal perfusion pressure due to a decrease in BP, stenosis collapse, or coronary steal.[36]

PERFUSION IMAGING PROTOCOLS

Patients should be instructed to fast for 4 to 6 hours before the test to minimize nausea and vomiting.[3,4] The methylxanthines competitively inhibit the adenosine receptors and may cause false-negative results.[4] Current imaging guidelines recommend holding caffeinated products for 12 hours and dipyridamole, dipyridamole-containing medications (Aggrenox), or aminophylline for 24 hours prior to the test.[3,4] Pentoxifylline can be continued prior to adenosine, and oral dipyridamole can be continued prior to intravenous dipyridamole.[3,4] Some recommend holding antianginal medications for 24 to 48 hours prior to dobutamine and even vasodilator stress due to the ameliorating effect of these medications on perfusion defects.[3,37] An intravenous line with a dual-port Y-connector for injecting the radiopharmaceutical and an infusion pump are needed for adenosine and dobutamine, whereas dipyridamole infusion does not require an infusion pump.[3,4] Continuous electrocardiographic (ECG) monitoring and BP recordings at 1-minute intervals are recommended.[4] The contraindications and endpoints of pharmacologic MPI are listed in Tables 15-5 and 15-6.

The acquisition protocols with the different stressors and radiotracers used (thallium, sestamibi, and tetrofosmin) are shown in Figure 15-3. The protocols used with technetium-labeled agents can be same-day stress/rest or rest/stress, 2-day stress/rest, or dual isotope.[3,4,38,39] The thallium protocol is stress/4-hour redistribution/reinjection. The images are acquired 10 minutes after thallium injection and 40 to 60 minutes after sestamibi or tetrofosmin injection.[3,4,38]

Adenosine is marketed as Adenoscan and is infused intravenously at a rate of 140 μg/kg/min over 5 to 6 minutes.[4,37,38] A 3- or 4-minute infusion is used in some laboratories.[4,37,38] The radiotracer is injected during the third minute of the infusion.[4] A modified adenosine protocol can be used in higher-risk patients such as those with history of hyperactive airway disease, liver cirrhosis with massive ascites, recent ischemic events, or low

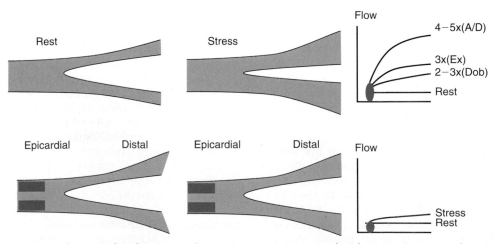

Figure 15-2 Comparison of a normal and a stenosed coronary artery at rest and with stress. In a normal artery, the myocardial blood flow increases distally with the different stressors used. In the stenosed coronary artery, the microcirculation is already dilated to compensate for the degree of stenosis. Any further stress fails to further augment the flow, compared to a normal vessel. This disparity in flow is the basis for stress-induced defects. A, adenosine; D, dipyridamole; Dob, dobutamine; Ex, exercise. *(From Zoghbi G, Iskandrian AE: Pharmacologic stress testing. In Garcia EV, Iskandrian AE [eds]: Nuclear Cardiac Imaging: Principles and Applications. New York: Oxford University Press, 2008, pp 293–315. With permission.)*

Table 15-5 Contraindications to Pharmacologic Stress Testing

Contraindications to Dipyridamole or Adenosine

- Severe obstructive lung disease
- Second- or third-degree AV block without a functioning pacemaker
- Acute MI or unstable coronary syndrome (<24 hours)
- Systolic blood pressure < 90 mm Hg
- Hypersensitivity to adenosine or dipyridamole
- Intake of xanthine-containing compounds within the last 12 hours

Contraindications to Dobutamine

- Acute coronary syndrome (<4 days)
- Severe aortic stenosis or hypertrophic obstructive cardiomyopathy
- Uncontrolled hypertension
- Uncontrolled atrial arrhythmias
- Uncontrolled heart failure
- Severe ventricular arrhythmias
- Large aortic aneurysms
- Narrow-angle glaucoma, myasthenia gravis, obstructive uropathy, or obstructive gastrointestinal disorders

AV, atrioventricular; MI, myocardial infarction. Reprinted from Zoghbi G, Iskandrian AE: *Coronary artery disease detection: Pharmacologic stress.* Zaret BL, Beller GA, eds. *Clinical Nuclear Cardiology: State of the Art and Future Directions,* 3rd ed. Philadelphia: Elsevier Mosby, 2005, pp 233–253 with permission from Elsevier.

Table 15-6 Endpoints in Pharmacologic Stress Testing

With Dipyridamole or Adenosine

- Severe side effects
- Severe hypotension (systolic BP < 90 mm Hg)
- Symptomatic second- or third-degree heart block

With Dobutamine

- Severe chest pain or intolerable side effects
- ST-segment depression > 2 mm
- ST-segment elevation > 1 mm in leads without a Q wave
- Significant ventricular or supraventricular arrhythmias
- Blood pressure ≥ 240/120 mm Hg
- Systolic blood pressure drop > 40 mm Hg
- Attaining target heart rate (220–age)
- Attaining a dobutamine infusion rate of 50 μg/kg/min

Reprinted from Zoghbi G, Iskandrian AE: *Coronary artery disease detection: Pharmacologic stress.* Zaret BL, Beller GA, eds. *Clinical Nuclear Cardiology: State of the Art and Future Directions,* 3rd ed. Philiadelphia: Elsevier Mosby, 2005, pp 233–253 with permission from Elsevier.

systolic BP.[3,4,37,38] The modified protocol starts at a rate of 50 μg/kg/min for 1 minute followed by 75, 100, and 140 μg/kg/min at 1-minute intervals if tolerated.[3,4,37,38] Low-level upright treadmill exercise at 1.7 mph and 0% grade during adenosine infusion can be used in patients without LBBB or a permanent pacemaker.[3,4,37,38]

Dipyridamole is injected intravenously at a dose of 0.56 mg/kg over a 4-minute period.[3,4,37,38] The radioactive tracer is injected 3 to 5 minutes after termination

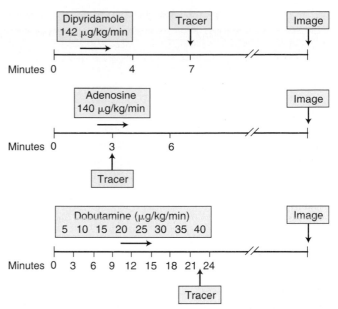

Figure 15-3 The different pharmacologic perfusion imaging protocols. The images are acquired 10 minutes after thallium injection and 40 to 60 minutes after sestamibi or tetrofosmin injection. *(Reprinted from Zoghbi G, Iskandrian AE: Coronary artery disease detection: Pharmacologic stress. Zaret BL, Beller GA, eds. Clinical Nuclear Cardiology: State of the Art and Future Directions, 3rd ed. Philadelphia: Elsevier Mosby, 2005, pp 233–253 with permission from Elsevier.)*

of the dipyridamole infusion.[3,4,37,38] Low-level upright treadmill exercise at 1.7 mph and 0% grade for 4 to 6 minutes shortly after completion of the dipyridamole infusion can be used in patients without a LBBB or permanent pacemaker.[3,4,37,38] The radiotracer is injected during the low-level exercise, which should be continued for 2 minutes after radiotracer injection.[3,4,37,38] A 50% higher dose of dipyridamole is sometimes used in Europe, but it is not certain whether the higher dose produces more coronary hyperemia.[21]

Dobutamine is administered intravenously at an initial dose of 5 to 10 μg/kg/min and is augmented by 10 μg/kg/min every 3 minutes until a maximum dose of 40 μg/kg/min is reached, target HR is achieved, or symptoms develop.[4,37,38] Atropine in 0.5- to 1-mg increments (up to 2 mg total) is administered intravenously if the peak HR is not reached with a maximal dobutamine dose.[3,40] Atropine is contraindicated in patients with myasthenia gravis, obstructive gastrointestinal tract, narrow-angle glaucoma, or uropathy.[3,40] The radioactive tracer is administered at peak HR, and the dobutamine infusion is continued for an additional 1 minute (see Fig. 15-3).[40]

SAFETY AND SIDE EFFECTS

Minor side effects occur more commonly with adenosine than with dipyridamole; however, they are short lived and better tolerated and rarely require reversal with theophylline.[4] Around 80% of patients developed minor symptoms during adenosine infusion and 50% during dipyridamole infusion.[4,6,41,42] Clinically significant side effects such as severe chest pain, hypotension, and bronchospasm occurred in 1.6% of patients receiving

Table 15-7 Side Effects of the Various Pharmacologic Stress Agents

	Dipyridamole N = 3911 (%)	Adenosine N = 9256 (%)	Dobutamine N = 1012 (%)	Regadenoson* N = 517 (%)	Binodenoson† N = 821 (%)
			Minor Event		
Chest pain	770 (20)	3207 (37)	309 (31)	41 (8)	312 (38)
Headache	476 (12)	1318 (14)	138 (14)	147 (28)	370 (45)
Dizziness	460 (12)	783 (9)	—	36 (7)	155 (19)
ST-T changes	292 (8)	531 (6)	—	73 (15)	
Nausea/GI discomfort	218 (6)	1325 (15)	81 (8.0)	61 (13)	
Hypotension	179 (5)	163 (2)	—	—	
Flushing	132 (3)	3377 (37)	104 (10)	88 (17)	288 (35)
Palpitations	127 (3)	—	98 (10)	—	
Pain (unspecified)	102 (3)	—	—	—	
Dyspnea	100 (3)	3260 (35)	123 (12)	128 (25)	358 (44)
Hypertension	59 (2)	—	—	—	
Paresthesias	49 (1)	—	—	2 (11)	
Extra systoles	204 (5)	—	137 (14)	—	
AV block	—	706 (8)	—	0 (0)	0 (0)
Arrhythmia	—	309 (3)	55 (18)	—	
			Major Event		
Death	2 (0.05)	0 (0)	0 (0)	0 (0)	
MI	2 (0.05)	1 (0)	0 (0)	0 (0)	
Bronchospasm	6 (0.15)	12 (0.1)	0 (0)	0 (0)	
Any Minor Side Effect	47 %	82%	85%	79%	

*Results from the phase III trial of the 400-μg bolus of regadenoson
†Results from the phase III trial of the 1.5 μg bolus of binodenoson
Adapted from Refs. 41, 42, 53 and modified from Ref. 3.

adenosine.[4,6,41,42] The most common side effects of adenosine and dipyridamole are listed in Table 15-7. Adenosine was better tolerated in men than women (except for flushing) and in older patients than younger patients, and was preferred over dipyridamole in the patients who received both stressors on separate days.[43,44] Reversal of side effects with theophylline was required in 12% of patients receiving dipyridamole but in fewer than 1% of patients receiving adenosine.[4] Chest pains during vasodilator stress are due to stimulation of the adenosine A1 receptor and thus could occur in patients with normal coronary arteries.[7,45] Dyspnea during vasodilator stress is rarely due to bronchospasm or pulmonary edema and more commonly due to carotid chemoreceptor stimulation that increases the depth and rate of respiration (tachypnea).[46] Adenosine and dipyridamole are well tolerated in smokers and in patients with compensated nonreactive airway disease.[38,41,46] To prevent bronchospasm during stress testing, prophylactic administration of inhaled β agonists before adenosine or dipyridamole infusions has been used in patients with moderate to severe obstructive lung disease.[47]

Atrioventricular (AV) blocks occur in 2% of patients undergoing dipyridamole stress and in 7.6% of patients undergoing adenosine stress and are usually intermittent, transient, well tolerated, may resolve even if the adenosine infusion is continued, and are not reasons to terminate the infusion.[3,37] Second- and third-degree AV blocks occurred in 4% and less than 1% of patients undergoing adenosine stress.[48] In patients with first-degree AV block at baseline undergoing adenosine stress,

second- and third-degree AV blocks occurred transiently in 37% and 14%, respectively, did not require any treatment, and usually resolved with decreasing or discontinuing the adenosine infusion.[37,48] Concomitant use of AV blocking agents with adenosine or increasing age did not influence the incidence of AV blocks.[48,49] AV block during adenosine infusion usually occurs in the first 2 to 3 minutes of the infusion, follows the hyperemic response, and does not require termination of the infusion in over 95% of cases.[3,37] The radiotracer can be injected when the AV block occurs while the adenosine dose is subsequently down-titrated.[3] Adenosine testing has been shown to be safe in elderly patients and in patients with significant aortic stenosis.[49,50]

Severe side effects with vasodilator stress agents occur rarely. In two large multicenter safety trials, the respective incidences of death and nonfatal myocardial infarction (MI) were 0 and 1/10,000 with adenosine and 1/10000 and 1.8/10,000 with dipyridamole.[41,51] Severe side effects, especially bronchospasm (incidence of 8/10000 with adenosine), can be promptly reversed with 50 to 100 mg of intravenous theophylline injected over 1 minute and repeated to a total dose of 250 to 300 mg.[3,37] Theophylline competitively inhibits the adenosine receptor, and its injection should be delayed for 1 to 2 minutes after tracer injection, if possible, to ensure adequate tracer uptake.[3] An exaggerated hypotensive response with adenosine stress may occur in patients with severe liver disease who are being evaluated for transplant surgery. The hypotension is likely due to overdosing, as the dry weight in these patients may be only 50% of their total weight because they often have massive ascites. A titration adenosine protocol is more prudent in these patients.

Side effects occur in around 75% of patients undergoing dobutamine stress.[52,53] The most common side effects are chest pains, palpitations, flushing, dyspnea, and arrhythmias (see Table 15-7).[54] Chest pain during dobutamine stress testing is not a predictor of ischemia as defined by reversible perfusion defects on SPECT imaging.[55] Premature ventricular complexes and nonsustained ventricular tachycardia occurred in 12% and 4.2% of patients who received dobutamine and in 31% and 6.3% of patients who received dobutamine-atropine.[10,53] Ventricular arrhythmias were more frequent in patients with LV dysfunction, fixed perfusion defects, resting wall-motion abnormalities, and history of prior ventricular arrhythmias.[10,11,40,53,54] In a dobutamine safety study that involved 1012 patients, there were no deaths, MIs, or malignant arrhythmias.[53] The side effects of dobutamine can be reversed by a short-acting β-blocker such as esmolol.[4] We believe that dobutamine should not be used shortly after acute MI and possibly also in patients with large aortic abdominal aneurysm and those with atrial fibrillation or history of serious ventricular arrhythmias.

HEMODYNAMIC EFFECTS

Vasodilators

Adenosine and dipyridamole cause modest decreases in systolic, diastolic, and mean BP and a modest increase in HR, with a greater effect observed with adenosine than dipyridamole.[38] Dipyridamole increased the HR by 11 ± 7 beats/min, decreased the mean BP by 10 ± 3 mm Hg, and increased the cardiac output by 34%.[56] Adenosine increased the HR by 14 to 17 beats/min and decreased the systolic BP by 10 to 18 mm Hg and the diastolic BP by 8-9 mm Hg.[41] In patients undergoing adenosine stress, the HR increased in 94% of patients, the systolic BP decreased in 85% of patients, and the diastolic BP decreased in 80% of patients.[6] The HR response to adenosine infusion was diminished in patients with diabetes mellitus (DM) and normal perfusion on SPECT imaging, most likely due to diabetes induced cardiovascular autonomic neuropathy.[57] The systolic BP decreased transiently to less than 80 mm Hg in 2.5% of patients and increased paradoxically in 13% of patients.[6] The pulmonary capillary wedge pressure slightly increased in normal subjects and more so in patients with CAD.[41] The decrease in BP is due to a drop in the systemic vascular resistance. The increase in the pulmonary capillary wedge pressure is due to an increase in venous return and preload, increased diastolic stiffness, and coronary turgor in normal patients, and also due to ischemia-induced diastolic and systolic LV dysfunction in patients with CAD.[36] The increase in cardiac output is primarily due to an increase in HR.[36] Adenosine and dipyridamole produce their coronary vasodilatory effects independent from their peripheral hemodynamic effects. Thus, CAD detection accuracy is independent of the vasodilator peripheral hemodynamic changes.[58,59]

Dobutamine

The hemodynamic effects of dobutamine are comparable to those observed with submaximal exercise.[3,10] A 40 µg/kg/min dobutamine dose increased the systolic BP by 27 mm Hg and the HR by 45 beats/min and decreased the diastolic BP by 17 mm Hg.[3,60] Incremental dobutamine doses progressively increased the HR while the BP increased and leveled at a dose of 20 µg/kg/min.[3,60] Hypotension during dobutamine stress, defined as ≥ 20 mm Hg drop in BP from baseline, occurred in 14% to 20% of patients and is due to peripheral vasodilatation, not to ischemia.[3,11] As such it is not predictive of the presence or extent of wall-motion abnormality or LV dysfunction and has no prognostic implications as seen with exercise-induced hypotension.[3,11] The hypotensive response occurs more commonly in patients with advanced age, high baseline systolic BP, dynamic LV outflow obstruction, and small hyperdynamic LV.[3,10,11] In one study, however, dobutamine-induced hypotension correlated with the number of ischemic segments on perfusion imaging in patients with previous MI.[10] *Dobutamine-related sinus node deceleration* is defined as an initial increase followed by a decrease in HR and occurs in 7% to 19% of patients.[3,10,11] It results from activation of cardioinhibitory receptors that activate the Bezold-Jarisch reflex.[10,11]

ISCHEMIC RESPONSE

Vasodilators

Adenosine or dipyridamole can cause ischemia by producing coronary steal that could be collateral dependent or transmural. Collateral-dependent steal results from decrease in collateral flow distal to a stenosed artery because of differential flow decrease in the donor vessel.[61,62] Transmural steal is less common and less severe and occurs from the subendocardial to subepicardial region, owing to the difference in residual vasodilatory reserve in the subendocardium and subepicardium.[61–63] Systemic hypotension that occurs due to systemic vasodilatation exacerbates the steal phenomenon.[62] Markers of ischemia are ST-segment depressions, typical angina pectoris, and regional wall-motion abnormalities.[61] Most perfusion defects, however, are not due to ischemia but rather to disparity in regional blood flow as a result of variations in hemodynamic severity of coronary stenoses.

Ischemic ST-segment changes due to vasodilator stress are usually depression and rarely elevation. Ischemic changes occurred in 15% to 40% of patients with CAD undergoing dipyridamole stress and in less than 10% of an unselected population.[64,65] ST depressions occurred in 7.6% of 959 patients who underwent adenosine stress and were more common in women (64%) compared to men (36%).[66] Adenosine-induced ischemic ST-segment changes have been correlated with higher baseline and peak systolic BP, greater increase in BP and HR, occurrence of typical angina during adenosine infusion, extensive CAD, presence of collaterals on coronary angiography, extensive and severe perfusion abnormalities, and transient ischemic dilation (TID) (Fig. 15-4).[66–68] ST depressions occur less commonly

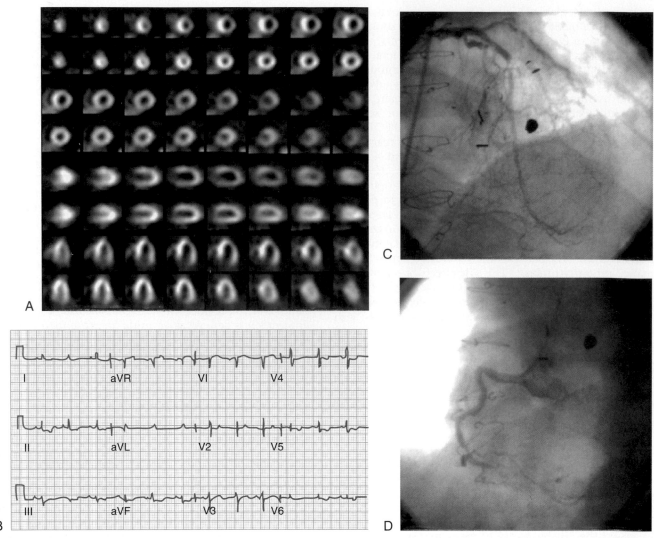

Figure 15-4 Significance of ischemic ECG changes during adenosine SPECT imaging. A 48-year-old male with diabetes mellitus presented with new-onset atypical chest pains. **A,** Adenosine SPECT images show a reversible perfusion defect with transient ischemic dilation suggestive of three-vessel disease *(stress images in the first row of paired rows).* **B,** ST-segment depression during adenosine infusion. **C,** Coronary angiography of the left coronary artery shows severe disease with collaterals to the RCA. **D,** Coronary angiography of the RCA shows a distal occlusion with right-to-right collaterals. *(Reprinted from Zoghbi G, Iskandrian AE: Coronary artery disease detection: Pharmacologic stress. Zaret BL, Beller GA, eds. Clinical Nuclear Cardiology: State of the Art and Future Directions, 3rd ed. Philiadelphia: Elsevier Mosby, 2005, pp 233–253 with permission from Elsevier.)*

than perfusion defects but have a specificity of 90% for CAD detection.[68] Adenosine-induced ischemic ECG changes with normal perfusion on MPI occurred in 1% to 2% of patients, of whom 80% to 88% were women.[69–71] A high event rate was reported in these patients in two studies but was not supported by another study from our own group.[69–71]

Dobutamine

ST-segment depressions occurred in up to 50% of patients with CAD undergoing dobutamine and had a 60% sensitivity and a 90% specificity.[10,11] ST-segment depressions were significantly related to the dobutamine dose and to the CAD extent.[10,11] ST-segment elevations occurred in 6% of patients and as such are markers of extensive perfusion abnormalities, severe CAD, and depressed LV function.[10,11]

LUNG THALLIUM UPTAKE

Increased thallium uptake, defined as a lung-to-heart ratio greater than 50%, is thought to occur because of increased LV filling pressure.[3] Increased lung thallium uptake was reported in 22% to 38% of patients who underwent dipyridamole-thallium imaging and in 30% to 52% of patients who underwent adenosine-thallium imaging.[72] Increased thallium uptake correlates with LV cavity dilation, poor LV function, prior MI, the extent and severity of ischemia, and multivessel disease and collaterals on coronary angiography.[56,65,73] Although increased lung thallium uptake and TID are both associated with severe and extensive CAD, there was no significant correlation between the two indices during dipyridamole-thallium MPI, signifying different pathophysiologic processes.[74] An increased lung-to-heart ratio has also been described with technetium tracers, but the absolute values are lower than with thallium.[73]

TRANSIENT ISCHEMIC DILATATION

Transient ischemic dilation is defined as the quantitative or visual increase in LV cavity size on the poststress images compared to the resting images.[3,75] TID results from subendocardial hypoperfusion or rarely from a true ischemia-mediated increase in LV end-diastolic volume.[65,76] TID occurs in up to a third of patients undergoing adenosine stress and in up to a fourth of patients undergoing dipyridamole stress.[65,76] The presence of TID has been associated with the presence of extensive and severe CAD on angiography, presence of collaterals, extensive and severe perfusion abnormalities on MPI, lower poststress LV function, and more wall-motion abnormalities.[77–80] In patients without prior MI who underwent dipyridamole MPI, the sensitivity and specificity of TID to detect severe multivessel CAD were 80% and 92%, respectively.[81] The accuracy of TID for detecting left main (LM) or severe three-vessel disease during adenosine MPI was 81%.[82] TID can occur in the absence of CAD, as a result of subendocardial ischemia (seen in patients with hypertensive heart disease or hypertrophic cardiomyopathy) or due to technical factors.[73]

POSTSTRESS LEFT VENTRICULAR DYSFUNCTION

Poststress LV dysfunction is defined as a poststress LV ejection fraction (EF) drop by more than 5% compared to rest.[83,84] *Poststress stunning* is defined as poststress worsening or new regional wall-motion or thickening abnormalities compared to rest.[83,84] Poststress LV dysfunction occurred in 33% of patients with CAD who underwent adenosine MPI and in 25% of patients who underwent dipyridamole MPI.[83,85,86] Poststress LV dysfunction with dipyridamole stress had a sensitivity and specificity of 35% and 93%, respectively, for the detection of severe CAD.[86] Poststress LV dysfunction has been correlated with abnormal segmental wall thickening, TID, large ischemic defects, end-systolic dilation and extensive CAD on coronary angiography.[83,86,87] Poststress LV dysfunction or wall motion abnormalities are thought to result from ischemia-induced stunning. A recent study suggested that poststress LV stunning resulted from artifacts of low count regions, since there was an overestimation of post-ischemic stunning on gated SPECT imaging compared to simultaneous poststress ECG.[84] Alternatively, poststress stunning might be more frequent if imaging is performed earlier, as suggested by PET experience. In patients with normal stress SPECT imaging, ATP stress or exercise stress had differential effects on LV volumes that were measured more than 30 minutes after stress, implying differential effects of stress methods on LV volumes.[88] In another study of patients with normal stress SPECT, adenosine stress resulted in a significant decrease in stress LVEF, while exercise stress resulted in a significant increase in stress LVEF compared to rest LVEF.[89]

DIAGNOSIS OF CORONARY ARTERY DISEASE

The accuracy of CAD diagnosis by stress MPI depends on several factors such as pretest and posttest referral biases, patient selection, definition of CAD and perfusion abnormalities, endpoints attained with dobutamine, use of attenuation correction and gating, radiotracer type, and the experience of the reader.[3] Most of the studies compared the results of MPI to coronary angiography, considered the gold standard. However, various studies using PET and pressure-based or Doppler-based catheter techniques have shown considerable variability between coronary angiography and the physiologic significance of coronary lesions (Fig. 15-5).[3,13,90] Even in patients with nonsevere lesions on coronary angiography and normal FFR, the presence of reversible perfusion defects was associated with a higher lesion plaque burden detected by intravascular ultrasound.[91]

Vasodilators

Most of the intravenous dipyridamole MPI studies were performed using planar thallium imaging and used qualitative analysis without gating and attenuation correction. The average sensitivity and specificity of planar thallium dipyridamole MPI were 82% and 75%, respectively, while those of dipyridamole-thallium SPECT were 89% and 78%, respectively.[92] The mean sensitivities and specificities of vasodilator SPECT for detecting CAD (≥50% stenosis) without correction for referral bias were 86% and 73%, respectively (Fig. 15-6).[92] In a study designed without referral bias, the sensitivity and specificity were 72% with pharmacologic SPECT compared to 78% and 85% with exercise SPECT, respectively.[93] The results of dipyridamole and adenosine MPI with the different radiotracers are shown in Figure 15-6. The results of a meta-analysis of adenosine and dipyridamole SPECT for detecting CAD and multivessel CAD are shown in Figure 15-7.[94] The normalcy rate of adenosine-sestamibi performed in patients with low likelihood of CAD was 90%.[94] The sensitivity of adenosine-thallium SPECT for the detection of one-vessel, two-vessel and three-vessel CAD was 83%, 91%, and 97%, respectively.[56] The respective sensitivities and specificities of adenosine thallium SPECT to detect over 50% stenosis were 60% and 90% for the left circumflex (LCX) artery, 75% and 96% for the right coronary artery (RCA), and 75% and 97% for the left anterior descending (LAD) artery, with an accuracy of 75% for the LCX, 86% for the RCA, and 85% for the LAD arteries.[6] Thallium and sestamibi-dipyridamole SPECT performed in the same patients had similar sensitivities of 100% and specificities of 75% for CAD detection.[95] Sestamibi had a higher sensitivity compared with tetrofosmin; however, the diagnostic accuracy and image quality were not different between the two tracers.[96]

The use of gating, attenuation correction, and imaging in the prone position have improved the specificity of

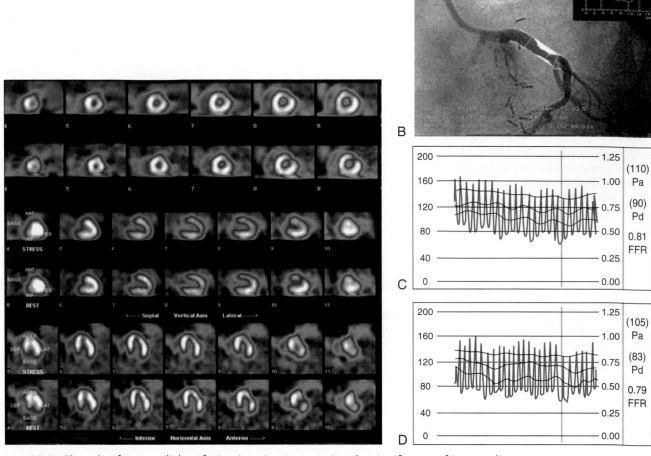

Figure 15-5 The role of myocardial perfusion imaging in assessing the significance of intermediate coronary stenoses. A 54-year-old patient presented with chest pains and had a normal adenosine myocardial perfusion imaging. Coronary angiography performed for recurrence of symptoms revealed a moderate distal left main stenosis. The patient developed a small non-ST elevation myocardial infarction a few months after coronary bypass grafting. **A,** Adenosine-sestamibi SPECT showed a small anterolateral scar with no ischemia *(stress images in the first row of paired rows).* **B,** Coronary angiography was CABG showed occluded grafts and a moderate distal left main stenosis (diameter stenosis 48% and area stenosis 72% by quantitative coronary analysis). **C** and **D,** Pressure wire measurements across the distal left main with wire placed in LAD and LCX showed respective FFRs of 0.81 and 0.79. The patient was left on medical treatment. CABG, coronary artery bypass graft; FFR, fractional flow reserve; LAD, left anterior descending; LCX, left circumflex. *(Reprinted from Zoghbi G, Iskandrian AE: Coronary artery disease detection: Pharmacologic stress. Zaret BL, Beller GA, eds. Clinical Nuclear Cardiology: State of the Art and Future Directions, 3rd ed. Philiadelphia: Elsevier Mosby, 2005, pp 233–253 with permission from Elsevier.)*

SPECT imaging without overall change in sensitivity.[92,97,98] Figure 15-8 shows the effects of attenuation correction and gating on the accuracy of adenosine SPECT.

Dobutamine

Most patients undergoing dobutamine stress tend to be sicker patients, resulting in an important selection bias. Dobutamine also directly affects sestamibi kinetics by affecting mitochondrial potentials, resulting in a lower tracer concentration at a given level of MBF compared to adenosine.[10] In a meta-analysis of 20 studies involving 1014 patients who underwent dobutamine SPECT, the weighted sensitivity, specificity, and accuracy for CAD detection were 88%, 74%, and 84%, respectively.[11] The sensitivity was 82% in studies that did not use atropine and was 90% in studies that used a maximum dobutamine

dose with atropine.[11] The sensitivity of dobutamine SPECT to detect one-, two-, and three-vessel disease 84%, 95%, and 100%, respectively.[11] The mean respective sensitivities and specificities to detect significant CAD were 50% and 94% for the LCX, 88% and 81% for the RCA, and 68% and 90% for the LAD arteries.[11]

Comparison of Pharmacologic Myocardial Perfusion Imaging

In a meta-analysis of 44 pharmacologic SPECT studies, the respective sensitivities and specificities for adenosine, dipyridamole, and dobutamine were 90% and 75%, 89% and 65%, and 82% and 75%.[94] In a study of 54 patients that compared adenosine and dipyridamole, adenosine produced more but shorter-lived side effects (83% versus 65%), a greater decrease in systolic

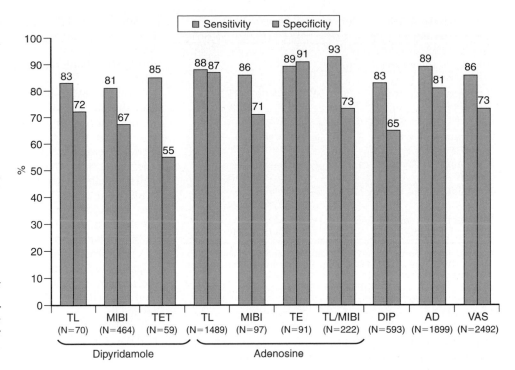

Figure 15-6 Average sensitivities and specificities for detection of greater than 50% coronary artery stenoses by dipyridamole and adenosine myocardial perfusion imaging, without correction for referral bias. MIBI, sestamibi; SPECT, single photon emission computed tomography; TL, thallium. *(From Zoghbi G, Iskandrian AE: Pharmacologic stress testing. In Garcia EV, Iskandrian AE [eds]: Nuclear Cardiac Imaging: Principles and Applications. New York: Oxford University Press, 2008, pp 293-315.)*

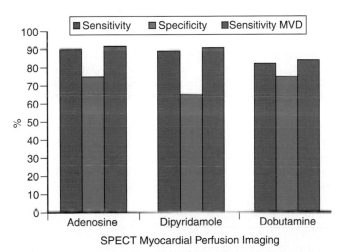

Figure 15-7 Weighted sensitivities of pharmacologic stress SPECT for detecting multivessel disease (MVD). *(From Zoghbi G, Iskandrian AE: Pharmacologic stress testing. In Garcia EV, Iskandrian AE [eds]: Nuclear Cardiac Imaging: Principles and Applications. New York: Oxford University Press, 2008, pp 293-315.)*

BP (−12 versus −5 mm Hg), a greater increase in HR (+18 versus +8 beats/min), and more reversible defects.[44] The sensitivity for CAD detection was 87% with dipyridamole and 91% with adenosine.[44] Dobutamine and vasodilator SPECT were compared in the same 157 patients.[11] The respective sensitivity and specificity for CAD detection were 77% and 78% with dobutamine compared to 90% and 85% with vasodilator SPECT.[11]

Adenosine, dobutamine, and arbutamine were evaluated in 40 patients undergoing tetrofosmin MPI.[99] There was a significant agreement for semiquantitative and visual segmental analysis among the three stressors despite differences in hemodynamic and side-effect profiles.[99]

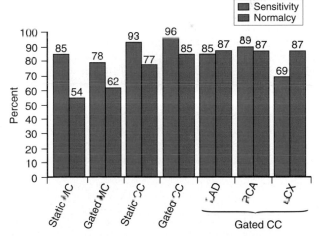

Figure 15-8 Diagnostic accuracy of attenuation correction and gating for the diagnosis of coronary artery disease (n = 66 subjects). CC, combined correction (motion correction + attenuation correction); MC, motion corrected. *(Reprinted from Zoghbi G, Iskandrian AE: Coronary artery disease detection: Pharmacologic stress. Zaret BL, Beller GA, eds. Clinical Nuclear Cardiology: State of the Art and Future Directions, 3rd ed. Philiadelphia: Elsevier Mosby, 2005, pp 233-253 with permission from Elsevier.)*

Comparison to Exercise

The results of vasodilator SPECT are comparable to those of maximal exercise SPECT and at least better than those of submaximal exercise SPECT. In two different multicenter trials involving 244 patients, the average sensitivity, specificity, and accuracy for CAD detection were 83%, 81%, and 82% with adenosine MPI and 82%, 77%, and 79% with exercise MPI, respectively.[100,101] In another study of 175 patients who performed exercise and adenosine MPI within 1 month, the visual and quantitative

Table 15-8 Selection of Stress Test

Condition	Test of Choice
If patient can achieve a good exercise	➢ Use TET
If patient has exercise limitations	➢ Use adenosine or dipyridamole
If patient has bronchospasm	➢ Use dobutamine
If patient has LBBB/pacemaker	➢ Use adenosine or dipyridamole
If patient is < 72 hours of acute MI	➢ Use adenosine or dipyridamole
If patient is < 24 hours of PCI	➢ Use adenosine or dipyridamole
If patient has a large AAA	➢ Use adenosine or dipyridamole

AAA, abdominal aortic aneurysm; LBBB, left bundle branch block; MI, myocardial infarction, PCI, percutaneous coronary intervention; TET, treadmill exercise test.

agreements between exercise and adenosine results were 83% and 86%, respectively.[102] The defect sizes were greater with adenosine, especially when the exercise stress was submaximal.[102] Bicycle exercise SPECT and adenosine were performed in the same 22 patients and showed a 100% agreement on the presence of an abnormal study and a 90% concordance rate in identifying abnormal segments.[103] Dipyridamole and exercise SPECT were performed in the same 16 patients, with myocardial bridging of the LAD by coronary angiography.[104] The prevalence of perfusion defects was similar between the two stressors, though there was a trend toward higher perfusion scores with exercise.[104] Dipyridamole and treadmill exercise N-13 ammonia PET MPI were performed in the same 26 patients.[105] The summed difference score (SDS), summed stress score (SSS), and total perfusion defect size were significantly larger with exercise stress compared to dipyridamole stress.[105] Dipyridamole, adenosine, and exercise sestamibi MPI were compared in the same 20 subjects and were found to have comparable defect sizes and severity.[106] Dipyridamole, adenosine, dobutamine, and exercise tetrofosmin MPI were compared in the same 38 patients.[107] Dipyridamole and dobutamine produced less defect severity, extent, and reversibility compared to exercise and adenosine.[107]

In summary, dipyridamole and adenosine have similar sensitivities for CAD detection as with exercise, though adenosine has a slightly higher specificity.[26] Table 15-8 shows the appropriate selection of a specific stress modality.

Results in Women

Most of the stress SPECT studies were performed in men. Women usually present at an older age, attain lower exercise endpoints, and undergo pharmacologic stress rather than exercise stress.[108] The diagnostic accuracy of stress SPECT in women is affected by the presence of smaller LV size and myocardial mass, and breast attenuation.[109] The diagnostic accuracy of CAD detection in women has improved with the use of vasodilator stress, higher-energy tracers, attenuation correction, and gating.[110]

Adenosine SPECT in women had a sensitivity, specificity, and positive predictive value of 93%, 78%, and 88%, respectively, and a normalcy rate of 93% for detecting ≥ 50% diameter stenosis.[111] Adenosine SPECT had a higher sensitivity for CAD detection in men compared to women (94% versus 84%).[112] Adenosine and exercise had similar sensitivity for multivessel disease detection in men and women, but the sensitivity of adenosine was higher than that of exercise in women with one-vessel disease.[112] Women who underwent dual-isotope adenosine SPECT had significantly smaller stress, rest, and reversible defects than had men.[97] In women who underwent stress SPECT with thallium and sestamibi, the respective sensitivity and specificity for detecting greater than 70% stenosis were 80% and 84% with sestamibi and 84% and 67% with thallium.[113] The specificity of sestamibi imaging improved to 94% with the addition of gating, which was not used in the thallium images.[113] Exercise or dobutamine tetrofosmin SPECT had a sensitivity, specificity, and accuracy of 83%, 80%, and 82%, respectively, to detect greater than 50% CAD in women.[109] The sensitivity was 72% for single-vessel CAD and 93% for multivessel CAD.[109]

Detection of Left Main or Three-Vessel Disease

Left main (LM) or three-vessel disease has no specific pathognomonic perfusion abnormality pattern. Abnormal perfusion in more than one vascular territory is seen in 30% to 70% of patients with LM or three-vessel disease, and rarely no perfusion abnormalities are detected.[112,114] The use of tracers with better extraction fraction and newer quantitative techniques that assess perfusion reserve ratio may improve the ability to more reliably detect individual diseased vessels and eliminate false-negative results. Stepwise discriminant analysis identified multivessel thallium abnormality, increased lung thallium uptake, and ST depression as predictors of LM or three-vessel disease in patients who underwent adenosine-thallium SPECT.[114] A model consisting of magnitude of ST depression, summed reversibility score, and increased lung uptake had incremental power over clinical variables to detect severe LM or three-vessel disease.[115] Severe LM or three-vessel disease was present in the 57% of the predicted high-risk patients and in 9% of the predicted low-risk patients.[115] The SSS and the pre-scan likelihood of CAD were the independent multivariate predictors of severe LM or multivessel CAD in women who underwent adenosine SPECT.[116] A SSS of greater than 8 had a sensitivity of 91% and a specificity of 70% for identifying women with severe CAD.[116] In a study of 101 patients with greater than 50% LM CAD who underwent gated exercise or adenosine stress sestamibi SPECT MPI, moderate to severe defects (>10% myocardium at stress) were identified in only 56% of patients visually and 59% quantitatively.[117] Non-significant perfusion defects (<5% myocardium) were seen in 13% of patients visually and 15% quantitatively.[117] Combining perfusion and nonperfusion abnormalities, especially TID, identified 83% of patients as high risk.

HYBRID PROTOCOLS

Abbreviated Adenosine Protocols

Abbreviated adenosine infusion times have been used in some laboratories to reduce adenosine side effects and costs. Studies that compared a 3-minute to a 6-minute adenosine protocol showed less AV block, hypotension, tachycardia, and other side effects in the 3-minute group.[118,119] Dysrhythmias occurred within 2 minutes from initiation of the 3-minute and 6-minute infusions.[118] The sensitivity for CAD detection was similar between the two groups, although perfusion defect size was slightly smaller in the 3-minute group in one study, and the redistribution was higher in the 6-minute group in another study.[118,119]

In a study that compared a 4-minute to a 6-minute adenosine infusion protocol, side effects occurred in a similar frequency in both groups but were of shorter duration in the 4-minute group.[120] Premature discontinuation of the infusion was more common in the 6-minute group.[120] Ischemic ST changes and chest discomfort occurred less frequently in the 4-minute group, although the accuracies for CAD detection were similar between the two groups.[120] In a study that compared a 4-minute adenosine infusion in conjunction with low-level treadmill exercise to a 6-minute adenosine infusion protocol, the 4-minute protocol with exercise had better image quality and fewer side effects.[121]

Vasodilators and Exercise

Adenosine or dipyridamole stress has been combined with handgrip, submaximal, or maximal exercise during or shortly after the vasodilator infusion but before tracer injection.[4] The reported benefits of the combination protocols include an increase in the double-product and the incidence of ischemic ECG changes, improved image quality, improved target-to-background ratio (decreased hepatic activity), reduced hypotension and other side effects, and a trend to produce more ischemic defects.[122–128] As discussed earlier, the addition of exercise did not increase MBF above that achieved with dipyridamole or adenosine alone.[21]

Modified Dobutamine Protocols

Dobutamine was used in combination with dipyridamole as an additional 10 and 20 µg/kg/min each for 3 minutes at the end of the 4 minute 0.56 mg/kg dipyridamole infusion.[129] The systolic BP, double-product, summed stress and reversibility scores, ECG changes, angina, and abnormal perfusion images were greater in the combination protocol compared to the dipyridamole-only protocol.[129] Side effects were similar between the two groups.[129]

Patients who fail to attain their target HR by the end of the 40 µg/kg/min dobutamine infusion are routinely given 0.5 to 1.0 mg of atropine.[4] The atropine-dobutamine regimen caused 94% of patients to achieve target HR or an ischemic endpoint.[54] The sensitivity of CAD detection improved from 82% with dobutamine alone to 90% with atropine-dobutamine.[11]

Low-level exercise supplementation for the last 2 minutes of a dobutamine infusion caused significantly higher heart-to-liver and heart-to-diaphragm thallium uptake ratios, with resultant improved image quality and no differences in the occurrence of side effects or ECG changes.[130] A leg-raising protocol was used in patients who did not reach their target HR by the end of the 30 µg/kg/min, and involved alternating leg raising to 45 degrees up to 3 minutes as tolerated while dobutamine was increased and maintained at 40 µg/kg/min.[131] Compared to the conventional dobutamine with atropine as-needed protocol, the leg-raising protocol caused significantly higher peak HR and double-product, lower time to reach peak HR, fewer side effects including arrhythmias, and 100% attainment in target HR.[131] Combination of handgrip exercise with dobutamine compared to dobutamine alone reduced the total dose of dobutamine required to achieve target HR and decreased the side effects associated with dobutamine.[132] Target HR was achieved in 97% of the patients in the combination protocol and in 82% of the dobutamine-alone protocol.[132] One study compared a standard progressive dobutamine protocol with increments of 10 µg/kg/min and atropine at the end of the 40 µg/kg/min infusion if target HR is not reached, to an accelerated protocol where atropine was administered at the end of the first stage of a progressive dobutamine protocol aiming at the same HR of the standard protocol.[133] The incidence of adverse effects was reduced in the accelerated (34.5%) compared to the standard protocol (54.8%; $P < 0.05$), as well as the dobutamine infusion duration (508 ± 130 versus 715 ± 142 sec; $P < 0.001$).[133] The maximal HR, percent of achieved maximal HR, rate-pressure product, ST changes, and perfusion scores were similar in the two groups.[133]

SPECIAL PATIENTS

Patients With Left Bundle Branch Block

Patients with LBBB can develop false anteroseptal ischemic perfusion defects on dobutamine or exercise SPECT in the absence of disease in the LAD territory.[134] Doppler flow wire studies in patients with LBBB and normal coronary arteries demonstrated a reduction in diastolic MBF in the LAD due to early diastolic compressive resistance resulting from the asynchronous and delayed systolic septal contraction.[134] The decreased diastolic MBF is further exacerbated during exercise by the tachycardia-induced reduction in the diastolic filling time.[134] False-positive perfusion abnormalities can occur in up to 50% of patients undergoing exercise SPECT and in 84% to 100% of patients undergoing dobutamine SPECT.[10,135]

In a study that compared exercise and adenosine thallium MPI in patients with LBBB, the specificity for detecting greater than 50% diameter stenosis in the LAD was 82% with adenosine and 42% with exercise.[135] Adenosine-tetrofosmin SPECT and coronary angiography were performed in patients with chest pain and LBBB.[136] A significant angiographic LAD disease was found in 25% of patients. The sensitivity and the specificity of adenosine SPECT were 75% and 89%, respectively, and the positive and negative predictive values were 70% and 91%, respectively.[136] The use of iterative reconstruction and attenuation correction in patients with spontaneous or pacemaker-induced LBBB resulted in more pronounced and less reversible apical-septal defect patterns compared with filtered projection.[137]

Vasodilators are the stressors of choice for patients with LBBB, and neither should be combined with exercise or dobutamine.[4] Perfusion defects in the RCA or LCX territory are predictive of disease in these vessels regardless of the stress modality.[3] Additionally, a normal perfusion study is meaningful regardless of stress modality.[3] Finally, anteroseptal fixed defects are predictors of prior MI and are not affected by stress modality.[3] Gated SPECT imaging in patients with LBBB may show septal wall motion abnormality despite normal perfusion, but the thickening is often normal.[3]

Patients with Permanent Ventricular Pacing

Permanent ventricular pacing, like LBBB, may produce false-positive reversible perfusion defects in the septum and also in the inferior wall and apex in the absence of coronary disease.[138,139] These perfusion defects are thought to arise from the asynchronous ventricular activation of pacing that alters regional perfusion and function.[139] Patients with right ventricular pacing who underwent exercise thallium MPI and coronary angiography developed false-positive perfusion defects in the inferoposterior (71%), apical (50%), and inferoseptal walls (28%).[140] In another study of patients with pacemakers who underwent exercise SPECT, false-positive perfusion defects occurred in 58% of patients and were associated with longer durations of pacing, apical wall motion abnormalities, and lower LVEF.[138] As with LBBB, it is recommended to use vasodilator stress in patients with pacemakers.[4]

Patients with Left Ventricular Hypertrophy or Cardiomyopathy

LV septal hypertrophy observed in some patients with end-stage renal disease, hypertension, or hypertrophic cardiomyopathy may downscale the lateral wall, mimicking a lateral wall perfusion abnormality due to lower lateral-to-septal count density ratio.[141] A racial difference in CFR and perfusion defects on dipyridamole-thallium MPI was demonstrated between whites and blacks who had normal coronary arteries and LV hypertrophy on echocardiography.[142] In blacks, the CFR decreased significantly as the severity of LV hypertrophy increased, whereas in whites the CFR and the frequency of perfusion defects did not significantly differ in the presence or absence of LV hypertrophy. The frequency of abnormal scans in blacks was 59% in those with LV hypertrophy and 31% in those without hypertrophy.[142] Exercise SPECT in patients with LV hypertrophy on echocardiography had a sensitivity and a specificity of 84% and 82%, respectively.[143] The sensitivity,

specificity, and accuracy for CAD detection were similar between hypertensive patients with and without LV hypertrophy and between hypertensive and normotensive patients who underwent exercise SPECT.[144] LV hypertrophy should not affect the results of perfusion imaging, as long as the "hot spot" artifact is recognized as a normal variant.

Patients with hypertrophic, ischemic, or nonischemic cardiomyopathies may develop reversible or fixed perfusion in the septum or elsewhere, even in the absence of CAD.[145] These defects are likely due to supply-demand imbalances, metabolic abnormalities, MBF regional differences, and microscarring.[145] The relationship between the extent of adenosine-tetrofosmin SPECT defect and the presence of significant CAD as cause of cardiomyopathy was statistically significant in patients with LVEF between 35% and 50% but not significant in those with LVEF ≤ 35%.[146]

EFFECT OF ANTI-ISCHEMIA MEDICATIONS

The effect of anti-ischemia medications on stress SPECT has been studied in patients on therapy compared to patients without therapy (parallel studies) or in the same patients before and after treatment (serial studies).[147] The lipid-lowering and anti-angina medications such as calcium channel blockers, β-blockers, and nitrates have been shown to improve perfusion abnormalities in some studies.[147] β-blockers and some of the calcium channel blockers attenuate the double-product of dobutamine or exercise stress.[3] Calcium channel blockers and nitrates dilate the epicardial, resistive, and collateral circulation and decrease the epicardial-to-endocardial flow ratio and the heterogeneity of MBF.[3] These effects are thought to attenuate the effects of vasodilators. Additionally, nitrates decrease preload, afterload, and oxygen demand and subsequently improve subendocardial flow.[3,148] β-blockers improve the vasodilatory capacity of coronary arteries by decreasing the extravascular compressive forces and improving diastolic relaxation.[149]

Intravenous propranolol administration before dobutamine SPECT caused lower peak HR and BP despite infusing higher doses of dobutamine.[150] The perfusion defects were smaller after propranolol infusion, and myocardial ischemia was abolished in 23% of patients.[150] The accuracy of dobutamine MPI was not altered when atropine was given to augment the submaximal chronotropic response.[150]

The effects of anti-ischemia medications on vasodilator stress MPI have been variable. Treatment with atenolol or placebo prior to dipyridamole MPI did not cause a difference in the overall perfusion results between the groups.[151] However, the sizes of the perfusion defects were larger in 25% of patients after atenolol.[151] Acute administration of metoprolol before dipyridamole SPECT decreased the sensitivity of CAD detection from 86% to 71% and reduced the extent and severity of ischemia by 25% to 30%.[152] In a retrospective study of patients who underwent adenosine SPECT while on β-blockers, the extent, severity, and reversibility of perfusion defects were not significantly different from a group of patients with gender, age, pretest symptoms, and history of CAD who underwent adenosine SPECT while off β-blockers.[153] The effects of amlodipine, nitroglycerin, and metoprolol were studied in patients with CAD (>70% stenosis) who randomly underwent dipyridamole MPI PET while on and off these medications (>5 half-lives).[154] Amlodipine did not have a significant effect on resting or dipyridamole-induced hyperemic MBF. Nitroglycerin increased the resting MBF, and metoprolol decreased the resting and hyperemic MBF.[154] The effects of nitrates, calcium channel blockers, or both were studied in patients who underwent dipyridamole with low-level exercise MPI with and without these medications.[148] Anti-angina medication use before dipyridamole-exercise MPI decreased the defect size by 30%, decreased individual vessel sensitivity from 92% to 62% (especially LAD and LCX) with no effect on specificity and had no hemodynamic effects.[148]

In patients who underwent adenosine ^{13}N-ammonia PET, pretreatment with β-blockers for 12 weeks significantly improved the hyperemic MBF in stenosis-dependent segments to a similar level in stenosis-independent segments.[149] In patients with CAD who underwent adenosine and exercise SPECT on two different occasions, treatment with β-blockers caused less severe and less extensive reversible perfusion defects with exercise stress compared with adenosine stress.[155]

Lipid-lowering medications, particularly statins, improve perfusion defects on stress MPI by their beneficial effects on endothelial integrity and function, decreasing vascular inflammation, improving intrinsic coronary wall elasticity, improving coronary reserve and arterial wall responsiveness to vasodilators, and to a lesser extent by mild regression of fixed stenoses.[147] Lipid-lowering medications have been shown to improve the perfusion abnormality of exercise and vasodilator SPECT or PET in several studies.[156–163] The improvement occurred as early as 2 months in some studies and more definitely beyond 6 months of lipid-lowering therapy.[147]

Combined anti-ischemia medications, including calcium channel blockers, β-blockers, nitrates, and statins, decreased perfusion defect size and severity with dipyridamole and adenosine SPECT.[148,164] In a study of stable patients after MI who underwent sequential adenosine SPECT studies, intensive medical therapy was comparable to coronary revascularization for suppressing ischemia, as demonstrated by before-and-after treatment.[165]

In summary, acute or chronic administration of nitrates has been shown to decrease the size and severity of exercise-induced myocardial perfusion defects.[147] β-blockers ameliorate the perfusion pattern of exercise and dobutamine MPI, but the results are inconsistent with vasodilator MPI. The changes are likely due to alterations in MBF.[147] Calcium channel blockers improve myocardial perfusion during exercise in patients with CAD.[147] Their effects on vasodilator MPI have not been studied. In patients with known CAD who are undergoing exercise MPI and are on anti-anginal medications, it is important to continue these medications until the day of the exercise study to determine the protective effects of such medications. In patients with suspected but unproven CAD, it may be useful to discontinue such medications for 24 to 48 hours, especially if exercise perfusion imaging is used.[5] We still believe that such medications have fewer effects on the results of vasodilator imaging and may be continued until the day of the study. Thus vasodilator imaging is not the most appropriate stress modality to study drug effect, unless these medications are given in very high doses.[5]

The effects of caffeine on adenosine appear to be related to the dose of caffeine and could be overcome by a higher dose of adenosine. In a study of 10 patients with CAD, FFR was not significantly different before and after the infusion of 4 mg/kg intravenous caffeine (mean caffeine level of 3.7 ± 1.8 mg/L).[166] In a study of 30 patients with ischemia on adenosine SPECT perfusion imaging done while off caffeine, the ingestion of an 8-oz cup of coffee 1 hour before adenosine SPECT did not affect the results.[167] The respective total quantitative perfusion defect and the SDS were $12 \pm 10\%$ and 3.8 ± 1.9 before caffeine and $12 \pm 10\%$ ($P =$ ns) and 3.9 ± 2.3 ($P =$ ns) after caffeine (mean level of 3.1 ± 1.6 mg/L).[167] In another study of 30 patients, 2 cups of coffee (200 mg of caffeine) attenuated the results of 140 µ/kg/min infusion of adenosine with exercise (SDS of 12.0 ± 4.4 at baseline versus SDS of 4.1 ± 2.1 after caffeine [mean level of 6.2 ± 2.6 mg/L], $P < 0.001$) but did not have any effect on the results of a 210 µ/kg/min infusion of adenosine with exercise (SDS of 7.7 ± 4.0 at baseline versus 7.8 ± 4.2 after caffeine [mean level of 5.7 ± 2.0], $P = 0.7$)[168] (Fig. 15-9).

NEW AGENT DEVELOPMENT

Compared to adenosine, the selective adenosine A2A receptor agonists can be administered as a single bolus and are more specific for the A2A receptor, causing selective coronary vasodilatation with lesser side effects.[169] Apadenoson (BMS068645 or ATL146e), regadenoson (CVT-Lexiscan), and binodenoson (MRE-0470 and WRC-0470) are selective A2A agonists that have been clinically tested.[169,170] Lexiscan was approved by the U. S. Food and Drug Administration in April 2008. The three selective agonists differ in their affinity to the A2A receptor, onset and duration of hyperemia, and mode of administration as fixed-dose or weight-based boluses.[170] Regadenoson is administered as a fixed bolus, whereas the other two agonists are weight-based.[170] Binodenoson has higher receptor affinity and thus has longer duration of hyperemia than regadenoson and adenosine.[170] The clinical results of apadenoson have not yet been published.

Binodenoson

In a study that used a Doppler flow wire to study the coronary hemodynamic response to five different binodenoson doses, the 1.5 µg/kg intravenous bolus produced coronary hyperemia similar to intravenous adenosine, with lower side effects than the 3.0 µg/kg bolus dose.[171] The 1.5 µg/kg dose produced coronary

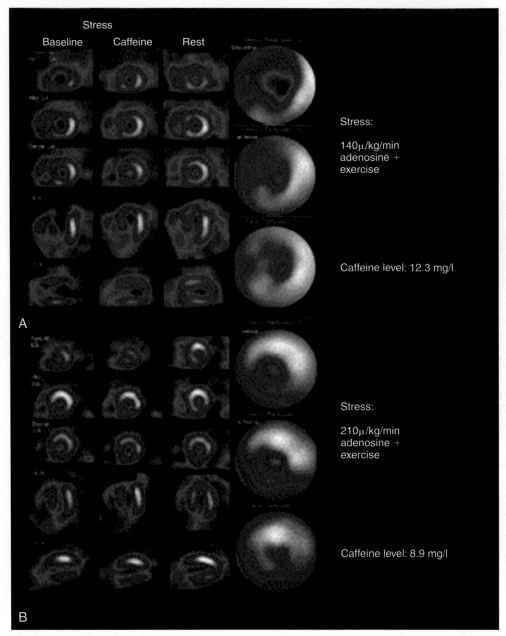

Figure 15-9 **A,** Standard-dose adenosine SPECT images before and after two cups of coffee. **B,** High-dose adenosine SPECT images before and after two cups of coffee. *(Modified from Reyes E, Loong CY, Harbinson M, Donovan J, Anagnostopoulos C, Underwood SR: High-dose adenosine overcomes the attenuation of myocardial perfusion reserve caused by caffeine, J Am Coll Cardiol 52:2008-2016, 2008.)*

hyperemia within seconds that reached its maximal effect by 4.5 ± 3.7 minutes and was sustained for 7.4 ± 6.9 minutes. This was accompanied by modest changes in BP, HR, and double-product and produced no adverse ECG changes.[171] In the phase II clinical trial, binodenoson had dose-dependent side effects (Table 15-9) and comparable ischemia detection to adenosine.[172] There were no second- or third-degree AV blocks, bronchospasm, or hypotension. Chest pain, flushing, and dyspnea occurred less commonly with binodenoson compared to adenosine.[172] There was very good to excellent agreement between binodenoson and adenosine with respect to the extent and severity of reversible perfusion defects.[172] The results of the phase III study, a

double-blind, double-dummy MPI of 1.5 μg/kg binodenoson bolus along with a 6-minute placebo infusion compared with placebo bolus along with a 6-minute 140 μg/kg/min adenosine infusion, were recently presented during the 2008 American College of Cardiology late-breaking clinical trials. The mean paired summed difference score difference of binodenoson versus adenosine images was −0.09 with 61% concordance between the two agents, and 3% complete discordance. The incidence of second- or third-degree AV blocks was 0% with binodenoson and 3% with adenosine. Compared to adenosine, binodenoson caused less flushing (50% versus 32%; $P < 0.05$), chest pain (61% versus 38%; $P < 0.05$), and dyspnea (51% versus 42%; $P < 0.05$) with

Table 15-9 Hemodynamics and Side Effects of the Selective Adenosine Agonists.

	Adenosine 140 μg/kg/min N = 267%	Regadenoson 400 μg bolus N = 517%	Adenosine 140 μg/kg/min N = 226%	BINODENOSON 0.5 μg/kg bolus N = 48%	1.0 μg/kg bolus N = 56%	1.5 μg/kg bolus N = 48%
Max HR ↑ beats/min	20 ± 10	25 ± 11*	23 ± 12	19 ± 10	26 ± 10	31 ± 13
Max SBP ↓ mm Hg	−14 ± 13	−13 ± 14	22 ± 16	19 ± 13	22 ± 17	22 ± 16
Max DBP ↓ mm Hg	−10 ± 8	−10 ± 8	14 ± 9	12 ± 9	11 ± 8	12 ± 7
Hypotension[†]	—	—		0 (0)	0 (0)	0 (0)
AV block (second- or third-degree)	3 (1)	0 (0)	7–(3)	0 (0)	0 (0)	0 (0)
ST depression	38 (15)	73 (15)	—	—	—	—
Bronchospasm	0 (0)	0 (0)	0 (0)	0 (0)	0 (0)	0 (0)
Death/MI/CHF/Stroke	0 (0)	0 (0)	—	—	—	—
Subjective Symptoms						
Chest pain	34 (13)	41 (8)	138 (61)	12 (21)	24 (40)	24 (45)
Angina pectoris	22 (8)	39 (8)	—	—	—	—
Dyspnea	49 (18)	128 (25)	130 (5)	9 (16)	32 (53)	22 (42)
Flushing	63 (24)	88 (17)	128 (57)	10 (17)	17 (28)	18 (34)
Headache	41 (15)	147 (28)	—	—	—	—
Abdominal pain	5 (2)	32 (7)	—	—	—	—
Nausea	12 (5)	29 (6)	—	—	—	—
Dizziness	12 (3)	36 (7)	—	—	—	—
Any event	209 (78)	408 (79)	207 (92)	19 (33)	44 (73)	38 (72)
Any severe event	15 (6)	25 (5)	—	—	—	—
Flushing score	0.4 ± 0.04	0.2 ± 0.02				
Chest pain score	0.5 ± 0.05	0.3 ± 0.03				
Dyspnea score	0.2 ± 0.03	0.3 ± 0.03				
Total score	1.1 ± 0.08	0.9 ± 0.05*				

From the phase II trial of binodenoson compared to adenosine and the phase III trial of regadenoson compared to adenosine.
*$P < 0.05$.
†Hypotension: systolic blood pressure < 70 mm Hg.
AV, atrioventricular; CHF, congestive heart failure; DBP, diastolic blood pressure; HR, heart rate; Max, maximum; MI, myocardial infarction; SBP, systolic blood pressure.
From Zoghbi G, Iskandrian AE: Pharmacologic stress testing. In Garcia EV, Iskandrian AE (eds): *Nuclear Cardiac Imaging: Principles and Applications.* New York: Oxford University Press, 2008, pp 293-315, with permission.

lower patient-rated intensities. Binodenoson caused higher maximal changes in HR (25.3 versus 22.5 beats/min, $P < 0.001$) and similar changes in BP compared to adenosine. However, the Cardiovascular and Renal Drugs Advisory Committee that met in July 2009 did not recommend binodenoson for approval by the FDA due to design, endpoint and analysis related issues in the phase III trial.

Regadenoson

In a study that used a Doppler flow wire to study the coronary hemodynamic response, regadenoson increased peak blood flow velocity by up to 3.4-fold in a dose-dependent manner.[173] Regadenoson (400 to 500 μg) caused a mean duration of CFR ≥ 2.5 for 2.3 to 2.4 minutes, increased HR by up to 21 ± 6 beats/min, decreased systolic BP by up to −24 ± 16 mm Hg, and decreased diastolic BP by up to 15 ± 14 mm Hg.[173] Aminophylline at 100 mg attenuated the increase in peak blood flow velocity but not the tachycardia caused by 400 μg of regadenoson.[173] The hemodynamic and side effects of

regadenoson from the phase III trial are listed in Table 15-9.[174] Regadenoson was better tolerated and preferred over adenosine and caused a greater and faster increase in HR, a similar drop in diastolic and systolic BP, and a slower recovery of BP and HR to baseline.[174] There was good concordance for ischemia detection extent and severity between adenosine and regadenoson.[174] Regadenoson was efficacious in detecting ischemia regardless of age, gender, body mass index, and presence of diabetes mellitus.[175]

In summary, despite the selectivity of the newer agents to the A2A receptor, subjective side effects such as flushing, dyspnea, and chest pain still occur with variable frequencies though are more transient and less severe.[3,174] This might be due to the dose-dependent effects used in these clinical trials that might have rendered them less selective for the A2A receptor.[3,174] Moreover, chest pain and dyspnea might be induced by A2A sympathetic receptor stimulation, as evidenced by rapid and sustained increase in HR in the face of slight drop in BP.[3,174] However, the more serious side effects such as hypotension, AV blocks, and bronchospasm have not been observed so far, leading to optimism about the future role of these agents as stressors with ease of bolus administration and less serious adverse effects.[3,174] In a pilot safety study of 48 patients with mild or moderate asthma who had bronchial reactivity to adenosine monophosphate, regadenoson was safe and well tolerated.[176] In another pilot study of 49 outpatients with moderate or severe chronic obstructive pulmonary disease, regadenoson was overall safe when compared to placebo.[177] New-onset wheezing was observed in 6% and 12% after regadenoson and placebo, respectively ($P = 0.33$).[177] Mean maximum decline in FEV_1 was similar between the two groups. No patient required acute treatment with bronchodilators or oxygen.[177]

Regadenoson is marketed as Lexiscan and is administered as a single 0.4-mg peripheral intravenous bolus (<10 seconds) followed immediately by a 5-mL saline solution flush. The radiotracer is injected 10 to 20 seconds after the saline flush and may be injected directly into the same catheter as Lexiscan (see Fig. 15-3).[174]

SUMMARY

Pharmacologic stress produces coronary hyperemia comparable to that achieved by maximal exercise. Pharmacologic stress SPECT is widely used for diagnosis and prognosis of CAD in patients unable to exercise. The diagnostic accuracy of CAD detection is comparable or exceeds that of exercise SPECT. Newer selective adenosine A2A agonists have the potential of ease of administration and fewer side effects.

REFERENCES

1. Hendel RC, Jamil T, Glover DK: Pharmacologic stress testing: New methods and new agents, *J Nucl Cardiol* 10:197–204, 2003.
2. Orlandi C: Pharmacology of coronary vasodilation: a brief review, *J Nuc Cardiol* 3:S27–S30, 1996.
3. Zoghbi G, Iskandrian AE: Chapter 16: Pharmacologic Stress Testing. In Garcia EV, Iskandrian AE, editors: *Nuclear Cardiac Imaging: Principles and Applications*, New York, 2008, Oxford University Press, pp 293–315.
4. Henzlova MJ, Cerqueira MD, Mahmarian JJ, Yao SS: Stress protocols and tracers, *J Nucl Cardiol* 13:e80–e90, 2006.
5. Zoghbi GJ, Iskandrian AE: Chapter 14: Coronary Artery Disease detection: Pharmacologic Stress. In Zaret BL, Beller GA, editors: *Clinical Nuclear Cardiology: State of the Art and Future Directions*, Philadelphia, 2005, Mosby, Inc, pp 233–253.
6. Abreu A, Mahmarian JJ, Nishimura S, Boyce TM, Verani MS: Tolerance and safety of pharmacologic coronary vasodilation with adenosine in association with thallium-201 scintigraphy in patients with suspected coronary artery disease, *J Am Coll Cardiol* 18:730–735, 1991.
7. Bertolet BD, Belardinelli L, Franco EA, Nichols WW, Kerensky RA, Hill JA: Selective attenuation by N-0861 (N6-endonorboran-2-yl-9-methyladenine) of cardiac A1 adenosine receptor-mediated effects in humans, *Circulation* 93:1871–1876, 1996.
8. Sato A, Terata K, Miura H, Toyama K, Loberiza FR Jr, Hatoum OA, Saito I, Sakuma I, Gutterman DD: Mechanism of vasodilation to adenosine in coronary arterioles from patients with heart disease, *Am J Physiol Heart Circ Physiol* 288:H1633–H1640, 2005.
9. Hendel RC, Wackers FJ, Berman DS, Ficaro E, Depuey EG, Klein L, Cerqueira M: American society of nuclear cardiology consensus statement: reporting of radionuclide myocardial perfusion imaging studies, *J Nucl Cardiol* 10:705–708, 2003.
10. Elhendy A, Bax JJ, Poldermans D: Dobutamine stress myocardial perfusion imaging in coronary artery disease, *J Nucl Med* 43:1634–1646, 2002.
11. Geleijnse ML, Elhendy A, Fioretti PM, Roelandt JR: Dobutamine stress myocardial perfusion imaging, *J Am Coll Cardiol* 36:2017–2027, 2000.
12. Meuwissen M, Siebes M, Chamuleau SA, van Eck-Smit BL, Koch KT, de Winter JG, Tijssen JG, Spaan JA, Piek JJ: Hyperemic stenosis resistance index for evaluation of functional coronary lesion severity, *Circulation* 106:441–446, 2002.
13. Ogilby JD: Role of adenosine in the cardiac catheterization laboratory, *Am J Cardiol* 79:15–19, 1997.
14. Chareonthaitawee P, Kaufmann PA, Rimoldi O, Camici PG: Heterogeneity of resting and hyperemic myocardial blood flow in healthy humans, *Cardiovasc Res* 50:151–161, 2001.
15. Czernin J, Muller P, Chan S, Brunken RC, Porenta G, Krivokapich J, Chen A, Chan A, Phelps ME, Schelbert HR: Influence of age and hemodynamics on myocardial blood flow and flow reserve, *Circulation* 88:62–69, 1993.
16. Kaufmann PA, Gnecchi-Ruscone T, Schafers KP, Luscher TF, Camici PG: Low density lipoprotein cholesterol and coronary microvascular dysfunction in hypercholesterolemia, *J Am Coll Cardiol* 36:103–109, 2000.
17. Yokoyama I, Momomura S, Ohtake T, Yonekura K, Nishikawa J, Sasaki M, Omata M: Reduced myocardial flow reserve in non-insulin-dependent diabetes mellitus, *J Am Coll Cardiol* 30:1472–1477, 1997.
18. Wilson RF, Wyche K, Christensen BV, Zimmer S, Laxson DD: Effects of adenosine on human coronary arterial circulation, *Circulation* 82:1595–1606, 1990.
19. Rossen JD, Quillen JE, Lopez AG, Stenberg RG, Talman CL, Winniford MD: Comparison of coronary vasodilation with intravenous dipyridamole and adenosine, *J Am Coll Cardiol* 18:485–491, 1991.
20. Chan SY, Brunken RC, Czernin J, Porenta G, Kuhle W, Krivokapich J, Phelps HR, Schelbert HR: Comparison of maximal myocardial blood flow during adenosine infusion with that of intravenous dipyridamole in normal men, *J Am Coll Cardiol* 20:979–985, 1992.
21. Czernin J, Auerbach M, Sun KT, Phelps M, Schelbert HR: Effects of modified pharmacologic stress approaches on hyperemic myocardial blood flow, *J Nucl Med* 36:575–580, 1995.
22. Krivokapich J, Huang SC, Schelbert HR: Assessment of the effects of dobutamine on myocardial blood flow and oxidative metabolism in normal human subjects using nitrogen-13 ammonia and carbon-11 acetate, *Am J Cardiol* 71:1351–1356, 1993.
23. Skopicki HA, Abraham SA, Picard MH, Alpert NM, Fischman AJ, Gewirtz H: Effects of dobutamine at maximally tolerated dose on myocardial blood flow in humans with ischemic heart disease. *Circulation* 96:3346–3352, 1997.
24. Tadamura E, Iida H, Matsumoto K, Mamede M, Kubo S, Toyoda H, Shiozaki T, Mukai T, Magata Y, Konishi J: Comparison of myocardial blood flow during dobutamine-atropine infusion with that after dipyridamole administration in normal men, *J Am Coll Cardiol* 37:130–136, 2001.
25. Muller P, Czernin J, Choi Y, Aguilar F, Nitzsche EU, Buxton DB, Sun K, Phelps SC, Huang SC, Schelbert HR: Effect of exercise supplementation during adenosine infusion on hyperemic blood flow and flow reserve, *Am Heart J* 128:52–60, 1994.
26. Beller GA, Zaret BL: Contributions of nuclear cardiology to diagnosis and prognosis of patients with coronary artery disease, *Circulation* 101:1465–1478, 2000.
27. Gould KL: Noninvasive assessment of coronary stenoses by myocardial perfusion imaging during pharmacologic coronary vasodilatation. I. Physiologic basis and experimental validation, *Am J Cardiol* 41:267–278, 1978.
28. Uren NG, Melin JA, De Bruyne B, Wijns W, Baudhuin T, Camici PG: Relation between myocardial blood flow and the severity of coronary-artery stenosis, *N Engl J Med* 330:1782–1788, 1994.
29. Wilson RF, Marcus ML, White CW: Prediction of the physiologic significance of coronary arterial lesions by quantitative lesion geometry in patients with limited coronary artery disease, *Circulation* 75:723–732, 1987.
30. Krivokapich J, Czernin J, Schelbert HR: Dobutamine positron emission tomography: absolute quantitation of rest and dobutamine myocardial blood flow and correlation with cardiac work and percent diameter stenosis in patients with and without coronary artery disease, *J Am Coll Cardiol* 28:565–572, 1996.
31. Jagathesan R, Barnes E, Rosen SD, Foale RA, Camici PG: Comparison of myocardial blood flow and coronary flow reserve during dobutamine and adenosine stress: Implications for pharmacologic stress testing in coronary artery disease, *J Nucl Cardiol* 13:324–332, 2006.
32. Kaul S: The role of capillaries in determining coronary blood flow reserve: Implications for stress-induced reversible perfusion defects, *J Nucl Cardiol* 8:694–700, 2001.
33. Okada RD, Glover DK, Nguyen KN, Johnson G 3rd, : Technetium-99m sestamibi kinetics in reperfused canine myocardium, *Eur J Nucl Med* 22:600–607, 1995.
34. Voudris V, Manginas A, Vassilikos V, Koutelou M, Kantzis J, Cokkinos DV: Coronary flow velocity changes after intravenous dipyridamole infusion: measurements using intravascular Doppler guide wire. A documentation of flow inhomogeneity, *J Am Coll Cardiol* 27:1148–1155, 1996.

35. Deychak YA, Segal J, Reiner JS, Rohrbeck SC, Thompson MA, Lundergan AM, Ross AM, Wasserman AG: Doppler guide wire flow-velocity indexes measured distal to coronary stenoses associated with reversible thallium perfusion defects, *Am Heart J* 129:219–227, 1995.
36. Ogilby JD, Iskandrian AS, Untereker WJ, Heo J, Nguyen TN, Mercuro J: Effect of intravenous adenosine infusion on myocardial perfusion and function, Hemodynamic/angiographic and scintigraphic study, *Circulation* 86:887–895, 1992.
37. Boger LA, Volker LL, Hertenstein GK, Bateman TM: Best patient preparation before and during radionuclide myocardial perfusion imaging studies, *J Nucl Cardiol* 13:98–110, 2006.
38. Hansen CL, Goldstein RA, Berman DS, Churchwell KB, Cooke CD, Corbett JG, Cullom SJ, Dahlberg ST, Galt JR, Garg RK, Heller GV, Hyun LL, Johnson LL, Mann A, McCallister BD, Taillefer R, Ward RP: Myocardial perfusion and function SPECT, *J Nucl Cardiol* 13:e89–114, 2006.
39. Tadehara F, Yamamoto H, Tsujiyama S, Hinoi T, Matsuo S, Matsumoto Y, Sato Y, Kohno N: Feasibility of a rapid protocol of 1-day single-isotope rest/adenosine stress Tc-99m sestamibi ECG-gated myocardial perfusion imaging, *J Nucl Cardiol* 15:35–41, 2008.
40. Elhendy A, van Domburg RT, Bax JJ, Nierop PR, Valkema R, Geleijnse JD, Kasprzak JD, Liqui-Lung AF, Cornel JH, Roelandt JR: Dobutamine-atropine stress myocardial perfusion SPECT imaging in the diagnosis of graft stenosis after coronary artery bypass grafting, *J Nucl Cardiol* 5:491–497, 1998.
41. Cerqueira MD, Verani MS, Schwaiger M, Heo J, Iskandrian AS: Safety profile of adenosine stress perfusion imaging: results from the Adenoscan Multicenter Trial Registry, *J Am Coll Cardiol* 23:384–389, 1994.
42. Ranhosky A, Kempthorne-Rawson J: The safety of intravenous dipyridamole thallium myocardial perfusion imaging. Intravenous Dipyridamole Thallium Imaging Study Group, *Circulation* 81:1205–1209, 1990.
43. Iskandrian AS: Adenosine myocardial perfusion imaging, *J Nucl Med* 35:734–736, 1994.
44. Taillefer R, Amyot R, Turpin S, Lambert R, Pilon C, Jarry M: Comparison between dipyridamole and adenosine as pharmacologic coronary vasodilators in detection of coronary artery disease with thallium 201 imaging, *J Nucl Cardiol* 3:204–211, 1996.
45. Crea F, Pupita G, Galassi AR, el-Tamimi H, Kaski JC, Davies G, Maseri A: Role of adenosine in pathogenesis of anginal pain, *Circulation* 81:164–172, 1990.
46. Balan KK, Critchley M: Is the dyspnea during adenosine cardiac stress test caused by bronchospasm? *Am Heart J* 142:142–145, 2001.
47. Johnston DL, Scanlon PD, Hodge DO, Glynn RB, Hung JC, Gibbons RJ: Pulmonary function monitoring during adenosine myocardial perfusion scintigraphy in patients with chronic obstructive pulmonary disease, *Mayo Clin Proc* 74:339–346, 1999.
48. Alkoutami GS, Reeves WC, Movahed A: The safety of adenosine pharmacologic stress testing in patients with first-degree atrioventricular block in the presence and absence of atrioventricular blocking medications, *J Nucl Cardiol* 6:495–497, 1999.
49. Alkoutami GS, Reeves WC, Movahed A: The frequency of atrioventricular block during adenosine stress testing in young, middle-aged, young-old, and old-old adults, *Am J Geriatr Cardiol* 10:159–161, 2001.
50. Samuels B, Kiat H, Friedman JD, Berman DS: Adenosine pharmacologic stress myocardial perfusion tomographic imaging in patients with significant aortic stenosis. Diagnostic efficacy and comparison of clinical, hemodynamic and electrocardiographic variables with 100 age-matched control subjects, *J Am Coll Cardiol* 25:99–106, 1995.
51. Lette J, Tatum JL, Fraser S, Miller DD, Waters DD, Heller G, Stanton EB, Bom J, Leppo J, Nattel S: Safety of dipyridamole testing in 73,806 patients: the Multicenter Dipyridamole Safety Study, *J Nucl Cardiol* 2:3–17, 1995.
52. Cerqueira MD, Lawrence A: Nuclear cardiology update, *Radiol Clin North Am* 39:931–946, vii–viii, 2001.
53. Dakik HA, Vempathy H, Verani MS: Tolerance, hemodynamic changes, and safety of dobutamine stress perfusion imaging, *J Nucl Cardiol* 3:410–414, 1996.
54. Elhendy A, Valkema R, van Domburg RT, Bax JJ, Nierop PR, Cornel JH, Geleijnse AE, Reijs AE, Krenning EP, Roelandt JR: Safety of dobutamine-atropine stress myocardial perfusion scintigraphy, *J Nucl Med* 39:1662–1666, 1998.
55. Lee JH, Abuannadi M, Jones PG, Bateman T, Thompson R, O'Keefe JH: Dobutamine-induced chest pain does not predict ischemic findings on myocardial perfusion imaging, *J Nucl Cardiol* 15:526–529, 2008.
56. Mahmarian JJ, Verani MS: Myocardial perfusion imaging during pharmacologic stress testing, *Cardiol Clin* 12:223–245, 1994.
57. Bravo PE, Hage FG, Woodham RM, Heo J, Iskandrian AE: Heart rate response to adenosine in patients with diabetes mellitus and normal myocardial perfusion imaging, *Am J Cardiol* 102:1103–1106, 2008.
58. Aksut SV, Pancholy S, Cassel D, Cave V, Heo J, Iskandrian AS: Results of adenosine single photon emission computed tomography thallium-201 imaging in hemodynamic nonresponders, *Am Heart J* 130:67–70, 1995.
59. Amanullah AM, Berman DS, Kiat H, Friedman JD: Usefulness of hemodynamic changes during adenosine infusion in predicting the diagnostic accuracy of adenosine technetium-99m sestamibi single-photon emission computed tomography (SPECT), *Am J Cardiol* 79:1319–1322, 1997.
60. Hays JT, Mahmarian JJ, Cochran AJ, Verani MS: Dobutamine thallium-201 tomography for evaluating patients with suspected coronary artery disease unable to undergo exercise or vasodilator pharmacologic stress testing, *J Am Coll Cardiol* 21:1583–1590, 1993.
61. Iskandrian AS: Myocardial ischemia during pharmacological stress testing, *Circulation* 87:1415–1417, 1993.
62. Nishimura S, Kimball KT, Mahmarian JJ, Verani MS: Angiographic and hemodynamic determinants of myocardial ischemia during adenosine thallium-201 scintigraphy in coronary artery disease, *Circulation* 87:1211–1219, 1993.
63. Werner GS, Fritzenwanger M, Prochnau D, Schwarz G, Ferrari M, Aarnoudse NH, Pijls NH, Figulla HR: Determinants of coronary steal in chronic total coronary occlusions donor artery, collateral, and microvascular resistance, *J Am Coll Cardiol* 48:51–58, 2006.
64. Chambers CE, Brown KA: Dipyridamole-induced ST segment depression during thallium-201 imaging in patients with coronary artery disease: angiographic and hemodynamic determinants, *J Am Coll Cardiol* 12:37–41, 1988.
65. Iskandrian AE, Heo J: Myocardial perfusion imaging during adenosine-induced coronary hyperemia, *Am J Cardiol* 79:20–24, 1997.
66. Gulati M, Pratap P, Kansal P, Calvin JE Jr, Hendel RC: Gender differences in the value of ST-segment depression during adenosine stress testing, *Am J Cardiol* 94:997–1002, 2004.
67. Amanullah AM, Aasa M: Significance of ST segment depression during adenosine-induced coronary hyperemia in angina pectoris and correlation with angiographic, scintigraphic, hemodynamic, and echocardiographic variables, *Int J Cardiol* 48:167–176, 1995.
68. Marshall ES, Raichlen JS, Kim SM, Intenzo CM, Sawyer DT, Brody EA, Tighe CH, Park CH: Prognostic significance of ST-segment depression during adenosine perfusion imaging, *Am Heart J* 130:58–66, 1995.
69. Abbott BG, Afshar M, Berger AK, Wackers FJ: Prognostic significance of ischemic electrocardiographic changes during adenosine infusion in patients with normal myocardial perfusion imaging, *J Nucl Cardiol* 10:9–16, 2003.
70. Hage FG, Dubovsky EV, Heo J, Iskandrian AE: Outcome of patients with adenosine-induced ST-segment depression with normal perfusion on tomographic imaging, *Am J Cardiol* 98:1009–1011, 2006.
71. Klodas E, Miller TD, Christian TF, Hodge DO, Gibbons RJ: Prognostic significance of ischemic electrocardiographic changes during vasodilator stress testing in patients with normal SPECT images, *J Nucl Cardiol* 10:4–8, 2003.
72. Verani MS: Pharmacologic stress myocardial perfusion imaging, *Curr Probl Cardiol* 18:481–525, 1993.
73. Kumar SP, Brewington SD, O'Brien KF, Movahed A: Clinical correlation between increased lung to heart ratio of tecnetium-99m sestamibi and multivessel coronary artery disease, *Int J Cardiol* 101:219–222, 2005.
74. Hansen CL, Cen P, Sanchez B, Robinson R: Comparison of pulmonary uptake with transient cavity dilation after dipyridamole Tl-201 perfusion imaging, *J Nucl Cardiol* 9:47–51, 2002.
75. McLaughlin MG, Danias PG: Transient ischemic dilation: a powerful diagnostic and prognostic finding of stress myocardial perfusion imaging, *J Nucl Cardiol* 9:663–667, 2002.
76. Mazzanti M, Germano G, Kiat H, Kavanagh PB, Alexanderson E, Friedman R, Hachamovitch R, Van Train KF, Berman DS: Identification of severe and extensive coronary artery disease by automatic measurement of transient ischemic dilation of the left ventricle in dual-isotope myocardial perfusion SPECT, *J Am Coll Cardiol* 27:1612–1620, 1996.
77. Abidov A, Bax JJ, Hayes SW, Hachamovitch R, Cohen I, Gerlach J, Kang JD, Friedman JD, Germano G, Berman DS: Transient ischemic dilation ratio of the left ventricle is a significant predictor of future cardiac events in patients with otherwise normal myocardial perfusion SPECT, *J Am Coll Cardiol* 42:1818–1825, 2003.
78. Abidov A, Berman DS: Transient ischemic dilation associated with poststress myocardial stunning of the left ventricle in vasodilator stress myocardial perfusion SPECT: true marker of severe ischemia? *J Nucl Cardiol* 12:258–260, 2005.
79. Emmett L, Magee M, Freedman SB, Van der Wall H, Bush V, Trieu J, Van Gaal W, Allman KC, Kritharides L: The role of left ventricular hypertrophy and diabetes in the presence of transient ischemic dilation of the left ventricle on myocardial perfusion SPECT images, *J Nucl Med* 46:1596–1601, 2005.
80. Hung GU, Lee KW, Chen CP, Lin WY, Yang KT: Relationship of transient ischemic dilation in dipyridamole myocardial perfusion imaging and stress-induced changes of functional parameters evaluated by Tl-201 gated SPECT, *J Nucl Cardiol* 12:268–275, 2005.
81. Chouraqui P, Rodrigues EA, Berman DS, Maddahi J: Significance of dipyridamole-induced transient dilation of the left ventricle during thallium-201 scintigraphy in suspected coronary artery disease, *Am J Cardiol* 66:689–694, 1990.
82. Takeishi Y, Tono-oka I, Ikeda K, Komatani A, Tsuiki K, Yasui S: Dilatation of the left ventricular cavity on dipyridamole thallium-201 imaging: a new marker of triple-vessel disease, *Am Heart J* 121:466–475, 1991.

83. Tanaka H, Chikamori T, Hida S, Usui Y, Harafuji K, Igarashi Y, Yamashina A: Comparison of post-exercise and post-vasodilator stress myocardial stunning as assessed by electrocardiogram-gated single-photon emission computed tomography, *Circ J* 69:1338–1345, 2005.

84. Ward RP, Gundeck EL, Lang RM, Spencer KT, Williams KA: Overestimation of postischemic myocardial stunning on gated SPECT imaging: correlation with echocardiography, *J Nucl Cardiol* 13:514–520, 2006.

85. D'Antono B, Dupuis G, Fortin C, Arsenault A, Burelle D: Detection of exercise-induced myocardial ischemia from symptomatology experienced during testing in men and women, *Can J Cardiol* 22:411–417, 2006.

86. Hung GU, Lee KW, Chen CP, Yang KT, Lin WY: Worsening of left ventricular ejection fraction induced by dipyridamole on Tl-201 gated myocardial perfusion imaging predicts significant coronary artery disease, *J Nucl Cardiol* 13:225–232, 2006.

87. Druz RS, Akinboboye OA, Grimson R, Nichols KJ, Reichek N: Postischemic stunning after adenosine vasodilator stress, *J Nucl Cardiol* 11:534–541, 2004.

88. Ohtaki Y, Chikamori T, Igarashi Y, Hida S, Tanaka H, Hatano T, Usui Y, Miyagi A, Yamashina A: Differential effects comparing exercise and pharmacologic stress on left ventricular function using gated Tc-99m sestamibi SPECT, *Ann Nucl Med* 22:185–190, 2008.

89. Brinkman N, Dibbets-Schneider P, Scholte AJ, Stokkel MP: Myocardial perfusion scintigraphy with adenosine: does it impair the left ventricular ejection fraction obtained with gated SPECT? *Clin Nucl Med* 33:89–93, 2008.

90. Pijls NH, De Bruyne B, Peels K, Van Der Voort PH, Bonnier HJ, Bartunek JJ, Koolen JJ: Measurement of fractional flow reserve to assess the functional severity of coronary-artery stenoses, *N Engl J Med* 334:1703–1708, 1996.

91. Rodes-Cabau J, Candell-Riera J, Angel J, de Leon G, Pereztol O, Castell-Conesa J, Soto A, Anivarro I, Aguade S, Vazquez M, Domingo E, Tardif J, Soler-Soler J: Relation of myocardial perfusion defects and nonsignificant coronary lesions by angiography with insights from intravascular ultrasound and coronary pressure measurements, *Am J Cardiol* 96:1621–1626, 2005.

92. Klocke FJ, Baird MG, Lorell BH, Bateman TM, Messer JV, Berman DS, O'Gara BA, Carabello BA, Russell RO Jr, Cerqueira MD, St John Sutton AN, DeMaria AN, Udelson JE, Kennedy JW, Verani MS, Williams EM, Antman EM, Smith SC Jr, Alpert JS, Gregoratos G, Anderson LF, Hiratzka LF, Faxon DP, Hunt SA, Fuster V, Jacobs AK, Gibbons RO, Russell RO: ACC/AHA/ASNC guidelines for the clinical use of cardiac radionuclide imaging—executive summary: a report of the American College of Cardiology/American Heart Association Task Force on Practice Guidelines (ACC/AHA/ASNC Committee to Revise the 1995 Guidelines for the Clinical Use of Cardiac Radionuclide Imaging), *J Am Coll Cardiol* 42:1318–1333, 2003.

93. Johansen A, Hoilund-Carlsen PF, Christensen HW, Vach W, Jorgensen A, Veje A, Haghfelt T: Diagnostic accuracy of myocardial perfusion imaging in a study population without post-test referral bias, *J Nucl Cardiol* 12:530–537, 2005.

94. Kim C, Kwok YS, Heagerty P, Redberg R: Pharmacologic stress testing for coronary disease diagnosis: A meta-analysis, *Am Heart J* 142:934–944, 2001.

95. Tartagni F, Dondi M, Limonetti P, Franchi R, Maiello L, Monetti N, Magnani B: Dipyridamole technetium-99m-2-methoxy isobutyl isonitrile tomoscintigraphic imaging for identifying diseased coronary vessels: comparison with thallium-201 stress-rest study, *J Nucl Med* 32:369–376, 1991.

96. Soman P, Taillefer R, DePuey EG, Udelson JE, Lahiri A: Enhanced detection of reversible perfusion defects by Tc-99m sestamibi compared to Tc-99m tetrofosmin during vasodilator stress SPECT imaging in mild-to-moderate coronary artery disease, *J Am Coll Cardiol* 37:458–462, 2001.

97. Berman DS, Kang X, Hayes SW, Friedman JD, Cohen I, Abidov A, Shaw AM, Amanullah AM, Germano G, Hachamovitch R: Adenosine myocardial perfusion single-photon emission computed tomography in women compared with men. Impact of diabetes mellitus on incremental prognostic value and effect on patient management, *J Am Coll Cardiol* 41:1125–1133, 2003.

98. Nishina H, Slomka PJ, Abidov A, Yoda S, Akincioglu C, Kang X, Cohen SW, Hayes SW, Friedman JD, Germano G, Berman DS: Combined Supine and Prone Quantitative Myocardial Perfusion SPECT: Method Development and Clinical Validation in Patients with No Known Coronary Artery Disease, *J Nucl Med* 47:51–58, 2006.

99. Wright DJ, Williams SG, Lindsay HS, Sheard KL, Thorley PJ, Sivananthan UM: Assessment of adenosine, arbutamine and dobutamine as pharmacological stress agents during (99m)Tc-tetrofosmin SPECT imaging: a randomized study, *Nucl Med Commun* 22:1305–1311, 2001.

100. Coyne EP, Belvedere DA, Vande Streek PR, Weiland FL, Evans RB, Spaccavento LJ: Thallium-201 scintigraphy after intravenous infusion of adenosine compared with exercise thallium testing in the diagnosis of coronary artery disease, *J Am Coll Cardiol* 17:1289–1294, 1991.

101. Gupta NC, Esterbrooks DJ, Hilleman DE, Mohiuddin SM: Comparison of adenosine and exercise thallium-201 single-photon emission computed tomography (SPECT) myocardial perfusion imaging. The GE SPECT Multicenter Adenosine Study Group, *J Am Coll Cardiol* 19:248–257, 1992.

102. Nishimura S, Mahmarian JJ, Boyce TM, Verani MS: Equivalence between adenosine and exercise thallium-201 myocardial tomography: a multicenter, prospective, crossover trial, *J Am Coll Cardiol* 20:265–275, 1992.

103. Cuocolo A, Soricelli A, Pace L, Nicolai E, Castelli L, Nappi A, Imbriaco C, Morisco C, Ell PJ, Salvatore M: Adenosine technetium-99m-methoxy isobutyl isonitrile myocardial tomography in patients with coronary artery disease: comparison with exercise, *J Nucl Med* 35:1110–1115, 1994.

104. Vallejo E, Morales M, Sanchez I, Sanchez G, Alburez JC, Bialostozky D: Myocardial perfusion SPECT imaging in patients with myocardial bridging, *J Nucl Cardiol* 12:318–323, 2005.

105. Chow BJ, Beanlands RS, Lee A, DaSilva JN, deKemp RA, Alkahtani A, Ruddy TD: Treadmill exercise produces larger perfusion defects than dipyridamole stress N-13 ammonia positron emission tomography, *J Am Coll Cardiol* 47:411–416, 2006.

106. Santos-Ocampo CD, Herman SD, Travin MI, Garber CE, Ahlberg AW, Messinger GV, Heller GV: Comparison of exercise, dipyridamole, and adenosine by use of technetium 99m sestamibi tomographic imaging, *J Nucl Cardiol* 1:57–64, 1994.

107. Levine MG, Ahlberg AW, Mann A, White MP, McGill CC, Mendes de Leon JM, Piriz JM, Waters D, Heller GV: Comparison of exercise, dipyridamole, adenosine, and dobutamine stress with the use of Tc-99m tetrofosmin tomographic imaging, *J Nucl Cardiol* 6:389–396, 1999.

108. Mieres JH, Shaw LJ: Stress myocardial perfusion imaging in the diagnosis and prognosis of women with suspected coronary artery disease, *Cardiol Rev* 11:330–336, 2003.

109. Elhendy A, Schinkel AF, Bax JJ, van Domburg RT, Valkema R, Biagini HH, Feringa HH, Poldermans D: Accuracy of stress Tc-99m tetrofosmin myocardial perfusion tomography for the diagnosis and localization of coronary artery disease in women, *J Nucl Cardiol* 13:629–634, 2006.

110. Shaw LJ, Bairey Merz CN, Pepine CJ, Reis SE, Bittner V, Kelsey SF, Olson BD, Johnson BD, Mankad S, Sharaf BL, Rogers WJ, Wessel CB, Arant CB, Pohost GM, Lerman A, Quyyumi AA, Sopko G: Insights from the NHLBI-Sponsored Women's Ischemia Syndrome Evaluation (WISE) Study: Part I: gender differences in traditional and novel risk factors, symptom evaluation, and gender-optimized diagnostic strategies, *J Am Coll Cardiol* 47:S4–S20, 2006.

111. Amanullah AM, Kiat H, Friedman JD, Berman DS: Adenosine technetium-99m sestamibi myocardial perfusion SPECT in women: diagnostic efficacy in detection of coronary artery disease, *J Am Coll Cardiol* 27:803–809, 1996.

112. Iskandrian AE, Heo J, Nallamothu N: Detection of coronary artery disease in women with use of stress single-photon emission computed tomography myocardial perfusion imaging, *J Nucl Cardiol* 4:329–335, 1997.

113. Taillefer R, DePuey EG, Udelson JE, Beller GA, Latour Y, Reeves F: Comparative diagnostic accuracy of Tl-201 and Tc-99m sestamibi SPECT imaging (perfusion and ECG-gated SPECT) in detecting coronary artery disease in women, *J Am Coll Cardiol* 29:69–77, 1997.

114. Iskandrian AS, Heo J, Lemlek J, Ogilby JD, Untereker WJ, Iskandrian V, Cave V: Identification of high-risk patients with left main and three-vessel coronary artery disease by adenosine-single photon emission computed tomographic thallium imaging, *Am Heart J* 125:1130–1135, 1993.

115. Ho KT, Miller TD, Christian TF, Hodge DO, Gibbons RJ: Prediction of severe coronary artery disease and long-term outcome in patients undergoing vasodilator SPECT, *J Nucl Cardiol* 8:438–444, 2001.

116. Amanullah AM, Berman DS, Hachamovitch R, Kiat H, Kang X, Friedman JD: Identification of severe or extensive coronary artery disease in women by adenosine technetium-99m sestamibi SPECT, *Am J Cardiol* 80:132–137, 1997.

117. Berman DS, Kang X, Slomka PJ, Gerlach J, de Yang L, Hayes SW, Friedman LE, Thomson LE, Germano G: Underestimation of extent of ischemia by gated SPECT myocardial perfusion imaging in patients with left main coronary artery disease, *J Nucl Cardiol* 14:521–528, 2007.

118. Villegas BJ, Hendel RC, Dahlberg ST, McSherry BA, Leppo JA: Comparison of 3- versus 6-minute infusions of adenosine in thallium-201 myocardial perfusion imaging, *Am Heart J* 126:103–107, 1993.

119. Treuth MG, Reyes GA, He ZX, Cwajg E, Mahmarian JJ, Verani MS: Tolerance and diagnostic accuracy of an abbreviated adenosine infusion for myocardial scintigraphy: a randomized, prospective study, *J Nucl Cardiol* 8:548–554, 2001.

120. O'Keefe JH Jr, Bateman TM, Handlin LR, Barnhart CS: Four- versus 6-minute infusion protocol for adenosine thallium-201 single photon emission computed tomography imaging, *Am Heart J* 129:482–487, 1995.

121. Elliott MD, Holly TA, Leonard SM, Hendel RC: Impact of an abbreviated adenosine protocol incorporating adjunctive treadmill exercise on adverse effects and image quality in patients undergoing stress myocardial perfusion imaging, *J Nucl Cardiol* 7:584–589, 2000.

122. Pennell DJ, Mavrogeni SI, Forbat SM, Karwatowski SP, Underwood SR: Adenosine combined with dynamic exercise for myocardial perfusion imaging, *J Am Coll Cardiol* 25:1300–1309, 1995.

123. Samady H, Wackers FJ, Joska TM, Zaret BL, Jain D: Pharmacologic stress perfusion imaging with adenosine: role of simultaneous low-level treadmill exercise, *J Nucl Cardiol* 9:188–196, 2002.

124. Thomas GS, Prill NV, Majmundar H, Fabrizi RR, Thomas JJ, Hayashida S, Kothapalli S, Payne JL, Payne MM, Miyamoto MI: Treadmill exercise during adenosine infusion is safe, results in fewer adverse reactions, and improves myocardial perfusion image quality, *J Nucl Cardiol* 7:439–446, 2000.

125. Casale PN, Guiney TE, Strauss HW, Boucher CA: Simultaneous low level treadmill exercise and intravenous dipyridamole stress thallium imaging, *Am J Cardiol* 62:799–802, 1988.

126. Ignaszewski AP, McCormick LX, Heslip PG, McEwan AJ, Humen DP: Safety and clinical utility of combined intravenous dipyridamole/symptom-limited exercise stress test with thallium-201 imaging in patients with known or suspected coronary artery disease, *J Nucl Med* 34:2053–2061, 1993.

127. Holly TA, Satran A, Bromet DS, Mieres JH, Frey MJ, Elliott MD, Heller RC, Hendel RC: The impact of adjunctive adenosine infusion during exercise myocardial perfusion imaging: Results of the Both Exercise and Adenosine Stress Test (BEAST) trial, *J Nucl Cardiol* 10:291–296, 2003.

128. Thomas GS, Miyamoto MI: Should simultaneous exercise become the standard for adenosine myocardial perfusion imaging?*Am J Cardiol* 94:3D–10D, 2004 discussion 10D-11D.

129. Shehata AR, Ahlberg AW, White MP, Mann A, Fleming IA, Levine JF, Mather JF, Waters D, Heller GV: Dipyridamole-dobutamine stress with Tc-99m sestamibi tomographic myocardial perfusion imaging, *Am J Cardiol* 82:520–523, 1998.

130. Aydin M, Caner B, Yildirir A, Sari O, Tokgozoglu L: Dobutamine combined with low-level exercise for myocardial perfusion scintigraphy, *Nucl Med Commun* 21:1015–1020, 2000.

131. Bokhari S, Pinsky DJ, Bergmann SR: An improved dobutamine protocol for myocardial perfusion imaging, *Am J Cardiol* 88:1303–1305, 2001.

132. Nadig MR, Patel CD, Malhotra A: Comparison between dobutamine stress and combination of handgrip exercise with dobutamine stress in myocardial perfusion SPECT, *Nucl Med Commun* 28:301–304, 2007.

133. Leao Lima Rde S, De Lorenzo A, Issa A: Reduced adverse effects with an accelerated dobutamine stress protocol compared with the conventional protocol: a prospective, randomized myocardial perfusion scintigraphy study, *Int J Cardiovasc Imaging* 24:55–59, 2008.

134. Skalidis EI, Kochiadakis GE, Koukouraki SI, Parthenakis FI, Karkavitsas PE, Vardas PE: Phasic coronary flow pattern and flow reserve in patients with left bundle branch block and normal coronary arteries, *J Am Coll Cardiol* 33:1338–1346, 1999.

135. O'Keefe JH Jr, Bateman TM, Barnhart CS: Adenosine thallium-201 is superior to exercise thallium-201 for detecting coronary artery disease in patients with left bundle branch block, *J Am Coll Cardiol* 21:1332–1338, 1993.

136. Feola M, Biggi A, Vado A, Ribichini F, Ferrero V, Leonardi G, Uslenghi E: The usefulness of adenosine 99mTc tetrofosmin SPECT for the diagnosis of left anterior descending coronary artery disease in patients with chest pain and left bundle branch block, *Nucl Med Commun* 25:265–269, 2004.

137. Hoefflinghaus T, Husmann L, Valenta I, Moonen C, Gaemperli O, Schepis M, Namdar M, Koepfli P, Siegrist PT, Kaufmann PA: Role of attenuation correction to discriminate defects caused by left bundle branch block versus coronary stenosis in single photon emission computed tomography myocardial perfusion imaging, *Clin Nucl Med* 33:748–751, 2008.

138. Tse HF, Lau CP: Long-term effect of right ventricular pacing on myocardial perfusion and function, *J Am Coll Cardiol* 29:744–749, 1997.

139. Tse HF, Yu C, Wong KK, Tsang V, Leung YL, Ho WY, Lau CP: Functional abnormalities in patients with permanent right ventricular pacing: the effect of sites of electrical stimulation, *J Am Coll Cardiol* 40:1451–1458, 2002.

140. Lakkis NM, He ZX, Verani MS: Diagnosis of coronary artery disease by exercise thallium-201 tomography in patients with a right ventricular pacemaker, *J Am Coll Cardiol* 29:1221–1225, 1997.

141. DePuey EG, Guertler-Krawczynska E, Perkins JV, Robbins WL, Whelchel SD, Clements SD: Alterations in myocardial thallium-201 distribution in patients with chronic systemic hypertension undergoing single-photon emission computed tomography, *Am J Cardiol* 62:234–238, 1988.

142. Houghton JL, Prisant LM, Carr AA, Flowers NC, Frank MJ: Racial differences in myocardial ischemia and coronary flow reserve in hypertension, *J Am Coll Cardiol* 23:1123–1129, 1994.

143. Vaduganathan P, He ZX, Mahmarian JJ, Verani MS: Diagnostic accuracy of stress thallium-201 tomography in patients with left ventricular hypertrophy, *Am J Cardiol* 81:1205–1207, 1998.

144. Elhendy A, van Domburg RT, Sozzi FB, Poldermans D, Bax JJ, Roelandt JR: Impact of hypertension on the accuracy of exercise stress myocardial perfusion imaging for the diagnosis of coronary artery disease, *Heart* 85:655–661, 2001.

145. Yao SS, Qureshi E, Nichols K, Diamond GA, Depuey EG, Rozanski A: Prospective validation of a quantitative method for differentiating ischemic versus nonischemic cardiomyopathy by technetium-99m sestamibi myocardial perfusion single-photon emission computed tomography, *Clin Cardiol* 27:615–620, 2004.

146. Her SH, Yoon HJ, Lee JM, Jin SW, Youn HJ, Seung KB, Kim JH: Adenosine Tc-99m tetrofosmin SPECT in differentiation of ischemic from nonischemic cardiomyopathy in patients with LV systolic dysfunction, *Clin Nucl Med* 33:459–463, 2008.

147. Zoghbi GJ, Dorfman TA, Iskandrian AE: The effects of medications on myocardial perfusion, *J Am Coll Cardiol* 52:401–416, 2008.

148. Sharir T, Rabinowitz B, Livschitz S, Moalem I, Baron J, Kaplinsky E, Chouraqui P: Underestimation of extent and severity of coronary artery disease by dipyridamole stress thallium-201 single-photon emission computed tomographic myocardial perfusion imaging in patients taking antianginal drugs, *J Am Coll Cardiol* 31:1540–1546, 1998.

149. Koepfli P, Wyss CA, Namdar M, Klainguti M, von Schulthess GK, Luscher PA, Kaufmann PA: Beta-adrenergic blockade and myocardial perfusion in coronary artery disease: differential effects in stenotic versus remote myocardial segments, *J Nucl Med* 45:1626–1631, 2004.

150. Shehata AR, Gillam LD, Mascitelli VA, Herman SD, Ahlberg AW, White C, Chen C, Waters DD, Heller GV: Impact of acute propranolol administration on dobutamine-induced myocardial ischemia as evaluated by myocardial perfusion imaging and echocardiography, *Am J Cardiol* 80:268–272, 1997.

151. Bridges AB, Kennedy N, McNeill GP, Cook B, Pringle TH: The effect of atenolol on dipyridamole 201Tl myocardial perfusion tomography in patients with coronary artery disease, *Nucl Med Commun* 13:41–46, 1992.

152. Taillefer R, Ahlberg AW, Masood Y, White CM, Lamargese I, Mather CC, McGill CC, Heller GV: Acute beta-blockade reduces the extent and severity of myocardial perfusion defects with dipyridamole Tc-99m sestamibi SPECT imaging, *J Am Coll Cardiol* 42:1475–1483, 2003.

153. Lakkireddy D, Aronow WS, Bateman T, McGhee I, Nair C, Khan IA: Does beta blocker therapy affect the diagnostic accuracy of adenosine single-photon-emission computed tomographic myocardial perfusion imaging?*Am J Ther* 15:19–23, 2008.

154. Bottcher M, Refsgaard J, Madsen MM, Randsbaek F, Kaltoft A, Botker TT, Nielsen TT: Effect of antianginal medication on resting myocardial perfusion and pharmacologically induced hyperemia, *J Nucl Cardiol* 10:345–352, 2003.

155. Muller-Suur R, Eriksson SV, Strandberg LE, Mesko L: Comparison of adenosine and exercise stress test for quantitative perfusion imaging in patients on beta-blocker therapy, *Cardiology* 95:112–118, 2001.

156. Gould KL, Martucci JP, Goldberg DI, Hess MJ, Edens RP, Latifi R, Dudrick SJ: Short-term cholesterol lowering decreases size and severity of perfusion abnormalities by positron emission tomography after dipyridamole in patients with coronary artery disease. A potential noninvasive marker of healing coronary endothelium, *Circulation* 89:1530–1538, 1994.

157. Mostaza JM, Gomez MV, Gallardo F, Salazar ML, Martin-Jadraque R, Plaza-Celemin L, Gonzalez-Maqueda I, Martin-Jadraque L: Cholesterol reduction improves myocardial perfusion abnormalities in patients with coronary artery disease and average cholesterol levels, *J Am Coll Cardiol* 35:76–82, 2000.

158. Treasure CB, Klein JL, Weintraub WS, Talley JD, Stillabower ME, Kosinski J, Zhang J, Boccuzzi SJ, Cedarholm JC, Alexander RW: Beneficial effects of cholesterol-lowering therapy on the coronary endothelium in patients with coronary artery disease, *N Engl J Med* 332:481–487, 1995.

159. Schwartz RG, Pearson TA, Kalaria VG, Mackin ML, Williford DJ, Awasthi A, Shah A, Rains A, Guido JJ: Prospective serial evaluation of myocardial perfusion and lipids during the first six months of pravastatin therapy: coronary artery disease regression single photon emission computed tomography monitoring trial, *J Am Coll Cardiol* 42:600–610, 2003.

160. Guethlin M, Kasel AM, Coppenrath K, Ziegler S, Delius W, Schwaiger M: Delayed response of myocardial flow reserve to lipid-lowering therapy with fluvastatin, *Circulation* 99:475–481, 1999.

161. Huggins GS, Pasternak RC, Alpert NM, Fischman AJ, Gewirtz H: Effects of short-term treatment of hyperlipidemia on coronary vasodilator function and myocardial perfusion in regions having substantial impairment of baseline dilator reverse, *Circulation* 98:1291–1296, 1998.

162. Yokoyama I, Momomura S, Ohtake T, Yonekura K, Yang W, Kobayakawa T, Aoyagi T, Sugiura S, Yamada N, Ohtomo K, Sasaki Y, Omata Y, Yazaki Y: Improvement of impaired myocardial vasodilatation due to diffuse coronary atherosclerosis in hypercholesterolemics after lipid-lowering therapy, *Circulation* 100:117–122, 1999.

163. Yokoyama I, Yonekura K, Inoue Y, Ohtomo K, Nagai R: Long-term effect of simvastatin on the improvement of impaired myocardial flow reserve in patients with familial hypercholesterolemia without gender variance, *J Nucl Cardiol* 8:445–451, 2001.

164. Dakik HA, Kleiman NS, Farmer JA, He ZX, Wendt JA, Pratt CM, Verani JJ, Mahmarian JJ: Intensive medical therapy versus coronary angioplasty for suppression of myocardial ischemia in survivors of acute myocardial infarction: a prospective, randomized pilot study, *Circulation* 98:2017–2023, 1998.

165. Mahmarian JJ, Dakik HA, Filipchuk NG, Shaw LJ, Iskander SS, Ruddy F, Keng F, Henzlova MJ, Allam A, Moye LA, Pratt CM: An initial strategy of intensive medical therapy is comparable to that of coronary revascularization for suppression of scintigraphic ischemia in high-risk but stable survivors of acute myocardial infarction, *J Am Coll Cardiol* 48:2458–2467, 2006.

166. Aqel RA, Zoghbi GJ, Trimm JR, Baldwin SA, Iskandrian AE: Effect of caffeine administered intravenously on intracoronary-administered adenosine-induced coronary hemodynamics in patients with coronary artery disease, *Am J Cardiol* 93:343–346, 2004.

167. Zoghbi GJ, Htay T, Aqel R, Blackmon L, Heo J, Iskandrian AE: Effect of caffeine on ischemia detection by adenosine single-photon emission computed tomography perfusion imaging, *J Am Coll Cardiol* 47:2296–2302, 2006.

168. Reyes E, Loong CY, Harbinson M, Donovan J, Anagnostopoulos C, Underwood SR: High-dose adenosine overcomes the attenuation of myocardial perfusion reserve caused by caffeine, *J Am Coll Cardiol* 52:2008–2016, 2008.

169. Cerqueira MD: Advances in pharmacologic agents in imaging: new A2A receptor agonists, *Curr Cardiol Rep* 8:119–122, 2006.

170. Iskandrian AE: A new generation of coronary vasodilators in stress perfusion imaging, *Am J Cardiol* 99:1619–1620, 2007.

171. Hodgson JM, Dib N, Kern MJ, Bach RG, Barrett RJ: Coronary circulation responses to binodenoson, a selective adenosine A2A receptor agonist, *Am J Cardiol* 99:1507–1512, 2007.

172. Udelson JE, Heller GV, Wackers FJ, Chai A, Hinchman D, Coleman V, Dilsizian V, DiCarli M, Hachamovitch R, Johnson JR, Barrett RJ, Gibbons RJ: Randomized, controlled dose-ranging study of the selective adenosine A2A receptor agonist binodenoson for pharmacological stress as an adjunct to myocardial perfusion imaging, *Circulation* 109:457–464, 2004.

173. Lieu HD, Shryock JC, von Mering GO, Gordi T, Blackburn B, Olmsted L, Belardinelli L, Kerensky RA: Regadenoson, a selective A2A adenosine receptor agonist, causes dose-dependent increases in coronary blood flow velocity in humans, *J Nucl Cardiol* 14:514–520, 2007.

174. Iskandrian AE, Bateman TM, Belardinelli L, Blackburn B, Cerqueira RC, Hendel RC, Lieu H, Mahmarian JJ, Olmsted A, Underwood J, Vitola J, Wang W: Adenosine versus regadenoson comparative evaluation in myocardial perfusion imaging: results of the ADVANCE phase 3 multicenter international trial, *J Nucl Cardiol* 14:645–658, 2007.

175. Cerqueira MD, Nguyen P, Steahr P, Underwood R, Iskandrian AE: on behalf of the ADVANCE-MPI trial investigators. Effects of age, gender, obesity, and diabetes on the efficacy and safety of the selective A2A agonist regadenoson versus adenosine in myocardial perfusion imaging: integrated ADVANCE-MPI trial results, *JACC Cardiovasc Imaging* 1:307–316, 2008.

176. Leaker BR, O'Connor B, Hansel TT, Barnes PJ, Meng L, Mathur VS, Lieu HD: Safety of regadenoson, an adenosine A2A receptor agonist for myocardial perfusion imaging, in mild asthma and moderate asthma patients: a randomized, double-blind, placebo-controlled trial, *J Nucl Cardiol* 15:329–336, 2008.

177. Thomas GS, Tammelin BR, Schiffman GL, Marquez R, Rice DL, Milikien V, Mathur V: Safety of regadenoson, a selective adenosine A2A agonist, in patients with chronic obstructive pulmonary disease: A randomized, double-blind, placebo-controlled trial (RegCOPD trial), *J Nucl Cardiol* 15:319–328, 2008.

Chapter 16

Prognostic Implications of MPI Stress SPECT

RORY HACHAMOVITCH AND DANIEL S. BERMAN

INTRODUCTION

At a time when other modalities—specifically cardiac computed tomography (CT), cardiac magnetic resonance (CMR), and positron emission tomography (PET)—are increasingly being used in the assessment and management of patients with known or suspected coronary artery disease (CAD),[1] the question of why stress myocardial perfusion single-photon emission computed tomography (SPECT), or MPS, continues to be the most commonly utilized of these modalities must be asked. Cardiac CT and CMR have superior resolution, hence can successfully image coronary arteries, left ventricular size, shape, and wall thickness, as well as valves, pericardium, and other clinically relevant structures. Further, coronary CT angiography (CCTA) has the promise of imaging atherosclerotic plaque burden, morphology, and composition. In this era of newer, advanced modalities, will MPS still have a home?

This chapter addresses what is likely the most important application of stress MPS: its proven ability for prognostication, risk stratification, estimation of patient risk and, potentially, identification of which patients may benefit from medical therapy alone as opposed to referral to catheterization for consideration of revascularization.

PRINCIPLES OF RISK STRATIFICATION: PATIENT SELECTION AND METRICS OF RISK

Several concepts define the basis of risk stratification after stress imaging; generally speaking, these principals hold true for all testing modalities. First, with respect to appropriate selection of patients for testing, the basic concept underlying the use of nuclear testing for risk stratification is that only those patients who can be successfully further stratified (or restratified) in a cost-effective manner would be appropriate patients for stress MPS.[2] While MPS has

been shown to successfully risk stratify multiple, diverse populations,[3] it is cost-effective only when applied to intermediate and high-risk patients,[3–6] and its use should be limited to these populations.[7]

Practically, optimal risk stratification is based on the hypothesis that the risk associated with a normal stress imaging study is sufficiently low that aggressive CAD management and therapeutics will not further improve patient outcomes.[3,8,9] Hence, for example, it is commonly held that invasive coronary angiography and coronary interventions are less frequently performed in patients with normal stress imaging studies than in symptomatic patients in whom these studies are not performed.[6]

On the other hand, patients with abnormal stress imaging results are at greater risk of adverse events, thus resulting in risk stratification in its most basic form relative to normal MPS results (Fig. 16.1). Also, these patients are potential candidates for intervention,[10–12] and the magnitude of their risk is related to the extent and severity of the imaging abnormalities. Based on this premise, outcomes data from an imaging modality should initially be examined for two patterns: (1) risk of adverse events after a normal study and (2) relationship between risk and increasing test abnormality.[2]

To date, examination of MPS test performance has focused on significant clinical events as endpoints—all cause death, cardiac death, and nonfatal myocardial infarction. In this chapter, we will focus on studies evaluating the association of MPS with major events. For purposes of risk assessment, it has been proposed that *low risk* be defined as a less than 1% annual cardiac mortality rate, *intermediate risk* defined by the range of 1% to 3% per year, and *high risk* as greater than 3% per year.[13] It is likely that in the future, studies will increasingly use endpoints related to resource utilization (hospitalization of cardiac causes, emergency department visits, referral to downstream interventions and procedures) to better capture the association of MPS with the global cardiac outcomes, thus better defining its role in patient care.[2]

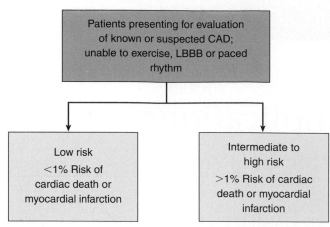

Figure 16-1 Diagram outlining an example of the most basic risk stratification by means of stress MPS in patients with known or suspected CAD.

The use of metrics and thresholds to define the success of risk stratification by testing is challenging. Historically in nuclear cardiology, risk stratification was considered successful if patients with normal scans had either a hard event rate or a mortality rate (varying with publication) of less than 1% per year of follow-up, while patients with abnormal scans have rates exceeding 1%. As will be discussed, the use of thresholding to define levels of risk is problematic. The effectiveness of stratification may also be judged by the ratio of risk in patients with abnormal, compared to those with normal, scans (as measured by a relative risk or odds ratio); increasing relative risks indicate increasing effectiveness in risk stratification.[2]

Risk of Adverse Events After a Normal Imaging Study

To date, there is extensive literature that supports the concept that a normal stress SPECT study is associated with a low risk of hard events (cardiac death or nonfatal myocardial infarction). A pooled analysis from 19 series in the literature comprising 39,173 patients with normal stress SPECT studies, followed for an average of 2.3 years, showed an annual death or myocardial infarction rate of 0.6%.[8] Further, an American Society of Nuclear Cardiology position statement on normal SPECT results reported the very low likelihood (<1%) of adverse events such as cardiac death or myocardial infarction for at least 12 months, independent of gender, age, symptom status, past history of CAD, presence of anatomic CAD, imaging technique, or isotope.[14]

A closer scrutiny of the published literature reveals inconsistency in the message of the statements in the previous paragraph. In general, these studies have suggested that this low risk is independent of imaging type (SPECT versus planar), the type of stress performed (exercise versus pharmacologic), the radiopharmaceutical used, patients' clinical characteristics, patients' prior history of CAD, the results of stress testing, as well as many other factors. However, studies in patients undergoing pharmacologic stress, a population at higher risk

and with more comorbidities than patients undergoing exercise stress, have reported hard event rates of 1.3% to 2.7% per year, suggesting that underlying clinical risk and previous CAD may influence event rates after a normal MPS.[15–21]

These studies encompass cohorts undergoing dipyridamole stress,[15] patients aged 70 years or older,[22] [Hachamovitch, 2003 #11] patients with stable chest pain undergoing dipyridamole stress,[18] patients with diabetes mellitus undergoing adenosine stress,[19,21,19–21] and patients undergoing dobutamine stress.[17] This paradigm is particularly challenged with diabetic patients. Diabetic patients have been found to have strikingly higher event rates after normal MPS,[23] with a number of studies reporting annual hard event rates of 2.0% or more. Interestingly, the event rates in diabetics after stress echocardiography are even greater.[24]

The issue of variability in risk after a normal MPS and the temporal characteristics of this risk (e.g., its "warranty" period) was addressed by a series of 7376 patients with normal stress MPS.[21] This study identified a number of variables: the use of pharmacologic stress, the presence of known CAD, diabetes mellitus (in particular, female diabetics), and advanced age as markers of increased risk and shortened time to risk (e.g., risk in the first year of follow-up was less than in the second year). This study attributed the increased risk after normal MPS in a small subset of patients to the presence of comorbidities that increased the baseline risk of these patients (diabetes mellitus, age, inability to exercise, previous CAD). The more of these characteristics present, the greater the risk after a normal MPS test (Figs. 16-2 and 16-3).

A review by Kalamesh et al.[24] addresses the issue of event rates exceeding the threshold of 1% risk per year in specific patient subsets and posed the question of whether it is a failure of the test or a characteristic of the patient. If it is a failure of the test, the implication

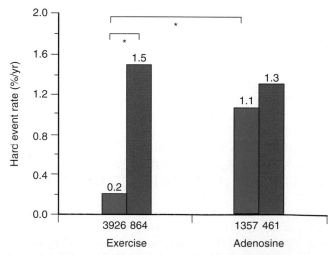

Figure 16-2 Hard event rates (% per year) in patients without history of known coronary artery disease (*blue bars*) versus with history of known coronary artery disease (*pink bars*) undergoing exercise (*left*) or adenosine (*right*) stress. Numbers under bars represent number of patients within category.[21] *$P < 0.001$.

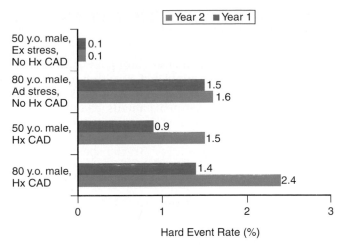

Figure 16-3 Predicted hard event rates, based on Cox proportional hazards modeling, in four patient examples: a 50-year-old male without prior CAD referred to exercise stress, an 80-year-old male without prior CAD referred to adenosine pharmacologic stress, a 50-year-old male with a history of prior CAD referred to MPS, and an 80-year-old male with a history of prior CAD referred to MPS. *blue bars* represent predicted hard event rate in the first year after MPS; *green bars* predicted hard event risk in the second year of follow-up. *(From Hachamovitch R, Hayes S, Friedman JD, et al: Determinants of risk and its temporal variation in patients with normal stress myocardial perfusion scans: What is the warranty period of a normal scan? J Am Coll Cardiol 41:1329-1340, 2003.)*

would be that the test should not be relied on in certain patient subsets (e.g., diabetic patients with suspected CAD should not go to MPS). If the higher event rates after a normal study result from a characteristic of the patient, then it becomes important to set aside generalized thresholds and define what patient-specific event rates are acceptable after a normal study. An alternative answer is that the failure is of the paradigm of defining risk by a single threshold. Given the diversity of patients presenting for evaluation for risk of cardiac events and their wide pretest range of risk of adverse events, the definition of low risk after testing (i.e., the posttest risk) needs to take into account the patient's pretest risk as well as the characteristics of the test, similar to the methods applied to calculate the pretest and posttest likelihood of CAD. Thus, although normal MPS results are associated with low absolute risk in most patient cohorts, care must be taken in assessing post-MPS risk in patients with comorbidities and risk factors.

Relationship Between Risk and the Extent and Severity of Imaging Results

In general, it is safe to say that a close relationship exists between the extent and severity of perfusion abnormalities on stress MPS and subsequent risk of adverse outcomes (Fig. 16-4).[11,12,25] Several characteristics of abnormal studies are worth highlighting. First, even after first stratifying a cohort by their pre-MPS risk, MPS results will still achieve further risk stratification in all levels of pre-MPS risk (Figs. 16-5 and 16-6).[2,12] This

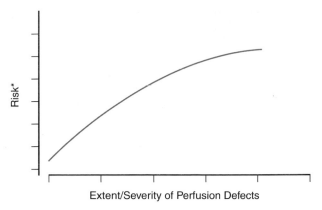

*Adjusted or unadjusted

Figure 16-4 A generalized schematic representing the relationship between the extent and severity of MPS defects and post-MPS risk. The shape of this curve (flattening of the curve at high levels of defect extent and severity) is related to the use of revascularization in higher-risk patients, thus reducing the observed risk in MPS populations.[2,5] This curve is shifted up or down (change in risk for any MPS result) by the patients' baseline (pre-MPS) risk. *(From Hachamovitch R, Di Carli MF: Contemporary reviews in cardiovascular medicine: Methods and limitations of assessing new noninvasive tests II. Outcomes-based validation and reliability assessment of noninvasive testing. Circulation 117:2793-2801, 2008.)*

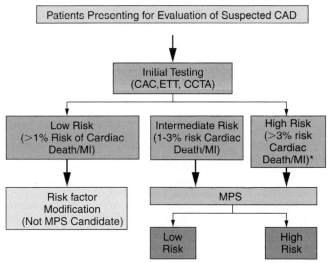

Figure 16-5 A schematic depicting enhanced stratification by MPS results after initial stratification by pre-MPS data. Patients referred to an initial test (CAC: coronary artery calcium scoring; ETT: exercise treadmill testing; CCTA: coronary CT angiography) that stratifies them into low-risk, intermediate-risk, and high-risk groups. Low-risk patients are not candidates for MPS and should be managed medically, but patients at intermediate and high risk can be further stratified (identification of low-risk patients from among the higher-risk patients) by MPS. *Depending on symptoms and the degree of abnormality of the initial test, in some patients it may be appropriate to go directly to invasive coronary angiography. MI, myocardial infarction.

pattern of results can be considered to be a demonstration of clinical incremental prognostic value.[12] In a similar relationship, nonperfusion SPECT imaging variables such as transient ischemic dilation of the left ventricle and variables reflecting regional and global LV function

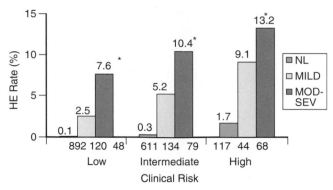

Figure 16-6 Hard event (HE) rates by category of MPS results in patients with baseline low, intermediate, and high clinical risk. Even after initial stratification by clinical risk, MPS results further stratify patients within each clinical risk group. Numbers under bars represent number of patients within category. *P < 0.01 across MPS results within each clinical risk group. NL, normal MPS; MOD-SEV, moderately to severely abnormal MPS. *(From Hachamovitch R, Berman DS, Kiat H, et al: Exercise myocardial perfusion SPECT in patients without known coronary artery disease: Incremental prognostic value and use in risk stratification. Circulation 93:905-914, 1996.)*

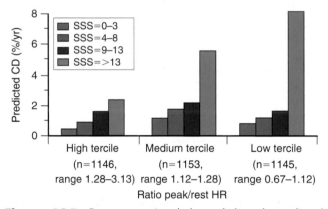

Figure 16-7 Cox proportional hazards-based predicted cardiac death rates by terciles of peak heart rate–to–rest heart rate ratio and summed stress score categories. Overall P < 0.001 across categories. *(From Abidov A, Hachamovitch R, Hayes SW, et al: Prognostic impact of hemodynamic response to adenosine in patients older than age 55 years undergoing vasodilator stress myocardial perfusion study, Circulation 107:2894-2899, 2003.)*

add useful prognostic information to sole assessment of extent and severity of perfusion defects.[3] Further, in patients undergoing vasodilator stress, the presence of a lower baseline heart rate and a greater peak heart rate were both associated with decreased risk (Fig. 16-7).[26]

Added Value of Gated SPECT

Since gated SPECT has become routine only recently, there are several reports of its incremental value over perfusion in assessing prognosis. The first report showed that poststress LVEF and LV end-systolic volume (ESV), as measured by gated SPECT, provided incremental information over the perfusion defect assessment in the prediction of cardiac death.[27] The results of these studies were in large part confirmed by reports from other centers.[28,29]

USE OF MPS IN SPECIFIC PATIENT POPULATIONS

A principal strength of nuclear cardiology is that large databases have been accumulated, resulting in evidence documenting the effectiveness of MPS for risk stratification of appropriately selected patients comprising the full spectrum of patients with suspected or chronic CAD. This evidence has resulted in many class I indications for the use of stress MPS.[8] Several specific lines of evidence are described in the following sections.

Patient Cohorts Defined by CAD Likelihood and ECG Criteria

Patients With an Intermediate Likelihood of CAD or Indeterminate Treadmill Test

A number of studies support a role for MPS for risk stratification in patients with either intermediate post-ETT likelihood of CAD or patients with uninterpretable ETT results.[8] An initial report from Cedars-Sinai demonstrated that MPS was effective in risk stratification and driving management of patients with an intermediate Duke Treadmill Score (DTS).[12] Subsequent studies revealed that the cost-effectiveness of a strategy utilizing MPS is cost saving versus a strategy of direct referral to catheterization in these patients.[4,30] Similar results were shown in subsequent multicenter studies reporting event rates and catheterization rates.[8]

Patients With Normal Resting ECG Able to Exercise

Patients with normal resting electrocardiograms (ECGs) have been a problematic group with respect to their appropriateness for stress imaging. On the one hand, in clinical practice, these patients represent a large subgroup regularly referred to MPS when, taking into account various clinical factors, the post-ETT risk is not low. On the other hand, patients with a normal resting ECG in general are likely (92% to 96%) to have normal LV function[31,32] and to have an excellent prognosis.[4,33] The reticence of many writers of guidelines to embrace the use of MPS in these patients is based in part on a study from the Mayo Clinic.[34] Although these investigators demonstrated that MPS was able to reclassify the likelihood of anatomically severe CAD after considering clinical and ETT data, so few patients were reclassified with respect to their likelihood that MPS was not cost-effective. Hence, previous guidelines did not recommend the use of MPS in these patients,[13] and use of MPS is controversial.

More recently, however, a study designed to parallel the study mentioned was reported, with the important distinction that it employed a prognostic rather than anatomic endpoint.[4] Contrary to findings of the prior study using the anatomic definition of high risk, this study reported that selective use of MPS in patients with intermediate to high post-ETT CAD likelihood yielded significant risk stratification, statistical incremental value, and cost-effectiveness in predicting hard events (Fig. 16-8). A subsequent report has shown that patients with a high clinical risk (based on a clinical score combining age,

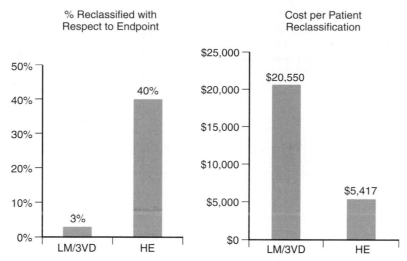

Figure 16-8 Comparison of two studies examining clinical and cost-effectiveness of MPS in patients with normal rest ECG and no prior history of CAD, one using an anatomic endpoint (presence of left main or three vessel CAD; 411 patients)[34] and a second a prognostic endpoint (hard events; 3058 patients with a 1.6-year follow-up).[4] On the *left*, the percent of patients reclassified with respect to their likelihood of the endpoint; on the *right*, the cost per patient reclassified. In the first study, very few patients were reclassified with respect to their risk of severe anatomic CAD, thus the cost per reclassification was unacceptably high. On the other hand, the use of a prognostic endpoint in this population resulted in considerably more patients reclassified with respect to the endpoint, thus a much lower cost per reclassification.

sex, prior MI, and diabetic state) are at too high pretest risk to be classified as low risk by nonimaging exercise testing alone. The authors suggested that initial stress MPS testing might be appropriate in this group.[35]

Thus, while referral of *functionally* capable patients with a normal ECG to MPS is considered inappropriate according to the ACC appropriateness criteria,[7] recent studies indicate that there are patient groups able to exercise with normal rest ECG (such as those with a high pretest likelihood of CAD[5] and the elderly) in which MPS may be indicated.

Patients With Normal Resting ECG Unable to Exercise

In patients unable to exercise to a target heart rate, there is a clear consensus supporting MPS using pharmacologic stress as the initial test in symptomatic male and female patients with intermediate or high pretest likelihood of CAD.[8,36] As shown in multiple previous studies, the inability to exercise per se is itself an incremental predictor of adverse outcomes[8,11,21,37] on par with prior CAD, abnormal MPS, or other high-risk markers. Despite the higher event rates for any test result, for patients who have a normal resting ECG and an intermediate to high likelihood of CAD but are unable to exercise, vasodilator stress MPS has been shown to be effective for both CAD diagnosis and risk stratification.[8,20,38] The relative effectiveness of risk identification tends to be superior with pharmacologic versus exercise stress (due to the considerably greater event rates in the setting of abnormal MPS with pharmacologic stress).

Patients With High Pretest Likelihood of CAD

Historically, symptomatic patients without known CAD who have a high likelihood of CAD based on age, sex, symptoms, and risk factors were considered candidates for direct referral to revascularization. This was based on

the argument that a normal ETT or MPS result would not be sufficient to reclassify the patient as having a low likelihood of CAD, hence precluding the ability for the clinician to confidently exclude the presence of angiographically significant CAD, resulting in diagnostic uncertainty. However, prognostically, it might be possible to classify such patients as low risk. A study assessing the clinical and cost effectiveness of MPS in 1270 patients with a high CAD likelihood (=0.85) revealed that the majority of these patients had a normal MPS study (which had an associated hard event rate of 1.3%).[5] A strategy incorporating initial testing with MPS in these patients to guide decision for coronary angiography was shown to be cost-effective.[5,6] The ACC appropriateness criteria support MPS in high-likelihood patients who have an interpretable or uninterpretable ECG, as well as for those able or unable to exercise.[7]

Patients With Left Bundle Branch Block (See Chapter 5)

At the current time, the guidelines support the use of MPS in symptomatic patients with left bundle branch block, since ETT is not an option in these patients,[8] and the rate of false-positive perfusion defects is observed less frequently with vasodilator stress. This is further supported by the finding of a greater specificity associated with vasodilator stress compared to exercise stress in these patients with similar sensitivities.[39] This approach has also been found to be prognostically valuable and predictive of adverse outcomes in LBBB patients.[40,41] Whereas patients with LBBB and normal MPS have relatively low event rates, patients with LBBB and abnormal MPS results tend to have greater event rates for any defect size compared to other patients.

Patients With LVH or Atrial Fibrillation

In patients with LVH, exertional ST-segment depression is frequently associated without significant CAD. MPS has been shown to be similarly effective in patients with and without LVH for identifying obstructive disease and for risk stratification. In one report, patients with LVH and a low-risk MPS had a less than 1% annual risk of cardiac death or nonfatal myocardial infarction, while the annual cardiac death or nonfatal myocardial infarction rates ranged from 4.9% for mildly abnormal scans to 10.3% for those with moderate to severely abnormal MPS.[42]

In asymptomatic patients with new-onset atrial fibrillation, the use of stress MPS in patients with a high pretest risk is considered appropriate[7] in view of a higher baseline clinical risk, resulting in higher expected cardiac events. A study on the prognostic value of MPS in patients with atrial fibrillation reported an annualized cardiac death rate of 1.6% in the setting of a normal MPS result versus 0.4% for a normal MPS in patients without AF ($P < 0.001$).[43] These authors also reported that a mildly abnormal MPS study in patients with atrial fibrillation is associated with a higher risk than in those without atrial fibrillation, potentially implying the need for a different threshold for determining the appropriateness of referral of these patients catheterization.

Patient Cohorts Defined by Risk Factors and Demographics

Asymptomatic Patients

The diagnostic and prognostic value of stress MPS in asymptomatic populations has been previously examined. The routine use of any test for detection of CAD in a population at low risk/low prevalence of CAD is unlikely to be effective and will be associated with high cost-effectiveness ratios and low positive predictive values. Nonetheless, these evaluations are often performed in patients with high-risk occupations (e.g., pilots, firefighters).[8] However, specific asymptomatic populations who are at intermediate to high risk will be candidates for MPS. For example, asymptomatic siblings of patients with manifest CAD have been found to be at elevated risk of developing CAD and at higher risk of adverse outcomes subsequently.[44] Similarly, certain diabetic patients and women, the former often asymptomatic and the latter with atypical or noncardiac symptoms, also fall into the asymptomatic category but may well be MPS candidates, depending on their estimated risk. The ACCF/ASNC appropriateness criteria consider the use of MPS in asymptomatic patients with a high Framingham risk and those classified as CAD risk equivalent (diabetics) to be appropriate.[7]

Nuclear Imaging in Patients With Diabetes Mellitus

Multiple reports, to date, have supported the value of MPS for risk stratification of diabetic patients.[3] Event rates associated with any MPS result are greater in diabetic compared to nondiabetic patients (Fig. 16-9).[19,20,45] These findings were confirmed in a multicenter series.[46] In the latter study, diabetic women had the worst outcome for any given extent of myocardial infarction. In patients with normal MPS results, survival worsened sooner in diabetic compared to nondiabetic patients,

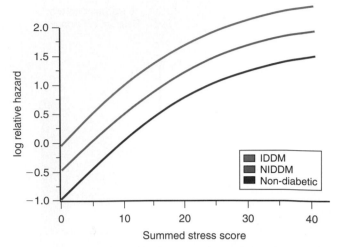

Figure 16-9 Relationship between log relative hazard for predicted cardiac mortality and summed stress score in insulin-dependent diabetes mellitus (IDDM), non–insulin dependent diabetes mellitus (NIDDM), and nondiabetics as a function of summed stress score. Results based on Cox proportional hazards modeling. $P < 0.001$ across the three groups. *(From Berman DS, Kang X, Hayes SW, et al: Adenosine myocardial perfusion single-photon emission computed tomography in women compared with men. Impact of diabetes mellitus on incremental prognostic value and effect on patient management, J Am Coll Cardiol 41:1125-1133, 2003.)*

suggesting that retesting of diabetics with normal studies might be needed earlier than in nondiabetics.[21] In a study of 1430 diabetic patients (701 asymptomatic) followed for a mean of 2.1 years after MPS, Zellweger et al.[47] reported that significant risk stratification was seen when comparing normal and abnormal MPS results in asymptomatic diabetic patients. They observed 1.6% and 3.4% annual hard event rates in those with normal and abnormal MPS scans, respectively. Of interest, this same report revealed that while risk stratification was also observed in the diabetics with angina and shortness of breath, the event rates for both the normal and abnormal scan groups were higher in these groups than in the asymptomatic diabetics (Fig. 16-10). It has been shown that 22% of asymptomatic diabetic patients have ischemia by adenosine MPS,[48] but the preponderance of these patients with abnormal MPS had mildly abnormal studies. Nonetheless, another recent large study has shown that 59% of asymptomatic diabetics have abnormal stress MPS studies, including 20% with a "high-risk" scan.[49] A further study by this latter group showed that ECG Q waves and/or evidence of peripheral artery disease identified the most suitable diabetic candidates for screening with MPS.[50] The differences in these studies is likely explained by differences in underlying risk of the patients studied. Given the diversity of pretest risk in these various diabetic groups, some investigators recommend atherosclerosis testing rather than MPS as a more cost-effective approach to the initial screening tool of diabetics.[51,52] A more recent statement from the American Diabetes Association recommended that testing for atherosclerosis or ischemia for patients with type 2 diabetes, perhaps with cardiac CT as the initial test, be reserved for those in

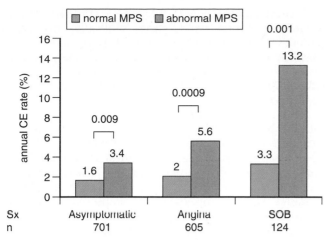

Figure 16-10 Annualized rates of cardiac events (CE) in diabetic patients presenting asymptomatically, with angina, and with dyspnea (shortness of breath [SOB]) in the setting of normal *(blue bars)* and abnormal *(pink bars)* MPS results. The numbers under the bars represent the number of patients in the group. *P* values for the comparison of event rates between normal and abnormal MPS are shown above the bars. *(From Zellweger MJ, Hachamovitch R, Kang X, et al: Prognostic relevance of symptoms versus objective evidence of coronary artery disease in diabetic patients, Eur Heart J 25:543-550, 2004.)*

whom medical treatment goals cannot be met. Similar recommendations were made for selected asymptomatic diabetics in whom there is strong clinical suspicion of very-high-risk CAD.[53]

Gender-Based Differences in the Prognostic Value of MPS

The historical limitations of MPS, related to breast tissue artifact and smaller left ventricular chamber size, has been ameliorated in large part with the advent of ^{99m}Tc agents. This is related to both enhanced image quality and the ability to gate SPECT images; prone imaging and/or the use of validated attenuation correction algorithms has further aided efforts.[36,54]

With respect to the prognostic value of MPS, the low risk associated with normal MPS is similar in men and women.[8] This is limited, however, in female diabetics where event rates tend to be far greater.[21] High-risk findings (e.g., >10% ischemic myocardium) elevated a woman's risk by nearly 10-fold, with annual rates of major cardiac events of 6.3% for all women and 10.9% for diabetic subsets of women.[55]

Endothelial dysfunction and microvascular disease have been proposed as mechanisms for false-positive stress testing results, suggesting that some of these studies may represent true perfusion abnormalities without large-vessel CAD. Recent evidence suggests that these MPS perfusion findings may be associated with increased near-term risk of major cardiac events, more so in women than in men,[56,57] suggesting that prognostically important coronary disease states not involving obstructive CAD occur more frequently in women than in men, and MPS could provide a tool for detection of this process.

Nuclear Imaging in Elderly Patients

The importance of MPS in an elderly population has grown because of two distinct factors: (1) the aging of the U.S. population and (2) the difficulty in assessing CAD in an elderly population in light of the frequency of asymptomatic and atypical presentations.[58,59] This is further confounded by the reduced value of indices such as the DTS[60] in an elderly population. Although a relatively smaller proportion of the elderly population is able to achieve adequate exercise on a treadmill, in those who are able to exercise, MPS provides effective risk stratification in elderly men and elderly women.[61] This suggests the possibility that exercise MPS may replace ETT as the initial test in an elderly population.

Pharmacologic stress testing is increasingly being applied in the elderly, who frequently are unable to exercise adequately; this population accounts for a high proportion of patients undergoing pharmacologic stress imaging. For elderly patients, as well as for those with functional limitations, similar risk assessment is possible with pharmacologic stress SPECT.[62-64] Consistent with data on other functionally impaired patients, the prognostic value of MPS is associated with higher cardiac event rates for normal to severely abnormal test results.

MPS in Patients With Chronic Kidney Disease

There is an increasing recognition of the cardiovascular implications of chronic kidney disease (CKD), and examination of the role of MPS in these patients. CKD is associated with hypertension and dyslipidemia, both promoters of atherosclerosis and further renal damage.[65] Because diabetic nephropathy is the leading cause of CKD in the United States, diabetes is often present as well. In addition, CKD is also associated with activation of both inflammatory mediators and the renin-angiotensin system. These factors all contribute to accelerated atherosclerosis and early development of CAD in these patients. Additionally, CKD is associated with worsening risk for the entire spectrum of cardiovascular disease—for example, increased risk of thromboembolism in atrial fibrillation (AF), independent of other risk factors.[66] As a result, patients with CKD are exposed to increased morbidity and mortality due to cardiovascular events.[65,67] Indeed, the cardiovascular mortality rate in CKD patients is 15 to 30 times the age-adjusted cardiovascular mortality rate in the general population.[65,68,69]

Determining the role of MPS in this patient population is challenging. On the one hand, successful risk stratification of these patients by MPS results has been reported by a number of investigators.[70-74] As we have touched on earlier, post-MPS risk is contextual, resulting in worsening event rates at every level of MPS abnormalities.[21,75] In fact, the presence of CKD has been shown to increase risk at any level of MPS results. Hakeem and colleagues followed 1652 patients who underwent stress MPS for more than 2 years, finding that both stress perfusion defects and CKD were independent and incremental predictors of cardiac death after accounting for baseline data, risk factors, left ventricular dysfunction, type of stress used, and symptom status. Hence, MPS results add incrementally and risk-stratify these patients.

As important, for any MPS result, normal or abnormal, cardiac mortality is far greater in CKD patients, and the degree of renal dysfunction is predictive of adverse outcome, even after adjusting for MPS data.[74] However, in light of the relatively high event rates after a normal MPS, it remains unclear whether and how MPS results can guide the management of CKD patients. Is the risk associated with normal MPS in CKD patients amenable to treatment? Is it lower than the baseline risk of patients with kidney disease in the United States? Does therapeutic action based on abnormal MPS data result in improved patient outcomes?

In patients with CKD, known to be higher-risk patients, MPS has been shown to achieve risk stratification. In these patients, the added value of MPS is present at all levels of renal function. Additional information is needed to assist clinicians in the decision-making process.

MPS in Ethnic Minority Patients

Limited studies to date, have evaluated the impact of patient race on the association of MPS results and patient outcomes. This question is challenging in that defining this relationship necessitates the separation of socioeconomic and risk-factor components from patient race per se. The rate of cardiac death or nonfatal myocardial infarction in African Americans with a normal MPS is approximately 2% per year.[8] Whether this is a function of inherent risk (as has been the case with other disease entities such as chronic renal failure[76]) or whether this is due to aggregation of risk factors and/or depressed socioeconomic conditions associated with patient race is unclear.

Evidence Supporting Nuclear Imaging for Obese Patients

Despite the potential obfuscation of scan interpretation in obese patients by attenuation artifact, MPS remains a highly useful test for diagnosis and prognosis in these patients. The use of both attenuation correction hardware and software in combination with quantitation and ECG gating, a well as prone imaging of stress images as a part of ^{99m}Tc protocols as an alternative to attenuation correction, have been associated with improvements in diagnostic test performance in obese cohorts.[77]

Several studies, to date, have demonstrated the value of MPS in the risk stratification of obese patients.[78–80] Early data using PET imaging have also been associated with risk stratification in these patients.[81] Whether normal MPS is associated with a "low" event rate in an obese cohort is unclear.[80,81]

MPS After Other Noninvasive Testing

MPS After Coronary Calcium Screening or Coronary CT Angiography *(See Chapter 20)*

A recent revision of ACC/AHA guidelines supports the use of CT-derived coronary calcium scores (CCS) as a means to evaluate asymptomatic patients with multiple risk factors for detection of early subclinical coronary atherosclerosis.[82] Referral of patients first for CCS and

then subsequently for MPS if extensive coronary atherosclerosis is found would seem clinically intuitive— patients with a high CCS would likely be at sufficient likelihood of CAD to justify MPS. Conversely, it may also be helpful to evaluate symptomatic patients with normal MPS and multiple risk factors for CCS determination to assess coronary atherosclerosis.

With respect to the former, however, the CCS thresholds resulting in sufficiently high likelihood of an abnormal MPS to warrant referral for MPS will vary with the population examined and the means by which the patients were recruited. For example, if asymptomatic patients routinely referred to CCS are recruited to undergo MPS, as opposed to symptomatic patients referred to MPS recruited for CCS, the profile of frequencies of MPS abnormality as a function of CCS will vary significantly.

In an early study addressing this question, 46% of patients with CCS $\geq$ 400 had an abnormal MPS.[83] These patients were selected from a large population presenting for CCS where patients with abnormal CCS were encouraged to undergo MPS. A subsequent study reported 1195 asymptomatic patients who underwent MPS and also had CCS, either on the basis of self-referral to CCS (8%), physician referral to CCS (65%), or recruitment into ongoing research (27%).[84] In this study, CCS $\geq$ 400 was associated with a 29% frequency of any MPS ischemia and an 11% frequency of moderate to severe ischemia. Interestingly, a CCS threshold of $\geq$ 1000 was associated with only a 19.9% frequency of MPS ischemia (Fig. 16-11). Finally, a more recent report of 695 symptomatic patients referred for adenosine stress PET who underwent CCS as part of routine image acquisition reported a 48.5% frequency of abnormal stress PET in patients with CCS $\geq$ 400, with an only slightly greater frequency (49.4%) of abnormal PET with a CCS $\geq$ 1000.[85] Interestingly, 16% of patients with no measurable calcium had PET-identified ischemia (negative predictive value 84%) (Fig. 16-12).

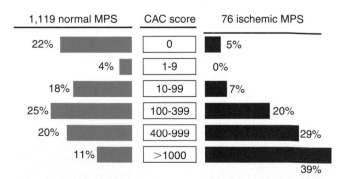

1,119 normal MPS	CAC score	76 ischemic MPS
22%	0	5%
4%	1-9	0%
18%	10-99	7%
25%	100-399	20%
20%	400-999	29%
11%	>1000	39%

Figure 16-11 Distribution of coronary artery calcium scores (CAC) in 1199 patients with normal MPS *(left)* and 76 patients with ischemic MPS. Patients with normal MPS have a wide distribution of CAC values, whereas patients with ischemic MPS tend toward higher CAC values. This distribution exemplifies the challenge of determining a specific threshold of CAC defining intermediate likelihood of abnormal MPS. *(From Berman DS, Wong ND, Gransar H, et al: Relationship between stress-induced myocardial ischemia and atherosclerosis measured by coronary calcium tomography, J Am Coll Cardiol 44:923-930, 2004.)*

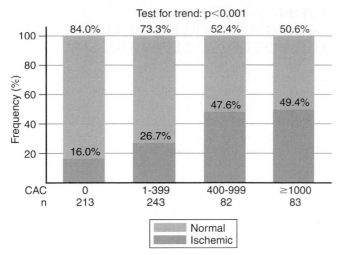

Figure 16-12 Bar graph illustrating the relative frequencies of normal *(orange bars)* versus ischemic *(blue bars)* vasodilator stress PET results as a function of coronary artery calcium score (CAC) category. A significant trend is present ($P < 0.01$), with increasing frequencies of ischemic PET with increasing coronary artery calcium score. This increase appears to plateau at a coronary artery calcium score of 400. *(From Schenker MP, Dorbala S, Hong EC, et al: Interrelation of coronary calcification, myocardial ischemia, and outcomes in patients with intermediate likelihood of coronary artery disease: A combined positron emission tomography/computed tomography study. Circulation 117:1693-700, 2008.)*

The discrepancies in the reported frequencies of abnormal MPS in patients with high CCS appear to be largely explained by differences in the underlying patient risk. Recent subset analyses have supported this concept, indicating that the threshold of CCS warranting referral for MPS will vary further as a function of underlying patient risk. In this regard, the frequency of abnormal MPS for any level of CCS has been reported to be higher in patients with type 2 diabetes,[51,86] in patients with the metabolic syndrome,[87] in patients with a family history of premature CAD,[86] and in patients with a high likelihood of CAD.[88] Although no validated threshold is currently recognized, in patient cohorts at greater risk for developing early atherosclerosis, it has been suggested that a threshold CCS of 100 might be appropriate for these patients. Nonetheless, the ACC appropriateness criteria support the use of MPS in patients with a high-risk CCS, or = 400.[7]

MPS in Patients with Prior CAD

Patients After Percutaneous Coronary Intervention

MPS is frequently utilized in patients after percutaneous coronary intervention (PCI). Potentially, MPS can aid in identification of restenosis, de novo disease, periprocedural myocardial injury, side-branch compromise, or functionally significant angiographic disease in nonrevascularized vessels. Further, the ability of MPS to assess jeopardized myocardium yields a role for this modality in staged PCI strategies, albeit limited by the potential for underestimation of CAD by MPS techniques.

Despite these potential applications and the clear superiority of MPS to ETT techniques, a number of limitations exist in the use of MPS in these settings. First, the absolute risk of patients after PCI is relatively low (~1%), suggesting no need for routine testing despite the predictive value of abnormal MPS for adverse events.[89,90] Given the relatively low prevalence of post-stent restenosis, the use of routine MPS post-PCI would be associated with the likelihood of a false-positive MPS exceeding the likelihood of a true-positive MPS.[91] Indeed, due to the relatively low prevalence of clinically significant silent restenosis in the era of drug eluting stents, routine poststent MPS is not currently recommended.[7,8]

In general, however, when symptoms develop after PCI or in high-risk subgroups, MPS can be helpful in defining the culprit vessel and assessing the extent of ischemic abnormality. The ACC/AHA 2002 Guideline Update for Exercise Testing favors selective stress imaging in patients considered to be at particularly high risk (e.g., patients with decreased LV function, multivessel CAD, proximal LAD disease, previous sudden death, diabetes mellitus, hazardous occupations, and suboptimal PCI results). Whenever moderate to severe ischemia is found by nuclear testing, consideration should be given to repeat catheterization, even in the absence of symptoms.

Evidence Supporting Nuclear Testing for Patients After CABG

MPS is frequently used in patients with prior coronary artery bypass grafting (CABG) to assess graft patency, the development of silent graft disease or progression of underlying graft disease, and to determine the importance of new symptoms. As more than 50% of vein grafts can be expected to be occluded by 10 years post-CABG, an intermediate likelihood of vein graft disease can be considered to be present at this time point.[92]

A number of studies have investigated the prognostic value of MPS in patients with prior CABG in various circumstances. MPS was prognostically valuable both when performed early (<2 years post-CABG)[93] and later (≥5 years).[89,94,95] MPS yielded incremental value with respect to death and nonfatal myocardial infarction even in asymptomatic, stable patients with prior CABG.[96]

USE OF MPS IN GUIDING DECISIONS FOR CATHETERIZATION

While assessing the prognostic performance characteristics of MPS is key in understanding its optimal application, it is equally important to examine how referring physicians actually use MPS in daily practice. This is particularly the case with respect to examining what aspects of MPS results trigger further testing, whether there are any distinct referral biases leading to over- or under-referral of distinct patient subgroups, and what the confounders of the referral to post-MPS care may be.

Several studies have shown that MPS results heavily influence post-MPS clinical decision making. Among patients with normal scans, only a small proportion undergo early post-MPS cardiac catheterization, usually as a result of persisting or worsening clinical symptomatology.[11,12] Post-MPS referral to catheterization is overwhelmingly driven by the extent and severity of present on MPS.[11,12] In patients without prior CAD, the relationship between the percent ischemic myocardium ischemic and the likelihood of referral to catheterization and/or revascularization after MPS is highly nonlinear and takes on a distinct shape (Fig. 16-13).[11] Although the likelihood of this referral is very low in the absence of ischemia, in the range of small to medium amounts of ischemia, the slope of the relationship is very steep, particularly in the setting of anginal symptoms. This steep slope indicates that within this critical range of small to medium amounts of ischemia, small changes in reported ischemia yield large changes in the likelihood of physician action. Interestingly, once a threshold of ischemia is exceeded, there is no further increase in the likelihood of referral to revascularization (plateau phase).[11] Importantly, referring physicians' actions are not triggered by MPS results alone but factors such as ST-segment change on the electrocardiogram during stress, anginal symptoms on presentation, cardiovascular risk factors, and other clinical information also modulate the level of aggressiveness of post-MPS care.

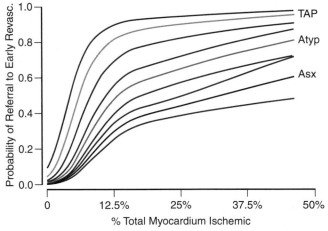

Figure 16-13 Relationship between percent myocardium ischemic and likelihood of referral to early revascularization (<60 days post-MPS). Results based on multivariable modeling in 10,647 patients. Logistic regression modeling identified percent myocardium ischemic as most strongly associated with referral to revascularization (83% of all information used for decision making). This process was also influenced by patients' presenting symptoms, as evidenced by greater likelihood of referral at any level of ischemia with typical versus atypical versus asymptomatic patients. *(From Hachamovitch R, Hayes SW, Friedman JD, Cohen I, Berman DS: Comparison of the short-term survival benefit associated with revascularization compared with medical therapy in patients with no prior coronary artery disease undergoing stress myocardial perfusion single photon emission computed tomography, Circulation 107:2900-2907, 2003.)*

ESTIMATING THE TRUE PROGNOSTIC VALUE OF MPS AND POSTTEST REFERRAL BIAS

An important consequence of the referral pattern described is the widely recognized post-MPS referral bias (partial verification bias) that has been widely described.[97] This bias—the high referral rate to catheterization after abnormal MPS, the low referral rates to catheterization after normal MPS—results in a significant lowering of test specificity and a slight increase in test sensitivity. What is less widely understood is that this same pattern of post-MPS resource utilization introduces a referral bias that affects our abilities to assess the *prognostic* value of testing.[98]

Prognostic analyses performed, to date, are predominantly based on data from patients who underwent MPS and were then treated medically.[97] This is the result of the accepted methodology; prognostic analyses of noninvasive testing using observational data series typically remove or censor patients undergoing early revascularization after testing, owing to the relationship between the referral to revascularization and the test results (since the test results drive the revascularization, an intervention that alters the natural history of the disease, the patients with the most abnormal test results are most likely to have their risk reduced). With increasing physician acceptance of and dependence on MPS to guide patient management, progressive increases in early revascularization rates in the setting of ischemia occur, accompanied by progressive decreases in patient risk after abnormal MPS (owing to the revascularization). Hence, studies evaluating medically treated patients will underestimate the prognostic value of MPS.[2,3] The impact of this bias has been quantified by a recent study.[5]

This finding indicates that prognostic studies of MPS in medically treated patients drawn from routine practice may be misleading, particularly in the absence of information regarding post-MPS referral patterns to revascularization (the latter defining the amount of potential bias). This suggests that to avoid this bias, future studies of MPS (or the assessment of any modality in active use) include both patients treated medically and those referred to early revascularization. The implications of including the latter patients can be handled statistically to permit more accurate estimates of patient risk.[2,11,99]

Other more complicated biases can develop as well when data elements associated with risk and those associated with referral to revascularization become disparate.[2,11,98,99] For example, if post-MPS referral to revascularization is based on one variable (e.g., ischemia) but not on a second (e.g., scar), a referral bias will result in underestimation of risk associated with the first variable (blunted increase in risk as a function of ischemia) but no such finding with respect to the second variable (appropriate increase in risk as a function of increasing scar). It is important to note that this type of bias is actually ubiquitous in prognostic research. Since, as was discussed earlier, revascularization referral is heavily based on ischemia, prognostic studies conducted in medically treated patients will underestimate the value of MPS ischemia in comparison to other factors. As noted, this bias can be overcome in two ways, either by utilizing MPS results obtained outside of conventional patient care pathways (e.g., research studies only) or statistical adjustment of observational patient data utilizing both medically treated and revascularized patients.[2] Finally, the use of validated prognostic scores, such as the DTS, can also overcome this bias by including and appropriately weighting non-MPS factors, as well as basing the score on both medically treated and revascularization patients. Importantly, estimations of risk with both medical therapy and revascularization will need to be generated.

INCREMENTAL PROGNOSTIC VALUE OF PRE-MPS DATA

Understanding and Estimating Posttest Risk

In the previous discussion and in many reviews and reports of MPS, post-MPS risk is expressed as an annualized event rate, either for a general MPS result category (normal, abnormal MPS) or for a specific category of defect type (e.g., >20% myocardium ischemic). Most clinicians consider their patients' post-MPS risk in this context and possibly make their clinical management decisions based on this approach as well. As seen in Figure 16-14, a wide range of posttest risk exists for any

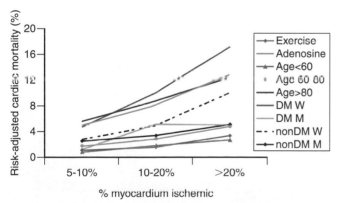

Figure 16-14 Rates of risk-adjusted cardiac mortality in medically treated patients as a function of percent myocardium ischemic (5% to 10%, 10% to 20%, and > 20%): exercise versus adenosine stress; patients aged < 60 years, 60 to 80 years, and > 80 years; diabetic men versus women and nondiabetic men and women. Although predicted cardiac mortality increases with increasing percent myocardium ischemic, the rates at any level of ischemia vary widely at any level of ischemia as a function of clinical information.[45] DM W, diabetic women; DM M, diabetic men; nonDM W, nondiabetic women; NonDM M, nondiabetic men. *(From Hachamovitch R, Hayes SW, Friedman JD, Cohen I, Berman DS: Comparison of the short-term survival benefit associated with revascularization compared with medical therapy in patients with no prior coronary artery disease undergoing stress myocardial perfusion single photon emission computed tomography, Circulation 107:2900-2907, 2003.)*

level of test abnormality. The risk of cardiac death associated with a moderate amount of ischemia, 10% to 20% of the myocardium, varies widely (from 2% to 10%) according to the patient subset examined. Patients with a higher clinical risk profile (increased age, pharmacologic stress, diabetic) will have higher risk than patients with lower clinical risk profiles (younger, exercise stress, nondiabetic). As noted previously, this same phenomenon also holds true after normal MPS.[21]

The Need for Imaging Scores in Risk Estimation and Reporting

With this in mind, it can be appreciated that a significant challenge facing physicians is how to incorporate pre-imaging data into their postimaging estimates of patient risk. A diversity of data potentially impacts on post-MPS risk—clinical, historical, stress test, perfusion, and function data—and must be considered in formulating estimates of risk. The optimal solution to this dilemma is the use of validated scores to generate an estimate of likelihood of CAD or risk of adverse events for an individual patient that could be incorporated into MPS reporting.

Recently such a score was developed for patients undergoing adenosine stress.[100] The first such score was developed in 5873 patients studied by adenosine stress who experienced 387 cardiac deaths on follow-up (6.6%). Using a combination of split-set validation and bootstrapping techniques, the authors derived three scores, including both a simplified score and a more complex score (with an eye to incorporation into MPS software). The complex score presented by these authors was as follows: (age [decades] × 5.19) + (% myocardium ischemic [per 10%] × 4.66) + (% myocardium fixed [per 10%] × 4.81) + (diabetes mellitus × 3.88) + (if patient treated with early revascularization, 4.51) + (if dyspnea was a presenting symptom, 5.47) + (resting heart rate [per 10 beats] × 2.88) − (peak heart rate [per 10 beats] × 1.42) + (ECG score × 1.95)—if patient treated with early revascularization, % myocardium ischemic [per 10%] × 4.47). Separate scores can be calculated for both the use of medical therapy and revascularization, and patient risk can be determined by use of Figure 16-15. This approach can be extended to incorporate a variety of information (clinical, imaging, biochemical, etc.) but will require validation in a variety of populations to ensure generalizability.

When applied to patient care, several important concepts emerge. First, two patients with similar clinical characteristics and MPI defect sizes, but one with ischemia and the other with fixed defects, may have similar risk but very different potential benefit with revascularization, hence very different optimal management approaches. Further, even in a patient with extensive ischemia, where there is a clear potential benefit associated with the use of revascularization, postrevascularization risk is not "low" but at least intermediate to high. Hence, we cannot assume that revascularization will always eliminate risk, only lower it.

Thus, conceptually, the major contribution of this work is that physicians need to focus not on estimates

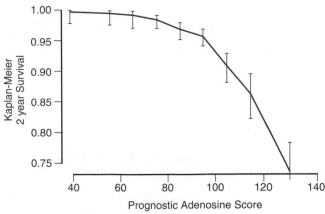

Figure 16-15 Relationship between prognostic adenosine score and 2-year Kaplan-Meier survival free of cardiac death. With lower scores, patient risk is relatively low with narrower confidence intervals. As scores increase, particularly over 50, risk increases more rapidly and confidence intervals increase as well. This score and the figure can be applied as follows: For a given patient, the adenosine score is calculated yielding two values, one for treatment with medical therapy and a second for treatment with revascularization. There are two lines shown on this slide in addition to the curve relating survival to the prognostic adenosine score. *(From Hachamovitch R, Hayes S, Friedman J, Cohen I, Berman DS: A prognostic score for prediction of cardiac mortality risk after adenosine stress myocardial perfusion scintigraphy, J Am Coll Cardiol 45:722-729, 2005.)*

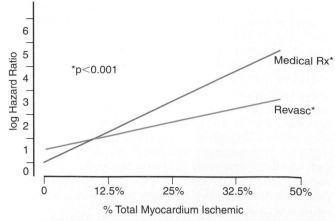

Figure 16-16 Relationship between percent total myocardium ischemic and log of the hazard ratio in 10,647 patients treated either with medical therapy *(green line)* or early revascularization (<60 days post-MPS; *orange line),* based on Cox proportional hazards modeling. In the setting of little or no ischemia, medical therapy is associated with greater survival. However, with increasing amounts of ischemia, a progressive survival benefit with revascularization over medical therapy is present.

of risk, but on those of potential benefit, to maximally impact patient care. It must always be recognized, however, that clinical judgment is paramount in the application of these approaches because of imperfections in the data derived from populations in defining all variables that might be operative in determining the risk of an individual patient as well as limitations of the tests themselves.

USING MPS FOR MEDICAL DECISION MAKING: IDENTIFYING RISK VERSUS IDENTIFYING POTENTIAL SURVIVAL BENEFIT

Based on the previous discussion, it appears that the natural evolution the role of stress imaging is to play a part in the identification of which therapeutic strategy is associated with enhanced patient *benefit*, rather than the estimation of patient risk. To date, limited single-site observational data support this paradigm.

A recent study in 10,627 patients without prior myocardial infarction or revascularization who underwent stress MPS compared post-MPS outcomes with revascularization versus medical therapy using multivariable modeling with a propensity score. This study identified a survival benefit for patients undergoing medical therapy versus revascularization in the setting of no or mild ischemia, whereas patients undergoing revascularization had an increasing survival benefit over patients undergoing medical therapy when moderate to severe ischemia was present (>10% of the total myocardium

ischemic) (Fig. 16-16).[11] This survival benefit was particularly striking in higher-risk patients (elderly, requiring adenosine stress, and women, especially diabetics) (Fig. 16-17). These results have been extended to incorporate gated MPS EF information.[99] Comparing the roles in risk assessment of perfusion and function data—although EF, percent myocardium ischemic, and the percent myocardium fixed are all predictors of

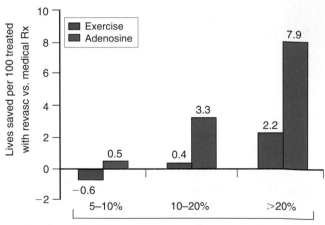

Figure 16-17 Lives saved per 100 treated with revascularization versus medical therapy in patients undergoing exercise *(blue bars)* versus adenosine stress *(pink bars)* as a function of percent myocardium ischemic. Results based on Cox proportional hazards model. Statistical significance as per model. Revasc, revascularization. *(From Hachamovitch R, Hayes SW, Friedman JD, Cohen I, Berman DS: Comparison of the short-term survival benefit associated with revascularization compared with medical therapy in patients with no prior coronary artery disease undergoing stress myocardial perfusion single photon emission computed tomography, Circulation 107:2900-2907, 2003.)*

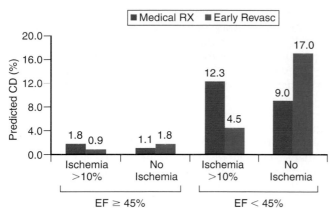

Figure 16-18 Predicated cardiac death (CD) rates (based on Cox proportional hazards modeling) as a function of gated SPECT ejection fraction (≥45% versus <45%) and presence of significant ischemia (>10% myocardium ischemic versus no ischemia; <10% myocardium ischemic) in patients treated medically *(pink bars)* and with early (<60 days post-MPS) revascularization *(blue bars). (From Hachamovitch R, Rozanski A, Hayes SW, et al: Predicting therapeutic benefit from myocardial revascularization procedures: Are measurements of resting left ventricular ejection fraction and stress-induced myocardial ischemia both necessary? J Nucl Cardiol 13:768-778, 2006.)*

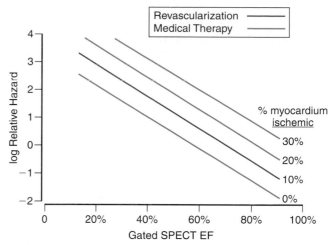

Figure 16-19 Relationship between gated SPECT LV ejection fraction and log of the hazard ratio based on Cox proportional hazards modeling in 5366 patients. *Green lines* represent predicted survival for 0%, 10%, 20%, and 30% myocardium ischemic in patients treated medically. *Pink lines* represent predicted survival for patients treated with revascularization for all values of percent myocardium ischemic (note pink line is superimposed on green line at 10% myocardium ischemic). Overall, risk increased with decreasing ejection fraction. For any value of ejection fraction, however, risk also increased as percent myocardium ischemic increased, indicating an incremental value for percent myocardium ischemic over ejection fraction. Compared to risk in patients treated medically, risk in patients undergoing early revascularization was independent of the percent myocardium ischemic present (as evidenced by a *single pink line* representing survival after revascularization for all degrees of ischemia). Risk in the early revascularization patients was similar to the risk of medically treated patients with 10% myocardium ischemic, throughout the range of ejection fraction.

cardiac death—the former is by far the best predictor of cardiac mortality. On the other hand, only inducible ischemia identified patients who would benefit from revascularization in comparison to medical therapy (Fig. 16-18). With increasing amounts of ischemia, increasing survival benefit for revascularization over medical therapy was found, irrespective of EF (Fig. 16-19). As shown by previous RCTs, the absolute benefit to be gained from a therapeutic strategy for any level of ischemia present is proportional to underlying patient risk. Thus, in assessing treatment options in an individual patient, cardiac risk factors, comorbidities, and EF all have to be considered along with ischemia in order to determine the potential advantages of a specific therapeutic strategy.

Imaging in the Post-COURAGE Era

In this context, the results of the recent COURAGE trial[101] comparing strategies of PCI and medical therapy versus medical therapy alone in stable patients with known CAD must be mentioned as well. Since in this RCT, no survival advantage was present with the addition of PCI, the question must be raised as to whether stress imaging has a role in the future. After all, if patients will not benefit from revascularization, catheterization is not needed, so no stress imaging will be needed to identify the potential catheterization candidate. Several issues, however, stand in the way of this new paradigm.

First, does COURAGE really suggest that revascularization does not aid in reducing patient risk, or does it suggest that PCI may have limited prognostic impact? Also, the use of CABG would have yielded different results. Further, it is very important to recognize that

COURAGE was a trial of patients *with known CAD.* Hence, these results cannot be generalized to patients presenting for evaluation of suspected CAD but without prior CAD. Of note, the observational data suggesting the potential use of MPS to identify patients with a survival benefit with one therapeutic approach versus another was limited to those patients without prior CAD.[11,99]

Finally, COURAGE included many patients with prior myocardial infarction and, possibly, scar without jeopardized myocardium. More recently, the results of the FAME (Fractional Flow Reserve Versus Angiography for Multivessel Evaluation) study revealed that guiding PCI by means of physiologic data (fractional flow reserve) was associated with a significantly lower incidence of major adverse cardiac events compared with routine angiography-guided PCI in patients with multivessel disease, without a significant increase in the procedure time.[102] Whether the use of ischemia imaging in COURAGE to identify patients with jeopardized myocardium, hence enhanced benefit from revascularization, would have substantively altered the results of this trial is unknown. It is also unclear how much ischemia was present in the COURAGE patients, and whether the absence of demonstrable therapeutic benefit is related to insufficient amounts of ischemia in recruited patients. It must be noted that the results of COURAGE are generalizable to patients with known CAD but not to patients being evaluated with suspected CAD, a patient group with very different hazard function in whom very different results may have occurred.

New Paradigm: The Added Value Of a Modality Is Its Ability to Identify Candidates for Expensive Rx Resulting in Enhanced Clinical and Cost-Effectiveness

The application of MPS defined herein is one example of a new paradigm for cardiovascular imaging, the use of a modality to identify potential patient benefit, hence, aiding in the allocation of more expensive therapeutic options. Thus the finding of jeopardized myocardium (ischemic and/or hibernating) identifies candidates for PCI or CABG. This approach is readily applied to other current (and potential) roles of imaging techniques (Fig. 16-20).

- The use of imaging, possibly radionuclide ventriculography, CMR, or echocardiography, to derive indices of dyssynchrony may aid in the identification of optimal pacemaker candidates.
- Potentially, the use of MIBG imaging may, in the future, aid in the identification of AICD candidates.
- Can CCTA or CMR, by imaging atherosclerotic plaque presence, composition, and morphology, identify the level of aggressiveness of cholesterol reduction therapy?
- In patients presenting to the emergency department with chest pain, can either CCTA or BMIPP (an agent with "ischemic memory") better guide

the triage of patients to admission, the catheterization laboratory, versus discharge for follow-up?
- If, as recent studies suggest, the requisite data to guide preoperative risk assessment is to exclude severe LV dysfunction or significant valvular disease, will CMR or CCTA be the first-line test in this setting?

In each of the given examples, patients who are potential candidates for an expensive intervention (revascularization, AICD, hospitalization, etc.) instead undergo cardiac imaging to determine whether they may gain sufficient benefit from the intervention that it will enhance their status and, if applied, enhance cost-effectiveness. For any of these applications to be valid, extensive outcomes data, preferably in the form of RCT, will be needed. Although this may be an expensive proposition, the potential cost savings (since these interventions are expensive and the number of potential patient candidates large) will likely outweigh the costs.

Where and When Will MPS be Used?

Asymptomatic patients: In the future, many asymptomatic patients with low likelihood of CAD may be evaluated for atherosclerosis to aid in their medical management with CAC scoring or carotid intimal-medial thickness (IMT) measurements. Those low-likelihood patients with evidence of extensive atherosclerosis may be referred on to MPS. These patients are frequently not ideal candidates for CCTA, owing to extensive coronary calcification and the fact that in the absence of symptoms, revascularization most likely would not be indicated without extensive ischemia.

Symptomatic patients: Patients with severe anginal symptoms are likely to go directly to invasive coronary angiography, although the COURAGE data suggest that there might be a role for MPS. Those with moderate to severe ischemia and symptoms would then by common practice undergo invasive coronary angiography. Those with mild ischemia or no objective ischemia may be equally well served by an initial strategy of aggressive medical management.

For the remaining patients without known CAD but with symptoms raising suspicion of CAD, the diagnostic pathways remain controversial. Many advocate the use of CCTA as the initial test in this subset. CCTA would be used to determine whether primary or secondary prevention measures are appropriate and whether further testing for the extent and severity of ischemia is needed. Thus, CCTA would be serving as a gatekeeper before MPS. In this scenario, MPS would be positioned after CCTA as a test to identify revascularization candidates in need of invasive coronary angiography.

Alternatively, the approach that remains in place according to guidelines is based on stress-induced ischemia. In this regard, symptomatic patients with intermediate likelihood of CAD might be defined as two distinct groups, a low-intermediate likelihood (15% to 50%) group and a high-intermediate likelihood group (50% to 85%). All patients with low-intermediate likelihood unable to exercise or with an uninterpretable ECG

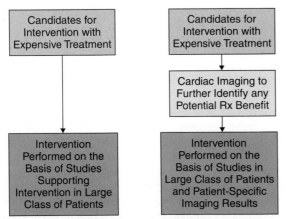

Figure 16-20 Schematic comparing conventional patient selection for many newer technologies *(left)* and with the use of cardiac imaging *(right)*. When applied to a large group of patients who are potential candidates for an expensive intervention, the use of cardiac imaging has the potential to identify individuals within this pool of patients who are likely to benefit from the procedure versus those patients unlikely to benefit. This paradigm has long been in place for the use of viability imaging (identification of patients more likely to benefit from revascularization, owing to the presence of jeopardized myocardium).

would go to MPS as their initial test. Otherwise, under a conventional strategy, the patients would undergo ETT as their initial test, with those patients with intermediate to high post-ETT likelihood going on to MPS and the low post-ETT likelihood to medical management.

Patients with intermediate pretest likelihood of CAD in the 50% to 85% range would be candidates for MPS as their initial test. This direct MPS approach can be justified, since if ETT is performed as the initial test in these patients, a negative test is unlikely to reclassify them as low likelihood (or risk). In patients referred to MPI, a normal MPS will indicate the potential for medical management. Patients with greater than 10% myocardium ischemic on MPS are potential candidates for referral to catheterization. Patients with normal MPS or abnormal MPS but with only mild ischemia are candidates for medical management. In some of these patients, CAC testing or CCTA might be of value to assess the presence and extent of coronary atherosclerosis as a guide to preventive and antianginal therapy, as well as to rule out severe proximal coronary stenosis that might be underestimated by MPS due to "balanced reduction" of flow.

In patients with a high pretest likelihood of CAD, MPS may be the test of choice, based on data showing its cost-effectiveness in this group as an alternative to direct coronary angiography. Those with ischemia would likely be sent for invasive coronary angiography, particularly if moderate to severe ischemia is found. It is widely held that CCTA is not likely to prove cost-effective in this patient group, since a large proportion of patients would be expected to have CCTA findings that are sufficiently abnormal that further assessment for the magnitude of ischemia would be required. However, when MPS is used in this subset, just as with the patients with an intermediate likelihood of CAD, the possible supplemental role of CCTA remains for patients in whom balanced reduction of flow is suspected.

In symptomatic patients with known CAD, the value of CCTA is untested, and the little data that exist suggest that MPI is far more cost-effective. In contrast, MPS remains a mainstay of the assessment of myocardial ischemia and myocardial viability in these patients, providing a useful guide to patient management.

Important Questions to Help Define the Role and Value of MPS

A number of factors that play important roles in our understanding the optimal utilization and performance characteristics of MPS are at this time unclear.

First, as already noted, it is recognized that MPS is susceptible to issues of "balanced reduction" of flow, potentially resulting in underestimation or even missing the presence of CAD entirely (Fig. 16-21). While it is likely that the frequency of this occurring is in part dependent on the patient profile of any given laboratory, the frequency of this phenomenon is unclear. If it is found to be significant, despite the use of various ancillary markers (TID, lung uptake of tracer, etc.), adjunct CT (for either CAC or CCTA) might be helpful. Alternatively, PET might be useful in this setting to assess coronary flow reserve, but whether this assessment will be

sufficiently specific for cost-effective application has not yet been shown; that is, if no or mild perfusion abnormality is seen on myocardial perfusion PET but abnormal coronary flow reserve is seen, will this finding be sufficiently associated with severe ischemia to warrant invasive coronary angiography? Importantly, however, recent data indicate that PET without flow reserve can also circumvent "balanced reduction" by assessment of peak pharmacologic stress versus rest left ventricular ejection fraction.[103]

Despite the lack of evidence regarding its specificity, the future role of flow reserve as an adjunct to perfusion imaging is an important question for the future of nuclear cardiology. The ability to assess this measure not only may reduce concern regarding "balanced reduction," but may also more fully characterize CAD beyond angiographic assessments. Prognostic assessment of the incremental value of flow reserve over perfusion imaging is awaited, as is evidence that this assessment can be successfully used to guide therapy. The ability to assess flow reserve also provides an entrée into functional assessment of atherosclerosis and microvascular disease.

An important question with respect to the future use of SPECT is where it will fit into testing strategies relative to CCTA. The comparison of these two modalities strikes at the heart of whether anatomic or physiologic data are needed to best mange CAD patients. Each of these modalities, however, has its own advantages and disadvantages.

The clear advantage of CCTA is its ability to exclude the presence of coronary atherosclerosis and, in most cases, to exclude the presence of obstructive CAD because of its very high negative predictive value. The disadvantage of CCTA is that multiple limitations of the technology remain, including inability to characterize stenosis in areas with dense coronary calcification, dependence on slow heart rate and regular rhythm, and a tendency to overestimate stenosis severity. Additionally, the ability of CCTA to accurately identify the presence of hemodynamically significant stenosis is limited with current technology (Fig. 16-22).

The primary advantage of MPS is its being based on functional assessment of disease. The primary justification of stress imaging for prognostic assessment is based on the role of ischemia assessment in the management of the CAD patient. It is hypothesized (although not proven) that this will translate into identification of which patients may benefit from a revascularization strategy. Although with its advantages—avoidance of excess catheterizations, their associated cost and risk, and the potential "occulostenotic reflex,"[6] differentiation of high-risk patients into those with extensive scar versus extensive ischemia,[84] etc.—only indirect evidence supports its use inasmuch as no RCT to date compare medical therapy to revascularization on the basis of non invasive ischemia estimates in stable patients.

As mentioned, the recently presented FAME study supports the concept that evaluation of the hemodynamic significance of CAD enhances the identification of what is optimal therapy for a given patient.[102] These results are similar to older data showing that

Patient A

78 year old male presenting with atypical chest pain
No prior CAD, risk factors: ↑cholesterol, hypertension, diabetes; normal rest ECG

ETT: 4:05 minutes, HR 136 (96% PMHR)

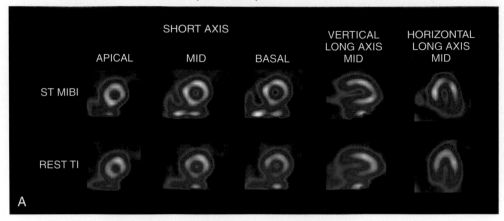

Catheterization Results

LM: 90% mid & distal
LAD: 80% proximal
LCX: 80% 1st obtuse marginal
RCA: 90% ostial

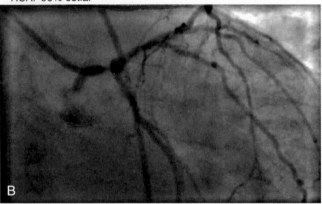

Disposition: CABG (2/10/05; 9 days post-MPS)

Figure 16-21 A, Patient A: clinical details and results of exercise dual-isotope stress MPS. Note the absence of any perfusion defects on the stress images compared to the rest images. **B,** Results of cardiac catheterization in Patient A, identifying the presence of subtotal left main and significant three-vessel CAD, despite the absence of perfusion defects (catheterization performed 13 days after the MPS study). The patient was subsequently treated with CABG. This case illustrates the failure of MPS to detect perfusion defects in the setting of extensive CAD when there is "balanced reduction" of flow.

Continued

revascularization in patients with three-vessel CAD was associated with enhanced survival only in those patients with ischemic ETT results, whereas medical therapy was a superior initial therapy in patients without this finding.[104] In the FAME study, data also parallel the results reported using MPS in patients without prior CAD in whom there was accrued survival benefit from revascularization over medical therapy only when significant ischemia was present,[11] with the absolute benefit varying with underlying patient risk and LVEF.[11,99]

CONCLUSIONS

Considerable evidence exists supporting the use of stress SPECT for prognostic applications. As reviewed, the prognostic value of MPS has been demonstrated in multiple patient subsets. Increasing evidence suggests that estimates of patient risk are feasible, and identification of which patients may benefit from revascularization will be the new basis of judging testing in the future. Given the numerous new applications of SPECT, the future role of MPS may evolve considerably.

Patient B

85 year old female presenting with atypical chest pain and dyspnea
Prior MI, risk factors: ↑cholesterol, hypertension.

ETT: 4:05 minutes, HR 136 (96% PMHR)

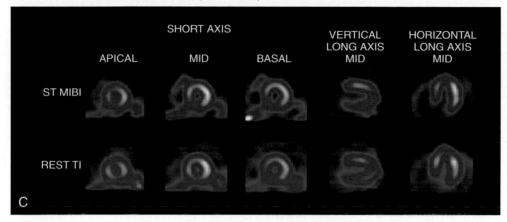

Catheterization Results

LAD: 85% proximal
LCX: 75% 2nd obtuse marginal
RCA: subtotal occlusion

LV angiogram: normal

Disposition: CABG

D

Figure 16-21 Cont'd C, Patient B: clinical details and results of exercise dual-isotope stress MPS. Note the presence of a reversible defect of the basal, mid, and distal inferior wall and the basal inferoseptum, consistent with disease of the PDA. **D,** Results of cardiac catheterization in Patient B, identifying the presence of significant three-vessel CAD. The RCA lesion was correctly identified, but the less severe obstructions in the LAD and LCX were not. This case illustrates a second potential presentation of "balanced reduction": the most severe lesion results in the most severe flow mismatch, while the defects associated with the other lesions have insufficient reduction in flow to be differentiated from the normal myocardium.

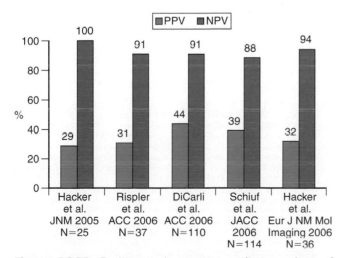

Figure 16-22 Positive and negative predictive values of CCTA for the identification of inducible ischemia, based on myocardial perfusion imaging in five initial studies. While CCTA appears to have an excellent to outstanding negative predictive value, its positive predictive value is relatively low.

REFERENCES

1. Di Carli MF, Hachamovitch R: New technology for non-invasive evaluation of coronary artery disease, *Circulation* 115:1464–1480, 2007.
2. Hachamovitch R, Di Carli MF: Contemporary reviews in cardiovascular medicine: Methods and limitations of assessing new noninvasive tests II. Outcomes-based validation and reliability assessment of noninvasive testing, *Circulation* 117:2793–2801, 2008.
3. Berman DS, Hachamovitch R, Shaw LJ, Germano G, Hayes S: Nuclear Cardiology. In Fuster VAR, King S, O'Rourke RA, Wellens HJJ, [eds]: Hurst's The Heart, New York, NY, 2004, McGraw-Hill Companies 2004, pp 525–565.
4. Hachamovitch R, Berman DS, Kiat H, Cohen I, Friedman JD, Shaw LJ: Value of stress myocardial perfusion single photon emission computed tomography in patients with normal resting electrocardiograms: an evaluation of incremental prognostic value and cost-effectiveness, *Circulation* 105:823–829, 2002.
5. Hachamovitch R, Hayes S, Friedman J, Cohen I, Berman D: Stress myocardial perfusion SPECT is clinically effective and cost-effective in risk-stratification of patients with a high likelihood of CAD but no known CAD, *J Am Coll Cardiol* 43:200–208, 2004.
6. Shaw LJ, Hachamovitch R, Berman DS, Marwick TH, Lauer MS, Heller AE, Iskandrian AE, Kesler KL, Travin MI, Lewin HC, Hendel S, Borges-Neto S, Miller DD: The economic consequences of available diagnostic and prognostic strategies for the evaluation of stable angina patients: an observational assessment of the value of pre-catheterization ischemia. Economics of Noninvasive Diagnosis (END) Multicenter Study Group., *J Am Coll Cardiol* 33:661–669, 1999.

7. Brindis RG, Douglas PS, Hendel RC, Peterson ED, Wolk MJ, Allen JM, Patel IE, Raskin IE, Bateman TM, Cerqueira MD, Gibbons RJ, Gillam JA, Gillespie JA, Iskandrian AE, Jerome SD, Krumholz HM, Messer JA, Spertus JA, Stowers SA: ACCF/ASNC appropriateness criteria for single-photon emission computed tomography myocardial perfusion imaging (SPECT MPI): a report of the American College of Cardiology Foundation Quality Strategic Directions Committee Appropriateness Criteria Working Group and the American Society of Nuclear Cardiology endorsed by the American Heart Association, *J Am Coll Cardiol* 46:1587–1605, 2005.

8. Klocke FJ, Baird MG, Bateman TM, Berman DS, Carabello BA, Cerqueira MD, et al: ACC/AHA/ASNC Guidelines for the clinical use of cardiac radionuclide imaging: A report of the American 1995 guidelines for the clinical use of radionuclide imaging, *Circulation* 2003.

9. Hachamovitch R, Beller GA: Critical review of imaging approaches for diagnosis and prognosis of CAD. In Di Carli MF, Kwong R, editors: *Novel Techniques for Imaging the Heart: Cardiac MR and CT*, Oxford, 2008, Blackwell Publishing.

10. Hachamovitch R, Shaw L, Berman DS: Methodological considerations in the assessment of noninvasive testing using outcomes research: pitfalls and limitations, *Prog Cardiovasc Dis* 43:215–230, 2000.

11. Hachamovitch R, Hayes SW, Friedman JD, Cohen I, Berman DS: Comparison of the short-term survival benefit associated with revascularization compared with medical therapy in patients with no prior coronary artery disease undergoing stress myocardial perfusion single photon emission computed tomography, *Circulation* 107:2900–2907, 2003.

12. Hachamovitch R, Berman DS, Kiat H, Cohen I, Cabico JA, Friedman J, Diamond GA: Exercise myocardial perfusion SPECT in patients without known coronary artery disease: incremental prognostic value and use in risk stratification, *Circulation* 93:905–914, 1996.

13. Gibbons RJ, Abrams J, Chatterjee K, Daley J, Deedwania PC, Douglas TB, Ferguson TB Jr, Fihn SD, Fraker TD Jr, Gardin JM, O'Rourke RA, Pasternak RC, Williams SV: ACC/AHA 2002 guideline update for the management of patients with chronic stable angina—summary article: a report of the American College of Cardiology/American Heart Association Task Force on practice guidelines (Committee on the Management of Patients With Chronic Stable Angina), *J Am Coll Cardiol* 41:159–168, 2003.

14. Bateman TM: Clinical relevance of a normal myocardial perfusion scintigraphic study, *J Nucl Cardiol* 4:172–173, 1997.

15. Heller GV, Herman SD, Travin MI, Baron JI, Santos-Ocampo C, McClellan JR: Independent prognostic value of intravenous dipyridamole with technetium-99m sestamibi tomographic imaging in predicting cardiac events and cardiac-related hospital admissions, *J Am Coll Cardiol* 26:1202–1208, 1995.

16. Parisi AF, Hartigan PM, Folland ED: Evaluation of exercise thallium scintigraphy versus exercise electrocardiography in predicting survival outcomes and morbid cardiac events in patients with single- and double-vessel disease. Findings from the Angioplasty Compared to Medicine (ACME) study, *J Am Coll Cardiol* 30:1256–1263, 1997.

17. Calnon DA, McGrath PD, Doss AL, Harrell FEJ, Watson DD, Beller GA: Prognostic value of dobutamine stress technetium-99msestamibi single-photon emission computed tomography myocardial perfusion imaging: stratification of a high-risk population, *J Am Coll Cardiol* 38:1511–1517, 2001.

18. Stratmann HG, Tamesis BR, Younis LT, Wittry MD, Miller DD: Prognostic value of dipyridamole technetium-99m sestamibi myocardial tomography in patients with stable chest pain who are unable to exercise, *Am J Cardiol* 73:647–652, 1994.

19. Kang X, Berman DS, Lewin HC, Cohen I, Friedman JD, Germano G, Hachamovitch LJ, Shaw LJ: Incremental prognostic value of myocardial perfusion single photon emission computed tomography in patients with diabetes mellitus, *Am Heart J* 138:1025–1032, 1999.

20. Berman DS, Kang X, Hayes SW, Friedman JD, Cohen I, Abidov A, Shaw AM, Amanullah AM, Germano G, Hachamovitch R: Adenosine myocardial perfusion single-photon emission computed tomography in women compared with men. Impact of diabetes mellitus on incremental prognostic value and effect on patient management, *J Am Coll Cardiol* 41:1125–1133, 2003.

21. Hachamovitch R, Hayes S, Friedman JD, Cohen I, Shaw LJ, Germano G, Berman DS: Determinants of risk and its temporal variation in patients with normal stress myocardial perfusion scans: what is the warranty period of a normal scan?*J Am Coll Cardiol* 41:1329–1340, 2003.

22. Shaw L, Chaitman BR, Hilton TC, Stocke KS, Younis LT, Caralis DG, Kong DD, Miller DD: Prognostic value of dipyridamole thallium-201 imaging in elderly patients, *J Am Coll Cardiol* 19:1390–1398, 1992.

23. Bax JJ, Young LH, Frye RL, Bonow RO, Steinberg HO, Barrett EJ: ADA. Screening for coronary artery disease in patients with diabetes, *Diabetes Care* 30:2729–2736, 2007.

24. Kamalesh M, Feigenbaum DH, Sawada S: Challenge of identifying patients with diabetes mellitus who are at low risk for coronary events by use of cardiac stress imaging, *Am Heart J* 147:561–563, 2004.

25. Berman DS, Hachamovitch R, Kiat H, Cohen I, Cabico JA, Wang FP, Friedman G, Germano G, Van Train K, Diamond GA: Incremental

value of prognostic testing in patients with known or suspected ischemic heart disease: a basis for optimal utilization of exercise technetium-99m sestamibi myocardial perfusion single-photon emission computed tomography [published erratum appears in *J Am Coll Cardiol* 27(3):756, 1996], *J Am Coll Cardiol* 26:639–647, 1995.

26. Abidov A, Hachamovitch R, Hayes SW, Ng CK, Cohen I, Friedman JD, Germano DS, Berman DS: Prognostic impact of hemodynamic response to adenosine in patients older than age 55 years undergoing vasodilator stress myocardial perfusion study, *Circulation* 107:2894–2899, 2003.

27. Sharir T, Berman DS, Lewin HC, Friedman JD, Cohen I, Miranda R, Agafitei G, Germano G: Incremental prognostic value of rest-redistribution (201)Tl single-photon emission computed tomography, *Circulation* 100:1964–1970, 1999.

28. Thomas GS, Miyamoto MI, Morello AP 3rd, Majmundar H, Thomas JJ, Sampson R, Hachamovitch R, Shaw LJ: Technetium 99m sestamibi myocardial perfusion imaging predicts clinical outcome in the community outpatient setting. The Nuclear Utility in the Community (NUC) Study, *J Am Coll Cardiol* 43:213–223, 2004.

29. Travin MI, Heller GV, Johnson LL, Katten D, Ahlberg AW, Isasi CR, Kaplan RC, Taub CC, Demus D: The prognostic value of ECG-gated SPECT imaging in patients undergoing stress Tc-99m sestamibi myocardial perfusion imaging, *J Nucl Cardiol* 11:253–262, 2004.

30. Shaw LJ, Miller DD, Romeis JC, Younis LT, Gillespie KN, Kimmey JR, Chaitman BR: Prognostic value of noninvasive risk stratification in younger and older patients referred for evaluation of suspected coronary artery disease, *J Am Geriatr Soc* 44:1190–1197, 1996.

31. O'Keefe JH Jr, Zinsmeister AR, Gibbons RJ: Value of normal electrocardiographic findings in predicting resting left ventricular function in patients with chest pain and suspected coronary artery disease, *Am J Med* 86:658–662, 1989.

32. Christian TF, Miller TD, Chareonthaitawee P, Hodge DO, O'Connor RJ, Gibbons RJ: Prevalence of normal resting left ventricular function with normal rest electrocardiograms, *Am J Cardiol* 79:1295–1298, 1997.

33. Ladenheim ML, Kotler TS, Pollock BH, Berman DS, Diamond GA: Incremental prognostic power of clinical history, exercise electrocardiography and myocardial perfusion scintigraphy in suspected coronary artery disease, *Am J Cardiol* 59:270–277, 1987.

34. Christian TF, Miller TD, Bailey KR, Gibbons RJ: Exercise tomographic thallium-201 imaging in patients with severe coronary artery disease and normal electrocardiograms, *Ann Intern Med* 121:825–832, 1994.

35. Poornima IG, Miller TD, Christian TF, Hodge DO, Bailey KR, Gibbons RJ: Utility of myocardial perfusion imaging in patients with low-risk treadmill scores, *J Am Coll Cardiol* 43:194–199, 2004.

36. Mieres JH, Shaw LJ, Arai A, Budoff MJ, Flamm SD, Hundley WG, Marwick L, Mosca L, Patel AR, Quinones MA, Redberg RF, Taubert AJ, Taylor AJ, Thomas GS, Wenger NK: Role of noninvasive testing in the clinical evaluation of women with suspected coronary artery disease: Consensus statement from the Cardiac Imaging Committee, Council on Clinical Cardiology, and the Cardiovascular Imaging and Intervention Committee, Council on Cardiovascular Radiology and Intervention, American Heart Association, *Circulation* 111:682–696, 2005.

37. Hachamovitch R, Berman DS, Shaw LJ, Kiat H, Cohen I, Cabico JA, Friedman GA, Diamond GA: Incremental prognostic value of myocardial perfusion single photon emission computed tomography for the prediction of cardiac death: differential stratification for risk of cardiac death and myocardial infarction, *Circulation* 97:535–543, 1998.

38. Hachamovitch R, Hayes S, Friedman J, Cohen I, Berman DS: A prognostic score for prediction of cardiac mortality risk after adenosine stress myocardial perfusion scintigraphy, *J Am Coll Cardiol* 45:722–729, 2005.

39. Vaduganathan P, He ZX, Raghavan C, Mahmarian JJ, Verani MS: Detection of left anterior descending coronary artery stenosis in patients with left bundle branch block: exercise, adenosine or dobutamine imaging? *J Am Coll Cardiol* 28:543–550, 1996.

40. Nallamothu N, Bagheri B, Acio ER, Heo J, Iskandrian AE: Prognostic value of stress myocardial perfusion single photon emission computed tomography imaging in patients with left ventricular bundle branch block, *J Nucl Cardiol* 4:487–493, 1997.

41. Wagdy HM, Hodge D, Christian TF, Miller TD, Gibbons RJ: Prognostic value of vasodilator myocardial perfusion imaging in patients with left bundle-branch block, *Circulation* 97:1563–1570, 1998.

42. Amanullah AM, Berman DS, Kang X, Cohen I, Germano G, Friedman JD: Enhanced prognostic stratification of patients with left ventricular hypertrophy with the use of single-photon emission computed tomography, *Am Heart J* 140:456–462, 2000.

43. Abidov A, Hachamovitch R, Rozanski A, Hayes SW, Santos MM, Sciammarella I, Cohen I, Gerlach J, Friedman JD, Germano G, Berman DS: Prognostic implications of atrial fibrillation in patients undergoing myocardial perfusion single-photon emission computed tomography, *J Am Coll Cardiol* 44:1062–1070, 2004.

44. Blumenthal RS, Becker DM, Moy TF, Coresh J, Wilder LB, Becker LC: Exercise thallium tomography predicts future clinically manifest

coronary heart disease in a high-risk asymptomatic population, *Circulation* 93:915–923, 1996.

45. Hachamovitch R, Berman DS: The use of nuclear cardiology in clinical decision making, *Semin Nucl Med* 35:62–72, 2005.

46. Giri S, Shaw LJ, Murthy DR, Travin MI, Miller DD, Hachamovitch R, Borges-Neto S, Berman DS, Waters DD, Heller GV: Impact of diabetes on the risk stratification using stress single-photon emission computed tomography myocardial perfusion imaging in patients with symptoms suggestive of coronary artery disease, *Circulation* 105:32–40, 2002.

47. Zellweger MJ, Hachamovitch R, Kang X, Hayes SW, Friedman JD, Germano ME, Pfisterer ME, Berman DS: Prognostic relevance of symptoms versus objective evidence of coronary artery disease in diabetic patients, *Eur Heart J* 25:543–550, 2004.

48. Wackers FJ, Young LH, Inzucchi SE, Chyun DA, Davey JA, Barrett EJ, Taillefer SD, Wittlin SD, Heller GV, Filipchuk N, Engel S, Ratner RE, Iskandrian AE: Detection of silent myocardial ischemia in asymptomatic diabetic subjects: the DIAD study, *Diabetes Care* 27:1954–1961, 2004.

49. Miller TD, Rajagopalan N, Hodge DO, Frye RL, Gibbons RJ: Yield of stress single-photon emission computed tomography in asymptomatic patients with diabetes, *Am Heart J* 147:890–896, 2004.

50. Rajagopalan N, Miller TD, Hodge DO, Frye RL, Gibbons RJ: Identifying high-risk asymptomatic diabetic patients who are candidates for screening stress single-photon emission computed tomography imaging, *J Am Coll Cardiol* 45:43–49, 2005.

51. Anand DV, Lim E, Hopkins D, Corder R, Shaw LJ, Sharp P, Lipkin D, Lahiri A: Risk stratification in uncomplicated type 2 diabetes: prospective evaluation of the combined use of coronary artery calcium imaging and selective myocardial perfusion scintigraphy, *Eur Heart J* 27:713–721, 2006.

52. Berman D, Hachamovitch R, Shaw LJ, Friedman JD, Hayes SW, Thomson DS, Fieno DS, Germano G, Slomka PJ, Wong ND, Kang X, Rozanski A: Roles of nuclear cardiology, cardiac computed tomography, and cardiac magnetic resonance: noninvasive risk stratification and a conceptual framework for the selection of noninvasive imaging tests in patients with known or suspected coronary artery disease, *J Nucl Med* 47:1107–1118, 2006.

53. Bax JJ, van der Wall EE: Assessment of coronary artery disease in patients with (a)symptomatic diabetes, *Eur Heart J* 27:631–632, 2006.

54. Slomka PJ, Nishina H, Abidov A, Hayes SW, Friedman JD, Berman DS, Germano G: Combined quantitative supine-prone myocardial perfusion SPECT improves detection of coronary artery disease and normalcy rates in women, *J Nucl Cardiol* In press, 2006.

55. Shaw LJ, Iskandrian AE: Prognostic value of gated myocardial perfusion SPECT, *J Nucl Cardiol* 11:171–185, 2004.

56. Shaw LJ, Bairey Merz CN, Pepine CJ, Reis SE, Bittner V, Kelsey SF, Olson BD, Johnson BD, Mankad S, Sharaf BL, Rogers WJ, Wessel TR, Arant CB, Pohost GM, Lerman A, Quyyumi AA, Sopko G: Insights from the NHLBI-Sponsored Women's Ischemia Syndrome Evaluation (WISE) Study: Part I: gender differences in traditional and novel risk factors, symptom evaluation, and gender-optimized diagnostic strategies, *J Am Coll Cardiol* 47:S4–S20, 2006.

57. Buglardini R, Bairey Merz CN: Angina with "normal" coronary arteries: a changing philosophy, *JAMA* 293:477–484, 2005.

58. Nadelmann J, Frishman WH, Ooi WL, et al: Prevalence, incidence, and prognosis of recognized and unrecognized myocardial infarction in persons aged 75 years or older: the Bronx Aging Study, *Am J Cardiol* 66:533–537, 1990.

59. Sigurdsson E, Thorgeirsson G, Sigvaldason H, Sigfusson N: Unrecognized myocardial infarction: epidemiology, clinical characteristics, and the prognostic role of angina pectoris. The Reykjavik Study, *Ann Intern Med* 122:96–102, 1995.

60. Kwok JM, Miller TD, Hodge DO, Gibbons RJ: Prognostic value of the Duke Treadmill Score in the elderly, *J Am Coll Cardiol* 39:1475–1481, 2002.

61. Valeti US, Miller TD, Hodge DO, Gibbons RJ: Exercise single-photon emission computed tomography provides effective risk stratification of elderly men and elderly women, *Circulation* 111:1771–1776, 2005.

62. Zafrir N, Mats I, Solodky A, Ben-Gal T, Sulkes J, Battler A: Prognostic value of stress myocardial perfusion imaging in octogenarian population, *J Nucl Cardiol* 12:671–675, 2005.

63. Schinkel AF, Elhendy A, Biagini E, van Domburg RT, Valkema R, Rizello C, Pedone C, Simoons M, Bax JJ, Poldermans D: Prognostic stratification using dobutamine stress 99mTc-tetrofosmin myocardial perfusion SPECT in elderly patients unable to perform exercise testing, *J Nucl Med* 46:12–18, 2005.

64. Lima RS, De Lorenzo A, Pantoja MR, Siqueira A: Incremental prognostic value of myocardial perfusion 99m-technetium-sestamibi SPECT in the elderly, *Int J Cardiol* 93:137–143, 2004.

65. Schiffrin EL, Lipman ML, Mann JFE: Chronic kidney disease: Effects on the cardiovascular system, *Circulation* 116:85–97, 2007.

66. Go AS, Fang MC, Udaltsova N, et al: Impact of proteinuria and glomerular filtration rate on risk of thromboembolism in atrial fibrillation: The Anticoagulation and Risk Factors in Atrial Fibrillation (ATRIA) Study, 2009.

67. Verma A, Anavekar NS, Meris A, Thune JJ, Arnold JM, Ghali JK, Velazquez JJ, McMurray JJ, Pfeffer MA, Solomon SD: The relationship between renal function and cardiac structure, function, and prognosis after myocardial infarction: the VALIANT Echo Study, *J Am Coll Cardiol* 50:1238–1245, 2007.

68. Go AS, Chertow GM, Fan D, McCulloch CE, Hsu CY: Chronic kidney disease and the risks of death, cardiovascular events, and hospitalization, *N Engl J Med* 351:1296–1305, 2004.

69. Tonelli M, Wiebe N, Culleton B, House A, Rabbat C, Fok M, McAlister AX, Garg AX: Chronic kidney disease and mortality risk: a systematic review, *J Am Soc Nephrol* 17:2034–2047, 2006.

70. Al-Mallah M, Hachamovitch R, Dorbala S, Kwong R, Hainer J, Di Carli MF: Prognostic value of myocardial perfusion imaging in patients with impaired renal function, *J Nucl Cardiol* 14:S125, 2007 (abs).

71. Patel AD, Abo-Auda WS, Davis JM, Zoghbi GJ, Deierhoi MH, Heo J, Iskandrian AE: Prognostic value of myocardial perfusion imaging in predicting outcome after renal transplantation, *Am J Cardiol* 92:146–151, 2003.

72. Dahan M, Viron BM, Faraggi M, Himbert DL, Lagallicier BJ, Kolta AM, Pessione D, Le Guludec D, Gourgon R, Mignon FE: Diagnostic accuracy and prognostic value of combined dipyridamole-exercise thallium imaging in hemodialysis patients, *Kidney Int* 54:255–262, 1998.

73. Venkataraman R, Hage FG, Dorfman T, Heo J, Aqel RA, de Mattos AM, Iskandrian AE: Role of myocardial perfusion imaging in patients with end-stage renal disease undergoing coronary angiography, *Am J Cardiol* 102:1451–1456, 2008.

74. Hakeem A, Bhatti S, Dillie KS, Cook JR, Samad Z, Roth-Cline MD, Chang SM: Predictive value of myocardial perfusion single-photon emission computed tomography and the impact of renal function on cardiac death, *Circulation* 118:2540–2549, 2008.

75. Berman DS, Kang X, Hayes SW, Friedman JD, Cohen I, Abidov A, Shaw AM, Amanullah AM, Germano G, Hachamovitch R: Adenosine myocardial perfusion single-photon emission computed tomography in women compared with men. Impact of diabetes mellitus on incremental prognostic value and effect on patient management, *J Am Coll Cardiol* 41:1125–1133, 2003.

76. Suthanthiran M, Li B, Song JO, Ding R, Sharma VK, Schwartz JF, August P: Transforming growth factor-beta 1 hyperexpression in African-American hypertensives: A novel mediator of hypertension and/or target organ damage, *Proc Natl Acad Sci U S A* 97:3479–3484, 2000.

77. Nishina H, Slomka PJ, Abidov A, Yoda S, Akincioglu C, Kang X, Cohen SW, Hayes SW, Friedman JD, Germano G, Berman DS: Combined supine and prone quantitative myocardial perfusion SPECT: method development and clinical validation in patients with no known coronary artery disease, *J Nucl Med* 47:51–58, 2006.

78. Kang X, Shaw LJ, Hayes SW, Hachamovitch R, Abidov A, Cohen I, Friedman LE, Thomson LE, Polk D, Germano G, Berman DS: Impact of body mass index on cardiac mortality in patients with known or suspected coronary artery disease undergoing myocardial perfusion single-photon emission computed tomography, *J Am Coll Cardiol* 47:1418–1426, 2006.

79. Elhendy A, Schinkel AF, van Domburg RT, Bax JJ, Valkema R, Biagini E, Poldermans D: Prognostic stratification of obese patients by stress 99mTc-tetrofosmin myocardial perfusion imaging, *J Nucl Med* 47:1302–1306, 2006.

80. Duvall WL, Croft LB, Corriel JS, Einstein AJ, Fisher JE, Haynes PS, Rose MJ, Henzlova MJ: SPECT myocardial perfusion imaging in morbidly obese patients: image quality, hemodynamic response to pharmacologic stress, and diagnostic and prognostic value, *J Nucl Cardiol* 13:202–209, 2006.

81. Yoshinaga K, Chow BJ, Williams KA, Chen L, deKemp RA, Garrard L, Lok-Tin Szeto A, Aung M, Davies RA, Ruddy TD, Beanlands RS: What is the prognostic value of myocardial perfusion imaging using rubidium-82 positron emission tomography? *J Am Coll Cardiol* 48:1029–1039, 2006.

82. Greenland P, Bonow RO, Brundage BH, Budoff MJ, Eisenberg MJ, Grundy MS, Lauer MS, Post WS, Raggi P, Redberg RF, Rodgers GP, Shaw LJ, Taylor AJ, Weintraub WS: Computed tomography: ACC/AHA writing committee to update the 2000 clinical expert consensus document on electron-beam computed tomography for the diagnosis and prognosis for coronary artery disease, *J Am Coll Cardiol* 47:998–1004, 2006.

83. He ZX, Hedrick TD, Pratt CM, Verani MS, Aquino V, Roberts R, Mahmarian JJ: Severity of coronary artery calcification by electron beam computed tomography predicts silent myocardial ischemia, *Circulation* 101:244–251, 2000.

84. Berman DS, Wong ND, Gransar H, Miranda-Peats R, Dahlbeck J, Arad SW, Hayes SW, Friedman JD, Kang X, Polk D, Hachamovitch R, Rozanski A: Relationship between stress-induced myocardial ischemia and atherosclerosis measured by coronary calcium tomography, *J Am Coll Cardiol* 44:923–930, 2004.

85. Schenker MP, Dorbala S, Hong EC, Rybicki FJ, Hachamovitch R, Kwong RF, Di Carli MF: Interrelation of coronary calcification, myocardial ischemia, and outcomes in patients with intermediate

likelihood of coronary artery disease: a combined positron emission tomography/computed tomography study, *Circulation* 117: 1693–1700, 2008.

86. Blumenthal RS, Becker DM, Yanek LR, Moy TF, Michos ED, Fishman LC, Becker LC: Comparison of coronary calcium and stress myocardial perfusion imaging in apparently healthy siblings of individuals with premature coronary artery disease, *Am J Cardiol* 97: 328–333, 2006.

87. Wong ND, Rozanski A, Gransar H, Miranda-Peats R, Kang X, Hayes S, Shaw J, Friedman J, Polk D, Berman DS: Metabolic syndrome and diabetes are associated with an increased likelihood of inducible myocardial ischemia among patients with subclinical atherosclerosis, *Diabetes Care* 28:1445–1450, 2005.

88. Rozanski A, Gransar H, Wong ND, Shaw LJ, Miranda-Peats R, Hayes JD, Friedman JD, Berman DS: Use of coronary calcium scanning for predicting inducible myocardial ischemia: Influence of patients' clinical presentation, *J Nucl Cardiol* 14:669–679, 2007.

89. Zellweger MJ, Berman D, Shaw L, et al: Evaluation of patients after intervention. In Poshost G, et al: editor: *Imaging in Cardiovascular Medicine*, Philadelphia, 2000, Lippincott Williams & Wilkins.

90. Ho KT, Miller TD, Holmes DR, Hodge DO, Gibbons RJ: Long-term prognostic value of Duke treadmill score and exercise thallium-201 imaging performed one to three years after percutaneous transluminal coronary angioplasty, *Am J Cardiol* 84:1323–1327, 1999.

91. Garzon PP, Eisenberg MJ: Functional testing for the detection of restenosis after percutaneous transluminal coronary angioplasty: a meta-analysis, *Can J Cardiol* 17:41–48, 2001.

92. Grondin CM, Campeau L, Lespérance J, Enjalbert M, Bourassa MG: Comparison of late changes in internal mammary artery and saphenous vein grafts in two consecutive series of patients 10 years after operation, *Circulation* 70(3 Pt 2):I208–I212, 1984.

93. Miller TD, Christian TF, Hodge DO, Mullan BP, Gibbons RJ: Prognostic value of exercise thallium-201 imaging performed within 2 years of coronary artery bypass graft surgery, *J Am Coll Cardiol* 31:848–854, 1998.

94. Zellweger MJ, Lewin HC, Lai S, Dubois EA, Friedman JD, Germano G, Kang T, Sharir T, Berman DS: When to stress patients after coronary artery bypass surgery? Risk stratification in patients early and late post-CABG using stress myocardial perfusion SPECT: implications of appropriate clinical strategies., *J Am Coll Cardiol* 37: 144–152, 2001.

95. Palmas W, Bingham S, Diamond GA, Denton TA, Kiat H, Friedman D, Scarlata D, Maddahi J, Cohen I, Berman DS: Incremental prognostic value of exercise thallium-201 myocardial single-photon emission computed tomography late after coronary artery bypass surgery, *J Am Coll Cardiol* 25:403–409, 1995.

96. Lauer MS, Lytle B, Pashkow F, Snader CE, Marwick TH: Prediction of death and myocardial infarction by screening with exercise-thallium testing after coronary-artery-bypass grafting, *Lancet* 351:615–622, 1998.

97. Hachamovitch R, Di Carli MF: Contemporary reviews in cardiovascular medicine: Methods and limitations of assessing new noninvasive tests: I. Anatomy-based validation of noninvasive testing, *Circulation* 117:2684–2690, 2008.

98. Hachamovitch R, Hayes SW, Friedman JD, Cohen I, Kang X, Germano G, Berman DS: Is there a referral bias against revascularization of patients with reduced LV ejection fraction? Influence of ejection fraction and inducible ischemia on post-SPECT management of patients without history of CAD, *J Am Coll Cardiol* 42:1286–1294, 2003.

99. Hachamovitch R, Rozanski A, Hayes SW, Thomson LEJ, Germano G, Friedman JD, Cohen I, Berman DS: Predicting therapeutic benefit from myocardial revascularization procedures: Are measurements of resting left ventricular ejection fraction and stress-induced myocardial ischemia both necessary? *J Nucl Cardiol* 13(6):768–778, 2006.

100. Hachamovitch R, Hayes SW, Friedman JD, Cohen I, Berman DS: A prognostic score for prediction of cardiac mortality risk after adenosine stress myocardial perfusion scintigraphy, *J Am Coll Cardiol* 45:722–729, 2005.

101. Boden WE, O'Rourke RA, Teo KK, Hartigan PM, Maron DJ, Kostuk WJ, et al: Optimal medical therapy with or without PCI for stable coronary disease, *N Engl J Med* 356, 2007.

102. Fractional Flow Reserve Versus Angiography for Multivessel Evaluation (FAME): Presented at TCT 2008, 2008.

103. Dorbala S, Vangala D, Sampson UK, Limaye A, Kwong R, Di Carli MF: Value of vasodilator left ventricular ejection fraction reserve in evaluating the magnitude of myocardium at risk and the extent of angiographic coronary artery disease: a 82Rb PET/CT study, *J Nucl Med* 48:349–358, 2007.

104. Weiner DA, Ryan TJ, McCabe CH, Chaitman BR, Sheffield LT, Fisher F, Tristani F: The role of exercise testing in identifying patients with improved survival after coronary artery bypass surgery, *J Am Coll Cardiol* 8:741–748, 1986.

Chapter 17

Myocardial Perfusion: Magnetic Resonance Imaging

AMIT R. PATEL AND CHRISTOPHER M. KRAMER

INTRODUCTION

The presence of a hemodynamically significant coronary stenosis can be detected by studying its influence on the downstream microcirculation. As the stenosis worsens, myocardial perfusion is preserved via autoregulatory mechanisms that result in dilation of the arteriolar bed.[1] When challenged with vasodilators, blood flow will not increase in myocardial segments supplied by a significantly stenosed coronary artery because the perfusion reserve has already been exhausted by autoregulation, whereas perfusion will increase substantially in territories supplied by normal coronary arteries. Myocardial perfusion imaging can therefore identify the presence of a flow-limiting coronary stenosis by detecting regional variations in perfusion reserve.

Although myocardial perfusion can be studied using multiple imaging modalities, cardiac magnetic resonance (CMR) has several important advantages. Specifically, it does not require the use of ionizing radiation, has excellent spatial and temporal resolution, and has the potential to fully quantify myocardial blood flow. Additionally, a comprehensive CMR study that includes hyperemic and resting perfusion assessment, quantitative left ventricular volume and function determination, and scar and viability imaging can be performed in less than 45 minutes.

The diagnostic performance of perfusion CMR was recently evaluated in a meta-analysis of 14 studies including a total of 1183 patients.[2] When compared to x-ray angiography, the sensitivity and specificity for detecting significant coronary artery disease were 91% and 81%, respectively (Fig. 17-1). In addition to its ability to identify patients with flow-limiting coronary disease, perfusion CMR readily differentiates low-risk from high-risk patients (Fig. 17-2). Three recent studies have prospectively studied the ability of perfusion CMR to identify low-risk patients. In these studies, only 4 of the 625 patients with no evidence of ischemia had a major adverse cardiac event after 1 year of follow-up.[3-5] Stress testing in the MR environment is safe. Bernhardt et al. reported on the safety of performing an adenosine stress test in a MRI scanner.[6] Of the 3174 patients studied, only one had a major complication (grand mal seizure). Minor side effects were experienced by 35% of the patients (e.g., chest pain, dyspnea, transient AV block, nausea). In this chapter, we will discuss the basic principle of perfusion CMR image acquisition and review various approaches used for image analysis.

BASIC PRINCIPLE OF IMAGE PREPARATION AND ACQUISITION

Regardless of the imaging modality used for assessing myocardial perfusion, the signal measured must adequately differentiate normally perfused myocardial segments from abnormally perfused segments. Contrast-enhanced CMR was initially used to estimate the perfusion reserve by Miller et al. in 1989.[7] Atkinson et al. developed a technique a year later in 1990[8] that enabled a more dynamic evaluation of perfusion using first-pass imaging. Images are serially acquired in one or more preselected imaging planes as an intravenously administered bolus of a gadolinium chelate transits the vasculature and eventually the myocardium. As gadolinium migrates through the right-sided cardiac chambers, the pulmonary vasculature, the left-sided chambers, and ultimately the myocardium, a bright signal is generated. The rate of signal increase as the contrast agent initially perfuses a tissue is a gauge of blood flow.[9]

The signal generated and how closely it correlates to myocardial blood flow is also a function of the specific CMR pulse sequence parameters used. In order to

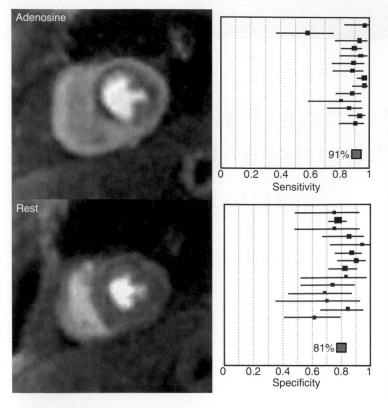

Figure 17-1 Perfusion CMR images are shown. The patient has critical left main stenosis. The image on the *top left* was acquired during hyperemia, and a large circumferential perfusion defect is present on the subendocardial border of the left ventricular short axis. No defect is present on the corresponding resting perfusion image shown on *bottom*. On the *right*, a Forest plot from a meta-analysis of 14 studies shows that the mean sensitivity and specificity were, respectively, 91% and 81%. *(Adapted from Nandalur KR, Dwamena BA, Choudhri AF, et al: Diagnostic performance of stress cardiac magnetic resonance imaging in the detection of coronary artery disease: A meta-analysis, J Am Coll Cardiol 50:1343-1353, 2007.)*

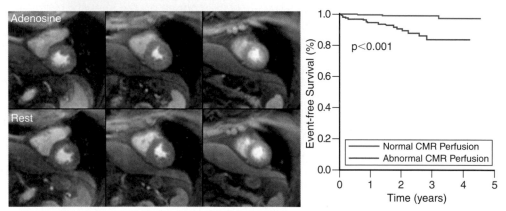

Figure 17-2 This is an example of a normal perfusion CMR study. The three left ventricular short-axis slices shown are from peak enhancement during the first-pass perfusion of gadolinium under both hyperemic and resting conditions. There is no evidence of ischemia because all of the myocardium enhances homogenously. A Kaplan-Meier curve based on the results of perfusion CMR performed on 461 patients is on the *right*. The absence of ischemia identified a cohort of patients with a very high event-free survival. *(Adapted from Jahnke C, Nagel E, Gebker R, et al: Prognostic value of cardiac magnetic resonance stress tests: Adenosine stress perfusion and dobutamine stress wall motion imaging, Circulation 115:1769-1776, 2007.)*

generate a signal using magnetic resonance, the magnetization must be manipulated by applying a brief radiofrequency pulse to flip the proton alignment into the transverse plane. Once the radiofrequency pulse is completed, the protons return to their previous alignment. The rate at which the proton alignment recovers determines the longitudinal relaxation time, T1, of the tissue. Gadolinium is a paramagnetic contrast agent that shortens the T1 of neighboring protons, ultimately causing increased signal intensity in a concentration-dependent manner for T1-weighted images. In addition to the gadolinium concentration, the magnitude of

the T1-weighted signal is dependent on the type of magnetization preparation used. The initial perfusion CMR studies were performed using an inversion recovery sequence.[8] Because inversion recovery can be used to null the signal from tissues that are not exposed to gadolinium, a large signal contrast exists between hypoperfused and normally perfused tissues. However, magnetization preparation using inversion recovery is less robust in the presence of arrhythmias and is time-consuming, which compromises temporal resolution and limits the number of left ventricular slices that can be acquired during one cardiac cycle.

A more commonly used magnetization preparation scheme is saturation recovery.[10] Saturation recovery is insensitive to arrhythmias, has a shorter acquisition window than inversion recovery, and more readily allows multislice coverage with an improved temporal resolution at the expense of reduced signal contrast between normally perfused and hypoperfused tissues. In experimental models and in clinical practice, the resultant contrast is sufficient to make a diagnosis.[11] The amount of signal generated by a given concentration of gadolinium also depends on the time delay between magnetization preparation and image acquisition.[12] Specifically, shorter delays allow for improved discrimination of higher concentrations of gadolinium, whereas longer delays allow for improved differentiation between lower concentrations of gadolinium.

Another important component of the CMR pulse sequence is the method of image acquisition. Currently, three approaches are most commonly used: gradient recalled echo (GRE),[8] hybrid GRE and echoplanar imaging (GRE-EPI),[13] and balanced steady-state free precession (SSFP).[14] Each approach has its unique set of advantages and disadvantages. No consensus exists as to the best technique for image acquisition. The use of parallel imaging shortens the time necessary to acquire an image and likely reduces blurring and improves image quality of all three approaches.[15,16]

Of the three techniques, SSFP-based approaches have the highest contrast-to-noise ratio, and the signal is most linearly related to the underlying gadolinium concentration.[17] However, the technique also requires a longer imaging duration, resulting in more blurring and motion artifact; SSFP also suffers most from susceptibility artifact. GRE-EPI has the most extensive spatial coverage and the shortest imaging duration, which results in less blurring and better image quality at higher heart rates. The signal is also linearly correlated with the concentration of gadolinium, but higher gadolinium concentrations are underestimated, and the overall CNR is less than that for SSFP-based images. GRE-based techniques have the lowest contrast-to-noise ratio and the poorest relationship between signal and gadolinium

concentration. Its image duration is similar to SSFP, but the image quality may be better than SSFP at higher heart rates.

An important challenge of perfusion CMR is the so-called "dark rim artifact," which mimics a hypoperfused segment on the subendocardial border of the myocardium.[18,19] The etiology of the artifact is not clearly defined but appears to be related to cardiac motion, partial volume effects between the left ventricular cavity and the myocardium, and sudden changes in the concentration of contrast agent in the left ventricular blood pool and the myocardium. Whatever the etiology, the artifact is less pronounced when the hybrid GRE-EPI pulse sequence and parallel imaging are used.

APPROACHES TO IMAGE ANALYSIS

Because of its dynamic nature and versatility, perfusion CMR images can be analyzed qualitatively or quantitatively using time-intensity curves generated as the contrast agent perfuses the myocardium. Because qualitative interpretation can be performed immediately after image acquisition and does not require extensive postprocessing, it has been the most accepted in clinical practice. Atkinson et al. initially used CMR to visually detect first pass of gadolinium in humans in 1990.[8] Since then, significant improvements in hardware and pulse sequence development allow for multislice imaging with high temporal resolution. Typically, complete images for at least three left ventricular short-axis slices are acquired during each cardiac cycle. As the contrast agent traverses the cardiac chambers and the myocardium, serial images are acquired for approximately 50 beats. Myocardial segments that are supplied by a severe coronary stenosis have a slower rise in signal intensity and become hypointense compared to normal segments (Fig. 17-3).[9] The hypointensity is typically present in a coronary distribution and is most pronounced in the subendocardium and can extend into the midmyocardium.

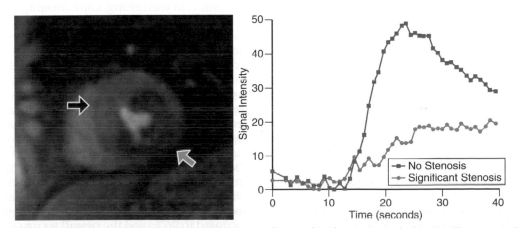

Figure 17-3 An image of the left ventricular short axis acquired at peak enhancement during the first pass of gadolinium is shown on the *left*. The *purple arrow* points to a segment perfused by a normal coronary artery. The *orange arrow* points to a region perfused by a significantly stenosed coronary artery. Time-intensity curves derived from the two regions are shown. In the presence of a significantly stenosed coronary artery, the signal increases more gradually and plateaus at a lower threshold.

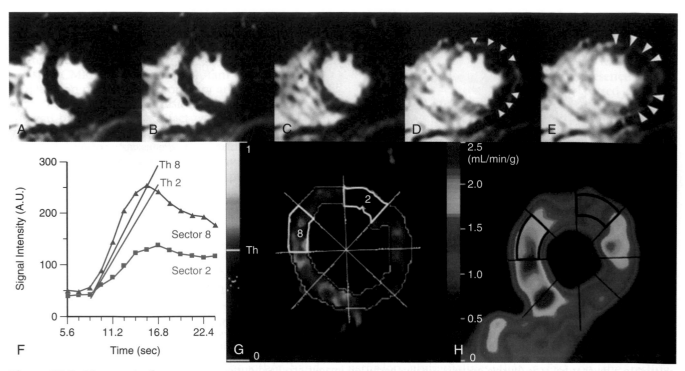

Figure 17-5 The transit of contrast over time is shown in images **A** through **E**. Note the hypointensity in the anterior and lateral walls of the ventricle. This patient has significant stenoses in the left anterior descending and the right coronary arteries. Image **F** shows the difference in upslope between the normal sector 8 and the abnormal sector 2. On the parametric map shown in image **G**, regions colored in shades of red have a normal perfusion reserve index, whereas blue regions are abnormal. Note the corresponding perfusion defects seen by positron emission tomography on image **H**. *(Adapted from Schwitter J, Nanz D, Kneifel S, et al: Assessment of myocardial perfusion in coronary artery disease by magnetic resonance: A comparison with positron emission tomography and coronary angiography, Circulation 103:2230-2235, 2001.)*

underestimated) the perfusion reserve as measured by PET. Additionally, the upslope technique was more closely related to PET than to x-ray angiography. Rieber et al. investigated the ability of perfusion CMR to accurately identify physiologically significant coronary artery disease by comparing the MPRi to invasive fractional flow reserve (FFR) in 43 patients.[39] Those patients with a coronary stenosis greater than 50% and an FFR less than 0.75 had significantly lower MPRi than those patients with a coronary stenosis greater than 50% and an FFR greater than 0.75. The presence of MPRi less than 1.5 had a sensitivity of 88% and a specificity of 90% (area under the curve of 0.93) for detecting hemodynamically significant stenoses. Only a moderate correlation between diameter stenosis and MPRi existed. In addition to being reduced in the presence of a hemodynamically significant coronary stenosis, the upslope parameter improves substantially following revascularization.[40] Patients revascularized with a stent have a greater improvement in the MPRi than those revascularized by balloon angioplasty.[41]

Fully Quantitative Perfusion CMR

Absolute measures of myocardial blood flow during a myocardial perfusion imaging study would be desirable. In an ideal situation, this can be determined by measuring how quickly a contrast agent flows out of a region of interest (washout or tissue impulse response). However, an accurate measurement requires that the entire

contrast bolus arrives instantaneously into the region of interest. Such circumstances necessitate that the contrast agent be injected directly into the coronary artery. When injected peripherally, upstream dispersion distorts the contrast bolus into a bell-shaped curve, preventing the entire bolus from arriving instantaneously into the region of interest. As the "bell-shaped" bolus travels through the myocardium, the concentration of contrast agent entering the tissue initially increases; therefore, as the initial low-concentration part of the contrast agent bolus is washing out, a higher concentration of contrast is simultaneously entering the tissue. Effectively, the changing bolus concentration (AIF, or arterial input function) masks the actual tissue impulse response. In fact, the signal (or time-intensity curve) that is actually generated as the bolus transits the myocardium (TF, or tissue function) is a fusion (or convolution) of the AIF and the tissue impulse response. Using a constrained Fermi function deconvolution, the tissue impulse response can be extracted from the AIF and TF. The amplitude of the tissue impulse response is a measure of absolute myocardial blood flow (Fig. 17-6).[42,43] Therefore, a fully quantitative perfusion reserve (PR) is simply a ratio of the impulse response amplitudes obtained during hyperemia and during resting conditions. PR determined using a Fermi function deconvolution measures perfusion more accurately than other simpler methods such as peak contrast enhancement technique or signal upslope technique. The latter methods significantly underestimate higher myocardial blood

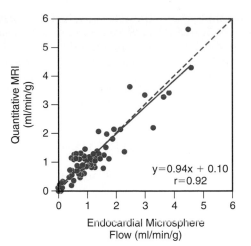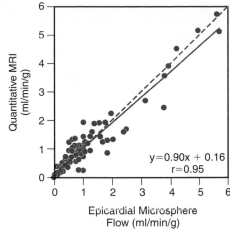

Figure 17-6 Myocardial blood flow measured using Fermi function deconvolution is highly correlated to gold-standard measurements made using radiolabeled microspheres. Because of its excellent spatial resolution, perfusion CMR can accurately resolve subendocardial from subepicardial blood flow. *(Adapted from Christian TF, Rettmann DW, Aletras AH, et al: Absolute myocardial perfusion in canines measured by using dual-bolus first-pass MR imaging, Radiology 232:677-684, 2004.)*

flows (those > 1.5 to 2 mL/kg/min) as determined by gold-standard radiolabeled microspheres.[44]

Using a deconvolution technique, Cullen et al. showed that CMR-measured myocardial perfusion reserve was inversely correlated with the severity of underlying coronary stenosis ($r = -0.81$; $P < 0.01$).[45] Futamatsu et al. prospectively compared the diagnostic performance of deconvolution analysis of perfusion CMR to semiquantitative and visual interpretation.[46] Using FFR as the reference standard, perfusion reserve measured using deconvolution most accurately identified the presence of hemodynamically significant coronary stenoses.[47] Other fully quantitative techniques have compared favorably to coronary flow reserve measurements made using intracoronary Doppler flow wire.[48]

An accurate assessment of myocardial blood flow requires precise measurement of the gadolinium concentration in both the left ventricular cavity and the myocardium. This is typically accomplished by using a low concentration of gadolinium; however, a low concentration of gadolinium is suboptimal for visual interpretation of the tissue perfusion. To solve this problem, Christian et al. proposed using a dual-bolus technique in which the arterial input function is separately measured using a very low dose of gadolinium and the tissue function is measured using a full dose.[44] When compared to the standard single-bolus technique, the dual technique also resulted in reduced measurement variability.[49] Alternatively, dual-contrast techniques simultaneously acquire low-resolution images that do not underestimate the AIF, and high-resolution and higher signal images that provide adequate contrast enhancement for the tissue perfusion.[50]

Using the dual-bolus technique, our group studied 30 patients referred for an x-ray angiogram.[51] By selecting the appropriate perfusion reserve cutoff value, the dual-bolus technique can be optimized to detect the desired severity of coronary stenosis. A higher perfusion reserve cutoff value is better for detecting coronary stenoses greater than 50%, and a lower cutoff value is optimal for detecting stenoses greater than 70%. Furthermore, when compared to fully quantitative perfusion reserve analysis, visual interpretation significantly underestimated the ischemic burden in patients with three-vessel

coronary artery disease and did not adequately differentiate single-vessel disease from three-vessel disease.

In addition to accurately defining the ischemic burden of coronary disease, quantitative perfusion analysis can provide new insights into the pathophysiology of ischemic heart disease. Selvanayagam et al. studied 27 patients with known coronary disease and wall-motion abnormalities prior to revascularization.[52] They found that the resting myocardial blood flow was impaired in regions of hibernating myocardium and preserved in normal myocardial segments. Following revascularization, both resting myocardial blood flow and regional contraction improved. In another study, the same group evaluated the effects of distal embolization on myocardial perfusion reserve following percutaneous coronary intervention.[53] Regions of myocardium that had new late gadolinium enhancement following revascularization had no improvement in perfusion reserve immediately following revascularization. Myocardial segments that were not complicated by distal embolization during revascularization had an acute improvement in the perfusion reserve.

Others have used fully quantitative perfusion CMR to demonstrate that the myocardial perfusion reserve is also reduced in asymptomatic patients with coronary artery calcification[54] and other coronary risk factors.[55] An important advantage of perfusion CMR is that it has the spatial resolution to resolve transmural differences in blood flow. Under normal circumstances, the resting myocardial blood flow is higher on the subendocardial border than on the subepicardial border, but in disease states such as hypertrophic cardiomyopathy[56] and transplant arteriopathy,[57] perfusion on the subendocardial border is disproportionately affected. This heterogeneity in myocardial blood flow is readily differentiated using CMR.

FUTURE DIRECTIONS

Unique to CMR perfusion imaging is the ability to determine perfusion without the use of exogenous contrast agents. One approach, arterial spin labeling (ASL), uses endogenous water as a freely diffusible tracer.[58]

Although numerous implementations are possible, in some approaches, protons in water molecules located proximal to the desired imaging plane are inverted or labeled. As these labeled protons enter the desired imaging slice, an apparent change in the T1 of the imaging slice occurs. Using specific variants of ASL, quantification of myocardial blood flow is feasible.[59] An important limitation of ASL is that a large increase in flow results in a relatively small increase in signal. Despite this limitation, when combined with vasodilator stress testing, territories supplied by a stenotic coronary artery have a measurably lower perfusion reserve than segments supplied by normal coronary arteries.[60]

An alternative approach, blood oxygen level–dependent (BOLD) imaging, takes advantage of the fact that deoxygenated hemoglobin changes proton signals in such a way as to reflect blood oxygenation.[61] In normal volunteers, Li et al. used BOLD imaging to detect alterations in the relationship between myocardial oxygen supply and demand caused by vasodilators and inotropes.[62] Segments of myocardium distal to a significant stenosis can only maintain adequate tissue oxygenation by increasing myocardial blood volume.[63] As the myocardial blood volume increases, the amount of deoxygenated hemoglobin present increases. As such, Wacker et al. showed that under resting conditions, myocardial segments supplied by a stenosed coronary had a significantly lower BOLD signal than normal segments, and this difference could be amplified using vasodilators.[64] An important limitation of BOLD imaging is that significant changes in perfusion result in relatively small changes in signal.[65] Newer multislice techniques with a more robust signal response are currently under development.[66] In addition to its ability to estimate myocardial blood flow without the use of exogenous contrast agents, some investigators have combined ASL with BOLD imaging to quantify the rate of regional myocardial oxygen consumption.[67,68]

Nephrogenic Systemic Fibrosis

An important consideration in the use of gadolinium-based contrast agents for myocardial perfusion imaging is the potential complication of nephrogenic systemic fibrosis (NSF). NSF is a potentially life threatening and highly debilitating condition (initially described in 1997) that has some similarities to progressive systemic sclerosis and can involve the skin, pleura, pericardium, lungs, joints, and striated muscle. It has been associated with the use of gadolinium in patients with advanced renal disease.[69] NSF is rare[70] and is most likely to occur in patients on dialysis or those with a glomerular filtration rate less than 15 mL/min/1.73 m^2.[71] Current recommendations focus on minimizing the use of gadolinium in patients at risk for NSF. If possible, the use of gadolinium should be avoided in patients with a glomerular filtration rate less than 30 mL/min/1.73 m^2. If gadolinium-based contrast agents must be used, then the lowest dose needed to reliably provide the sought-after diagnostic information should be utilized. Some have advocated that dialysis patients who have received gadolinium should be dialyzed within 2 hours and possibly again on the next day to help clear any residual contrast agent; however, no conclusive data to support this recommendation currently exist.[72] Given that myocardial perfusion imaging can be performed using several alternative techniques, the authors currently recommend that gadolinium-based myocardial perfusion be avoided in patients at risk for NSF.

CONCLUSIONS

In this chapter, we have reviewed the basic principles of image acquisition and interpretation as they apply to perfusion CMR imaging. Myocardial blood flow can be accurately measured without the use of ionizing radiation. Its high spatial resolution and the absence of attenuation artifact make it a valuable clinical tool for the evaluation of suspected coronary artery disease. Image interpretation can be performed qualitatively, semiquantitatively, or fully quantitatively. The ability to accurately quantify perfusion, function, and scar during a single study could lead to an improved understanding of ischemic heart disease as well as other cardiac disorders. The clinical role of perfusion CMR will be better defined as larger multicenter studies are performed.

REFERENCES

1. Chilian WM, Layne SM, Klausner EC, et al: Redistribution of coronary microvascular resistance produced by dipyridamole, *Am J Physiol Heart Circ Physiol* 256:H383–H390, 1989.
2. Nandalur KR, Dwamena BA, Choudhri AF, et al: Diagnostic performance of stress cardiac magnetic resonance imaging in the detection of coronary artery disease: A meta-analysis, *J Am Coll Cardiol* 50:1343–1353, 2007.
3. Ingkanisorn WP, Kwong RY, Bohme NS, et al: Prognosis of negative adenosine stress magnetic resonance in patients presenting to an emergency department with chest pain, *J Am Coll Cardiol* 47:1427–1432, 2006.
4. Jahnke C, Nagel E, Gebker R, et al: Prognostic value of cardiac magnetic resonance stress tests: adenosine stress perfusion and dobutamine stress wall motion imaging, *Circulation* 115:1769–1776, 2007.
5. Pilz G, Jeske A, Klos M, et al: Prognostic value of normal adenosine-stress cardiac magnetic resonance imaging, *Am J Cardiol* 101(10):1408–1412, 2008.
6. Bernhardt P, Levenson B, Engels T, et al: Contrast-enhanced adenosine-stress magnetic resonance imaging: Feasibility and practicability of a protocol for detection or exclusion of ischemic heart disease in an outpatient setting, *Clin Res Cardiol* 95:461–467, 2006.
7. Miller DD, Holmvang G, Gill JB, et al: MRI detection of myocardial perfusion changes by gadolinium-DTPA infusion during dipyridamole hyperemia, *Magn Reson Med* 10:246–255, 1989.
8. Atkinson DJ, Burstein D, Edelman RR: First-pass cardiac perfusion: evaluation with ultrafast MR imaging, *Radiology* 174:757–762, 1990.
9. Manning WJ, Atkinson DJ, Grossman W, et al: First-pass nuclear magnetic resonance imaging studies using gadolinium-DTPA in patients with coronary artery disease, *J Am Coll Cardiol* 18:959–965, 1991.
10. Tsekos NV, Zhang Y, Merkle H, et al: Fast anatomical imaging of the heart and assessment of myocardial perfusion with arrhythmia insensitive magnetization preparation, *Magn Reson Med* 34:530–536, 1995.
11. Wilke N, Jerosch-Herold M, Wang Y, et al: Myocardial perfusion reserve: assessment with multisection, quantitative, first-pass MR imaging, *Radiology* 204:373–384, 1997.
12. Bertschinger KM, Nanz D, Buechi M, et al: Magnetic resonance myocardial first-pass perfusion imaging: parameter optimization for signal response and cardiac coverage, *J Magn Reson Imaging* 14:556–562, 2001.
13. Ding S, Wolff SD, Epstein FH: Improved coverage in dynamic contrast-enhanced cardiac MRI using interleaved gradient-echo EPI, *Magn Reson Med* 39:514–519, 1998.
14. Judd RM, Reeder SB, Atalar E, et al: A magnetization-driven gradient echo pulse sequence for the study of myocardial perfusion, *Magn Reson Med* 34:276–282, 1995.

15. Kellman P, Epstein FH, McVeigh ER: Adaptive sensitivity encoding incorporating temporal filtering (TSENSE), *Magn Reson Med* 45: 846–852, 2001.
16. Griswold MA, Jakob PM, Heidemann RM, et al: Generalized autocalibrating partially parallel acquisitions (GRAPPA), *Magn Reson Med* 47: 1202–1210, 2002.
17. Lyne JC, Gatehouse PD, Assomull RG, et al: Direct comparison of myocardial perfusion cardiovascular magnetic resonance sequences with parallel acquisition, *J Magn Reson Imaging* 26:1444–1451, 2007.
18. Storey P, Chen Q, Li W, et al: Band artifacts due to bulk motion, *Magn Reson Med* 48:1028–1036, 2002.
19. Di Bella EVR, Parker DL, Sinusas AJ: On the dark rim artifact in dynamic contrast-enhanced MRI myocardial perfusion studies, *Magn Reson Med* 54:1295–1299, 2005.
20. Wolff SD, Schwitter J, Coulden R, et al: Myocardial first-pass perfusion magnetic resonance imaging: a multicenter dose-ranging study, *Circulation* 110:732–737, 2004.
21. McCrohon JA, Lyne JC, Rahman SL, et al: Adjunctive role of cardiovascular magnetic resonance in the assessment of patients with inferior attenuation on myocardial perfusion SPECT, *J Cardiovasc Magn Reson* 7:377–382, 2005.
22. Ishida N, Sakuma H, Motoyasu M, et al: Noninfarcted myocardium: correlation between dynamic first-pass contrast-enhanced myocardial MR imaging and quantitative coronary angiography, *Radiology* 229:209–216, 2003.
23. Sakuma H, Suzawa N, Ichikawa Y, et al: Diagnostic accuracy of stress first-pass contrast-enhanced myocardial perfusion MRI compared with stress myocardial perfusion scintigraphy, *AJR Am J Roentgenol* 185:95–102, 2005.
24. Schwitter J, Wacker CM, van Rossum AC, et al: MR-IMPACT: comparison of perfusion-cardiac magnetic resonance with single-photon emission computed tomography for the detection of coronary artery disease in a multicentre, multivendor, randomized trial, *Eur Heart J* 29:480–489, 2008.
25. Paetsch I, Jahnke C, Wahl A, et al: Comparison of dobutamine stress magnetic resonance, adenosine stress magnetic resonance, and adenosine stress magnetic resonance perfusion, *Circulation* 110:835–842, 2004.
26. Klem I, Heitner JF, Shah DJ, et al: Improved detection of coronary artery disease by stress perfusion cardiovascular magnetic resonance with the use of delayed enhancement infarction imaging, *J Am Coll Cardiol* 47:1630–1638, 2006.
27. Cury RC, Cattani CA, Gabure LA, et al: Diagnostic performance of stress perfusion and delayed-enhancement MR imaging in patients with coronary artery disease, *Radiology* 240:39–45, 2006.
28. Kwong RY, Schussheim AE, Rekhraj S, et al: Detecting acute coronary syndrome in the emergency department with cardiac magnetic resonance imaging, *Circulation* 107:531–537, 2003.
29. Plein S, Greenwood JP, Ridgway JP, et al: Assessment of non-ST-segment elevation acute coronary syndromes with cardiac magnetic resonance imaging, *J Am Coll Cardiol* 44:2173–2181, 2004.
30. Bunce NH, Reyes E, Keegan J, et al: Combined coronary and perfusion cardiovascular magnetic resonance for the assessment of coronary artery stenosis, *J Cardiovasc Magn Reson* 6:527–539, 2004.
31. Plein S, Kozerke S, Suerder D, et al: High spatial resolution myocardial perfusion cardiac magnetic resonance for the detection of coronary artery disease, *Eur Heart J* 29(17):2148–2155, 2008.
32. Cheng AS, Pegg TJ, Karamitsos TD, et al: Cardiovascular magnetic resonance perfusion imaging at 3-tesla for the detection of coronary artery disease: a comparison with 1.5-tesla, *J Am Coll Cardiol* 49: 2440–2449, 2007.
33. Nagel E, Klein C, Paetsch I, et al: Magnetic resonance perfusion measurements for the noninvasive detection of coronary artery disease, *Circulation* 108:432–437, 2003.
34. Wilke N, Simm C, Zhang J, et al: Contrast-enhanced first pass myocardial perfusion imaging: correlation between myocardial blood flow in dogs at rest and during hyperemia, *Magn Reson Med* 29:485–497, 1993.
35. Epstein FH, London JF, Peters DC, et al: Multislice first-pass cardiac perfusion MRI: validation in a model of myocardial infarction, *Magn Reson Med* 47:482–491, 2002.
36. Giang TH, Nanz D, Coulden R, et al: Detection of coronary artery disease by magnetic resonance myocardial perfusion imaging with various contrast medium doses: first European multi-centre experience, *Eur Heart J* 25:1657–1665, 2004.
37. Schwitter J, Nanz D, Kneifel S, et al: Assessment of myocardial perfusion in coronary artery disease by magnetic resonance: a comparison with positron emission tomography and coronary angiography, *Circulation* 103:2230–2235, 2001.
38. Ibrahim T, Nekolla SG, Schreiber K, et al: Assessment of coronary flow reserve: comparison between contrast-enhanced magnetic resonance imaging and positron emission tomography, *J Am Coll Cardiol* 39: 864–870, 2002.
39. Rieber J, Huber A, Erhard I, et al: Cardiac magnetic resonance perfusion imaging for the functional assessment of coronary artery disease:
40. Lauerma K, Virtanen KS, Sipila LM, et al: Multislice MRI in assessment of myocardial perfusion in patients with single-vessel proximal left anterior descending coronary artery disease before and after revascularization, *Circulation* 96:2859–2867, 1997.
41. Al Saadi N, Nagel E, Gross M, et al: Improvement of myocardial perfusion reserve early after coronary intervention: assessment with cardiac magnetic resonance imaging, *J Am Coll Cardiol* 36:1557–1564, 2000.
42. Jerosch-Herold M, Wilke N, Stillman AE: Magnetic resonance quantification of the myocardial perfusion reserve with a Fermi function model for constrained deconvolution, *Med Phys* 25:73–84, 1998.
43. Axel L: Tissue mean transit time from dynamic computed tomography by a simple deconvolution technique, *Invest Radiol* 18:94–99, 1983.
44. Christian TF, Rettmann DW, Aletras AH, et al: Absolute myocardial perfusion in canines measured by using dual-bolus first-pass MR imaging, *Radiology* 232:677–684, 2004.
45. Cullen JHS, Horsfield MA, Reek CR, et al: A myocardial perfusion reserve index in humans using first-pass contrast-enhanced magnetic resonance imaging, *J Am Coll Cardiol* 33:1386–1394, 1999.
46. Futamatsu, Wilke, Klassen, et al: Evaluation of cardiac magnetic resonance imaging parameters to detect anatomically and hemodynamically significant coronary artery disease, *Am Heart J* 154:298–305, 2007.
47. Costa MA, Shoemaker S, Futamatsu H, et al: Quantitative magnetic resonance perfusion imaging detects anatomic and physiologic coronary artery disease as measured by coronary angiography and fractional flow reserve, *J Am Coll Cardiol* 50:514–522, 2007.
48. Kurita T, Sakuma H, Onishi K, et al: Regional myocardial perfusion reserve determined using myocardial perfusion magnetic resonance imaging showed a direct correlation with coronary flow velocity reserve by Doppler flow wire, *Eur Heart J* 30(4):444–452, 2009.
49. Utz W, Greiser A, Niendorf T, et al: Single- or dual-bolus approach for the assessment of myocardial perfusion reserve in quantitative MR perfusion imaging, *Magn Reson Med* 59(6):1373–1377, 2008.
50. Gatehouse PD, Elkington AG, Ablitt NA, et al: Accurate assessment of the arterial input function during high-dose myocardial perfusion cardiovascular magnetic resonance, *J Magn Reson Imaging* 20:39–45, 2004.
51. Patel AR, Antkowiak P, Nandalur KR, et al: Differentiating moderate from severe coronary artery stenosis using quantitative myocardial perfusion imaging, *J Cardiovasc Magn Reson* 11:239, 2008.
52. Selvanayagam JB, Jerosch-Herold M, Porto I, et al: Resting myocardial blood flow is impaired in hibernating myocardium: A magnetic resonance study of quantitative perfusion assessment, *Circulation* 112:3289–3296, 2005.
53. Selvanayagam JB, Cheng ASH, Jerosch-Herold M, et al: Effect of distal embolization on myocardial perfusion reserve after percutaneous coronary intervention: A quantitative magnetic resonance perfusion study, *Circulation* 116:1458–1464, 2007.
54. Wang L, Jerosch-Herold M, Jacobs DR Jr, et al: Coronary artery calcification and myocardial perfusion in asymptomatic adults: The MESA (Multi-Ethnic Study of Atherosclerosis), *J Am Coll Cardiol* 48: 1018–1026, 2006.
55. Wang L, Jerosch-Herold M, Jacobs DR Jr, et al: Coronary risk factors and myocardial perfusion in asymptomatic adults: The Multi-Ethnic Study of Atherosclerosis (MESA), *J Am Coll Cardiol* 47: 565–572, 2006.
56. Petersen SE, Jerosch-Herold M, Hudsmith LE, et al: Evidence for microvascular dysfunction in hypertrophic cardiomyopathy. New insights from multiparametric magnetic resonance imaging, *Circulation* 115:2418–2425, 2007.
57. Muehling OM, Wilke NM, Panse P, et al: Reduced myocardial perfusion reserve and transmural perfusion gradient in heart transplant arteriopathy assessed by magnetic resonance imaging, *J Am Coll Cardiol* 42:1054–1060, 2003.
58. Williams DS, Detre JA, Leigh JS, et al: Magnetic resonance imaging of perfusion using spin inversion of arterial water, *Proc Natl Acad Sci U S A* 89:212–216, 1992.
59. Reeder SB, Atalay MK, McVeigh ER, et al: Quantitative cardiac perfusion: a noninvasive spin-labeling method that exploits coronary vessel geometry, *Radiology* 200:177–184, 1996.
60. Wacker CM, Fidler F, Dueren C, et al: Quantitative assessment of myocardial perfusion with a spin-labeling technique: preliminary results in patients with coronary artery disease, *J Magn Reson Imaging* 18: 555–560, 2003.
61. Ogawa S, Lee TM, Kay AR, et al: Brain magnetic resonance imaging with contrast dependent on blood oxygenation, *Proc Natl Acad Sci U S A* 87:9868–9872, 1990.
62. Li D, Dhawale P, Rubin PJ, et al: Myocardial signal response to dipyridamole and dobutamine: demonstration of the BOLD effect using a double-echo gradient-echo sequence, *Magn Reson Med* 36:16–20, 1996.
63. Lindner JR, Skyba DM, Goodman NC, et al: Changes in myocardial blood volume with graded coronary stenosis, *Am J Physiol* 272: H567–H575, 1997.

64. Wacker CM, Hartlep AW, Pfleger S, et al: Susceptibility-sensitive magnetic resonance imaging detects human myocardium supplied by a stenotic coronary artery without a contrast agent, *J Am Coll Cardiol* 41:834–840, 2003.

65. Friedrich MG, Niendorf T, Schulz-Menger J, et al: Blood oxygen level-dependent magnetic resonance imaging in patients with stress-induced angina, *Circulation* 108:2219–2223, 2003.

66. Fieno DS, Shea SM, Li Y, et al: Myocardial perfusion imaging based on the blood oxygen level–dependent effect using T2-prepared steady-state free-precession magnetic resonance imaging, *Circulation* 110:1284–1290, 2004.

67. Reeder SB, Holmes AA, McVeigh ER, et al: Simultaneous noninvasive determination of regional myocardial perfusion and oxygen content in rabbits: Toward direct measurement of myocardial oxygen consumption at MR imaging, *Radiology* 212:739–747, 1999.

68. McCommis KS, Zhang H, Herrero P, et al: Feasibility study of myocardial perfusion and oxygenation by noncontrast MRI: comparison with PET study in a canine model, *Magn Reson Imaging* 26:11–19, 2008.

69. Cowper SE, Su LD, Bhawan J, et al: Nephrogenic fibrosing dermopathy, *Am J Dermatopathol* 23(5):383–393, 2001.

70. Janus N, Launay-Vacher V, Karie S, et al: Prevalence of nephrogenic systemic fibrosis in renal insufficiency patients: Results of the FINEST study, *Eur J Radiol* 2009.

71. Perez-Rodriguez J, Lai S, Ehst BD, et al: Nephrogenic systemic fibrosis: incidence, associations, and effect of risk factor assessment—report of 33 cases, *Radiology* 250(2):371–377, 2009.

72. Shellock FG, Spinazzi A: MRI safety update 2008: part 1, MRI contrast agents and nephrogenic systemic fibrosis, *Am J Roentgenol* 191(4):1129–1139, 2008.

Myocardial Perfusion Imaging with Contrast Echocardiography

JONATHAN R. LINDNER AND SANJIV KAUL

INTRODUCTION

Radionuclide imaging is presently the most widely used method for myocardial perfusion imaging. Other non-invasive imaging techniques are now being developed for the assessment of myocardial perfusion, including myocardial contrast echocardiography (MCE). In this chapter, we will review the basic principles of MCE. We will provide an overview of microbubble contrast agents and the specific detection methods developed to improve microbubble signal. We will also discuss microvascular anatomy and physiology pertinent to MCE and describe some of the clinical experience with this method.

ULTRASOUND CONTRAST AGENTS

MCE is performed by combining ultrasound imaging with simultaneous intravascular injection of microbubbles that produce ultrasonic backscatter. Microbubbles undergo oscillation in an acoustic field whereby they compress and expand at the pressure peaks and nadirs, respectively (Fig. 18-1).[1,2] Radial oscillation of microbubbles results in the generation of acoustic signals that greatly exceed backscatter produced solely by reflection or alteration in acoustic impedance. The ultrasound frequency required to produce backscatter depends on both the compressibility and size of the microbubble and fortuitously is within the range of frequencies routinely used for diagnostic ultrasound.[2]

There has been substantial progress in the formulation of microbubble contrast agents that can be used to opacify the left heart after intravenous administration. These advancements have resulted from the development of stable encapsulated microbubbles with a narrow size distribution, typically between 2 and 6 μm in diameter, that are able to pass freely through pulmonary and systemic capillaries (Table 18-1). The stability and size optimization for these newer agents has occurred from the modification of the microbubble gas content and shell. Inert biologically safe gases have been used that have low diffusion coefficients and low solubility in water or blood, which reduces bubble collapse.[3,4] These include octafluoropropane (C_3F_8), decafluorobutane (C_4F_{10}), dodecafluoropentane (C_5F_{12}) and sulfur hexafluoride (SF_6). Shells are typically composed of protein (albumin), lipid surfactants, or biopolymers (e.g., lactide polymers). In addition to controlling size, the presence of a shell reduces outward diffusion and surface tension, thereby improving in vivo stability as well as shelf life. The use of air or nitrogen alone rather than high-molecular-weight gases in microbubble contrast agents is still possible, provided that the shell is relatively impermeable to low-molecular-weight gases. Strategies to decrease permeability can adversely affect the compressibility of microbubbles and, hence, their signal generation in an acoustic field.[5]

Since microbubbles can be directly visualized by microscopy, their in vivo behavior in the microcirculation can be assessed by intravital microscopy (Fig. 18-2). Studies have demonstrated that after intravenous injection, microbubbles transit the microcirculation of normal muscle beds unimpeded. These agents do not coalesce or aggregate, do not affect microvascular hemodynamics, and have a velocity profile similar to erythrocytes in arterioles, venules, and capillaries.[6,7] After venous injection, any microbubbles larger than the average capillary dimension become entrapped by the pulmonary circulation. The extent of retention is directly related to the proportion of microbubbles that are larger than approximately 5 μm, which is relatively low (<1% to 2%) for most commercial microbubble agents. Moreover,

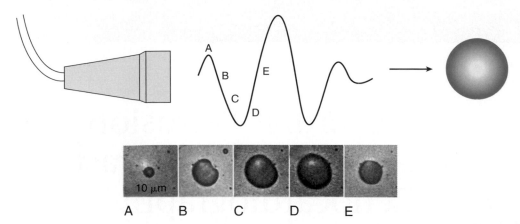

Figure 18-1 Microbubble oscillation during an acoustic pulse. The *top* figure schematically illustrates pressure fluctuations during ultrasound imaging. The microscopy images at the *bottom* obtained 330 ns apart illustrate volumetric oscillation of a microbubble during exposure to ultrasound (at 500 KHz). Bubble compression and expansion occur during high- and low-pressure phases, respectively, represented schematically by the location of frames **A-E**. *(Microbubble images courtesy of M. Postema, A. Bouakaz, and N. de Jong, Erasmus University.)*

Table 18-1 Commercially-Produced Microbubble Contrast Agents

Name	Shell	Gas	Mean Size (μm)
Optison	Albumin	Octafluoropropane	2–4.5
Definity/Luminity	Lipid/surfactant	Octafluoropropane	1.1–3.3
Sonovue	Lipid	Sulfur hexafluoride	2–3
Levovist	Lipid/galactose	Air	2–4
Sonazoid	Lipid/surfactant	Decafluorobutane	—
Imagify	PLGA polymer	Decafluorobutane	—

PLGA, polylactide *co*-glycolide.

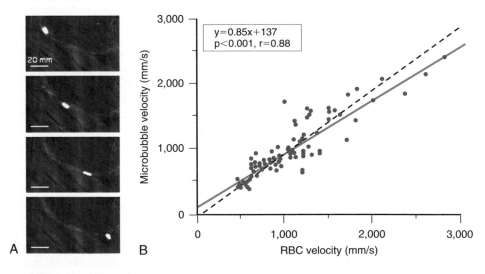

Figure 18-2 Capillary transit for microbubbles. **A,** Sequential intravital microscopy images of the microcirculation of skeletal muscle obtained 30 ms apart used to measure the capillary velocity of fluorescently-labeled microbubbles. **B,** Relation between RBC velocity and velocity of lipid-shelled microbubbles in capillaries (*dashed line* represents the line of identity). *(From Lindner JR, Song J, Jayaweera AR, et al: Microvascular rheology of Definity microbubbles following intra-arterial and intra-venous administration, J Am Soc Echocardiogr 15:396–403, 2002.)*

entrapment of microbubbles in pulmonary capillaries or very small arterioles is transient, owing to gradual gas loss and deformability of the microbubbles, which allow their eventual release.[6] As a result, venous injection at clinically relevant doses produces no significant alterations in pulmonary or hemodynamics or myocardial blood flow.[7,8]

Concerns regarding the safety of ultrasound contrast agents were raised with the announcement of a safety warning by the U.S. Food and Drug Administration

(FDA) in 2007 that included a temporary placement of new contraindications to microbubble agents. These actions were prompted based on the report of several deaths that occurred within 30 minutes of contrast administration. These events, however, occurred mostly in critically ill patients against a background of more than 2 million doses administered in the United States. The FDA action triggered multiple large safety studies that have in aggregate examined hundreds of thousands of patients in whom ultrasound contrast agents have been administered. These studies indicate an excellent safety profile with no significant mortality risk with ultrasound contrast agents.[9] Based on these findings and their own internal review, the FDA withdrew the contraindications in 2008.

Microbubble contrast agents have the potential to activate complement at their surface, similar to liposomal drugs and almost any therapy or diagnostic procedure that involves microparticle or nanoparticle administration. This response is in part responsible for clearance of microparticles. For lipid-encapsulated ultrasound contrast agents, the extent of complement activation is influenced by the net charge and presence of protective polymers such as polyethylene glycol, on the shell surface.[10] This complement activation is likely responsible for reports of anaphylactoid reactions in patients receiving microbubble contrast agents, although the incidence of these reactions is very small (1 in 10,000),[11] resulting in a safety profile that is favorable compared to most other contrast agents and cardiovascular diagnostic procedures.

IMAGING MICROBUBBLES IN TISSUE

As stated earlier, the ability of microbubbles to compress and expand in the alternating pressure environment of an acoustic field forms the basis for their use as contrast agents. The magnitude of bubble vibration is dependent on the compressibility and density of the gas, the viscosity and density of the surrounding medium, the frequency and power of ultrasound applied, and initial microbubble radius.[12,13] The degree of signal enhancement and signal-to-noise ratio during MCE is not, however, simply related to the degree of vibration in a monotonic fashion. When exposed to ultrasound at sufficient power and within the diagnostic frequency range for echocardiography, oscillation of microbubbles will occur in a nonlinear fashion in relation to acoustic pressure, meaning that even a small acoustic input will produce a large effect. At very high power, exaggerated microbubble oscillation will lead to microbubble disruption.[2,14] Nonlinear oscillation and microbubble destruction produce a broad band of acoustic frequencies that occur outside the bandwidth of the transmission (fundamental) frequency. This broadband signal includes intensity peaks at the harmonic frequencies (multiples of the transmit frequency) and, in certain circumstances, subharmonics (even fractions of the transmit frequency) (Fig. 18-3). Because these harmonic signals emanate preferentially from microbubbles rather than tissue, the signal-to-noise ratio during MCE is improved when receiving at harmonic or subharmonic frequencies.[14,15] In a similar fashion, it is also possible to improve signal-to-noise for ultrasound contrast agents by filtering for signals between the harmonic peaks where the difference between bubble and tissue signal is even greater.

Imaging at low to intermediate acoustic powers produces nonlinear oscillation without microbubble destruction. This response produces harmonic signals at a low amplitude so that it becomes desirable to

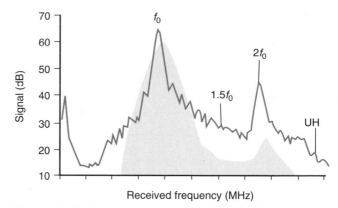

Figure 18-3 Frequency versus amplitude histogram for ultrasound signal returning from microbubbles *(solid line)* illustrating signal peaks at the transmission frequency *(f_0)* and at the second harmonic *($2f_0$)*. Microbubble signal relative to tissue *(shaded region)* is optimal at the second harmonic, between the first and second harmonics *($1.5f_0$)*, or beyond the second harmonic. UH, ultraharmonics. *(Microbubble signal represents actual data courtesy of P. Burns, University of Toronto.)*

eliminate all tissue signal in order to maximize signal-to-noise ratio. Signal processing techniques have been developed for this purpose. One technique termed *pulse-inversion* or *phase-inversion* is depicted schematically in Figure 18-4.[15] For each transmitted line, two successive pulses of ultrasound (A and B) are sent that are phase-inverted. Tissue produces linear signals that have equal amplitudes and 180-degree phase shifted for the two pulses. Thus summing these up results in no signal. In contradistinction, microbubbles produce nonlinear signals, and their summation does not cancel the signal, resulting in signal only from bubbles and not from tissue. Tissue signal can also be eliminated by alternating acoustic power rather than phase, termed *amplitude or power modulation* (Fig. 18-5).[15] Successive

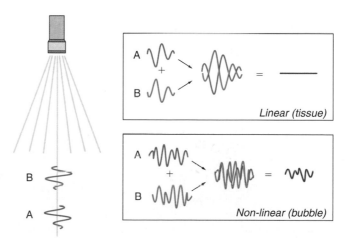

Figure 18-4 Schematic depicting pulse-(phase-)inversion imaging. Two or more sequential pulses are transmitted for each line that are phase-inverted or shifted 180 degrees. By summing the returning signals, tissue signal, which is a linear scatterer at low power, is eliminated. Nonlinear signals from microbubbles contain multiple frequency components and are not eliminated. *(From Kaul S: Myocardial contrast echocardiography: Basic principles, Prog Cardiovasc Dis 44:1–11, 2001.)*

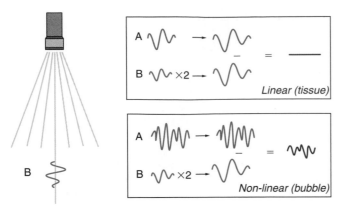

Figure 18-5 Schematic depicting amplitude modulation imaging. Two or more sequential pulses that differ in their amplitude are transmitted for each line (a full-amplitude low-power pulse and a half-amplitude pulse). By doubling the returning signals from the half-amplitude pulse and subtracting from those from the full-amplitude pulse, linear tissue signal is eliminated, whereas nonlinear microbubble signal is not. *(From Kaul S: Myocardial contrast echocardiography: Basic principles, Prog Cardiovasc Dis 44:1–11, 2001.)*

in-phase pulses are transmitted for each line, alternating between intermediate power and half amplitude or low power. Linear signals that return from tissue are similar in phase and frequency. Accordingly, these can be eliminated by doubling the half-amplitude signal and subtracting this from the intermediate power signal. Since microbubbles produce a nonlinear signal at only the intermediate power, doubling the low-power linear signal will not result in complete cancellation of signal. Signals that are not cancelled are displayed according to amplitude, and since non-cancellation occurs even at the fundamental frequency, receive bandwidth can be broadened to include relatively stronger fundamental frequencies.

A final method for amplifying microbubble signal-to-noise relative to tissue relies on multipulse decorrelation analysis (Fig. 18-6).[15] With these methods, a series of high-power pulses are transmitted for each line of ultrasound. The initial pulse(s) will return with nonlinear microbubble signal. Subsequent pulses return with less or no microbubble signal because of destruction from the initial pulse(s). The decorrelation or degree of difference between pulses is determined either by subtraction

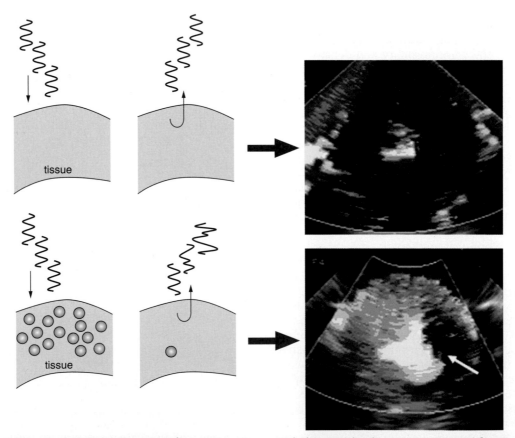

Figure 18-6 Schematic depicting power Doppler imaging. Sequential ultrasound pulses are transmitted for each line, and the amplitude of decorrelation of the returning signals, caused by microbubble destruction with the initial pulse(s), is used to detect the absence *(top panel)* or presence *(bottom panel)* of contrast. The myocardial territory denoted by the *white arrow* in the lower short-axis MCE image represents a perfusion defect during coronary occlusion where microbubbles are absent. *(From Kaul S: Myocardial contrast echocardiography: Basic principles, Prog Cardiovasc Dis 44:1–11, 2001.)*

of the radiofrequency pulse (rate subtraction imaging) or by demodulation from Doppler processing (termed *power Doppler imaging*). The amplitude of decorrelation is displayed as pixel brightness and reflects the number of microbubbles present in tissue that were destroyed.

Because of the limited dynamic range of ultrasound transducers, the relation between microbubble concentration and signal intensity is linear only at low to medium concentrations (Fig. 18-7).[16] The flat portion of the relation at higher concentrations is due in part to saturation by the upper limit of the dynamic range. Since ultrasound backscatter has to be displayed on a signal screen with an even smaller dynamic range (30 to 40 dB) than the received signal, some compression of the received signal must occur. Accordingly, direct assessment of digital data and imaging modalities that have a broad dynamic range (such as acoustic densitometry) are generally used during perfusion imaging when quantitative information on perfusion is desired.

QUANTIFICATION OF MYOCARDIAL BLOOD FLOW

Quantification of myocardial blood flow with MCE takes advantage of two key features of microbubbles: the rheology of microbubbles is identical to that of erythrocytes and the ability to destroy microbubbles with ultrasound. At steady state, when microbubble concentration in the blood pool is constant, the numbers of microbubbles entering or leaving any microcirculation within the ultrasound beam profile are equal; hence, the acoustic intensity from microbubbles or amount of myocardial contrast enhancement reflects myocardial blood volume (MBV).[17] Microbubbles within the ultrasound beam can then be destroyed by high-power ultrasound, after which their rate of replenishment, measured by the rate of increase in acoustic signal, reflects blood velocity or transfer rate through tissue. Perfusion at the microvascular level can be derived by the product of microvascular blood velocity and MBV.[17]

This concept is diagrammatically represented in Figure 18-8. The elevation (or thickness) of the ultrasound beam is represented by a rectangle with a thickness of *E (panel A)*. After microbubbles are destroyed at t_0 by a pulse of ultrasound *(panel A)*, new microbubbles will begin to replenish the ultrasound beam elevation. As the pulsing interval (PI) is increased *(panels B to E)*, there is more time for replenishment to occur between each destructive pulse of ultrasound, and the degree of microbubble replenishment into the elevation increases. Signal intensity will progressively increase at longer PIs

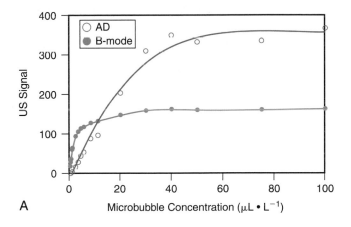

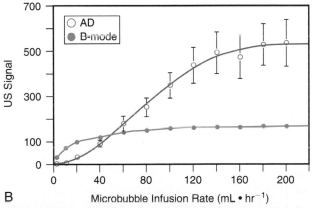

Figure 18-7 Relation between microbubble concentration and signal intensity for an ultrasound imaging system. Panel **A** shows in vitro data, and panel **B** shows in vivo data. All data were captured using both B-mode echo and acoustic densitometry (AD). It is obvious that with AD, the relation between microbubble concentration and signal intensity is linear over a wider range of microbubble concentration, but in both cases, the relation becomes nonlinear at higher concentrations. *(From Le DE, Bin JP, Coggins M, Lindner J, Wei K, Kaul S: Relation between myocardial oxygen consumption and myocardial blood volume: A study using myocardial contrast echocardiography. J Am Soc Echocardiogr 15:857–863, 2002.)*

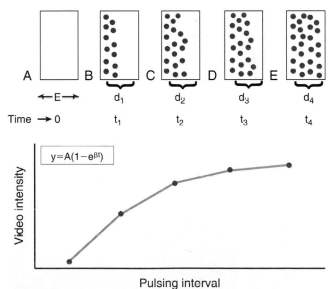

Figure 18-8 Schematic depicting microbubble replenishment of the ultrasound beam elevation (E) for different pulsing intervals. If all the microbubbles in the elevation are destroyed by a single pulse of ultrasound at t_0, then replenishment of the beam elevation *(panels B to E)* will depend on the velocity of microbubbles and the ultrasound pulsing interval *t*. *(From Wei K, Jayaweera AR, Firoozan S, et al: Ultrasound induced destruction of intravenously administered microbubbles: A novel method for the quantification of myocardial blood flow with echocardiography. Circulation 97:473–483, 1998.)*

(panel F). The rate of rise of signal intensity depicts myocardial blood flow velocity.[17] When the PI is long enough for the entire ultrasound beam elevation to be completely replenished with microbubbles *(panel E)*, the PI versus signal intensity relation plateaus. Steady state plateau signal intensity represents MBV, which is largely capillary blood volume. The PI versus signal intensity relation can be fitted to an exponential function: $y = A(1-e^{-\beta t})$, where y is myocardial VI at a PI of t, A is the plateau VI representing MBV, and β is the rate constant representing the mean microbubble velocity. MCE can therefore determine both specific components of blood flow—flow velocity (β) and MBV.

The plateau intensity, or the A-value, derived from replenishment curves described does not represent the MBV in absolute terms, since it is dependent on the concentration of microbubbles in blood and on regional attenuation. However, it is possible to normalize signal intensity values from the myocardium to that from adjacent parts of the left ventricular (LV) cavity to derive MBV fraction.[18] This approach requires that the microbubble concentration in the LV cavity is still within the linear range, a condition that is difficult to ensure by visual inspection. The product of MBV fraction and microbubble velocity provides a quantitative assessment of myocardial blood flow (MBF). This has been validated in animals using radiolabeled microspheres and in humans using positron emission tomography.[18,19]

Figures 18-9 and 18-10 illustrate examples of how separate analysis of MBF velocity and MBV can provide better pathophysiologic insights into disease than simply measuring total MBF. Figure 18-9 illustrates time versus acoustic intensity (AI) curves that are obtained at rest during normal *(panel A)* and reduced MBF *(panels B to D)*, where the reduction in MBF can be either due to decrease in MBV alone (such as non-transmural infarction when the infarct-related artery is patent with minimal stenosis, *panel B*), a decrease in blood velocity alone (such as during subtotal occlusion or total coronary occlusion with collateral-flow hibernating myocardium, *panel C*), or a combination of both a decrease in MBV and blood velocity, such as that seen in an infarcted myocardium supplied either by an artery with a very severe flow-limiting stenosis or by collaterals *(panel D)*.

Figure 18-10 illustrates time versus AI curves obtained from the normal myocardium during rest and different forms of stress. *Panel A* depicts curves before and during intracoronary infusion of adenosine, where MBV remains constant, and blood flow velocity increases.[20] At rest, the myocardium replenishes in 4 to 5 seconds after microbubble destruction. In the presence of intracoronary adenosine, MBF increases 4 to 5 times, solely because of an increase in MBF velocity without any change in MBV. Therefore, instead of taking 4 to 5 seconds to replenish, the myocardium now replenishes in 1 second.

Panel B shows curves before and during intracoronary infusion of dobutamine (where both MBV and velocity increase[21]). *Panel C* illustrates curves obtained before and during venous administration of either a vasodilator or dobutamine. The increase in MBV during intravenous compared to intracoronary administration of adenosine occurs from increase in myocardial oxygen demand that results from mild systemic hypotension and resultant reflex tachycardia.[22] Similar curves can also be obtained during supine bicycle exercise.[23]

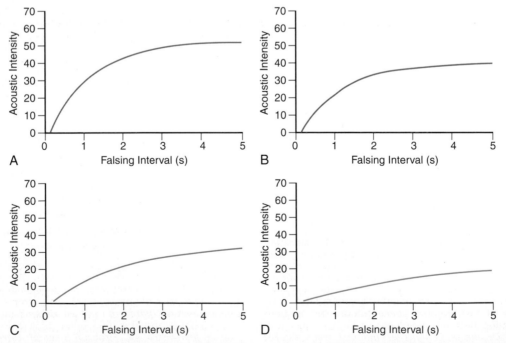

Figure 18-9 Time versus acoustic intensity curves obtained at rest from **A,** normal myocardium, **B,** non-transmural infarcted myocardium supplied by a nonstenotic coronary artery, **C,** chronically ischemic (hibernating myocardium), and **D,** infracted myocardium supplied by an artery with a flow-limiting stenosis or collaterals. *(From Kaul S: Myocardial contrast echocardiography: A 25-year retrospective, Circulation 118:291–308, 2008.)*

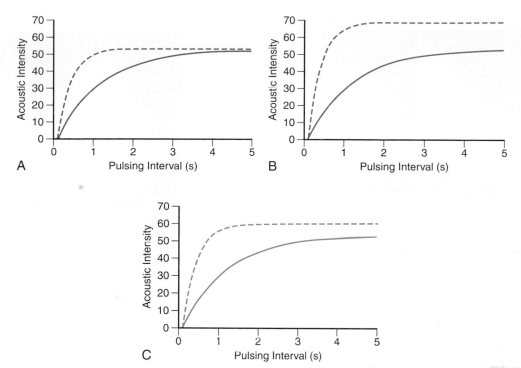

Figure 18-10 Time versus acoustic intensity curves obtained at rest *(solid line)* and stress *(dotted line)* during **A,** intracoronary administration of adenosine, **B,** intracoronary administration of dobutamine, and **C,** intravenous adenosine or dobutamine. *(From Kaul S: Myocardial contrast echocardiography: A 25-year retrospective, Circulation 118:291–308, 2008.)*

MYOCARDIAL CONTRAST ECHOCARDIOGRAPHY FOR CAD DETECTION

In the absence of prior infarction, the detection of coronary artery disease (CAD) on myocardial perfusion imaging is based on the occurrence of reversible perfusion defects during pharmacologic or exercise stress. Experimental studies had previously demonstrated the ability of MCE to detect coronary stenosis and to quantify the degree of MBF mismatch during pharmacologic stress.[17] Studies also showed that coronary stenosis can be detected[24,25] and abnormal coronary blood flow reserve can be accurately measured[20] with MCE in humans using venous administration of microbubbles.

The conventional wisdom had been that a reversible perfusion defect results from MBF mismatch that is seen at stress and not at rest. Using MCE it has been shown that reversible perfusion defects are actually caused by a decrease in MBV distal to a stenosis during stress.[32] When flow increases through a stenosis during stress, the coronary perfusion pressure falls. In order to maintain a constant capillary hydrostatic pressure, capillary derecruitment occurs, leading to a decrease in MBV. In the case of nuclear tracers, the resultant decrease in capillary surface area causes less tracer uptake and hence a perfusion defect.[26] Thus the site of abnormal flow reserve in CAD is not at the level of the stenosis but actually at the level of the microcirculation.

The decrease in MBV during stress is seen only with moderate to severe stenosis. With less severe stenosis, the only abnormality seen on MCE is the inability of the MBF velocity to increase by the desired amount. As shown Figure 18-10, MBF velocity increases 4 to 5 times in the normal myocardium during stress. The inability of the MBF velocity to increase by this amount during stress indicates a reduction in MBF reserve. What discriminates the attenuation of flow reserve in the presence of a stenosis compared to other causes such as hyperlipidemia, and so forth, is its regional nature.[20]

Figures 18-11 and 18-12 demonstrate normal perfusion *(top panel)* and either a reversible (Fig. 18-11) or a fixed (Fig. 18-12) defect *(bottom panel)* in patients undergoing dipyridamole stress imaging. The imaging protocol is based on the principles depicted in Figure 18-10. At rest, microbubble replenishment should occur in 4 to 5 seconds if MBF is normal. Therefore, the rest images *(left panels)* are captured at the fourth heartbeat after bubble destruction. If MBF reserve is normal, then at stress the myocardium should replenish within 1 second. Hence the stress images are captured at the first heartbeat after bubble destruction *(right panels)*. In the normal setting, these two images (rest and stress) should look similar *(panel A in both figures)*. If there is a significant stenosis in the absence of prior infarction, the stress image should show a relative defect compared to the rest image (indicated by *arrows in panel B in* Fig. 18-11). In the presence of infarction, where MBV is markedly reduced due to capillary loss, a fixed defect (present at both rest and stress) should be noted (indicated by *arrows in panel B in* Fig. 18-12). The images shown here were obtained using power Doppler, described earlier, with each wall in each view imaged separately because of the narrow imaging sector necessary for a high pulse-repetition frequency required to minimize motion artifacts.

Rest   Stress

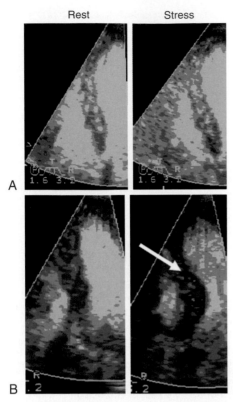

Rest   Stress

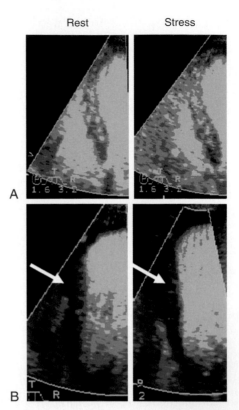

Figure 18-11 **A,** High MI intermittent power Doppler images obtained at rest *(left panel)* and stress *(right panel)* showing normal myocardial perfusion. **B,** High MI intermittent power Doppler images obtained at rest *(left panel)* and stress *(right panel)* showing a reversible defect *(arrow)*. *(From Kaul S: Myocardial contrast echocardiography: A 25-year retrospective, Circulation 118:291–308, 2008.)*

Figure 18-12 **A,** High MI intermittent power Doppler images obtained at rest *(left panel)* and stress *(right panel)* showing normal myocardial perfusion. **B,** High MI intermittent power Doppler images obtained at rest *(left panel)* and stress *(right panel)* showing a fixed defect *(arrow)*. *(From Kaul S: Myocardial contrast echocardiography: A 25-year retrospective, Circulation 118:291–308, 2008.)*

Diagnosis of CAD with echocardiography conventionally relies on the detection of abnormal wall-motion in response to exercise or pharmacologic stress. Perfusion imaging with MCE has the potential to enhance sensitivity for detection of single-vessel and multivessel CAD. The relationship between MBF and wall thickening during peak inotropic stress has been shown to be nonlinear.[27] In the presence of a mild to moderate stenosis, there is little impairment in wall thickening during peak dobutamine infusion, despite a substantial reduction in flow reserve. Accordingly, perfusion imaging has been shown in animal models to improve the sensitivity for detecting moderate stenosis, to detect stenosis at lower workload, to more accurately define the ischemic territory, and to detect multivessel disease more accurately.[27] Clinical studies have recently confirmed that MCE during dobutamine stress can detect the presence of significant CAD even when wall-motion response is normal.[28]

MCE IN ACUTE MYOCARDIAL INFARCTION

Clinical predictors for the diagnosis of acute myocardial infarction (AMI) have well-recognized limitations in terms of their sensitivity and specificity.[29–31] Although the use of cardiac-specific troponins has improved diagnosis of AMI and ability to assess higher risk, these tests may not be elevated at time of presentation of a patient in the emergency department and can be nonspecific in certain populations or disease conditions such as pulmonary embolism, pericarditis, myocarditis, and the like. MCE has been used to risk stratify patients with chest pain and nondiagnostic ECG in the emergency department.[32,33] In these studies, MCE improved accuracy for detecting acute coronary syndromes and for predicting risk for short-term and long-term cardiac events, compared to conventional clinical information.[33] A particular strength of this approach is its negative predictive value. Normal wall motion and perfusion during or soon after resolution of symptoms accurately exclude myocardial ischemia and portend an excellent prognosis. The positive predictive value is most accurate in those without prior ischemic events in whom a wall-motion abnormality or perfusion defect may not reflect a new event.

Even in patients with recognized AMI, assessment of the risk area size and extent may be helpful in risk assessment and treatment decision. The risk area is the region of the myocardium subtended an occluded coronary artery that is destined to undergo necrosis in the absence of reperfusion. The assessment of myocardial perfusion rather than wall motion is more accurate for defining the risk area, owing to contractile dysfunction that occurs in regions that are supplied by collateral perfusion.[27] Since MCE can be performed rapidly and at the patient bedside, it is possible to measure risk area in patients who present with acute coronary syndromes prior to reperfusion therapy. It has provided important information in clinical trials testing the efficacy of therapies aimed at improving microvascular salvage by measuring the final infarct size proportional to the original area at risk.[34]

Implicit in the ability to measure the risk area with MCE is the ability to evaluate the extent of collateral blood flow. Myocardial necrosis does not occur unless MBF is less than about 25% of normal resting flow (approximately 0.20 to 0.25 mL/min/g).[35,36] Sufficient flow for maintaining viability can be achieved through collateral circuits. However, perfusion in collateral-supplied regions is usually not normal, and these regions are usually characterized by slow microvascular blood velocity.[37] An example of slow collateral blood flow is illustrated in Figure 18-13, where a perfusion defect in

the territory of an occluded left circumflex is seen at low pulsing intervals *(panel A)* but is not seen at higher pulsing intervals *(panel B)* because of slow microbubble replenishment velocities through collateral circuits. As shown in the figure, the extent of collateral flow is important for predicting ultimate infarct size. Regions with adequate collateral flow did not exhibit infarction 6 hours later, while the region with very reduced flow *(arrows in panels B and C)* showed necrosis. In patients presenting with acute ST-elevation MI undergoing primary percutaneous intervention (PCI), myocardial salvage and functional recovery can be expected in areas supplied by collaterals that are detected by MCE prior to PCI.[38] Because slow microvascular velocity can also represent resting hypoperfusion from a critical stenosis with antegrade flow, the presence of collateral flow is best determined by combining MCE data with the information on coronary anatomy.

In the setting of AMI, clinical indicators of reperfusion offer little spatial information on salvage. The excellent spatial resolution and bedside capabilities of

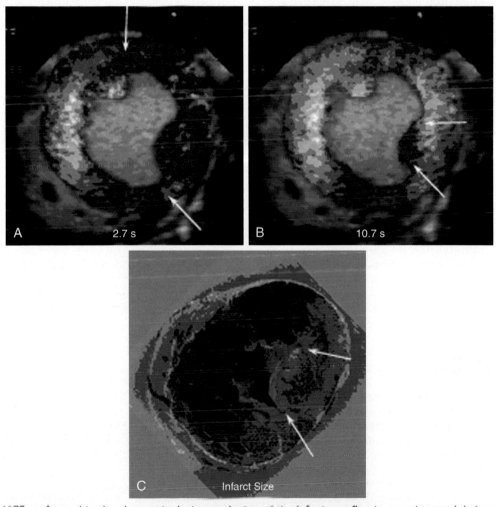

Figure 18-13 MCE performed in the short axis during occlusion of the left circumflex in a canine model. A perfusion defect is seen at short pulsing intervals *(arrows* in A) that almost completely resolves with further prolongation of the pulsing interval *(arrows* in B), indicative of slow-velocity collateral blood flow. Only the region not showing adequate perfusion at a long pulsing interval (B) shows necrosis on postmortem examination 6 hours after coronary occlusion (C). *(From Coggins MP, Sklenar J, Le DE, et al: Noninvasive prediction of ultimate infarct size at the time of acute coronary occlusion based on the extent and magnitude of collateral-derived myocardial blood flow. Circulation 2001;104:2471–2477.)*

MCE make it a practical method to assess the success of reperfusion. It is particularly valuable because flow is assessed at the capillary level. The spatial extent where capillary perfusion is absent is predictive of the eventual infarct zone, although the extent of reperfusion in the first few hours after reflow may not accurately estimate the ultimate infarct size due to temporal variation of flow and hyperemia in areas ultimately destined to undergo necrosis.[39–41]

ASSESSMENT OF MYOCARDIAL VIABILITY

In patients with recent AMI, wall motion does not recover in regions with poor microvascular flow after reperfusion therapy, and almost all segments that recover function have myocardial perfusion.[42–45] The presence of perfusion on MCE does not, however, guarantee that resting contractile function will always recover.[38,43,44,46,47] This seeming lack of "positive predictive value" is because segments with patchy or subendocardial infarction that have detectable perfusion will not regain resting wall motion if there is subendocardial necrosis. However, these segments do demonstrate contractile reserve during low-dose dobutamine challenge.[38] Spatial patterns of flow by MCE have recently been shown to correlate well with delayed-enhanced gadolinium magnetic resonance imaging, which is also characterized by excellent spatial resolution in terms of discriminating viable from nonviable myocardial tissue.[48] It is therefore not surprising that MCE in patients with recent acute MI can identify patients with a sufficient amount of myocardial salvage to protect against subsequent left ventricular remodeling.[49] Patients with low or no reflow, regardless of thrombolysis in myocardial infarction (TIMI) score, have poor functional recovery of left ventricular function and greater infarct expansion, remodeling, and left ventricular dilation.[50,51] Moreover, patients with poor microvascular reperfusion have a significantly higher incidence of cardiac events, including cardiac death, nonfatal myocardial infarction, and congestive heart failure, over a 1-year follow-up period.[51]

In patients with chronic CAD, determining the extent of myocardial viability is valuable for determining prognosis and deciding whether revascularization is warranted. A consistent, causative link exists between the extent of viability and survival, symptoms (angina and heart failure), exercise tolerance, and likelihood for remodeling after revascularization.[52–55] Traditionally, echocardiographic evaluation of myocardial viability relies on the assessment of contractile reserve. This approach is limited both because of the confounding influence of ischemia on wall-motion response and the traditional use of low-dose dobutamine protocols to evaluate contractile response, which predominately tests viability of the endocardial segment. MCE has been applied to determine the spatial extent of myocardial viability in patients with chronic CAD at rest. In patients undergoing myocardial biopsy at the time of surgical revascularization, microvascular perfusion patterns on MCE reliably differentiate the presence of scar, which contains a paucity of microvessels,

from viable muscle.[56] When using recovery of resting function as an endpoint, MCE is characterized by an excellent sensitivity but somewhat low specificity.[57–59] The low specificity finding is consistent with the idea that MCE can detect viability in regions other than the endocardium that do not necessarily contribute to resting function. Integration of perfusion data with DSE has been shown to improve both the sensitivity and specificity of viability diagnosis.[60]

SUMMARY

Methods for assessing perfusion and myocardial viability have been developed for essentially all forms of noninvasive cardiac imaging that are used in clinical practice. The specific methods used to assess perfusion are quite varied, depending on the behavior of the contrast agents and the methods used to acquire their signal. These techniques differ in terms of practical issues (cost, ease of operation, spatial resolution, robustness of data, speed). Equally important are the differences by which tracer signal is related to flow at rest or during stress. MCE is based on the detection of the two basic components of perfusion: the myocardial blood volume at the capillary level and the rate of flux of that volume through tissue. Hence, it is the most direct measurement of flow at the microvascular level. Despite these advantages, practical considerations, including lack of a contrast agent specifically approved for MCE, lack of general expertise in its routine clinical application, and lack of reimbursement, have not allowed MCE to reach its full potential so far.

REFERENCES

1. Dayton PA, Morgan KE, Klibanov AL, et al: Optical and acoustical observations of the effects of ultrasound on contrast agents, *IEEE Trans Ultrason Ferroelect Freq Contr* 46:220–232, 1999.
2. deJong N, Ten Cate FJ, Lancee CT, et al: Principles and recent developments in ultrasound contrast agents, *Ultrasonics* 29:324–330, 1991.
3. Epstein PS, Plesset MS: On the stability of gas bubbles in liquid-gas solutions, *J Chem Phys* 18:1505–1509, 1950.
4. Kabalnov A, Klein D, Pelura T, Schutt E, Weers J: Dissolution of multi-component microbubbles in the bloodstream: 1. Theory, *Ultrasound Med Biol* 24(5):739–749, 1998.
5. Leong-Poi H, Song J, Rim SJ, Christiansen J, Kaul S, Lindner JR: Influence of microbubble shell on ultrasound signal during real-time myocardial contrast echocardiography, *J Am Soc Echocardiogr* 15:1269–1276, 2002.
6. Lindner JR, Song J, Jayaweera AR, et al: Microvascular rheology of Definity microbubbles following intra-arterial and intravenous administration, *J Am Soc Echocardiogr* 15:396–403, 2002.
7. Skyba DM, Camarano G, Goodman NC, et al: Hemodynamic characteristics, myocardial kinetics and microvascular rheology of FS-069, a second generation contrast agent capable of producing myocardial opacification from a venous injection, *J Am Coll Cardiol* 28:1292–1300, 1996.
8. Lindner JR, Firschke C, Wei K, et al: Myocardial perfusion characteristics and hemodynamic profile of MRX-115, a venous echocardiographic contrast agent, during acute myocardial infarction, *J Am Soc Echocardiogr* 11:36–46, 1998.
9. Main ML, Ryan AC, Davis TE, Albano MP, Kusnetzky LL, Hibberd M: Acute mortality in hospitalized patients undergoing echocardiography with and without an ultrasound contrast agent (multicenter registry results in 4,300,966 consecutive patients), *Am J Cardiol* (e-publication).
10. Fisher NG, Christiansen JP, Klibanov AL, et al: Influence of surface charge on capillary transit and myocardial contrast enhancement, *J Am Coll Cardiol* 40:811–819, 2002.

11. Wei K, Mulvagh SL, Carson L, et al: The safety of Definity and Optison for ultrasound image enhancement: a retrospective analysis of 78,383 administered contrast doses, *J Am Soc Echocardiogr* 21:1202–1206, 2008.

12. Forsberg F, Shi WT: Physics of contrast microbubbles. In Goldberg BB, Raichlen JS, Forsberg JS, editors: *Ultrasound contrast agents*, 2nd ed., London, 2001, Martin Dunitz, pp 15–24.

13. DeJong N, Hoff L, Skotland T, Bom N: Absorption and scatter of encapsulated gas filled microspheres: theoretical considerations and some measurements, *Ultrasonics* 30(2):95–103, 1992.

14. Wei K, Skyba DM, Firschke C, et al: Interactions between microbubbles and ultrasound: in vitro and in vivo observations, *J Am Coll Cardiol* 29:1081–1088, 1997.

15. Kaul S: Myocardial contrast echocardiography: Basic principles, *Prog Cardiovasc Dis* 44:1–11, 2001.

16. Le DE, Bin JP, Coggins M, Lindner J, Wei K, Kaul S: Relation between myocardial oxygen consumption and myocardial blood volume: A study using myocardial contrast echocardiography, *J Am Soc Echocardiogr* 15:857–863, 2002.

17. Wei K, Jayaweera AR, Firoozan S, et al: Ultrasound-induced destruction of intravenously administered microbubbles: a novel method for the quantification of myocardial blood flow with echocardiography, *Circulation* 97:473–483, 1998.

18. Yano A, Ito H, Iwakura K, et al: Myocardial contrast echocardiography with a new calibration method can estimate myocardial viability in patients with myocardial infarction, *J Am Coll Cardiol* 43:1799–1806, 2004.

19. Vogel R, Indermuhle A, Reinhardt J, et al: The quantification of absolute myocardial perfusion in humans by contrast echocardiography: algorithm and validation, *J Am Coll Cardiol* 45:754–762, 2005.

20. Wei K, Ragosta M, Thorpe J, Coggins M, Moos S, Kaul S: Noninvasive quantification of coronary blood flow reserve in humans using myocardial contrast echocardiography, *Circulation* 103:2560–2565, 2001.

21. Bin JP, Le DE, Jayaweera AR, Coggins MP, Wei K, Kaul S: Direct effects of dobutamine on the coronary microcirculation: comparison with adenosine using myocardial contrast echocardiography, *J Am Soc Echocardiogr* 16:871–879, 2003.

22. Bin JP, Pelberg RA, Coggins MP, Wei K, Kaul S: Mechanism of inducible regional dysfunction during dipyridamole stress, *Circulation* 106:112–117, 2002.

23. Miszalski-Jamka T, Kuntz-Hehner S, Schmidt H, et al: Real time myocardial contrast echocardiography during supine bicycle stress and continuous infusion of contrast agent: cutoff values for myocardial contrast replenishment discriminating abnormal myocardial perfusion, *Echocardiography* 24:638–648, 2007.

24. Kaul S, Senior R, Dittrich H, Raval U, Khattar R, Lahiri A: Detection of coronary artery disease using myocardial contrast echocardiography: comparison with 99mTc-sestamibi single photon emission computed tomography, *Circulation* 96:785–792, 1997.

25. Porter TR, Li S, Jiang L, Grayburn P, Deligonul U: Real-time visualization of myocardial perfusion and wall thickening in human beings with intravenous ultrasonographic contrast and accelerated intermittent harmonic imaging, *J Am Soc Echocardiogr* 12:266–271, 1999.

26. Wei K, Ragosta M, Thorpe J, Moos S, Kaul S: Noninvasive measurement of coronary blood flow reserve myocardial contrast echocardiography, *Circulation* 103:2560–2565, 2001.

27. Leong-Poi H, Rim SJ, Le DE, Fisher NG, Wei K, Kaul S: Perfusion versus function: the ischemic cascade in demand ischemia: implications of single-vessel versus multivessel stenosis, *Circulation* 105:987–992, 2002.

28. Elhendy A, O'Leary EL, Xie F, McGrain AC, Anderson JR, Porter TR: Comparative accuracy of real-time myocardial contrast perfusion imaging and wall motion analysis during dobutamine stress echocardiography for the diagnosis of coronary artery disease, *J Am Coll Cardiol* 44:2185–2191, 2004.

29. Sabia P, Afrookteh A, Touchstone DA, Keller MW, Esquivel L, Kaul S: Value of regional wall motion abnormality in the emergency room diagnosis of acute myocardial infarction. A prospective study using two-dimensional echocardiography, *Circulation* 84(3 Suppl):I85–I92, 1991.

30. Short D: The earliest electrocardiographic evidence of myocardial infarction, *Br Heart J* 32:6–15, 1970.

31. Zarling EJ, Sexton H, Milnor P Jr, : Failure to diagnose acute myocardial infarction. The clinicopathologic experience at a large community hospital, *JAMA* 250:1177–1181, 1983.

32. Rinkevich D, Kaul S, Wang XQ, et al: Regional left ventricular perfusion and function in patients presenting to the emergency department with chest pain and no ST-segment elevation, *Eur Heart J* 26:1606–1611, 2005.

33. Tong KL, Kaul S, Wang XQ, et al: Myocardial contrast echocardiography versus Thrombolysis In Myocardial Infarction score in patients presenting to the emergency department with chest pain and a non-diagnostic electrocardiogram, *J Am Coll Cardiol* 46:920–927, 2005.

34. Micari A, Belcik TA, Balcells EA, et al: Improvement in microvascular reflow and reduction of infarct size with adenosine in patients undergoing primary coronary stenting, *Am J Cardiol* 96:1410–1415, 2005.

35. Schaper W, Frenzel H, Hort W: Experimental coronary artery occlusion. I. Measurement of infarct size, *Basic Res Cardiol* 74:46–53, 1979.

36. Gewirtz H, Fischman AJ, Abraham S, Gilson M, Strauss HW, Alpert NM: Positron emission tomographic measurements of absolute regional myocardial blood flow permits identification of nonviable myocardium in patients with chronic myocardial infarction, *J Am Coll Cardiol* 23:851–859, 1994.

37. Coggins MP, Sklenar J, Le DE, Wei K, Lindner JR, Kaul S: Noninvasive prediction of ultimate infarct size at the time of acute coronary occlusion based on the extent and magnitude of collateral-derived myocardial blood flow, *Circulation* 104:2471–2477, 2001.

38. Balcells E, Powers ER, Lepper W, et al: Detection of myocardial viability by contrast echocardiography in acute infarction predicts recovery of resting function and contractile reserve, *J Am Coll Cardiol* 41:827–833, 2003.

39. Villanueva FS, Glasheen WP, Sklenar J, Kaul S: Assessment of risk area during coronary occlusion and infarct size after reperfusion with myocardial contrast echocardiography using left and right atrial injections of contrast, *Circulation* 88:596–604, 1993.

40. Ragosta M, Camarano G, Kaul S, Powers ER, Sarembock IJ, Gimple LW: Microvascular integrity indicates myocellular viability in patients with recent myocardial infarction. New insights using myocardial contrast echocardiography, *Circulation* 89:2562–2569, 1994.

41. Sakuma T, Okada T, Hayashi Y, Otsuka M, Hirai Y: Optimal time for predicting left ventricular remodeling after successful primary coronary angioplasty in acute myocardial infarction using serial myocardial contrast echocardiography and magnetic resonance imaging, *Circ J* 66:685–690, 2002.

42. Kamp O, Lepper W, Vanoverschelde JL, et al: Serial evaluation of perfusion defects in patients with a first acute myocardial infarction referred for primary PTCA using intravenous myocardial contrast echocardiography, *Eur Heart J* 22:1485–1495, 2001.

43. Swinburn JM, Lahiri A, Senior R: Intravenous myocardial contrast echocardiography predicts recovery of dyssynergic myocardium early after acute myocardial infarction, *J Am Coll Cardiol* 38:19–25, 2001.

44. Andrassy P, Zielinska M, Busch R, Schomig A, Firschke C: Myocardial blood volume and the amount of viable myocardium early after mechanical reperfusion of acute myocardial infarction: prospective study using venous contrast echocardiography, *Heart* 87:350–355, 2002.

45. Janardhanan R, Swinburn JM, Greaves K, Senior R: Usefulness of myocardial contrast echocardiography using low-power continuous imaging early after acute myocardial infarction to predict late functional left ventricular recovery, *Am J Cardiol* 92:493–497, 2003.

46. Lepper W, Hoffmann R, Kamp O, et al: Assessment of myocardial reperfusion by intravenous myocardial contrast echocardiography and coronary flow reserve after primary percutaneous transluminal coronary angioplasty [correction of angiography] in patients with acute myocardial infarction, *Circulation* 101:2368–2374, 2000.

47. Main ML, Magalski A, Chee NK, Coen MM, Skolnick DG, Good TH: Full-motion pulse inversion power Doppler contrast echocardiography differentiates stunning from necrosis and predicts recovery of left ventricular function after acute myocardial infarction, *J Am Coll Cardiol* 38:1390–1394, 2001.

48. Janardhanan R, Moon JC, Pennell DJ, Senior R: Myocardial contrast echocardiography accurately reflects transmurality of myocardial necrosis and predicts contractile reserve after acute myocardial infarction, *Am Heart J* 149:355–362, 2005.

49. Jeetley P, Swinburn J, Hickman M, Bellenger NG, Pennell DJ, Senior R: Myocardial contrast echocardiography predicts left ventricular remodelling after acute myocardial infarction, *J Am Soc Echocardiogr* 17:1030–1036, 2004.

50. Ito H, Maruyama A, Iwakura K, et al: Clinical implications of the 'no reflow' phenomenon. A predictor of complications and left ventricular remodeling in reperfused anterior wall myocardial infarction, *Circulation* 93:223–228, 1996.

51. Sakuma T, Hayashi Y, Sumii K, Imazu M, Yamakido M: Prediction of short- and intermediate-term prognoses of patients with acute myocardial infarction using myocardial contrast echocardiography one day after recanalization, *J Am Coll Cardiol* 32:890–897, 1998.

52. Pasquet A, Robert A, D'hondt AM, Dion R, Melin JA, Vanoverschelde JL: Prognostic value of myocardial ischemia and viability in patients with chronic left ventricular ischemic dysfunction, *Circulation* 100:141–148, 1999.

53. Afridi I, Grayburn PA, Panza JA, Oh JK, Zoghbi WA, Marwick TH: Myocardial viability during dobutamine echocardiography predicts survival in patients with coronary artery disease and severe left ventricular systolic dysfunction, *J Am Coll Cardiol* 32:921–926, 1998.

54. Senior R, Kaul S, Lahiri A: Myocardial viability on echocardiography predicts long-term survival after revascularization in patients with ischemic congestive heart failure, *J Am Coll Cardiol* 33:1848–1854, 1999.

55. Samady H, Elefteriades JA, Abbott BG, Mattera JA, McPherson CA, Wackers FJ: Failure to improve left ventricular function after coronary revascularization for ischemic cardiomyopathy is not associated with worse outcome, *Circulation* 100:1298–1304, 1999.

56. Shimoni S, Frangogiannis NG, Aggeli CJ, et al: Microvascular structural correlates of myocardial contrast echocardiography in patients with coronary artery disease and left ventricular dysfunction: implications for the assessment of myocardial hibernation, *Circulation* 106: 950–956, 2002.

57. Shimoni S, Frangogiannis NG, Aggeli CJ, et al: Identification of hibernating myocardium with quantitative intravenous myocardial contrast echocardiography: comparison with dobutamine echocardiography and thallium-201 scintigraphy, *Circulation* 107: 538–544, 2003.

58. Nagueh SF, Vaduganathan P, Ali N, et al: Identification of hibernating myocardium: comparative accuracy of myocardial contrast echocardiography, rest-redistribution thallium-201 tomography and dobutamine echocardiography, *J Am Coll Cardiol* 29:985–993, 1997.

59. Korosoglou G, Hansen A, Hoffend J, et al: Comparison of real-time myocardial contrast echocardiography for the assessment of myocardial viability with fluorodeoxyglucose-18 positron emission tomography and dobutamine stress echocardiography, *Am J Cardiol* 94: 570–576, 2004.

60. Meza MF, Ramee S, Collins T, et al: Knowledge of perfusion and contractile reserve improves the predictive value of recovery of regional myocardial function postrevascularization: a study using the combination of myocardial contrast echocardiography and dobutamine echocardiography, *Circulation* 18(96):3459–3465, 1997.

Diagnosis and Prognosis in Cardiac Disease Using Cardiac PET Perfusion Imaging

MARIA CECILIA ZIADI, ROBERT A. DEKEMP,
KEIICHIRO YOSHINAGA AND ROB S. BEANLANDS

INTRODUCTION

There is a worldwide rising concern about the increasing morbidity and mortality rates related to coronary artery disease (CAD). This has motivated remarkable advances in the field of cardiovascular imaging that we have witnessed within the last 2 decades. The latest evidence underscores that functional imaging remains essential for an appropriate selection of therapy and for improving patient outcomes.[1] The introduction of positron emission tomography (PET) represented a major breakthrough that ultimately has shed light on the pathophysiology and diagnosis of heart diseases. More recently, the concept of dual-modality imaging technology emerged,[2] mainly spurred by the use of computed tomography (CT) to achieve accurate attenuation correction (AC). Currently, hybrid PET/CT systems allow simultaneous assessment of cardiac and coronary arterial structure together with myocardial perfusion and metabolism.

At first PET was regarded a powerful investigative tool that contributed to the understanding of several diseases.[3,4] Nevertheless, the leading role of PET imaging in the field of oncology, along with the U.S. Food and Drug Administration (FDA) approval of radiotracers and changes in reimbursement, have all contributed to move the state-of-the-art technology from the research laboratory to the clinical arena. Currently, cardiac PET constitutes a well-developed means for detecting and tracking the progression of CAD, diagnosing microvascular dysfunction, and for the follow-up of different therapies, offering a comprehensive approach for the workup of CAD.

Cardiac PET has potential advantages in patients with multivessel CAD as well as in subjects with large body habitus, prone to attenuation artifacts. Taking into account risk stratification, a normal PET study indicates an excellent prognosis,[5-8] and the risk of hard cardiac events increases with higher summed stress scores (SSS) and lower LVEF.[3,9,10]

Three-dimensional (3D)-mode PET imaging is becoming the standard with the latest brands of PET/CT systems. 3D-mode combines improved image quality and reduced patient radiation exposure, but this method increases scatter and presents certain technical challenges for cardiac PET.[11-13]

In this chapter, we will overview PET perfusion imaging from basic aspects to clinical applications. Another important application for PET flow studies, guiding patient management and detection of early atherosclerosis, will be discussed. Continued research is needed to understand the full potential advantage of these new approaches and how they impact our patients' well-being.

PRACTICAL ASPECTS OF IMAGING AND ANALYSIS

General Principles of PET Imaging

PET imaging is based on the use of radiotracers that decay by positron emission. A positron (a positively charged electron) is emitted from the nuclei of unstable isotopes during radioactive decay.[14] Then, both the positron and an electron undergo a process known as *positron annihilation* and are converted into two coincident gamma-ray photons of 511 keV that travel in opposite directions. The distance traveled by the positron prior to annihilation constitutes the *positron range*. Detectors placed on either side of the active volume are connected in a coincidence circuit, so that if both detectors record an event within a very short interval, it is assumed that positron annihilation has occurred.[12] This constitutes the basis of PET.

PET utilizes biological radiotracers labeled with positron-emitting isotopes such as carbon (^{11}C), oxygen (^{15}O), rubidium (^{82}Rb), and fluorine (^{18}F) that mimic natural substances. Thus, PET enables the measurement of several biological processes, including cardiac tissue blood flow, metabolism, and neurohormonal and receptor function. Many of the isotopes used for PET imaging have short physical half-lives ($T_{1/2}$),[14] making them readily applicable in studies requiring repetitive measurements in the same session.[15]

Attenuation effects are significantly higher with PET than with SPECT. Attenuation correction (AC) is relatively straightforward with PET because the length of the path of attenuation for the pair of 511-keV photons is constant and known for PET, whereas it is variable with SPECT.[13] Traditionally, external transmission sources, such as germanium-68 (^{68}Ge) or cesium-137 (^{137}Cs), have been used as established means for AC of the PET emission data.[13] Today this has been replaced exclusively by x-ray transmission scanning in the current generation of PET/CT systems, shortening the total transmission imaging time to under a minute. Since fast helical CT scans acquire images at a single point in the respiratory cycle, whereas PET data are averaged over many respiratory cycles, respiratory motion mismatch artifacts can be produced.[11] These artifacts, when present, typically affect the anterior and anterolateral segments of the LV.[16,17]

In recent years, PET instrumentation has shown substantial evolution. New crystal materials, such as lutetium oxyorthosilicate (LSO) and gadolinium oxyorthosilicate (GSO) have become available.[13] These crystals are attractive for PET, owing to faster light decay time and higher light yield than bismuth germanate (BGO) crystals.[18] Furthermore, there is an increasing trend to apply 3D-imaging acquisition mode (septa out) instead of the traditional two-dimensional (2D) mode (septa in), with the potential to improve image quality and reduce injected doses but at the expense of increased background counts and higher reliance on scatter-correction accuracy.[11,19] Notably, several new PET/CT scanners operate only in 3D mode.[13] *The current role of 3D mode versus 2D-mode will be fully described elsewhere in this textbook.*

Cardiac PET has several technical advantages over traditional SPECT that should be appreciated:

1. Accurate depth-independent AC
2. High spatial resolution (4 to 5 mm[18,20] versus SPECT, 10 mm)[18,21,22]
3. High temporal resolution (5 to 10 seconds)
4. Tracers with higher extraction fractions and shorter half-lives than SPECT radiotracers
5. Less equivocal results because of superior image quality in comparison with the standard SPECT[23]

Myocardial PET Perfusion Tracers

According to their physical properties, myocardial PET blood flow tracers fall into two basic categories: (1) inert, freely diffusible tracers like $H_2^{15}O$ and (2) physiologically retained tracers like $^{13}NH_3$ and ^{82}Rb.[4,14] The main aspects of PET flow tracers have been summarized in Tables 19-1, 19-2, and 19-3.

Nitrogen-13 Ammonia

$^{13}NH_3$ ($T_{1/2}$ = 9.96 minutes) requires an on-site cyclotron and radiochemistry synthesis capability.[3,22] In the bloodstream, neutral $^{13}NH_3$ is in equilibrium with the ionic form, ammonium (NH_4^+). $^{13}NH_3$ diffuses freely across capillary and cell membranes and is retained in myocardial tissue,[24] whereby it can be either incorporated into synthesis of ^{13}N-glutamine, or it can diffuse back into the vascular space. The initial extraction is high, even at high flow rates. As such, the uptake rate constant K_1 is a good estimate for quantitative blood flow (Fig. 19-1).

The net tissue retention is approximately 90% in the resting state. For $^{13}NH_3$, the direct relationship between net tissue retention and blood flow is preserved for values of blood flow up to 2.5 mL/min/g, but at higher flow rates this linear relationship is lost (Fig. 19-2).[25] Therefore, it is necessary to correct for flow-dependent changes in net tissue retention.

Myocardial retention of $^{13}NH_3$ may be heterogeneous,[26] and the lateral LV wall uptake can be 10% lower than that of other segments. Also, image quality can be hampered by the occasional intense liver activity, which could interfere with the evaluation of the inferior wall. Finally, in patients with severe left ventricular ejection fraction (LVEF) impairment, chronic obstructive pulmonary disease (COPD), or smoking, the sequestration of $^{13}NH_3$ in the lungs can be abnormally increased. Then it would be necessary to delay the time between injection and image acquisition to enhance image quality.[13]

Rubidium-82

^{82}Rb is produced from a strontium-82 (^{82}Sr)/^{82}Rb generator, which can be eluted every 10 minutes.[27] The $T_{1/2}$ of ^{82}Sr is 25.5 days, which results in a generator life of 6 to 8 weeks. The short $T_{1/2}$ of ^{82}Rb (76 seconds) allows repeated and sequential perfusion studies but requires rapid image acquisition shortly after tracer administration.[3,12] ^{82}Rb is a monovalent cationic analog of potassium and has similar biological activity to thallium-201 (^{201}Tl). Myocardial uptake of ^{82}Rb requires active transport via the sodium/potassium adenosine triphosphate transporter. In animal models, the net retention is approximately 50% at rest and decreases to 30% at peak flow. The retention fraction can be altered by acidosis and acute hypoxia.[4]

A small and mobile generator infusion system is used for eluting ^{82}Rb every 10 to 15 minutes with low radiation exposure.[27] Quantitative assessment with ^{82}Rb is quite feasible and clinically practical with this generator as compared to cyclotron-produced compounds (Figs. 19-3, 19-4, and 19-5).[28–31]

Table 19-1 Myocardial PET Flow Tracers

Pharmaceutical	Radioisotope	Physical Half-life	Production Method	Parent Compound Physical Half-life	Physiology	Primary Application	Average Positron Energy (MeV)**	RMS Positron Range (mm)
Water	^{15}O	122 sec	Cyclotron	-	Diffusible	Perfusion	0.74	1.02
Ammonia	^{13}N	10 min	Cyclotron	-	Diffusible/retained	Perfusion	0.49	0.57
Acetate	^{11}C	20 min	Cyclotron	-	Extracted/metabolized	Oxidative metabolism	0.39	0.39
FBnTP	^{13}F	110 min	Cyclotron	-	Extracted/retained	Perfusion	0.25	0.23
BMS-747158-02	^{18}F	110 min	Cyclotron	-	Extracted/retained	Perfusion	0.25	0.23
Rubidium	^{82}Rb	76 sec	$^{82}Sr/^{82}Rb$ generator	^{82}Sr = 25.5 days	Extracted/retained	Perfusion	1.48	2.60
PTSM ETS	^{62}Cu	9.7 min	$^{62}Zn/^{62}Cu$ generator	^{62}Zn = 9.2 hours	Extracted/retained	Perfusion	1.32	2.2
Gallium-Complexes*	^{67}Ga	68 min	$^{68}Ge/^{63}Ga$ generator	^{68}Ge = 271 days	Extracted/washout	Perfusion	0.84	1.2

*Data based on studies using ^{67}Ga;
**from: www.nndc.bnl.gov/mird (May 2008).

Table 19-2 Myocardial PET Perfusion Tracers: Principal Features

Radioisotope	Patient Throughput	Availability	Static Image Quality	Liver/Visceral Uptake	Myocardial Blood Flow Quantification
$H_2^{15}O$	++++	+	NA	NA	
$^{13}NH_3$	++	++	+++	+++	
^{82}Rb	++++	(++++)	+++	++	
^{62}Cu compounds	++	(+++)	++	++++	
^{11}C-acetate	++	+	+	+	
^{18}F agents	+	(+++)	++++*	+	?

+, low; ++, good; +++, moderate; ++++, possible; ?, might be feasible but not in clinical practice; NA, not available; ( ), potential availability; *, based on animal imaging.

Table 19-3 PET/CT Studies and Effective Doses

Study	Primary Application	Injected Activity MBq (mCi)	Effective Dose mSv
^{82}Rb	Perfusion	2200 (60)	1.4
$H_2^{15}O$	Perfusion	1500 (40)	1.7
$^{13}NH_3$	Perfusion	750 (20)	1.5
^{11}C-acetate	Oxidative metabolism	370 (10)	1.3
^{18}F-FDG	Glucose metabolism	370 (10)	7.0
Low-dose CTAC	Attenuation correction	—	0.5
Prospective-gated CCS	Coronary calcium score	—	2.2
Retrospective-gated CTA	Coronary angiogram	—	16

CCS, coronary calcium score; CTA, computed tomography angiogram; CTAC, computed tomography attenuation correction.

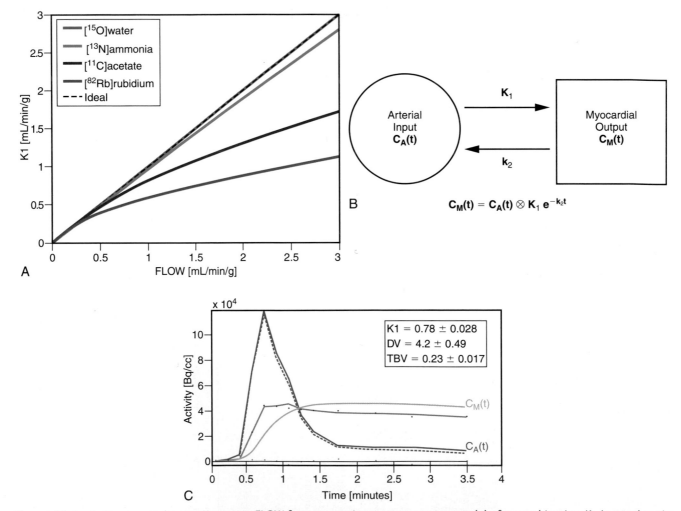

Figure 19-1 A, Tracer uptake rate K_1 versus FLOW from a one-tissue-compartment model of tracer kinetics. K_1 is equal to the product of FLOW times the unidirectional extraction fraction. **B,** One-tissue-compartment model diagram and equation. The myocardial curve $C_M(t)$ is equal to the arterial input curve $C_A(t)$ convolved with a single decaying exponential function $K_1 e^{-k_2 t}$. **C,** The model parameters K_1, DV (=K_1/k_2), and a partial-volume correction parameter (1-TBV) are estimated by nonlinear least-squares fitting of the model *(dark blue line)* to the measured PET data *(blue dots)*.

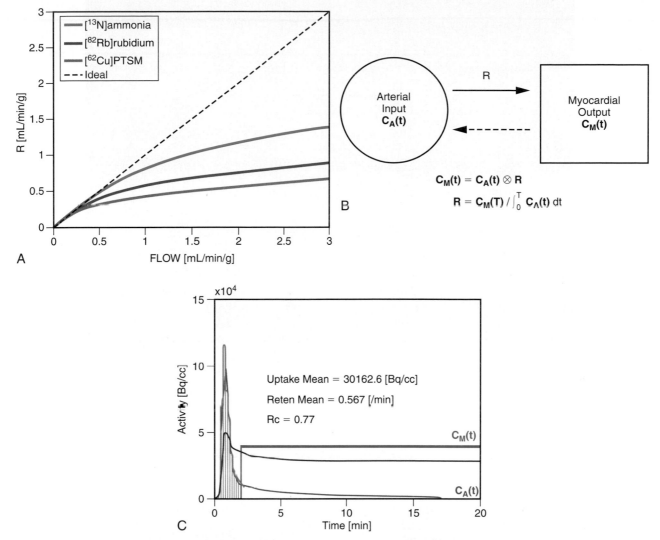

Figure 19-2 A, Tracer retention rate R versus FLOW from a net retention model of tracer kinetics. R is equal to the product of FLOW times the net retention fraction. **B,** Net retention model diagram and equation. The myocardial curve $C_M(t)$ is equal to the arterial input curve $C_A(t)$ convolved with a constant retention rate R, assuming there is no washout *(dotted line)* from the myocardium. **C,** The model parameter R is computed simply as the ratio of the myocardial uptake activity *(dark blue)* after time T (e.g., 2 min) divided by the integral area *(green)* under the arterial input curve, and assuming a constant partial-volume correction factor Rc.

Oxygen-15 Water

$H_2{}^{15}O$ ($T_{1/2}$ = 2.04 minutes) is a cyclotron product and is considered the gold standard for absolute flow quantification.[14] Since $H_2{}^{15}O$ is a freely diffusible agent, the extraction fraction is not affected by flow rates and is independent of the metabolic state of the myocardium.[22] Cardiac imaging with $H_2{}^{15}O$ can be demanding because of its high concentration in the blood pool, entailing subtraction of the blood pool counts from the original image to visualize the myocardium.[32] As such, it does not usually produce clinically interpretable perfusion images. Despite the success of $H_2{}^{15}O$ for research purposes, its clinical applications remain limited.[18,22]

Carbon-11-Acetate

Currently, PET using ^{11}C-acetate ($T_{1/2}$ = 20.4 minutes), a cyclotron product, is considered to be the most accurate and commonly used noninvasive method for measuring myocardial oxygen consumption ($M\dot{V}O_2$). As well, ^{11}C-acetate has been proposed as a potential myocardial blood flow tracer[33] because of its relatively high initial extraction fraction. Van den Hoff et al.[34] reported that good MBF estimates can be obtained by fitting a simple compartmental model to regional acetate kinetics, providing similar quantitative accuracy relative to $^{13}NH_3$-based blood flow methods. In addition, a potential advantage of ^{11}C-acetate is its ability to simultaneously assess MBF and oxidative metabolism under resting conditions in a single tracer administration.[35]

Cu-62 PTSM, Cu-62 ETS

^{62}Cu pyruvaldehyde bis (N^4 methylthiosemicarbazone) (PTSM) ($T_{1/2}$ = 9.7 minutes[36]) is another generator-produced PET perfusion tracer and is produced from $^{62}Zn/^{62}Cu$ generator.[37,38] ^{62}Cu-PTSM is a promising tracer for assessing myocardial and cerebral perfusion.[36,39]

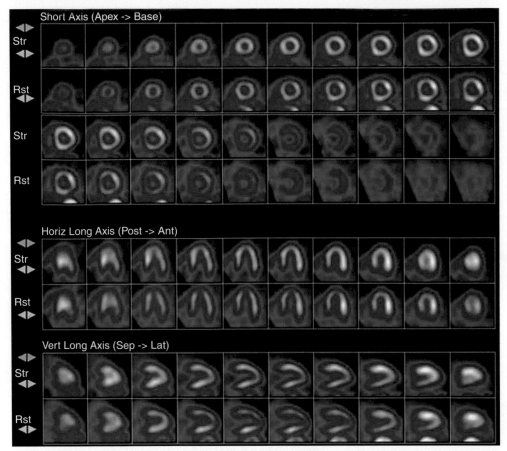

Figure 19-3   4DM display of ^{82}Rb PET MPI in a patient with normal perfusion.

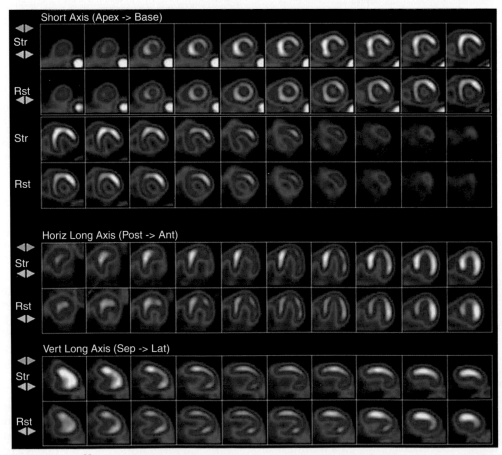

Figure 19-4   4DM display of ^{82}Rb PET MPI shows a severe perfusion defect in the inferior and inferolateral walls that partially improves at rest. There was a reversible wall-motion abnormality on the gated images. The findings are consistent with mostly moderate ischemia and nontransmural scar in the distribution of the LCX territory.

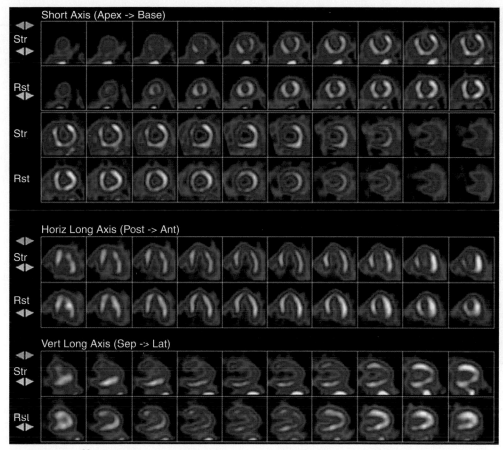

Figure 19-5 4DM display of ^{82}Rb PET MPI of a high risk scan. Images show a severe perfusion defect in the anterior wall and apex with significant improvement on rest images. This is consistent with severe ischemia in the distribution of the LAD territory. In addition, there is transient ischemic dilation and Gated images showed stress induced wall motion abnormalities.

Approximately 5% to 10% of the injected dose of ^{62}Cu-PTSM remains in the circulation due to binding to red blood cells. Therefore, the quantitative measurement of regional MBF using the microsphere model requires correction of the arterial blood time-activity curve for blood-pool binding.[40]

The generator parent ^{62}Zn $T_{1/2}$ is 9.3 hours. This means daily distribution is required. This may be best suited for labs without large numbers of patients requiring perfusion imaging, where they do not perform perfusion imaging daily.

Liver uptake may be problematic, but this appears less with newer related compounds such as ^{62}Cu-ETS. Also, ^{62}Cu has high positron energy similar to ^{82}Rb, which may reduce image resolution.[41,42]

Recent Advances in PET Imaging: Novel Myocardial Blood Flow Tracers

The development of novel tracers could help circumvent some of the current limitations observed with the conventional radioisotopes, such as the "roll-off phenomenon" from incomplete retention and short half-lives that entail on-site production, which ultimately increase costs. The principal characteristics of a new class of radiotracers have been evaluated. Despite promising preliminary results, further research is necessary to elucidate whether these agents will have clinical application in humans.

^{18}F-labeled compounds have relatively long physical $T_{1/2}$ (110 minutes). Among these, *^{18}F-p-fluorobenzyl triphenyl phosphonium cation (^{18}F-FBnTP)* is a member of a new class of positron-emitting lipophilic cations that may act as myocardial perfusion PET tracers.[43,44] *^{18}F-BMS-747158-02* constitutes another emerging agent that is an analog of the insecticide pyridaben, an inhibitor of mitochondrial complex I (MC-1).[45] Mitochondria constitute 20% to 30% of the myocardial intracellular volume. Consequently, molecules that target mitochondrial proteins may be enriched and retained selectively in the myocardium. With the longer ^{18}F $T_{1/2}$, these compounds have the potential for wide distribution. However, they may require reinjection or 2-day stress/rest imaging protocol similar to technetium-99 (^{99m}Tc) SPECT agents. On the other hand, this feature may enable routine exercise stress, which has not been widely developed with PET imaging to date. Recent data suggest kinetics may be suitable for quantification (Fig. 19-6).[46]

A ^{60}Ge/^{60}Ga generator can provide a convenient source of PET tracers because of the long physical half-life of ^{68}Ge ($T_{1/2}$ = 271 days) and a suitable daughter half-life (^{68}Ga; $T_{1/2}$ = 67.7 minutes). Recently, a ligand has been successfully labeled and tested with ^{67}Ga for SPECT.[47] The biodistribution of this novel complex has

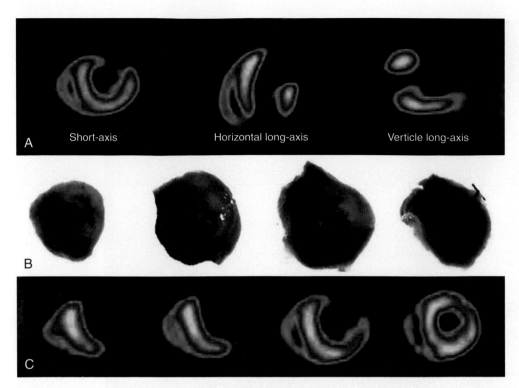

Figure 19-6 Cardiac images in rat model of left coronary ligation. **A,** Cardiac PET short- and long-axis images with BMS-747158-02 at 5 to 15 minutes after injection. The no-flow region is clearly identified. **B,** Ex vivo histologic images of heart short-axis slices from apex to base stained with blue dye. *Blue areas* indicate well-perfused zones, and *no-blue areas* indicate no-flow zones. **C,** In vivo cardiac PET short-axis images from apex to base. The *dark areas* in the left ventricular wall of PET images with BMS-747158-02 **C,** match closely with the no-flow zones identified by blue stain ex vivo **B.** (Reprinted with permission from Yu M, Guaraldi MT, Mistry M, Robinson SP, et al: BMS-747158-02: A novel PET myocardial perfusion imaging agent, J Nucl Cardiol 14:789–798, 2007.)

been assessed in normal and infarcted rat models, whereby it showed a high heart uptake, albeit low cardiac retention and high liver uptake. Further studies of other gallium complexes may improve the feasibility of measuring regional myocardial perfusion using similar ligands labeled with the PET isotope [68]Ge.

MYOCARDIAL IMAGING PROTOCOLS AND ACQUISITION

Patient Preparation

Patients should be instructed to fast for at least 6 hours, to abstain from caffeine-containing products at least 12 hours, and to avoid theophylline-containing medications for 48 hours prior to the test.[13] Diabetic patients should be guided on how to administer insulin before the study. Patients undergoing dobutamine stress tests should discontinue beta-blockers 48 hours prior to the test (only for diagnostic purposes and if it is clinically safe to do so).

Stress Testing Protocols

PET perfusion imaging is usually performed with pharmacologic stress. *Adenosine, dipyridamole,* and *adenosine triphosphate* block transport of adenosine into the cells and/or increase extracellular levels of adenosine, which causes coronary vasodilatation by interacting with the adenosine A_2 receptors in the cell membrane.[13] Adenosine and dipyridamole increase MBF without increasing oxygen demand. Side effects are somewhat greater with adenosine than with dipyridamole, but the latter more often require reversal with aminophylline (which is routine in some laboratories). More selective agonism of the adenosine A_{2A} receptor subtype should theoretically result in a similar degree of coronary vasodilation with fewer and less severe side effects. *Binodenoson,*[48] *regadenoson,*[49] and *apadenoson*[50] are highly selective agonists for the adenosine A_{2A} receptor and are under investigation for clinical use for vasodilator stress imaging.

Dobutamine stress is a feasible alternative in those situations where adenosine, dipyridamole, or ATP are contraindicated.[13,51] Dobutamine increases MBF to meet increasing myocardial oxygen demand. In segments supplied by diseased vessels, the increase in flow is attenuated during high-dose dobutamine administration (20 to 40 µg/kg/min).

Exercise stress may be a valid alternative and provide clinical information unobtainable with pharmacologic stress that is helpful in decision making, particularly for patients unable to tolerate pharmacologic stress. [13]NH_3 can be used in conjunction with treadmill exercise (TEX) or upright bicycle test. The tracer is administrated at peak exercise, and exercise should be continued for an additional 30 to 60 seconds after tracer injection. The patient is then repositioned in the PET camera to start the acquisition within 4 to 6 minutes.[52] Accurate repositioning is of key importance to minimize artifact due to incorrect AC. Exercise stress is also available for the [82]Rb imaging[13,53,54] but can be logistically demanding; patients must be moved to and positioned in the scanner within 3 minutes of completing exercise.

Myocardial Perfusion Imaging Protocols

Common protocols used for imaging myocardial perfusion with dedicated PET or PET/CT systems involve the following steps:

1. *Scout scanning* to ensure that the patient is correctly positioned. With PET/CT systems, the CT scout scan is routinely used.
2. *Transmission scan* for AC purposes.
3. *Emission scans* (both at rest and stress) whereby images are acquired in three different ways: *ECG gated imaging, multiframe or dynamic imaging,* and *list-mode imaging.* In patients undergoing a PET/CT study, it is also possible to estimate coronary calcium score, and with >16 slice MDCT PET/CT systems, to also obtain a coronary CT angiogram (CTA) (Fig. 19-7).[3,13]

The most widely applied tracers in clinical practice are[13]NH$_3$ and [82]Rb.

[13]N Ammonia

For relative perfusion imaging, [13]NH$_3$ is injected as a bolus of 370 to 740 MBq (10 to 20 mCi), and static images are acquired 2 to 3 minutes after tracer administration for an imaging time of 5 to 15 minutes.[3,13] For patients undergoing PET/CT, *two* separate CT-based transmission scans should be performed for correction of rest and stress (after each emission scan is preferred to prevent misregistration artifacts).[3]

For flow quantification, a dynamic acquisition is required. This can be accomplished by performing separate dynamic and gated acquisitions with the same injection or through a single list-mode acquisition. From the dynamic images, time-activity curves are generated for the myocardium and the blood pool.[13] Global and regional MBF can be measured with use of one- or two-tissue-compartment tracer kinetic modeling fit to myocardial activity data and corrected for spillover from the arterial input function.[22]

[82]Rubidium

A larger amount of tracer can be administered with similar absorbed dose to the patient because of the short physical half-life of [82]Rb. In 2D acquisition mode, approximately 1500 to 2200 MBq (40 to 60 mCi) of [82]Rb can be injected as an infusion over 30 seconds, with serial dynamic imaging acquisition starting at onset of the infusion. Between 70 and 150 seconds after completion of tracer infusion, a 3- to 7.5-minute image acquisition is initiated.[8,13] Alternatively, newer-generation PET cameras can acquire data in 3D mode,[28] which enables lower doses of [82]Rb (750 to 1100 MBq [20 to 30 mCi]).

For quantitative assessment of global and regional MBF, one- and two-tissue-compartment models have been used. These account for activity in the vascular space and within the tissue compartment.[55] Following bolus injection of the tracer, predominantly unidirectional transport is assumed from the vascular space into the tissue space.[56] A simplified approach using tracer retention that involves a summed late image corrected for the input function, which can subsequently be corrected for the net retention,[57,58] and similar methods have been developed for [13]NH$_3$.[59] This approach enables a robust means to quantify perfusion that may be easier to apply in the clinical setting (see Figs. 19-1 and 19-2).[28,30]

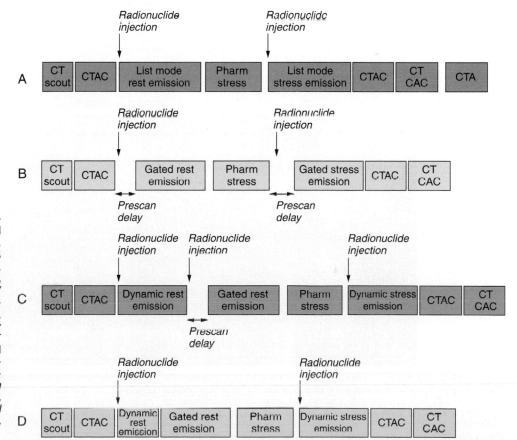

Figure 19-7 Protocols for clinical cardiac PET/CT. **A,** Hybrid list-mode PET + CTA protocol. List mode enables simultaneous gating and dynamic acquisition. **B,** Gated PET/CT protocol. **C,** Multiframe (dynamic) [82]Rb PET/CT + CAC protocol. **D,** Multiframe (dynamic) [13]NH$_3$ PET/CT, + CAC protocol. CAC, coronary artery calcium scan; CTA, CT angiography; CTAC, CT-based attenuation correction (transmission scan); pharm, pharmacologic. *(Reprinted with permission from Di Carli MF, Dorbala S, Moore S, et al: Clinical myocardial perfusion PET/CT, J Nucl Med 48:783–793, 2007.)*

Image Evaluation for Technical Sources of Errors: Quality Control

This step is of extreme importance for an accurate interpretation of the images. Patient body movements can lead to blurring of contours. Acquisition of a brief scan or scout image may facilitate accurate patient positioning. Body motion or respiratory movement can lead to transmission-emission misalignment and potential AC-induced artifacts (Fig. 19-8). However, most PET/CT systems should include software tools to correct transmission-emission misalignments. Finally, other potential sources of reconstruction artifacts encompass streak artifacts seen in large patients with arms-down imaging, metal implants, and IV contrast, as well as residual radioactivity in the IV line within the field of view (FOV).[3,13]

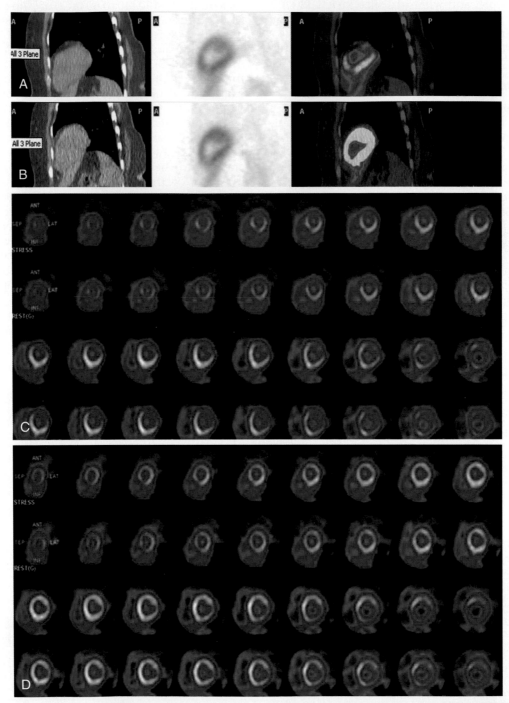

Figure 19-8 **A,** PET/CT misregistration: The area of myocardium superimposed on the lung has an attenuation value lower than soft tissue (myocardium), thus the PET perfusion exam is undercorrected. **B,** Correct PET/CT registration using repeat CT attenuation scan. **C,** PET/CT misregistration: apparent hypoperfusion of the anterolateral wall. **D,** Correct PET/CT registration: shows normal perfusion. Recent software developments now enable realignment of the PET/CT image prior to reprocessing without needing to repeat the CT acquisition. This has reduced the frequency of misalignment at the time of interpretation. Careful QC continues to be required. *(Images reproduced with permission and courtesy of Kevin Berger, MD, Michigan State University.)*

Image Analysis and Interpretation of Perfusion Images

Myocardial perfusion defects are usually identified by visual analysis of the reconstructed slices and compared between stress and rest images. Perfusion defect description, including extent, severity, reversibility, location, and specific coronary territories, should be reported routinely.[60] Defects are typically defined as *fixed*, suggesting scar formation; *reversible*, indicating ischemia; or *partly reversible*, indicating a mixture of scar and ischemia. ACC/AHA/ASNC guidelines recommend semiquantitative analysis using a 17-segment model.[13,61] Using this approach, summed perfusion defect score can be calculated, and this score is useful for cardiac risk stratification.[61,62]

Gated images are also acquired and interpreted. Contour definitions used for EF and volume estimates should be confirmed prior to interpreting gated EF data. The change in EF may have diagnostic value in terms of the extent of disease (discussed later).[63] Wall-motion abnormalities at rest represent myocardial injury, either scar or otherwise, as may occur in a dilated cardiomyopathy. Wall-motion abnormalities that appear or are worse on stress imaging indicate ischemia-induced wall-motion abnormalities. This is in contrast to post-stress SPECT imaging acquired at least 30 minutes after the tracer injection, whereby wall-motion abnormalities are not reflecting concurrent ischemia but rather postischemic dysfunction or stunning. PET wall motion is acquired shortly after tracer injection, and thus changes reflect ischemic wall-motion abnormalities.

ABSOLUTE MYOCARDIAL BLOOD FLOW QUANTIFICATION

Advantages of Absolute Quantitative Analysis

Atherosclerotic vascular disease has become a leading cause of death worldwide, and there is a need to identify the presence of CAD before the onset of symptoms. PET technology has the potential to image and measure pathophysiologic and molecular processes in vivo and is now recognized as the best noninvasive means by which to quantify MBF in absolute terms (mL/min/g) and CFR. Table 19-4 describes normal values of MBF and CFR in healthy subjects.

Parkash et al. demonstrated the clinical importance of CFR over conventional visual analysis in patients with three-vessel CAD using ^{82}Rb PET. In this study, the perfusion defect sizes were larger using quantification in comparison with the conventional relative uptake evaluation.[29] Yoshinaga and colleagues compared the clinical value of CFR by PET to the relative assessment of MPI by SPECT in a population of 27 patients with overt CAD. Approximately two-thirds of regions with angiographic lesions more than 50% showed normal SPECT perfusion scans but significant impaired CFR by PET.[70] Further investigations in larger sample size populations are needed to fully understand the clinical utility and added value of this approach. Only a few studies have assessed the prognostic value of abnormal MBF and CFR.[73,74]

Table 19-4 Normal Values in Baseline Myocardial Blood Flow and Coronary Flow Reserve in Normal Subjects

Author	Tracer	Stress Agent	Number of Subjects	Age (Years)	MBF at Rest	MBF at Hyperemia	CFR
Camici[64]	^{13}NH$_3$	Dipy	12	51±8	1.0±0.2	2.7±0.2	2.9±1.0
Chan[65]	^{13}NH$_3$	ADO	20	35±16	1.1±0.2	4.4±0.9	4.4±1.5
Chan[65]	^{13}NH$_3$	Dipy	20	35±16	1.1±0.2	4.3±1.3	4.3±1.9
Czernin[66]	^{13}NH$_3$	Dipy	22	64±9	0.9±0.3	2.7±0.6	3.0±0.7
Beanlands[67]	^{13}NH$_3$	ADO	5	27±4	0.62±0.09	2.51±0.27	4.1±0.7
Beanlands[67]	^{13}NH$_3$	ADO	7	53±6	0.68±0.15	2.58±0.68	3.7±0.4
Laine[68]	H$_2$^{15}O	Dipy	19	35±3	0.8±0.2	3.8±1.4	4.9±2.5
Kaufmann[69]	H$_2$^{15}O	ADO	61	45±7	0.8±0.1	3.6±1.0	4.2±1.2
Yoshinaga[70]	H$_2$^{15}O	ATP	11	57±12	0.9±0.1	3.6±1.2	3.8±1.2
Furuyama[15]	H$_2$^{15}O	ATP	12	26±3	0.79±0.1	3.8±1.0	4.9±1.3
Lin[71]	^{82}Rh	Dipy	11	44	1.15±0.46	2.50±0.54	(-)
Wassenar[19]	^{82}Rh	Dipy	15	34±6	0.95±0.35	3.0±0.70	3.2±0.8
Lortie[72]	^{82}Rh	Dipy	14	31±7	0.69±0.14	2.83±0.81	4.25±1.37
Total	Weighted Mean		Total 229	42.4	0.89	3.43	3.83
	Mean			41.3	0.88	3.26	3.97

ADO, adenosine; ATP, adenosine triphosphate; CFR, coronary flow reserve; Dipy, dipyridamole; MBF, myocardial blood flow.
Reprinted with permission of Current Pharmaceutical Design.

Models for Flow Quantification

Absolute measurements of physiologic or biochemical function are obtained using tracer kinetic modeling. The time course of radioactivity of the arterial blood input function Ca (t) can usually be measured from image regions within the LV cavity and combined with the myocardial response function Cm (t) to estimate a quantitative rate of transport.

A mathematical model is constructed with parameters that represent the flux of the radiotracer between the compartments. Various tracer kinetic models have been applied and validated for MBF quantification with $H_2^{15}O$, $^{13}NH_3$, ^{82}Rb, and ^{11}C-acetate. Simple one-tissue-compartment models can be applied for flow quantification with each,[25,32,34,56,75,76] providing a reasonable approach for estimating absolute tissue perfusion (see Fig. 19-1).[11]

A further simplified retention model assumes that the tracer is retained completely without subsequent washout. A flow-dependent correction for net tracer retention is required to obtain quantitative perfusion estimates from the retention rates. The net retention model has been shown to produce precise estimates with $^{13}NH_3$[77] and ^{82}Rb[62,78] in normal subjects and in patients with CAD, but the results depend in part on the time at which the model is evaluated and on the accuracy of retention measurement.[11] 3D PET studies in normal subjects have yielded retention fractions similar to those reported in 2D mode[11,59,62] with $^{13}NH_3$ and ^{82}Rb.[11,57]

Three-Dimensional Imaging Mode for Absolute Blood Flow Quantification

It is important to realize that MBF quantification studies have generally applied 2D-mode PET technology. However, with the widespread application of PET/CT for oncology imaging, there has been a shift from 2D to 3D imaging also being applied to cardiac imaging. Currently, the available evidence supports the use of 3D cardiac PET for flow quantification, which offers the potential to measure MBF simultaneously with routine ECG-gated perfusion imaging. The ideal requirements for clinical 3D-mode imaging include a wide dynamic-range scanner along with robust tracer kinetic models, regional partial volume correction and lastly, simultaneous dynamic, static, and ECG-gated imaging through list-mode acquisition and processing.[11]

Radiotracers and Myocardial Blood Flow Quantification

Oxygen-15-Water

The biological behavior of $H_2^{15}O$ can be modeled with a simple one-compartment model as originally described by Kety et al.[32,79]

Iida et al.[80] proposed a mathematical model to correct the input function for the tissue-to-blood spillover and partial volume effect. This model permits estimation of the perfusable tissue fraction, defined as the water-perfusable tissue divided by total extravascular anatomic tissue. Katoh et al. developed an automatic algorithm to calculate regional MBF using a semiautomatic region of interest algorithm and uniform input function.[81]

Nitrogen-13-Ammonia

The most common approach assumes a two-tissue-compartment model with the compartments being the extravascular and metabolic spaces.[25] The initial unidirectional extraction is assumed to be 100%.[82] K_1 representing the transport of the tracer from the vascular space into the extravascular space, is an accurate estimate of MBF. These PET measurements have been well validated with microsphere measurements in experimental preparations confirming that regional MBF can be quantitatively measured over a wide blood-flow range using $^{13}NH_3$ and the compartmental approach.[83–85] Simplified approaches have been used to quantify regional MBF with $^{13}NH_3$ as described earlier.[86] The simplest method is the net retention approximation of the "microsphere model" that requires one static scan and arterial input function and correction for the net retention fraction,[59] but the quantitative value is quite variable, depending on the time of measurement after tracer administration. To reduce this effect, Patlak graphic analysis of the early uptake phase has been applied for the quantitative estimation of MBF with parametric imaging.[87]

Rubidium-82

A few groups have examined the possibility of quantifying MBF with ^{82}Rb. The use of a retention model along with an extraction correction to obtain estimates of MBF has been proposed.[58,78] Other investigators[55,88] have applied a two-compartment model to describe the kinetics of ^{82}Rb in myocardium. Although the two-compartment model was found to provide acceptable estimates of MBF under noise-free conditions, large estimation errors prevented adequate differentiation of flow at more realistic noise levels. Coxson et al.[88] suggested that clinically relevant differences in flow could be detected with a simple one-compartment model. Moreover, fits to experimental data obtained with the two-compartment and the one-compartment models were of comparable quality. A recent study by Lortie et al.[76] has shown that it is possible to obtain accurate estimates of MBF in normal myocardium by using a one-tissue-compartment model of ^{82}Rb kinetics and a nonlinear extraction function. This has been subsequently confirmed in CAD patients.[56]

Physiologic Parameters for Absolute Quantification

The coronary circulation is a dynamic vascular bed that can accommodate marked increases in blood flow through changes in arteriolar resistance in response to increasing metabolic tissue demands and during periods of activation of the sympathetic nervous system. Vasodilators induce a mixed response with both smooth muscle vasodilation and endothelial-dependent vasodilation at the resistance vessels. The magnitude of the flow response, that is, the CFR, is defined as the ratio of near-maximal MBF during pharmacologically induced hyperemia to MBF at rest (effectively, the relative flow reserve).[4,89] The MBF difference, also termed the *absolute flow reserve*, represents the difference in stress/rest flow and may also be a useful parameter.[29,90]

MBF and CFR are considered to reflect the functional status of both the macrocirculation and the microcirculation. Normal values of CFR with PET range between 2 and 5.[4,14] $H_2^{15}O$ and $^{13}NH_3$ have been validated in animal studies by microspheres and shown comparable results.[85,91] The CFR measured by PET is well correlated with intracoronary Doppler guide wire.[92]

$H_2^{15}O$ and $^{13}NH_3$ have good short-term and long-term reproducibility at both rest and hyperemic MBF in normal controls.[93,94] Using an appropriate noise-reduction approach, MBF measured by ^{82}Rb has shown good correlation with $H_2^{15}O$.[94] Recent data also suggest a good correlation between ^{82}Rb and $H_2^{15}O$ MBF measured using the one-compartment approach.[95-97]

FUSION OF STRUCTURE AND FUNCTION: INSIGHTS OF INTEGRATED PET/CT SYSTEMS

Combining images from different modalities could offer significant diagnostic advantages. This has given rise to sophisticated software techniques that allow a true integration of cardiac structure and function. State-of-the-art PET/CT enables simultaneous assessment of cardiac and coronary arterial structure together with myocardial perfusion and metabolism (Fig. 19-9).[21] The synergistic effect of dual-modality imaging potentially offers a more in-depth evaluation for patients with suspected CAD, and may ultimately facilitate appropriate selection of therapy to optimize patient outcomes. Of note, ischemia measured on PET imaging is observed less frequently than stenoses are observed on CTA. CTA tends to define stenoses as more severe relative to quantitative coronary angiography or perfusion imaging. As such, PET can be used to assess the functional significance of CTA findings and to determine the presence of ischemia in patients with high coronary calcium scores. Figures 19-8, 19-9, and 19-10 show examples of hybrid PET/CT imaging. For more details on hybrid PET/CT imaging in this textbook, see Chapter 23.

CLINICAL APPLICATIONS FOR MYOCARDIAL PERFUSION IMAGING WITH PET

Cardiac PET MPI provides accurate regional myocardial perfusion information in patients with suspected or established CAD.[98] PET MPI may be useful for obese patients, women, patients with nondiagnostic findings using other diagnostic tests, and patients with poor LV function.[13,61] Although SPECT MPI remains the traditional approach, there is increasing interest in the use of PET for this purpose.

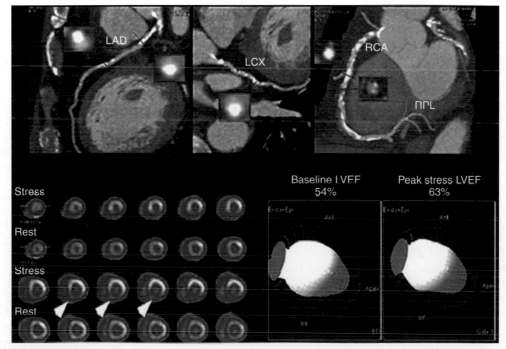

Figure 19-9 Integrated PET/CTA. The left anterior descending (LAD) and circumflex (LCX) coronary arteries show severe calcified plaque in their proximal and mid segments. The dominant right coronary artery (RCA) shows multiple calcified plaques, with a severe predominantly noncalcified plaque in its mid segment; however, the rest and peak adenosine stress myocardial perfusion PET study *(lower left panel)* demonstrates only moderate ischemia in the inferior wall *(arrowheads)*. In addition, left ventricular ejection fraction (LVEF) demonstrated a normal rise during peak stress, effectively excluding the presence of flow-limiting three-vessel coronary artery disease (CAD). *(Reprinted with permission from Di Carli MF, Hachamovitch R: New technology for noninvasive evaluation of coronary artery disease, Circulation 115:1464–1480, 2007.)*

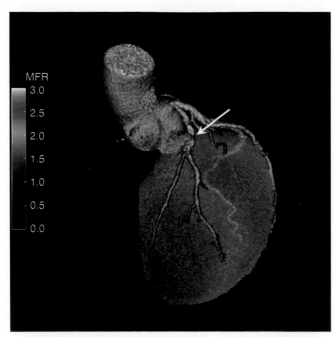

Figure 19-10 Example of fusion of CT with MBF.

Selection of Patients

ACC/AHA/ASNC clinical guidelines from 2003 and the joint position statement by CCS/CAR/CANM/CNCS/CanSCMR from 2007 agree that diagnosis and risk stratification of CAD patients with nondiagnostic or equivocal previous tests are important indications for PET MPI (class 1 indication and evidence level B).[9,61]

Left bundle branch block (LBBB) or ventricular pacing rhythm may also benefit from PET MPI (ACC/AHA/ASNC class IIa and CCS: Class I [level of evidence B]).[9,61] Obese patients or other patients prone to equivocal results could take advantage of PET imaging evaluation as well (CCS et al. Class I [level of evidence B]).[9]

PET MPI can also be used as the initial first test for detection of the extent and location of ischemia. (ACC/AHA/ASNC 2003 class IIa and more recent evaluation by CCS 2007: Class I [level of evidence B]).[9,61]

Diagnosis of Coronary Artery Disease

The mean sensitivity and specificity of PET MPI for diagnosis of CAD have been found to be 89% and 90%, with ranges from 83% to 100% and 73% to 100%, respectively (Table 19-5).[9,23,82,99–113,115]

Previous studies comparing CAD diagnostic accuracy demonstrated superiority of ^{82}Rb or ^{13}NH$_3$ PET MPI over ^{201}Tl SPECT imaging.[82,101,104,105] More recently, Bateman et al.[23] showed greater diagnostic accuracy using ^{82}Rb PET versus gated ^{99m}Tc-sestamibi SPECT (89% versus 79%, $P = 0.03$). This study also demonstrated a significant improvement in diagnostic certainty in favor of PET. Husmann et al.[113] also showed superiority of PET compared to SPECT regarding sensitivity. Namdar et al.[114] evaluated the diagnostic accuracy of ^{13}NH$_3$ using hybrid PET/CT systems for detecting disease

in 100 coronary lesions in 25 patients with CAD. The sensitivity and specificity of PET/CT were 90% and 98%, while PPV and NPV were 82% and 99%, respectively. Sampson et al.[115] reported that ^{82}Rb PET/CT MPI correctly identified CAD in patients with sensitivity of 93% and specificity of 83%. However, the agreement between stress PET MPI findings and coronary stenosis in assessing the anatomic CAD showed relatively low agreement in patients with multivessel disease (58%). Thus PET MPI has excellent ability to define patients with underlying CAD, but conventional relative perfusion approaches (as also used with SPECT) may have limitations in defining extent of disease. MBF quantification provides additional information that may improve diagnostic accuracy in this setting.[29,116] The Study of Perfusion versus Anatomy's Role in CAD (SPARC) is expected to clarify the relative value of the new approaches in relation to SPECT and CT angiography imaging (see examples in Figs. 19-3 through 19-5 and 19-9).[117]

PET is able to estimate LV function at baseline and during peak stress.[21,63] An increase in LVEF of more than 5% yielded an NPV of 97% for ruling out three-vessel CAD.[63] In addition, a recent study suggested that the magnitude of LVEF increase is determined in part by stress perfusion/reversible perfusion defects ($r = -0.25$; $P = 0.009$).[10]

Prognosis of Coronary Artery Disease

SPECT MPI has well-established utility for determining prognosis of patients with known or suspected CAD. Patients with normal stress perfusion imaging have a low hard cardiac event rate and hence an excellent prognosis.[61] There have been some limited data assessing the prognostic value of PET MPI. An early report by Marwick et al. reported that the results of PET perfusion imaging yielded incremental prognostic information in comparison with clinical and angiographic findings alone.[6] Chow et al. described a very low hard cardiac event rate (0.09%/year) in a group of patients with normal ^{82}Rb PET scans.[5] Yoshinaga et al. reported that a normal ^{82}Rb PET MPI scan also indicates an excellent prognosis, and cardiac events are associated with stress perfusion defect severity (Fig. 19-11).[8] This study also reported that ^{82}Rb PET MPI has prognostic value in patients whose diagnosis remains uncertain after SPECT MPI and in obese patients (Table 19-6). Further studies of the prognostic value of PET MPI are underway.

POTENTIAL CLINICAL APPLICATIONS OF PET ABSOLUTE QUANTIFICATION

Clinical applications of MBF and CFR measurements can be categorized into four main areas: (1) early detection of atherosclerotic disease, (2) established CAD, (3) non-atherosclerotic microvascular disease, and (4) assessment of therapeutic approaches.[4,89]

Table 19-5 PET CAD Diagnosis

Author	Year	Number	Stress	Tracer	Reference Cor. Angio	SENSITIVITY			SPECIFICITY		
						+ve test	Pt. w. CAD	%	-ve test	Pt. w.o. CAD	%
Schelbert[82]	1982	45	Dipyridamole	^{13}NH$_3$	>50%	31	32	97%	13	13	100%
Tamaki[99]	1985	25	Exercise	^{13}NH$_3$	N/R	18	19	95%	6	6	100%
Yonekura[100]	1987	50	Exercise	^{13}NH$_3$	>75%	37	38	97%	12	12	100%
Tamaki[101]	1988	51	Exercise	^{13}NH$_3$	>50%	47	48	98%	3	3	100%
Gould (@)[102]	1986	50	Dipyridamole	^{82}Rb/^{13}NH$_3$	QCA SFR < 3	—	—	—	—	—	—
Demer (@)[103]	1989	193	Dipyridamole	^{82}Rb /^{13}NH$_3$	QCA SFR < 4	126	152	83%	39	41	95%
Go[104]	1990	202	Dipyridamole	^{82}Rb	>50%	142	152	93%	39	50	78%
Stewart[105]	1991	81	Dipyridamole	^{82}Rb	QCA >50%*	50	60	83%	18	21	86%
Marwick[106]	1992	74	Dipyridamole	^{82}Rb	>50%	63	70	90%	4	4	100%
Grover-McKay[107]	1992	31	Dipy/adenosine	^{82}Rb	>50%	16	16	100%	11	15	73%
Laubenbacher[108]	1993	34	Dipy/adenosine	^{13}NH$_3$	QCA >50%*	14	16	88%	15	18	83%
Wallhaus[109]	2001	45	Dipyridamole	^{64}Cu-PTSM	>50%	21	25	84%	20	20	100%
Bateman†[23]	2006	112	Dipyridamole	^{82}Rb	>50%*	64	74	86%	38	38	100%
Walsh[110]	1988	33	Dipyridamole	H$_2$^{15}O	QCA	22	24	92%	—	—	—
Williams**[111]	1994	287	Dipyridamole	^{82}Rb	>67%	88	101	87%	99	112	88%
Simone**[112]	1992	225	Dipyridamole	^{82}Rb	>67%	**	**	83%	**	**	91%
Sampson‡[115]	2007	102	Dipy/aden/dbt-CTAC	^{82}Rb	>70%	41	44	93%	48	58	83%
Husmann[113]	2007	70	Dipyridamole	^{13}NH$_3$	>50%	51	53	96%	***	***	***
Totals + weighted mean		1660				831	924	90%	365	411	89%

@Study reported that 50 patients in Gould et al. 1986 were included. Thus Gould et al. not included in mean calculations.
*Other cutoffs reported; > 50% noted here.
**Retrospective study; MFI influenced CAG decision; mixed patient and region method for sensitivity/specificity; patients with/without disease could not be easily determined.
***Specificity reported for lesion only, not for patient diagnosis.
†Electronic database, matched cohort design; values derived from reported population, sensitivity, and specificity.
‡Specificity was determined from combination of patients with low likelihood of disease and those with negative angiogram.
aden, adenosine; CAG, coronary angiogram; CTAC, computed tomography attenuation correction; dbt, dobutamine; Dipy, dipyridamole; QCA, quantitative coronary angiography; SFR, stenosis flow reserve based on QCA data.

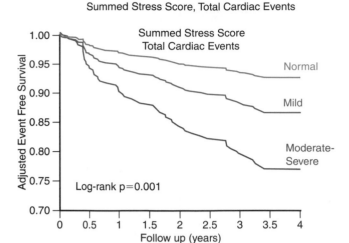

Kaplan-Meier survival curve
Summed Stress Score, Total Cardiac Events

Figure 19-11 Prognostic value of PET MPI. Risk-adjusted survival, free from any (total) cardiac events, as a function of summed stress score (SSS). *(Reprinted with permission from Yoshinaga K, Chow BJ, deKemp RA, Beanlands RS, et al: What is the prognostic value of myocardial perfusion imaging using rubidium-82 positron emission tomography? J Am Coll Cardiol 48:1029–1039, 2006. Color added to the figure.)*

Preclinical Diagnosis of Cardiovascular Disease

Significance of Endothelial and Microvessel Dysfunction

Microvascular disease underlies the involvement of the small coronary arteries in early phases of several cardiovascular conditions that usually precede the onset of symptoms. Microvascular disease or dysfunction is considered to be an independent prognostic value.[120] Coronary endothelial vasodilator dysfunction has been observed in patients with traditional cardiovascular risk factors.

Endothelial cells protect the coronary artery as mechanical barriers and produce vasoactive substances, cytokines, and other active biological compounds to maintain vascular homeostasis.[121] The biochemical hallmark of *coronary endothelial dysfunction* is a reduction in the synthesis or bioactivity of NO, with reduced endothelium-dependent vasodilatation.

Methods to Assess Microvascular Structure and Function

Several techniques are available to estimate endothelial function, such as coronary angiography, ultrasonographic evaluation of brachial arteries, or PET.[122] Clinical studies of endothelial function involve local infusion of acetylcholine, with measurement of the change in vessel diameter by quantitative coronary angiography or Doppler flow wires. These catheter-based approaches are considered the gold standard, but being invasive limits their routine use and their use in repeated testing for serial follow-up.

The cold pressor test induces a mixed vascular response with adrenergically mediated vasoconstrictor and vasorelaxant effects. In healthy individuals, the adrenergically mediated coronary vasoconstriction is offset by flow-mediated endothelium-dependent relaxation, whereas in patients with endothelial dysfunction, cold-induced flow responses can be diminished, absent, or even paradoxical. Several observations support the validity of noninvasively measured changes in MBF during CPT as indicators of endothelium-dependent coronary vasomotion.[89,123,124] The protocol for CPT involves immersing the patient's foot or forearm in ice water for at least 3 to 4 minutes.[15] MBF increases 30% to 60% of baseline in normal volunteers.[15] Reduced MBF response or reductions in flow indicate endothelial dysfunction.[15]

Mental stress also induces catecholamine release from the adrenal medulla and cardiac nerve terminals. Schoder et al. reported that during mental stress, MBF increases by about 30% in normal, healthy individuals, using measured $^{13}NH_3$ and correlated with changes in cardiac work. The increase in MBF under mental stress is reduced in patients with CAD but to a lesser degree (14%).[125]

The methods discussed consider the global impairments in flow or flow reserve measured using PET in response to a stressor. Johnson and Gould have also observed that heterogeneity of resting flow with improvement during dipyridamole, and base-to-apex perfusion gradient suggests the presence of microvascular dysfunction and early atherosclerosis.[126,127] These may also become useful parameters for microvascular disease characterization in addition to flow quantification.

Functional Significance of Cardiovascular Risk Factors on MBF and CFR

Various coronary risk factors may cause reduction of CFR despite angiographically normal coronary arteries. PET has been extensively used to investigate the correlation of CFR and coronary risk factors.

Dayanikli et al.[128] first described a linear relationship between coronary flow measurement and serum cholesterol levels in asymptomatic patients at risk for developing CAD. Yokoyama et al.[129] confirmed these results by describing reduction of CFR in asymptomatic patients with familial hypercholesterolemia.

Czernin et al.[130] evaluated the acute effect of smoking on myocardial vasculature reactivity to vasodilator stimulation. Campisi et al. demonstrated an altered response of MBF during a CPT despite normal CFR in long-term smokers, suggesting endothelial dysfunction.[124]

PET studies have shown that individuals with diabetes mellitus have consistently higher MBF at rest[131] than controls. Diabetic patients do have altered myocardial vasodilation responses to either pharmacologic agents[131] or CPT.[132] It has been suggested that chronic hyperglycemia may play a leading role in the pathogenesis of vascular dysfunction in diabetic patients.

Arterial hypertension with or without LVH can reduce CFR by altering the coronary vasculature and resistance.[12] This reduction of CFR may be dependent on impaired maximal vasodilator capacity. It has been proposed that hemodynamic pressure overload and local vasoactive substances may play a key role in the genesis of regional perfusion abnormalities.[89]

Table 19-6 PET CAD Prognosis

Author	Year	Patient Number	Stress	Tracer	Outcomes	Follow-up Time (years)	NORMAL SCAN ANNUAL EVENT RATE (%/YR)		ABNORMAL SCAN ANNUAL EVENT RATE (%/YR)	
							Hard Events	Total Events	Hard Events	Total Events
Yoshinaga[8]	2006	367	Dipyridamole	[82]Rb	Death, MI, Rev, Hosp	3.1	0.4	1.7	Mild: 2.3 mod/sev: 7.0	Mild: 12.9 mod/ sev: 13.2
Chow[5]	2005	629	Dipyridamole	[82]Rb	Death, MI, Rev, CAG	2.3	0.09	0.98	ECG +ve Normal MP:0.6	ECG +ve Normal MP: 1.9
Marwick[5]	1997	581	Dipyridamole	[82]Rb	Death, MI, Rev, UAP	3.4	0.9	4	4	7
Marwick,[118]	1995	Prediction of perioperative and late cardiac events before vascular surgery								
MacIntrye,[119]	1993	Outcomes in patients with false-negative thallium-201 SPECT								

CAG, coronary angiogram; MI, myocardial infarction; Rev, revascularization; UAP, unstable angina.
Reprinted with permission of the Canadian Journal of Cardiology.

Myocardial Blood Flow Parameters in Established Cardiovascular Disease

The assessment of MBF parameters represents a more physiologic evaluation of cellular perfusion than coronary angiography.[133] Gould et al.[134] described the value of CFR as an index of the functional severity of CAD. MBF at rest remains normal until there is an 80% to 85% diameter coronary stenosis, while hyperemic coronary flow measured after maximal vasodilatation begins to decrease progressively if the stenosis is more than about 40%.

Demer et al.[135] first reported a significant relationship between the severity of relative perfusion abnormalities on PET perfusion images and CFR measurements from quantitative coronary angiography. Uren et al.[98] showed a relationship between coronary artery stenosis on angiography and CFR data obtained by $H_2^{15}O$ PET perfusion studies. Similar results were obtained with $^{13}NH_3$ PET perfusion data.[67] Notably, since multiple factors other than lesion diameter influence the measured CFR, interpretation of CFR may require consideration of dynamic characteristics of both epicardial coronary artery and resistance vessels[22] and/or the concomitant definition of coronary anatomy.

MBF and CFR can also help detect extensive epicardial disease, since overt perfusion defects diagnostic of multivessel CAD may be apparent in only a third of these patients due to the "balanced ischemia" phenomenon.[136] Finally, quantitative PET can assist distinguishing the presence of collaterals[29] and early hibernating myocardium.[137]

Myocardial Blood Flow Parameters in Nonatherosclerotic Microvascular Disease

In patients with *hypertrophic cardiomyopathy* (HCM), Camici et al. reported that CFR is markedly impaired not only in the hypertrophied septum but also in the less hypertrophied LV free wall.[138] In the absence of coronary stenoses, this is indicative of a diffuse microvascular dysfunction, which is associated with poor clinical outcomes.[139] This study was the first to evaluate the prognostic value of PET blood flow measurements.

Rajappan et al. observed that the subendocardial CFR was lower than subepicardial CFR in patients with *aortic valve stenosis* (AS), despite normal coronary arteries.[20] Burwash et al. reported that very low CFR in patients with AS had an accuracy of 85% for distinguishing true low-flow AS from pseudoaortic stenosis.[88,140] This study suggested CFR would be a useful parameter for the differential diagnosis of truly severe, compared to pseudo-severe, AS in patients with poor LV function.

Myocardial Blood Flow Parameters as Surrogate Markers

MBF and CFR for the Follow-up of Current Medical Managements

PET offers useful information for monitoring disease progression and the effects of treatment, both in clinical trials and clinical practice.

Guethlin et al.[141] evaluated the CFR before, at 3 months, and at 6 months after initiation of therapy with fluvastatin. The investigator verified that CFR increased only after 6 months of therapy. Combined therapy with conventional lipid-lowering therapy and the insulin sensitizer pioglitazone improved resting MBF in patients with familial combined hyperlipidemia.[142] On the other hand, Ling et al.[143] observed that simvastatin improved endothelial function measured using brachial blood flow but did not significantly improve MBF measured using dipyridamole PET imaging. This was possibility related to dose and/or the patient population or the imaging parameter used. This is exemplified by Sdringola et al., who recently demonstrated that the severity of quantified myocardial perfusion defects on PET imaging did not improve after 6 months of atorvastatin versus placebo. However, visual change scores did significantly improve compared to placebo.[144]

Short-term intravenous angiotensin-converting enzyme inhibitor (ACEI) treatment improves stress flow and flow reserve in ischemic regions.[145] Akinboboye et al.[146] compared the long-term effects of the ACEI, lisinopril and the angiotensin receptor blocker (ARB) losartan. The ACEI improved hyperemic MBF, but the ARB did not. In contrast, another ARB, olmesartan, reduced coronary resistance during the cold pressor test, indicating olmesartan may benefit coronary endothelial function.[90] The discrepancies between the two studies may be due to the method of coronary microcirculation assessment. The latter study by Naya et al. evaluated coronary microcirculation using the cold pressor test, and the former study used pharmacologic stress. Pharmacologic stress evaluates mixed vascular function, including endothelial function and vascular smooth cell function.[4,147] Thus, detailed coronary microvascular evaluation in the ideal setting may require both the cold pressor test and vasodilator stress. This has been and will continue to be a limitation to its routine and clinical use.

Diabetes mellitus patients have an increased coronary event risk, and clinical trials have shown the possibility of risk reduction by appropriate therapeutic interventions. Pitkänen et al. reported reduced CFR even in young men with insulin-dependent diabetes mellitus (IDDM) with or without minimum microvascular complications.[148] Di Carli et al. compared the coronary vascular function between type 1 diabetes and type 2 diabetes. Both groups showed similar vascular dysfunction.[149] Yokoyama et al. found that CFR reduction was inversely correlated with the over-5-year average hemoglobin A_{1c} ($r = -0.55$; $P < 0.01$) but not age.[150] These studies may indicate the importance of the glycemic control for coronary vascular dysfunction. In patients with diabetes mellitus, perindopril improved endothelial function measured using CPT/PET imaging.[151] The insulin sensitizer pioglitazone improved glycemic control in patients with insulin-dependent type 2 diabetes. However, pioglitazone did not lead to improvement in either adenosine-induced hyperemia or CFR.[152]

Yoshinaga et al. evaluated the effect of exercise training effect on regional MBF in patients with stable CAD. The exercise training increased hyperemic MBF in diseased segments compared to the sedentary lifestyle group.[31] Furthermore, Sdringola et al. has also applied relative PET perfusion imaging to demonstrate that combined intensive lifestyle and target-driven lipid-lowering drug therapy reduce perfusion abnormalities as well as cardiac events when compared to usual care or cholesterol-lowering drugs.[153]

MBF and CFR for the Assessment of Interventional Therapies

Van Tosh et al.[154] demonstrated that abnormal CFR after angioplasty on PET imaging identifies increased risk for future coronary restenosis. Scott et al. used PET perfusion imaging to demonstrate the benefit of stent therapy in acute myocardial infarction.[155] Such surrogate endpoint data have helped lead to larger clinical trials that support the routine use of PCI in STEMI.[155]

Rechavia et al.[156] demonstrated higher resting MBF with reduction of CFR in patients with cardiac transplantation. Chan et al.[157] described a decrease in hyperemic flow with an increase in resting flow in excess of cardiac work in patients with transplant rejection. During a follow-up study after successful treatment, patients with transplant rejection had significant improvement of vascular function, suggesting the role and possible importance of serial noninvasive flow measurements by PET.[158]

Studies that investigated the effect of cardiac resynchronization therapy (CRT) on MBF[159,160] demonstrated a more homogeneous resting blood flow distribution and a significant increase in LVEF after 3 months of CRT, compared with baseline.

Myocardial Blood Flow Parameters and Novel Therapeutic Approaches

The emergent development of new treatments for improving advanced heart disease have created a need for noninvasive imaging tools to provide specific disease-related biological insights.

PET is well suited for tracking of transplanted cells by use of labeling with radionuclides or reporter-genes. Preliminary investigations have been performed by either FDG PET or SPECT MPI.[161,162] Reporter-gene approaches[163] are expected to shed more light on mechanisms of therapy on the tissue level, but significant advances in this technology are still required.

PET perfusion imaging and flow quantification is likely to play a key role in the evaluation of these cell- and gene-based therapies. Recently, in a randomized trial, Ruel et al. applied $^{13}NH_3$ PET quantification and was able to demonstrate that the combination of vascular endothelial growth factor angiogenesis and endothelium modulator L-arginine improved perfusion in patients with surgical multivessel CAD and severe diffuse disease in the LAD.[164]

The utility of PET perfusion and flow quantification to evaluate the effects of a multitude of therapies is well demonstrated. It is also capable of defining microvascular disease and early and late diffuse atherosclerosis. These approaches hold tremendous promise for being able to provide additional clinically relevant data over and above what is currently available from routine relative PET MPI. Further research is needed to determine

their ultimate clinical utility. This will be judged by whether or not the added information influences clinical decisions that can positively affect the outcomes of our patients.

Hybrid Imaging: Fusion Images of CTA and MBF

Hybrid PET/CT systems would afford mechanistic insights into atherothrombotic processes and may also enable identification of vulnerable plaques by enabling image fusion of structure and function (see Fig. 19-10). Sites with these capabilities are now exploring the role of such a comprehensive evaluation that includes traditional relative uptake perfusion images at stress and rest, gated studies for regional and global function, flow and reserve quantification, and combining these with calcium scoring and coronary CT angiography. Further discussion on hybrid methodologies is found in Chapter 23.

SUMMARY AND CONCLUSIONS

The introduction of PET technology more than 26 years ago marked the commencement of a new era in the field of cardiovascular imaging. The role of PET MPI is now well established for the diagnosis of CAD. In addition, recent data have shown the prognostic value of PET MPI in patients with suspected CAD.

Clinical use of state-of-the-art technology has been limited by issues related to cost, access to radiotracers, and infrastructure requirements. Clinical application of PET cardiac imaging is increasing as the cost reduction of PET instrumentation and cyclotrons occurs. Generator-produced radiotracers also now contribute to the wider and increasing access to PET studies.

PET imaging is the most validated noninvasive method for absolute flow quantification. PET imaging also has been applied for endothelial function measurements capable of defining the early stage of coronary arteriosclerosis. Currently, integrated PET/CT provides new means for AC but also the capability to evaluate coronary function and anatomy in a single setting. More studies are needed to determine whether this approach will help optimize the clinical decision-making process and whether this will improve patient outcomes. PET remains an ideal research tool for the study of the pathophysiology of CAD and other heart diseases. PET has and will continue to play a central role for the evaluation of treatment as new therapies continue to develop.

The routine clinical role of PET MPI in CAD evaluation is now well established. The added value of hybrid data combining PET with coronary calcium scores and/or CT angiography and the clinical utility of MBF quantification in defining early and late atherosclerosis, microvascular disease, and treatment evaluation are matters of ongoing investigation. The utility of these emerging methodologies will be judged by whether or not the added information influences clinical decisions that can positively shape the outcomes of our patients.

REFERENCES

1. Shaw LJ, Berman DS, Hartigan PH, et al: Differential improvement in stress myocardial perfusion ischemia following percutaneous coronary intervention as compared with optimal medical therapy alone: nuclear substudy results from the clinical outcomes using revascularization and aggressive drug evaluation (COURAGE) trial, *Circulation* 116:2628, 2007.
2. Townsend DW, Cherry SR: Combining anatomy and function: the path to true image fusion, *Eur Radiol* 11:1968–1974, 2001.
3. Di Carli MF, Dorbala S, Moore S, et al: Clinical myocardial perfusion PET/CT, *J Nucl Med* 48:783–793, 2007.
4. Yoshinaga K, Chow B, deKemp RA, Beanlands RS, et al: Application of cardiac molecular imaging using positron emission tomography in evaluation of drug and therapeutics for cardiovascular disorders, *Curr Pharm Des* 11:903–932, 2005.
5. Chow BJ, Williams K, Yoshinaga K, et al: Prognostic significance of dipyridamole-induced ST depression in patients with normal [82]Rb PET myocardial perfusion imaging, *J Nucl Med* 46:1095–1101, 2005.
6. Marwick T, Go RT, Patel S, et al: Incremental value of rubidium-82 positron emission tomography for prognostic assessment of known or suspected coronary artery disease, *Am J Cardiol* 80:865–870, 1997.
7. Yoshinaga K, Chow B, deKemp RA, et al: Prognostic value of rubidium-82 perfusion positron emission tomography: Preliminary results from 153 consecutive patients, *J Am Coll Cardiol* 43:338A, 2004.
8. Yoshinaga K, Chow BJ, deKemp RA, Beanlands RS, et al: What is the prognostic value of myocardial perfusion imaging using rubidium-82 positron emission tomography? *J Am Coll Cardiol* 48:1029–1039, 2006.
9. Beanlands R, Chow BJ, Dick A, et al: CCS / CAR / CANM / CNCS / CanSCMR Joint Position Statement on Advanced Non-invasive Cardiac Imaging using Positron Emission Tomography, Magnetic Resonance Imaging and Multi-Detector Computed Tomographic Angiography in the Diagnosis and Evaluation of Ischemic Heart Disease Abbreviated Report, *Can J Cardiol* 23:107–119, 2007.
10. Brown TL, Bengel FM, Merrill J, Volokh L: Determinants of the response of left ventricular ejection fraction to vasodilator stress in electrocardiographically gated 82rubidium myocardial perfusion PET, *Eur J Nucl Med Mol Imaging* 35:336–342, 2008.
11. deKemp RA, Yoshinaga K, Beanlands RS: Will 3-dimensional PET-CT enable the routine quantification of myocardial blood flow? *J Nucl Cardiol* 14:380–397, 2007.
12. Machac J: Cardiac positron emission tomography imaging, *Semin Nucl Med* 35:17–36, 2005.
13. Machac J, Beanlands RS, Di Carli MF, et al: Positron emission tomography perfusion and glucose metabolism imaging, *J Nucl Cardiol* 13:e121–e151, 2006.
14. Camici PG: Positron emission tomography and myocardial imaging, *Heart* 83:475–480, 2000.
15. Furuyama H, Katoh C, Odagawa Y, et al: Assessment of coronary function in children with a history of Kawasaki disease using (15) O-water positron emission tomography, *Circulation* 105:2878–2884, 2002.
16. Loghin C, Gould KL, Sdringola S: Common artifacts in PET myocardial perfusion images due to attenuation-emission misregistration: clinical significance, causes, and solutions, *J Nucl Med* 45:1029–1039, 2004.
17. Martinez-Moller A, Schwaiger M, Souvatzoglou M, et al: Artifacts from misaligned CT in cardiac perfusion PET/CT studies: frequency, effects, and potential solutions, *J Nucl Med* 48:188–193, 2007.
18. Schwaiger M, Ziegler S, et al: PET/CT: Challenge for nuclear cardiology, *J Nucl Med* 46:1664–1678, 2005.
19. Wassenaar RW, Beanlands RS, deKemp RA, Ruddy TD: Three dimensional cardiac positron emission tomography, *Res Adv Nuc Med* 1:51–60, 2002.
20. Rajappan K, Dutka DP, Rimoldi OE, et al: Mechanisms of coronary microcirculatory dysfunction in patients with aortic stenosis and angiographically normal coronary arteries, *Circulation* 105:470–476, 2002.
21. Di Carli MF, Hachamovitch R: New Technology for Noninvasive evaluation of coronary artery disease, *Circulation* 115:1464–1480, 2007.
22. Yoshinaga K: Principles and Practice in Positron Emission Tomography. In Wahl R, editor: *Chapter 8: Cardiac Applications*, ed 2, 2007.
23. Bateman TM, Friedman JD, Heller GV, McGhie AI, et al: Diagnostic accuracy of rest/stress ECG-gated Rb-82 myocardial perfusion PET: comparison with ECG-gated Tc-99m sestamibi SPECT, *J Nucl Cardiol* 13:24–33, 2006.
24. Krivokapich J, Huang SC, MacDonald NS, Phelps ME, et al: Dependence of 13NH3 myocardial extraction and clearance on flow and metabolism, *Am J Physiol* 242:H536–H542, 1982.
25. Hutchins GD, Krivokapich J, Rosenspire KC, Schelbert H, Schwaiger M, et al: Noninvasive quantification of regional blood flow in the human heart using N-13 ammonia and dynamic positron emission tomographic imaging, *J Am Coll Cardiol* 15:1032–1042, 1990.
26. Beanlands RS, Hutchins GD, Muzik O, et al: Heterogenicity of regional nitrogen 13-labeled ammonia tracer distribution in the normal human heart: comparison with rubidium 82 and copper 62-labeled PTSM, *J Nucl Cardiol* 1:225–235, 1994.
27. Alvarez-Diez TM, Beanlands RS, deKemp R, Vincent J: Manufacture of strontium-82/rubidium-82 generators and quality control of rubidium-82 chloride for myocardial perfusion imaging in patients using positron emission tomography, *Appl Radiat Isot* 50:1015–1023, 1999.
28. deKemp RA, Hewitt T, Ruddy TD, Beanlands RS, et al: Detection of serial changes in absolute myocardial perfusion with 82Rb PET, *J Nucl Med* 41:1426–1435, 2000.
29. Parkash R, deKemp RA, Ruddy TD, Beanlands RS, et al: Potential utility of rubidium 82 PET quantification in patients with 3-vessel coronary artery disease, *J Nucl Cardiol* 11:440–449, 2004.
30. Scott N, deKemp R, LeMay M, et al: Evaluation of myocardial perfusion using rubidium-8/82 positron emission tomography after myocardial infarction in patients receiving primary stent implantation or thrombolytic therapy, *Am J Cardiol* 88:886–889, 2001.
31. Yoshinaga K, deKemp RA, Beanlands RS, et al: Effect of exercise training on myocardial blood flow in patients with stable coronary artery disease, *Am Heart J* 151(1324):e11–e18, 2006.
32. Bergmann SR, Fox KAA, Rond AL, et al: Quantification of regional myocardial blood flow in vivo with $H_2^{15}O$, *Circulation* 70:724–733, 1984.
33. Gropler RJ, Geltman EM, Siegel BA: Myocardial uptake of carbon-11-acetate as an indirect estimate of regional myocardial blood flow, *J Nucl Med* 32:245–251, 1991.
34. van den Hoff J, Börner AR, Burchert W, et al: [1–11C]acetate as a quantitative perfusion tracer in myocardial PET, *J Nucl Med* 42:1174–1182, 2001.
35. Sun KT, Buxton DB, Yeatman LA, et al: Simultaneous measurement of myocardial oxygen consumption and blood flow using 11-carbon acetate, *J Nucl Med* 39:272–280, 1998.
36. Beanlands RS, Mintun M, Muzik O, et al: The kinetics of copper-62-PTSM in the normal human heart, *J Nucl Med* 33:684–690, 1992.
37. Green MA, Mathias CJ, Welch MJ, et al: Copper-62-labeled pyruvaldehyde bis(N4-methylthiosemicarbazonato)copper(II): synthesis and evaluation as a positron emission tomography tracer for cerebral and myocardial perfusion, *J Nucl Med* 31:1989–1996, 1990.
38. Shelton ME, Bergmann SR, Green MA, Mathias CJ, Welch MJ: Assessment of regional myocardial and renal blood flow with copper-PTSM and positron emission tomography, *Circulation* 82:990–997, 1990.
39. Wallhaus TR, Green MA, Nickles RJ, Stone CK, et al: Human biodistribution and dosimetry of the PET perfusion agent copper-62-PTSM, *J Nucl Med* 39:1958–1964, 1998.
40. Mathias CJ, Bergmann SR, Green MA: Development and validation of a solvent extraction technique for determination of Cu-PTSM in blood, *Nucl Med Biol* 20:343–349, 1993.
41. Haynes NG, Lacy JL, Nayak N, et al: Performance of a 62Zn/62Cu generator in clinical trials of PET perfusion agent 62Cu-PTSM, *J Nucl Med* 41:309–314, 2000.
42. Ackerman LJ, Green MA, Mathias CJ, West DX: Synthesis and evaluation of copper radiopharmaceuticals with mixed bis (thiosemicarbazone) ligands, *Nucl Med Biol* 26:551–554, 1999.
43. Madar I, Du Y, Hilton J, Volokh L, et al: Characterization of uptake of the new PET imaging compound18F-fluorobenzyl triphenyl phosphonium in dog myocardium, *J Nucl Med* 47:1359–1366, 2006.
44. Madar I, DiPaula A, Ravert H, et al: Assessment of severity of coronary artery stenosis in a canine model using the PET agent ^{18}F-fluorobenzyl triphenyl phosphonium: Comparison with ^{99m}Tc-tetrofosmin, *J Nucl Med* 48:1021–1030, 2007.
45. Yalamanchili P, Hayes M, Wexler e, et al: Mechanism of uptake and retention of F-18 BMS-747158–02 in cardiomyocytes: a novel PET myocardial imaging agent, *J Nucl Cardiol* 14:782–788, 2007.
46. Yu M, Guaraldi MT, Mistry M, Robinson SP, et al: BMS-747158–02: A novel PET myocardial perfusion imaging agent, *J Nucl Cardiol* 14:789–798, 2007.
47. Plössla K, Chandraa R, Qua W, et al: A novel gallium bisaminothiolate complex as a myocardial perfusion imaging agent, *Nucl Med Biol* 35:83–90, 2008.
48. Udelson JE, Heller GV, Wackers FJ, et al: Randomized, controlled dose-ranging study of the selective adenosine A2A receptor agonist binodenoson for pharmacological stress as an adjunct to myocardial perfusion imaging, *Circulation* 109:457–464, 2004.
49. Iskandrian AE, Bateman TM, Hendel RC, et al: Adenosine versus regadenoson comparative evaluation in myocardial perfusion imaging: Results of the ADVANCE phase 3 multicenter international trial, *J Nucl Cardiol* 14:645–658, 2007.
50. Cerqueira MD: Advances in pharmacologic agents in imaging: new A2A receptor agonists, *Curr Cardiol Rep* 8:119–122, 2006.
51. American Society of Nuclear Cardiology: Imaging guidelines for nuclear cardiology procedures, part 2, *J Nucl Cardiol* 6:G47–G84, 1999.
52. Chow BJ, Lee A, Beanlands RS, et al: Treadmill exercise produces larger perfusion defects than dipyridamole stress N-13 ammonia positron emission tomography, *J Am Coll Cardiol* 47:411–416, 2006.

53. Chow BJ, Ananthasubramaniam K, deKemp RA, Beanlands RS, et al: Feasibility of exercise rubidium-82 positron emission tomography myocardial perfusion imaging, *J Am Coll Cardiol* 41:428A, 2003.

54. Chow BJ, deKemp RA, Ruddy TD, Beanlands RS, et al: Comparison of treadmill exercise versus dipyridamole stress with myocardial perfusion imaging using rubidium-82 positron emission tomography, *J Am Coll Cardiol* 45:1227–1234, 2005.

55. Herrero P, Bergmann SR, Markham J, Shelton ME: Implementation and evaluation of a two-compartment model for quantification of myocardial perfusion with rubidium-82 and positron emission tomography, *Circ Res* 70:496–507, 1992.

56. Lortie M, Beanlands R, DaSilva J, deKemp R: Quantification of myocardial blood flow in subjects with coronary artery disease with 82Rb dynamic PET imaging, *J Nucl Med* 48:2007.

57. Renaud J, Beanlands RS, deKemp RA, Lortie M, et al: Quantifying the normal range of myocardial blood flow with ^{13}N-ammonia and ^{82}Rb dynamic PET imaging, *J Nucl Med* 47:67P, 2006.

58. Yoshida K, Gould KL, Mullani N: Coronary flow and flow reserve by PET simplified for clinical applications using rubidium-82 or nitrogen-13-ammonia, *J Nucl Med* 37:1701–1712, 1996.

59. Bellina C, Camici P, Parodi O, Salvadori PA, et al: Simultaneous in vitro and in vivo validation of nitrogen-13-ammonia for the assessment of regional myocardial blood flow, *J Nucl Med* 31:1335–1343, 1990.

60. Hendel RC, Berman DS, Wackers FJ, et al: American Society of Nuclear Cardiology consensus statement: reporting of radionuclide myocardial perfusion imaging studies, *J Nucl Cardiol* 10:705–708, 2003.

61. Klocke FJ, Baird MG, Lorell BH, et al: ACC/AHA/ASNC guidelines for the clinical use of cardiac radionuclide imaging: executive summary-a report of the American College of Cardiology/American Heart Association Task Force on Practice Guidelines (ACC/AHA/ASNC Committee to Revise the 1995 Guidelines for the Clinical Use of Cardiac Radionuclide Imaging), *J Am Coll Cardiol* 42:1318–1333, 2003.

62. Yoshinaga K, Chow BJ, deKemp RA, Beanlands RS, et al: Prognostic value of rubidium-82 perfusion positron emission tomography in patients referred after SPECT imaging, *J Nucl Cardiol* 12:S43, 2005.

63. Dorbala S, Di Carli MF, Kwong R, et al: Value of left ventricular ejection fraction in assessment of severe left main/three-vessel coronary artery disease: a rubidium-82 PET-CT Study, *J Nucl Med* 48:349–358, 2007.

64. Camici P, Chiriatti G, Lorenzoni R, et al: Coronary vasodilation is impaired in both hypertrophied and nonhypertrophied myocardium of patients with hypertrophic cardiomyopathy: a study with nitrogen-13 ammonia and positron emission tomography, *J Am Coll Cardiol* 17:879–886, 1991.

65. Chan SY, Brunken RC, Czernin J, et al: Comparison of maximal myocardial blood flow during adenosine infusion with that of intravenous dipyridamole in normal men, *J Am Coll Cardiol* 20:979–985, 1992.

66. Czernin J, Chan S, Muller P, et al: Influence of age and hemodynamics on myocardial blood flow and flow reserve, *Circulation* 88:62–69, 1993.

67. Beanlands RS, Hutchins GD, Schwaiger M, et al: Noninvasive quantification of regional myocardial flow reserve in patients with coronary atherosclerosis using nitrogen-13 ammonia positron emission tomography: determination of extent of altered vascular reactivity, *J Am Coll Cardiol* 26:1465–1475, 1995.

68. Laine H, Niinikoski H, Raitakari OT, et al: Early impairment of coronary flow reserve in young men with borderline hypertension, *J Am Coll Cardiol* 32:147–153, 1998.

69. Kaufmann PA, Gnecchi-Ruscone T, Schafers KP, et al: Low density lipoprotein cholesterol and coronary microvascular dysfunction in hypercholesterolemia, *J Am Coll Cardiol* 36:103–109, 2000.

70. Yoshinaga K, Katoh C, Noriyasu K, et al: Reduction of coronary flow reserve in areas with and without ischemia on stress perfusion imaging in patients with coronary artery disease: a study using oxygen 15-labeled water PET, *J Nucl Cardiol* 10:275–283, 2003.

71. Lin JW, Chou RL, Laine AF, Sciacca RR, et al: Quantification of myocardial perfusion in human subjects using 82Rb and wavelet-based noise reduction, *J Nucl Med* 42:201–208, 2001.

72. Lortie M, Kelly C, Mostert K, et al: Quantification of myocardial blood flow with rubidium-82 dynamic PET imaging, *J Nucl Med* 46:60P, 2005.

73. Cecchi F, Camici PG, Gistri R, Olivotto I, et al: Coronary microvascular dysfunction and prognosis in hypertrophic cardiomyopathy, *N Engl J Med* 349:1027–1035, 2003.

74. Neglia D, Michelassi C, Pratali L, Trivieri MG, et al: Prognostic role of myocardial blood flow impairment in idiopathic left ventricular dysfunction, *Circulation* 105:186–193, 2002.

75. DeGrado TR, Hanson MW, Turkington TG, Vallee JP, et al: Estimation of myocardial blood flow for longitudinal studies with 13N-labeled ammonia and positron emission tomography, *J Nucl Cardiol* 3:494–507, 1996.

76. Lortie M, Beanlands RS, Yoshinaga K, deKemp RA, et al: Quantification of myocardial blood flow with ^{82}Rb dynamic PET imaging, *Eur J Nucl Med Mol Imaging* 34:1765–1774, 2007.

77. Choi Y, Huang SC, Hawkins RA, Kim JY, Kim BT, Hoh CK, et al: Quantification of myocardial blood flow using ^{13}N-ammonia and PET: comparison of tracer models, *J Nucl Med* 40:1045–1055, 1999.

78. Herrero P, Bergmann SR, Markham J, Shelton ME, et al: Noninvasive quantification of regional myocardial perfusion with rubidium-82 and positron emission tomography: exploration of a mathematical model, *Circulation* 82:1377–1386, 1990.

79. Kety SS: The theory and applications of the exchange of inert gas at the lungs and tissues, *Pharmacol Rev* 3:1–41, 1951.

80. Iida H, Kanno I, Takahashi A, et al: Measurement of absolute myocardial blood flow with H215O and dynamic positron-emission tomography. Strategy for quantification in relation to the partial-volume effect, *Circulation* 78:104–115, 1988.

81. Katoh C, Morita K, Shiga T, Tamaki N, et al: Improvement of algorithm for quantification of regional myocardial blood flow using ^{15}O-water with PET, *J Nucl Med* 45:1908–1916, 2004.

82. Schelbert HR, Phelps ME, Wisenberg G, et al: Noninvasive assessment of coronary stenoses by myocardial imaging during pharmacologic coronary vasodilation. VI. Detection of coronary artery disease in human beings with intravenous N-13 ammonia and positron computed tomography, *Am J Cardiol* 49:1197–1207, 1982.

83. Bol A, Melin JA, Vanoverschelde JL, et al: Direct comparison of [13N] ammonia and [15O]water estimates of perfusion with quantification of regional myocardial blood flow by microspheres, *Circulation* 87:512–525, 1993.

84. Kuhle WG, Huang SC, Porenta G, et al: Quantification of regional myocardial blood flow using ^{13}N-ammonia and reoriented dynamic positron emission tomographic imaging, *Circulation* 86:1004–1017, 1992.

85. Muzik O, Beanlands RS, Hutchins GD, Mangner TJ, et al: Validation of nitrogen-13-ammonia tracer kinetic model for quantification of myocardial blood flow using PET, *J Nucl Med* 34:83–91, 1993.

86. Choi Y, Hawkins RA, Huang SC, et al: A simplified method for quantification of myocardial blood flow using nitrogen-13-ammonia and dynamic PET, *J Nucl Med* 34:488–497, 1993.

87. Tadamura E, Tamaki N, Yonekura Y, et al: Assessment of coronary vasodilator reserve by N-13 ammonia PET using the microsphere method and Patlak plot analysis, *Ann Nucl Med* 9:109–118, 1995.

88. Burwash I, deKemp R, Pibarot P, et al: Myocardial blood flow in patients with low flow gradient aortic stenosis: differences between true and pseudo severe aortic stenosis. Results from the multicenter TOPAS study [abstract], *Circulation* 112:718, 2005.

89. Kaufmann PA, Camici PG: Myocardial blood flow measurement by PET: Technical aspects and clinical applications, *J Nucl Med* 46:75–88, 2005.

90. Naya M, Katoh C, Morita K, Tsukamoto T, et al: Olmesartan, but not amlodipine, improves endothelium-dependent coronary dilation in hypertensive patients, *J Am Coll Cardiol* 50:1144–1149, 2007.

91. Schafers KP, Camici PG, Spinks TJ, et al: Absolute quantification of myocardial blood flow with H215O and 3-dimensional PET: an experimental validation, *J Nucl Med* 43:1031–1040, 2002.

92. De Bruyne B, Baudhuin T, Melin JA, et al: Coronary flow reserve calculated from pressure measurements in humans. Validation with positron emission tomography, *Circulation* 89:1013–1022, 1994.

93. Nagamachi S, Czernin J, Kim AS, et al: Reproducibility of measurements of regional resting and hyperemic myocardial blood flow assessed with PET, *J Nucl Med* 37:1626–1631, 1996.

94. Kaufmann PA, Camici PG, Gnecchi-Ruscone T, Rimoldi O, et al: Assessment of the reproducibility of baseline and hyperemic myocardial blood flow measurements with ^{15}O-labeled water and PET, *J Nucl Med* 42:1848–1856, 1999.

95. Lortie M, Mostert K, Renaud J, et al: Myocardial blood flow quantification with Rb-82 and N-13-ammonia PET in healthy volunteers, *Can J Cardiol* 2004.

96. Yoshinaga K, Beanlands RS, deKemp RA, et al: Measurement of coronary endothelial function with rubidium-82 PET. Comparison with oxygen 15-labeled water PET, *J Nucl Med* 49(Suppl 1):75P, 2008.

97. Prior JO, Allenbach G, Valenta L, et al: Myocardial blood flow quantification using Rb-82: Validation to O-15-Water in healthy volunteer and CAD patients, *J Nucl Med* 2008. In press.

98. Uren NG, De Bruyne B, Camici PG, Melin JA: Relation between myocardial blood flow and the severity of coronary artery stenosis, *N Engl J Med* 330:1782–1788, 1994.

99. Tamaki N, Senda M, Yonekura Y, et al: Myocardial positron computed tomography with 13N-ammonia at rest and during exercise, *Eur J Nucl Med* 11:246–251, 1985.

100. Yonekura Y, Senda M, Tamaki N, et al: Detection of coronary artery disease with ^{13}N ammonia and high resolution positron-emission computed tomography, *Am Heart J* 113:645–654, 1987.

101. Tamaki N, Koide H, Saji H, Yamashita K, et al: Value and limitation of stress thallium 201 single photon emission computed tomography: comparison with nitrogen-13 ammonia positron tomography, *J Nucl Med* 29:1181–1188, 1988.

102. Gould KL, Goldstein RA, Mullani NA, et al: Noninvasive assessment of coronary stenoses by myocardial perfusion imaging during pharmacologic coronary vasodilation. VIII. Clinical feasibility of positron

cardiac imaging without a cyclotron using generator-produced rubidium-82, *J Am Coll Cardiol* 7:775–789, 1986.

103. Demer LL, Gould KL, Goldstein RA, et al: Assessment of coronary artery disease severity by positron emission tomography. Comparison with quantitative arteriography in 193 patients, *Circulation* 79:825–835, 1989.

104. Go RT, Marwick TH, MacIntyre WJ, et al: A prospective comparison of rubidium-82 PET and thallium-201 SPECT myocardial perfusion imaging utilizing a single dipyridamole stress in the diagnosis of coronary artery disease, *J Nucl Med* 31:1899–1905, 1990.

105. Stewart RE, Molina E, Popma J, Squicciarini S, et al: Comparison of rubidium-82 positron emission tomography and thallium-201 SPECT imaging for detection of coronary artery disease, *Am J Cardiol* 67:1303–1310, 1991.

106. Marwick TH, Nemec JJ, Salcedo EE, Stewart WJ: Diagnosis of coronary artery disease using exercise echocardiography and positron emission tomography: comparison and analysis of discrepant results, *J Am Soc Echocardiogr* 5:231–238, 1992.

107. Grover-McKay M, Ratib O, Schwaiger M, et al: Detection of coronary artery disease with positron emission tomography and rubidium 82, *Am Heart J* 123:646–652, 1992.

108. Laubenbacher C, Rothley J, Sitomer J, et al: An automated analysis program for the evaluation of cardiac PET studies: initial results in the detection and localization of coronary artery disease using nitrogen-13-ammonia, *J Nucl Med* 34:968–978, 1993.

109. Wallhaus TR, Lacy J, Stewart R, Stone CK, et al: Copper-62-pyruvaldehyde bis(N-methyl-thiosemicarbazone) PET imaging in the detection of coronary artery disease in humans, *J Nucl Cardiol* 8:67–74, 2001.

110. Walsh MN, Bergmann SR, Kenzora JL, Steele RL, et al: Delineation of impaired regional myocardial perfusion by positron emission tomography with $^{15}OH_2O$, *Circulation* 78:612–620, 1988.

111. Williams BR, Jansen DE, Mullani NA, et al: A retrospective study of the diagnostic accuracy of a community hospital-based PET center for the detection of coronary artery disease using rubidium-82, *J Nucl Med* 35:1586–1592, 1994.

112. Simone GL, Mullani NA, Page DA, et al: Utilization statistics and diagnostic accuracy of a nonhospital-based positron emission tomography center for the detection of coronary artery disease using rubidium-82, *Am J Physiol Imaging* 7:203–209, 1992.

113. Husmann L, Kaufmann PA, Valenta L, Wiegand M, et al: Diagnostic accuracy of myocardial perfusion imaging with single photon emission computed tomography and positron emission tomography: a comparison with coronary angiography, *Int J Cardiovasc Imaging* 2007. In press.

114. Namdar M, Hany TF, Koepfli P, et al: Integrated PET/CT for the assessment of coronary artery disease: a feasibility study, *J Nucl Med* 46:930–935, 2005.

115. Sampson UK, Di Carli MF, Dorbala S, Kwong R, et al: Diagnostic accuracy of rubidium-82 myocardial perfusion imaging with hybrid positron emission tomography/computed tomography in the detection of coronary artery disease, *J Am Coll Cardiol* 49:1052–1058, 2007.

116. Yoshinaga K, Katoh C, Noriyasu K, et al: Reduction of coronary flow reserve in areas with and without ischemia on stress perfusion imaging in patients with coronary artery disease: a study using oxygen 15-labeled water PET, *J Nucl Cardiol* 10:275–283, 2003.

117. Study of Myocardial Perfusion and Coronary Anatomy Imaging Roles in CAD (SPARC): Web page Available at: http://www.sparctrial.org.

118. Marwick TH, Go RT, Lauer MS, MacIntyre WJ, et al: Use of positron emission tomography for prediction of perioperative and late cardiac events before vascular surgery, *Am Heart J* 130:1196–1202, 1995.

119. MacIntyre WJ, Go RT, King JL, et al: Clinical outcome of cardiac patients with negative thallium-201 SPECT and positive rubidium-82 PET myocardial perfusion imaging, *J Nucl Med* 34:400–404, 1993.

120. Schächinger V, Britten M, Zeiher AM: Prognostic impact of coronary vasodilator dysfunction on adverse long-term outcome of coronary heart disease, *Circulation* 101:1899–1906, 2000.

121. Deanfield E, Halcox JP, Rabelink TJ: Contemporary reviews in cardiovascular medicine. Endothelial function and dysfunction testing and clinical relevance, *Circulation* 115:1285–1295, 2007.

122. Struijker-Boudier HA, Bruneval P, Camiri PG, Rosei A, et al: Evaluation of the microcirculation in hypertension and cardiovascular disease, *Eur Heart J* 28:2834–2840, 2007.

123. Iwado Y, Yoshinaga K, Furuyama H, et al: Decreased endothelium-dependent coronary vasomotion in healthy young smokers, *Eur J Nucl Med Mol Imaging* 29:984–990, 2002.

124. Campisi R, Czernin J, Schoder H, et al: Effects of long-term smoking on myocardial blood flow, coronary vasomotion, and vasodilator capacity, *Circulation* 98:119–125, 1998.

125. Schoder H, Campisi R, Silverman DH, et al: Effect of mental stress on myocardial blood flow and vasomotion in patients with coronary artery disease, *J Nucl Med* 41:11–16, 2000.

126. Gould KL, Nakagawa K, Parker N, et al: Frequency and clinical implications of fluid dynamically significant diffuse coronary artery disease manifest as graded, longitudinal, base-to-apex myocardial perfusion abnormalities by noninvasive positron emission tomography, *Circulation* 101:1931–1939, 2000.

127. Johnson NP, Gould KL: Clinical evaluation of a new concept: Resting myocardial perfusion heterogeneity quantified by Markovian analysis of PET identifies coronary microvascular dysfunction and early atherosclerosis in 1,034 subjects, *J Nucl Med* 46:1427–1437, 2005.

128. Dayanikli F, Grambow D, Muzik O, Schwaiger M, et al: Early detection of abnormal coronary flow reserve in asymptomatic men at high risk for coronary artery disease using positron emission tomography, *Circulation* 90:808–817, 1994.

129. Yokoyama I, Murakami T, Ohtake T, et al: Reduced coronary flow reserve in familial hypercholesterolemia, *J Nucl Med* 37:1937–1942, 1996.

130. Czernin J, Brunken R, Schelbert H, Sun K, et al: Effect of acute and long-term smoking on myocardial blood flow and flow reserve, *Circulation* 91:2891–2897, 1995.

131. Di Carli MF, Grunberger G, Janisse J, et al: Role of chronic hyperglycemia in the pathogenesis of coronary microvascular dysfunction in diabetes, *J Am Coll Cardiol* 41:1387–1393, 2003.

132. Schindler TH, Facta AD, Prior JO, Schelbert HR, et al: Improvement in coronary vascular dysfunction produced with euglycaemic control in patients with type 2 diabetes, *Heart* 93:345–349, 2007.

133. Muzik O, Beanlands RSB, Duvernoy C, Sawada S, et al: Assessment of diagnostic performance of quantitative flow measurements in normal subjects and patients with angiographically documented coronary artery disease by means of nitrogen-13 ammonia and positron emission tomography, *J Am Coll Cardiol* 31:534–540, 1998.

134. Gould KL, Hamilton GW, Lipscomb K: Physiologic basis for assessing critical coronary stenosis. Instantaneous flow response and regional distribution during coronary hyperemia as measures of coronary flow reserve, *Am J Cardiol* 33:87–94, 1974.

135. Demer LL, Goldstein RA, Gould KL, et al: Assessment of coronary artery disease severity by positron emission tomography. Comparison with quantitative arteriography in 193 patients, *Circulation* 79:825–835, 1989.

136. Seth R, deKemp RA, Hart B, Ruddy TD, et al: Quantification of absolute perfusion reserve using 82Rb positron emission tomography defines greater extent of disease in three vessel coronary atherosclerosis, *J Am Coll Cardiol* 37:387A, 2001.

137. Beanlands RS, deKemp R, Iwanochko RM, Ruddy T, et al: Positron emission tomography and recovery following revascularization (PARR-1): the importance of scar and the development of a prediction rule for the degree of recovery of left ventricular function, *J Am Coll Cardiol* 40:1735–1743, 2002.

138. Camici PG, Lorenzoni R, Marraccini P, et al: Coronary hemodynamics and myocardial metabolism in patients with syndrome X: response to pacing stress, *J Am Coll Cardiol* 17:1461–1470, 1991.

139. Knaapen P, Camici PG, Germans T, et al: Determinants of coronary microvascular dysfunction in symptomatic hypertrophic cardiomyopathy, *Am J Physiol Heart Circ Physiol* 294:H986–H993, 2008.

140. Burwash IG, Beanlands RS, deKemp RA, Lortie M, et al: Myocardial blood flow in patients with low Flow, low gradient aortic stenosis: Differences between true and pseudo-severe aortic stenosis. Results from the multicenter TOPAS (Truly or Pseudo-Severe Aortic Stenosis) Study, *Heart* In press.

141. Guethlin M, Coppenrath K, Kasel AM, Schwaiger M, Ziegler S, et al: Delayed response of myocardial flow reserve to lipid-lowering therapy with fluvastatin, *Circulation* 99:475–481, 1999.

142. Naoumova RP, Camici PG, Kindler H, et al: Pioglitazone improves myocardial blood flow and glucose utilization in nondiabetic patients with combined hyperlipidemia, *J Am Coll Cardiol* 50:2051–2058, 2007.

143. Ling MC, deKemp RA, Ruddy TD, et al: Early effects of statin therapy on endothelial function and microvascular reactivity in patients with coronary artery disease, *Am Heart J* 149(1137):e9–e16, 2005.

144. Sdringola S, Gould KL, Zamarka LG, et al: A 6 month randomized, double blind, placebo controlled, multi-center trial of high dose atorvastatin on myocardial perfusion abnormalities by positron emission tomography in coronary artery disease, *Am Heart J* 155:245–253, 2008.

145. Schneider CA, Moka D, Voth E, et al: Improvement of myocardial blood flow to ischemic regions by angiotensin-converting enzyme inhibition with quinaprilat IV: a study using [15O] water dobutamine stress positron emission tomography, *J Am Coll Cardiol* 34:1005–1011, 1999.

146. Akinboboye OO, Bergmann SR, Chou RL: Augmentation of myocardial blood flow in hypertensive heart disease by angiotensin antagonists: a comparison of lisinopril and losartan, *J Am Coll Cardiol* 40:703–709, 2002.

147. Camici PG, Crea F: Coronary microvascular dysfunction, *N Engl J Med* 356:830–840, 2007.

148. Pitkänen OP, Nuutila P, Raitakari OT, et al: Coronary flow reserve is reduced in young men with IDDM, *Diabetes* 47:248–254, 1998.

149. Di Carli MF, Ager J, Grunberger G, et al: Role of chronic hyperglycemia in the pathogenesis of coronary microvascular dysfunction in diabetes, *J Am Coll Cardiol* 41:1387–1393, 2003.

150. Yokoyama I, Momomura S, Ohtake T, et al: Reduced myocardial flow reserve in non-insulin-dependent diabetes mellitus, *J Am Coll Cardiol* 30:1472–1477, 1997.

151. Kjaer A, Meyer C, Nielsen FS, Parving HH, et al: Dipyridamole, cold pressor test, and demonstration of endothelial dysfunction: a PET study of myocardial perfusion in diabetes, *J Nucl Med* 44:19–23, 2003.

152. McMahon GT, Di Carli MF, Plutzky J, et al: Effect of a peroxisome proliferator-activated receptor agonist on myocardial blood flow in type 2 diabetes, *Diabetes Care* 28:1145–1150, 2005.

153. Sdringola S, Nakagawa K, Nakagawa Y, Gould KL, et al: Combined intense lifestyle and pharmacologic lipid treatment further reduce coronary events and myocardial perfusion abnormalities compared with usual-care cholesterol-lowering drugs in coronary artery disease, *J Am Coll Cardiol* 41:263–272, 2003.

154. van Tosh A, Garza D, Roberti R, et al: Serial myocardial perfusion imaging with dipyridamole and rubidium-82 to assess restenosis after angioplasty, *J Nucl Med* 36:1553–1560, 1995.

155. Scott NS, Beanlands RS, de Kemp R, Ruddy TD, et al: Evaluation of myocardial perfusion using rubidium-82 positron emission tomography after myocardial infarction in patients receiving primary stent implantation or thrombolytic therapy, *Am J Cardiol* 88:886–889, 2001.

156. Rechavia E, Araujo LI, De Silva R, et al: Dipyridamole vasodilator response after human orthotopic heart transplantation: quantification by oxygen-15-labeled water and positron emission tomography, *J Am Coll Cardiol* 19:100–106, 1992.

157. Chan SY, Kobashigawa J, Stevenson LW, Schelbert HR, et al: Myocardial blood flow at rest and during pharmacological vasodilation in cardiac transplants during and after successful treatment of rejection, *Circulation* 90:204–212, 1994.

158. Zanco P, Gambino A, Livi U, et al: Changes in myocardial blood flow and coronary reserve evaluated by PET early and late heart transplant, *J Nucl Med* 41:41P, 2000.

159. Knaapen P, van Campen LM, de Cock CC, et al: Effects of cardiac resynchronization therapy on myocardial perfusion reserve, *Circulation* 110:646–651, 2004.

160. Lindner O, Kammeier A, Vogt J, et al: Effect of cardiac resynchronization therapy on global and regional oxygen consumption and myocardial blood flow in patients with non-ischaemic and ischaemic cardiomyopathy, *Eur Heart J* 26:70–76, 2005.

161. Chang GY, Xie X, Wu JC: Overview of stem cells and imaging modalities for cardiovascular diseases, *J Nucl Cardiol* 13:554–569, 2006.

162. Zhou R, Acton PD, Ferrari VA: Imaging stem cells implanted in infarcted myocardium, *J Am Coll Cardiol* 48:2094–2106, 2006.

163. Bengel FM, Anton M, Richter T, et al: Noninvasive imaging of transgene expression by use of positron emission tomography in a pig model of myocardial gene transfer, *Circulation* 108:2127–2133, 2003.

164. Ruel M, Beanlands RS, deKemp RA, Lortie M, et al: Concomitant treatment with oral L-arginine improves the efficacy of surgical angiogenesis in patients with severe diffuse coronary artery disease: the Endothelial Modulation in Angiogenic Therapy randomized controlled trial, *J Thorac Cardiovasc Surg* 135:762–770, 2008.

Coronary Artery Calcification: Pathogenesis, Imaging, and Risk Stratification

SHREENIDHI VENURAJU, AJAY KUMAR YERRAMASU,
DENNIS A. GOODMAN AND AVIJIT LAHIRI

INTRODUCTION

Assessing atherosclerotic plaque burden has long been the goal of cardiologists, considering that the initial presentation of a significant percentage of previously asymptomatic patients is with myocardial infarction (MI) or sudden cardiac death.[1] Large epidemiologic studies have identified a host of "conventional" risk factors that are able to predict only about two-thirds of those patients who will eventually go on to develop coronary artery disease (CAD).[2] Nearly a third of patients dying of CAD in the United States are classified as being at low risk with the Framingham Risk Index score.[3]

It is now well known that most of the acute coronary events result from the rupture and/or erosion of non-stenotic but vulnerable plaques.[4,5] To date, invasive coronary angiography remains the gold standard for imaging the coronary arteries and intravascular ultrasonography (IVUS) is the investigation of choice to accurately assess the total atherosclerotic plaque burden and plaque morphology. With the attending risk (though small) involved with an non-invasive technique to image the coronary arteries and accurately assess the total atherosclerotic plaque burden. The exponential improvements in imaging technology in the last 2 decades, most notably the improvements in computed tomography (CT) and the rapid growth of computer technology, have made this goal a reality. There has been a plethora of articles published on the subject of detection of coronary artery calcification (CAC) using electron beam CT (EBCT) and multislice CT (MSCT) and its value in prognosis and risk

stratification, particularly in asymptomatic patients or in those patients with a low to intermediate probability of developing CAD.

TYPES OF ARTERIAL CALCIFICATION

Two distinct types of arterial calcification have been described: medial arterial calcification and calcification associated with atherosclerotic plaque.[6] These two types of calcification differ in terms of their pathophysiology, morphologic features, and clinical significance. In atherosclerotic plaque, calcium deposits are typically found in the intima. In contrast, medial calcification, also known as *Mönckeberg's sclerosis*, occurs independently of atherosclerosis. Medial arterial calcification (MAC) occurs in the small and medium sized muscular arteries. It is typically noted in the arteries of the abdominal viscera, breast and the thyroid gland. Medial calcification of the coronary arteries, though rare, has been noted in patients with advanced diabetes and/or chronic kidney disease. MAC is not associated with luminal stenosis but causes stiffening and decreased compliance of the arteries.

PATHOGENESIS OF CORONARY ARTERY CALCIFICATION

Atherosclerosis is known to be a chronic inflammatory process where various components of the immune system are implicated.[7,8] In the majority of cases, the presence of a high plasma lipid concentration fuels the process of atherosclerosis. Endothelial cells, leukocytes, and intimal smooth muscle cells, as well as other contributory factors such as smoking, hypertension, diabetes, and in some cases, high homocysteine levels, all play an important part in the process of atherosclerosis, but the exact nature of their interactions with each other is yet to be fully unraveled.

There have been different views regarding the mechanism of calcium deposition in atherosclerotic plaques.[9] Some initial theories suggest that calcification results from passive adsorption of Gla-containing proteins with a high affinity for calcium phosphate and hydroxyapatite, whose only known function is to bind calcium.[10,11] This seems unlikely in light of the fact that calcification occurs in only those vessels with atherosclerosis and is absent in normal arteries.[12] Other evidence suggests that coronary calcification is an actively regulated process rather than passive adsorption and precipitation.[13] In fact, several intriguing similarities have been noted between coronary calcification and bone formation.[14]

Calcium deposition within an atherosclerotic plaque lesion starts as early as the second decade of life, when the plaque lesion is no more than a fatty streak[15] (type III plaque lesion). When calcification becomes widespread, it is then classified as a type IV lesion, which contains granules of calcium within the smooth muscle cells and the extracellular matrix. The process of calcification starts in the damaged intracellular organelles of smooth muscle cells that subsequently become apoptotic and act as niduses of further calcification.[16] The extracellular accumulation of lipids within the plaque deep within the intima appears to be the starting point for this process.[17] The small granules of calcium fuse together to form larger deposits in the form of lumps and plates. These are progressively classified as type V, VI, and VII plaque lesions, with increasing quantities of calcium. The stages in the progression of atherosclerotic plaque have been illustrated in Figure 20-1.

Clinical Relevance of Coronary Artery Calcification

The amount of coronary calcium correlates well with the segmental atherosclerotic plaque burden[18] and is clearly illustrated in Figure 20-2. Histologic study by Rumberger et al. showed that on average, calcium represents about a fifth of the total atherosclerotic burden.[19] However, the amount of calcium does not correlate with the severity of angiographic luminal stenosis, and this is most likely due to the remodeling process, whereby there is an increase in size of the arteries, compensating for the

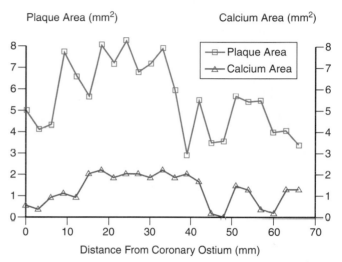

Figure 20-2 Correlation between plaque area and area of calcium in the plaque. Good correlation between the total atherosclerotic plaque area and the area of calcium within the plaque irrespective of the distance of the lesion from the ostium of the vessel. *(From Rumberger JA, Simons DB, Fitzpatrick LA, et al: Coronary artery calcium area by electron-beam computed tomography and coronary atherosclerotic plaque area. A histopathologic correlative study, Circulation 92: 2157-2162, 1995.)*

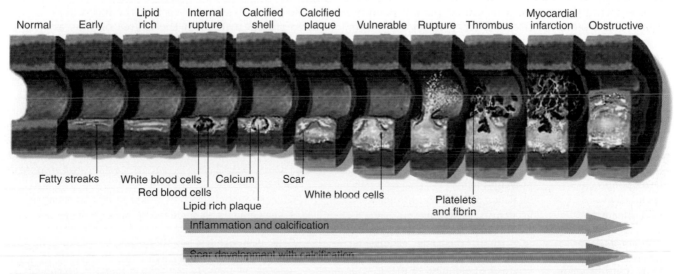

Figure 20-1 Stages in the evolution of an atherosclerotic plaque lesion. Schematic representation of different stages in the natural history of atherosclerotic plaque, progressing from fatty streak to advanced vulnerable plaque that is prone to rupture and precipitate occlusive thrombus.

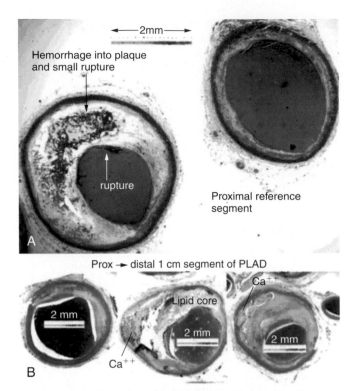

Figure 20-3 Complex plaque lesion and vessel wall remodeling. Cross-section through an atherosclerotic plaque lesion: (**A**) Overall vessel diameter is greater at the level of the lesion as a result of positive remodeling, as compared to the proximal segment, but with a much narrower lumen diameter. Lesion also indicates hemorrhage into the plaque lesion. Similarly, panel (**B**) shows changes in overall vessel diameter, luminal diameter, and degree of stenosis in a reference segment *(left)*, lipid rich plaque *(middle)*, and calcified plaque *(right)*. *(From Burke AP, Kolodgie FD, Farb A, et al: Morphological predictors of arterial remodeling in coronary atherosclerosis, Circulation 105:297-303, 2002.)*

atherosclerotic plaque (Fig. 20-3).[20] Furthermore, presence and extent of calcification do not predict the future risk of plaque rupture. In fact, there are conflicting theories regarding the effect of calcium on plaque stability. It has been suggested that calcified plaques are much stiffer and hence less likely to rupture than cellular plaques. Culprit lesions revealed by IVUS were found to contain less calcium than stable lesions,[21] lending

credibility to the notion that calcification stabilizes a plaque. There have also been studies suggesting that calcification is a result of subclinical plaque rupture, a sort of protective mechanism of the plaque, to stabilize and prevent further plaque rupture.

On the contrary, Abedin et al. suggest that the vessel is rendered less vulnerable to rupture only when extensive calcification has occurred, whereas the early stages of calcification may actually enhance plaque vulnerability.[22] It has been shown that calcified atherosclerotic plaque is at least 4 to 5 times stiffer than cellular plaque.[23] In the initial stages of calcification, plaques are most prone to rupture at areas of interface between high- and low-density tissue.[24] As the degree of calcification increases, the number of interfaces between rigid and distensible plaque initially would increase until the point at which the rigid plaques coalesce. Calcification beyond this point may be associated with decreasing risk of plaque rupture. However, further research is needed to unravel the association between calcification and plaque vulnerability.

Biochemical Factors Implicated in Coronary Calcification

Current opinion suggests that coronary artery calcification is an active process mediated by the production of ectopic bone matrix proteins by either vascular pericyte-like cells, smooth muscle cells or macrophage-derived foam cells.[25,26] Fitzpatrick and colleagues have identified the mRNA of the matrix protein Osteopontin in coronary artery specimens with calcification.[27] The bone matrix proteins implicated in the development of coronary artery calcification so far are shown in Table 20-1.

Osteoprotegerin (OPG) in particular appears to have garnered a fair share of attention. Anand and colleagues showed that OPG levels correlated significantly with increased CAC scores in a cohort of asymptomatic diabetics with an unadjusted odds ratio of 3.08 (95% CI: 2.42 to 3.92, $P < 0.001$).[28] More recently, in a very high-risk population of patients with chronic kidney disease (CKD), it was shown that the levels of OPG correlated significantly with the degree of CAC as well as survival. In a multivariate logistic regression model, OPG independently predicted all-cause mortality in CKD patients.[29]

Table 20-1 Biochemical Factors Implicated in Coronary Artery Calcification

Biomarker	Class	Action/Role
Osteopontin	Glycoprotein	Cell attachment
Osteonectin	Calcium-binding glycoprotein	Binds strongly to both hydroxyapatite and collagen
Osteocalcin	Gamma-carboxylated protein	Responsible for mineralization, only produced by osteoblasts
Osteoprotegerin	Cytokine of the tumor necrosis factor family (glycoprotein)	Osteoclastogenesis inhibitory factor, inhibiting the differentiation of macrophages into osteoclasts
Bone morphogenetic protein (BMP) 2a	Cytokine belonging to the transforming growth factor beta superfamily of proteins	Induces the pericyte-like cells to undergo osteogenic differentiation leading to production of bonelike matrix

CORONARY ARTERY CALCIUM IMAGING USING ELECTRON BEAM COMPUTED TOMOGRAPHY/MULTISLICE COMPUTED TOMOGRAPHY

Though conventional fluoroscopy was the first technique for imaging coronary artery calcification, the advent of EBCT, with its superior temporal and spatial resolution, soon became the method of choice. The guiding principle of CT scanners is the differential attenuation of x-rays passing through various tissues of the body. Unlike the conventional CT scanners, EBCT scanners do not have the disadvantage of having a mechanically rotating gantry. An electron gun shoots the electrons, which are then guided electromagnetically to tungsten target rings. The x-rays thus produced then pass through the patient and are detected on two parallel rings housed within the gantry of the scanner. Usually it takes 100 milliseconds (ms) for one sweep of the target rings. Considering that it requires 30 to 40 slices for an average 3-mm (range 1.5 to 6 mm) thickness to image the entire coronary tree, the entire heart can be imaged in 30 to 40 seconds, which is a realistic goal for one breath hold. The radiation burden and motion artifacts are reduced by prospective gating, whereby the image acquisition is triggered at 60% to 80% of the R-R interval on the ECG, corresponding to the end of diastole. The total radiation delivered during one study is approximately 0.8 to 1.3 mSv. Stable heart rate and rhythm are essential for prospective triggering during image acquisition.

Recent MSCT scanners have an isotropic resolution of 0.4 mm, although for CAC scoring, a reconstructed slice thickness of 3 mm is still usually chosen. Unlike the EBCT, MSCT scanners use a mechanically rotating gantry. The gantry speed has improved through successive scanner generations. The current state-of-the-art scanners can complete one rotation in 330 ms. Further acceleration is likely to be difficult, owing to problems in handling the huge gravitational force generated by the rapid movement of a relatively heavy gantry. The presence of the mechanical gantry makes the temporal resolution of MSCT lower than that of EBCT, except in the newer dual-source CT scanners, which have two x-ray sources and detector arrays incorporated into the gantry, allowing for a twofold improvement in temporal resolution. Images can be acquired by using either prospective or retrospective ECG gating. Retrospective gating requires the retrospective analysis of the entire data set to select the optimum cardiac phase, and also results in larger data sets. The other disadvantage of retrospectively gated image acquisition is the increase in radiation exposure, which can be reduced by ECG-gated tube current modulation (the tube current is reduced substantially during the less informative phases of cardiac cycle). Prospectively gated image acquisition reduces the radiation burden but can result in longer examination times if the heart rate is not regular. CAC scoring using MSCT confers a higher radiation burden than the EBCT scanners, and this is usually in the range of 1 to 5 mSv; however, prospective gating can reduce the radiation dose to 1 to 2 mSv.

A few studies have compared the data variability between these two imaging modalities (EBCT and MSCT scanners), and they show good correlation between the scanners in terms of accuracy and reproducibility. Knez et al. showed an excellent correlation between MSCT and EBCT for quantification of coronary calcium in 99 patients ($r = 0.994$; $P = 0.01$).[30] Becker et al. compared the two modalities in 100 patients and found a good correlation between the two types of scanners.[31]

ALGORITHMS FOR QUANTIFICATION OF CORONARY CALCIUM

Agatston Score

The calcium scoring system first described by Agatston et al.[32] in 1990 is widely used even today. They described a scoring algorithm that takes into consideration the area and density of the calcified plaque. Calcified foci within the outline of epicardial coronary arteries with a threshold area of 1 mm^2 and a threshold attenuation value of 130 Hounsfield units are scored. CAC score is calculated as maximal computed tomographic number (MCTN) multiplied by area of calcification in mm^2. The MCTN is obtained from the maximal Hounsfield intensity within the area of interest, as shown in Table 20-2. For example, if the peak x-ray density of a calcified lesion is 400 Hounsfield units, and the total area occupied is 10 mm^2, then the CAC score using this method is: $4 \times 10 = 40$ Agatston units (Au). The score for each lesion in a given patient is measured, and all the scores are added to give the total CAC score for the patient.

The Agatston method is susceptible to partial volume effects, and the reported variability of repeated EBCT scanning ranges from 22% to 49%.[33-35] In a study by Bielak et al.,[36] hyperattenuating foci less than 2 mm^2 showed less than 50% reproducibility in 256 subjects who underwent two sequential electron beam CT examinations several minutes apart. The factors mainly responsible for poor reproducibility are cardiac, respiratory, and patient motion; arrhythmias; image noise; and image gaps due to discontinuous acquisition of image data. There are a few other factors that can also

Table 20-2 Calculating Maximum Computed Tomographic Number*

Attenuation Density of Coronary Plaque (Hounsfield Units)	Maximum Computed Tomographic Number
130–200	1
201–300	2
301–400	3
>400	4

*Used in coronary artery calcium scoring using the Agatston method.

cause artifacts and difficulty in scan analysis, such as the presence of pacing or ICD wires and coronary stents.

Volume Score

One of the ways of improving reproducibility is to use volume-based calcium quantification, as reported by Callister et al.[37] An important limitation of the Agatston scoring algorithm is that it is based on the area (rather than the volume) of the calcified plaque. This means only the length and breadth of a plaque are taken into account, and the depth is ignored. Volume-based calcium quantification uses isotropic interpolation, and thus the value obtained is the volume of calcium present and not an abstract number. The absence of a Hounsfield units–dependent factor makes this system less susceptible to the effects of partial-volume averaging. This is particularly useful with the newer spiral scanners, which use overlapping image reconstruction, since the volume score is independent of the image overlap and the slice thickness used.

Detrano et al.[38] evaluated the effect of scanner type and scoring algorithm on the reproducibility of CAC measurements among the participants of the Multi-Ethnic Study of Atherosclerosis (MESA), a multicenter observational study of 6814 asymptomatic subjects. Three of the study centers used EBCT, and the other three centers used MSCT. Each participant underwent two scans 2 minutes apart. EBCT and MSCT scanners showed equivalent reproducibility for measuring coronary artery calcium. Calcium volume scores showed slightly better reproducibility compared to Agatston scores.

Mass Score

It has also been suggested that calculating absolute calcium mass is a reliable method of quantification of coronary artery calcium. If appropriate calibration is used, either with an external standard or a calibration phantom, the reliability is improved and is independent of the CT hardware or the differing scanning protocols.[39] Calcium mass is calculated as a product of lesion volume, average CT density of the lesion in Hounsfield units, and a calibration factor. These newer methods of calcium quantification are not widely being used, because there is no standardized reference database for them as yet. Since the majority of the large-scale trials have used the Agatston score, this method continues to be the clinical standard used in most centers.

The age/sex percentile rank and diagrammatic representation of the coronary arteries with CAC lesions (depicted in *black*) in a typical CAC score report is shown in Figure 20-4.

Coronary Artery Calcium Score: What Does It Mean?

Age and sex of a patient play an important role in determining the prevalence and extent of CAC. In both the sexes, prevalence of CAC increases with age.[40] CAC scores vary greatly, so even in subjects of similar age groups, an age/sex nomogram is required to standardize

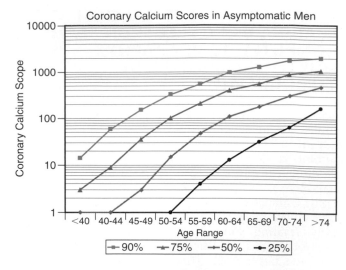

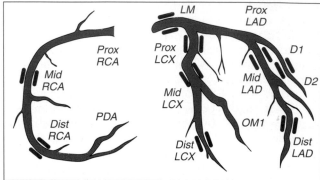

Figure 20-4 Typical coronary artery calcification (CAC) report. **A,** The CAC scores obtained are plotted on this age- and sex-specific nomogram, with CAC scores divided by quartiles. The *red star* represents the percentile rank for this particular patient. This example has been generated by the TeraRecon (San Mateo, California) workstation. **B,** Diagrammatic representation of distribution of calcium in the coronary arteries.

an individual patient value against that of a matched population—or in essence, to suggest a "coronary age."[41,42] Hoff et al. analyzed 35,246 self-referred, predominantly white, asymptomatic subjects between the ages of 30 and 90 years and categorized them according to percentiles.[43] The total CAC scores in this study group were decidedly non-Gaussian. The age/sex nomogram generated from this study is particularly useful in the risk stratification of individuals, depending on their CAC scores. For example, a calcium score of 15 Au in a male subject younger than 40 years of age, though not alarming in itself, places him above the 90th percentile when ranked with the nomogram. From these data, it is also clear that CAC measured in men is similar to the scores measured in women who are 15 years older.

However, a recent study by Budoff and colleagues[44] demonstrated that absolute CAC score groups were a better predictor of incident CHD events than age/sex and ethnicity-based percentile rank in the MESA cohort of patients. This is clearly illustrated in Figure 20-5. The Kaplan-Meier curves based on absolute CAC scores appear to have a better separation than those based on age-sex-race/ethnicity percentile ranks, indicative of better risk

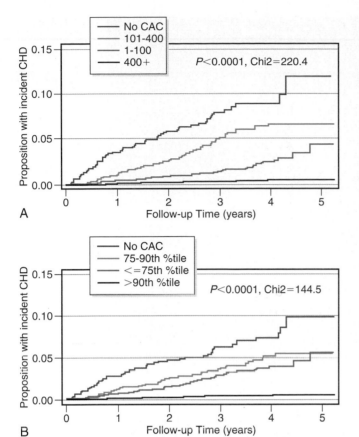

Figure 20-5 Incident coronary artery disease (CAD) events with different categories of coronary artery calcification (CAC). The Kaplan-Meier curves for absolute CAC categories (**A**) offer more separation, indicating better risk-stratifying ability compared to the curves for CAC categories based on age-sex-ethnicity percentile rank (**B**). (*From Budoff MJ, Nasir K, McClelland RL, et al. Coronary artery calcium predicts coronary events better with absolute calcium scores than age-sex-race/ethnicity percentiles: (MESA) Multi Ethnic Study of Atherosclerosis, J Am Coll Cardiol 53:345-352, 2009.*)

stratification capability in the short term. What this suggests is that patients in the lower absolute CAC score group are at low risk of CHD events irrespective of their age-sex-race/ethnicity percentile rank. This appears to be true for prediction of obstructive CAD as well in both asymptomatic and symptomatic patients.[45]

Severity of CAC score is arbitrarily classified as minimal, mild, moderate, severe, and extensive based on the absolute score, as shown in Table 20-3. Snapshots

Table 20-3 Categories of Coronary Artery Calcification

CAC Score (Agatston Units)	Coronary Calcification Category
0	Absent
1–10	Minimal
11–100	Mild
101–400	Moderate
401–1000	Severe
>1000	Extensive

of the varying degrees of severity of CAC score in a typical scan are clearly illustrated in Figure 20-6.

ROLE OF CAC IMAGING IN RISK STRATIFICATION

The Significance of Risk Stratification in Coronary Artery Disease

In approximately 50% of patients with newly diagnosed CAD, the first presentation is either MI or sudden cardiac death.[1] Nearly half a million sudden deaths occur in the United States each year, and approximately 70% of them are due to CAD.[46] Although the overall mortality of cardiovascular diseases has decreased in the United States, mortality due to SCD has remained largely unchanged.[47] Conventional cardiovascular risk factors account for a large proportion of CAD burden[48]; early identification and timely intervention to lower risk in asymptomatic individuals could prevent or postpone a majority of CAD events.[49] Risk stratification is an important initial step in the clinical management of cardiovascular risk factors. Risk stratification should start with simple evaluation of clinical risk markers, including age, sex, history of hypertension, diabetes, smoking, hypercholesterolemia, and family history of premature cardiovascular disease. Commonly used risk algorithms include the Framingham Risk Score (FRS),[50] PROCAM score,[51] or the European risk prediction system called *SCORE*[52] (systemic cardiovascular risk evaluation). These risk scores predict the 10-year absolute risk of cardiovascular events and are helpful in selecting the most appropriate candidates for risk-reduction treatments. Such office-based, clinically derived risk scores, though practical, inexpensive, and easy to calculate, have significant limitations[53] and are not uniformly applicable in different populations.[54-57] CAC imaging, by virtue of its ability to detect and accurately quantify subclinical atherosclerosis in coronary arteries, offers promise to refine the current risk stratification strategies.

Correlation Between Coronary Artery Calcium and Conventional Cardiovascular Risk Factors

The prevalence of coronary calcification is significantly higher in subjects with traditional cardiovascular risk factors such as hypertension, diabetes, obesity, infrequent exercise, previous smoking, and hypercholesterolemia.[58] There was a significant, continuous graded relationship between prevalence of coronary calcium, mean CAC scores, and the number of risk factors. The prevalence of CAC deposits was 40% in asymptomatic men aged younger than 60 years with no risk factors, as opposed to 74% in those with three or more risk factors. However, in older men (>60 years of age), the prevalence of CAC deposits was more than 80% regardless of the number of risk factors present. Multiple logistic regression analysis showed age (relative risk [RR] = 2.82 per 10 years), female gender (RR = 0.34),

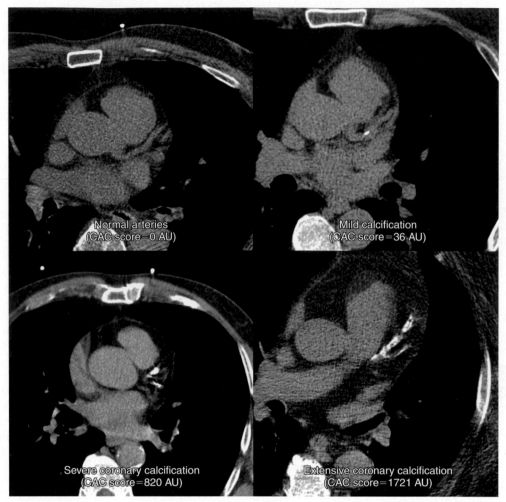

Figure 20-6 Severity of coronary artery calcification. *Clockwise from top left;* calcium score of 0, mild calcification in proximal LAD with a CAC score of 36 Au, severe calcification in proximal LAD and LCX with a CAC score of 820 Au, and extensive calcification in proximal LAD and diagonal with a CAC score of 1720 Au. Au, agatson units; CAC, coronary artery calcification; LAD, left anterior descending; LCX, left circumflex.

history of hypertension (RR = 1.53), diabetes (RR = 2.32), obesity (RR = 2.22), and hypercholesterolemia (RR = 1.63) to be significant independent predictors of the presence of coronary calcium. In a recent study, Parikh et al.[59] performed CAC measurements in the second- and third-generation descendents of original Framingham cohorts and showed that parental premature cardiovascular disease was associated with a significantly high likelihood of coronary calcification in the offspring, after adjustment for other cardiovascular risk factors.

The Coronary Artery Risk Development in Young Adults (CARDIA) Study[60] observed the effect of cardiovascular risk factors in young adults on subsequent development of coronary calcification. The study involved over 3000 adults, aged between 18 and 30 years, who underwent risk assessment at years 0, 3, 5, 7, 10, and 15, followed by CAC measurement in year 15. Individuals with above-average baseline risk were significantly more likely to develop coronary atherosclerosis as indicated by the presence of CAC, underscoring the importance of risk assessment in younger individuals.

Who Should Undergo CAC Screening?

The fundamental principle of preventive cardiology is that the intensity of risk-reduction measures should match the baseline risk of disease,[61] so that the benefits of intervention outweigh the risks. Accordingly, the National Cholesterol Educational Programme (NCEP) Expert Panel[62] recommends that individuals with multiple cardiovascular risk factors that confer a CAD risk greater than 20% in 10 years should be targeted for intensive lipid-lowering therapy, with a target LDL cholesterol level of under 100 mg/dL, similar to those with established CAD or CAD risk equivalents such as diabetes, peripheral artery disease, and symptomatic carotid artery disease. Hence, high-risk individuals should be targeted for aggressive risk-reduction measures without need for additional risk assessment tests. At the other end of the spectrum, in low-risk individuals (10-year absolute CAD risk < 10%), the likelihood of adverse cardiovascular events is too low to justify any interventions beyond simple lifestyle changes.

In individuals at intermediate risk, it is difficult to make decisions regarding the administration of

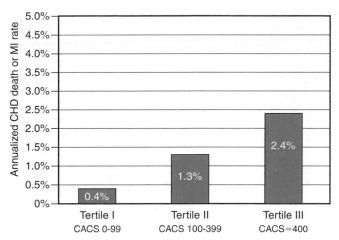

Figure 20-7 Independent and incremental prognostic value of CAC score in intermediate Framingham risk patients. Annual CAD death/MI rates shown by tertile of the Agatston score in patients at intermediate CAD event risk using definitions of an intermediate Framingham Risk Score (FRS) of greater than 1 cardiac risk factor. CAC, coronary artery calcification; CAD, coronary artery disease; MI, myocardial infarction. *(Reproduced from Greenland P, Bonow RO, Brundage BH, et al: ACCF/AHA 2007 Clinical Expert Consensus document on coronary artery calcium scoring by computed tomography in global cardiovascular risk assessment and in evaluation of patients with chest pain: A report of the American College of Cardiology Foundation Clinical Expert Consensus Task Force, J Am Coll Cardiol 49:378-402, 2007.)*

risk-reduction treatments. Subclinical disease markers such as CAC imaging are most likely to be effective in this group by reclassifying them into either low- or high-risk groups, thereby influencing management decisions. In a prospective observational study,[63] Greenland et al. demonstrated that asymptomatic individuals at intermediate risk according to Framingham criteria but with CAC scores above 300 had an annualized hard cardiac event rate of 2.8% (10-year absolute risk > 20%) and therefore would have to be reclassified as high-risk patients. This information would then mandate a more intensive approach to modification of risk factors, including goals for reducing LDL cholesterol. Furthermore, in low-risk (<10% over 10 years) and high-risk (>20% over 10 years) individuals, CAC measurements did not change the risk prediction substantially enough to alter their prognosis and clinical management.

As a caveat, estimation of lifetime risk of cardiovascular disease (CVD) should be considered as an adjunct to 10-year risk calculation in adults younger than 50 years of age. A significant percentage of adults younger than 50 are placed in the low-risk category for developing CVD over a 10-year period, despite a high lifetime risk of developing CVD. Estimation of lifetime risk for CVD has been elucidated by Lloyd-Jones et al. previously.[64] Berry et al.[65] studied 2988 subjects aged younger than 50 years at study entry into the MESA cohort and at year 15 of follow-up of the CARDIA trial, respectively, and divided them into three distinct groups. The first group was composed of subjects with low (<10%) 10-year risk of CVD and low lifetime risk (<39%) of developing CVD, the second group was composed of subjects with

low 10-year risk but high lifetime risk (>39%) for CVD, and finally those with high 10-year risk or diagnosed diabetes mellitus (DM). In the cohort of subjects with low 10-year risk of CVD, those with a high lifetime risk had a significantly higher prevalence of CAC in men and women, as well as greater carotid intima media thickness. Subjects with a higher lifetime risk also showed greater CAC progression than those with lower lifetime risk. This was true for subjects in both the CARDIA and the MESA trials.

The ACC/AHA expert committee task force analysis[66] of intermediate FRS patients from four studies[63,67–69] reported annual CAD death/MI rates of 0.4%, 1.3%, and 2.5% for CAC score categories of less than 100, 100 to 400, and =400, respectively. This is illustrated in Figure 20-7 and reflects the discriminatory ability of CAC in this important intermediate-risk group, which represents a third of the U.S. population aged 60 years or older, according to data from the third National Health and Nutrition Examination Survey (NHANES III).[70]

THE PROGNOSTIC VALUE OF CAC: AVAILABLE EVIDENCE

A screening test should add to the prognostic information provided by the clinical and demographic data, and the test should be readily available and affordable. This additional prognostic value can be quantified statistically as the increase in the area under the curve of the receiver operating characteristic (ROC), also expressed as C-statistic, after the addition of a new test result. In the past decade, several studies reported on the independent and incremental prognostic value of CAC measurement for the prediction of CAD events in univariable and multivariable models containing data from measured or reported risk factors and CRP measurements.

A meta-analysis[71] of 4 studies[72–75] showed that CAC scores remained predictive of coronary events, even after adjustment for established cardiovascular risk factors. The event rates in individuals with even mild coronary calcification (CAC scores of 1 to 100) were twice as high compared to those with no detectable coronary calcium (RR = 2.1). CAC scores over 400 were associated with very high relative risks (RR = 4.3 to 17) after adjustment for age, sex, and other cardiovascular risk. However, the meta-analysis showed a significant heterogeneity in the quality of these studies, most of which used self-reported or historical as opposed to measured risk factor data and did not use blinded outcome adjudication, which could have overestimated the predictive accuracy of CAC measurements. Selection bias was also an issue, since most of these studies recruited self-referred or physician-referred individuals, who are not necessarily representative of the general population. Furthermore, earlier studies included "soft" endpoints, including coronary revascularization, which could have overestimated the predictive ability of CAC, since CAC results per se could influence the decision to undertake revascularization.

More recent studies have focused on the prediction of "hard" cardiac events (myocardial infarction, CAD death) and are less likely to be subjective. One such study conducted by Ostrom and colleagues[76] included 2538 consecutive patients referred for CT coronary angiography. Correlation of mortality and absolute CAC score groups (1 to 9, 10 to 99, 100 to 399 and > 400) was assessed in the 1060 patients diagnosed with non-obstructive CAD. The survival rates for different CAC score groups over a follow-up period of 78 ± 12 months were 99.2%, 99%, 96.9%, and 96.1%, respectively. The risk factor adjusted RR of 5.1 ($P = 0.003$) and 6.2 ($P = 0.001$) for CAC scores of 100 to 399 and over 400, respectively, elegantly demonstrated the independent and incremental value of the CAC score.

A recent meta-analysis reported as part of the ACC/AHA 2007 Expert Consensus statement[66] on CAC imaging included six studies[63,67-69,77,78] published between 2003 and 2005, involving a total of 27,622 patients with 395 hard cardiac events. CAC score of zero was associated with a very low risk (0.4%; 49 events in 11,815 individuals) of CAD death or MI over 3 to 5 years of observation, and presence of *any detectable coronary calcium* increased the risk fourfold ($P < 0.0001$). The summary RR increased significantly in those with more severe coronary calcification (7.2 for CAC score of 400 to 1000, and 10.8 for CAC scores >1000, compared to zero CAC score), establishing a continuous graded relationship between CAC scores and risk of coronary events.

A subsequent large observational study[79] published in 2007 evaluated the effect of CAC on all-cause mortality in a cohort of 25,253 patients followed for 6.8 ± 3 years. The study conclusively established the independent and incremental prognostic ability of CAC to predict all-cause mortality. The 10-year cumulative survival was 99.4% for a CAC score of zero and reduced to 87.8% for a score of over 1000 ($P < 0.0001$) (Fig. 20-8). ROC analysis showed a significant increase in the area under the curve when CAC score was added to risk factors and age. The improved strength and quality of available evidence were enough for the 2007 Expert Consensus Committee of the AHA/ACC to recommend CAC imaging as a reasonable choice for refining the risk stratification in asymptomatic individuals with intermediate Framingham Risk Score,[66] which is a significant change from the earlier recommendation made in 2000 by the same body.[80]

Limitations of CAC Imaging as a Screening Tool in the General Population

For a screening program to be successful, both the disease to be screened and the screening test should satisfy certain criteria.[81] The disease should be of considerable public health importance and should have a prolonged latent, preclinical stage, and early identification of preclinical patients should lead to treatments that can reduce the risk of subsequent adverse clinical events. The screening test should be practical, safe, acceptable, available, and affordable, and should accurately differentiate between high-risk and low-risk patients. CAD remains the most deadly and the also most expensive disease in most industrialized nations. Autopsy studies[82] showed atherosclerotic lesions in men in their 20s and

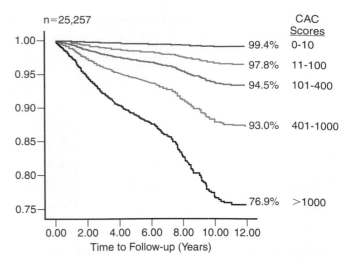

Figure 20-8 Survival rates in subjects in progressive quintiles of coronary artery calcification (CAC) scores. The graph shows progressively significant differences in survival rates in quintiles of CAC scores (<10, 11-100, 101-400, 401-1000, and >1000) after 12 years of follow-up. The increased separation of the curves elucidates the significant survival predictive ability of CAC. (*From Budoff MJ, Shaw LJ, Liu ST, et al: Long-term prognosis associated with coronary calcification: Observations from a registry of 25,253 patients, J Am Coll Cardiol 49:1860-1870, 2007.*)

30s, indicating a long subclinical asymptomatic stage. Studies have consistently shown that institution of aggressive risk-reduction treatments in high-risk asymptomatic individuals is associated with a significant reduction in mortality and morbidity. Although CAD appears to be an ideal disease for screening, CAC imaging as a universal screening test for CAD has certain limitations.

Although CAC imaging is a safe, noninvasive test and generally acceptable, currently its availability is limited, especially outside the United States. The current cost of a CAC scan (approximately $500 per scan)[83] makes it a relatively expensive test for screening the general population. Also, it involves exposure to radiation, which, though very low for an individual patient, might have consequences when applied in the general population.[84] Perhaps the most important limitation for CAC screening is its limited ability to accurately differentiate between individuals who are likely to have events from those who will not.[85] In most of the outcome analysis studies performed to date, in spite of the positive correlation between CAC scores and likelihood of events, 85% to 95% of those with high CAC scores remained event free over 2 to 7 years of follow-up, and absence of coronary calcium did not always preclude events.[86] Calcium is just one of the components of the atherosclerotic plaque and tends to develop late in the natural course of an individual plaque. Thus a CAC score of zero, though it may indicate a low risk of coronary events, by no means excludes the possibility of acute coronary events, since such events can result from the rupture of plaques that have not yet calcified or accumulated enough calcium to exceed the threshold for detection by Agatston method. The study by Cheng and colleagues[87] showed that 6.5% of patients with zero CAC had evidence of noncalcified coronary plaque on

CT angiography, though only a small minority (0.5%) had evidence of significant (= 50%) luminal stenosis.

When individuals were stratified according to FRS, CAC results did not cause substantial change in treatment targets in low- and high-risk groups.[63] Also, there are no prospective data to show that the use of CAC screening can reduce CAD-associated mortality and morbidity. Therefore, even after a cumulative experience of nearly 400,000 patient years of observation in various prospective and observational studies, CAC is not approved as a screening tool for CAD in the general population, unlike other established screening strategies for abdominal aortic aneurysm,[88] colon cancer, and breast cancer.[89,90]

Role of CAC Imaging in the Diagnosis of CAD in Symptomatic Patients

Several studies evaluating the role of CAC imaging in the diagnosis of symptomatic patients with suspected CAD reported reasonable diagnostic accuracy, with the cutoff CAC score chosen in a particular study determining the relative sensitivity and specificity. The 2000 ACC/AHA Expert Consensus document[80] on EBCT reported a meta-analysis of 16 studies[32,36,91-104] published before 1999, involving a total of 3683 patients without prior CAD who underwent EBCT and diagnostic angiography. The weighted average sensitivity and specificity were 80.4% and 39.9%, respectively. For non-zero CAC scores, the summary odds of having significant obstructive CAD elevated 20-fold. However, there was heterogeneity in the included studies in terms of the use coronary calcium score thresholds, patient entry criteria, and angiographic stenosis thresholds to define significant obstructive CAD. Subsequent studies established the ability of CAC scoring to improve diagnostic discrimination over conventional risk factors in the identification of patients with angiographic coronary disease.[105-110]

Haberl et al. studied 1764 patients with suspected CAD from a single center.[107] CAC score greater than 0 Au had very high sensitivity (99% in men and 100% in women) and negative predictive value (97% in men and 100% in women) in detecting the equivalent of 50% angiographic stenosis. However, the specificity was poor (23% in men and 40% in women), and the positive predictive value was moderate (62% in men and 66% in women). Importantly, in the absence of detectable coronary calcium, angiographically significant stenosis was a rare finding, even in the presence of symptoms (n = 5, of whom only 2 patients needed intervention). There was no evidence of coronary calcium in 11% of men and 22% of women with high pretest probability of CAD. Calcium scoring can therefore identify a subset of patients with a very low risk of significant CAD in whom invasive diagnostic procedures may be omitted; it can thus act as a potential gatekeeper before more invasive tests. In another large multicenter trial, Budoff and colleagues evaluated 1851 patients who underwent angiography for clinical indications.[108] The overall sensitivity and specificity of non-zero CAC score to predict obstructive CAD were 95% and 40%, respectively. Increasing the cutoff CAC score to 20, 80,

and 100 Au decreased the sensitivity to 90%, 79%, and 76%, whereas the specificity increased to 58%, 72%, and 75%, respectively. CAC scores demonstrated independent and incremental power to predict obstructive CAD when added to age and sex (area under the curve increased from 0.67 to 0.84; $P < 0.001$). CAC scores, when added to clinically derived pretest probabilities, dramatically changed the posttest probability of obstructive coronary disease across a wide range of patients; the greatest change was noted in patients with intermediate (20% to 70%) pretest probabilities. These earlier studies were subjected to verification bias, which could increase sensitivity and reduce specificity.

In a more recent large, angiographically correlated study[109] involving 2115 symptomatic patients, Knez et al. used volumetric calcium scores for prediction of obstructive CAD. In symptomatic patients with no detectable coronary calcium, the likelihood of angiographic stenosis was very low (<1%). Similar to the previous studies, this finding reinforces the reliability of a calcium score of zero to essentially rule out obstructive disease in symptomatic subjects. The presence of any calcium was highly sensitive (99%) for diagnosis of obstructive coronary disease, but the high sensitivity was achieved at the expense of a high percentage of false-positive results and a low specificity (28%), which may lead to unnecessary additional investigations; hence, the use of calcium score percentiles was suggested. For CAC equal to 75%, the overall predictive accuracy was 80% to 82%, which is comparable to stress echocardiography and scintigraphy.

Keelan et al. followed 288 symptomatic patients who underwent EBCT and coronary angiography within 4 weeks of each other, for a mean duration of 6.9 years.[110] Only 1 of the 87 patients in this cohort with a CAC score less than 20 Au experienced a hard coronary event, in spite of the presence of symptoms (the patient also had a normal coronary angiogram). In the stepwise Cox proportional hazards model that included risk factors, CAD event history, CAC scores, and angiographic measures of disease, only age and CAC scores were predictive of hard coronary events (risk ratios 1.72 and 1.88, respectively; $P < 0.05$). CAC scores provided more prognostic information than angiography in symptomatic patients. Although regarded as the gold-standard investigation for diagnosis of obstructive CAD, the angiogram is essentially a "lumenogram" and provides no information on plaque burden or the likelihood of vulnerable plaque.[111] Budoff et al. evaluated the ability of EBCT to noninvasively differentiate between ischemic and nonischemic etiologies of cardiomyopathy.[112] EBCT was performed within 3 months of coronary angiography in 125 patients with cardiomyopathy. EBCT-derived CAC measurements were 99% sensitive and 83% specific in detecting an ischemic etiology.

From the available evidence, it is tempting to conclude that in patients with typical angina and/or a definite evidence of myocardial ischemia on conventional stress tests, there is no indication for EBCT calcium screening because of the extremely high pretest likelihood of significant stenosis. However, in patients with atypical chest pain, calcium scoring—in view of its high negative predictive value—can act as a potential filter to reduce the number of invasive procedures that do not lead to intervention. Being a fast, safe, highly reproducible, and operator-independent test, CAC imaging is particularly appealing for this purpose.

COMPARISON OF CAC WITH OTHER DIAGNOSTIC TESTS

To secure its place in the diagnostic armamentarium of a cardiologist, CAC imaging should prove its cost and clinical effectiveness in comparison to other diagnostic tests that are well established and readily available. Earlier studies comparing EBCT with stress electrocardiography (ECG) and scintigraphy indicated that CAC scores were at least as good if not better in predicting angiographically confirmed obstructive coronary disease.[113,114] The anatomic information obtained by CAC imaging can complement the functional information from stress testing and improve the overall diagnostic accuracy for obstructive CAD.

CAC and Stress Electrocardiography

The clinical advantage of CAC imaging lies in its remarkably high negative predictive value.[107–110] In the study by Lamont et al.,[115] the absence of coronary calcium in symptomatic patients with abnormal stress ECG result correlated very well with the absence of obstructive CAD. Only 2 out of 112 patients with angiographic CAD had a zero CAC score. Thus the absence of coronary calcium by EBCT in symptomatic patients with a positive stress ECG test accurately identified those with a false-positive treadmill test. In a similar study by Shavelle et al.,[113] when stress ECG results were combined with CAC scores, the specificity of stress ECG increased from 47% to 83% ($P < 0.005$). The relative risk of obstructive angiographic CAD for an abnormal test was higher for EBCT (RR = 4.53) than either stress ECG (RR = 1.72) or stress single-photon emission computed tomography (SPECT) (RR = 1.96). The study by Schmermund et al.[116] showed that addition of CAC result was most beneficial in patients with equivocal stress ECG due to either inadequate exercise or nondiagnostic ECG changes. When CAC scores were added to a negative or equivocal stress ECG result, 84% of false-negative results were correctly classified as having obstructive CAD.

CAC and Myocardial Perfusion Scintigraphy: Role of Synergistic Imaging

For over 3 decades, myocardial perfusion scintigraphy (MPS) by SPECT has been extensively validated for the diagnosis of patients with suspected CAD, and has played a key role in formulating management decisions regarding revascularization or medical therapy in symptomatic patients with established obstructive CAD.[117–124] Attempts have been made to integrate a newer, evolving technology such as CAC imaging with SPECT in investigating patients with suspected or known CAD. Berman et al.[125] observed the relationship between CAC scores and stress MPS results in 1195 individuals who underwent both these tests within 7.2 + 44.8 days of each other. While only 2% of patients with CAC scores under 100 Au had evidence of ischemia on MPS, 20% of those with CAC scores over 1000 Au had ischemic MPS, indicating significant relationship between these two clinical markers of atherosclerosis and ischemia, respectively. This relationship is elucidated in (Figure 20-9). After multivariable logistic regression analysis, CAC score was found to be the most potent predictor of ischemia. However, 56% of all normal MPS results were noted in those with significant subclinical atherosclerosis, as indicated by CAC score over 100 Au. Furthermore, even among patients with CAC score over 1000 Au, 85% of asymptomatic and 68% of symptomatic individuals had normal MPS.

In another study to assess the predictive ability of CAC score for the presence of ischemia, Schenker et al.[126] looked at 621 patients who had no known CAD but were clinically referred to have a PET scan. The frequency of myocardial ischemia showed significant correlation with the severity of coronary calcification; patients with CAC over 400 Au were more likely to have an abnormal scan than those with CAC 1 to 399 Au (48.5% compared to 21.7%; $P < 0.001$) (Fig. 20-10). But what was interesting was that even in patients with a zero CAC score, 16% had abnormal scans. At the other end of the spectrum, in patients with a CAC score over 1000 Au, 50.6% had a normal perfusion scan. In the same study, CAC score was found to be strongly predictive of survival in patients with abnormal PET scans and also in those with normal scans. In the presence of a normal PET scan, annualized event rates in patients with a CAC score over 1000 Au and those with no CAC were 12.3% and 2.6%, respectively. Similarly, in those patients with demonstrable ischemia on PET scan, CAC scores of over 1000 Au and under 1000 Au were associated with annualized event rates of 22.1% and 8.1%, respectively.

This disparity between CAC and MPS results reflects the fundamental difference in the nature of information provided by these two tests. Coronary calcium allows detection of atherosclerotic lesions, both obstructive and nonobstructive. Secondary to expansive remodeling of the vessel wall, a considerable amount of plaque can accumulate before luminal encroachment starts. Stress scintigraphy (as with all stress imaging methods), in contrast, requires the presence of a hemodynamically significant obstructive lesion, either fixed or dynamic, before an abnormality becomes evident. The study by Ramakrishna et al.[127] also showed a weak correlation between CAC scores and summed stress scores by SPECT; however, the two tests were complementary in predicting mortality. CAC and MPS appear to have different but complementary roles in risk prediction and diagnosis. While MPS is an excellent tool for predicting short-term risk, thereby guiding decisions regarding revascularization, CAC is a better predictor of long-term risk and hence more useful in the determination of the need for aggressive medical prevention measures. Absence of ischemia on MPS is associated with a low short-term risk of coronary events, even when the CAC scores are high (>1000 Au).[128]

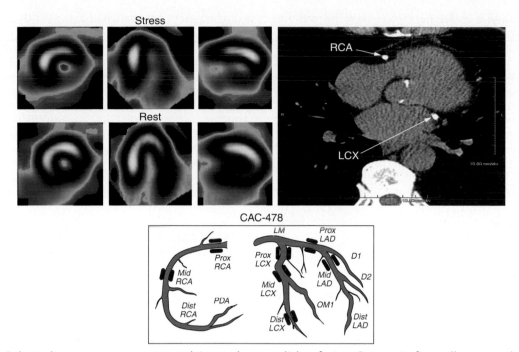

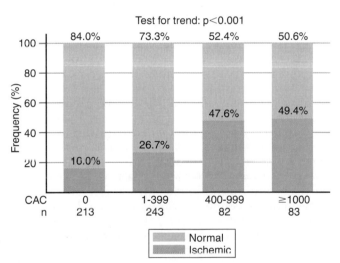

Figure 20-9 Relation between coronary artery calcium and myocardial perfusion. Composite figure illustrating the advantage of a sequential screening approach, with initial coronary artery calcification (CAC) imaging followed by myocardial perfusion scan if the CAC score is high. These are the scans of a 44-year-old asymptomatic man. On the *right* is a diagrammatic representation of the CAC score as well as an actual image of his CAC scan showing calcification in the right coronary and left circumflex arteries. On the *left* is an image of this patient's myocardial perfusion scan showing extensive reversible ischemia.

Figure 20-10 Increasing CAC score predicts myocardial ischemia with PET. Bar graph demonstrates increasing frequency of myocardial ischemia with PET, with progressively increasing absolute CAC score categories. CAC, coronary artery calcification; PET, positron emission tomography. *(From Schenker MP, Dorbala S, Hong ECT, et al. Interrelation of coronary calcification, myocardial ischemia, and outcomes in patients with intermediate likelihood of coronary artery disease: A combined positron emission tomography/computed tomography study, Circulation 117:1693-1700, 2008.)*

The high sensitivity and negative predictive value of CAC scoring can be combined with relatively high specificity and positive predictive value of MPS to achieve high overall diagnostic accuracy. CAC scores less than 100 Au are typically associated with a low probability

(> 2%) of abnormal perfusion on nuclear stress tests[125] and less than 3% probability of significant obstruction on cardiac catheterization.[107–108] He et al.[129] evaluated the relationship between the severity of coronary calcification and stress-induced myocardial ischemia in a large cohort of asymptomatic subjects with risk factors for CAD. CAC score was the best predictor of an abnormal SPECT. Nearly half of those with scores over 400 Au had evidence of ischemia, compared to only 6.6% of those with scores under 400 Au.

In the study by Anand et al.,[130] CAC imaging and MPS were synergistic for the prediction of short-term cardiovascular events in 510 asymptomatic diabetic subjects without prior cardiovascular disease. Those with CAC scores over 100 Au (n = 127) and a random sample of the remaining participants with a CAC score of 100 Au (n = 53) underwent MPS and were followed up. In the multivariable model, CAC score was the only predictor of myocardial perfusion abnormality ($P < 0.001$); CAC score and extent of myocardial ischemia were the only independent predictors of outcome. Twenty cardiovascular events were noted over a median follow-up of 2.2 years, of which 15 were in those with CAC score over 400 Au, and no events were noted in those with scores less than 10 Au. The CAC score predicted events more accurately than the UKPDS (UK Prospective Diabetes Study) and Framingham Risk Scores (area under the curves were 0.92, 0.74, and 0.60 for CAC, UKPDS, and FRS, respectively; $P < 0.0001$). In a similar study by Wong et al.,[131] CAC scores below 100 Au were associated with a very low risk (<3%) of ischemic MPS, even in patients with metabolic syndrome and diabetes. The strong and independent relationship between CAC scores and ischemic MPS persisted, even in patients receiving comprehensive medical therapy with adequate control of risk factors.[132]

In view of this association between the presence of CAC, especially above a threshold value of 400 Au, and abnormal myocardial perfusion study in a wide variety of populations, a sequential screening approach with initial CAC scoring followed by MPS in those with high CAC scores was suggested for maximizing the yield of MPS and improving cost-effectiveness.[133] Using CAC imaging prior to MPS seems logical from a pathophysiologic point of view as well, since the development of coronary atherosclerosis almost always precedes the onset of myocardial ischemia in the ischemic cascade. The incremental value of an integrated approach is clearly shown in Figure 20-11.

CAC and Other Stress Tests

CAC scores also showed a weak but statistically significant correlation with wall-motion abnormalities on stress echocardiography.[134] The proportion of patients with abnormal exercise Wall Motion Score Index (WMSI) was higher with increasing CAC scores; but even in patients with severe coronary calcification, the majority of patients had a normal WMSI. Symptoms, age, and CAC score were independently associated with abnormal exercise WMSI. More recently, Wang et al. explored the correlation between CAC scores and myocardial perfusion reserve in a subgroup of MESA cohorts

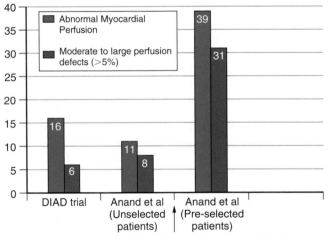

Figure 20-11 Preselection of asymptomatic diabetic subjects by electron beam computed tomography improves the yield of perfusion abnormalities detected by myocardial perfusion imaging. *Left,* Myocardial perfusion imaging was performed in asymptomatic diabetic subjects (n = 522) in the DIAD study. In the study of Anand et al,[130] myocardial perfusion imaging was performed in asymptomatic diabetic subjects with coronary artery calcium scores of greater than 100: unselected patients (*middle*) and patients selected based on electron beam computed tomography (coronary calcium scores >100 Agatston units) (*right*). (Reproduced from Wackers FJ, Young LH, Inzucchi SE, et al: Detection of silent myocardial ischemia in asymptomatic diabetic subjects: The DIAD Study, Diabetes Care 27:1954-1961, 2004; and Lim E, Lahiri A: The importance of the link between coronary artery calcification and myocardial ischemia: A developing argument, J Nucl Cardiol 14:272-274, 2007.)

using magnetic resonance imaging (MRI) at rest and during adenosine-induced hyperemia.[135] Higher CAC scores were associated with low myocardial perfusion reserve independent of the coronary risk factors. The study suggests that subclinical coronary atherosclerosis can impair coronary vasoreactivity and myocardial perfusion reserve in the absence of clinical CAD. Another study using CAC measurements and tagged MRI showed a positive correlation between subclinical atherosclerosis, as indicated by CAC score in a particular coronary artery, and subclinical regional ventricular dysfunction, as indicated by myocardial strain and strain rate in the corresponding perfusion territory.[136]

PROPOSED ALGORITHM FOR SEQUENTIAL SCREENING

Based on the available evidence, a diagnostic algorithm was proposed for assessing patients at risk of CAD and those with atypical symptoms (Fig. 20-12).[133] CAC scoring can be used in those subjects assessed to be at intermediate or high risk after an initial clinical evaluation using established risk-assessment systems such as FRS. In individuals with CAC scores above 400 Au, the frequency of ischemia is usually substantial, and MPS is thus likely to be cost-effective. This threshold could be lowered perhaps to 200 Au in diabetic subjects, but more data are required before an exact cutoff value can be agreed upon. In individuals with CAC scores in the intermediate range of 100 to 400 Au, the need for MPS should be determined on the basis of overall risk profile and the likelihood of CAD. The severity of perfusion abnormality on MPS determines the need for angiography. When less than 10% of the myocardium is involved, optimum medical therapy was shown to be better than revascularization; hence, coronary angiography can be avoided in these patients. Patients with more extensive ischemia (>10% myocardial involvement) could be referred for angiography and possible revascularization. Finally, those individuals with severe coronary calcification and normal MPS were shown to have a low frequency of hard coronary events (<1% per year) over 3 years of follow-up[128]; therefore, these patients can be targeted for aggressive medical treatments and spared from invasive interventions.

CAC IMAGING IN PATIENTS WITH DIABETES MELLITUS AND CARDIOMETABOLIC SYNDROME

CAD accounts for 70% of the deaths among patients with DM.[137] Diabetic patients face a two- to fourfold higher risk of cardiac events than their nondiabetic counterparts, and in fact, diabetes is now treated as CAD equivalent[138] in risk stratifying patients. CAD is often asymptomatic and is associated with worse prognosis in diabetic patients, thus posing a major dilemma in identifying those at increased risk.[139] CAC imaging

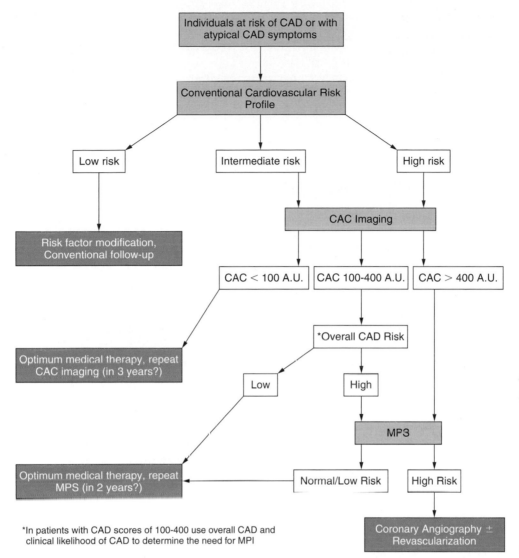

Figure 20-12 Proposed diagnostic algorithm. Sequential screening approach starting with conventional cardiovascular risk profiling, followed by coronary artery calcification (CAC) imaging in those at intermediate or high risk, and myocardial perfusion imaging in those with high CAC scores or high clinical risk with moderate CAC scores. *(Modified from Yerramasu A, Maggae SV, Lahiri A, Anand DV: Cardiac computed tomography and myocardial perfusion imaging for risk stratification in asymptomatic diabetic patients: A critical review, J Nucl Cardiol 15:13-22, 2008.)*

in diabetic patients promises to be an effective test for early detection of silent CAD.

Mielke et al.[140] showed that the median CAC score was higher in diabetic subjects compared to their nondiabetic counterparts. In a large study comparing the CAC scores in self-referred diabetic (n = 1075) and nondiabetic subjects (n = 29,829) with no known previous CAD, Hoff et al.[141] reported that diabetes was the strongest predictor for having a CAC score in the highest quartile, irrespective of sex.

The PREDICT trial[142] researchers prospectively studied 589 asymptomatic diabetic patients who were followed up for a median of 4 years with first-incident stroke or CAD events as primary endpoints. Similar to previous large observational studies, CAC score was an independent predictor of primary endpoint events, inclusion of which increased the ROC area under the curve from 0.63 to 0.73, using Framingham CAD risk,

and from 0.67 to 0.75 for UKPDS CAD risk prediction. What was interesting was that the doubling of CAC score was associated with a 32% increased risk for primary endpoint events. The authors were able to demonstrate this by using a base 2 logarithm (CAC score + 1), as seen in Figure 20-13.

Diabetic patients with coronary calcification have worse prognosis than nondiabetic subjects with the same extent of coronary calcification (Fig. 20-14).[143] Furthermore, in the presence of low CAC scores, the risk of coronary events is low even in diabetic patients. The study by Raggi et al.[143] showed that diabetic patients with no detectable coronary calcium had excellent 5-year survival that was not significantly different from nondiabetic subjects (survival 98.8% versus 99.4%, respectively, $P = 0.49$). The South Bay Heart Watch Study,[144] in which 1312 diabetic and nondiabetic patients were screened with CAC scoring using an EBCT

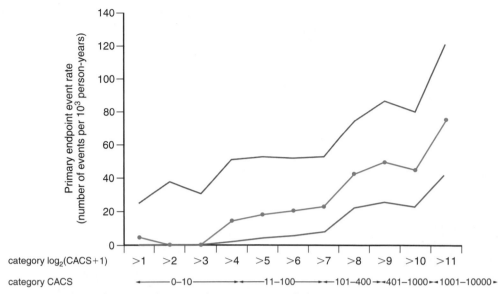

Figure 20-13 Increasing CAD and stroke primary endpoint events in diabetics. Y-axis represents primary endpoint events per 1000 person years, and x-axis represents CAC score variables represented in log 2 (CACS + 1) values. Each unit increase in log 2 (CACS + 1) represents a doubling of CAC score. The traditional CAC score categories of 0-10, 11-100, 101-400, 401-1000, and 1001-10,000, as well as equivalent log transformed value categories of 1-4, 4-7, 7- 9, 9-10, and 11, are shown on the x-axis. The *dotted lines* on either side represent the 95% confidence intervals. CAC, coronary artery calcification; CAD, coronary artery disease. *(From Elkeles RS, Godsland IF, Feher MD, et al: Coronary artery calcium measurement improves prediction of cardiovascular events in asymptomatic patients with type 2 diabetes: The PREDICT Study, Eur Heart J 29:2244-2251, 2008.)*

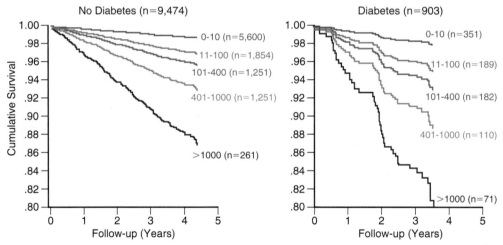

Figure 20-14 Comparison of cumulative survival in diabetics and nondiabetics. Cumulative survival is significantly greater across all quintiles of CAC scores in nondiabetics as compared to diabetics over a follow-up period of 5 years. *(From Raggi P, Shaw LJ, Berman DS, Callister TQ: Prognostic value of coronary artery calcium screening in subjects with and without diabetes, J Am Coll Cardiol 43:1663-1669, 2004.)*

scanner and followed up for 6.3 ± 1.4 years, with the endpoints of coronary death, nonfatal MI, coronary revascularization, or stroke, demonstrated a nearly four-fold increase in event rates in diabetics with a higher CAC than in the nondiabetics with a lower CAC.

One of the theories put forth to explain the increased mortality in diabetic patients as compared to nondiabetics with similar CAC scores is the increased prevalence of noncalcified plaque lesions and the presence of a greater volume of necrotic core with a thin-cap fibroatheroma. Plaque lesions with the aforementioned characteristics are deemed vulnerable for rupture and

consequently thrombosis and acute coronary syndromes and/or death.

In patients with diabetes, the presence of metabolic abnormalities increases the likelihood of an abnormal myocardial perfusion scan.[145] Wong et al.[146] examined 4468 asymptomatic individuals who underwent CAC imaging. The prevalence of CAC ranged from 51% in men and 35% in women with neither DM nor cardiometabolic syndrome (CMS) to 75% in men and 58% in women with both DM and CMS. These data concur with the results of the NHANES study[147] that reported the highest prevalence of CAD in patients with both DM and CMS in the United States. The same study also reported higher prevalence of CAD in women with CMS without DM compared to those with DM without CMS (13.9% and 7.5%, respectively).

So far, there are no data to suggest that patients with CMS but no diabetes benefit from aggressive risk-factor modification, as do patients with overt diabetes.[148] This makes a good case for CAC imaging screening of asymptomatic diabetic patients, as well as those with CMS but without overt diabetes, to better guide their clinical management. Metabolic syndrome alone is not a robust marker for 10-year cardiovascular risk, but the presence of metabolic syndrome even in the absence of DM should prompt a reassessment of cardiovascular risk, ideally with imaging for the presence of subclinical atherosclerosis.

EFFECT OF ETHNICITY ON PREVALENCE AND PROGNOSTIC SIGNIFICANCE OF CORONARY CALCIUM

CVD-associated morbidity and mortality varies widely across different ethnic groups, and it is likely that these differences are related to genetic as well as environmental factors. Most of the studies that investigated the prevalence and prognostic significance of coronary calcium were based on a predominantly white population. Earlier studies based on necropsy reports[149,150] and cine-fluoroscopy,[151] and more recent studies using EBCT-derived CAC measurements,[152–154] found higher prevalence of coronary calcium in Caucasians compared to African Americans. Using EBCT and coronary angiography, Budoff et al. reported a higher prevalence of coronary atherosclerosis in Caucasians compared to African Americans or Hispanics.[155] On the contrary, the CARDIA study[156] showed no significant difference in the prevalence of coronary calcification in 443 young black and white adults aged between 28 and 40 years. However, the prevalence of CAC was low in this young cohort. Also, the threshold area for CAC detection was 2.06 mm^2, twice the threshold area used in most of the other studies. In another smaller study of 128 black and 733 white asymptomatic postmenopausal women (mean age, 63 ± 8 years), a similar distribution of CAC scores was found in both the ethnic groups.[157]

The Dallas Heart Study evaluated the prevalence and severity of CAC in a multiethnic population-based sample in which blacks were systematically oversampled to make the final sample 50% black.[158] The prevalence of subclinical atherosclerosis was similar in the black and white participants, as were the mean FRSs.[159] However, this study used a score of greater than 10 Au (as opposed to > 0 Au) as the minimum score to define CAC prevalence. Also, greater obesity in black women could have resulted in increased noise, which could be misinterpreted as calcium. In a more recent larger study[160] involving over 16,000 asymptomatic individuals, Budoff and colleagues reported that African American men were least likely to have any coronary calcium, after adjusting for age and risk factors. African American

women, on the other hand, had significantly higher odds of having non-zero CAC scores. Caucasians and Hispanics have a significantly higher prevalence of CAC when compared to African and Asian men. Similarly, in the MESA cohort, white men had the highest prevalence of coronary calcification (70.4%), followed by Chinese (59.2%), Hispanic (55.6%), and black men (52.1%). The weight of evidence points to higher prevalence and severity of CAC in Caucasians compared to ethnic minorities, but it is not yet clear if this is due to differences in the plaque burden or due to differing degrees of plaque calcification among different ethnicities.

Two recent studies evaluated the influence of ethnicity on the predictive value of CAC. Nasir et al. reported the prevalence and the prognostic value of CAC in predicting all-cause mortality in a large, ethnically diverse population of over 14,000 asymptomatic individuals with no prior history of CHD.[161] After a mean follow-up of 6.8 years, CAC score was the best predictor of time to death among all ethnic groups. Compared to non-Hispanic whites, ethnic minorities have lower odds of having any, as well as increasing, CAC burden ($P < 0.0001$). Higher CAC scores were associated with greater mortality among ethnic minorities. However, in the MESA study, no interaction was noted between ethnicity and the risk associated with increasing calcium score.[162] Following a median follow-up of 3.9 years, CAC scores were independently predictive of the risk of major coronary events in all ethnic groups; no major differences in the predictive value of calcium scores were detected among different ethnic groups.

The recently concluded London Life Sciences Population (LOLIPOP) study[163] evaluated the ethnic differences in the prevalence of subclinical atherosclerosis among 2398 asymptomatic participants with no known previous CAD, recruited from the primary care practices in west London, UK. In comparison to the Europeans (n = 1031), Indian Asians (n = 1367) had approximately twofold higher prevalence of hypertension and type 2 diabetes, higher waist-hip ratio and triglycerides, and lower HDL cholesterol. However, there was no difference in CAC prevalence or mean CAC scores between Indian Asians and Europeans either before or after adjustment for the measured cardiovascular risk factors. In the same study, 262 patients with CAC over 100 Au underwent myocardial perfusion scan. There was no difference in prevalence of silent myocardial ischemia between the two ethnic groups, following adjustment for conventional risk factors. These results contrast with an almost twofold higher risk of MI and CAD mortality in Asians compared to Europeans, and indicate the need for more studies to conclusively establish the relationship between ethnicity and CAD.

PROGRESSION OF CORONARY CALCIUM—CAUSES AND CONSEQUENCES

There is a wealth of published data highlighting the prognostic significance of CAC scoring, but there have been very few trials studying the factors responsible for the progression of CAC scores. Yoon et al.[164] showed that the baseline CAC score was the most important determinant of rate of calcium progression. This study showed that neither age nor sex significantly correlated with progression of CAC. But from more robust data from the MESA cohort,[165] annual CAC progression had a linear correlation with age irrespective of race and showed a similar trend in both sexes. Among the 2948 participants (51.2%) without detectable CAC at baseline, 475 (16.1%) went on to develop incident CAC over an average of 2.4 years of follow-up. Thus, the estimated incidence rate was 6.6% per year. The incidence was less than 5% per year at younger ages and more than 12% per year at the highest ages. It is important to note that this study did not control for baseline CAC score, since CAC progression is assumed to be a continuous spectrum of change from the initial focus of calcification in the atherosclerotic plaque lesion; therefore, to control for baseline CAC score would be to ignore the effect of causative factors from initiation untill the baseline scan. The study showed that the age differences were similar across gender and race/ethnicity subgroups. Black women had the highest yearly incident rates at 6.3%. Hispanic, white, and Chinese women had yearly rates of 6%, 5.6%, and 4.7%, respectively. These ethnic differences in yearly incident rates were non significant when adjusted for age. With the exception of Chinese participants, men had higher incidence rates than women ($P < 0.001$). The yearly incidence rates in decreasing order are 10.3% for white men, 8.2% for black men, 7.2% for Hispanic men, and 4.4% for Chinese men. In the same cohort, after adjusting for age, gender, race, and smoking, systolic blood pressure (SBP) and serum glucose were found to be strong predictors of progression of CAC. Serum glucose level was strongly associated with progression even in patients with no diabetes.

Anand et al.[166] reported a similar finding in a cohort of 398 asymptomatic diabetic subjects. The study revealed that whereas traditional risk factors except smoking and hyperlipidemia were all univariate predictors of CAC progression, suboptimal glycemic control was one of the strongest predictors of CAC progression. Anand et al. also demonstrated that patients with minimal CAC scores did not progress significantly, but those who already had evidence of increased CAC earlier showed considerable CAC progression despite treatment. Though presence of cardiometabolic syndrome with or without diabetes was associated with a higher prevalence of CAC scores, in the recent Rancho Bernardo study,[167] only hypertension and fasting plasma glucose levels significantly predicted the progression of CAC, whereas metabolic syndrome did not.

Yoon et al. also showed that hypertension and diabetes were independent predictors of progression of CAC.[164] In a few studies it has been shown that family history of CAD is a strong predictor for the progression of CAC scores, pointing to hitherto undiscovered genetic factors at play in the progression of CAC scores.[168,169] Surprisingly, most of the studies looking at progression did not find any significant correlation between levels of LDL and progression of CAC.

It has been shown that increased rate of progression of CAC is associated with increased cardiac event rates, as demonstrated by Shemesh et al.[170] in a cohort of high-risk hypertensive patients. The percentage change in CAC score in the three groups of their study population of asymptomatic patients, patients with stable CAD, and patients who suffered a cardiovascular event during the 3 years of follow-up were 118%, 124%, and 180% ($P < 0.05$). Similarly, Raggi et al.[171] also showed that in asymptomatic patients, higher progression rate of calcium volume score was significantly associated with increased risk of coronary events. In a study population of 1310 subjects undergoing sequential EBCT scanning with at least a 1-year interval between scans and average follow up of 2.2 to 2.7 years, 49 subjects suffered from an MI; 90% of the diabetics (n = 9) and 71% of nondiabetics (n = 24) who suffered from an MI had greater than 15% annualized change in their calcium volume score.

It is important to know how frequently a patient should be imaged in order to monitor the progression of CAC, especially when the score is zero. In an interesting study by Gopal et al.,[172] 710 physician-referred patients with an initial CAC of zero were followed up differentially: 35% for 1 to 3 years, 36% for 3 to 5 years, and 29% for over 5 years. A CAC change/year of zero was found in 61% of the study population; in fact 97% of the subjects had a change in CAC/year of less than 10 Au. Only 1% had a CAC change/year of more than 50 Au, and 2% were in the intermediate group of 10 to 50 Au. They concluded that with a baseline score of zero, there was no evidence to suggest repeating the scan before 5 years. These data are supported by an earlier study by Budoff et al., who reported that only 2% of their study population with an initial score of zero had a CAC score of greater than 10 Au at repeat scanning after 1 to 6 years.[173]

EFFECT OF TREATMENT ON PROGRESSION OF CORONARY CALCIUM

The evidence for the importance of CAC imaging as a prognostic indicator and as a method of risk stratification has already been elucidated. Logically, identification of high-risk patients based on CAC imaging would lead to the institution of more intense risk-reduction measures. Some trials have suggested targets for LDL as low as 70 mg/dL for additional benefit in selected populations.[174-176] However, the evidence for the effect of aggressive HMG-CoA reductase inhibitor therapy on the rate of progression of CAC is conflicting. Earlier studies[177,178] that showed slowing of progression of CAC score with HMG-CoA reductase inhibitor therapy are not supported by the data from more recent, larger prospective trials.[179-181] Houslay et al.[181] showed that despite aggressive therapy with atorvastatin 80 mg compared with placebo, leading to significant reduction in both LDL (more than half of baseline) and CRP, there was no significant correlation with the progression of CAC. The annualized change in CAC in the atorvastatin group was 26%/year, and in the placebo group it was

18%/year ($P =$ NS). Owing to progression in CAC despite aggressive LDL lowering, they also concluded that there was no significant correlation between LDL levels and progression of CAC. In the special case of familial hypercholesterolemia, it has been shown in a very small study group of 8 patients (7 male and 1 female), that LDL apheresis with an extracorporeal device on a weekly or twice-weekly basis in addition to 80 mg of atorvastatin resulted in a significant reduction in coronary calcium scores ($26 \pm 14\%$, $P < 0.01$) during a 29-month follow-up period.[182] It is postulated that the reduction in cholesterol levels reduced the exposure of macrophages to the toxic effects of oxidized LDL, thus reducing cell death and denying a focus for calcium deposition.

In a larger observational study, Hecht et al.[183] studied a group of 182 asymptomatic patients who were treated with an HMG-CoA reductase inhibitor, either alone or in combination with niacin. The study population was divided into those who had achieved an LDL of lower than 80 mg/dL and those who had an LDL level of higher than 80 mg/dL. Repeat scan after 1.2 years did not show any significant difference in the annualized progression rates of the calcium score between the two groups (9.3% in the group with LDL < 80 mg/dL and 9.1% in the group with LDL > 80 mg/dL). Similar annual progression was noted in the group of patients given an HMG-CoA reductase inhibitor alone and the group given a combination of HMG-CoA reductase inhibitor and niacin (12.2% and 12.1%, respectively). Similarly, in the St. Francis Heart Study,[179] treatment with 20 mg of atorvastatin, 1g of vitamin C, and 1000 units of vitamin E (alpha tocopherol) induced a significant reduction in LDL but no significant reduction in CAC progression, compared to treatment with placebo. Interestingly, in subjects with a CAC score of over 400, treatment reduced the incidence of atherosclerotic cardiovascular disease events by 42% ($P = 0.046$). This discrepancy between the effect of HMG-CoA reductase inhibitors on cardiovascular event rates and CAC progression could be due to the fact that they stabilize the plaque by reducing the free lipid core and inducing a fibrovascular transformation of the thin fibrous cap.[184] HMG-CoA reductase inhibitor therapy also reduces the number of macrophages in the plaque,[185] therefore attenuating the inflammatory impetus rendering the plaque vulnerable,[186] consequently reducing the plaque vulnerability and cardiovascular mortality in general. This effect of HMG-CoA reductase inhibitor therapy on stabilization of the plaque has very little effect on the calcium component of the atherosclerotic plaque lesion or in some cases, an increase in the proportion of calcification in the plaque even as the total volume of the lesion regresses.[187]

COST-EFFECTIVENESS OF CAC IMAGING

In the current era of inflation beating health care costs and increasing budgetary constraints, imaging services are under growing scrutiny to prove their cost and clinical effectiveness before they can be accepted as part of routine clinical care. Cardiovascular disease already imposes a huge economic burden on the society, costing in excess of $329 billion per year in the United States,[188] and can increase substantially in the future as a result of an aging population and growing prevalence of risk factors. Approximately 300,000 EBCT CAC are scans are performed annually in 79 centers in the United States. In the last 2 decades, the number of cardiac imaging procedures has grown markedly while prevalence of CAD has remained steady.[189] The American College of Cardiology and the American Heart Association now recommend CAC imaging as a reasonable choice in intermediate Framingham risk patients.[66] The 34th Bethesda Conference[190] on Atherosclerosis Imaging estimated that applying CAC screening to the 34 million intermediate-risk individuals in the United States could result in direct imaging costs of approximately $1 billion, with additional downstream costs from the ensuing tests and treatments. It is estimated that using CAC screening with a cutoff value of above 75% of age- and gender-adjusted percentile, 25% of intermediate-risk individuals could be reclassified into the high-risk group,[191] which will have a significant impact on the extra cost of additional aggressive risk-reduction treatments.

To make sense economically, a screening or diagnostic test should provide "incremental" information to clinical history, physical examination, and other low-cost tests (such as lipid analysis and hs-CRP). The incremental cost-effectiveness ratio (ICER, incremental cost/incremental benefit) is usually expressed as cost per quality adjusted life year (QALY) saved, and the U.S. Public Health Service set a threshold of less than $50,000 per QALY for any intervention or investigation to be recommended for routine clinical use. A number of European countries have used lower thresholds of approximately $20,000 per life year saved. However, in the case of CAC imaging, cost per QALY is difficult to assess, since the survival benefit of the test is indirect, dictated largely by the effectiveness of ensuing treatment. Hence, cost to identify CAD death or nonfatal MI was proposed as an intermediate outcome measure.

Most of the evidence for cost effectiveness of CAC imaging comes from analysis based on decision modeling rather than actual trial data. The cost-effectiveness of CAC scoring depends largely on the population being screened. Cost-effectiveness analysis based on a decision model[192] estimated that the cost to identify a CAD event was $73,070 for low-risk and $37,260 for intermediate-risk individuals ($P < 0.00001$). When the costs and benefits of resulting treatment were taken into account, the cost was $500,000 per life year saved in the low-risk group, whereas in intermediate-risk individuals, cost-effectiveness ratios were much more favorable, ranging between $30,000 and $42,000 per life year saved. Similarly, when CAC imaging is used as a diagnostic test in symptomatic patients, cost-effectiveness depends largely on the disease prevalence and the cutoff CAC score. In a decision tree model,[83] CAC scan with a cutoff score of 168 Au represented the most cost-effective initial test in population groups with low/intermediate disease prevalence (<70%), compared to other investigations such as stress ECG, stress echo, stress scintigraphy, or direct angiography. CAC scan with a cutoff score of greater than 0 proved to be the least cost-effective noninvasive strategy in the same group. In high-prevalence groups, initial angiography with no prior noninvasive testing proved to be the most cost-effective diagnostic strategy. However, an inherent problem with these decision models is that they either are too simplistic in their assumptions or make too many assumptions. Thus, there is a need for prospective studies evaluating the cost performance and economic implications of CAC scoring in the screening and diagnosis of CAD.

FUTURE DIRECTIONS: CAN CT CORONARY ANGIOGRAPHY REPLACE CAC IMAGING?

CAC imaging is already being used extensively in the United States and some European countries, mainly for reclassifying patients who have a 10-year intermediate cardiovascular risk based on conventional risk factors. Despite the extensive research and the wide availability of CT scanners, there is still a reluctance to integrate CAC imaging into the burgeoning investigative arsenal at the disposal of cardiologists today. With the introduction of successive generations of MSCT scanners and gradual improvements in temporal and spatial resolution, it is now possible to make a more comprehensive assessment of coronary atherosclerotic plaques, both calcified and noncalcified. It is well known that although CAC correlates well with the overall atherosclerotic burden, it does not represent the atherosclerotic plaque in its entirety. More important, CAC imaging provides no information regarding the degree of luminal stenosis caused by an individual plaque. CT coronary angiography can provide important information regarding the location,[193] extent, and morphology of the plaque,[194] vessel wall remodelling,[195,196] and the degree of luminal

compromise caused by an individual lesion (Fig. 20-15).[197] Although there is not enough evidence currently to advocate the use of CTA as a screening tool in asymptomatic patients, aggressive marketing strategies and mass media have, on occasions, prompted self-referral from the public, posing additional dilemmas to the physician. A recent study by Choi et al.[198] evaluated the use of CTA as a screening tool in 1000 middle-aged asymptomatic subjects (age 50 ± 9 years; 63% men). Interestingly, 40 participants (4%) had exclusively noncalcified plaque; 10 of these subjects had significant stenosis on CTA (defined as > 50%), and 5 of them had severe stenosis (defined as > 70%). Midterm follow-up of the study population revealed 15 events; however, only one of these events was ACS, and the rest were revascularizations, mostly prompted by the results of the scan. The study showed that the prevalence of significant noncalcified atherosclerotic lesions in asymptomatic individuals is low (1%) but non-negligible. With the additional costs and risks involved with CTA, there is (1) a need for more robust data to prove that CTA can provide prognostic information that is independent of and incremental to CAC imaging and (2) a need to lower the radiation burden significantly before it can replace the latter as a tool for CAD screening and risk stratification.

There is active ongoing research in the field of atherosclerosis imaging, with an intense pursuit for imaging modalities that can assess not only the extent and severity of the plaque but also its composition and vulnerability.[199] Newer imaging modalities are in various stages of development and mostly rely on the use of specific antibodies and ligands with high affinity for various components of atherosclerotic plaque. Since inflammation plays an important role in all stages of atherosclerosis, macrophages have been an attractive target for most of these modalities. MRI studies using targeted immunomicelles showed strong correlation with macrophage content in atherosclerotic plaques[200]; however, these

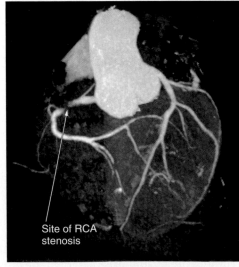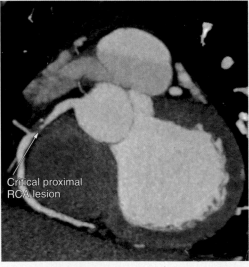

Figure 20-15 Computed tomography coronary angiography (CTCA) for comprehensive evaluation of coronary atherosclerosis. *Left*, CT coronary angiogram showing the outline of coronary arteries in a 45-year-old man with atypical chest pain and equivocal exercise ECG test. Severe stenosis was noted in proximal right coronary artery (RCA). *Right*, Curved multiplanar reformation showing a large, predominantly noncalcified plaque at the site of stenosis. Coronary artery calcification (CAC) imaging showed minimal coronary calcification (<10 Au) in this patient.

studies were mostly limited to extracardiac vessels. Also, positron emission tomography (PET) studies using fluoro-deoxyglucose (FDG) demonstrated increased FDG uptake in atherosclerotic plaques, and there was a significant correlation between the PET signal from carotid plaques and the macrophage staining from corresponding histologic sections ($r = 0.70$; $P < 0.0001$).[201] Similarly, in rabbits, specific uptake of an iodine-containing contrast agent by macrophages allows atherosclerotic lesions to be detected using CT.[202] Pending further clinical trials, this contrast agent may become an important adjunct to the clinical evaluation of coronary arteries with CT. These evolving techniques, when successfully validated for use in humans, can potentially transform cardiovascular imaging from a method of diagnosis in symptomatic patients to a tool for noninvasive detection of early subclinical abnormalities. Until such time, CAC imaging, by virtue of its established efficacy and ease of use, remains the method of choice for noninvasive detection of coronary atherosclerosis.

REFERENCES

1. Myerburg RJ, Kessler KM, Castellanos A: Sudden cardiac death: epidemiology, transient risk, and intervention assessment, *Ann Intern Med* 119:1187–1197, 1993.
2. Kannel WB, Neaton JD, Wentworth D, et al: Overall and coronary heart disease mortality rates in relation to major risk factors in 325,348 men screened for the MRFIT: Multiple Risk Factor Intervention Trial, *Am Heart J* 112:825–836, 1986.
3. Taylor AJ, Burke AP, O'Malley PG, et al: A comparison of Framingham Risk Index, Coronary Artery Calcification and culprit plaque morphology in sudden cardiac death, *Circulation* 101:1243–1248, 2000.
4. Little WC, Constantinescu M, Applegate RJ, et al: Can coronary angiography predict the site of a subsequent myocardial infarction in patients with mild-to-moderate coronary artery disease? *Circulation* 78:1157–1166, 1988.
5. Giroud D, Li JM, Urban P, et al: Relation of the site of acute myocardial infarction to the most severe coronary arterial stenosis at prior angiography, *Am J Cardiol* 71:257–258, 1993.
6. Proudfoot D, Shanahan CM: Biology of calcification in vascular cells: intima versus media, *Herz* 26:245–251, 2001.
7. Ross R: The pathogenesis of atherosclerosis: a perspective for the 1990s, *Nature* 362:801–809, 1993.
8. Libby P: Inflammation in atherosclerosis, *Nature* 420:868–874, 2002.
9. Doherty TM, Fitzpatrick LA, Inoue D, et al: Molecular, endocrine, and genetic mechanisms of arterial calcification, *Endocr Rev* 25:629–672, 2004.
10. Vermeer C: Gamma-carboxyglutamate-containing proteins and the vitamin K-dependent carboxylase, *Biochem J* 266:625–636, 1990.
11. Price PA: Gla-containing proteins of bone, *Connect Tissue Res* 21:51–60, 1989.
12. Simons DB, Schwartz RS, Edwards WD, et al: Noninvasive definition of anatomic coronary artery disease by ultrafast computed tomographic scanning: a quantitative pathologic comparison study, *J Am Coll Cardiol* 20:1118–1126, 1992.
13. Doherty TM, Detrano RC: Coronary arterial calcification as an active process: a new perspective on an old problem, *Calcif Tissue Int* 54:224–230, 1994.
14. Doherty TM, Asotra K, Fitzpatrick LA, et al: Calcification in atherosclerosis: bone biology and chronic inflammation at the arterial crossroads, *Proc Natl Acad Sci U S A* 100:11201–11206, 2003.
15. Stary HC: The sequence of cell and matrix changes in atherosclerotic lesions of coronary arteries in the first forty years of life, *Eur Heart J* 11(Suppl E):3–19, 1990.
16. Proudfoot D, Skepper JN, Hegyi L, et al: The role of apoptosis in the initiation of vascular calcification, *Z Kardiol* 90(Suppl 3):43–46, 2001.
17. Proudfoot D, Davies JD, Skepper JN, et al: Acetylated low-density lipoprotein stimulates human vascular smooth muscle cell calcification by promoting osteoblastic differentiation and inhibiting phagocytosis, *Circulation* 106:3044–3050, 2002.
18. Sangiorgi G, Rumberger JA, Severson A, et al: Arterial calcification and not lumen stenosis is highly correlated with atherosclerotic plaque burden in humans: a histologic study of 723 coronary artery segments using nondecalcifying methodology, *J Am Coll Cardiol* 31:126–133, 1998.
19. Rumberger JA, Simons DB, Fitzpatrick LA, et al: Coronary artery calcium area by electron-beam computed tomography and coronary atherosclerotic plaque area. A histopathologic correlative study, *Circulation* 92:2157–2162, 1995.
20. Clarkson TB, Prichard RW, Morgan TM, et al: Remodelling of coronary arteries in human and non-human primates, *JAMA* 279:289–294, 1994.
21. Ehara S, Kobayashi Y, Yoshiyama M, et al: Spotty calcification typifies the culprit plaque in patients with acute myocardial infarction: an intravascular ultrasound study, *Circulation* 110:3424–3429, 2004.
22. Abedin M, Tintut Y, Demer LL: Vascular calcification: mechanisms and clinical ramifications, *Arterioscler Thromb Vasc Biol* 24:1161–1170, 2004.
23. Lee RT, Grodzinsky AJ, Frank EH, et al: Structure-dependent dynamic mechanical behavior of fibrous caps from human atherosclerotic plaques, *Circulation* 83:1764–1770, 1993.
24. Richardson PD, Davies MJ, Born GV: Influence of plaque configuration and stress distribution on fissuring of coronary atherosclerotic plaques, *Lancet* 2:941–944, 1989.
25. Johnson RC, Leopold JA, Loscalzo J: Vascular calcification: pathobiological mechanisms and clinical implications, *Circ Res* 99:1044–1059, 2006.
26. Doherty TM, Fitzpatrick LA, Inoue D, et al: Molecular, endocrine, and genetic mechanisms of arterial calcification, *Endocr Rev* 25:629–672, 2004.
27. Fitzpatrick LA, Severson A, Edwards WD, Ingram RT: Diffuse calcification in human coronary arteries: association of osteopontin with atherosclerosis, *J Clin Invest* 94:1597–1604, 1994.
28. Anand DV, Lahiri A, Lim E, et al: The relationship between osteoprotegerin levels and coronary artery calcification in uncomplicated type 2 diabetic subjects, *J Am Coll Cardiol* 47(9):1850–1857, 2006.
29. Mesquita M, Demulder A, Damry N, et al: Plasma osteoprotegerin is an independent risk factor for mortality and an early bio-marker of coronary vascular calcification in chronic kidney disease, *Clin Chem and Lab Med* (Epub ahead of print).
30. Knez A, Becker C, Becker A, et al: Determination of coronary calcium with multi-slice spiral computed tomography: a comparative study with electron-beam CT, *Int J Cardiovasc Imaging* 18:295–303, 2002.
31. Becker CR, Kleffel T, Crispin A: Coronary artery calcium measurement: agreement of multirow detector and electron beam CT, *AJR Am J Roentgenol* 176:1295–1298, 2001.
32. Agatston AS, Janowitz WR, Hildner FJ: Quantification of coronary artery calcium using ultrafast computed tomography, *J Am Coll Cardiol* 15:827–832, 1990.
33. Becker CR, Jakobs TF, Aydemir S: Helical and single slice conventional CT versus EBCT for the quantitation of coronary artery calcification, *AJR Am J Roentgenol* 174:543–547, 2000.
34. Bielak LF, Sheedy PF 2nd, Peyser PA: Coronary artery calcification measured at EBCT: agreement in dual scan runs and change over time, *Radiology* 218:224–229, 2001.
35. Yoon HC, Greaser LE 3rd, Mather R: Coronary artery calcium: alternate methods for accurate and reproducible quantitation, *Acad Radiol* 4:666–673, 1997.
36. Bielak LF, Kaufmann RB, Moll PP: Small lesions identified in the heart by EBCT: calcification or noise? *Radiology* 192:631–636, 1994.
37. Callister TQ, Cooil B, Raya SP, et al: Coronary artery disease: Improved reproducibility of calcium scoring with an EBCT volumetric method, *Radiology* 208:807–814, 1998.
38. Detrano RC, Anderson M, Nelson J, et al: Coronary calcium measurements: effect of CT scanner type and calcium measure on rescan reproducibility—MESA study, *Radiology* 236:477–484, 2005.
39. Hong C, Becker CR, Schoepf UJ, et al: Coronary artery calcium: absolute quantification in non-enhanced and contrast enhanced multi-detector row CT studies, *Radiology* 223:474–480, 2002.
40. Shisen J, Leung DY, Juergens CP: Gender and age differences in the prevalence of coronary artery calcification in 953 Chinese subjects, *Heart Lung Circ* 14:69–73, 2005.
41. Shaw LJ, Raggi P, Berman DS, Callister TQ: Coronary artery calcium as a measure of biologic age, *Atherosclerosis* 188:112–119, 2006.
42. Anand DV, Lipkin D, Lahiri A: Finding the age of the patient's heart, *BMJ* 326:1045–1046, 2003.
43. Hoff JA, Chomka EV, Krainik AJ, et al: Age and gender distributions of coronary artery calcium detected by EBCT in 35246 adults, *Am J Cardiol* 87:1335–1339, 2001.
44. Budoff MJ, Nasir K, McClelland RL, et al: Coronary artery calcium predicts coronary events better with absolute calcium scores than age-sex-race/ethnicity percentiles: (MESA) Multi Ethnic Study of Atherosclerosis, *J Am Coll Cardiol* 53:345–352, 2009.
45. Akram K, Voros S: Absolute coronary artery calcium scores are superior to MESA percentile rank in predicting obstructive coronary artery disease, *Int J Cardiovasc Imaging* 24:743–749, 2008.
46. Centers for Disease Control and Prevention (CDC): State-specific mortality from sudden cardiac death–United States, 1999, *MMWR Morb Mortal Wkly Rep* 51:123–126, 2002.

47. Goraya TY, Jacobsen SJ, Kottke TE, et al: Coronary heart disease death and sudden cardiac death: a 20-year population-based study, *Am J Epidemiol* 157:763–770, 2003.

48. EUROASPIRE II Study Group: Lifestyle and risk factor management and use of drug therapies in coronary patients from 15 countries; principal results from EUROASPIRE II Euro Heart Survey Programme, *Eur Heart J* 22:554–572, 2001.

49. Stampfer MJ, Hu FB, Manson JE, et al: Primary prevention of coronary heart disease in women through diet and lifestyle, *N Engl J Med* 343:16–22, 2000.

50. Truett J, Cornfield J, Kannel W: A multivariate analysis of the risk of coronary heart disease in Framingham, *J Chronic Dis* 20:511–524, 1967.

51. Assmann G, Cullen P, Schulte H: Simple scoring scheme for calculating the risk of acute coronary events based on the 10-year follow-up of the prospective cardiovascular Münster (PROCAM) study, *Circulation* 105:310–315, 2002.

52. Conroy RM, Pyorala K, Fitzgerald AP, et al: Estimation of ten-year risk of fatal cardiovascular disease in Europe: the SCORE project, *Eur Heart J* 24:987–1003, 2003.

53. Hemann BA, Bimson WF, Taylor AJ: The Framingham Risk Score: an appraisal of its benefits and limitations, *Am Heart Hosp J* 5:91–96, 2007.

54. Coleman RL, Stevens RJ, Retnakaran R, Holman R: Framingham, SCORE, and DECODE risk equations do not provide reliable cardiovascular risk estimates in type 2 diabetes, *Diabetes Care* 30:1292–1293, 2007.

55. Brindle P, Emberson J, Lampe F, et al: Predictive accuracy of the Framingham coronary risk score in British men: prospective cohort study, *BMJ* 327:1267, 2003.

56. Eichler K, Puhan MA, Steurer J, Bachmann LM: Prediction of first coronary events with the Framingham score: a systematic review, *Am Heart J* 153:722–731, 2007.

57. Empana JP, Ducimetière P, Arveiler D, et al: PRIME Study Group. Are the Framingham and PROCAM coronary heart disease risk functions applicable to different European populations? The PRIME Study, *Eur Heart J* 24:1903–1911, 2003.

58. Wong ND, Kouwabunpat D, Vo AN, et al: Coronary calcium and atherosclerosis by ultrafast computed tomography in asymptomatic men and women: relation to age and risk factors, *Am Heart J* 127:422–430, 1994.

59. Parikh NI, Hwang SJ, Larson MG, et al: Parental occurrence of premature cardiovascular disease predicts increased coronary artery and abdominal aortic calcification in the Framingham offspring and third-generation cohorts, *Circulation* 116:1473–1481, 2007.

60. Loria CM, Liu K, Lewis CE, et al: Early adult risk factor levels and subsequent coronary artery calcification: the CARDIA Study, *J Am Coll Cardiol* 49:2013–2020, 2007.

61. 27th Bethesda Conference: Matching the Intensity of Risk Factor Management with the Hazard for Coronary Disease Events. September 14 to 15, 1995, *J Am Coll Cardiol* 27:957–1047, 1996.

62. Executive Summary of the Third Report of the National Cholesterol Education Program (NCEP): Expert Panel on Detection, Evaluation, and Treatment of High Blood Cholesterol in Adults (Adult Treatment Panel III), *JAMA* 285:2486–2497, 2001.

63. Greenland P, LaBree L, Azen SP, et al: Coronary artery calcium score combined with Framingham score for risk prediction in asymptomatic individuals, *JAMA* 291:210–215, 2004.

64. Lloyd-Jones D, Leip EP, Larson MG, et al: Prediction of lifetime risk for cardiovascular disease by risk factor burden at 50 years of age, *Circulation* 117:791–798, 2006.

65. Berry JD, Liu K, Folsom AR, et al: Prevalence and progression of subclinical atherosclerosis in younger adults with low short term but high lifetime estimated risk for cardiovascular disease: The Coronary Artery Risk Development in Young Adults Study and Multi-Ethnic Study of Atherosclerosis, *Circulation* 119:382–389, 2009.

66. Greenland P, Bonow RO, Brundage BH, et al: ACCF/AHA 2007 Clinical Expert Consensus document on coronary artery calcium scoring by computed tomography in global cardiovascular risk assessment and in evaluation of patients with chest pain: A report of the American College of Cardiology Foundation Clinical Expert Consensus Task Force, *J Am Coll Cardiol* 49:378–402, 2007.

67. Arad Y, Goodman KJ, Roth M, et al: Coronary calcification, coronary disease risk factors, C-reactive protein, and atherosclerotic cardiovascular disease events: the St. Francis Heart Study, *J Am Coll Cardiol* 46:158–165, 2005.

68. Vliegenthart R, Oudkerk M, Hofman A, et al: Coronary calcification improves cardiovascular risk prediction in the elderly, *Circulation* 112:572–577, 2005.

69. LaMonte MJ, FitzGerald SJ, Church TS, et al: Coronary artery calcium score and coronary heart disease events in a large cohort of asymptomatic men and women, *Am J Epidemiol* 162:421–429, 2005.

70. Ford ES, Giles WH, Mokdad AH: The distribution of 10-year risk for coronary heart disease among U.S. adults: findings from the National Health and Nutrition Examination Survey III, *J Am Coll Cardiol* 43:1791–1796, 2004.

71. Pletcher MJ, Tice JA, Pignone M, Browner WS: Using the coronary artery calcium score to predict coronary heart disease events: a systematic review and meta-analysis, *Arch Intern Med* 164:1285–1292, 2004.

72. Yang T, Doherty TM, Wong ND, Detrano RC: Alcohol consumption, coronary calcium, and coronary heart disease events, *Am J Cardiol* 84:802–806, 1999.

73. Arad Y, Spadaro LA, Goodman K, et al: Prediction of coronary events with electron beam computed tomography, *J Am Coll Cardiol* 36:1253–1260, 2000.

74. Wong ND, Hsu JC, Detrano RC, et al: Coronary artery calcium evaluation by electron beam computed tomography and its relation to new cardiovascular events, *Am J Cardiol* 86:495–498, 2000.

75. Raggi P, Cooil B, Callister TQ: Use of electron beam tomography data to develop models for prediction of hard coronary events, *Am Heart J* 141:375–382, 2001.

76. Ostrom MP, Gopal A, Ahmadi N, et al: Mortality incidence and the severity of coronary atherosclerosis assessed by computed tomography angiography, *J Am Coll Cardiol* 52:1335–1343, 2008.

77. Taylor AJ, Bindeman J, Feuerstein I, et al: Coronary calcium independently predicts incident premature coronary heart disease over measured cardiovascular risk factors: mean three-year outcomes in the Prospective Army Coronary Calcium (PACC) Project, *J Am Coll Cardiol* 46:807–814, 2005.

78. Kondos GT, Hoff JA, Sevrukov A, et al: Electron-beam tomography coronary artery calcium and cardiac events: a 37-month follow-up of 5635 initially asymptomatic low- to intermediate-risk adults, *Circulation* 107:2571–2576, 2003.

79. Budoff MJ, Shaw LJ, Liu ST, et al: Long-term prognosis associated with coronary calcification: observations from a registry of 25,253 patients, *J Am Coll Cardiol* 49:1860–1870, 2007.

80. O'Rourke RA, Brundage BH, Froelicher VF, et al: American College of Cardiology/American Heart Association Expert Consensus document on electron-beam computed tomography for the diagnosis and prognosis of coronary artery disease, *Circulation* 102:126–140, 2000.

81. Criteria for appraising the viability, effectiveness and appropriateness of a screening programme. http://www.nsc.nhs.uk/uk_nsc/uk_nsc_ind.htm. Accessed 23 April 2008.

82. Virmani R, Robinowitz M, McAllister HA Jr, : Coronary heart disease in 48 autopsy patients 30 years old and younger, *Arch Pathol Lab Med* 107:535–540, 1983.

83. Rumberger JA, Behrenbeck T, Breen JF, Sheedy PF II: Coronary calcification by electron beam computed tomography and obstructive coronary artery disease: a model for costs and effectiveness of diagnosis as compared with conventional cardiac testing methods, *J Am Coll Cardiol* 33:453–462, 1999.

84. Nickoloff EL, Alderson PO: Radiation exposures to patients from CT: reality, public perception, and policy, *AJR Am J Roentgenol* 177:285–287, 2001.

85. Mozaffarian D: Electron-beam computed tomography for coronary calcium: a useful test to screen for coronary heart disease? *JAMA* 294:2897–12890, 2005.

86. Doherty TM, Wong ND, Shavelle RM, et al: Coronary heart disease deaths and infarctions in people with little or no coronary calcium, *Lancet* 353:41–42, 1999.

87. Cheng VY, Lepor NE, Madyoon H, et al: Presence and severity of noncalcified coronary plaque on 64-slice computed tomographic coronary angiography in patients with zero and low coronary artery calcium, *Am J Cardiol* 99:1183–1186, 2007.

88. Fleming C, Whitlock EP, Beil TL, Lederle FA: Screening for abdominal aortic aneurysm: a best-evidence systematic review for the U.S. Preventive Services Task Force, *Ann Intern Med* 142:203–211, 2005.

89. Pignone M, Rich M, Teutsch SM, et al: Screening for colorectal cancer in adults at average risk: a summary of the evidence for the U.S. Preventive Services Task Force, *Ann Intern Med* 137:132–141, 2002.

90. Humphrey LL, Helfand M, Chan BK, Woolf SH: Breast cancer screening: a summary of the evidence for the U.S. Preventive Services Task Force, *Ann Intern Med* 137:347–360, 2002.

91. Tanenbaum SR, Kondos GT, Veselik KE, et al: Detection of calcific deposits in coronary arteries by ultrafast computed tomography and correlation with angiography, *Am J Cardiol* 63:870–872, 1989.

92. Detrano R, Hsiai T, Wang S, et al: Prognostic value of coronary calcification and angiographic stenoses in patients undergoing coronary angiography, *J Am Coll Cardiol* 27:285–290, 1996.

93. Schmermund A, Baumgart D, Adamzik M, et al: Comparison of electron-beam computed tomography and intracoronary ultrasound in detecting calcified and noncalcified plaques in patients with acute coronary syndromes and no or minimal to moderate angiographic coronary artery disease, *Am J Cardiol* 81:141–146, 1998.

94. Breen JF, Sheedy PF, Schwartz RS, et al: Coronary artery calcification detected with ultrafast CT as an indication of coronary artery disease, *Radiology* 185:435–439, 1992.

95. Kaufmann RB, Sheedy PF, Maher JE, et al: Quantity of coronary artery calcium detected by electron beam computed tomography in asymptomatic subjects and angiographically studied patients, *Mayo Clin Proc* 70:223–232, 1995.

96. Devries S, Wolfkiel C, Shah V, Chomka E, Rich S: Reproducibility of the measurement of coronary calcium with ultrafast computed tomography, *Am J Cardiol* 75:973–975, 1995.

97. Kajinami K, Seki H, Takekoshi N, Mabuchi H: Quantification of coronary artery calcification using ultrafast computed tomography: reproducibility of measurements, *Coron Artery Dis* 4:1103–1108, 1993.

98. Rumberger JA, Sheedy PF, Breen JF, Schwartz RS: Coronary calcium, as determined by electron beam computed tomography, and coronary disease on arteriogram: effect of patient's sex on diagnosis, *Circulation* 91:1363–1367, 1995.

99. Braun J, Oldendorf M, Moshage W, et al: Electron beam computed tomography in the evaluation of cardiac calcification in chronic dialysis patients, *Am J Kidney Dis* 27:394–401, 1996.

100. Budoff MJ, Georgiou D, Brody A, et al: Ultrafast computed tomography as a diagnostic modality in the detection of coronary artery disease: a multicenter study, *Circulation* 93:898–904, 1996.

101. Fallavollita JA, Brody AS, Bunnell IL, et al: Fast computed tomography detection of coronary calcification in the diagnosis of coronary artery disease: comparison with angiography in patients, 50 years old, *Circulation* 89:285–290, 1994.

102. Baumgart D, Schmermund A, Goerge G, et al: Comparison of electron beam computed tomography with intracoronary ultrasound and coronary angiography for detection of coronary atherosclerosis, *J Am Coll Cardiol* 30:57–64, 1997.

103. Schmermund A, Baumgart D, Goörge G, et al: Coronary artery calcium in acute coronary syndromes: a comparative study of electron-beam computed tomography, coronary angiography, and intracoronary ultrasound in survivors of acute myocardial infarction and unstable angina, *Circulation* 96:1461–1469, 1997.

104. Kennedy J, Shavelle R, Wang S, et al: Coronary calcium and standard risk factors in symptomatic patients referred for coronary angiography, *Am Heart J* 135:696–702, 1998.

105. Schmermund A, Bailey KR, Rumberger JA, et al: An algorithm for noninvasive identification of angiographic three-vessel and/or left main coronary artery disease in symptomatic patients on the basis of cardiac risk and electron-beam computed tomographic calcium scores, *J Am Coll Cardiol* 33:444–452, 1999.

106. Guerci AD, Spadaro LA, Goodman KJ, et al: Comparison of electron beam computed tomography scanning and conventional risk factor assessment for the prediction of angiographic coronary artery disease, *J Am Coll Cardiol* 32:673–679, 1998.

107. Haberl R, Becker A, Leber A, et al: Correlation of coronary calcification and angiographically documented stenoses in patients with suspected coronary artery disease: results of 1,764 patients, *J Am Coll Cardiol* 37:451–457, 2001.

108. Budoff MJ, Diamond GA, Raggi P, et al: Continuous probabilistic prediction of angiographically significant coronary artery disease using electron beam tomography, *Circulation* 105:1791–1796, 2002.

109. Knez A, Becker A, Leber A, et al: Relation of coronary calcium scores by electron beam tomography to obstructive disease in 2,115 symptomatic patients, *Am J Cardiol* 93:1150–1152, 2004.

110. Keelan PC, Bielak LF, Ashai K, et al: Long-term prognostic value of coronary calcification detected by electron-beam computed tomography in patients undergoing coronary angiography, *Circulation* 104:412–417, 2001.

111. Topol EJ, Nissen SE: Our preoccupation with coronary luminology: the dissociation between clinical and angiographic findings in ischemic heart disease, *Circulation* 92:2333–2342, 1995.

112. Budoff MJ, Shavelle DM, Lamont DH, et al: Usefulness of electron beam computed tomography scanning for distinguishing ischemic from nonischemic cardiomyopathy, *J Am Coll Cardiol* 32:1173–1178, 1998.

113. Shavelle DM, Budoff MJ, LaMont DH, et al: Exercise testing and electron beam computed tomography in the evaluation of coronary artery disease, *J Am Coll Cardiol* 36:32–38, 2000.

114. Kajinami K, Seki H, Takekoshi N, Mabuchi H: Noninvasive prediction of coronary atherosclerosis by quantification of coronary artery calcification using electron beam computed tomography: comparison with electrocardiographic and thallium exercise stress test results, *J Am Coll Cardiol* 26:1209–1221, 1995.

115. Lamont DH, Budoff MJ, Shavelle DM, et al: Coronary calcium scanning adds incremental value to patients with positive stress tests, *Am Heart J* 143:861–867, 2002.

116. Schmermund A, Baumgart D, Sack S, et al: Assessment of coronary calcification by electron-beam computed tomography in symptomatic patients with normal, abnormal or equivocal exercise stress test, *Eur Heart J* 21:1674–1682, 2000.

117. Ladenheim ML, Pollock BH, Rozanski A, et al: Extent and severity of myocardial hypoperfusion as predictors of prognosis in patients with suspected coronary artery disease, *J Am Coll Cardiol* 7:464–471, 1986.

118. Staniloff HM, Forrester JS, Berman DS, Swan HJ: Prediction of death, myocardial infarction, and worsening chest pain using thallium scintigraphy and exercise electrocardiography, *J Nucl Med* 27:1842–1848, 1986.

119. Brown KA: Prognostic value of thallium-201 myocardial perfusion imaging. A diagnostic tool comes of age, *Circulation* 83:363–381, 1991.

120. Iskandrian AS, Chae SC, Heo J, et al: Independent and incremental prognostic value of exercise single photon emission computed tomographic (SPECT) thallium imaging in coronary artery disease, *J Am Coll Cardiol* 22:665–670, 1993.

121. Heller GV, Herman SD, Travin MI, et al: Independent prognostic value of intravenous dipyridamole with technetium-99m sestamibi tomographic imaging in predicting cardiac events and cardiac-related hospital admissions, *J Am Coll Cardiol* 26:1202–1208, 1995.

122. Hachamovitch R, Berman DS, Kiat H, et al: Exercise myocardial perfusion SPECT in patients without known coronary artery disease: incremental prognostic value and use in risk stratification, *Circulation* 93:905–914, 1996.

123. Hachamovitch R, Berman DS, Shaw LJ, et al: Incremental prognostic value of myocardial perfusion single photon emission computed tomography for the prediction of cardiac death: differential stratification for risk of cardiac death and myocardial infarction, *Circulation* 97:535–543, 1998.

124. Hachamovitch R, Hayes SW, Friedman JD, et al: Stress myocardial perfusion SPECT is clinically effective and cost-effective in risk-stratification of patients with a high likelihood of CAD but no known CAD, *J Am Coll Cardiol* 43:200–208, 2004.

125. Berman DS, Wong ND, Gransar H, et al: Relationship between stress-induced myocardial ischemia and atherosclerosis measured by coronary calcium tomography, *J Am Coll Cardiol* 44:923–930, 2004.

126. Schenker MP, Dorbala S, Hong ECT, et al: Interrelation of coronary calcification, myocardial ischemia, and outcomes in patients with intermediate likelihood of coronary artery disease: A combined positron emission tomography/computed tomography study, *Circulation* 117:1693–1700, 2008.

127. Ramakrishna G, Miller TD, Breen JF, et al: Relationship and prognostic value of coronary artery calcification by electron beam computed tomography to stress-induced ischemia by single photon emission computed tomography, *Am Heart J* 153:807–814, 2007.

128. Rozanski A, Gransar H, Wong ND, et al: Clinical outcomes after both coronary calcium scanning and exercise myocardial perfusion scintigraphy, *J Am Coll Cardiol* 49:1352–1361, 2007.

129. He ZX, Hedrick TD, Pratt CM, et al: Severity of coronary artery calcification by electron beam computed tomography predicts silent myocardial ischemia, *Circulation* 101:244–251, 2000.

130. Anand DV, Lim E, Hopkins D, et al: Risk stratification in uncomplicated type 2 diabetes: prospective evaluation of the combined use of coronary artery calcium imaging and selective myocardial perfusion scintigraphy, *Eur Heart J* 27:713–721, 2006.

131. Wong ND, Rozanski A, Gransar H, et al: Metabolic syndrome and diabetes are associated with an increased likelihood of inducible myocardial ischemia among patients with subclinical atherosclerosis, *Diabetes Care* 28:1445–1450, 2005.

132. Ho J, FitzGerald S, Stolfus L, et al: Severe coronary artery calcifications are associated with ischemia in patients undergoing medical therapy, *J Nucl Cardiol* 14:341–346, 2007.

133. Yerramasu A, Maggae SV, Lahiri A, Anand DV: Cardiac computed tomography and myocardial perfusion imaging for risk stratification in asymptomatic diabetic patients: a critical review, *J Nucl Cardiol* 15:13–22, 2008.

134. Ramakrishna G, Breen JF, Mulvagh SL, et al: Relationship between coronary artery calcification detected by electron-beam computed tomography and abnormal stress echocardiography: association and prognostic implications, *J Am Coll Cardiol* 48:2125–2131, 2006.

135. Wang L, Jerosch-Herold M, Jacobs DR, et al: Coronary artery calcification and myocardial perfusion in asymptomatic adults: The MESA (Multi-Ethnic Study of Atherosclerosis), *J Am Coll Cardiol* 48:1018–1026, 2006.

136. Edvardsen T, Detrano R, Rosen BD, et al: Coronary artery atherosclerosis is related to reduced regional left ventricular function in individuals without history of clinical cardiovascular disease: the Multiethnic Study of Atherosclerosis, *Arterioscler Thromb Vasc Biol* 26:206–211, 2006.

137. Gu K, Cowie CC, Harris MI: Mortality in adults with and without diabetes in a national cohort of the US population, 1971–1993, *Diabetes Care* 21:1138–1145, 1998.

138. Haffner SM, Lehto S, Rönemaa T, et al: Mortality from coronary heart disease in subjects with type 2 diabetes and in nondiabetic subjects with and without prior myocardial infarction, *N Engl J Med* 339:229–234, 1998.

139. Donnan PT, Boyle DI, Broomhall J, Hunter K, et al: Prognosis following first acute myocardial infarction in type 2 diabetes: A comparative population study, *Diabet Med* 19:448–455, 2002.

140. Mielke CH, Shields JP, Broemeling LD: Coronary artery calcium, coronary artery disease, and diabetes, *Diabetes Res Clin Pract* 53:55–61, 2001.

141. Hoff JA, Quinn L, Sevrukov A, et al: The prevalence of CAD among diabetic individuals without known CAD, *J Am Coll Cardiol* 41:1008–1012, 2003.

142. Elkeles RS, Godsland IF, Feher MD, et al: Coronary artery calcium measurement improves prediction of cardiovascular events in asymptomatic patients with type 2 diabetes: the PREDICT study, *Eur Heart J* 29:2244–2251, 2008.

143. Raggi P, Shaw LJ, Berman DS, Callister TQ: Prognostic value of coronary artery calcium screening in subjects with and without diabetes, *J Am Coll Cardiol* 43:1663–1669, 2004.

144. Qu W, Le TT, Azen SP, et al: Value of coronary artery calcium scanning by computed tomography for predicting coronary heart disease in diabetic subjects, *Diabetes Care* 26:905–910, 2003.

145. Wong ND, Rozanski A, Gransar H, et al: Metabolic syndrome and diabetes are associated with an increased likelihood of inducible myocardial ischaemia among patients with sub-clinical atherosclerosis, *Diabetes Care* 28:1445–1450, 2005.

146. Wong ND, Gransar H, Shaw LJ, et al: Comparison of atherosclerotic calcification burden in persons with cardiometabolic syndrome and diabetes, *J Cardiometab Syndr* 1:90–94, 2006.

147. Alexander CM, Landsman PB, Teutsch SM, et al: Third National Health and Nutritional Survey (NHANES III); National Cholesterol Education Programme (NCEP). NCEP defined metabolic syndrome, diabetes and prevalence of coronary heart disease among NHANES III participants age 50 years and older, *Diabetes* 26:3160–3167, 2003.

148. Budoff MJ, Yu D, Nasir K, et al: Diabetes and the progression of coronary calcium under the influence of statin therapy, *Am Heart J* 149:695–700, 2005.

149. Strong JP, Oalmann MC, Newman WP, et al: Coronary heart disease in young black and white males in New Orleans: community pathology study, *Am Heart J* 108:747–759, 1984.

150. Eggen DA, Stong JP, McGill HC: Coronary calcification: relationship to clinically significant coronary lesions and race, sex and topographic distribution, *Circulation* 32:948–955, 1965.

151. Tang W, Detrano RC, Brezden OS, et al: Racial differences in coronary calcium prevalence among high-risk adults, *Am J Cardiol* 75:1088–1091, 1995.

152. Lee TC, O'Malley PG, Feuerstein I, Taylor AJ: The prevalence and severity of coronary artery calcification on coronary artery computed tomography in black and white subjects, *J Am Coll Cardiol* 41:39–44, 2003.

153. Newman AB, Naydeck BL, Whittle J, et al: Racial differences in coronary artery calcification in older adults, *Arterioscler Thromb Vasc Biol* 122:424–430, 2002.

154. Doherty TM, Tang W, Detrano RC: Racial differences in the significance of coronary calcium in asymptomatic black and white subjects with coronary risk factors, *J Am Coll Cardiol* 34:787–794, 1999.

155. Budoff MJ, Yang TP, Shavelle RM, et al: Ethnic differences in coronary atherosclerosis, *J Am Coll Cardiol* 39:408–441, 2002.

156. Bild DE, Folsom AR, Lowe LP, et al: Prevalence and correlates of coronary calcification in black and white young adults: the Coronary Artery Risk Development in Young Adults (CARDIA) Study, *Arterioscler Thromb Vasc Biol* 21:852–857, 2001.

157. Khurana C, Rosenbaum CG, Howard BV, et al: Coronary artery calcification in black women and white women, *Am Heart J* 145:724–729, 2003.

158. Victor RG, Haley RW, Willett D, et al: A population-based probability sample for the multidisciplinary study of ethnic disparities in cardiovascular disease: recruitment and validation in the Dallas Heart study, *Am J Cardiol* 93:1473–1480, 2004.

159. Jain T, Peshock R, McGuire DK, et al: Dallas Heart Study Investigators. African Americans and Caucasians have a similar prevalence of coronary calcium in the Dallas Heart Study, *J Am Coll Cardiol* 44:1011–1017, 2004.

160. Budoff MJ, Nasir K, Mao S, et al: Ethnic differences of the presence and severity of coronary atherosclerosis, *Atherosclerosis* 187:343–350, 2006.

161. Nasir K, Shaw LJ, Liu ST, et al: Ethnic differences in the prognostic value of coronary artery calcification for all-cause mortality, *J Am Coll Cardiol* 50:953–960, 2007.

162. Detrano R, Guerci AD, Carr JJ, et al: Coronary calcium as a predictor of coronary events in four racial or ethnic groups, *N Engl J Med* 358:1336, 2008.

163. Jain P, Chambers JC, Elliott P, et al: Coronary artery calcification as a predictor of increased coronary heart disease risk in UK Indian Asians [abstract], *Heart* 94(Suppl II):A77, 2008.

164. Yoon HC, Emerick AM, Hill JA, et al: Calcium begets calcium: progression of coronary artery calcification in asymptomatic subjects, *Radiology* 224:236–241, 2002.

165. Kronmal RA, McClelland RL, Detrano R, et al: Risk factors for the progression of coronary artery calcification in asymptomatic subjects: results from the Multi-Ethnic Study of Atherosclerosis (MESA), *Circulation* 115:2722–2730, 2007.

166. Anand DV, Lim E, Darko D, et al: Determinants of progression of coronary artery calcification in type 2 diabetes role of glycemic control and inflammatory/vascular calcification markers, *J Am Coll Cardiol* 50:2218–2225, 2007.

167. Kramer CK, von Muhlen D, Gross JL, et al: Blood pressure and fasting plasma glucose rather than metabolic syndrome predict progression of coronary artery calcium: Rancho Bernardo study, *Diabetes Care* 32:141–146, 2009.

168. Peyser PA, Bielak LF, Chu JS, et al: Heritability of coronary artery calcium quantity measured by electron beam computed tomography in asymptomatic adults, *Circulation* 106:304–308, 2002.

169. Cassidy-Bushrow AE, Bielak LF, Sheedy PF 2nd, et al: Coronary artery calcification progression is heritable, *Circulation* 116:25–31, 2007.

170. Shemesh J, Apter S, Stolero D, et al: Annual progression of coronary artery calcium by spiral computed tomography in hypertensive patients without myocardial ischemia but with prominent atherosclerotic risk factors, in patients with previous angina pectoris or healed acute myocardial infarction, and in patients with coronary events during follow-up, *Am J Cardiol* 87:1395–1397, 2001.

171. Raggi P, Cooil B, Ratti C, et al: Progression of coronary artery calcium and occurrence of myocardial infarction in patients with and without diabetes mellitus, *Hypertension* 46:238–243, 2005.

172. Gopal A, Nasir K, Liu ST, et al: Coronary calcium progression rates with a zero initial score by electron beam tomography, *Int J Cardiol* 117:227–231, 2007.

173. Budoff MJ, Lane KL, Bakhsheshi H, et al: Rates of progression of coronary calcium by electron beam tomography, *Am J Cardiol* 86:8–11, 2000.

174. Nissen SE, Tuzcu EM, Schoenhagen P, et al: Effect of intensive compared with moderate lipid lowering therapy on progression of coronary atherosclerosis: a randomized controlled trial, *JAMA* 291:1071–1080, 2004.

175. O'keefe JH Jr, Cordain L, Harris WH, et al: Optimal LDL is 50–70 mgs/dl: lower is better and physiologically normal, *J Am Coll Cardiol* 43:2142–2146, 2004.

176. Larosa JC, Grundy SM, Waters DD, et al: Intensive lipid lowering with atorvastatin in patients with stable coronary disease, *N Engl J Med* 352:1425–1435, 2005.

177. Callister TQ, Raggi P, Cooil B, et al: Effect of HMG-CoA reductase inhibitors on coronary artery disease as assessed by electron-beam computed tomography, *N Engl J Med* 339:1972–1978, 1998.

178. Achenbach S, Ropers D, Pohle K, et al: Influence of lipid-lowering therapy on the progression of coronary artery calcification: a prospective evaluation, *Circulation* 106:1077–1082, 2002.

179. Arad Y, Spadaro LA, Roth M, et al: Treatment of asymptomatic adults with elevated coronary calcium scores with atorvastatin, vitamin C, and vitamin E: the St. Francis Heart Study randomized clinical trial, *J Am Coll Cardiol* 46:166–172, 2005.

180. Raggi P, Davidson M, Callister TQ, et al: Aggressive versus moderate lipid-lowering therapy in hypercholesterolemic postmenopausal women: Beyond Endorsed Lipid Lowering with EBT Scanning (BELLES), *Circulation* 112:563–571, 2005.

181. Houslay ES, Cowell SJ, Prescott RJ, et al: Progressive coronary calcification despite intensive lipid lowering treatment, *Heart* 92:1207–1212, 2006.

182. Hoffmann U, Derfler K, Haas M, et al: Effects of combined LDL apheresis and aggressive statin therapy on coronary calcified plaque as measured by computed tomography, *Am J Cardiol* 91:461–463, 2003.

183. Hecht HS, Harman SM: Relation of aggressiveness of lipid-lowering treatment to changes in calcified plaque burden by EBCT, *Am J Cardiol* 92:334–336, 2003.

184. Crisby M, Nordin-Fredriksson G, Shah PK, et al: Pravastatin treatment increases collagen content and decreases lipid content, inflammation, metalloproteinases, and cell death in human carotid plaques: implications for plaque stabilization, *Circulation* 103:926–933, 2001.

185. Aikawa M, Rabkin E, Sugiyama S, et al: An HMG-CoA reductase inhibitor, cerivastatin, suppresses growth of macrophages expressing matrix metalloproteinases, and tissue factor in vivo, and in vitro, *Circulation* 103:276–283, 2001.

186. Kwak BR, Mulhaupt F, Mach F: Atherosclerosis: anti-inflammatory and immunomodulatory activities of statins, *Autoimmun Rev* 2:332–338, 2003.

187. Trion A, Schutte-Bart C, Bax WH: Modulation of calcification of vascular smooth muscle cells in culture by calcium antagonists, statins, and their combination, *Mol Cell Biochem* 308:25–33, 2008.

188. Weinstein MC, Stason WB: Cost-effectiveness of interventions to prevent or treat coronary heart disease, *Annu Rev Public Health* 6:41–63, 1985.

189. Lucas FL, DeLorenzo MA, Siewers AE, Wennberg DE: Temporal trends in the utilization of diagnostic testing and treatments for cardiovascular disease in the United States, 1993–2001, *Circulation* 113:374–379, 2006.

190. Mark DB, Shaw LJ, Lauer MS, O'Malley PG, Heidenreich P: 34th Bethesda Conference: Task Force #5—Is atherosclerosis imaging cost effective, *J Am Coll Cardiol* 4:1906–1917, 2003.

191. Lakoski SG, Cushman M, Blumenthal RS, et al: Implications of C-reactive protein or coronary artery calcium score as an adjunct to global risk assessment for primary prevention of CHD, *Atherosclerosis* 193:401–407, 2007.

192. Shaw LJ, Raggi P, Berman DS, Callister TQ: Cost effectiveness of screening for cardiovascular disease with measures of coronary calcium, *Prog Cardiovasc Dis* 46:171–184, 2003.

193. Sheth T, Amlani S, Ellins ML, et al: Computed tomographic coronary angiographic assessment of high-risk coronary anatomy in patients with suspected coronary artery disease and intermediate pretest probability, *Am Heart J* 155:918–923, 2008.

194. Carrascosa PM, Capuñay CM, Garcia-Merletti P, et al: Characterization of coronary atherosclerotic plaques by multidetector computed tomography, *Am J Cardiol* 97:598–602, 2006.

195. Achenbach S, Ropers D, Hoffmann U, et al: Assessment of coronary remodeling in stenotic and nonstenotic coronary atherosclerotic lesions by multidetector spiral computed tomography, *J Am Coll Cardiol* 43:842–847, 2004.

196. Schmid M, Pflederer T, Jang IK, et al: Relationship between degree of remodeling and CT attenuation of plaque in coronary atherosclerotic lesions: an in-vivo analysis by multi-detector computed tomography, *Atherosclerosis* 197:457–464, 2008.

197. Leber AW, Johnson T, Becker A, et al: Diagnostic accuracy of dual-source multi-slice CT-coronary angiography in patients with an intermediate pretest likelihood for coronary artery disease, *Eur Heart J* 28:2354–2360, 2007.

198. Choi EK, Choi SI, Rivera JJ, et al: Coronary computed tomography angiography as a screening tool for the detection of occult coronary artery disease in asymptomatic individuals, *J Am Coll Cardiol* 52:357–365, 2008.

199. Rudd JH, Fayad ZA: Imaging atherosclerotic plaque inflammation, *Nat Clin Pract Cardiovasc Med* 5(Suppl 2):S11–S17, 2008.

200. Amirbekian V, Lipinski MJ, Briley-Saebo KC, et al: Detecting and assessing macrophages in vivo to evaluate atherosclerosis noninvasively using molecular MRI, *Proc Natl Acad Sci U S A* 104:961–966, 2007.

201. Tawakol A, Migrino RQ, Bashian GG, et al: In vivo ^{18}F-fluorodeoxyglucose positron emission tomography imaging provides a noninvasive measure of carotid plaque inflammation in patients, *J Am Coll Cardiol* 48:1818–1824, 2006.

202. Hyafil F, et al: Noninvasive detection of macrophages using a nanoparticulate contrast agent for computed tomography, *Nature Med* 13:636–641, 2007.

Chapter 21

Coronary Artery Computed Tomography Angiography

PAOLO RAGGI, DALTON S. McLEAN AND
NIKOLAOS ALEXOPOULOS

INTRODUCTION

The technologic innovations of the past 15 years have made it possible for the clinician to perform an accurate, noninvasive assessment of the coronary anatomy with computed tomography angiographic (CTA) technologies. The test requires the injection of iodinated contrast through a peripheral vein and entails exposure to radiation, but its evolution has been extremely rapid, and the potential for a high-quality, low-radiation test is becoming more of a reality each day. In this chapter we review the state of the art of coronary artery CT angiography, with a look at the future advancements for the next 5 years from today.

COMPUTED TOMOGRAPHY CORONARY ARTERY ANGIOGRAPHY: TECHNOLOGIC CONSIDERATIONS

The main challenge in imaging the coronary arteries with CT is the complex and continuous motion of these small targets. Therefore, both high temporal and spatial resolution are of paramount importance to obtain diagnostic quality images. The field of noninvasive coronary angiography started with the introduction of electron beam CT (EBCT; Imatron, San Francisco, CA) that operated at a temporal resolution varying between 50 and 100 milliseconds (ms) per tomographic image. This was a fourth-generation CT scanner that utilized a beam of electrons directed toward a tungsten ring; the impact of the electrons against the tungsten created a fan of x-rays moved along an arc of 210 degrees around the gantry (Fig. 21-1). The issuance of the electron beam, followed by the generation of the x-ray fan, was timed at 60% to 80% of the R-R interval on the surface electrocardiogram (ECG), and the patient was moved

in small increments of 3 mm through the stationary gantry at each heartbeat while holding his breath. This step-and-shoot prospective (i.e., ECG triggered) acquisition required a 20- to 30-second breath hold to cover the entire z-axis (cranial-caudal distance) of the heart. The benefits of the EBCT scanner were the very high temporal resolution and the relatively low radiation dose provided to the patient because of the intermittent (once per heartbeat) exposure to x-rays. However, there were also important drawbacks to the technology, such as the low spatial resolution, a significant partial volume effect due to the thick tomographic slices, and the fact that the axial acquisition of the slices with a small interslice gap often created a stair-step artifact in the reconstructed images. Finally, the prospective ECG-triggered acquisition forced patients with slow heart rates to maintain long breath holds, often inducing artifacts when the patients breathed in the middle of the test. In the early 2000s, the field witnessed an important evolution with the introduction of the first 4-slice mechanical CT. A dual-slice helical CT (Elscint, Haifa, Israel) had been in use for a few years[1–3] but had not received much attention in cardiovascular circles. The development of multislice CT (also known as *multidetector CT* [MDCT]) was made possible by the introduction of the *slip-ring technology* that permitted the continuous revolution of the x-ray source-detector pair in the CT gantry, allowing a perpetual spiraling motion around the patient. With this new technology, an x-ray tube generates a beam of x-rays that is split, collimated, and detected by several rows of detectors positioned on the other side of the patient's table (Figs. 21-2 and 21-3).

Several limitations of the EBCT technology were overcome with the introduction of MDCT, such as the low spatial resolution and the significant partial volume averaging effect seen with EBCT. In fact, the continuous spiral acquisition without interslice gap utilized in MDCT imaging permits the collection of true isotropic volumes of data, with a typical slice thickness of

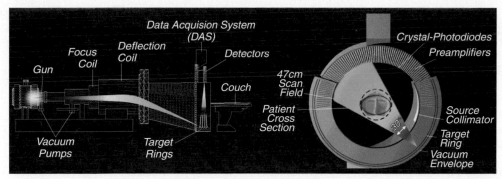

Figure 21-1 Schematic representation of an electron beam computed tomography scanner. The *picture on the left* demonstrates how the electron beam is generated by a gun and projected toward a tungsten ring surrounding the patient's couch. The electron beam is swept along an arc of 210 degrees, and the impact of the electrons against the tungsten ring produces a fan of x-rays *(right side of figure)*. The gantry does not move in this design; the patient is advanced in small increments across the x-ray fan.

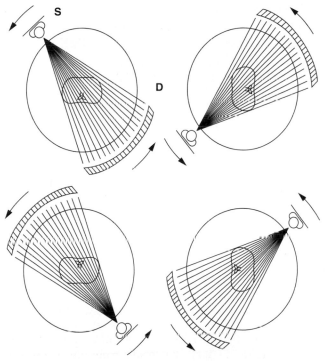

Figure 21-2 Schematic representation of the function of a multidetector computed tomography scanner. An x-ray source (S) is coupled with multiple rows of detectors (D), and together they revolve in a spiral motion around the patient lying on the radiologic couch.

0.7 mm to 0.4 mm (with the most recent models) and a pixel of similar size. However, the 4-slice MDCTs operated at an unsatisfactory low temporal resolution (about 500 ms per 360-degree revolution of the source-detector pair), and the gain in spatial resolution was offset by a significant degradation in image quality due to motion artifact with heart rates above 60 to 65 beats/min. Several steps can be implemented to partially overcome the limitation of low temporal resolution with MDCT. First, patients with heart rates above 70 beats/min should receive β-blockade. Furthermore, a tomographic image is reconstructed utilizing data acquired during a portion of the 360-degree revolution (a *segment* of the full circle), and each detector row is responsible for acquiring data around an angle of 150 to 160 degrees. This is called *segmental reconstruction*, which reduces the effective temporal resolution to 150 to 180 ms per tomographic image with the most recent MDCT models. A *multi segmental reconstruction* is also possible if the information collected by multiple detector rows during shorter rotation spans and over different cardiac cycles is utilized for image reconstruction. Although this reduces the temporal resolution further, the need to collate information from several detector rows during different heart cycles introduces the potential for severe artifact. Finally, since several hundred images are obtained during the continuous spiral acquisition of the tube-detector pair, off-line reconstruction of

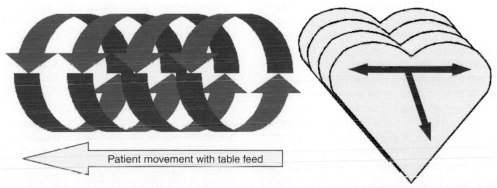

Patient movement with table feed

Figure 21-3 The image acquisition proceeds in a spiral (helical) motion while the patient, lying on the couch, is advanced through the gantry. This cartoon represents the schematic of a four-row multidetector computed tomography scanner.

the coronary arteries is performed by choosing the images showing the least motion artifact at different percentages of the R-R interval on the simultaneously recorded surface ECG (*phase reconstruction*).

As can be deduced from the preceding discussion, the introduction of scanners with more than 4 rows (16 to 64), despite better spatial resolution, did not fully improve the temporal resolution limitation of MDCT. As a result, even when using most current MDCT technology, β-blockade is still necessary to limit motion artifacts if the heart rate is greater than 70 beats/min. Nonetheless, by increasing the distance covered in the z-axis during a single rotation of the gantry, they shortened the acquisition time. This weakness of MDCT was partially overcome with the introduction of dual-source 64-row MDCT scanners (Siemens, Forcheim, Germany).[4-6] These scanners utilize two x-ray tubes and two sets of detector rows set at 90 degrees from each other that operate simultaneously, reducing the effective temporal resolution to about 83 ms per tomographic slice. Furthermore, the two tubes can issue x-rays of different energy spectra (*dual-energy* systems), with potential advantages for the study of tissues with different x-ray absorption characteristics, as discussed later in this chapter.

The temporal resolution of the dual-source MDCT is similar to that of EBCT, and no β-blockade appears to be necessary when imaging, reportedly even in the presence of atrial fibrillation.[7,8]

More recently a 320-row MDCT has been introduced on the market (Toshiba AquilionOne Dynamic Volume CT, Tochigi-ken, Japan). The spatial resolution of this scanner is 0.5 mm, and the rotation time for a 360-degree revolution is 350 ms. The advantage offered by this technology is that the z-axis coverage is so wide (160 mm) that a single rotation may be sufficient to cover the entire heart span. The large z-axis coverage also eliminates the need for spiral acquisition, allowing true axial imaging with the elimination of the stair-step artifact sometimes seen with MDCT. Finally, the obvious advantage of the 320-row MDCT is the potential for substantial radiation dose reduction. In fact, since the gantry rotates at 350 ms, only a portion of a single rotation is used—typically in end-diastole—for image acquisition. There are, however, some potential drawbacks to this technology; in the presence of a high heart rate, the diastolic time may be too short for good quality imaging. This renders a single-beat acquisition problematic and will force the performance of multiple rotations, with loss of the radiation dosing advantage, so the administration of β-blockers may be required even with this equipment. Finally, the acquisition of the entire heart volume in a fraction of one rotation will not allow the collection of sufficient data to perform wall motion and left ventricular volume and function analyses that are possible with other MDCTs. Newer MDCT technologies on the horizon include a high-definition scanner (GE Healthcare, Milwaukee, WI) with substantially improved spatial resolution and a 256-row MDCT (Philips, Highland Heights, OH). The latter two scanners are not yet available in the marketplace, and no further data can be shared at this time.

Although invasive coronary angiography will retain its role in guiding the need for surgical and catheter-based revascularization of high-grade stenoses, noninvasive CT angiography may be of great value to the practicing cardiologist in excluding the presence of obstructive lesions in several clinical scenarios, as will be discussed in this chapter. The diagnosis of in-stent stenosis and the interference caused by large calcium deposits, however, remain problematic with the current MDCT technology, and further advances will be necessary to improve on these aspects. Finally, the radiation exposure provided by MDCT is a source of concern and an issue that requires further investigation and improvement if this technology is to become readily available to the practicing physician.

COMPARISON OF CORONARY COMPUTED TOMOGRAPHY ANGIOGRAPHY WITH INVASIVE ANGIOGRAPHY FOR THE DETECTION OF LUMINAL STENOSIS

Native Coronary Arteries
(Figs. 21-4 and 21-5)

The initial results of coronary CT angiography with EBCT were encouraging but also demonstrated the limitations of the technology. Achenbach et al[9] reported a sensitivity and specificity of 92% and 94% for EBCT angiography compared to invasive coronary angiography for the detection of a luminal obstruction greater than 50% in 125 patients. However, 25% of the coronary segments were not evaluable, owing to technical limitations such as motion artifacts, calcium overlay, high image noise, and so forth. Similar results were obtained with 4-slice MDCT technology. Leber et al.[10] reported a sensitivity and specificity of 82% and 96% for 4-slice MDCT with 25% to 30% nonevaluable coronary segments, and similar results were also shown by other investigators.[11] A recent meta-analysis, including 22 studies of 4-slice MDCT versus invasive angiography, yielded a sensitivity of 87% and specificity of 87% on a per-vessel basis and 91% and 83% on a per-patient basis, respectively.[12]

The newer generations of MDCT scanners, starting with the 16-slice MDCTs, have shown improved accuracy compared to 4-slice MDCT. Each advance in technology with increased spatial and temporal resolution has been accompanied by improved results. Better spatial resolution leads to improved ability to assess coronary stents and calcified coronary artery segments (decreased partial volume effect) and improved ability to assess smaller arteries and side branches. As discussed, 16-slice MDCT typically has a spatial resolution of 0.7 mm and a temporal resolution of about 200 ms,[13] whereas 64-slice MDCTs typically have a spatial resolution of 0.5 mm and a temporal resolution of 165 ms,[14] except for the dual-source 64-slice MDCT that has a temporal resolution of 83 ms.[15]

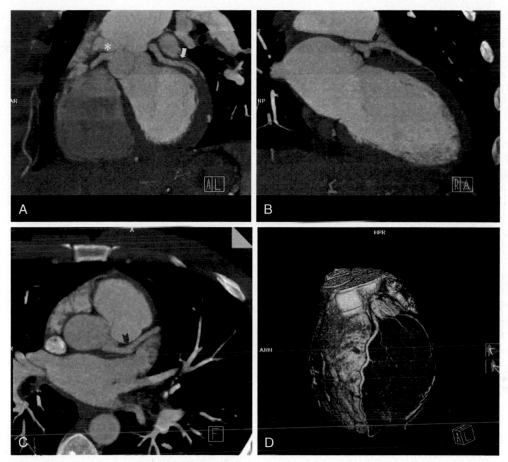

Figure 21-4 **A-C,** Maximum intensity projection reformatted images of the coronary artery tree in a patient with patent coronary arteries. **D,** Volume-rendered image of the heart and coronary arteries in the same patient. In panel **A,** the asterisk (*) indicates the origin of the right coronary artery and the *yellow arrow* points at a bifurcation point of the circumflex and obtuse marginal vessel. In quadrant **B-D,** the *red arrow head* points at the proximal mid-left anterior descending coronary artery.

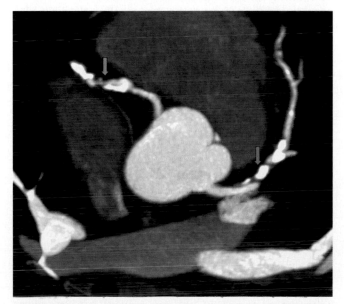

Figure 21-5 Maximum intensity projection reformatted image showing the right coronary artery to the *left* of the figure and the left anterior descending coronary artery to the *right* of the figure. The *orange arrow* points at an area of severe stenosis in the right coronary artery amidst an area of dense calcification. The *blue arrow* points at areas of bright "blooming" artifact produced by dense calcification in the proximal left anterior descending coronary artery.

These technical characteristics need to be compared to those of invasive angiography with a spatial resolution of 0.2 mm and temporal resolution of 5 to 20 ms.[13]

A number of relatively small studies compared 16-slice[16–29] and 64-slice MDCT[30–47] to invasive coronary angiography as the gold standard for detection of obstructive coronary artery disease (CAD) defined as either =50% or =70% luminal artery stenosis. These studies had limitations: they tended to be small (most enrolled less than 100 patients) single-center studies and involved mostly men. To date, there have been three multicenter trials comparing 64-slice MDCT to invasive coronary angiography.[48–50] The published estimates of accuracy are somewhat variable because of the use of different scanning protocols and different hardware. Many of the earlier studies excluded unassessable coronary artery segments from statistical analysis, which resulted in artificially elevated measurements of accuracy.[12] Most studies included only coronary segments over 1.5 to 2 mm in diameter, although a few evaluated all segments, including small side branches, leading to lower estimates of accuracy. Finally, some of the investigators reported results only on a coronary artery segment or vessel basis, rather than on a patient basis. A segment-by-segment analysis obviously provides more statistical power for the investigation, but a patient-based analysis tends to be more relevant to clinical practice and to the current use of CTA, which revolves around the decision as to whether a patient should be sent to the invasive catheterization laboratory or not.[51]

Three meta-analyses summarized several studies comparing the diagnostic accuracy of coronary MDCT angiography versus invasive angiography as the reference standard.[12,51,52] Vanhoenacker et al.[12] included 22 4-slice MDCT studies, 26 16-slice studies, and 6 64-slice studies. Each study in this meta-analysis assessed the ability of MDCT angiography to detect =50% coronary stenosis on invasive angiography. Analyses were performed on three levels: per patient (1474 total patients), in which the presence of any stenosis in any coronary artery was considered a positive result; per vessel (2692 vessels); and per coronary artery segment, based on the American Heart Association approved 15-segment model (30,775 segments). On a per-patient basis, the 4-slice MDCTs, 16-slice MDCTs, and 64-slice MDCTs demonstrated the following sensitivity and specificity: 91% and 83%, 97% and 81%, and 99% and 93%, respectively. Thus, with an increasing number of detectors, the diagnostic performance of MDCT for detection of obstructive CAD seems to have increased. Additionally, there were fewer unassessable segments with 16- and 64-slice MDCT in comparison to 4-slice MDCT.

A second meta-analysis[51] comparing 4-, 8-, 16-, and 64-slice MDCT to invasive angiography reached similar conclusions. In this analysis, the authors used 41 single-center studies published between 1997 and 2006 and analyzed data per patient (2515) and per segment (21,821). Diagnostic accuracy improved with each newer generation of scanner. On a per-patient basis, 4- and 8-slice MDCT (combined analysis) showed a sensitivity and specificity of 97% and 81%, respectively, 16-slice MDCT had a sensitivity and specificity of 99% and 83%, and 64-slice MDCT had a sensitivity and specificity of 98% and 92%.

In the third meta-analysis,[52] the authors compared 64-slice MDCT alone to invasive angiography. Twenty-seven studies including 1740 patients were reviewed, including four studies with patients who had undergone coronary artery bypass grafting (CABG) and five studies of patients with coronary stents. Of the 18,920 coronary segments, only 4% were unassessable and thus excluded from analysis. A positive study by MDCT or invasive angiography was defined as =50% coronary stenosis. For stenoses in the native coronary artery on a per-patient basis, 64-slice MDCT showed a sensitivity of 97.5%, specificity of 91%, positive predictive value (PPV) of 93%, and negative predictive value (NPV) of 96.5%, consistent with findings in the other two meta-analyses. For post-CABG patients, sensitivity was 98.5%, specificity 96%, PPV 92%, and NPV 99%. Accuracy was considerably less for detection of in-stent restenosis, with a sensitivity of 87%, specificity 96%, PPV 83.5%, and NPV 97%.[52]

The more recent prospective multicenter trials conducted utilizing 64-slice CT, however, did not completely confirm the very optimistic results reported in the earlier meta-analyses. Budoff et al. compared coronary CTA using 64-slice MDCT to invasive coronary angiography in 230 patients.[48] As reported in the meta-analyses, this study showed a high NPV (99%) of coronary 64-slice MDCT for the detection of =50% or =70% coronary luminal stenoses, but a lower specificity and PPV (83% and 99%, respectively, for both per-patient and per-vessel analyses). The authors further noted a substantial decrease in specificity of MDCT in the presence of a coronary artery calcium (CAC) score over 400. The study by Meijboom et al. again illustrated the high NPV of 64-slice MDCT (97% and 99% for patient and segmental analyses) but also the lower than expected specificity and PPV of 64-slice MDCT (64% and 86% for patient and 90% and 47% for segmental analyses).[49] In this study of 360 patients with stable or unstable angina, the authors reported a high false-positive rate for MDCT: 41 patients with only mild CAD on invasive angiography were classified by MDCT as having obstructive CAD. However, the investigators did not exclude any coronary segment from evaluation, and heavily calcified segments were considered to harbor obstructive stenoses. Finally, Miller et al.[50] reported the results of a nine-center study conducted with Toshiba 64-slice scanners involving 291 patients. Patients with a CAC score over 600 and vessels with a diameter less than 1.5 mm were excluded. The overall area under the curve for detection of more than 50% stenosis by MDCT was 0.93 for patient and 0.91 for vessel analyses. Although the specificities were high (90% and 93%), the NPVs were lower than previously reported (83% and 89%) for both patient and vessel analyses.

Dual-source 64-slice MDCT (Siemens, Forcheim, Germany) has improved temporal resolution, with fewer motion artifacts,[53] and the initial clinical experience has shown excellent diagnostic performance of this scanner.[4-6]

Finally, the new 320-slice MDCT scanner (Toshiba, Tochigi-ken, Japan) has undergone a very initial evaluation.[54] The attractiveness of this technology is the potential to limit radiation exposure by allowing whole-heart coverage with a single rotation, although this cannot be obtained for high heart rates, as explained earlier in this chapter. In a study of 40 patients, only one of 1166 coronary artery segments was unassessable, and 89% of the segments showed excellent image quality. Four of the 40 patients underwent invasive angiography. There were seven coronary stenoses =50% noted on 320-row MDCT, and all were confirmed by invasive angiography.[54] The average radiation dose was 6.8 ± 1.4 mSv for the single-rotation protocol, although several patients required more rotations, with a substantial increase in radiation dose.

In aggregate, the various studies conducted so far, with the exception of one outlying study showing an NPV of only 83%,[50] have consistently shown a high NPV of CTA (in every other case >97% and often close to 100%). It is therefore appropriate to assume that at this stage of development, CTA is especially useful to exclude the presence of obstructive CAD, rather than conclusively demonstrating its presence. In fact, as illustrated by the most recent randomized studies,[48,49,50] MDCT does appear to carry a significant false-positive risk for prediction of obstructive luminal disease on invasive angiography.

Coronary CTA for Evaluation of Bypass Grafts (Fig. 21-6)

Coronary CTA is useful for the evaluation of bypass grafts. Saphenous vein grafts are larger than coronary arteries and less mobile, making them easier to image. Arterial grafts are smaller in caliber than vein grafts but can be evaluated accurately by coronary CTA. Coronary CTA has shown excellent diagnostic performance for the evaluation of coronary grafts compared to invasive angiography, with 64-slice MDCT being more accurate than 16-slice MDCT.[36,55-62] Several studies have quoted a sensitivity and specificity of 100% for evaluation of patency of the body of the grafts. Difficulty can arise, however, in evaluation of the anastomotic site and of the native coronary arteries distal to the anastomosis. A clear visibility of the anastomotic site to the native coronary artery is often hampered by the presence of surgical clips that cause significant image artifact. The distal segments of the native coronary arteries after the anastomosis are often small, diseased, and at times heavily calcified. These factors limit the ability of CTA to accurately detect for full spectrum of disease in patients submitted to CABG. Another potentially useful application of coronary CTA is planning for repeat bypass surgery, as shown in a publication by Gasparovic et al.[63] The clear three-dimensional (3D) reconstruction of the chest cavity and visualization of the course of previous grafts, mammary arteries, location of an aortic aneurysm with respect to other vital organs, and so forth, provide an accurate in-space orientation and may be of great aid to the surgeon planning an often difficult and at times dangerous reoperation.

Coronary CTA for Evaluation of Coronary Stent Patency (Fig. 21-7)

In-stent restenosis occurs at a relatively high rate, and patients with prior stent placement comprise a good proportion of patients referred for invasive coronary angiography. Therefore, the development of a noninvasive modality that can accurately detect in-stent restenosis would be very clinically useful. Coronary stent evaluation, however, continues to be limited with coronary CTA. The main problem encountered is the "blooming artifact" (see artificial overexpansion of the borders of the stent in Fig. 21-7) caused by the high-density material of the struts that makes assessment of stent lumen patency difficult. The size of the stent[64] and the coexistence of calcification in the vicinity of the stent further complicate the performance of diagnostic-quality CTA imaging. Some improvement in diagnostic quality can be obtained by reconstructing angiographic images with a sharper kernel, as shown in Figure 21-7. Naturally, the evaluation of large stents, such as those in the left main coronary artery, is more accurate.[65,66]

In an earlier study, 64 patients with 102 stents were assessed with 64-slice MDCT, and the results were compared to those of invasive quantitative coronary angiography.[67] Only 58% of the stents were assessable, and these were larger than the stents that could not be accurately viewed (average diameter 3.28 versus 3.03 mm; $P = 0.0002$), yielding an overall sensitivity and specificity of 50% and 57%, respectively. For the assessable stents, the sensitivity and specificity rose to 86% and 98%, respectively. The authors further reported that paclitaxel-eluting stents (Boston Scientific, Maple Grove, MN) with 0.13-mm strut thickness were more likely to be assessable than sirolimus-eluting stents (Cordis Corporation, Miami Lakes, FL) with 0.14-mm strut thickness ($P < 0.001$ for frequency of assessability). Two more

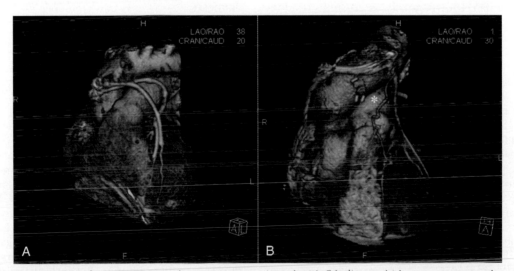

Figure 21-6 Two examples of coronary artery bypass surgery viewed with 64-slice multidetector computed tomography angiography. The patient in panel **A** underwent a dual saphenous vein bypass grafting to the left anterior descending coronary artery and diagonal vessel. The patient in panel **B** underwent bypass grafting of the left anterior descending coronary artery via the left internal mammary artery (*asterisk*).

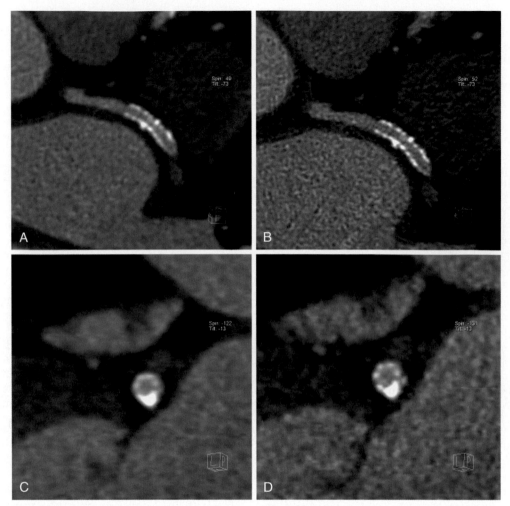

Figure 21-7 A and **C** show axial and cross-sectional images of a stent in the middle portion of the left circumflex coronary artery obtained with a 64-slice multidetector computed tomography scanner (multiplanar reformatted images). Note the hazy appearance of the lumen, especially in the vicinity of a calcified focus, as shown in panel *C*. The same images were reconstructed using a sharper kernel (**B** and **D**), with a slight improvement in resolution.

recent publications addressed the ability of 64-slice MDCT to establish the diagnosis of in-stent restenosis.[68,69] Cademartiri et al.[68] evaluated 182 patients who had received 192 stents larger than 2.5 mm in diameter and reported that 7.3% of the stents could not be evaluated. For the remaining stents, 64-slice MDCT demonstrated excellent test characteristics as follows: sensitivity 95%, specificity 93%, PPV 63%, and NPV 99%. Schuijf et al.[69] performed a similar analysis in 50 patients who had received 76 stents (2.25 to 4.0 mm in diameter and 8 to 33 mm in length); of these, 14% could not be evaluated, mostly due to motion artifacts (mean heart rate in patients with nonevaluable stents versus evaluable stents: 72+9 versus 55+2; $P = 0.002$). In the remaining 56 stents, 64-slice MDCT demonstrated both a sensitivity and specificity of 100%. The authors further reported that nonobstructive disease within the stent was clearly diagnosable in 71% of the cases. Dual-source 64-slice MDCT also been evaluated in a recent study of 35 patients with 48 stents.[70] All 48 stents were assessable by dual-source MDCT that showed a diagnostic performance versus invasive angiography as follows: sensitivity of 100%, specificity of 94%, PPV 89%, and NPV

100%. However, 67% of the stents were over 3 mm in diameter.

CORONARY COMPUTED TOMOGRAPHY ANGIOGRAPHY: COMPARISON WITH NUCLEAR MYOCARDIAL PERFUSION IMAGING

For many years, the most common and readily available noninvasive modality for the diagnosis of CAD was myocardial perfusion imaging (MPI) by single-photon emission computed tomography (SPECT) and more recently positron emission tomography (PET). The well-defined diagnostic utility and prognostic value of myocardial ischemia in a variety of clinical settings are well known and have been highlighted in this textbook in several other chapters. Because of the very nature of these tests, coronary CTA and MPI serve separate purposes: CTA is mostly used to identify stenotic lesions and—to a degree—burden of atherosclerosis; MPI is used to demonstrate the existence of hemodynamically significant coronary lesions. There are, however, several important questions to be asked at this stage: *What is the correlation between CTA and MPI? What CTA findings warrant further investigation with MPI? Can CTA be used to assess myocardial perfusion?*

In an early study, 114 patients at intermediate pretest likelihood of CAD underwent CTA (mostly by 64-slice MDCT) and MPI.[71] Of the 114 patients, 58 also underwent invasive angiography, based on the results of imaging studies and clinical data, once again introducing a bias due to the presence of an abnormal test guiding the performance of the subsequent test. All patients with a normal CTA had a normal invasive angiogram, and 90% had a normal MPI, emphasizing the ability of a normal CTA to rule out obstructive CAD in an intermediate-risk population. All patients with obstructive or nonobstructive disease on CTA had CAD on invasive angiography, but only 59% had an abnormal MPI. Of the patients with obstructive CAD on CTA, 82% had obstructive disease on invasive angiography, and 50% had an abnormal MPI. Di Carli et al.,[72] Hacker et al.,[73] and Gaemperli et al.[74] reached the same conclusion: There is often a substantial discrepancy between severity of stenosis assessed by CTA and MPI results. Lin et al.[75] proposed a method for improving detection of perfusion abnormalities in patients with atherosclerotic disease on CTA. Taking advantage of the ability of CTA to detect the presence and extent of obstructive and nonobstructive atherosclerosis along the coronary arteries, the authors devised a variety of scores based not only on the severity of stenosis but also the location, extent, and composition of all visualized plaques. They utilized data from 163 patients submitted to sequential CTA and MPI, and were able to show that a score based on the sum of all stenoses, or one based on the presence of mixed plaque (calcified and noncalcified), as well as the proximity of plaques to the coronary ostia, predicted an abnormal result on MPI with high accuracy. Hence, plaque location and morphology may provide additional data that improve the physician's ability to predict based on abnormal MPI results.

An elegant method to potentially overcome the partial limitations of both CTA and MPI and improve the diagnostic accuracy of these tools is image fusion. The existence of hybrid imaging equipment, such as PET/CT and SPECT/CT scanners, and the implementation of postprocessing software to merge data obtained from separate MPI and CTA equipment allow superimposing the coronary artery tree over perfusion maps of the left ventricle (Figs. 21-8 and 21-9).[76,77] Fusion imaging appears to provide a more precise co-localization of perfusion defects in a specific area of the myocardium with coronary artery stenoses, and to improve the overall diagnostic accuracy of either tool taken separately.

The preceding discussion clearly demonstrates that MPI and CTA provide complementary information, since a stenotic lesion on CTA or invasive angiography is not necessarily associated with a hemodynamic abnormality, and an abnormal MPI is not necessarily accompanied by a critical luminal stenosis on CTA. An abnormal CTA in the presence of a normal MPI, however, indicates the presence of subclinical atherosclerosis that should prompt more aggressive medical therapy even in the absence of hemodynamic alterations. The discrepancy between severity of stenosis on CTA and invasive angiography (described in the first section of this chapter), as well as the discrepancy between severity of stenosis on CTA and inducibility of myocardial ischemia on MPI, should not come as a complete surprise. Indeed, it is important to remember that with CTA, the clinician identifies more than the mere luminal stenosis of a vessel, as can be seen with invasive angiography. In fact, with CTA it is possible to identify the presence of outward and inward vessel wall remodeling, which increases the difficulty of clearly assessing the severity of luminal restriction. Furthermore, the presence of mere stenosis does not necessarily establish the presence of flow abnormalities. Neither invasive coronary angiography nor coronary CTA correlate well with the assessment of the hemodynamic significance of coronary stenoses by intracoronary fractional flow reserve measured by Doppler flow wires.[78,79] Finally, as said in other sections of this chapter, the presence of dense

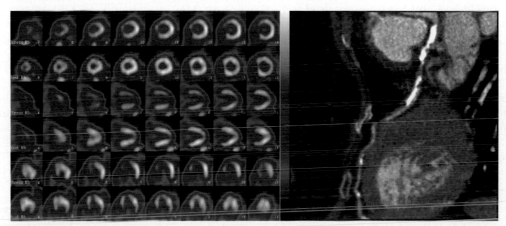

Figure 21-8 SPECT scan *(left)* and the corresponding computed tomography angiography image *(right)* of the left anterior descending coronary artery (curved multiplanar reformatted image). Note the luminal disease between two areas of dense calcification along the left anterior descending coronary artery. This was read as equivocal for obstructive coronary artery disease.

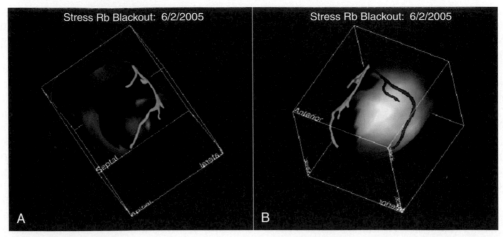

Figure 21-9 Fusion of SPECT and computed tomography angiography images shown in Fig. 21-8, in a patient with single-vessel coronary artery disease. In the fused display, the *black area* identifies a region of myocardial hypoperfusion during stress. The segment of the left anterior descending coronary artery rendered in *green* identifies the area of disease seen on CT angiography.

calcification causing blooming artifact (see Fig. 21-5) and the occurrence of motion artifacts render the interpretation of severity of stenosis very difficult. All of these factors mitigate the probability of a perfect match between anatomic and functional imaging.

Nicol et al.[80] addressed the question of what type of CTA results should prompt a referral to MPI. In a study of 52 symptomatic patients with low to intermediate pretest probability of disease, an abnormal MPI result was observed more often (86% versus 50%) in subjects with a CTA stenosis =70% than =50%. They concluded that CTA lesions narrowing the coronary lumen =70% should be considered "hemodynamically significant," and patients hosting this type of lesion should be referred for invasive angiography. Since the NPV of a CTA stenosis less than 50% was 100% for an abnormal MPI, no further testing should be recommended for these patients. Further MPI testing, however, should be considered for patients with stenosis severity graded as 50% to 69%. Similarly, Sato et al.[81] performed 64-slice CTA and MPI in 104 lean Japanese patients; once again the probability of an abnormal MPI was significantly greater for CTA stenosis =80% (PPV: 86%) compared to lower degrees of stenosis. It should be noted that both investigator groups (Nicol and Sato) emphasized ischemia detected by MPI as the primary target of investigation for CAD, a viewpoint that clinicians interested in the detection of preclinical coronary atherosclerosis may find arguable and oppose.

MPI and CTA have been compared in the setting of acute chest pain in the emergency room. In low-risk patients, the accuracy of CTA appears to be at least as good as MPI for the diagnosis of acute coronary syndrome (ACS).[82] In one study, a low-risk population of 85 patients with chest pain, negative serial cardiac enzymes, and normal ECG were submitted to both rest/stress MPI and CTA (64-slice MDCT). Patients with a reversible defect on MPI or =50% stenosis on CTA were referred for invasive angiography. The endpoints were accurate identification of greater than 70% stenosis by invasive angiography or a major adverse cardiac event within 30 days. Seven patients met a primary endpoint (all > 70% stenosis by invasive angiography). Sensitivity and specificity of MPI for predicting an endpoint were 71% and 90%, respectively, while sensitivity and specificity of 64-slice MDCT were 86% and 92%. In a similar emergency room setting, Goldstein et al.[83] randomized 99 low-risk patients to 64-slice CTA and 98 similar patients to MPI at a single medical center. The patients in whom CTA showed minimal or no disease were discharged home; if CTA showed over 70% stenosis in one or more vessels, they were sent directly to invasive angiography, and if the lesion was determined to be intermediate, they were referred for MPI. A standard protocol was followed for the patients referred to MPI first. Among the CTA patients, 68 were immediately discharged home, 8 were referred for invasive angiography, and 24 to MPI. Patients were managed equally well in the two imaging arms, and there were no untoward events at 6 months in either group. In the CTA group, however, the final diagnosis was reached in a significantly shorter time (3.4 versus 15 hours; $P < 0.001$), with a cost saving of about $300 per patient, and the patients required fewer recurrent evaluations for chest pain. It would appear, therefore, that in the emergency room setting, CTA may be an acceptable alternative to MPI in patients at low pretest likelihood of disease. Of interest, in a matched-cohort observational study of patients with new-onset chest pain undergoing coronary CTA or MPI, the 2-year mortality rate based on severity of CAD as assessed by coronary CTA was not significantly different from the rate based on severity of ischemia as assessed by MPI.[84] This isolated outcome study suggests that the noninvasive assessment of severity of anatomic stenosis or hemodynamic impediment to blood flow may have similar prognostic implications. Obviously, such data will need to be confirmed in larger prospective studies, but they constitute interesting hypothesis-generating information. Cury et al. recently reviewed the use of coronary CTA in the emergency department setting (Table 21-1).[85] This review confirmed the high NPV of CTA for the exclusion of acute coronary syndromes in patients at low to intermediate pretest probability of disease.

Table 21-1 Summary of Studies Validating Cardiac CT to Detect Patients with ACS in ED

Author (Journal, Year)	Scanner Type	TIMI Risk (Prevalence of ACS)	N	% Stenosis	Sensitivity (%)	Specificity (%)	PPV (%)	NPV (%)
Sato et al (Circ J, 2005)	16-Slice CT	Intermediate (71%)	31	>75	95	89	95	89
White et al. (AJR Am J Roentgenol, 2005)	16-Slice CT	Low to intermediate (21%)	69	>50	87	96	87	96
Hoffmann et al. (Circulation, 2006)	64-Slice CT	Low (14%)	103	>50	100	82	47	100
Gallagher et al. (Ann Emerg Med, 2007)	64-Slice CT	Very low (8%)	85	>50 (Ca > 400)	86	92	50	99
Rubinshtein et al. (Circulation, 2007)	64-Slice CT	Intermediate (34%)	58	>50	100	92	87	100
Goldstein et al.* (J Am Coll Cardiol, 2007)	64-Slice CT	Very low (8%)	99	>25	100	74	25	100
Total[†]			445	25-75	95	86	61	99

*In the study of Goldstein et al., 24 patients with intermediate stenosis (25%-70%) or nondiagnostic results were considered positive by multidetector computed tomography (MDCT) in this analysis; these patients needed further workup and could not be discharged from the ED based only on the cardiac CT results.
†Pooled sensitivity, specificity, positive predictive value (PPV), and negative predictive value (NPV) were calculated by combining all six studies.
ACS, acute coronary syndrome; Ca > 400, calcium score above 400; CT, computed tomography; ED, emergency department; TIMI, thrombolysis in myocardial infarction.
From Cury RC, Feutchner G, Pena CS, et al: Acute chest pain imaging in the emergency department with cardiac computed tomography angiography, J Nucl Cardiol 15:564-75, 2008.

CORONARY COMPUTED TOMOGRAPHY ANGIOGRAPHY TO PERFORM MYOCARDIAL PERFUSION IMAGING AND ASSESS VIABILITY

The option to utilize CTA to evaluate myocardial perfusion, infarct size, and viability has been recently explored. Although MDCT can be used for these applications, there is a substantial difference between CTA and MPI; with the former, one can obtain mostly perfusion information (i.e., presence or absence of blood flow in the coronary arteries and into the myocardium), the latter provides information on cellular and molecular function, which is, of course, dependent on coronary blood flow. During the arterial phase of CT angiography, reduced contrast enhancement may be due to severe epicardial coronary stenosis or occlusion, obstruction of the microcirculation, or myocardial scar. Chronic myocardial infarction can usually be identified as an area of reduced myocardial enhancement, but wall thickness and abnormal wall motion, differentiation of severe stenosis, acute myocardial infarction, or microvascular obstruction are problematic on resting CTA angiography. One of the major limiting factors for CTA is the rapid fading of contrast from the myocardium. MPI imaging is an "equilibrium imaging" acquired over several minutes, while CTA perfusion imaging is an instantaneous form of myocardial imaging, and the fleeting appearance of iodine contrast hampers the clear distinction of hypoperfused myocardium, normally perfused myocardium, and the blood pool. Pharmacologic stress testing prior to CTA to improve detection of myocardial ischemia with this tool has been applied in both

animal[86] and human experiments.[87] George et al.[86] created coronary artery stenoses in the LAD of eight anesthetized dogs and performed rest and adenosine stress CTA. They then compared the myocardial signal intensity (measured in Hounsfield units [HU]) of ischemic and remote nonischemic regions and measured myocardial blood flow (MBF) with infusion of microphages. They found a close correlation between MBF and myocardial signal intensity, both in ischemic and distant regions. Kurata et al.[87] performed rest and stress CTA in 12 patients. All 12 patients were also submitted to MPI and 9 of them to invasive coronary angiography. Adenosine triphosphate (ATP) stress CTA and MPI showed an agreement of 83% ($P < 0.05$ for concordance), with only a few discordant myocardial segments between the two techniques. Hence, it appears that stress CTA may perform fairly well for detection of myocardial ischemia. However, the performance of stress CTA implies not only a double exposure to a considerable amount of radiation but also a double dose of iodine contrast, rendering this technique unattractive at the current state of development. An interesting application of CTA for myocardial perfusion was recently proposed by Ruzsics et al.[53] In 35 patients with chest pain, the authors performed CTA utilizing a dual-source 64-slice MDCT (Siemens, Forcheism, Germany) with each x-ray tube operated at different x-ray energy spectra. The aim of the authors was to obtain simultaneous diagnostic information on coronary artery stenosis and myocardial perfusion from the same CT acquisition without the need to repeat two separate studies. The patients were also submitted to invasive coronary angiography and MPI for comparison. CT demonstrated an accuracy of 92% to detect both coronary artery obstructive disease and myocardial perfusion abnormalities

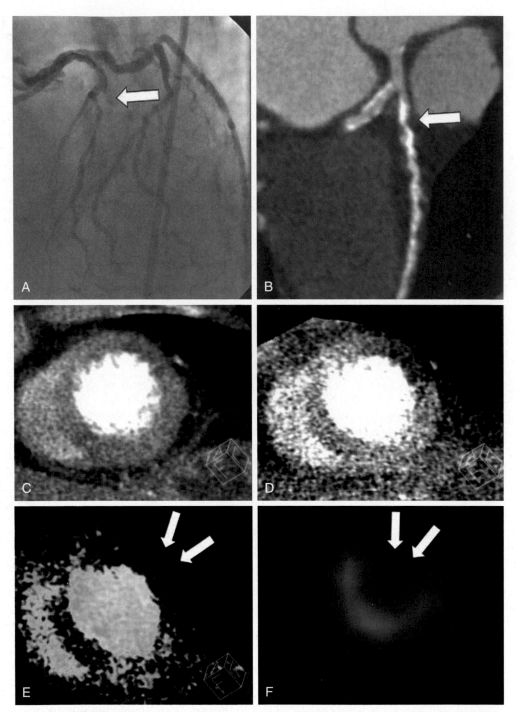

Figure 21-10 Comparison of dual-source computed tomography angiography perfusion and SPECT in a patient with obstructive disease of the left anterior descending coronary artery. **A-B,** Site of severe stenosis in the proximal left anterior descending coronary artery *(white arrow)* on invasive angiography *(A)* and coronary computed tomography angiography *(B)* (curved multiplanar reformatted image). **C-D,** Same short-axis section across the left ventricle obtained with 140 kV *(C)* and 80 kV *(D)*. **E,** Color-coded image of the iodine pool in the myocardium, obtained by merging the two images in *(C)* and *(D)*; figure shows good correspondence with a perfusion abnormality in the same area of the myocardium obtained with SPECT **(F)**. *(From Ruzsics B, Lee H, Zwerner PL, et al: Dual-energy CT of the heart for diagnosing coronary artery stenosis and myocardial ischemia: Initial experience, Eur Radiol 18:2414-2424, 2008. Reprinted with permission.)*

(Fig. 21-10). Since dual-energy imaging will become available in several CT systems in the near future, these findings suggest that the presence of perfusion defects may enhance the diagnostic accuracy of CTA for coronary stenoses, often hampered by the presence of severe artifacts (as discussed elsewhere in this chapter).

Numerous publications have addressed the ability of CTA to identify areas of acute myocardial infarction as well as areas of scar, as defined by the presence of delayed hyperenhancement. In fact, it appears that gadolinium and iodine contrast demonstrate similar molecular weight and volume of distribution in areas of myocardial infarction. The best time delay to evaluate presence of infarction by CTA is not yet defined. Investigators have used a time delay varying between 5 and 15 minutes, although there is some evidence that the best results are obtained when imaging at 5 minutes after contrast infusion.[88] Possible explanations for the accumulation of iodine contrast in areas of acute infarction include the accumulation of iodine in the extracellular matrix and/or the inability of necrotic myocardial cells to excrete the iodine due to sarcolemmal membrane dysfunction.[89] In the chronic phase of a myocardial infarction, the iodine contrast is accumulated in the extracellular matrix of a scar. Infarcted areas with microvascular obstruction due to cellular debris blockage of intramyocardial capillaries appear as subendocardial areas of hypoenhancement adjacent to the hyperenhanced areas.[89]

In animal experiments, myocardial infarction has been induced with ligation of a coronary artery[90] or via prolonged inflations of angioplasty balloons,[89,91] and the size of the infarct measured by means of postmortem triphenyltetrazolium chloride (TTC) myocardial staining. Hoffmann et al.[90] ligated the LAD and performed first-pass CTA in 5 pigs within 3 hours of inducing myocardial infarction. A distinct area of hypoenhancement, which correlated well with reduced blood flow measured by microspheres and size of infarction by TTC, was seen in all animals. Baks et al.[91] performed CTA imaging in pigs 5 days after inducing myocardial infarction with prolonged balloon inflation, while Lardo et al.[89] waited 8 weeks after inducing the infarction. Both groups of investigators showed a good correlation between the area of hyperenhancement detected on delayed CTA and infarct size on TTC staining. A hypoenhanced area on delayed CTA images was found to be a reliable indicator of microvascular obstruction (i.e., no-reflow phenomenon).[89] Finally, there was an excellent correlation between the area of delayed hyperenhancement found on CTA and MRI.[91] Very similar correlation results between CT and MRI were reported in humans by Gerber et al.[88] and Nieman et al.[92] In several small human studies, the extent of myocardial scarring, subendocardial to transmyocardial, was correlated with subsequent recovery of left ventricular function.[93-96]

From the preceding discussion, it would appear that CTA is well poised to provide useful information about presence and extent of myocardial infarction. However, this information must be obtained with a second radiation exposure, and where MRI is feasible, it may still represent the preferred approach.

ASSESSMENT OF LEFT VENTRICULAR FUNCTION AND MASS BY CARDIAC COMPUTED TOMOGRAPHY

The assessment of left ventricular volumes, function, and mass was shown to be feasible and very accurate with the older EBCT technique.[97-101] However, since EBCT used a step-and-shoot acquisition protocol for the coronary arteries (one image per heartbeat or every other beat), left ventricular function could only be obtained after the injection of a second dose of iodine contrast and the acquisition of a multiphase and multilevel scan; this of course increased the risk and discomfort for the patient. With MDCT scanners, the continuous helical acquisition of hundreds of slices throughout the cardiac cycle makes it possible to utilize the same scan used to assess CAD to evaluate left ventricular function. To assess left ventricular function, end-diastolic and end-systolic volumes are usually measured using the Simpson method or, more recently, using a threshold-based volumetric method that takes advantage of the high contrast-to-noise ratio between the left ventricular cavity filled with contrast and the myocardium.[102] The end-diastolic frames are obtained from a late-diastolic phase at 85% to 95% of the R-R interval on the surface ECG and the end-systolic frames from an early systolic phase at 25% to 30% of the R-R interval, respectively (Fig. 21-11). Magnetic resonance imaging (MRI), currently considered the noninvasive modality of reference for the assessment of global and regional left ventricular function, has been compared to MDCT in several publications. Whereas MDCT has a better spatial resolution than EBCT and MRI, its accuracy for the determination of left ventricular ejection fraction is affected by its lower temporal resolution, which usually results in the overestimation of end-systolic volumes and an underestimation of left ventricular ejection fraction. Despite this limitation, the left ventricular ejection fraction obtained with 4- and 16-slice cardiac MDCT showed a very good correlation with that obtained with invasive contrast ventriculography[103] and with MRI.[104-115] In several comparative studies, the MDCT and MRI left ventricular ejection fraction showed a correlation coefficient varying from 0.82 to 0.99. Although the majority of studies demonstrated an excellent correlation of 64-slice MDCT with MRI ($r = 0.92$ to 0.95),[111,112] Schlosser et al.[116] calculated a significantly lower left ventricular ejection fraction with 64-slice cardiac MDCT than MRI. So far, dual-source MDCT, with greater temporal resolution than other currently available 64-slice MDCT scanners, has shown mixed results, with an excellent[114] to modest[113] correlation with MRI (Table 21-2). Finally, Schepis et al.[110] compared 64-slice MDCT with gated SPECT and found a correlation coefficient of 0.82 for the measurement of left ventricular function. Mass can also be accurately assessed with MDCT, with a closer similarity to MRI than seen with measurement of left ventricular volumes and function.[109,115-118] However, Ferencik et al.[119] calculated a significantly lower left ventricular mass with 64-slice MDCT than echocardiography in heart transplant recipients. This systematic error between the techniques may be secondary to the very different assumptions made with 3D and 2D imaging techniques.

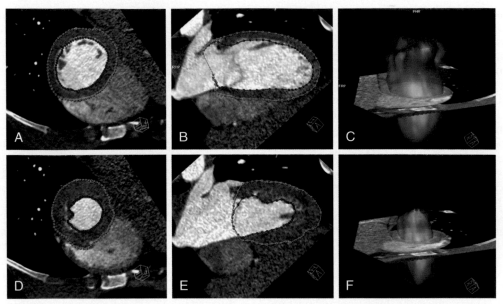

Figure 21-11 Example of calculation of left ventricular volumes and function with multidetector computed tomography angiography. The endocardial border is marked by the *red dotted line* and the epicardial border by the *green dotted line*. **A,** Short-axis left ventricular end-diastolic frame. **B,** Vertical long-axis left ventricular end-diastolic frame. **C,** End-diastolic volumetric reformation of the left ventricle. **D,** Short-axis left ventricular end-systolic frame. **E,** Vertical long-axis left ventricular end-systolic frame. **F,** End-systolic volumetric reformation of the left ventricle.

Table 21-2 Publications Addressing the Ability of Multidetector Computed Tomography Angiography to Assess Left Ventricular Volumes, Ejection Fraction, and Mass

Study	Multidetector Computed Tomography Type	Modality of Reference	Correlation Coefficient
Left Ventricular Volume and Ejection Fraction Calculation			
Juergens, 2002[104]	4-slice	Cine	0.80
Halliburton, 2003[105]	4-slice	MRI	0.82
Yamamuro, 2005[106]	8-slice	MRI	0.96
Mahnken, 2005[107]	16-slice	MRI	0.99
Sugeng, 2006[108]	16-slice	MRI	0.85
Raman, 2006[108]	16-slice	MRI	0.97
Gilard, 2006[103]	16-slice	Cine	0.79
Schepis, 2006[110]	64-slice	Gated SPECT	0.82
Annuar, 2008[111]	64-slice	MRI	0.92
Wu, 2008[112]	64-slice	MRI	0.97
Busch, 2008[113]	Dual source 64-slice	MRI	0.64
Puesken, 2008[114]	Dual source 64-slice	MRI	0.99
van der Vleuten, 2008[115]	Dual source 64-slice	MRI	0.90
Left Ventricular Mass Calculation			
Raman, 2006[109]	16-slice	MRI	0.95
Heuschmid, 2006[118]	16-slice	MRI	0.84
Schlosser, 2007[116]	64-slice	MRI	—*
Ferencik, 2007[119]	64-slice	2D Echocardiography	0.67
van der Vleuten, 2008[115]	Dual-source 64-slice	MRI	0.94
Bastarrika, 2008[117]	Dual-source 64-slice	MRI	0.97

*Left ventricular mass measurements did not differ between CT and MRI.
2D Echocardiography, two-dimensional echocardiography; Cine, cine ventriculography; CT, computed tomography; MRI, magnetic resonance imaging; Gated SPECT, gated single-photon emission computed tomography.

PROGNOSIS OF PATIENTS UNDERGOING COMPUTED TOMOGRAPHY ANGIOGRAPHY TO DIAGNOSE CORONARY ARTERY DISEASE

Because MDCT angiography is such a recently introduced imaging system, there are very few studies evaluating its prognostic value. These studies were performed in patients with chest pain, in patients with multiple risk factors for CAD, or in patients with known CAD.

Based on the findings of a CTA study, patients could be categorized as having (1) no disease, (2) nonobstructive disease, and (3) obstructive CAD. As expected, patients with no disease have the lowest risk for subsequent cardiovascular events or death. This has been clearly demonstrated in several studies. Gilard et al. followed 141 patients with normal CTA findings for a mean period of 14.7 months. These patients experienced 0% mortality, a 3.5% rate of subsequent conventional coronary angiography, and a 0.7% rate of myocardial infarction, which compared favorably with those following conventional coronary angiography with normal findings.[120] In two other recent studies, patients without abnormal findings on CTA had no major cardiovascular events (i.e., cardiac death, nonfatal myocardial infarction, unstable angina, revascularization) after an average follow-up of 12 months.[121,122] In the experience reported by Matsumoto et al.,[123] the annual rate of acute coronary syndromes (nonfatal myocardial infarction, unstable angina) and cardiac death was 0.66% and 0.21%, respectively, over a 3-year follow-up period.

The high NPV of CTA makes it an attractive alternative for low-risk patients in the emergency room setting. Rubinshtein et al.[124] discharged 35 patients from the emergency room after initial triage and CTA and showed that no patient died or had a myocardial infarction during a 15-month period, and only one underwent late percutaneous coronary intervention; despite this apparent mishap, the NPV of CTA was still 97%.

When the findings of CTA are indicative of atherosclerotic disease with nonobstructive lesions, this confers a moderately elevated risk for subsequent cardiovascular events. The risk of first-year major cardiovascular events (cardiac death, nonfatal myocardial infarction, unstable angina, and revascularization) in this group of patients is in the range of 3% to 8%.[121,122] In a 3-year follow-up, the annual event rate for any acute coronary syndrome or cardiac death in patients with mild to moderate stenoses on CTA (25% to 75%) was about 2%, significantly higher than the event rate in patients with no stenoses.[123]

One of the main advantages of CTA over conventional coronary angiography is its ability to visualize not only the lumen but also the plaque itself. In more than 50% of myocardial infarctions, the culprit lesion is a nonstenotic yet vulnerable lipid-rich plaque.[125] CTA is currently the only noninvasive technology capable of evaluating plaque morphology, and this specific advantage of CTA may be the source of the additional prognostic information provided by this imaging modality. Indeed, the presence of nonobstructive disease on invasive angiography has also been shown to be predictive of an adverse outcome in the Coronary Artery Surgery Study.[126]

Finally, patients with obstructive coronary artery disease on CTA have a very high risk for subsequent cardiovascular events and death. Depending on multiple factors beyond the anatomic findings per se, this risk may be as high as 63% for the first year.[122] However, it is well known that the location and extent of CAD play an important role in determining prognosis. These findings are in line with the findings from conventional coronary angiography that have been widely used for risk stratification and management of patients with CAD. The presence of either obstructive or nonobstructive plaques in the left main (LM) coronary artery, the left anterior descending (LAD) coronary artery, and in the proximal segment of any of the three major coronary arteries confers an unfavorable prognosis. Another factor that affects prognosis is the number of segments with plaques.[121]

In the study of Pundziute et al.,[122] multivariate analyses revealed that the presence of obstructive CAD, obstructive CAD in left main or left anterior descending coronary artery, the number of segments with plaques, the number of segments with obstructive plaques, and the number of segments with mixed plaques were independent predictors of events.

In an attempt to assess the association of all-cause mortality with the extent and severity of CAD, Min et al.[127] followed 1127 patients with chest pain symptoms for 15 months after undergoing CTA. They applied several methods of estimating CAD severity and extent: (1) assessment of moderate (=50% of the vessel diameter) or severe (=70% of the vessel diameter) stenosis in the three coronary arteries and the left main trunk, (2) the Duke prognostic CAD index[128] and one modification of it in patients with <50% stenosis, and (3) three different clinical plaque scores measuring plaque burden and distribution. Each one of these methods gave important prognostic information.

The findings of all aforementioned studies highlight the potentially useful prognostic role of CTA in patients with chest pain or high-risk features for CAD. Patients with a negative CTA study (no evidence of obstructive or nonobstructive disease) have a very good prognosis. The presence of nonobstructive plaques confers a generally good prognosis, although worse than the absence of atherosclerotic plaques. Hence, by assessing presence of plaque and plaque characteristics, CTA may provide additional useful prognostic information not obtainable with an MPI study or an invasive angiogram. Finally, patients with severe stenoses suffer a significantly higher rate of events than all others, confirming older data obtained with invasive angiography. The obvious weakness is the limited amount of data currently available with CTA, and although several large databases are being collected for further outcome analyses, the prognostic value of CTA requires clarification with prospective trials.

OTHER USES OF COMPUTED TOMOGRAPHY ANGIOGRAPHY

Noncalcified Atherosclerotic Plaque

The superior spatial resolution of MDCT allows the visualization of the noncalcified component of atherosclerotic plaques (Fig. 21-12).[129–131] However, the identification of areas of low attenuation along the course of the coronary arteries is at times challenging and much more difficult than the identification of calcified foci, owing to the similar attenuation of plaque and pericoronary fat. Furthermore, the spatial resolution of MDCT is not yet sufficient to visualize the finer components of a plaque, such as the lipid core or the fibrous cap. Therefore, the precise quantification and characterization of noncalcified plaques remains an elusive goal at this time. Nonetheless, there is obviously a high degree of interest in pursuing this imaging venue because of the well-known tenet that plaques more prone to rupture (i.e., vulnerable) contain a large lipid core and are covered by a thin fibrous cap and should therefore have a lower attenuation on CT imaging than more stable and fibrotic plaques. Several attempts were made at separating lipid-rich from fibrotic plaques by assessing the mean CT attenuation in areas of apparent noncalcified atherosclerosis, and the CT findings were compared to intravascular ultrasound (IVUS) data. Achenbach et al.[130] with 16-slice MDCT and Leber et al.[132] with 64-slice MDCT showed that CTA underestimates plaque volume compared to IVUS and has modest (53%) to good sensitivity (83%) for the identification of noncalcified plaques compared to the invasive technique. The mean CT attenuation of hypoechogenic plaques on IVUS (i.e., lipid rich) was significantly lower than that of hyperechogenic (i.e., fibrotic) plaques, with values ranging from 14 to 58 HU for the former and

90-120 HU for the latter.[129,131,133] Patients with acute coronary syndromes show less coronary calcification, larger areas and greater numbers of low attenuation plaques,[134,135] and more plaques with positive remodeling[136] than patients with stable angina. In Motoyama's report,[136] the simultaneous presence of positive remodeling, areas of low attenuation, and spotty calcification identified with 95% accuracy the plaque associated with the acute coronary syndrome (i.e., culprit plaque). Since the mean CT attenuation in plaques exhibiting positive remodeling is lower than in vessels without remodeling,[137] and the plaques with the lowest attenuation have been associated with the presence of a necrotic core on spectral analysis of IVUS images (i.e., virtual histology),[138,139] the combination of low attenuation and positive remodeling makes for a severely increased risk of unstable plaques. Attempts at assessing changes in noncalcified plaque volume with sequential CTA have been conducted in animals[140] as well as in humans.[141,142] There appears to be a significant change in volume over time without treatment,[141] although this trend seems to be reversible with treatment.[140,142] Although interesting, there are some limitations to the data presented so far: The studies were very small, and data on the prognostic value of noncalcified plaque are missing, with an isolated small exception.[122] Many investigators reported a substantial overlap between CT attenuation values of lipid-rich and fibrotic plaques, hence the mere measurement of plaque attenuation may not be sufficient to define its vulnerability. Additionally, a change in image filter (technically called *kernel*) may substantially affect the measurement of CT attenuation within the plaque.[143] To overcome some of these limitations, more work is ongoing in the field. The application of dual-energy CT imaging, to take advantage of the difference in radiation absorption of different tissues, has been proposed to improve the chance to detect and characterize noncalcified plaques.[144] Although accurate, to date, this application has been limited to ex vivo experiments.[144] Finally, in animal testing, iodine-containing nanoparticles selectively uptaken by macrophages have been used in a rabbit model of atherosclerosis to image inflammation within a noncalcified plaque.[145] It is obvious that although attractive, this field needs to further expand before becoming a clinical reality.

Coronary Artery Anomalies

Visualization of congenital anomalies of the coronary arteries is achievable with high accuracy with both EBCT and MDCT.[146–149] With the isotropic volumetric information acquired with cardiac CT, it is possible to clearly delineate the origin and the course of the anomalous coronary in 3D-rendered images, as shown in Figs. 21-13 and 21-14. Although MDCT could be particularly helpful in children for early diagnosis of coronary anomalies, the younger the patients, the greater the risk linked with radiation exposure; therefore, MRI is often the preferred noninvasive imaging method for children. However, many anomalies are found serendipitously in scans ordered because of atypical chest pain or other unrelated reasons in unsuspecting adult individuals.[150]

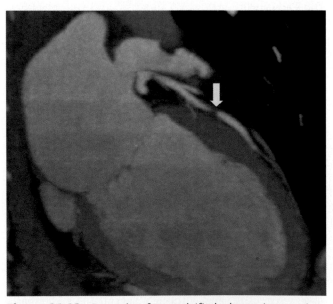

Figure 21-12 Example of noncalcified plaque in a patient with single-vessel disease. This multiplanar reformatted image shows a noncalcified plaque in the middle of the left anterior descending coronary artery *(yellow arrow)*.

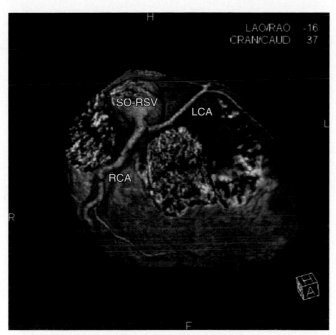

Figure 21-13 Example of anomalous left coronary artery (LCA) originating with the right coronary artery (RCA) from a single ostium from the right sinus of Valsalva (SO-RSV).

Guidance Prior to Attempting Angioplasty of a Chronic Total Occlusion

One of the main hurdles to performing a successful percutaneous angioplasty and one of the most frequent reasons for complications and restenosis after angioplasty of a chronic total occlusion is heavy calcification at the site of occlusion. Furthermore, it is often difficult for the operator to predict the length of the occlusion and the size and course of the occluded vessel. CTA has been reported to be of aide in the preoperative evaluation of patients scheduled to undergo angioplasty of totally occluded vessels. Mollet et al.[151] found two independent predictors of failure to complete the angioplasty: an occlusion length exceeding 15 mm and calcification involving more than 50% of the cross-sectional area of the coronary artery at the site of occlusion. Soon et al.[152] confirmed these findings. Yokoyama et al.[153] noted that the majority of calcification is usually located very proximal to the total occlusion, and the success rate (ability to cross the total occlusion with a guide wire) was 91% under MDCT guidance because of the visual guidance provided to the operator.

Presurgical Risk Stratification

Cardiac CT may be of value in excluding the presence of obstructive CAD prior to surgery in patients with a contraindication to cardiac catheterization or a very high risk for it. Gilard et al.[154] performed CTA with a 16-slice MDCT in 55 patients scheduled to undergo invasive coronary angiography prior to surgery for aortic valve stenosis. In cases with a CAC score <1000, 80% of the patients would not have needed an invasive angiogram, because the CT clearly excluded the presence of critical CAD. For patients with more extensive calcium scores, this proportion dropped to 6%.[154] Similar conclusions were reached by Holmström et al.,[155] who showed a sensitivity of 8-slice MDCT angiography of 63% but a NPV of 98% for obstructive CAD in 22 patients with severe aortic stenosis. A different result was reported by Scheffel et al.[156] in 50 patients awaiting surgery for aortic valve regurgitation. Given the much lower CAC score in these patients, CTA performed much better in comparison with invasive angiography to exclude obstructive disease with sensitivity, specificity, PPV and NPVs of 100%, 95%, 87%, and 100%, respectively. Accordingly, preoperative invasive angiography could have been avoided in 70% of the patients. Schlosser et al.[157] reviewed a small case series of 11 patients scheduled to undergo repair of a thoracic aorta aneurysm or

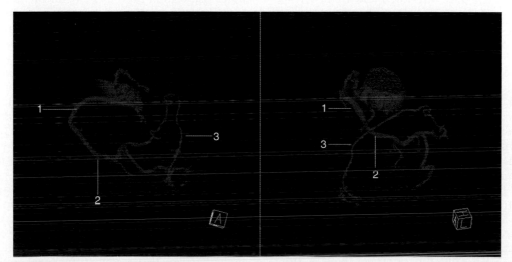

Figure 21-14 Three-dimensional reconstruction of the course of a single coronary artery originating from the right sinus of Valsalva. Numbers indicate different segments of the same vessel: 1, proximal right coronary artery; 2, distal right coronary artery, giving origin to posterior descending and posterolateral branches and continuing to the left atrioventricular groove to give origin to the left circumflex and a very thin left anterior descending coronary artery (3) running in the anterior interventricular groove.

aortic dissection in whom 64-slice CTA was performed instead of invasive angiography. They reported 100% success rate in excluding or confirming the presence of CAD, but they were also able to visualize and size the thoracic pathology of interest and clearly assess the calcification and mobility status of the mitral and aortic valves.

Assessment of Etiology of Left Ventricular Dysfunction

One of the most frequent etiologies of left ventricular dysfunction in Western countries is CAD, and invasive angiography is often performed at the time of first diagnosis of congestive heart failure. Cardiac CT can assist in excluding CAD as a cause of left ventricular dysfunction. The initial demonstration of the utility of CT in this field was provided several years ago by Budoff et al.,[158] who showed that absence of coronary artery calcium is associated with a very low probability of CAD in patients with recent diagnosis of left ventricular dysfunction. More recently, other investigators have shown that CTA is a valid alternative to invasive angiography for the exclusion of ischemic heart disease in patients with systolic dysfunction but otherwise no clinical suspicion of CAD.[159,160]

RADIATION EXPOSURE (See Chapter 10)

Despite the numerous helpful applications and the enthusiasm we witnessed in recent years, patients submitted to CTA should be carefully chosen because of the potential risks associated with the use of ionizing radiation, especially in young patients and women (added risk inherent with additional radiation to the breast and ovaries). The effective dose, expressed in millisieverts (mSv), is the dose parameter most frequently cited in the literature.[161] While coronary calcium screening delivers a relatively low radiation dose (effective dose of 0.7 mSv with EBCT and 1.0 to 4.1 mSv with MDCT), coronary CT angiography delivers much higher levels of radiation (effective dose of 9 to 20 mSv).[162] This should be compared to the radiation dose provided by MPI studies (effective dose range of 13 to 16 mSv), especially those conducted using thallium-201 or dual-isotope techniques (effective dose of 25 to 30 mSv)[163] or invasive diagnostic coronary catheterization (effective dose of 3 to 10 mSv).[164] The dose delivered depends both on the imaging protocol used and the patient's body habitus: the heavier the patient, the greater the photon flux needed to obtain a good-quality image and the greater the radiation dose. The effective dose can be decreased by using ECG-triggered tube current modulation. With this method, the x-ray tube current is decreased during systole and increased during diastole, since images typically are reconstructed from data obtained during diastole. Tube current modulation can decrease radiation dose by about a third, depending on the heart rate (the slower the heart rate, the longer the systolic phase during which current is reduced).[165–168] Prospective gating can also help reduce

radiation dose while performing coronary CTA. With standard retrospective gating, the patient moves through the gantry at a steady speed and images are obtained throughout the cardiac cycle. With prospective gating, the scans are initiated at a certain point on the cardiac cycle and typically obtained during the later portion of diastole. A limitation of this method is that systolic images are not obtained, and ventricular function cannot be assessed. Earls et al.[169] studied 82 patients with retrospective gating and 121 patients with prospective gating. They reported 83% reduction in effective dose with prospective gating compared to retrospective gating, with no difference in proportion of unassessable coronary segments and better image quality for prospective gating.[169]

Much of our knowledge on the carcinogenic effects of low doses of radiation (whole body exposures of 5 to 150 mSv) derives from follow-up data on the survivors of the atomic bombing during World War II. Although small, there appears to be an increase in incidence of cancer in subjects exposed to low doses of radiation—especially in children because of the higher radiation sensitivity and the long lifetime during which they can receive further radiation exposure and can develop cancer. There are several theories as to how risk should be estimated. The *linear no-threshold theory* assumes that risk increases linearly with dose. The *supralinear no-threshold* theory considers the risk increasing at a greater rate than the dose received. Finally, the *threshold theory* assumes that risk starts increasing only after a certain dose of radiation is absorbed. The linear no-threshold theory is the predominant view. Using this model and the organ-specific risk from Biological Effects of Ionizing Radiation (BEIR VII),[170] the data presented by Einstein et al.[171] indicate that the lifetime risk of cancer for a CTA in a 50-year-old individual is 0.4% for a man and 1.2% for a woman. Obviously these data should be interpreted in light of the overall clinical scenario for the patient under study, including the background risk of cancer incidence in the general population and any other risk factors such as diabetes mellitus, high blood pressure, or a family history of cancer or heart disease. According to statistics from the American Cancer Society, the lifetime risk of cancer at any site is 45% for men and 38% for women; the respective death rates are 23% and 20%.[172] Thus, the additive cancer risk may be negligible for a 50-year-old, hypertensive, diabetic man who might benefit substantially from the information collected with CTA. Hence, an appropriate selection of subjects to be submitted to CTA, as well as any other test utilizing ionizing radiation, will guarantee that the gain derived from the examination is greater than the added risk to the patient.

There are further limitations to the wide implementation of CTA that have been discussed in part in this chapter. Calcified lesions (and stents) cause partial volume and beam-hardening artifacts (see Fig. 21-5). A given voxel (volume unit) in the image can contain more than one tissue type. If the voxel contains calcium and another tissue type, the dense calcium signal will overwhelm the other tissue type, and the entire voxel will appear bright, making a calcified lesion appear larger than the actual size (see Fig. 21-5). This partial-volume or blooming artifact can induce a false-positive reading. A beam-hardening artifact typically causes a "shadow" adjacent to a densely calcified lesion that can be confused with a noncalcified plaque. Additionally, CTA requires use of iodinated contrast (50 to 120 mL per study) with risk of both nephrotoxicity and anaphylactic reactions. In patients with impaired renal function, the use of coronary CTA is limited, especially since an abnormal result may lead to further testing by MPI and/or invasive coronary angiography with additional radiation exposure and contrast use. Small vessels (<1.5 to 2 mm), including branches of main vessels, the distal segments of main vessels, or the native vessel distal to a graft anastomosis, are difficult to visualize. As explained in the introductory remarks, at the present state of technologic development, the heart rate should be less than 60 to 65 beats/min to obtain diagnostic-quality images with most scanners. Administration of β-blockers is therefore commonly required to lower the heart rate prior to CTA with a 16- or 64-slice MDCT, and this may limit the application of CTA to those patients who can tolerate β-blockade. Additionally, patients with atrial fibrillation or frequent ectopic beats may have decreased-quality studies.

WHEN SHOULD CORONARY COMPUTED TOMOGRAPHY BE UTILIZED?

Both the American College of Cardiology[173] and the European Society of Cardiology[174] in association with several other professional societies summarized the current appropriate indications for CTA. Table 21-3 summarizes the American recommendations, which for the most part are similar to those issued by the European Writing Group. Asymptomatic patients should not be exposed to ionizing radiation unnecessarily, so there is no current indication for CTA in these patients. Patients with unclear functional stress test results, patients experiencing chest discomfort with normal ECG and

Table 21-3 Appropriate Indications for Computed Tomography Angiography

Asymptomatic patients	No indications
Symptomatic patients	Indeterminate pretest probability of coronary artery disease with uninterpretable ECG or patient unable to exercise
	Intermediate pretest probability of coronary artery disease with normal ECG and cardiac enzymes
	Uninterpretable or equivocal stress test
	Suspected coronary anomaly
	Evaluation of coronary artery disease in new-onset congestive heart failure

Summarized from Hendel RC et al.[167]

no cardiac enzyme elevation, and cases of suspected coronary anomaly or exclusion of CAD in patients with new-onset congestive heart failure constitute the main indications. Owing to the consistently high NPV, coronary CTA is better suited to ruling out CAD than establishing a firm diagnosis of obstructive disease. This could be especially useful in the emergency department, where a quick and accurate diagnosis may be desirable for a rapid and cost-effective disposition of the patient.[175] Finally, to improve overall quality as well as reduce inappropriate uses of the technique, both the European[174] and American[173] professional associations called for specific training prior to pursuing CT credentials.

ACKNOWLEDGEMENTS

Nikolaos Alexopoulos, MD was supported by a scholarship from the Hellenic Cardiology Society.

REFERENCES

1. Shemesh J, Apter S, Rozenman J, Lusky A, Rath S, Itzchak Y, Motro M: Calcification of coronary arteries: detection and quantification with double-helix CT, *Radiology* 197(3):779–783, 1995.
2. Shemesh J, Stroh CI, Tenenbaum A, Hod H, Boyko V, Fisman EZ, Motro M: Comparison of coronary calcium in stable angina pectoris and in first acute myocardial infarction utilizing double helical computerized tomography, *Am J Cardiol* 81(3):271–275, 1998.
3. Broderick LS, Shemesh J, Wilensky RL, Eckert GJ, Zhou X, Torres WF, Balk MA, Rogers WJ, Conces DJ Jr, Kopecky KK: Measurement of coronary artery calcium with dual-slice helical CT compared with coronary angiography: evaluation of CT scoring methods, interobserver variations, and reproducibility, *AJR Am J Roentgenol* 167(2):439–444, 1996.
4. Scheffel H, Alkadhi H, Plass A, Vachenauer R, Desbiolles L, Gaemperli O, Schepis T, Frauenfelder T, Schertler T, Husmann L, Grunenfelder J, Genoni M, Kaufmann PA, Marincek B, Leschka S: Accuracy of dual-source CT coronary angiography: First experience in a high pre-test probability population without heart rate control, *Eur Radiol* 16(12):2739–2747, 2006.
5. Johnson TR, Nikolaou K, Wintersperger BJ, Leber AW, von Ziegler F, Rist C, Buhmann S, Knez A, Reiser MF, Becker CR: Dual-source CT cardiac imaging: initial experience, *Eur Radiol* 16(7):1409–1415, 2006.
6. Achenbach S, Ropers D, Kuettner A, Flohr T, Ohnesorge B, Bruder H, Theessen H, Karakaya M, Daniel WG, Bautz W, Kalender WA, Anders K: Contrast-enhanced coronary artery visualization by dual-source computed tomography—initial experience, *Eur J Radiol* 57(3):331–335, 2006.
7. Oncel D, Oncel G, Tastan A: Effectiveness of dual-source CT coronary angiography for the evaluation of coronary artery disease in patients with atrial fibrillation: initial experience, *Radiology* 245(3):703–711, 2007.
8. Strub WM, Vagal A, Meyer C: Optimizing coronary artery imaging in patients with atrial fibrillation with ECG-gated 64-MDCT, *AJR Am J Roentgenol* 189(1):W50–W51, 2007.
9. Achenbach S, Moshage W, Ropers D, Nossen J, Daniel WG: Value of electron-beam computed tomography for the noninvasive detection of high-grade coronary-artery stenoses and occlusions, *N Engl J Med* 339(27):1964–1971, 1998.
10. Leber AW, Knez A, Becker C, Becker A, White C, Thilo C, Reiser M, Haberl R, Steinbeck G: Non-invasive intravenous coronary angiography using electron beam tomography and multislice computed tomography, *Heart* 89(6):633–639, 2003.
11. Achenbach S, Ulzheimer S, Baum U, Kachelriess M, Ropers D, Giesler T, Bautz W, Daniel WG, Kalender WA, Moshage W: Noninvasive coronary angiography by retrospectively ECG-gated multislice spiral CT, *Circulation* 102(23):2823–2828, 2000.
12. Vanhoenacker PK, Heijenbrok-Kal MH, Van Heste R, Decramer I, Van Hoe LR, Wijns W, Hunink MG: Diagnostic performance of multidetector CT angiography for assessment of coronary artery disease: meta-analysis, *Radiology* 244(2):419–428, 2007.
13. Roberts WT, Bax JJ, Davies LC: Cardiac CT and CT coronary angiography: technology and application, *Heart* 94(6):781–792, 2008.
14. Nikolaou K, Becker CR, Muders M, Babaryka G, Scheidler J, Flohr T, Loehrs U, Reiser MF, Fayad ZA: Multidetector-row computed

tomography and magnetic resonance imaging of atherosclerotic lesions in human ex vivo coronary arteries, *Atherosclerosis* 174 (2):243–252, 2004.

15. Flohr TG, McCollough CH, Bruder H, Petersilka M, Gruber K, Suss C, Grasruck M, Stierstorfer K, Krauss B, Raupach R, Primak AN, Kuttner A, Achenbach S, Becker C, Kopp A, Ohnesorge BM: First performance evaluation of a dual-source CT (DSCT) system, *Eur Radiol* 16(2):256–268, 2006.
16. Achenbach S, Ropers D, Pohle FK, Raaz D, von Erffa J, Yilmaz A, Muschiol G, Daniel WG: Detection of coronary artery stenoses using multi-detector CT with 16 x 0.75 collimation and 375 ms rotation, *Eur Heart J* 26(19):1978–1986, 2005.
17. Aviram G, Finkelstein A, Herz I, Lessick J, Miller H, Graif M, Keren G: Clinical value of 16-slice multi-detector CT compared to invasive coronary angiography, *Int J Cardiovasc Intervent* 7(1):21–28, 2005.
18. Dewey M, Laule M, Krug L, Schnapauff D, Rogalla P, Rutsch W, Hamm B, Lembcke A: Multisegment and halfscan reconstruction of 16-slice computed tomography for detection of coronary artery stenoses, *Invest Radiol* 39(4):223–229, 2004.
19. Fine JJ, Hopkins CB, Hall PA, Delphia RE, Attebery TW, Newton FC: Noninvasive coronary angiography: agreement of multi-slice spiral computed tomography and selective catheter angiography, *Int J Cardiovasc Imaging* 20(6):549–552, 2004.
20. Garcia MJ, Lessick J, Hoffmann MH: Accuracy of 16-row multidetector computed tomography for the assessment of coronary artery stenosis, *JAMA* 296(4):403–411, 2006.
21. Hoffmann MH, Shi H, Schmitz BL, Schmid FT, Lieberknecht M, Schulze R, Ludwig B, Kroschel U, Jahnke N, Haerer W, Brambs HJ, Aschoff AJ: Noninvasive coronary angiography with multislice computed tomography, *JAMA* 293(20):2471–2478, 2005.
22. Kaiser C, Bremerich J, Haller S, Brunner-La Rocca HP, Bongartz G, Pfisterer M, Buser P: Limited diagnostic yield of non-invasive coronary angiography by 16-slice multi-detector spiral computed tomography in routine patients referred for evaluation of coronary artery disease, *Eur Heart J* 26(19):1987–1992, 2005.
23. Kuettner A, Trabold T, Schroeder S, Feyer A, Beck T, Brueckner A, Heuschmid M, Burgstahler C, Kopp AF, Claussen CD: Noninvasive detection of coronary lesions using 16-detector multislice spiral computed tomography technology: initial clinical results, *J Am Coll Cardiol* 44(6):1230–1237, 2004.
24. Martuscelli E, Romagnoli A, D'Eliseo A, Razzini C, Tomassini M, Sperandio M, Simonetti G, Romeo F: Accuracy of thin-slice computed tomography in the detection of coronary stenoses, *Eur Heart J* 25 (12):1043–1048, 2004.
25. Mollet NR, Cademartiri F, Krestin GP, McFadden EP, Arampatzis CA, Serruys PW, de Feyter PJ: Improved diagnostic accuracy with 16-row multi-slice computed tomography coronary angiography, *J Am Coll Cardiol* 45(1):128–132, 2005.
26. Morgan-Hughes GJ, Roobottom CA, Owens PE, Marshall AJ: Highly accurate coronary angiography with submillimetre, 16 slice computed tomography, *Heart* 91(3):308–313, 2005.
27. Nieman K, Cademartiri F, Lemos PA, Raaijmakers R, Pattynama PM, de Feyter PJ: Reliable noninvasive coronary angiography with fast submillimeter multislice spiral computed tomography, *Circulation* 106(16):2051–2054, 2002.
28. Ropers D, Baum U, Pohle K, Anders K, Ulzheimer S, Ohnesorge B, Schlundt C, Bautz W, Daniel WG, Achenbach S: Detection of coronary artery stenoses with thin-slice multi-detector row spiral computed tomography and multiplanar reconstruction, *Circulation* 107 (5):664–666, 2003.
29. Schuijf JD, Bax JJ, Salm LP, Jukema JW, Lamb HJ, van der Wall EE, de Roos A: Noninvasive coronary imaging and assessment of left ventricular function using 16-slice computed tomography, *Am J Cardiol* 95(5):571–574, 2005.
30. Cademartiri F, Maffei E, Palumbo A, Malago R, Alberghina F, Aldrovandi A, Brambilla V, Runza G, La Grutta L, Menozzi A, Vignali L, Casolo G, Midiri M, Mollet NR: Diagnostic accuracy of 64-slice computed tomography coronary angiography in patients with low-to-intermediate risk, *Radiol Med (Torino)* 112(7):969–981, 2007.
31. Ehara M, Surmely JF, Kawai M, Katoh O, Matsubara T, Terashima M, Tsuchikane E, Kinoshita Y, Suzuki T, Ito T, Takeda Y, Nasu K, Tanaka N, Murata A, Suzuki T, Sato K: Diagnostic accuracy of 64-slice computed tomography for detecting angiographically significant coronary artery stenosis in an unselected consecutive patient population: comparison with conventional invasive angiography, *Circ J* 70 (5): 564–571, 2006.
32. Fine JJ, Hopkins CB, Ruff N, Newton FC: Comparison of accuracy of 64-slice cardiovascular computed tomography with coronary angiography in patients with suspected coronary artery disease, *Am J Cardiol* 97(2):173–174, 2006.
33. Herzog C, Zwerner PL, Doll JR, Nielsen CD, Nguyen SA, Savino G, Vogl TJ, Costello P, Schoepf UJ: Significant coronary artery stenosis: comparison on per-patient and per-vessel or per-segment basis at 64-section CT angiography, *Radiology* 244(1):112–120, 2007.
34. Leber AW, Knez A, von Ziegler F, Becker A, Nikolaou K, Paul S, Wintersperger B, Reiser M, Becker CR, Steinbeck G, Boekstegers P: Quantification of obstructive and nonobstructive coronary lesions by 64-slice computed tomography: a comparative study with quantitative coronary angiography and intravascular ultrasound, *J Am Coll Cardiol* 46(1):147–154, 2005.
35. Leschka S, Alkadhi H, Plass A, Desbiolles L, Grunenfelder J, Marincek B, Wildermuth S: Accuracy of MSCT coronary angiography with 64-slice technology: first experience, *Eur Heart J* 26(15): 1482–1487, 2005.
36. Malagutti P, Nieman K, Meijboom WB, van Mieghem CA, Pugliese F, Cademartiri F, Mollet NR, Boersma E, de Jaegere PP, de Feyter PJ: Use of 64-slice CT in symptomatic patients after coronary bypass surgery: evaluation of grafts and coronary arteries, *Eur Heart J* 28(15): 1879–1885, 2007.
37. Meijboom WB, Mollet NR, Van Mieghem CA, Weustink AC, Pugliese F, van Pelt N, Cademartiri F, Vourvouri E, de Jaegere P, Krestin GP, de Feyter PJ: 64-Slice CT coronary angiography in patients with non-ST elevation acute coronary syndrome, *Heart* 93 (11):1386–1392, 2007.
38. Mollet NR, Cademartiri F, van Mieghem CA, Runza G, McFadden EP, Baks T, Serruys PW, Krestin GP, de Feyter PJ: High-resolution spiral computed tomography coronary angiography in patients referred for diagnostic conventional coronary angiography, *Circulation* 112 (15): 2318–2323, 2005.
39. Muhlenbruch G, Seyfarth T, Soo CS, Pregalathan N, Mahnken AH: Diagnostic value of 64-slice multi-detector row cardiac CTA in symptomatic patients, *Eur Radiol* 17(3):603–609, 2007.
40. Oncel D, Oncel G, Tastan A, Tamci B: Detection of significant coronary artery stenosis with 64-section MDCT angiography, *Eur J Radiol* 62(3):394–405, 2007.
41. Plass A, Grunenfelder J, Leschka S, Alkadhi H, Eberli FR, Wildermuth S, Zund G, Genoni M: Coronary artery imaging with 64-slice computed tomography from cardiac surgical perspective, *Eur J Cardiothorac Surg* 30(1):109–116, 2006.
42. Pugliese F, Mollet NR, Runza G, van Mieghem C, Meijboom WB, Malagutti P, Baks T, Krestin GP, deFeyter PJ, Cademartiri F: Diagnostic accuracy of non-invasive 64-slice CT coronary angiography in patients with stable angina pectoris, *Eur Radiol* 16(3):575–582, 2006.
43. Raff GL, Gallagher MJ, O'Neill WW, Goldstein JA: Diagnostic accuracy of noninvasive coronary angiography using 64-slice spiral computed tomography, *J Am Coll Cardiol* 46(3):552–557, 2005.
44. Ropers D, Rixe J, Anders K, Kuttner A, Baum U, Bautz W, Daniel WG, Achenbach S: Usefulness of multidetector row spiral computed tomography with 64- × 0.6-mm collimation and 330-ms rotation for the noninvasive detection of significant coronary artery stenoses, *Am J Cardiol* 97(3):343–348, 2006.
45. Schlosser T, Mohrs OK, Magedanz A, Nowak B, Voigtlander T, Barkhausen J, Schmermund A: Noninvasive coronary angiography using 64-detector-row computed tomography in patients with a low to moderate pretest probability of significant coronary artery disease, *Acta Radiol* 48(3):300–307, 2007.
46. Schuijf JD, Pundziute G, Jukema JW, Lamb HJ, van der Hoeven BL, de Roos A, van der Wall EE, Bax JJ: Diagnostic accuracy of 64-slice multi-slice computed tomography in the noninvasive evaluation of significant coronary artery disease, *Am J Cardiol* 98(2):145–148, 2006.
47. Shabestari AA, Abdi S, Akhlaghpoor S, Azadi M, Baharjoo H, Pajouh MD, Emami Z, Esfahani F, Firouzi I, Hashemian M, Kouhi M, Mozafari M, Nazeri I, Roshani M, Salevatipour B, Tavalla H, Tehrai M, Zarrabi A: Diagnostic performance of 64-channel multislice computed tomography in assessment of significant coronary artery disease in symptomatic subjects, *Am J Cardiol* 99 (12):1656–1661, 2007.
48. Budoff MJ, Dowe D, Jollis JG, Gitter M, Sutherland J, Halamert E, Scherer M, Bellinger R, Martin A, Benton R, Delago A, Min JK: Diagnostic performance of 64-multidetector row coronary computed tomographic angiography for evaluation of coronary artery stenosis in individuals without known coronary artery disease: results from the prospective multicenter ACCURACY (Assessment by Coronary Computed Tomographic Angiography of Individuals Undergoing Invasive Coronary Angiography) trial, *J Am Coll Cardiol* 52 (21):1724–1732, 2008.
49. Meijboom WB, Meijs MF, Schuijf JD, Cramer MJ, Mollet NR, van Mieghem CA, Nieman K, van Werkhoven JM, Pundziute G, Weustink AC, de Vos AM, Pugliese F, Rensing B, Jukema JW, Bax JJ, Prokop M, Doevendans PA, Hunink MG, Krestin GP, de Feyter PJ: Diagnostic accuracy of 64-slice computed tomography coronary angiography: a prospective, multicenter, multivendor study, *J Am Coll Cardiol* 52(25):2135–2144, 2008.
50. Miller JM, Rochitte CE, Dewey M, Arbab-Zadeh A, Niinuma H, Gottlieb I, Paul N, Clouse ME, Shapiro EP, Hoe J, Lardo AC, Bush DE, de Roos A, Cox C, Brinker J, Lima JA: Diagnostic performance of coronary angiography by 64-row CT, *N Engl J Med* 359 (22):2324–2336, 2008.

51. Janne d'Othee B, Siebert U, Cury R, Jadvar H, Dunn EJ, Hoffmann U: A systematic review on diagnostic accuracy of CT-based detection of significant coronary artery disease, *Eur J Radiol* 65(3):449–461, 2008.

52. Abdulla J, Abildstrom SZ, Gotzsche O, Christensen E, Kober L: Torp-Pedersen C. 64-multislice detector computed tomography coronary angiography as potential alternative to conventional coronary angiography: a systematic review and meta-analysis, *Eur Heart J* 28 (24):3042–3050, 2007.

53. Ruzsics B, Lee H, Zwerner PL, Gebregziabher M, Costello P, Schoepf UJ: Dual-energy CT of the heart for diagnosing coronary artery stenosis and myocardial ischemia-initial experience, *Eur Radiol,* 2008.

54. Rybicki FJ, Otero HJ, Steigner ML, Vorobiof G, Nallamshetty L, Mitsouras D, Ersoy H, Mather RT, Judy PF, Cai T, Coyner K, Schultz K, Whitmore AG, Di Carli MF: Initial evaluation of coronary images from 320-detector row computed tomography, *Int J Cardiovasc Imaging* 24(5):535–546, 2008.

55. Anders K, Baum U, Schmid M, Ropers D, Schmid A, Pohle K, Daniel WG, Bautz W, Achenbach S: Coronary artery bypass graft (CABG) patency: assessment with high-resolution submillimeter 16-slice multidetector-row computed tomography (MDCT) versus coronary angiography, *Eur J Radiol* 57(3):336–344, 2006.

56. Burgstahler C, Beck T, Kuettner A, Drosch T, Kopp AF, Heuschmid M, Claussen CD, Schroeder S: Non-invasive evaluation of coronary artery bypass grafts using 16-row multi-slice computed tomography with 188 ms temporal resolution, *Int J Cardiol* 106 (2):244–249, 2006.

57. Jabara R, Chronos N, Klein L, Eisenberg S, Allen R, Bradford S, Frohwein S: Comparison of multidetector 64-slice computed tomographic angiography to coronary angiography to assess the patency of coronary artery bypass grafts, *Am J Cardiol* 99(11):1529–1534, 2007.

58. Meyer TS, Martinoff S, Hadamitzky M, Will A, Kastrati A, Schomig A, Hausleiter J: Improved noninvasive assessment of coronary artery bypass grafts with 64-slice computed tomographic angiography in an unselected patient population, *J Am Coll Cardiol* 49(9):946–950, 2007.

59. Pache G, Saueressig U, Frydrychowicz A, Foell D, Ghanem N, Kotter E, Geibel-Zehender A, Bode C, Langer M, Bley T: Initial experience with 64-slice cardiac CT: non-invasive visualization of coronary artery bypass grafts, *Eur Heart J* 27(8):976–980, 2006.

60. Ropers D, Pohle FK, Kuettner A, Pflederer T, Anders K, Daniel WG, Bautz W, Baum U, Achenbach S: Diagnostic accuracy of noninvasive coronary angiography in patients after bypass surgery using 64-slice spiral computed tomography with 330-ms gantry rotation, *Circulation* 114(22):2334–2341, 2006, quiz 2334.

61. Schlosser T, Konorza T, Hunold P, Kuhl H, Schmermund A, Barkhausen J: Noninvasive visualization of coronary artery bypass grafts using 16-detector row computed tomography, *J Am Coll Cardiol* 44(6):1224–1229, 2004.

62. Stauder NI, Kuttner A, Schroder S, Drosch T, Beck T, Stauder H, Blumenstock G, Claussen CD, Kopp AF: Coronary artery bypass grafts: assessment of graft patency and native coronary artery lesions using 16-slice MDCT, *Eur Radiol* 16(11):2512–2520, 2006.

63. Gasparovic H, Rybicki FJ, Millstine J, Unic D, Byrne JG, Yucel K, Mihaljevic T: Three dimensional computed tomographic imaging in planning the surgical approach for redo cardiac surgery after coronary revascularization, *Eur J Cardiothorac Surg* 28(2):244–249, 2005.

64. Maintz D, Seifarth H, Raupach R, Flohr T, Rink M, Sommer T, Ozgun M, Heindel W, Fischbach R: 64-slice multidetector coronary CT angiography: in vitro evaluation of 68 different stents, *Eur Radiol* 16(4):818–826, 2006.

65. Gilard M, Cornily JC, Rioufol G, Finet G, Pennec PY, Mansourati J, Blanc JJ, Boschat J: Noninvasive assessment of left main coronary stent patency with 16-slice computed tomography, *Am J Cardiol* 95 (1):110–112, 2005.

66. Van Mieghem CA, Cademartiri F, Mollet NR, Malagutti P, Valgimigli M, Meijboom WB, Pugliese F, McFadden EP, Ligthart J, Runza G, Bruining N, Smits PC, Regar E, van der Giessen WJ, Sianos G, van Domburg R, de Jaegere P, Krestin GP, Serruys PW, de Feyter PJ: Multislice spiral computed tomography for the evaluation of stent patency after left main coronary artery stenting: a comparison with conventional coronary angiography and intravascular ultrasound, *Circulation* 114(7):645–653, 2006.

67. Rixe J, Achenbach S, Ropers D, Baum U, Kuettner A, Ropers U, Bautz W, Daniel WG, Anders K: Assessment of coronary artery stent restenosis by 64-slice multi-detector computed tomography, *Eur Heart J* 27(21):2567–2572, 2006.

68. Cademartiri F, Schuijf JD, Pugliese F, Mollet NR, Jukema JW, Maffei E, Kroft LJ, Palumbo A, Ardissino D, Serruys PW, Krestin GP, Van der Wall EE, de Feyter PJ, Bax JJ: Usefulness of 64-slice multislice computed tomography coronary angiography to assess in-stent restenosis, *J Am Coll Cardiol* 49(22):2204–2210, 2007.

69. Schuijf JD, Pundziute G, Jukema JW, Lamb HJ, Tuinenburg JC, van der Hoeven BL, de Roos A, Reiber JH, van der Wall EE, Schalij MJ, Bax JJ: Evaluation of patients with previous coronary stent implantation with 64-section CT, *Radiology* 245(2):416–423, 2007.

70. Oncel D, Oncel G, Tastan A, Tamci B: Evaluation of coronary stent patency and in-stent restenosis with dual-source CT coronary angiography without heart rate control, *AJR Am J Roentgenol* 191(1):56–63, 2008.

71. Schuijf JD, Wijns W, Jukema JW, Atsma DE, de Roos A, Lamb HJ, Stokkel MP, Dibbets-Schneider P, Decramer I, De Bondt P, van der Wall EE, Vanhoenacker PK, Bax JJ: Relationship between noninvasive coronary angiography with multi-slice computed tomography and myocardial perfusion imaging, *J Am Coll Cardiol* 48(12):2508–2514, 2006.

72. Di Carli MF, Dorbala S, Curillova Z, Kwong RJ, Goldhaber SZ, Rybicki FJ, Hachamovitch R: Relationship between CT coronary angiography and stress perfusion imaging in patients with suspected ischemic heart disease assessed by integrated PET-CT imaging, *J Nucl Cardiol* 14(6):799–809, 2007.

73. Hacker M, Jakobs T, Hack N, Nikolaou K, Becker C, von Ziegler F, Knez A, Konig A, Klauss V, Reiser M, Hahn K, Tiling R: Sixty-four slice spiral CT angiography does not predict the functional relevance of coronary artery stenoses in patients with stable angina, *Eur J Nucl Med Mol Imaging* 34(1):4–10, 2007.

74. Gaemperli O, Schepis T, Koepfli P, Valenta I, Soyka J, Leschka S, Desbiolles L, Husmann L, Alkadhi H, Kaufmann PA: Accuracy of 64-slice CT angiography for the detection of functionally relevant coronary stenoses as assessed with myocardial perfusion SPECT, *Eur J Nucl Med Mol Imaging* 34(8):1162–1171, 2007.

75. Lin F, Shaw LJ, Berman DS, Callister TQ, Weinsaft JW, Wong FJ, Szulc M, Tandon V, Okin PM, Devereux RB, Min JK: Multidetector computed tomography coronary artery plaque predictors of stress-induced myocardial ischemia by SPECT, *Atherosclerosis* 197(2): 700–709, 2008.

76. Rispler S, Keidar Z, Ghersin E, Roguin A, Soil A, Dragu R, Litmanovich D, Frenkel A, Aronson D, Engel A, Beyar R, Israel O: Integrated single-photon emission computed tomography and computed tomography coronary angiography for the assessment of hemodynamically significant coronary artery lesions, *J Am Coll Cardiol* 49(10):1059–1067, 2007.

77. Gaemperli O, Schepis T, Valenta I, Husmann L, Scheffel H, Duerst V, Eberli FR, Luscher TF, Alkadhi H, Kaufmann PA: Cardiac image fusion from stand-alone SPECT and CT: clinical experience, *J Nucl Med* 48 (5):696–703, 2007.

78. Christou MA, Siontis GC, Katritsis DG, Ioannidis JP: Meta-analysis of fractional flow reserve versus quantitative coronary angiography and noninvasive imaging for evaluation of myocardial ischemia, *Am J Cardiol* 99(4):450–456, 2007.

79. Meijboom WB, Van Mieghem CA, van Pelt N, Weustink A, Pugliese F, Mollet NR, Boersma E, Regar E, van Geuns RJ, de Jaegere PJ, Serruys PW, Krestin GP, de Feyter PJ: Comprehensive assessment of coronary artery stenoses: computed tomography coronary angiography versus conventional coronary angiography and correlation with fractional flow reserve in patients with stable angina, *J Am Coll Cardiol* 52(8): 636–643, 2008.

80. Nicol ED, Stirrup J, Reyes E, Roughton M, Padley SP, Rubens MB, Underwood SR: Sixty-four-slice computed tomography coronary angiography compared with myocardial perfusion scintigraphy for the diagnosis of functionally significant coronary stenoses in patients with a low to intermediate likelihood of coronary artery disease, *J Nucl Cardiol* 15(3):311–318, 2008.

81. Sato A, Hiroe M, Tamura M, Ohigashi H, Nozato T, Hikita H, Takahashi A, Aonuma K, Isobe M: Quantitative measures of coronary stenosis severity by 64-Slice CT angiography and relation to physiologic significance of perfusion in nonobese patients: comparison with stress myocardial perfusion imaging, *J Nucl Med* 49(4):564–572, 2008.

82. Gallagher MJ, Ross MA, Raff GL, Goldstein JA, O'Neill WW, O'Neil B: The diagnostic accuracy of 64-slice computed tomography coronary angiography compared with stress nuclear imaging in emergency department low risk chest pain patients, *Ann Emerg Med* 49(2): 125–136, 2007.

83. Goldstein JA, Gallagher MJ, O'Neill WW, Ross MA, O'Neil BJ, Raff GL: A randomized controlled trial of multi-slice coronary computed tomography for evaluation of acute chest pain, *J Am Coll Cardiol* 49 (8):863–871, 2007.

84. Shaw LJ, Berman DS, Hendel RC, Borges Neto S, Min JK, Callister TQ: Prognosis by coronary computed tomographic angiography: matched comparison with myocardial perfusion single-photon emission computed tomography, *J Cardiovasc Comput Tomogr* 2(2):93–101, 2008, Epub 2008 Jan 12.

85. Cury RC, Feuchtner G, Pena CS, Janowitz WR, Katzen BT, Ziffer JA: Acute chest pain imaging in the emergency department with cardiac computed tomography angiography, *J Nucl Cardiol* 15(4):564–75, 2008.

86. George RT, Silva C, Cordeiro MA, DiPaula A, Thompson DR, McCarthy WF, Ichihara T, Lima JA, Lardo AC: Multidetector

computed tomography myocardial perfusion imaging during adenosine stress, *J Am Coll Cardiol* 48(1):153–160, 2006.

87. Kurata A, Mochizuki T, Koyama Y, Haraikawa T, Suzuki J, Shigematsu Y, Higaki J: Myocardial perfusion imaging using adenosine triphosphate stress multi-slice spiral computed tomography: alternative to stress myocardial perfusion scintigraphy, *Circ J* 69(5):550–557, 2005.

88. Gerber BL, Belge B, Legros GJ, Lim P, Poncelet A, Pasquet A, Gisellu G, Coche E, Vanoverschelde JL: Characterization of acute and chronic myocardial infarcts by multidetector computed tomography: comparison with contrast-enhanced magnetic resonance, *Circulation* 113(6):823–833, 2006.

89. Lardo AC, Cordeiro MA, Silva C, Amado LC, George RT, Saliaris AP, Schuleri KH, Fernandes VR, Zviman M, Nazarian S, Halperin HR, Wu KC, Hare JM, Lima JA: Contrast-enhanced multidetector computed tomography viability imaging after myocardial infarction: characterization of myocyte death, microvascular obstruction, and chronic scar, *Circulation* 113(3):394–404, 2006.

90. Hoffmann U, Millea R, Enzweiler C, Ferencik M, Gulick S, Titus J, Achenbach S, Kwait D, Sosnovik D, Brady TJ: Acute myocardial infarction: contrast-enhanced multi-detector row CT in a porcine model, *Radiology* 231(3):697–701, 2004.

91. Baks T, Cademartiri F, Moelker AD, Weustink AC, van Geuns RJ, Mollet NR, Krestin GP, Duncker DJ, de Feyter PJ: Multislice computed tomography and magnetic resonance imaging for the assessment of reperfused acute myocardial infarction, *J Am Coll Cardiol* 48(1):144–152, 2006.

92. Nieman K, Shapiro MD, Ferencik M, Nomura CH, Abbara S, Hoffmann U, Gold HK, Jang IK, Brady TJ, Cury RC: Reperfused myocardial infarction: contrast-enhanced 64-section CT in comparison to MR imaging, *Radiology* 247(1):49–56, 2008.

93. Wada H, Kobayashi Y, Yasu T, Tsukamoto Y, Kobayashi N, Ishida T, Kubo N, Kawakami M, Saito M: Multi-detector computed tomography for imaging of subendocardial infarction: prediction of wall motion recovery after reperfused anterior myocardial infarction, *Circ J* 68(5):512–514, 2004.

94. Koyama Y, Matsuoka H, Mochizuki T, Higashino H, Kawakami H, Nakata S, Aono J, Ito T, Naka M, Ohashi Y, Higaki J: Assessment of reperfused acute myocardial infarction with two-phase contrast-enhanced helical CT: prediction of left ventricular function and wall thickness, *Radiology* 235(3):804–811, 2005.

95. Lessick J, Dragu R, Mutlak D, Rispler S, Beyar R, Litmanovich D, Engel A, Agmon Y, Kapeliovich M, Hammerman H, Ghersin E: Is functional improvement after myocardial infarction predicted with myocardial enhancement patterns at multidetector CT? *Radiology* 244(3):736–744, 2007.

96. Sato A, Hiroe M, Nozato T, Hikita H, Ito Y, Ohigashi H, Tamura M, Takahashi A, Isobe M, Aonuma K: Early validation study of 64-slice multidetector computed tomography for the assessment of myocardial viability and the prediction of left ventricular remodelling after acute myocardial infarction, *Eur Heart J* 29(4):490–498, 2008.

97. Reiter SJ, Rumberger JA, Feiring AJ, Stanford W, Marcus ML: Precision of measurements of right and left ventricular volume by cine computed tomography, *Circulation* 74(4):890–900, 1986.

98. Rich S, Chomka EV, Stagl R, Shanes JG, Kondos GT, Brundage BH: Determination of left ventricular ejection fraction using ultrafast computed tomography, *Am Heart J* 112(2):392–396, 1986.

99. Roig E, Georgiou D, Chomka EV, Wolfkiel C, LoGalbo-Zak C, Rich S, Brundage BH: Reproducibility of left ventricular myocardial volume and mass measurements by ultrafast computed tomography, *J Am Coll Cardiol* 18(4):990–996, 1991.

100. Feiring AJ, Rumberger JA, Reiter SJ, Skorton DJ, Collins SM, Lipton MJ, Higgins CB, Ell S, Marcus ML: Determination of left ventricular mass in dogs with rapid-acquisition cardiac computed tomographic scanning, *Circulation* 72(6):1355–1364, 1985.

101. Mao S, Takasu J, Child J, Carson S, Oudiz R, Budoff MJ: Comparison of LV mass and volume measurements derived from electron beam tomography using cine imaging and angiographic imaging, *Int J Cardiovasc Imaging* 19(5):439–445, 2003.

102. Juergens KU, Seifarth H, Maintz D, Grude M, Ozgun M, Wichter T, Heindel W, Fischbach R: MDCT determination of volume and function of the left ventricle: are short-axis image reformations necessary? *AJR Am J Roentgenol* 186(6 Suppl 2):S371–378, 2006.

103. Gilard M, Pennec PY, Cornily JC, Vinsonneau U, Le Gal G, Nonent M, Mansourati J, Boschat J: Multi-slice computer tomography of left ventricular function with automated analysis software in comparison with conventional ventriculography, *Eur J Radiol* 59(2):270–275, 2006.

104. Juergens KU, Grude M, Fallenberg EM, Opitz C, Wichter T, Heindel W, Fischbach R: Using ECG-gated multidetector CT to evaluate global left ventricular myocardial function in patients with coronary artery disease, *AJR Am J Roentgenol* 179(6):1545–1550, 2002.

105. Halliburton SS, Petersilka M, Schvartzman PR, Obuchowski N, White RD: Evaluation of left ventricular dysfunction using multiphasic reconstructions of coronary multi-slice computed

tomography data in patients with chronic ischemic heart disease: validation against cine magnetic resonance imaging, *Int J Cardiovasc Imaging* 19(1):73–83, 2003.

106. Yamamuro M, Tadamura E, Kubo S, Toyoda H, Nishina T, Ohba M, Hosokawa R, Kimura T, Tamaki N, Komeda M, Kita T, Konishi J: Cardiac functional analysis with multi-detector row CT and segmental reconstruction algorithm: comparison with echocardiography, SPECT, and MR imaging, *Radiology* 234(2):381–390, 2005.

107. Mahnken AH, Koos R, Katoh M, Spuentrup E, Busch P, Wildberger JE, Kuhl HP, Gunther RW: Sixteen-slice spiral CT versus MR imaging for the assessment of left ventricular function in acute myocardial infarction, *Eur Radiol* 15(4):714–720, 2005.

108. Sugeng L, Mor-Avi V, Weinert L, Niel J, Ebner C, Steringer-Mascherbauer R, Schmidt F, Galuschky C, Schummers G, Lang RM, Nesser HJ: Quantitative assessment of left ventricular size and function: side-by-side comparison of real-time three-dimensional echocardiography and computed tomography with magnetic resonance reference, *Circulation* 114(7):654–661, 2006.

109. Raman SV, Shah M, McCarthy B, Garcia A, Ferketich AK: Multidetector row cardiac computed tomography accurately quantifies right and left ventricular size and function compared with cardiac magnetic resonance, *Am Heart J* 151(3):736–744, 2006.

110. Schepis T, Gaemperli O, Koepfli P, Valenta I, Strobel K, Brunner A, Leschka S, Desbiolles L, Husmann L, Alkadhi H, Kaufmann PA: Comparison of 64-slice CT with gated SPECT for evaluation of left ventricular function, *J Nucl Med* 47(8):1288–1294, 2006.

111. Annuar BR, Liew CK, Chin SP, Ong TK, Seyfarth MT, Chan WL, Fong YY, Ang CK, Lin N, Liew HB, Sim KH: Assessment of global and regional left ventricular function using 64-slice multislice computed tomography and 2D echocardiography: a comparison with cardiac magnetic resonance, *Eur J Radiol* 65(1):112–119, 2008.

112. Wu YW, Tadamura E, Yamamuro M, Kanao S, Okayama S, Ozasa N, Toma M, Kimura T, Komeda M, Togashi K: Estimation of global and regional cardiac function using 64-slice computed tomography: a comparison study with echocardiography, gated-SPECT and cardiovascular magnetic resonance, *Int J Cardiol* 128(1):69–76, 2008.

113. Busch S, Johnson TR, Wintersperger BJ, Minaifar N, Bhargava A, Rist C, Reiser MF, Becker C, Nikolaou K: Quantitative assessment of left ventricular function with dual-source CT in comparison to cardiac magnetic resonance imaging: initial findings, *Eur Radiol* 18(3):570–575, 2008.

114. Puesken M, Fischbach R, Wenker M, Seifarth H, Maintz D, Heindel W, Juergens KU: Global left-ventricular function assessment using dual-source multidetector CT: effect of improved temporal resolution on ventricular volume measurement, *Eur Radiol* 18:2087–2094, 2008.

115. van der Vleuten PA, de Jonge GJ, Lubbers DD, Tio RA, Willems TP, Oudkerk M, Zijlstra F: Evaluation of global left ventricular function assessment by dual-source computed tomography compared with MRI, *Eur Radiol* 19:271–277, 2009.

116. Schlosser T, Mohrs OK, Magedanz A, Voigtlander T, Schmermund A, Barkhausen J: Assessment of left ventricular function and mass in patients undergoing computed tomography (CT) coronary angiography using 64-detector-row CT: comparison to magnetic resonance imaging, *Acta Radiol* 48(1):30–35, 2007.

117. Bastarrika G, Arraiza M, De Cecco CN, Mastrobuoni S, Ubilla M, Rabago G: Quantification of left ventricular function and mass in heart transplant recipients using dual-source CT and MRI: initial clinical experience, *Eur Radiol* 18(9):1784–1790, 2008.

118. Heuschmid M, Rothfuss JK, Schroeder S, Fenchel M, Stauder N, Burgstahler C, Franow A, Kuzo RS, Kuettner A, Miller S, Claussen CD, Kopp AF: Assessment of left ventricular myocardial function using 16-slice multidetector-row computed tomography: comparison with magnetic resonance imaging and echocardiography, *Eur Radiol* 16(3):551–559, 2006.

119. Ferencik M, Gregory SA, Butler J, Achenbach S, Yeh RW, Hoffmann U, Inglessis I, Cury RC, Nieman K, McNulty IA, Healy JA, Brady TJ, Semigran MJ, Jang IK: Analysis of cardiac dimensions, mass and function in heart transplant recipients using 64-slice multi-detector computed tomography, *J Heart Lung Transplant* 26(5):478–484, 2007.

120. Gilard M, Le Gal G, Cornily JC, Vinsonneau U, Joret C, Pennec PY, Mansourati J, Boschat J: Midterm prognosis of patients with suspected coronary artery disease and normal multislice computed tomographic findings: a prospective management outcome study, *Arch Intern Med* 167(15):1686–1689, 2007.

121. Gaemperli O, Valenta I, Schepis T, Husmann L, Scheffel H, Desbiolles L, Leschka S, Alkadhi H, Kaufmann PA: Coronary 64-slice CT angiography predicts outcome in patients with known or suspected coronary artery disease, *Eur Radiol* 18(6):1162–1173, 2008.

122. Pundziute G, Schuijf JD, Jukema JW, Boersma E, de Roos A, van der Wall EE, Bax JJ: Prognostic value of multislice computed tomography coronary angiography in patients with known or suspected coronary artery disease, *J Am Coll Cardiol* 49(1):62–70, 2007.

123. Matsumoto N, Sato Y, Yoda S, Nakano Y, Kunimasa T, Matsuo S, Komatsu S, Saito S, Hirayama A: Prognostic value of non-obstructive CT low-dense coronary artery plaques detected by multislice computed tomography, *Circ J* 71(12):1898–1903, 2007.

124. Rubinshtein R, Halon DA, Gaspar T, Jaffe R, Karkabi B, Flugelman MY, Kogan A, Shapira R, Peled N, Lewis BS: Usefulness of 64-slice cardiac computed tomographic angiography for diagnosing acute coronary syndromes and predicting clinical outcome in emergency department patients with chest pain of uncertain origin, *Circulation* 115(13):1762–1768, 2007.

125. Falk E, Shah PK, Fuster V: Coronary plaque disruption, *Circulation* 92 (3):657–671, 1995.

126. Mock MB, Ringqvist I, Fisher LD, Davis KB, Chaitman BR, Kouchoukos NT, Kaiser GC, Alderman E, Ryan TJ, Russell RO Jr., Mullin S, Fray D, Killip T 3rd, : Survival of medically treated patients in the coronary artery surgery study (CASS) registry, *Circulation* 66 (3):562–568, 1982.

127. Min JK, Shaw LJ, Devereux RB, Okin PM, Weinsaft JW, Russo DJ, Lippolis NJ, Berman DS, Callister TQ: Prognostic value of multidetector coronary computed tomographic angiography for prediction of all-cause mortality, *J Am Coll Cardiol* 50(12):1161–1170, 2007.

128. Mark DB, Nelson CL, Califf RM, Harrell FE Jr., Lee KL, Jones RH, Fortin DF, Stack RS, Glower DD, Smith LR, et al: Continuing evolution of therapy for coronary artery disease. Initial results from the era of coronary angioplasty, *Circulation* 89(5):2015–2025, 1994.

129. Schroeder S, Kopp AF, Baumbach A, Meisner C, Kuettner A, Georg C, Ohnesorge B, Herdeg C, Claussen CD, Karsch KR: Noninvasive detection and evaluation of atherosclerotic coronary plaques with multislice computed tomography, *J Am Coll Cardiol* 37(5):1430–1435, 2001.

130. Achenbach S, Moselewski F, Ropers D, Ferencik M, Hoffmann U, MacNeill B, Pohle K, Baum U, Anders K, Jang IK, Daniel WG, Brady TJ: Detection of calcified and noncalcified coronary atherosclerotic plaque by contrast-enhanced, submillimeter multidetector spiral computed tomography: a segment-based comparison with intravascular ultrasound, *Circulation* 109(1):14–17, 2004.

131. Leber AW, Knez A, Becker A, Becker C, von Ziegler F, Nikolaou K, Rist C, Reiser M, White C, Steinbeck G, Boekstegers P: Accuracy of multidetector spiral computed tomography in identifying and differentiating the composition of coronary atherosclerotic plaques: a comparative study with intracoronary ultrasound, *J Am Coll Cardiol* 43(7):1241–1247, 2004.

132. Leber AW, Becker A, Knez A, von Ziegler F, Sirol M, Nikolaou K, Ohnesorge B, Fayad ZA, Becker CR, Reiser M, Steinbeck G, Boekstegers P: Accuracy of 64-slice computed tomography to classify and quantify plaque volumes in the proximal coronary system: a comparative study using intravascular ultrasound, *J Am Coll Cardiol* 47(3):672–677, 2006.

133. Pohle K, Achenbach S, Macneill B, Ropers D, Ferencik M, Moselewski F, Hoffmann U, Brady TJ, Jang IK, Daniel WG: Characterization of non-calcified coronary atherosclerotic plaque by multidetector row CT: comparison to IVUS, *Atherosclerosis* 190(1):174–180, 2007.

134. Leber AW, Knez A, White CW, Becker A, von Ziegler F, Muehling O, Becker C, Reiser M, Steinbeck G, Boekstegers P: Composition of coronary atherosclerotic plaques in patients with acute myocardial infarction and stable angina pectoris determined by contrast-enhanced multislice computed tomography, *Am J Cardiol* 91(6): 714–718, 2003.

135. Schuijf JD, Beck T, Burgstahler C, Jukema JW, Dirksen MS, de Roos A, van der Wall EE, Schroeder S, Wijns W, Bax JJ: Differences in plaque composition in stable coronary artery disease versus acute coronary syndromes; non-invasive evaluation with multi-slice computed tomography, *Acute Card Care* 9(1):48–53, 2007.

136. Motoyama S, Kondo T, Sarai M, Sugiura A, Harigaya H, Sato T, Inoue K, Okumura M, Ishii J, Anno H, Virmani R, Ozaki Y, Hishida H, Narula J: Multislice computed tomographic characteristics of coronary lesions in acute coronary syndromes, *J Am Coll Cardiol* 50 (4):319–326, 2007.

137. Schmid M, Pflederer T, Jang IK, Ropers D, Sei K, Daniel WG, Achenbach S: Relationship between degree of remodeling and CT attenuation of plaque in coronary atherosclerotic lesions: an in-vivo analysis by multi-detector computed tomography, *Atherosclerosis* 197(1):457–464, 2008.

138. Pundziute G, Schuijf JD, Jukema JW, Decramer I, Sarno G, Vanhoenacker PK, Boersma E, Reiber JH, Schalij MJ, Wijns W, Bax JJ: Evaluation of plaque characteristics in acute coronary syndromes: non-invasive assessment with multi-slice computed tomography and invasive evaluation with intravascular ultrasound radiofrequency data analysis, *Eur Heart J* 29:2373–2381, 2008.

139. Choi B-J, Kang D-K, Tahk S-J, Choi S-Y, Yoon M-H, Lim H-S, Kang S-J, Yang H-M, Park J-S, Zheng M, Hwang G-S, Shin J-H: Comparison of 64-slice multidetector computed tomography with spectral analysis of intravascular ultrasound backscatter signals for characterizations of noncalcified coronary arterial plaques, *Am J Cardiol* 102:988–993, 2008.

140. Ibanez B, Cimmino G, Benezet-Mazuecos J, Gallego CG, Pinero A, Prat-Gonzalez S, Speidl WS, Fuster V, Garcia MJ, Sanz J, Badimon JJ: Quantification of serial changes in plaque burden using multi-detector computed tomography in experimental atherosclerosis, *Atherosclerosis* 202:185–191, 2009.

141. Schmid M, Achenbach S, Ropers D, Komatsu S, Ropers U, Daniel WG, Pflederer T: Assessment of changes in non-calcified atherosclerotic plaque volume in the left main and left anterior descending coronary arteries over time by 64-slice computed tomography, *Am J Cardiol* 101(5):579–584, 2008.

142. Burgstahler C, Reimann A, Beck T, Kuettner A, Baumann D, Heuschmid M, Brodoefel H, Claussen CD, Kopp AF, Schroeder S: Influence of a lipid-lowering therapy on calcified and noncalcified coronary plaques monitored by multislice detector computed tomography: results of the New Age II Pilot Study, *Invest Radiol* 42(3): 189–195, 2007.

143. Cademartiri F, La Grutta L, Runza G, Palumbo A, Maffei E, Mollet NR, Bartolotta TV, Somers P, Knaapen M, Verheye S, Midiri M, Hamers R, Bruining N: Influence of convolution filtering on coronary plaque attenuation values: observations in an ex vivo model of multislice computed tomography coronary angiography, *Eur Radiol* 17(7): 1842–1849, 2007.

144. Boll DT, Hoffmann MH, Huber N, Bossert AS, Aschoff AJ, Fleiter TR: Spectral coronary multidetector computed tomography angiography: dual benefit by facilitating plaque characterization and enhancing lumen depiction, *J Comput Assist Tomogr* 30(5):804–811, 2006.

145. Hyafil F, Cornily JC, Feig JE, Gordon V, Vucic E, Amirbekian V, Fisher EA, Fuster V, Feldman LJ, Fayad ZA: Noninvasive detection of macrophages using a nanoparticulate contrast agent for computed tomography, *Nat Med* 13(5):636–641, 2007.

146. Ropers D, Moshage W, Daniel WG, Jessl J, Gottwik M, Achenbach S: Visualization of coronary artery anomalies and their anatomic course by contrast-enhanced electron beam tomography and three-dimensional reconstruction, *Am J Cardiol* 87(2):193–197, 2001.

147. Schmitt R, Froehner S, Brunn J, Wagner M, Brunner H, Cherevatyy O, Gietzen F, Christopoulos G, Kerber S, Fellner F: Congenital anomalies of the coronary arteries: imaging with contrast-enhanced, multidetector computed tomography, *Eur Radiol* 15(6):1110–1121, 2005.

148. Schmid M, Achenbach S, Ludwig J, Baum U, Anders K, Pohle K, Daniel WG, Ropers D: Visualization of coronary artery anomalies by contrast-enhanced multi-detector row spiral computed tomography, *Int J Cardiol* 111(3):430–435, 2006.

149. Shi H, Aschoff AJ, Brambs HJ, Hoffmann MH: Multislice CT imaging of anomalous coronary arteries, *Eur Radiol* 14(12):2172–2181, 2004.

150. Cademartiri F, La Grutta L, Malago R, Alberghina F, Meijboom WB, Pugliese F, Maffei E, Palumbo AA, Aldrovandi A, Fusaro M, Brambilla V, Coruzzi P, Midiri M, Mollet NR, Krestin GP: Prevalence of anatomical variants and coronary anomalies in 543 consecutive patients studied with 64-slice CT coronary angiography, *Eur Radiol* 18(4):781–791, 2008.

151. Mollet NR, Hoye A, Lemos PA, Cademartiri F, Sianos G, McFadden EP, Krestin GP, Serruys PW, de Feyter PJ: Value of preprocedure multislice computed tomographic coronary angiography to predict the outcome of percutaneous recanalization of chronic total occlusions, *Am J Cardiol* 95(2):240–243, 2005.

152. Soon KH, Cox N, Wong A, Chaitowitz I, Macgregor L, Santos PT, Selvanayagam JB, Farouque HM, Rametta S, Bell KW, Lim YL: CT coronary angiography predicts the outcome of percutaneous coronary intervention of chronic total occlusion, *J Interv Cardiol* 20 (5):359–366, 2007.

153. Yokoyama N, Yamamoto Y, Suzuki S, Suzuki M, Konno K, Kozuma K, Kaminaga T, Isshiki T: Impact of 16-slice computed tomography in percutaneous coronary intervention of chronic total occlusions, *Catheter Cardiovasc Interv* 68(1):1–7, 2006.

154. Gilard M, Cornily JC, Pennec PY, Joret C, Le Gal G, Mansourati J, Blanc JJ, Boschat J: Accuracy of multislice computed tomography in the preoperative assessment of coronary disease in patients with aortic valve stenosis, *J Am Coll Cardiol* 47(10):2020–2024, 2006.

155. Holmström M, Sillanpaa MA, Kupari M, Kivisto S, Lauerma K: Eight-row multidetector computed tomography coronary angiography evaluation of significant coronary artery disease in patients with severe aortic valve stenosis, *Int J Cardiovasc Imaging* 22(5):703–710, 2006.

156. Scheffel H, Leschka S, Plass A, Vachenauer R, Gaemperli O, Garzoli E, Genoni M, Marincek B, Kaufmann P, Alkadhi H: Accuracy of 64-slice computed tomography for the preoperative detection of coronary artery disease in patients with chronic aortic regurgitation, *Am J Cardiol* 100(4):701–706, 2007.

157. Schlosser FJ, Mojibian HR, Dardik A, Verhagen HJ, Moll FL, Muhs BE: Simultaneous sizing and preoperative risk stratification for thoracic endovascular aneurysm repair: Role of gated computed tomography, *J Vasc Surg*, 2008.

158. Budoff MJ, Shavelle DM, Lamont DH, Kim HT, Akinwale P, Kennedy JM, Brundage BH: Usefulness of electron beam computed

tomography scanning for distinguishing ischemic from nonischemic cardiomyopathy, *J Am Coll Cardiol* 32(5):1173–1178, 1998.

159. Andreini D, Pontone G, Pepi M, Ballerini G, Bartorelli AL, Magini A, Quaglia C, Nobili E, Agostoni P: Diagnostic accuracy of multidetector computed tomography coronary angiography in patients with dilated cardiomyopathy, *J Am Coll Cardiol* 49 (20):2044–2050, 2007.

160. Ghostine S, Caussin C, Habis M, Habib Y, Clement C, Sigal-Cinqualbre A, Angel CY, Lancelin B, Capderou A, Paul JF: Non-invasive diagnosis of ischaemic heart failure using 64-slice computed tomography, *Eur Heart J* 2008.

161. Hunold P, Vogt FM, Schmermund A, Debatin JF, Kerkhoff G, Budde T, Erbel R, Ewen K, Barkhausen J: Radiation exposure during cardiac CT: effective doses at multi-detector row CT and electron-beam CT, *Radiology* 226(1):145–152, 2003.

162. Hausleiter J, Meyer T, Hadamitzky M, Huber E, Zankl M, Martinoff S, Kastrati A, Schomig A: Radiation dose estimates from cardiac multi-slice computed tomography in daily practice: impact of different scanning protocols on effective dose estimates, *Circulation* 113 (10):1305–1310, 2006.

163. Thompson RC, Cullom SJ: Issues regarding radiation dosage of cardiac nuclear and radiography procedures, *J Nucl Cardiol* 13 (1):19–23, 2006.

164. Einstein AJ, Moser KW, Thompson RC, Cerqueira MD, Henzlova MJ: Radiation dose to patients from cardiac diagnostic imaging, *Circulation* 116(11):1290–1305, 2007.

165. Gerber TC, Stratmann BP, Kuzo RS, Kantor B, Morin RL: Effect of acquisition technique on radiation dose and image quality in multidetector row computed tomography coronary angiography with submillimeter collimation, *Invest Radiol* 40(8):556–563, 2005.

166. Jakobs TF, Becker CR, Ohnesorge B, Flohr T, Suess C, Schoepf UJ, Reiser MF: Multislice helical CT of the heart with retrospective ECG gating: reduction of radiation exposure by ECG-controlled tube current modulation, *Eur Radiol* 12(5):1081–1086, 2002.

167. Sanz J, Rius T, Kuschnir P, Fuster V, Goldberg J, Ye XY, Wisdom P, Poon M: The importance of end-systole for optimal reconstruction protocol of coronary angiography with 16-slice multidetector computed tomography, *Invest Radiol* 40(3):155–163, 2005.

168. Trabold T, Buchgeister M, Kuttner A, Heuschmid M, Kopp AF, Schroder S, Claussen CD: Estimation of radiation exposure in 16-detector row computed tomography of the heart with retrospective ECG-gating, *Rofo* 175(8):1051–1055, 2003.

169. Earls JP, Berman EL, Urban BA, Curry CA, Lane JL, Jennings RS, McCulloch CC, Hsieh J, Londt JH: Prospectively gated transverse coronary CT angiography versus retrospectively gated helical technique: improved image quality and reduced radiation dose, *Radiology* 246 (3):742–753, 2008.

170. National Research Council (U.S.): *Committee to Assess Health Risks from Exposure to Low Level of Ionizing Radiation. Health risks from exposure to low levels of ionizing radiation : BEIR VII Phase 2*, Washington, DC, 2006, National Academies Press.

171. Einstein AJ, Henzlova MJ, Rajagopalan S: Estimating risk of cancer associated with radiation exposure from 64-slice computed tomography coronary angiography, *JAMA* 298(3):317–323, 2007.

172. Jemal A, Siegel R, Ward E, Murray T, Xu J, Thun MJ: Cancer statistics, 2007, *CA: Cancer J Clin* 57(1):43–66, 2007.

173. Hendel RC, Patel MR, Kramer CM, Poon M, Carr JC, Gerstad NA, Gillam LD, Hodgson JM, Kim RJ, Lesser JR, Martin ET, Messer JV, Redberg RF, Rubin GD, Rumsfeld JS, Taylor AJ, Weigold WG, Woodard PK, Brindis RG, Douglas PS, Peterson ED, Wolk MJ, Allen JM: ACCF/ACR/SCCT/SCMR/ASNC/NASCI/SCAI/SIR 2006 appropriateness criteria for cardiac computed tomography and cardiac magnetic resonance imaging: a report of the American College of Cardiology Foundation Quality Strategic Directions Committee Appropriateness Criteria Working Group, American College of Radiology, Society of Cardiovascular Computed Tomography, Society for Cardiovascular Magnetic Resonance, American Society of Nuclear Cardiology, North American Society for Cardiac Imaging, Society for Cardiovascular Angiography and Interventions, and Society of Interventional Radiology, *J Am Coll Cardiol* 48(7):1475–1497, 2006.

174. Schroeder S, Achenbach S, Bengel F, Burgstahler C, Cademartiri F, de Feyter P, George R, Kaufmann P, Kopp AF, Knuuti J, Ropers D, Schuijf J, Tops LF, Bax JJ: Cardiac computed tomography: indications, applications, limitations, and training requirements: report of a Writing Group deployed by the Working Group Nuclear Cardiology and Cardiac CT of the European Society of Cardiology and the European Council of Nuclear Cardiology, *Eur Heart J* 29(4):531–556, 2008.

175. Raff GL, Goldstein JA: Coronary angiography by computed tomography: coronary imaging evolves, *J Am Coll Cardiol* 49(18):1830–1833, 2007.

Chapter 22

PET/CT and SPECT/CT Hybrid Imaging

MARCELO F. DI CARLI

. . . .

INTRODUCTION

During the last 2 decades, we have witnessed a significant improvement in the prevention and management of atherosclerotic heart disease and its devastating consequences. Despite these efforts, however, coronary artery disease (CAD) remains highly prevalent, and it represents a health care burden in industrialized and developing countries. This has resulted in a continued expansion and refinement of our noninvasive armamentarium and an intense debate regarding the strengths and weaknesses of competing imaging technologies and their appropriate clinical use. The introduction and dissemination of new technology provide the potential for enhancing and expanding our understanding of disease processes (e.g., atherosclerosis, myocardial dysfunction) and hopefully extend our treatment options while providing a tool for monitoring therapeutic responses.

In this context, the integration of nuclear medicine cameras with multidetector computed tomography (CT) scanners (e.g., PET-CT and SPECT-CT) provides a unique opportunity to delineate cardiac and vascular anatomic abnormalities and their physiologic consequences in a single setting. For the evaluation of the patient with known or suspected CAD, it allows detection and quantification of the burden of the extent of calcified and noncalcified plaques (coronary artery calcium and coronary angiography), quantification of vascular reactivity and endothelial health, identification of flow-limiting coronary stenoses, and assessment of myocardial viability. Consequently, by revealing the burden of anatomic CAD and its physiologic significance, hybrid imaging can provide unique information that may improve noninvasive diagnosis, risk assessment, and management of CAD. In addition, by integrating the detailed anatomic information from CT with the high sensitivity of radionuclide imaging to evaluate targeted molecular and cellular abnormalities, hybrid imaging may play a key role in shaping the future of molecular diagnostics and therapeutics. The discussion that follows will review potential clinical applications of hybrid imaging in cardiovascular disease.

RATIONALE FOR INTEGRATING NUCLEAR IMAGING AND CT

For many decades, CT and nuclear imaging have followed separate and distinct developmental pathways. Both modalities have their strengths; CT scanners image cardiac and coronary anatomy with high spatial resolution, whereas nuclear imaging can identify a functional abnormality in, for example, myocardial perfusion, metabolism, or receptors. While it may seem that in many cases it would be equally effective to view separately acquired CT and nuclear images for a given patient on adjacent computer displays, with or without software registration, experience over the past 10 years with commercial positron emission tomography (PET)/CT scanners has highlighted the superiority of the hybrid technology for improved detection and staging of cancer. However, the concept of applying dual-modality imaging to the evaluation of patients with known or suspected cardiovascular disease is relatively new and not without controversy. In thinking about the potentially complementary aspects of dual-modality imaging, one must necessarily begin by reviewing the strengths and limitations of single-modality approaches.

Myocardial Perfusion Imaging (See Chapters 14–16)

Myocardial perfusion imaging is a robust approach to diagnosing obstructive CAD, quantifying the magnitude of myocardium at risk, assessing the extent of tissue viability, and guiding therapeutic management (i.e., selection of patients for revascularization). The extensive published literature on single-photon emission computed tomography (SPECT) suggests that its average sensitivity for detecting greater than 50% angiographic stenosis is 87% (range,

71% to 97%), whereas the average specificity is 73% (range, 36% to 100%).[1] With the use of attenuation-correction methods, the specificity improves, especially among patients undergoing exercise stress testing.[1] With PET perfusion imaging, the reported average sensitivity for detecting greater than 50% angiographic stenosis is 91% (range, 83% to 100%), whereas the average specificity is 89% (range, 73% to 100%).[2]

Despite its widespread use and acceptance, a recognized limitation of this approach is that it often uncovers only coronary territories supplied by the most severe stenosis, and consequently it is relatively insensitive to accurately delineate the extent of obstructive angiographic CAD, especially in the setting of multivessel CAD. For example, in a recent study of 101 patients with significant angiographic left main coronary stenosis, Berman et al. reported that by perfusion assessment alone, high-risk disease with moderate to severe perfusion defects (involving > 10% myocardium at stress) was identified in only 59% by quantitative analysis.[3] Conversely, absence of significant perfusion defect (>5% myocardium) was seen in 15% of patients. Similar results have been reported with PET imaging.[4]

Recent evidence suggests that two quantitative approaches may be able to help mitigate this limitation, at least in part. One of them relates to PET's unique ability to assess left ventricular function at rest and during peak stress (as opposed to post stress with SPECT).[4] The data suggest that in normal subjects, left ventricular ejection fraction (LVEF) increases during peak vasodilator stress.[4] In patients with obstructive CAD, however, the delta change in LVEF (from baseline to peak stress) is inversely related to the extent of obstructive angiographic CAD. Indeed, patients with multivessel or left main disease show a frank drop in LVEF during peak stress even in the absence of apparent perfusion defects. In contrast, those without significant CAD or with one-vessel disease show a normal increase in LVEF. Consequently, the diagnostic sensitivity of gated PET for correctly ascertaining the presence of multivessel disease increases from 50% to 79%.[4]

The second approach is based on the ability of PET to enable absolute measurements of myocardial blood flow (in mL/min/g) and coronary vasodilator reserve. In patients with so-called balanced ischemia or diffuse CAD, measurements of coronary vasodilator reserve would uncover areas of myocardium at risk that would generally be missed by performing only relative assessments of myocardial perfusion.[5] It is important to point out, however, that neither of these approaches has been tested in prospective clinical trials.

Another limitation of the myocardial perfusion imaging approach is that it fails to describe the presence and extent of subclinical atherosclerosis.[6,7] This is not unexpected, since the myocardial perfusion imaging method is designed and targeted on the identification of flow-limiting stenoses. This is potentially important, especially in patient subgroups with intermediate-high clinical risk in whom there may be extensive subclinical CAD, and may explain at least in part the limitations of perfusion imaging alone to identify low-risk patients among those with high clinical risk (e.g., diabetes, end-stage renal disease).[8]

Cardiac Computed Tomography (See Chapter 21)

Using state-of-the-art technology in carefully selected patients, it is possible to obtain high-quality images of the coronary arteries. The available evidence suggests that on a per-patient basis, the average weighted sensitivity for detecting at least one coronary artery with greater than 50% stenosis is 94% (range, 75% to 100%), whereas the average specificity is 77% (range, 49% to 100%).[9] The corresponding average positive predictive value (PPV) and negative predictive value (NPV) are 84% (range, 50% to 100%) and 87% (range, 35% to 100%), respectively, and the overall diagnostic accuracy is 89% (range, 68% to 100%).

Two multicenter, single-vendor trials evaluating the diagnostic accuracy of CTA-64 have been completed and recently published.[10,11] The results of these two studies confirm the robustness of CTA-64 for complete visualization of the coronary tree. The Assessment by Coronary Computed Tomographic Angiography of Individuals Undergoing Invasive Coronary Angiography (ACCURACY) trial enrolled 230 patients with a disease prevalence of 25%. On a patient-based model, the sensitivity, specificity, PPV and NPV to detect =50% or =70% stenosis were 95%, 83%, 64%, and 99%, respectively, and 94%, 83%, 48%, 99%, respectively. The study reported no differences in sensitivity and specificity for nonobese compared with obese subjects, whereas calcium scores ≥400 reduced specificity significantly. The Coronary Artery Evaluation Using 64-Row Multidetector Computed Tomography Angiography (CorE 64) trial[11] enrolled 291 patients with a disease prevalence of 56% and provides additional evidence that is somewhat discordant to the ACCURACY trial and to initial results from single-center studies. The CorE 64 study excluded patients with calcium scores over 600. On a per-patient basis, the sensitivity for detecting at least one coronary artery with ≥50% stenosis was 85%, considerably lower than in single-center studies and in the ACCURACY trial using similar technology, whereas the specificity was 90%, higher than previously reported. The corresponding average PPV and NPV were 91% and 83%, respectively, surprisingly different than most previous studies. On a per-vessel basis, the reported sensitivity for detecting coronary arteries with =50% stenosis was 75%, whereas the specificity was 93%. The corresponding PPV and NPV were 82% and 89%, respectively.

Except for the ACCURACY study, these reported accuracies of CTA to date should be interpreted in light of the relatively narrow range of CAD likelihood in patients examined (i.e., high or intermediate-high), as evidenced by the high prevalence of obstructive CAD in these series (56% to 62%).[9,11] Further, results are generally limited to relatively large vessel sizes (≥1.5 mm), excluding the results of smaller or uninterpretable vessels (generally distal vessels and side branches), the inclusion of which lowers sensitivity. An ongoing problem with CT is that high-density objects such as calcified coronary plaques and stent struts limit its ability to accurately delineate the degree of coronary luminal narrowing.[12,13] Of note, the CorE 64 trial excluded patients with high calcium scores (>600).[11] From a clinical perspective, a normal CTA is helpful inasmuch as it effectively excludes the presence of obstructive CAD and the need for further testing, defines a low clinical risk, and makes management decisions straightforward. Because of its limited accuracy to define stenosis severity and predict flow-limiting disease,[14,15] however, abnormal CTA results are more problematic to interpret and to use as the basis for defining the potential need of invasive coronary angiography and myocardial revascularization.

CLINICAL APPLICATIONS OF DUAL-MODALITY IMAGING

Attenuation Correction (See Chapters 6 and 7)

One of the most basic uses of CT in dual-modality imaging scanners (e.g., PET/CT and SPECT/CT) is for patient positioning and correction of the in homogeneity of the scintigraphic data caused by overlapping soft tissue (so-called attenuation correction). Unlike CT for calcium scoring or coronary angiography, acquisition parameters for CT-based transmission imaging vary with the configuration of the CT scanner (e.g., 8-, 16-, 64-multidetector CT) and clinical protocol, and several approaches have been proposed.[16,17] However, the general scan settings for CT transmission imaging adhere to the following principles: (1) a slow gantry rotation speed (e.g., 1 sec/revolution), combined with a relatively high pitch (e.g., 0.5 to 0.6:1), (2) nongated scan, (3) a high tube potential (e.g., 140 kVp) and a low tube current (~10 to 20 mA), and (4) a CT acquisition obtained during tidal expiration breath hold or shallow breathing.

Proper attenuation correction for SPECT increases diagnostic certainty and reduces the number of equivocal studies (Fig. 22-1).[18,19] However, CT-based attenuation correction also poses significant challenges for cardiac imaging.[20] Attenuation correction errors leading to artifacts have been reported in 30% to 60% of cases with both SPECT/CT and PET/CT (Fig. 22-2).[20,21] These artifacts are usually related to misalignments between the emission and CT transmission data sets caused by patient, cardiac, and/or respiratory motion,[20,22] leading to regional defects and frequent in homogeneity in quantitative tracer distribution.[23] Proper quality control and availability of registration software are crucial before interpretation of SPECT/CT and PET/CT images.

Localization of Targeted Molecular Imaging Agents

An emerging advantage of dual-modality imaging relates to the ability of CT to provide an anatomic roadmap that is critical for localization of targeted imaging agents. This has proven useful in both clinical and research applications in oncology imaging. For cardiovascular imaging, dual-modality approaches may be especially useful for imaging of atherosclerosis, where the CT can help delineate plaques and the localization of the targeted imaging probe in relation to those plaques (Fig. 22-3).[24] The proposed integration between PET and MRI may expand the possibilities for characterization of both myocardial tissue and vasculature.[25]

Integrating Calcium Scoring with Myocardial Perfusion Imaging

Voluminous plaques are more prone to calcification, and stenotic lesions frequently contain large amounts of calcium.[26] There is growing, consistent evidence that

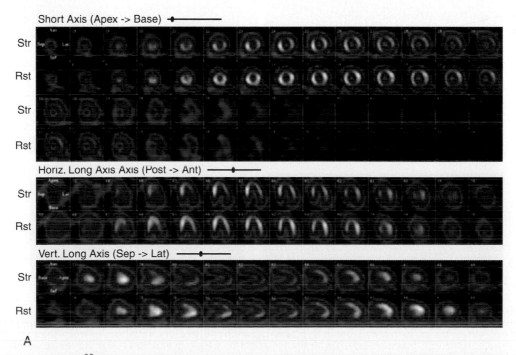

A

Figure 22-1 Rest and stress ^{99m}Tc-sestamibi myocardial perfusion imaging obtained with a hybrid SPECT/CT system fitted with a 6-slice multidetector CT in a 54-year-old woman with atypical angina. **A,** Images without attenuation correction show reversible perfusion defects in both the anterior and basal inferior walls.

Continued

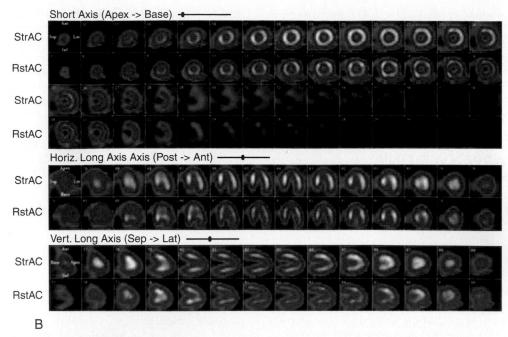

Short Axis (Apex -> Base)

StrAC

RstAC

StrAC

RstAC

Horiz. Long Axis Axis (Post -> Ant)

StrAC

RstAC

Vert. Long Axis (Sep -> Lat)

StrAC

RstAC

B

Figure 22-1—cont'd **B,** Images after CT-based attenuation correction show homogeneous perfusion throughout the left ventricle and complete resolution of the anterior and inferior stress defects, consistent with attenuation artifacts.

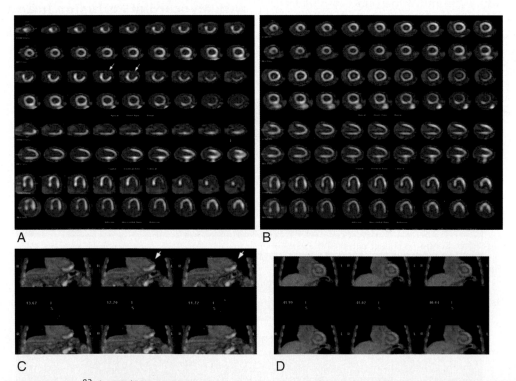

A   B

C   D

Figure 22-2 Rest and stress ^{82}Rb PET/CT in a 64-year-old man with atypical angina and dyspnea. **A,** Large and severe stress perfusion defect involving the anterior and anterolateral walls *(arrows)* with complete reversibility. **B,** Corresponding fused coronal PET and CT images showing classic misregistration (typically caused by respiratory variation between the two scans) such that the anterolateral wall on the PET images overlaps with the lung field on CT images *(arrows)*. During the reconstruction, this misregistration artifact leads to an attenuation correction error (undercorrection) that shows reduced tracer activity in the region overlapping the lung because of the low attenuation coefficient of air in the lungs. **C-D,** Correction of the misregistration error results in a normal myocardial perfusion scan.

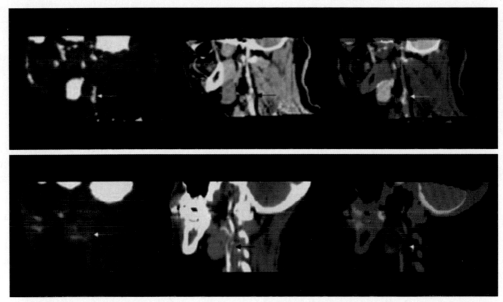

Figure 22-3 The *upper row (left to right)* shows PET, contrast CT, and coregistered PET/CT images in the sagittal plane, from a 63-year-old man who had experienced two episodes of left-sided hemiparesis. Angiography demonstrated stenosis of the proximal right internal carotid artery; this was confirmed on the CT image *(black arrow)*. The *white arrows* show [18]FDG uptake at the level of the plaque in the carotid artery. As expected, there was high [18]FDG uptake in the brain, jaw muscles, and facial soft tissues. The *lower row (left to right)* demonstrates a low level of [18]FDG uptake in an asymptomatic carotid stenosis. The *black arrow* highlights the stenosis on the CT angiogram, and the *white arrows* demonstrate minimal [18]FDG accumulation at this site on the [18]FDG PET and coregistered PET/CT images. *(Reproduced with permission from Rudd JH, Warburton EA, Fryer TD, et al: Imaging atherosclerotic plaque inflammation with [18F]-fluorodeoxyglucose positron emission tomography, Circulation 105:2708-2711, 2002.)*

coronary artery calcium (CAC) scores are generally predictive of a higher likelihood of ischemia (reflecting obstructive CAD) on myocardial perfusion imaging, and the available data support the concept of a threshold phenomenon governing this relationship.[27-29] Indeed, the frequency of myocardial ischemia increases significantly with increasing CAC scores, especially among patients with CAC ≥400 (Fig. 22-4).[27-29] A recent study reported that a CAC score ≥709 increased the sensitivity of SPECT MPI for detecting patients with obstructive CAD despite normal regional perfusion,[30] probably reflecting the ability of the CAC score to uncover the presence of extensive atherosclerosis in selected patients with balanced ischemia. Given the fact that CAC scores are not specific markers of

obstructive CAD,[31] however, one should be cautious in considering integrating this information into management decisions regarding coronary angiography, especially in patients with normal perfusion imaging. Conversely, CAC scores less than 400, especially in symptomatic patients with intermediate likelihood of CAD, may be less effective in excluding CAD, especially in young subjects and women.[32] In a recent study of symptomatic patients with intermediate likelihood of CAD, the absence of CAC only afforded an NPV of 84% to exclude ischemia.[29]

The potential to acquire and quantify rest and stress myocardial perfusion and non-contrast CT scan for CAC scoring from a single dual-modality study may offer a unique opportunity to expand the prognostic

Figure 22-4 Frequency of inducible ischemia by myocardial perfusion imaging in patients with Agatston CAC score ≥400. *(Reproduced from Schenker MP, Dorbala S, Hong EC, et al: Interrelation of coronary calcification, myocardial ischemia, and outcomes in patients with intermediate likelihood of coronary artery disease, Circulation 117:1693–1700, 2008.)*

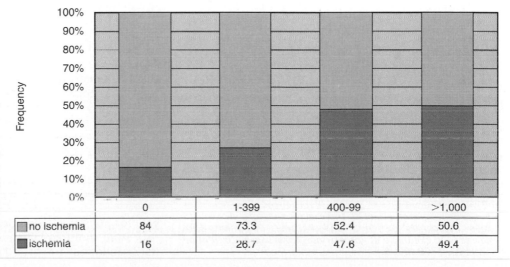

	0	1-399	400-99	>1,000
no ischemia	84	73.3	52.4	50.6
ischemia	16	26.7	47.6	49.4

value of stress nuclear imaging. The rationale for this integrated approach is predicated on the fact that the perfusion imaging approach is designed to uncover only obstructive atherosclerosis and is thus insensitive for detecting subclinical disease. The CAC score, reflecting the anatomic extent of atherosclerosis,[33] may offer an opportunity to improve the conventional models for risk assessment using nuclear imaging alone (especially in patients with normal perfusion), a finding that may serve as a more rational basis for personalizing the intensity and goals of medical therapy in a more cost-effective manner. For example, recent data suggest that quantification of CAC scores at the time of stress nuclear imaging using a dual-modality approach can enhance risk predictions in patients with suspected CAD.[29] In a consecutive series of 621 patients undergoing stress PET imaging and CAC scoring in the same clinical setting, risk-adjusted analysis demonstrated that for any degree of perfusion abnormality, there was a stepwise increase in adverse events (death and myocardial infarction) with increasing CAC scores. This finding was observed in patients with and without evidence of ischemia on PET MPI. Indeed, the annualized event rate in patients with normal PET MPI and no CAC was substantially lower than among those with normal PET MPI and a CAC ≥1000 (Fig. 22-5). Likewise, the annualized event rate

in patients with ischemia on PET MPI and no CAC was lower than among those with ischemia and a CAC ≥1000. Although CT coronary angiography as an adjunct to perfusion imaging could expand the opportunities to identify patients with noncalcified plaques at greater risk of adverse cardiovascular events, it is unclear how much added prognostic information there is in the contrast CT scan over the simple CAC scan.[34]

Integrating CT Coronary Angiography and Myocardial Perfusion Imaging for Diagnosis and Management of CAD

As discussed, CTA provides excellent diagnostic sensitivity for stenoses in the proximal and mid segments (>1.5 mm in diameter) of the main coronary arteries. Although the refinements implemented in the latest generation of CT technology have substantially reduced the number of nonevaluable coronary segments, the spatial resolution is still relatively limited compared to invasive angiography, and the sensitivity of this approach is reduced substantially in more distal coronary segments and side branches.[9] This limitation is unlikely to change, because a significant improvement in spatial resolution for CT will have to be coupled with a substantial increase in radiation dose in order to maintain noise constant. However, this limitation of CT can be offset by the MPI information that is generally unaffected by the location of coronary stenoses. First clinical results appear encouraging, and they support the notion that dual-modality imaging may offer superior diagnostic information with regard to identification of the culprit vessel.[35-37] For example, Rispler et al. reported a significant improvement in specificity (63% to 95%) and PPV (31% to 77%) without a change in sensitivity or NPV for detection of obstructive CAD as defined by quantitative coronary angiography in a cohort of 56 patients with known or suspected CAD undergoing hybrid SPECT/CTA imaging.[37] On the other hand, CTA improves the detection of multivessel CAD, which as discussed earlier is one of the main pitfalls of stress perfusion scintigraphy (Fig. 22-6). As noted, the incremental value seems most pronounced for coronary stenoses in distal segments and diagonal branches, and in vessels with extensive coronary lesions or heavy calcifications on CTA.

Nonetheless, one of the most compelling arguments supporting a clinical role of dual-modality imaging is its potential ability for optimizing management decisions. The importance of stress perfusion imaging in the integrated strategy is the ability of noninvasive estimates of jeopardized myocardium to identify which patients may benefit from revascularization—that is, differentiating high-risk patients with extensive scar versus those with extensive ischemia (Fig. 22-7). The advantages of this approach are clear: avoidance of unnecessary catheterizations that expose patients to risk and the potential for associated cost savings.[38] CTA is an excellent method to exclude CAD, but its ability to accurately assess the degree of luminal narrowing as a surrogate for physiologic significance is only modest. Recent data from multiple laboratories using either sequential (CTA followed by SPECT)[6,39-41] or hybrid imaging

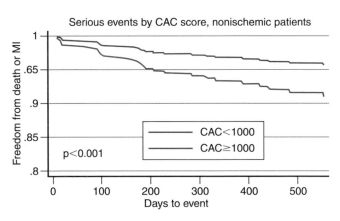

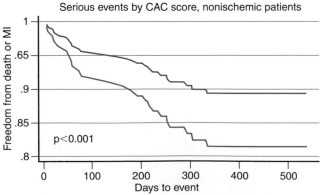

Figure 22-5 Adjusted survival curves for freedom from death or MI adjusted for age, sex, symptoms, and conventional CAD risk factors in patients without ischemia *(top panel)* and with ischemia *(lower panel)*. *(Reproduced from Schenker MP, Dorbala S, Hong EC, et al: Interrelation of coronary calcification, myocardial ischemia, and outcomes in patients with intermediate likelihood of coronary artery disease, Circulation 117:1693–1700, 2008.)*

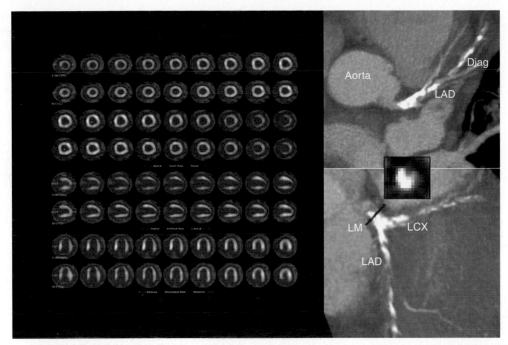

Figure 22-6 The *left panel* shows a stress and rest rubidium-82 PET/CTA study in a 68-year-old male referred for preoperative risk evaluation for atypical chest pain. There is normal relative myocardial perfusion on both the rest and stress images. The *right panel* demonstrates selected multiplanar reformats of his CT coronary angiogram demonstrating extensive calcified coronary plaque in the left main, left anterior descending, and left circumflex coronary arteries. Follow-up cardiac catheterization demonstrated severe left main disease.

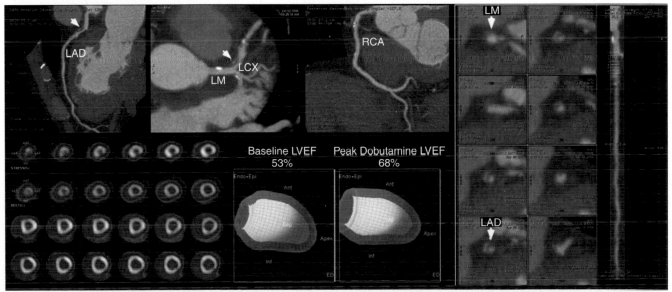

Figure 22-7 Integrated PET/CTA study. The CTA images demonstrate a noncalcified plaque *(arrow)* in the proximal LAD with 50% to 70% stenosis. However, the rest and peak dobutamine stress myocardial perfusion PET study *(lower left panel)* demonstrates only minimal inferoapical ischemia. In addition, LVEF was normal at rest and demonstrated a normal rise during peak dobutamine stress. CTA, computed tomography angiography; LAD, left anterior descending; LVEF, left ventricular ejection fraction; PET, positron emission tomography. *(Reproduced from Di Carli MF, Hachamovitch R: New technology for non-invasive imaging of coronary artery disease, Circulation 115:1464-1480, 2007.)*

(SPECT/CT or PET/CT)[7,19,42,43] suggest that the positive predictive value of CTA for identifying coronary stenoses producing objective evidence of stress-induced ischemia is suboptimal (Fig. 22-8).

The value of ischemia information for optimizing clinical decision making has been demonstrated by multiple studies. The nonrandomized Coronary Artery Surgery Study (CASS) registry reported that surgical revascularization in patients with CAD improved survival only among those with three-vessel disease with severe ischemia on exercise stress testing, while medical therapy was a superior initial therapy in patients

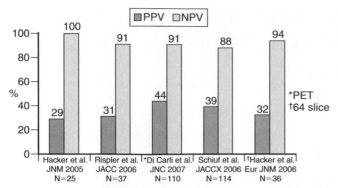

Figure 22-8 Frequency of inducible ischemia by myocardial perfusion imaging in territories supplied by stenosis greater than 50% on computed tomography coronary angiography. *(Data from Di Carli MF, Hachamovitch R: New technology for non-invasive imaging of coronary artery disease, Circulation 115:1464–1480, 2007.)*

without this finding.[44] Nonrandomized observational data using risk-adjustment techniques and propensity scores have also demonstrated the ability of stress perfusion imaging to identify which patients may accrue a survival benefit from revascularization.[45] The benefit of an ischemia-guided approach to management is further supported by invasive estimates of flow-limiting stenosis (e.g., fractional flow reserve [FFR]).[46] In the setting of an FFR above 0.75, revascularization can be safely deferred without increased patient risk, despite the presence of what visually appears to be a significant stenosis.[46] Indeed, cardiac event rates are extremely low in these patients, even lower than predicted if treated with PCI.[47] This differential risk appears to be sustainable in the long term.[48]

Further support came in a recent report from a randomized clinical trial evaluating the efficacy of revascularization decisions using an angiographically guided versus a functionally guided (as assessed by FFR) PCI in patients with multivessel CAD.[49] In this study, routine use of an FFR-guided approach significantly reduced the rate of the composite endpoint of death, nonfatal myocardial infarction, and repeat revascularization by 28% at 1 year

compared to the angiographically guided strategy. In addition, both groups have high and comparable rates of angina-free patients at 1 year.[49] Furthermore, in patients with visually defined left main coronary disease, an FFR above 0.75 was associated with excellent 3-year survival and freedom from major adverse cardiovascular events.[47] Conversely, event rates are increased when lesions with FFR less than 0.75 are not revascularized.[50]

Together, these data suggest that by identifying which patients have sufficient ischemia to merit revascularization, stress perfusion imaging may play a significant role in the selection of patients for catheterization within a strategy based on identification of patient benefit. From the previous discussion, this physiologic data would have greater clinical impact than visually defined coronary anatomy for revascularization decision making. In patients with multivessel CAD, the value of dual-modality imaging would allow better localization of the culprit stenosis and may offer a more targeted approach to revascularization (Fig. 22-9).

CHALLENGES, POTENTIAL OPPORTUNITIES, AND UNRESOLVED ISSUES FOR HYBRID IMAGING

Although intellectually appealing, the concept of a hybrid imaging approach is the subject of considerable debate within the cardiovascular imaging community. While it offers potential unique opportunities, there are also significant challenges and unresolved issues that one must consider.

Single-Setting Dual-Modality Versus Sequential Imaging

First, the cost of hybrid scanners integrating nuclear cameras (SPECT or PET) with advanced CT technology (64-slice CT) is considerably high, especially considering that throughput is vastly different for the nuclear test

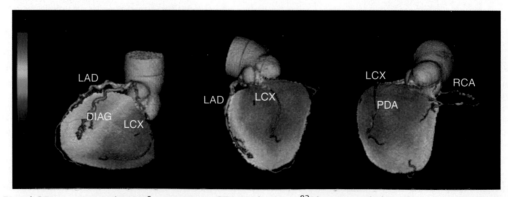

Figure 22-9 Fused 3D reconstructions of a coronary CTA and stress 82Rb myocardial perfusion study obtained in the same setting, assessed through integrated PET/CTA. The CTA demonstrated three-vessel CAD. The fused CTA-stress myocardial perfusion images demonstrate a large area of severe stress-induced perfusion abnormality *(deep blue color)* only in the territory of the dominant left circumflex (LCX) coronary artery. 3D, three-dimensional; CAD, coronary artery disease; CTA, computed tomography angiography; PET, positron emission tomography; 82Rb, rubidium-82. *(Reproduced with permission from Di Carli MF, Dorbala S, Meserve J, et al: Clinical myocardial perfusion PET/CT, J Nucl Med 48:783-793, 2007.)*

(slow) and the cardiac CT (very fast), making it difficult to develop a justifiable business model for both the practice and hospital settings. The development of ultrafast nuclear scanners or approaches that substantially shorten acquisition time may change the current economic reality for hybrid scanners in the future. In addition, the integrated scanner also makes it more difficult and expensive to integrate the rapid changes in technology, especially CT.

Second, we need to develop the evidence that would support which patients benefit from dual-modality testing from both diagnostic and prognostic perspectives. As discussed, there is some evidence that assessment CAC scores in combination with stress nuclear imaging may offer an opportunity to improve risk assessment, especially in symptomatic patients without prior CAD.[29] However, evaluation of CAC can be achieved without the need of advanced multidetector CT technology. For patients with equivocal stress nuclear test results, CT coronary angiography can be performed as a sequential test in a different scanner. Conversely, stress nuclear imaging is often used as a follow-up of patients with abnormal CTA studies to define hemodynamic significance of coronary stenosis. In such cases of sequential testing, the two data sets can be registered and fused off-line for interpretation and reporting.[40,51,52] Thus, the specific impact of hybrid imaging on treatment strategy and subsequently on outcome remains to be determined in prospective and long-term studies.

Radiation Dosimetry

The potential diagnostic appeal of a dual-modality approach must also be weighed against the challenges that it poses with regard to the added radiation dose to patients. This is a key issue as conventional spiral CTA protocols using retrospective ECG-gating have been shown to be associated with high total radiation doses between 9.4 and 21.4 mSv.[53,54] Hybrid cardiac imaging with CTA and SPECT MPI has been reported to expose patients to excessively high radiation doses up to 41.5 mSv,[37] which has prevented acceptance and the widespread use of this technology. However, this is changing rapidly. New low-dose CTA acquisition protocols with prospective electrocardiogram (ECG) triggering have recently been introduced and shown to offer a tremendous reduction of radiation dose to an average of 2.1 mSv[55-57] at maintained accuracy,[56] making this technique most suitable for hybrid imaging. Hybrid imaging with prospectively triggered CTA in conjunction with a stress-only SPECT MPI protocol may offer a significant reduction in dose.[56]

CONCLUSIONS

Innovation in noninvasive cardiovascular imaging is rapidly advancing our ability to image in great detail the structure and function in the heart and vasculature, and hybrid PET/CT and SPECT/CT represent clear examples of this innovation. By providing concurrent quantitative information about myocardial perfusion and metabolism with coronary and cardiac anatomy, hybrid imaging offers the opportunity for a comprehensive noninvasive evaluation of the burden of atherosclerosis and its physiologic consequences in the coronary arteries and the myocardium. This integrated platform for assessing anatomy and biology offers a great potential for translating advances in molecularly targeted imaging into humans. The goals of future investigation will be to refine these technologies, establish standard protocols for image acquisition and interpretation, address the issue of cost-effectiveness, and validate a range of clinical applications in large-scale clinical trials.

REFERENCES

1. Klocke FJ, Baird MG, Lorell BH, Bateman TM, Messer JV, Berman DS, O'Gara PT, Carabello BA, Russell RO Jr, Cerqueira MD, St John Sutton MG, DeMaria AN, Udelson JE, Kennedy JW, Verani MS, Williams KA, Antman EM, Smith SC Jr, Alpert JS, Gregoratos G, Anderson JL, Hiratzka LF, Faxon DP, Hunt SA, Fuster V, Jacobs AK, Gibbons RJ, Russell RO: ACC/AHA/ASNC guidelines for the clinical use of cardiac radionuclide imaging—executive summary: a report of the American College of Cardiology/American Heart Association Task Force on Practice Guidelines (ACC/AHA/ASNC Committee to Revise the 1995 Guidelines for the Clinical Use of Cardiac Radionuclide Imaging), *J Am Coll Cardiol* 42(7):1318–1333, 2003.
2. Di Carli MF, Dorbala S, Meserve J, El Fakhri G, Sitek A, Moore SC: Clinical myocardial perfusion PET/CT, *J Nucl Med* 48(5):783–793, 2007.
3. Berman DS, Kang X, Slomka PJ, Gerlach J, de Yang L, Hayes SW, Friedman JD, Thomson LE, Germano G: Underestimation of extent of ischemia by gated SPECT myocardial perfusion imaging in patients with left main coronary artery disease, *J Nucl Cardiol* 14(4):521–528, 2007.
4. Dorbala S, Vangala D, Sampson U, Limaye A, Kwong R, Di Carli MF: Value of vasodilator left ventricular ejection fraction reserve in evaluating the magnitude of myocardium at risk and the extent of angiographic coronary artery disease: a 82Rb PET/CT study, *J Nucl Med* 48(3):349–358, 2007.
5. Parkash R, deKemp RA, Ruddy Td T, Kitsilde A, Hart R, Beaushene L, Williams K, Davies RA, Labinaz M, Beanlands RS: Potential utility of rubidium 82 PET quantification in patients with 3-vessel coronary artery disease, *J Nucl Cardiol* 11(4):440–449, 2004.
6. Schuijf JD, Wijns W, Jukema JW, Atsma DE, de Roos A, Lamb HJ, Stokkel MP, Dibbets-Schneider P, Decramer I, De Bondt P, van der Wall EE, Vanhoenacker PK, Bax JJ: Relationship between noninvasive coronary angiography with multi-slice computed tomography and myocardial perfusion imaging, *J Am Coll Cardiol* 48(12):2508–2514, 2006.
7. Di Carli MF, Dorbala S, Curillova Z, Kwong RJ, Goldhaber SZ, Rybicki FJ, Hachamovitch R: Relationship between CT coronary angiography and stress perfusion imaging in patients with suspected ischemic heart disease assessed by integrated PET-CT imaging, *J Nucl Cardiol* 14(6):799–809, 2007.
8. Shaw LJ, Iskandrian AE: Prognostic value of gated myocardial perfusion SPECT, *J Nucl Cardiol* 11(2):171–185, 2004.
9. Di Carli MF, Hachamovitch R: New technology for noninvasive evaluation of coronary artery disease, *Circulation* 115(11):1464–1480, 2007.
10. Budoff MJ, Dowe D, Jollis JG, Gitter M, Sutherland J, Halamert E, Scherer M, Bellinger R, Martin A, Benton R, Delago A, Min JK: Diagnostic performance of 64-multidetector row coronary computed tomographic angiography for evaluation of coronary artery stenosis in individuals without known coronary artery disease: results from the prospective multicenter ACCURACY (Assessment by Coronary Computed Tomographic Angiography of Individuals Undergoing Invasive Coronary Angiography) trial, *J Am Coll Cardiol* 52(21):1724–1732, 2008.
11. Miller JM, Rochitte CE, Dewey M, Arbab-Zadeh A, Niinuma H, Gottlieb I, Paul N, Clouse ME, Shapiro EP, Hoe J, Lardo AC, Bush DE, de Roos A, Cox C, Brinker J, Lima JA: Diagnostic performance of coronary angiography by 64-row CT, *N Engl J Med* 359(22):2324–2336, 2008.
12. Hoffmann U, Moselewski F, Cury RC, Ferencik M, Jang IK, Diaz LJ, Abbara S, Brady TJ, Achenbach S: Predictive value of 16-slice multidetector spiral computed tomography to detect significant obstructive coronary artery disease in patients at high risk for coronary artery disease: patient-versus segment-based analysis, *Circulation* 110(17):2638–2643, 2004.
13. Mollet NR, Cademartiri F, Krestin GP, McFadden EP, Arampatzis CA, Serruys PW, de Feyter PJ: Improved diagnostic accuracy with 16-row

multi-slice computed tomography coronary angiography, *J Am Coll Cardiol* 45(1):128–132, 2005.

14. Leber AW, Becker A, Knez A, von Ziegler F, Sirol M, Nikolaou K, Ohnesorge B, Fayad ZA, Becker CR, Reiser M, Steinbeck G, Boekstegers P: Accuracy of 64-slice computed tomography to classify and quantify plaque volumes in the proximal coronary system: a comparative study using intravascular ultrasound, *J Am Coll Cardiol* 47(3): 672–677, 2006.

15. Raff GL, Gallagher MJ, O'Neill WW, Goldstein JA: Diagnostic accuracy of noninvasive coronary angiography using 64-slice spiral computed tomography, *J Am Coll Cardiol* 46(3):552–557, 2005.

16. Gould KL, Pan T, Loghin C, Johnson NP, Sdringola S: Reducing radiation dose in rest-stress cardiac PET/CT by single poststress cine CT for attenuation correction: quantitative validation, *J Nucl Med* 49(5): 738–745, 2008.

17. Lautamaki R, Brown TL, Merrill J, Bengel FM: CT-based attenuation correction in (82)Rb-myocardial perfusion PET-CT: incidence of misalignment and effect on regional tracer distribution, *Eur J Nucl Med Mol Imaging* 35(2):305–310, 2008.

18. Masood Y, Liu YH, Depuey G, Taillefer R, Araujo LI, Allen S, Delbeke D, Anstett F, Peretz A, Zito MJ, Tsatkin V, Wackers FJ: Clinical validation of SPECT attenuation correction using x-ray computed tomography-derived attenuation maps: multicenter clinical trial with angiographic correlation, *J Nucl Cardiol* 12(6):676–686, 2005.

19. Malkerneker D, Brenner R, Martin WH, Sampson UK, Feurer ID, Kronenberg MW, Delbeke D: CT-based attenuation correction versus prone imaging to decrease equivocal interpretations of rest/stress Tc-99m tetrofosmin SPECT MPI, *J Nucl Cardiol* 14(3):314–323, 2007.

20. Gould KL, Pan T, Loghin C, Johnson NP, Guha A, Sdringola S: Frequent diagnostic errors in cardiac PET/CT due to misregistration of CT attenuation and emission PET images: a definitive analysis of causes, consequences, and corrections, *J Nucl Med* 48(7):1112–1121, 2007.

21. Goetze S, Wahl RL: Prevalence of misregistration between SPECT and CT for attenuation-corrected myocardial perfusion SPECT, *J Nucl Cardiol* 14(2):200–206, 2007.

22. McQuaid SJ, Hutton BF: Sources of attenuation-correction artefacts in cardiac PET/CT and SPECT/CT, *Eur J Nucl Med Mol Imaging* 35(6): 1117–1123, 2008.

23. Slomka PJ, Le Meunier L, Hayes SW, Acampa W, Oba M, Haemer GG, Berman DS, Germano G: Comparison of myocardial perfusion 82Rb PET performed with CT- and transmission CT-based attenuation correction, *J Nucl Med* 49(12):1992–1998, 2008.

24. Rudd JH, Warburton EA, Fryer TD, Jones HA, Clark JC, Antoun N, Johnstrom P, Davenport AP, Kirkpatrick PJ, Arch BN, Pickard JD, Weissberg PL: Imaging atherosclerotic plaque inflammation with [18F]-fluorodeoxyglucose positron emission tomography, *Circulation* 105(23):2708–2711, 2002.

25. Judenhofer MS, Wehrl HF, Newport DF, Catana C, Siegel SB, Becker M, Thielscher A, Kneilling M, Lichy MP, Eichner M, Klingel K, Reischl G, Widmaier S, Rocken M, Nutt RE, Machulla HJ, Uludag K, Cherry SR, Claussen CD, Pichler BJ: Simultaneous PET-MRI: a new approach for functional and morphological imaging, *Nat Med* 14(4):459–465, 2008.

26. Wexler L, Brundage B, Crouse J, Detrano R, Fuster V, Maddahi J, Rumberger J, Stanford W, White R, Taubert K: Coronary artery calcification: pathophysiology, epidemiology, imaging methods, and clinical implications. A statement for health professionals from the American Heart Association. Writing Group, *Circulation* 94(5): 1175–1192, 1996.

27. He ZX, Hedrick TD, Pratt CM, Verani MS, Aquino V, Roberts R, Mahmarian JJ: Severity of coronary artery calcification by electron beam computed tomography predicts silent myocardial ischemia, *Circulation* 101:244–251, 2000.

28. Berman DS, Wong ND, Gransar H, Miranda-Peats R, Dahlbeck J, Arad Y, Hayes SW, Friedman JD, Kang X, Polk D, Hachamovitch R, Rozanski A: Relationship between stress-induced myocardial ischemia and atherosclerosis measured by coronary calcium tomography, *J Am Coll Cardiol* 44:923–930, 2004.

29. Schenker MP, Dorbala S, Hong EC, Rybicki FJ, Hachamovitch R, Kwong RY, Di Carli MF: Interrelation of coronary calcification, myocardial ischemia, and outcomes in patients with intermediate likelihood of coronary artery disease: a combined positron emission tomography/computed tomography study, *Circulation* 117(13): 1693–1700, 2008.

30. Schepis T, Gaemperli O, Koepfli P, Namdar M, Valenta I, Scheffel H, Leschka S, Husmann L, Eberli FR, Luscher TF, Alkadhi H, Kaufmann PA: Added value of coronary artery calcium score as an adjunct to gated SPECT for the evaluation of coronary artery disease in an intermediate-risk population, *J Nucl Med* 48(9): 1424–1430, 2007.

31. Nallamothu BK, Saint S, Bielak LF, Sonnad SS, Peyser PA, Rubenfire M, Fendrick AM: Electron-beam computed tomography in the diagnosis of coronary artery disease: a meta-analysis, *Arch Intern Med* 161(6): 833–838, 2001.

32. Knez A, Becker A, Leber A, White C, Becker CR, Reiser MF, Steinbeck G, Boekstegers P: Relation of coronary calcium scores by electron beam

tomography to obstructive disease in 2,115 symptomatic patients, *Am J Cardiol* 93(9):1150–1152, 2004.

33. Sangiorgi G, Rumberger JA, Severson A, Edwards WD, Gregoire J, Fitzpatrick LA, Schwartz RS: Arterial calcification and not lumen stenosis is highly correlated with atherosclerotic plaque burden in humans: a histologic study of 723 coronary artery segments using nondecalcifying methodology, *J Am Coll Cardiol* 31(1):126–133, 1998.

34. Mahmarian JJ: Computed tomography coronary angiography as an anatomic basis for risk stratification: deja vu or something new?*J Am Coll Cardiol* 50(12):1171–1173, 2007.

35. Gaemperli O, Schepis T, Koepfli P, Valenta I, Soyka J, Leschka S, Desbiolles L, Husmann L, Alkadhi H, Kaufmann PA: Accuracy of 64-slice CT angiography for the detection of functionally relevant coronary stenoses as assessed with myocardial perfusion SPECT, *Eur J Nucl Med Mol Imaging* 34(8):1162–1171, 2007.

36. Namdar M, Hany TF, Koepfli P, Siegrist PT, Burger C, Wyss CA, Luscher TF, von Schulthess GK, Kaufmann PA: Integrated PET/CT for the assessment of coronary artery disease: a feasibility study, *J Nucl Med* 46(6):930–935, 2005.

37. Rispler S, Keidar Z, Ghersin E, Roguin A, Soil A, Dragu R, Litmanovich D, Frenkel A, Aronson D, Engel A, Beyar R, Israel O: Integrated single-photon emission computed tomography and computed tomography coronary angiography for the assessment of hemodynamically significant coronary artery lesions, *J Am Coll Cardiol* 49(10):1059–1067, 2007.

38. Shaw LJ, Hachamovitch R, Berman DS, Marwick TH, Lauer MS, Heller GV, Iskandrian AE, Kesler KL, Travin MI, Lewin HC, Hendel RC, Borges-Neto S, Miller DD: The economic consequences of available diagnostic and prognostic strategies for the evaluation of stable angina patients: an observational assessment of the value of precatheterization ischemia. Economics of Noninvasive Diagnosis (END) Multicenter Study Group, *J Am Coll Cardiol* 33(3):661–669, 1999.

39. Hacker M, Jakobs T, Matthiesen F, Vollmar C, Nikolaou K, Becker C, Knez A, Pfluger T, Reiser M, Hahn K, Tiling R: Comparison of spiral multidetector CT angiography and myocardial perfusion imaging in the noninvasive detection of functionally relevant coronary artery lesions: first clinical experiences, *J Nucl Med* 46(8):1294–1300, 2005.

40. Gaemperli O, Schepis T, Kalff V, Namdar M, Valenta I, Stefani L, Desbiolles L, Leschka S, Husmann L, Alkadhi H, Kaufmann PA: Validation of a new cardiac image fusion software for three-dimensional integration of myocardial perfusion SPECT and stand-alone 64-slice CT angiography, *Eur J Nucl Med Mol Imaging* 34(7):1097–1106, 2007.

41. Gaemperli O, Schepis T, Valenta I, Husmann L, Scheffel H, Duerst V, Eberli FR, Luscher TF, Alkadhi H, Kaufmann PA: Cardiac image fusion from stand-alone SPECT and CT: clinical experience, *J Nucl Med* 48(5):696–703, 2007.

42. Rispler S, Roguin A, Keidar Z, Ghersin E, Aronson D, Dragu R, Engel A, Israel O, Beyar R: Integrated SPECT/CT for the assessment of hemodynamically significant coronary artery lesions, *J Am Coll Cardiol* 47: 115A, 2006.

43. Hacker M, Jakobs T, Hack N, Nikolaou K, Becker C, von Ziegler F, Knez A, Konig A, Klauss V, Tiling R: Combined use of 64-slice computed tomography angiography and gated myocardial perfusion SPECT for the detection of functionally relevant coronary artery stenoses. First results in a clinical setting concerning patients with stable angina, *Nuklearmedizin* 46(1):29–35, 2007.

44. Weiner DA, Ryan TJ, McCabe CH, Chaitman BR, Sheffield LT, Fisher LD, Tristani F: The role of exercise testing in identifying patients with improved survival after coronary artery bypass surgery, *J Am Coll Cardiol* 8(4):741–748, 1986.

45. Hachamovitch R, Hayes SW, Friedman JD, Cohen I, Berman DS: Comparison of the short-term survival benefit associated with revascularization compared with medical therapy in patients with no prior coronary artery disease undergoing stress myocardial perfusion single photon emission computed tomography, *Circulation* 107(23): 2900–2907, 2003.

46. Kern MJ, Lerman A, Bech JW, De Bruyne B, Eeckhout E, Fearon WF, Higano ST, Lim MJ, Meuwissen M, Piek JJ, Pijls NHJ, Siebes M, Spaan JAE: Physiological assessment of coronary artery disease in the cardiac catheterization laboratory: A scientific statement from the American Heart Association Committee on Diagnostic and Interventional Cardiac Catheterization, Council on Clinical Cardiology, *Circulation* 114:1321–1341, 2006.

47. Bech GJ, De Bruyne B, Pijls NH, de Muinck ED, Hoorntje JCA, Escaned J, Stella PR, Boersma E, Bartunek J, Koolen JJ, Wijns W: Fractional flow reserve to determine the appropriateness of angioplasty in moderate coronary stenosis: a randomized trial, *Circulation* 103:2928–2934, 2001.

48. Pijls NH, van Schaardenburgh P, Manahoran G, Boersma E, Bech JW, van't Veer M, Bar F, Hoorntjie J, Koolen J, Wijns W, De Bruyne B: Percutaneous coronary intervention of functionally nonsignificant stenosis: 5-year follow-up of the DEFER study 49:2105–2111, 2007.

49. Tonino PA, De Bruyne B, Pijls NH, Siebert U, Ikeno F, van' t Veer M, Klauss V, Manoharan G, Engstrom T, Oldroyd KG, Ver Lee PN, MacCarthy PA, Fearon WF: Fractional flow reserve versus angiography

for guiding percutaneous coronary intervention, *N Engl J Med* 360(3): 213–224, 2009.

50. Chamuleau SAJ, Meuwissen M, Koch KT, van Eck-Smit BLF, Tio RA, Tijssen JGP, Piek JJ: Usefulness of fractional flow reserve for risk stratification of patients with multivessel coronary artery disease and an intermediate stenosis, *Am J Cardiol* 89:377–380, 2002.

51. Santana CA, Garcia EV, Faber TL, Sirineni GK, Esteves FP, Sanyal R, Halkar R, Ornelas M, Verdes L, Lerakis S, Ramos JJ, Aguade-Bruix S, Cuellar H, Candell-Riera J, Raggi P: Diagnostic performance of fusion of myocardial perfusion imaging (MPI) and computed tomography coronary angiography, *J Nucl Cardiol* 2009.

52. Slomka PJ: Software approach to merging molecular with anatomic information, *J Nucl Med* 45(Suppl 1):36S–45S, 2004.

53. Mollet NR, Cademartiri F, de Feyter PJ: Non-invasive multislice CT coronary imaging, *Heart* 91(3):401–407, 2005.

54. Hausleiter J, Meyer T, Hadamitzky M, Huber E, Zankl M, Martinoff S, Kastrati A, Schomig A: Radiation dose estimates from cardiac multislice computed tomography in daily practice: impact of different scanning protocols on effective dose estimates, *Circulation* 113 (10):1305–1310, 2006.

55. Husmann L, Wiegand M, Valenta I, Gaemperli O, Schepis T, Siegrist PT, Namdar M, Wyss CA, Alkadhi H, Kaufmann PA: Diagnostic accuracy of myocardial perfusion imaging with single photon emission computed tomography and positron emission tomography: a comparison with coronary angiography, *Int J Cardiovasc Imaging* 24 (5):511–518, 2008.

56. Herzog BA, Husmann L, Landmesser U, Kaufmann PA: Low-dose computed tomography coronary angiography and myocardial perfusion imaging: cardiac hybrid imaging below 3 mSv, *Eur Heart J* 2008.

57. Javadi M, Mahesh M, McBride G, Voicu C, Epley W, Merrill J, Bengel FM: Lowering radiation dose for integrated assessment of coronary morphology and physiology: first experience with step-and-shoot CT angiography in a rubidium-82 PET-CT protocol, *J Nucl Cardiol* 15(6):783–790, 2008.

Comparison of Noninvasive Techniques for Myocardial Perfusion Imaging

GEORGE A. BELLER

INTRODUCTION

A variety of noninvasive techniques permit the assessment of regional myocardial perfusion at rest and during exercise or pharmacologic stress. These techniques include radionuclide imaging employing single-photon emission computed tomography (SPECT) or positron emission tomography (PET) methodologies, contrast echocardiography, computed tomography (CT), and cardiac magnetic resonance (CMR) imaging. All have particular strengths and weaknesses. The reader is directed to earlier chapters in this section of the book for detailed descriptions of the use of these perfusion imaging techniques for detecting functionally significant coronary artery stenoses or abnormal coronary flow reserve due to endothelial and microcirculatory abnormalities. In the paragraphs to follow, the major strengths and weaknesses of these diverse approaches to myocardial perfusion imaging (MPI) will be reviewed, with the understanding that advances in technology for all of these imaging methodologies are continuously being reported. Table 23-1 provides a summary of the strengths and limitations of these four diverse imaging technologies used for the assessment of myocardial perfusion under rest and stress conditions.

RADIONUCLIDE MYOCARDIAL PERFUSION IMAGING
(See Chapters 14 to 16)

Stress and rest SPECT myocardial perfusion imaging (MPI) is the most commonly performed imaging technique to detect CAD among patients presenting with chest pain or other symptoms thought to be secondary to ischemia. Table 23-1 shows the main strengths and limitations of radionuclide SPECT MPI relative to other noninvasive techniques for assessing myocardial perfusion. The sensitivity, specificity, and normalcy rate for SPECT MPI for detection of coronary artery disease (CAD) are 86%, 74%, and 89%, respectively.[1] The prognostic value of SPECT MPI has been proven with multiple studies reported in the literature (see Chapter 16).[2] For patients undergoing exercise stress SPECT imaging who have a normal perfusion scan, the annual death or myocardial infarction rate is 0.7% annually, compared to 5.6% for those with an abnormal scan.[2] Similarly, for pharmacologic stress SPECT MPI, the annual hard event rate with a normal scan is 1.2% per year versus 8.3% for patients with an abnormal scan.[2,3] The higher event rates with pharmacologic stress MPI are attributed to a higher pretest clinical risk in patients deemed unable to exercise. The greater the stress perfusion abnormalities, the higher the event rates.[3] The percentage of the left ventricle rendered ischemic with stress has proven clinically useful in separating patients who might benefit from coronary revascularization versus those who have a good outcome beginning medical therapy.[4] The percent left ventricular (LV) ischemia can also be used to serially evaluate response to therapy. The COURAGE nuclear substudy showed that patients who did not experience a 5% or more decrease in ischemic defect size after 1 year of therapy had a substantially higher cardiac event rate over 6 to 7 years of follow-up, compared to patients who showed a greater than 5% reduction in ischemic defect size.[5] Interestingly, those patients who had no residual ischemia had no future events during follow-up. Patients with diabetes[6] and those with chronic kidney disease[7] have higher cardiac event rates with ischemic SPECT studies than patients without diabetes or chronic kidney disease. Such patients also have a higher risk of cardiac death or nonfatal myocardial infarction with normal SPECT scans.[2]

Specificity of SPECT MPI is enhanced when gated images are obtained, since fixed defects due to

Table 23-1 High-Risk SPECT Imaging Variables

Multiple perfusion defects in > 1 coronary supply region (multivessel coronary artery disease scan pattern)

An extensive area of stress-induced hypoperfusion, even if confined to the territory of a single coronary artery (e.g., proximal left anterior descending coronary artery scan pattern)

A high ischemic burden reflected by multiple reversible defects

Transient ischemic left ventricular cavity dilation

Multiple abnormal regional wall-motion or thickening abnormalities, even if not associated with perfusion defects

A gated SPECT ejection fraction of < 40%

Increased diastolic and end-systolic volumes on quantitative SPECT, increased lung-to-heart ratio of thallium uptake when Tl-201 used for exercise imaging

SPECT, single-photon emission computed tomography.

attenuation artifacts can be distinguished from myocardial scar on stress and rest images.[8] Those due to scar (or severe ischemia) will show abnormal wall motion or abnormal wall thickening, whereas those due to attenuation artifacts, as with breast attenuation in women or inferobasilar wall attenuation in men, will show normal regional function. Gated SPECT MPI can provide functional information that contributes to the diagnostic and prognostic value of the test.[9] Functional variables include the left ventricular ejection fraction (LVEF), systolic and diastolic volumes at end-systole and end-diastole, and extent of regional wall-thickening or wall-motion abnormalities. Regional wall-motion or thickening abnormalities seen on SPECT images correlate well with measurements made on echocardiography and MRI. Transient ischemic cavity dilation from stress to rest images can also be identified and in most cases represents stress-induced subendocardial ischemia that resolves with rest. It is a scintigraphic marker of high-risk CAD.[10]

Attenuation correction algorithms have been introduced for clinical SPECT imaging and have enhanced the accuracy of CAD detection, chiefly by reducing false-positive studies that interpret attenuation artifacts as perfusion abnormalities.[11] Standardization of attenuation correction methods from one vendor to another has not yet been achieved. Another variable that may confound the interpretation of SPECT tomograms is high visceral activity, which may interfere with the evaluation of the inferior wall. This is more of an issue with vasodilator stress than with exercise stress. Image quality is also diminished with marked obesity, requiring 2-day stress/rest studies to optimize quality by having more activity injected with the rest image than is possible in same-day, low-dose rest and high-dose stress studies. The SPECT artifacts that interfere with accurate interpretation of MPI images are very well summarized in Chapters 6 and 7.

Stress myocardial perfusion imaging, employing the technetium (Tc)-99m-labeled tracers underestimates the extent of significant coronary artery stenoses.[12]

Some patients with left main and/or three-vessel CAD may have uniform tracer uptake on vasodilator stress perfusion SPECT images if coronary flow reserve is diffusely reduced in the supply regions of all three major coronary vessels. In the study by Lima et al., only a small percentage of patients with angiographic three-vessel disease had perfusion abnormalities in the distribution of all three affected coronary arteries[13]; on gated SPECT images, 23% had perfusion and/or regional wall-motion abnormalities in the myocardial supply zones of the three stenotic vessels (defined as =50% stenosis). Even using quantitative analysis of relative differences in regional counts on vasodilator stress SPECT, 12% of the patients in this study with three-vessel CAD had no perfusion or function abnormalities on their SPECT studies. Similarly, Berman et al.[14] reported that among 101 patients with left main CAD (=50% stenosis) and no clinical evidence of prior infarction, 40% had low-risk SPECT scans with less than 10% LV ischemia, and 15% had no ischemic defects.

The underestimation of the extent of CAD with SPECT is perhaps more common when ^{99m}Tc perfusion agents are used (sestamibi and tetrofosmin) rather than ^{201}Tl.[15] The first-pass myocardial extraction fraction is higher with ^{201}Tl (80%) than the other two tracers (55% to 60%), and myocardial uptake is more proportional to flow in the hyperemic flow ranges after vasodilator administration. But in fact all three perfusion agents plateau at high flows (Fig. 23-1). This particularly adversely affects the detection of mild to moderate stenoses.[16] Standard SPECT imaging normalizes counts to the region of the myocardium with the highest activity (regional counts). If diffuse multivessel disease is present, that "normal" area may also have subnormal perfusion in response to vasodilator infusion. In this situation, counts in that region may not be higher than in other perfusion zones, since flow reserve is diffusely diminished. When the activity is homogeneous throughout the myocardium in such patients, "balanced ischemia" is often present. If postischemic myocardial stunning or chronic hibernation is present,

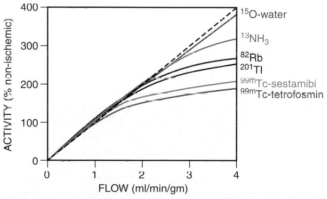

Figure 23-1 Myocardial uptake of various perfusion tracers (% nonischemic uptake) related to myocardial blood flow showing roll-off in myocardial extraction with hyperemic flows. *(From Glover DK, Gropler RJ: Journey to find the ideal PET flow tracer for clinical use: Are we there yet? J Nucl Cardiol 14:765-768, 2007.)*

or if the patient had a prior subendocardial infarction, abnormal regional function can be detected on gated images that would render the interpretation of the stress study as abnormal, despite the absence of focal perfusion abnormalities. Also, transient ischemic dilation of the LV cavity from stress to rest images can at times be observed with normal or minimally abnormal perfusion scans. This finding would hint at the possibility of more extensive underlying CAD.[17] A larger LV cavity post stress (compared to rest) is thought to be due to transient stress-induced subendocardial hypoperfusion.

Some attempts have been undertaken to quantitate coronary flow reserve with SPECT perfusion imaging.[18] This would address the limitation of standard SPECT in which only relative differences in perfusion from one area of the myocardium to another area are assessed. Estimation of coronary flow reserve (CFR) by SPECT[18] involves acquiring anterior planar list-mode images of the heart after intravenous tracer administration. Counts from a right pulmonary artery region of interest are quantified to estimate the arterial input function of the tracer. An estimate of myocardial tissue perfusion is determined by dividing myocardial counts on the SPECT images by the integrated arterial input function. Perfusion values for the stress studies are divided by the corresponding values from the rest studies to obtain myocardial perfusion reserve. Limitations of SPECT that do not allow absolute quantitation of regional myocardial blood flow in mL/min/g are factors such as scatter, attenuation, partial-volume effect, and low resolution. Nevertheless, just being able to evaluate CFR by measuring the ratios of tissue and arterial counts at rest and stress might enhance the detection of multivessel CAD. Figure 23-2 shows the relationship between SPECT-estimated CFR and intracoronary Doppler CFR measurements. Studies continue to be performed to try to achieve absolute quantitation of perfusion with dynamic SPECT imaging.[19] Using an experimental canine model, these investigators demonstrated that the kinetic analysis of quantitatively assessed myocardial ^{201}Tl accumulation provided myocardial blood flow measurements that agreed well with flows obtained using radioactive microspheres.

Recent advances have been made in SPECT technology, permitting high-speed imaging using a bank of independently controlled detector columns with large-hole tungsten collimators and multiple cadmium zinc telluride crystal arrays (see Chapter 9).[20] Using this high-speed camera, the entire stress/rest ^{99m}Tc sestamibi MPI procedure could be completed within 30 minutes. The stress and rest acquisition times were 16 and 12 minutes for conventional SPECT MPI and 4 and 2 minutes for high-speed SPECT. Image quality was high, and myocardial count rates were significantly higher versus conventional SPECT. Diagnostic performance for high-speed SPECT was as good as for conventional SPECT, with summed stress scores and summed reversibility scores correlating extremely well ($r = 0.93$). Introduction of this new technology will reduce the long procedure time for a full stress/rest study as currently performed with conventional SPECT.

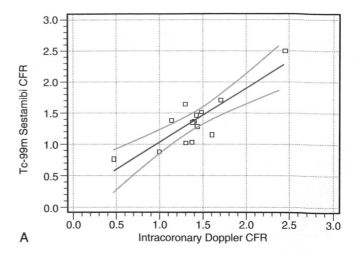

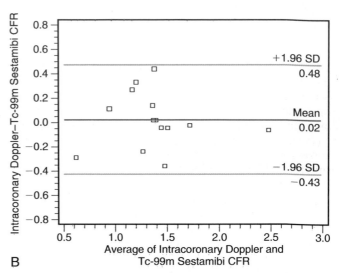

Figure 23-2 **A,** Relationship between SPECT-estimated coronary flow reserve (CFR) and intracoronary Doppler CFR. The *solid line* indicates the regression line, and the *dashed lines* indicate the 95% confidence intervals. **B,** Agreement between SPECT-estimated CFR and intracoronary Doppler CFR by Bland-Altman analysis. The differences between the two techniques are plotted against the means of the two techniques. The *solid line* indicates the mean difference between the techniques, and the *dashed lines* indicate the limits of agreements. *(From Petretta M, Soricelli A, Storto G, Cuocolo A: Assessment of coronary flow reserve using single photon emission computed tomography with technetium 99m-labeled tracers [review], J Nucl Cardiol 15:456-465, 2008.)*

POSITRON EMISSION TOMOGRAPHY (See Chapter 19)

PET MPI is an attractive alternative to SPECT for detecting CAD and determining its extent. PET perfusion tracers used clinically for MPI are rubidium (Rb)-82 and nitrogen (N)-13-ammonia. [82]Rb is eluted from a generator and has a short half-life of 78 seconds. It is only used with pharmacologic stress and not exercise, which is a limitation. ^{13}N-ammonia requires a cyclotron for production and has a half-life of 10 minutes. They both show a plateau in myocardial activity with increasing coronary flow, although the flow-uptake relationship is better than that of the ^{99m}Tc SPECT perfusion tracers (see Fig. 23-1). In the meta-analysis of clinical studies reported in the literature, the sensitivity and specificity of PET MPI are 89% and 86%, respectively.[1] When CT is used for attenuation correction, sensitivity is increased to 93% and 95% for detecting patients with multivessel disease.[21] Bateman et al.[22] compared SPECT with PET for CAD detection in different groups of patients studied in the same time period. They showed that the sensitivity and specificity were higher for PET (87% versus 82% and 93% versus 73%, respectively), as was the prediction of multivessel disease (71% versus 48%). Some reasons for the improved accuracy of PET over SPECT include higher spatial and contrast resolution and the fact that depth-independent attenuation correction is more easily performed, since it is intrinsic to PET methodology. Since the half-lives of the tracers used for PET MPI are so short, fast sequential evaluations of regional flow can be achieved. This promotes improved throughput of patients in clinical laboratories.

PET has the capability for rapid dynamic imaging of tracer kinetics, permitting absolute quantitation of myocardial blood flow not easily achieved by SPECT technology. This capability is one of the most important advantages of PET over SPECT and other noninvasive technologies for assessing myocardial perfusion. Quantitating regional myocardial blood flow in mL/min/g using tracer kinetic models with rapid dynamic imaging, and obtaining accurate values for CFR rather than just assessing relative differences in perfusion (myocardial counts) from one myocardial region to another, can be achieved. Oxygen 15 labeled water is a positron emitter that is metabolically inert, freely diffusible, and cyclotron-generated. There is virtually complete extraction of this tracer by the myocardium, independent of flow rate and myocardial metabolic state. This makes it the ideal radionuclide for quantitating absolute myocardial blood flow. Quantitation of blood flow with any of the PET tracers includes corrections for the partial volume effect (that causes an underestimation of myocardial tracer concentration), activity spillover from the blood pool to the myocardium, and physical decay. Parkash et al.[23] showed that quantitation of ^{82}Rb net retention and estimation of absolute perfusion at rest and with dipyridamole stress defined a greater extent of CAD in patients with three-vessel disease than using the standard approach of assessing relative differences in perfusion (69% of LV sectors versus 44%). The absolute stress-minus-rest perfusion difference in the myocardium is measured in this approach. Figure 23-3 shows an example of the comparison of the standard method for identification of perfusion defects with the quantification method in a patient with stenoses in the left anterior descending (LAD), right, and circumflex coronary arteries. A very good relationship was found between dipyridamole-induced myocardial blood flow in mL/min/g by ^{82}Rb quantitation and stenosis severity in patients with CAD.[24] The repeatability of rest and hyperemic myocardial blood flow measurements with ^{82}Rb PET is excellent.[25] Myocardial blood flow determinations were highly reproducible in this study

of 15 healthy volunteers who underwent two rest and pharmacologic stress studies 60 minutes apart.

PET can be used to assess CFR in the preclinical state in patients with CAD risk factors who may have endothelial and microvascular dysfunction.[26-28] Abnormal CFR by PET has been reported in patients with dyslipidemia, diabetic patients, smokers, and patients with hypertension. These risk factors are associated with abnormal vasodilator responses in the coronary circulation. Impaired coronary vasoreactivity may have prognostic implications. PET assessments of CFR with vasodilator stress can be undertaken before and after therapeutic interventions (e.g., statin treatment of hypercholesterolemia) to monitor improvement in myocardial perfusion reserve.[26] The normal CFR response to dipyridamole and adenosine is approximately 3.5 to 4.0.[29] This hyperemia is attenuated in patients with coronary atherosclerosis in the absence of critical stenoses. Additionally, PET measurement of myocardial blood flow responses to cold pressor testing, causing sympathetic stimulation, identifies a group of patients with an increased cardiac event rate who have normal coronary angiograms.[30]

Thus, as summarized in Table 23-1, PET has certain advantages over SPECT, particularly when quantitation of perfusion or CFR is accomplished. Disadvantages of PET are limited availability in most institutions for routine clinical imaging, inability to combine PET MPI with exercise stress for ^{82}Rb imaging, and higher cost than SPECT. For tracers other than ^{82}Rb, an on-site cyclotron is needed for tracer production. One exciting advance in PET MPI is the emergence of a new perfusion imaging agent, ^{18}F-BMS-747158-02, a novel pyridaben derivative that binds to the mitochondrial complex, ^{2}(MTC1), of the electron transport chain with very high affinity.[31,32] The first-pass extraction fraction of this ^{18}F-labeled PET perfusion tracer is similar to ^{201}Tl, and like sestamibi and tetrofosmin, it does not show redistribution. Extraction of this tracer is high at different flow rates, which makes it suitable for quantitation of absolute blood flow with dynamic PET imaging of tracer kinetics. In a pig model of transient coronary artery occlusion, uptake of ^{18}F-BMS showed a good correlation with regional flow measured by radioactive microspheres ($r = 0.88$), with flows ranging from 1 mL/min/g to 3 mL/min/g.[33] The 109-minute half-life of ^{18}F would permit the use of exercise stress imaging, since adequate time would be available between the time of tracer injection during peak exercise and acquisition of PET MPI images. ^{18}F is also widely available commercially and an in-house cyclotron is not necessary to produce it.

CARDIAC MAGNETIC RESONANCE PERFUSION IMAGING
(See Chapter 17)

Myocardial perfusion can be assessed at rest and during vasodilator stress, exploiting the first-pass kinetics of T1-weighted CMR imaging of gadolinium (Gd) chelates (e.g., Gd-DTPA) after bolus injection of the contrast

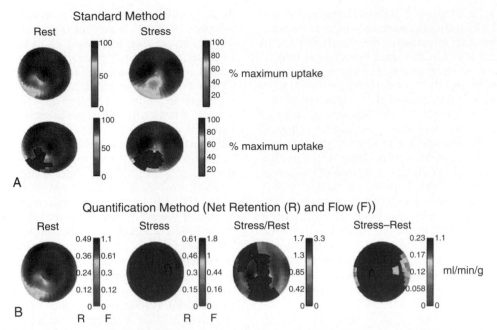

Figure 23-3 Polar maps of a patient with triple-vessel coronary artery disease (CAD). **A,** Standard method: rest and stress rubidium-82 uptake polar maps on a relative scale (0%-100% of maximum left ventricular uptake). The *lower panel* is the abnormal sector map. The *dark blue* segments represent sectors greater than 2 SDs below the mean of a normal population ($\leq$5% likelihood of CAD). Note that only the inferior wall is abnormal. **B,** Quantification method: rest and stress rubidium-82 uptake polar maps plus stress/rest (relative retention and flow reserve) and stress/rest (absolute retention and flow reserve). Retention scales (R) are *left* of color bar, and calculated flows (F) are *right* of the color bar. The *dark blue* segments represent sectors greater than 2 SDs below the mean of a normal population ($\leq$5% likelihood of CAD). Note that the absolute retention reserve (stress/rest in *B*) reveals that all abnormal perfusion is seen in the supply region of all three coronary arteries, whereas the standard method (stress polar map in *A*) suggests only right coronary artery disease. *(From Parkash R, deKemp RA, Ruddy TD, et al: Potential utility of rubidium 82 PET quantification in patients with 3-vessel coronary artery disease. J Nucl Cardiol 11:440-449, 2004.)*

agent.[34] The basic concept of CMR perfusion imaging by this approach is that signal intensity of the myocardium is proportional to myocardial blood flow as the contrast agent enters the microvasculature and the interstitial space. Normally perfused myocardium shows a fast signal increase per unit of time when contrast is injected during vasodilator stress. Areas perfused by stenotic vessels show a delay in the signal increase. The data acquisition for the first-pass contrast measurement can be obtained in only a few seconds during a single breath hold. The MRI data are collected with ECG gating, which eliminates cardiac motion. Because of the excellent spatial resolution of CMR, the transmurality of perfusion defects can be resolved. Most often, the stress-induced perfusion abnormalities are identified in the subendocardium. Figure 23-4 shows an example of a first-pass CMR perfusion imaging study, with associated time-intensity curves showing hypoperfusion in the stenotic region.[34] Late enhancement imaging after the first-pass data are acquired permits the differentiation between myocardial scar, which shows late Gd hyperenhancement, and transient ischemia, where the contrast washes out of the myocardium rather rapidly. It is also possible to measure coronary flow reserve with first-pass CMR by comparing rest and stress CMR data. Table 23-1 lists the strengths and limitations of CMR imaging of myocardial perfusion.

A meta-analysis of CMR perfusion imaging studies demonstrated a sensitivity of 91% and a specificity of 81% for CAD detection.[35] The prevalence of CAD in these studies averaged 57%. The MR-IMPACT study compared CMR perfusion imaging with SPECT for detection of CAD.[36] They found in a cohort of 241 patients who underwent adenosine stress Gd-DTPA-BMA (Omniscan, GE Healthcare) that perfusion CMR had a similar performance as SPECT by area under the receiver operating characteristic (ROC) curve analysis. The MR-IMPACT study compared the effect of five different contrast doses on image quality and diagnostic ability to detect CAD. The prognostic value of CMR perfusion imaging has not yet been ascertained, although one study[37] showed differences in event rates between patients with normal and abnormal scans.

CMR perfusion imaging has some advantages over SPECT and PET MPI:
1. No radiation exposure
2. Higher resolution, permitting identification of subendocardial ischemia
3. Shorter time to complete a study
4. Fewer artifacts
5. Ability to perform a rest study several minutes after a stress study because of the short physiologic half-life of the Gd contrast agent
6. Overall shorter duration for a complete stress/rest study (45 to 60 minutes)

Improvements in temporal resolution with CMR have permitted acquisition of several tomograms of the heart within one heartbeat. With CMR, myocardial viability, regional function, and global function can be evaluated during the same study in which first-pass perfusion

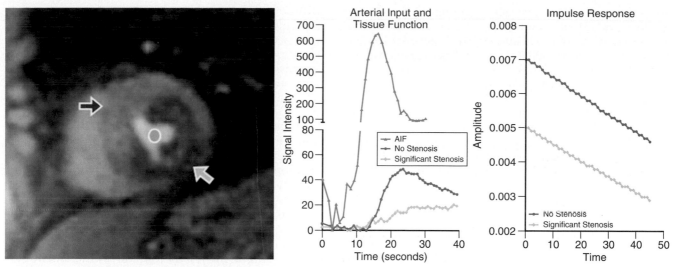

Figure 23-4 **Left,** Short-axis slice of left ventricle, shown at peak enhancement during first-pass CMR perfusion imaging. The *orange arrow* points to a large perfusion defect in the inferolateral wall, which is visually apparent, and the *purple arrow* points to a region with normal perfusion. The *green circle* is in the left ventricular cavity. *Middle,* Time-intensity curves generated as gadolinium traverses the left ventricular cavity and the normal and abnormal myocardial segments. By deconvolution of the tissue function *(purple and orange curves)* from the arterial input function (AIF) *(green curve)*, an impulse response is generated *(Right).* The initial amplitude of the impulse response (which is a measure of myocardial blood flow) is much higher for the normal *(purple)* sector than for the abnormal *(orange)* sector. *(From Patel AR, Epstein FH, Kramer CM: Evaluation of the microcirculation: Advances in cardiac magnetic resonance perfusion imaging. J Nucl Cardiol 15:698-708, 2008.)*

imaging is performed. The ability to quantitate flow in absolute terms is similar to PET MPI. Quantitative perfusion CMR with adenosine, in which the ratio between stress and rest myocardial blood flow determinations by the CMR time intensity curve analysis was derived, correlates well with fractional flow reserve of coronary stenoses determined at cardiac catheterization.[38] Thus, hemodynamic significance of coronary stenoses can be assessed by quantitative CMR perfusion imaging. As mentioned, SPECT MPI can underestimate three-vessel CAD because of "balanced ischemia" and diffuse abnormal flow reserve. In such patients, the SPECT perfusion study could show uniform tracer uptake at both rest and stress. With CMR perfusion imaging, diffuse subendocardial ischemia in the setting of three-vessel or left main CAD can be detected both visually and quantitatively because of the excellent spatial resolution of CMR. Absolute perfusion measurements are obtained by deconvolution of the tissue function and the arterial input function, similar to what is accomplished with PET. The microcirculation can also be assessed with CMR perfusion imaging. In patients with no-reflow after reperfusion following an acute myocardial infarction, a characteristic pattern on late Gd enhancement is identified.[39,40] Myocardial perfusion reserve abnormalities by CMR were reported in the subendocardium in patients with cardiac syndrome X.[41,42]

Limitations of CMR perfusion imaging are dark ring artifacts that must be distinguished from true perfusion defects, exclusion of patients with devices such as pacemakers and ICDs, claustrophobia in some patients, and the risk of nephrogenic systemic sclerosis in patients with advanced renal dysfunction. The combined cost of equipment, software, personnel, and contrast agents is relatively expensive.

Most CMR studies are performed with a 1.5 tesla (T)–strength magnet. A study by Cheng et al.[43] showed that for CMR perfusion imaging, a 3-T field strength was superior to 1.5 T with respect to sensitivity (89% versus 84%), specificity (76% versus 67%), and positive and negative predictive values for CAD detection. In this study, four short-axis images were acquired during every heartbeat using a saturation recovery fast-gradient echo sequence and 0.04 mmol/kg Gd-DTPA bolus injection. The 3-T system provides better signal-to-noise ratio and contrast enhancement, which improves spatial resolution and image quality. The authors of this paper suggested that 3-T may become the preferred CMR field strength for myocardial perfusion assessment in clinical practice.

COMPUTED TOMOGRAPHY PERFUSION IMAGING

Myocardial perfusion can be evaluated by multidetector CT (MDCT) scanning using first-pass, contrast-enhanced methodology similar in principle to first-pass imaging of myocardial perfusion.[44] However, for CT perfusion imaging, iodinated contrast agents are injected during vasodilator stress rather than a non–radiation producing agent like Gd-DTPA. With CT perfusion imaging, myocardial signal intensity correlates with myocardial blood flow. The first-pass myocardial extraction fraction of the contrast agent is rather low at 0.33, compared to 0.50 to 0.60 for first-pass CMR and 0.80 for [201]Tl. Significant diffusion of contrast moves into the extravascular space. Correction for this diffusion must be undertaken to get accurate measurements of absolute blood flow. In a LAD occlusion model, MDCT first-pass contrast-enhanced perfusion imaging correlated extremely well with microsphere-determined blood flow up to 8.0 mL/g/min ($P = 0.001$).[45] Figure 23-5 shows the data from this animal validation study. A few single-center patient studies of vasodilator stress CT perfusion imaging have been reported, and the findings show promise for using this first-pass perfusion imaging approach for detecting CAD.[46,47]

The strengths and limitations of CT scanning for myocardial perfusion during stress and rest are listed in Table 23-1. Perfusion imaging with CT may offer some advantages over other techniques so far discussed: high spatial resolution, rapid data acquisition, and the ability to assess coronary anatomy, perfusion, and regional and global ventricular function with one test.[48,49] The CT

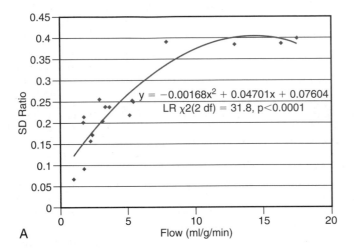

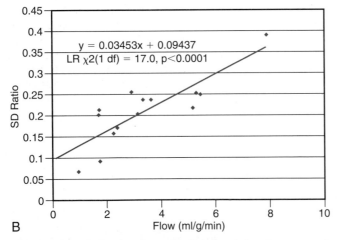

Figure 23-5 **A,** Regional myocardial signal density assessed by cardiac computed tomography divided by the left ventricular blood pool signal density (*y-axis*) versus microsphere-derived myocardial blood flow (*x-axis*) in both the stenosed left anterior descending artery territory and remote myocardial territory using a semiautomated volumetric analysis over the range of flows studied ($y = -0.00168x^2 + 0.04701x + 0.07604$, LR chi-square [2df] = 31.8, $P < 0.0001$). Note the roll-off of signal density with hyperemic flows. **B,** Data representing flows less than 8 mL/g/min from (**A**) are shown in (**B**) ($y = 0.03453x + 0.09437$, LR chi-square [1 degree of freedom] = 17.0, SE = 0.007, $P < 0.0001$) (n = 7). SD ratio = myocardial signal density/left ventricular blood pool signal density. *(From George RT, Silva C, Cordeiro MA, et al: Multidetector computed tomography myocardial perfusion imaging during adenosine stress, J Am Coll Cardiol 48:153-160, 2006.)*

perfusion imaging technique could prove useful in detecting regional myocardial hypoperfusion in patients with acute chest pain presenting to an emergency department. One study of 72 patients who underwent first-pass CT imaging for detection of hypoenhancement found that the technique detected more infarcts than SPECT imaging.[50] Like CMR, cardiac CT has the capability to quantitate perfusion and coronary flow reserve. CMR, however, has better temporal resolution than CT. Limitations of cardiac CT are lower-quality images with high heart rates, beam-hardening artifacts resulting in variations of signal intensity in the myocardium, and inability to use high doses of iodinated contrast in patients with renal dysfunction.[48] Radiation doses with rest and stress studies using dynamic imaging are quite high with current technology. For CMR perfusion imaging, no radiation exposure occurs. Obviously, CT perfusion imaging is in its infancy, and further studies are warranted to determine its worth over existing technologies that have less radiation exposure and can be undertaken with exercise stress.

PERFUSION IMAGING WITH MYOCARDIAL CONTRAST ECHOCARDIOGRAPHY
(See Chapter 18)

Myocardial contrast echocardiography (MCE) images the microcirculation at rest and with vasodilator stress in order to detect functionally significant CAD.[51,52,53,54] The gas-filled microbubbles remain in the intravascular space after intravenous administration. Approximately 90% of the microbubbles reside in the capillaries. In the presence of a critical coronary artery stenosis, hyperemia produced by vasodilator stress results in a decrease in capillary volume. This decrease is thought to be secondary to capillary derecruitment in the stenosed bed because of an imbalance between changes in coronary driving pressure and flow during vasodilation.[55] The capillaries derecruit to maintain capillary hydrostatic pressure. The resultant decrease in capillary volume in this situation is what produced the perfusion defects on MCE.

The technique now most often utilized for perfusion imaging with MCE is destroying the microbubbles that are infused to a steady state with high-energy ultrasound and then monitoring the rate of microbubble replenishment within the ultrasound beam (Fig. 23-6).[56] When fully replenished, the ultrasound signal represents relative blood volume within the beam. Usually the beam fills within 5 seconds but takes longer when flow is diminished and fills more rapidly with hyperemic flows. The volume of blood in the myocardium, reflected by the microbubbles, is normalized to the signal from the LV cavity. Myocardial blood flow is estimated by the product of the blood volume fraction and the myocardial blood flow velocity. The latter is estimated from rate of bubble reappearance in the myocardium after bubbles were destroyed.[56] Only end-systolic images at rest and stress are examined side by side so that the same region within the stress and rest images can be compared at the

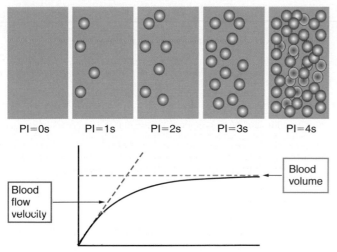

Figure 23-6 Schematic illustration of microbubble replenishment within the ultrasound beam after initial destruction *(top panels).* When fully replenished (PI = 4s) the ultrasound signal represents relative blood volume within the beam. Blood flow velocity is reflected by the rate of bubble reappearance in the myocardium after they were destroyed *(bottom graph and see text). (From Lepper W, Belcik T, Wei K, et al: Myocardial contrast echocardiography [review], Circulation 109:3132-3135, 2004.)*

same pulsing interval. Delayed subendocardial replenishment during hyperemia is reflective of an underlying coronary artery stenosis. Quantitative estimates of regional myocardial blood flow comprise fitting certain parameters to time-intensity curves derived from microbubble replenishment.[56]

Early studies for CAD detection with MCE showed sensitivities ranging from 75% to 96%, with specificities ranging from 55% to 100%. In most of these studies, SPECT was the gold standard.[55] A meta-analysis comparing SPECT to MCE that examined 9 studies comprising 588 patients revealed a concordance of 81% between the two techniques.[57] Another meta-analysis of 18 studies in the literature with more than a thousand patients demonstrated an average sensitivity of 82% and specificity of 80% for CAD detection.[57] A multicenter study comparing MCE with SPECT found no difference in sensitivity of (84% versus 82%), with similar specificities (56% versus 52%).[54] Agreement between MCE and SPECT for presence or absence of CAD was 73%.

There are certain advantages and limitations to the use of stress MCE for detection of CAD (see Table 23-1).[48] Advantages of MCE for the noninvasive assessment of myocardial perfusion include: no radiation exposure to the patient; better spatial resolution than SPECT for identifying subendocardial versus transmural hypoperfusion; ability to quantitate absolute flow; wide availability of echocardiography and lower cost than SPECT; CMR or CT for stress and rest perfusion imaging; and more versatile application in the acute setting (e.g., the emergency department). Disadvantages include: difficulty in obtaining high-quality images in some patients; attenuation artifacts, particularly in the lateral-basal myocardial areas of the left ventricle; and getting adequate spatial coverage of all areas of the LV myocardium.

Respiratory motion can also cause image-quality problems, as does the presence of chronic pulmonary disease. The technique is very operator dependent, particularly with the need for sustaining a constant image plane during replenishment of the myocardium by the microbubbles.

SUMMARY

In summary, five different approaches to the noninvasive assessment of regional myocardial perfusion and coronary flow reserve are reviewed. All have their strengths and their weaknesses. Gated SPECT and PET perfusion imaging have had the most validation, with multiple experimental clinical studies reported in the literature over many decades. These longstanding techniques are still being perfected with new imaging instrumentation, better software programs for image display and analysis, new imaging tracers, the ability to provide multimodality and hybrid imaging by combining perfusion data with CT-derived coronary anatomic data, and the continued demonstration of their diagnostic and prognostic value in a variety of patient populations with a host of different stressors. The field of radionuclide imaging must move toward quantitative myocardial flow measurements rather than the semiquantitative display of relative myocardial radionuclide uptake. CMR and cardiac CT are still in the midst of validation in research studies as the technology for both continues to improve. Although MCE has been in existence for many years, as of this writing no contrast agent has been FDA-approved for myocardial perfusion imaging. For CMR and CT, diagnostic and prognostic studies reported in the past several years are few but appear quite promising. These newer modalities will need to be compared with existing modalities in rigorous clinical trials (e.g., stress SPECT/PET or stress echocardiography) with respect to showing comparable or better accuracy and cost-effectiveness in the clinical setting.

REFERENCES

1. Schuijf JD, Poldermans D, Shaw LJ, Jukema JW, Lamb HJ, de Roos A, Wijns W, van der Wall EE, Bax JJ: Diagnostic and prognostic value of non-invasive imaging in known or suspected coronary artery disease, *Eur J Nucl Med Mol Imaging* 33(1):93–104, 2006, Review.
2. Shaw LJ, Iskandrian AE: Prognostic value of gated myocardial perfusion SPECT, *J Nucl Cardiol* 11(2):171–185, 2004, Review. No abstract available.
3. Navare SM, Mather JF, Shaw LJ, Fowler MS, Heller GV: Comparison of risk stratification with pharmacologic and exercise stress myocardial perfusion imaging: a meta-analysis, *J Nucl Cardiol* 11(5):551–561, 2004.
4. Hachamovitch R, Hayes SW, Friedman JD, Cohen I, Berman DS: Comparison of the short-term survival benefit associated with revascularization compared with medical therapy in patients with no prior coronary artery disease undergoing stress myocardial perfusion single photon emission computed tomography, *Circulation* 107(23): 2900–2907, 2003, Epub 2003 May 27.
5. Shaw LJ, Berman DS, Maron DJ, Mancini GB, Hayes SW, Hartigan PM, Weintraub WS, O'Rourke RA, Dada M, Spertus JA, Chaitman BR, Friedman J, Slomka P, Heller GV, Germano G, Gosselin G, Berger P, Kostuk WJ, Schwartz RG, Knudtson M, Veledar E, Bates ER, McCallister B, Teo KK, Boden WE: COURAGE Investigators. Optimal medical therapy with or without percutaneous coronary intervention to reduce ischemic burden: results from the Clinical Outcomes Utilizing Revascularization and Aggressive Drug Evaluation (COURAGE) trial nuclear substudy, *Circulation* 117(10):1283–1291, 2008, Epub 2008 Feb 11.

6. Anand DV, Lim E, Hopkins D, Corder R, Shaw LJ, Sharp P, Lipkin D, Lahiri A: Risk stratification in uncomplicated type 2 diabetes: prospective evaluation of the combined use of coronary artery calcium imaging and selective myocardial perfusion scintigraphy, *Eur Heart J* 27(6):713–721, 2006, Epub 2006 Feb 23.

7. Hakeem A, Bhatti S, Dillie KS, Cook JR, Samad Z, Roth-Cline MD, Chang SM: Predictive value of myocardial perfusion single-photon emission computed tomography and the impact of renal function on cardiac death, *Circulation* 118(24):2540–2549, 2008, Epub 2008 Dec 1.

8. Smanio PE, Watson DD, Segalla DL, Vinson EL, Smith WH, Beller GA: Value of gating of technetium-99m sestamibi single-photon emission computed tomographic imaging, *J Am Coll Cardiol* 30(7):1687–1692, 1997.

9. Travin MI, Heller GV, Johnson LL, Katten D, Ahlberg AW, Isasi CR, Kaplan RC, Taub CC, Demus D: The prognostic value of ECG-gated SPECT imaging in patients undergoing stress Tc-99m sestamibi myocardial perfusion imaging, *J Nucl Cardiol* 11(3):253–262, 2004.

10. Abidov A, Germano G, Berman DS: Transient ischemic dilation ratio: a universal high-risk diagnostic marker in myocardial perfusion imaging, *J Nucl Cardiol* 14(4):497–500, 2007, No abstract available.

11. Thompson RC, Heller GV, Johnson LL, Case JA, Cullom SJ, Garcia EV, Jones PG, Moutray KL, Bateman TM: Value of attenuation correction on ECG-gated SPECT myocardial perfusion imaging related to body mass index, *J Nucl Cardiol* 12(2):195–202, 2005.

12. Beller GA: Underestimation of coronary artery disease with SPECT perfusion imaging, *J Nucl Cardiol* 15(2):151–153, 2008, No abstract available.

13. Lima RS, Watson DD, Goode AR, Siadaty MS, Ragosta M, Beller GA, Samady H: Incremental value of combined perfusion and function over perfusion alone by gated SPECT myocardial perfusion imaging for detection of severe three-vessel coronary artery disease, *J Am Coll Cardiol* 42(1):64–70, 2003.

14. Berman DS, Kang X, Slomka PJ, Gerlach J, de Yang L, Hayes SW, Friedman JD, Thomson LE, Germano G: Underestimation of extent of ischemia by gated SPECT myocardial perfusion imaging in patients with left main coronary artery disease, *J Nucl Cardiol* 14(4):521–528, 2007.

15. Beller GA, Bergmann SR: Myocardial perfusion imaging agents: SPECT and PET, *J Nucl Cardiol* 11(1):71–86, 2004, Review. No abstract available.

16. Shanoudy H, Raggi P, Beller GA, Soliman A, Ammermann EG, Kastner RJ, Watson DD: Comparison of technetium-99m tetrofosmin and thallium-201 single-photon emission computed tomographic imaging for detection of myocardial perfusion defects in patients with coronary artery disease, *J Am Coll Cardiol* 31(2):331–337, 1998.

17. Abidov A, Bax JJ, Hayes SW, Hachamovitch R, Cohen I, Gerlach J, Kang X, Friedman JD, Germano G, Berman DS: Transient ischemic dilation ratio of the left ventricle is a significant predictor of future cardiac events in patients with otherwise normal myocardial perfusion SPECT, *J Am Coll Cardiol* 42(10):1818–1825, 2003.

18. Petretta M, Soricelli A, Storto G, Cuocolo A: Assessment of coronary flow reserve using single photon emission computed tomography with technetium 99m-labeled tracers, *J Nucl Cardiol* 15(3):456–465, 2008, Review.

19. Iida H, Eberl S, Kim KM, Tamura Y, Ono Y, Nakazawa M, Sohlberg A, Zeniya T, Hayashi T, Watabe H: Absolute quantitation of myocardial blood flow with (201)Tl and dynamic SPECT in canine: optimisation and validation of kinetic modelling, *Eur J Nucl Med Mol Imaging* 35 (5):896–905, 2008, Epub 2008 Jan 15.

20. Sharir T, Ben-Haim S, Merzon K, Prochorov V, Dickman D, Ben-Haim S, Berman DS: High-speed myocardial perfusion imaging: Initial clinical comparison with conventional dual detector Anger camera imaging, *JACC Cardiovasc Imaging* 1:156–163, 2008.

21. Sampson UK, Dorbala S, Limaye A, Kwong R, Di Carli MF: Diagnostic accuracy of rubidium-82 myocardial perfusion imaging with hybrid positron emission tomography/computed tomography in the detection of coronary artery disease, *J Am Coll Cardiol* 49(10):1052–1058, 2007, Epub 2007 Feb 26.

22. Bateman TM, Heller GV, McGhie AI, Friedman JD, Case JA, Bryngelson JR, Hertenstein GK, Moutray KL, Reid K, Cullom SJ: Diagnostic accuracy of rest/stress ECG-gated Rb-82 myocardial perfusion PET: comparison with ECG-gated Tc-99m sestamibi SPECT, *J Nucl Cardiol* 13(1):24–33, 2006.

23. Parkash R, deKemp RA, Ruddy TD, Kitsikis A, Hart R, Beauchesne L, Williams K, Davies RA, Labinaz M, Beanlands RS: Potential utility of rubidium 82 PET quantification in patients with 3-vessel coronary artery disease, *J Nucl Cardiol* 11(4):440–449, 2004.

24. Anagnostopoulos C, Almonacid A, El Fakhri G, Curillova Z, Sitek A, Roughton M, Dorbala S, Popma JJ, Di Carli MF: Quantitative relationship between coronary vasodilator reserve assessed by 82Rb PET imaging and coronary artery stenosis severity, *Eur J Nucl Med Mol Imaging* 35(9):1593–1601, 2008, Epub 2008 Apr 19.

25. Manabe O, Yoshinaga K, Katoh C, Naya M, deKemp RA, Tamaki N: Repeatability of rest and hyperemic myocardial blood flow measurements with 82Rb dynamic PET, *J Nucl Med* 50(1):68–71, 2009, Epub 2008 Dec 17.

26. Campisi R, Di Carli MF: Assessment of coronary flow reserve and microcirculation: a clinical perspective, *J Nucl Cardiol* 11(1):3–11, 2004, No abstract available.

27. Rimoldi OE, Camici PG: Positron emission tomography for quantitation of myocardial perfusion, *J Nucl Cardiol* 11(4):482–490, 2004, Review. No abstract available.

28. Neglia D, L'abbate A: Myocardial perfusion reserve in ischemic heart disease, *J Nucl Med* 50(2):175–177, 2009, Epub 2009 Jan 21. No abstract available.

29. Chareonthaitawee P, Kaufmann PA, Rimoldi O, Camici PG: Heterogeneity of resting and hyperemic myocardial blood flow in healthy humans, *Cardiovasc Res* 50(1):151–161, 2001.

30. Schindler TH, Nitzsche EU, Schelbert HR, Olschewski M, Sayre J, Mix M, Brink I, Zhang XL, Kreissl M, Magosaki N, Just H, Solzbach U: Positron emission tomography-measured abnormal responses of myocardial blood flow to sympathetic stimulation are associated with the risk of developing cardiovascular events, *J Am Coll Cardiol* 45(9): 1505–1512, 2005.

31. Yalamanchili P, Wexler E, Hayes M, Yu M, Bozek J, Kagan M, Radeke HS, Azure M, Purohit A, Casebier DS, Robinson SP: Mechanism of uptake and retention of F-18 BMS-747158-02 in cardiomyocytes: a novel PET myocardial imaging agent, *J Nucl Cardiol* 14(6):782–788, 2007, Epub 2007 Oct 22.

32. Yu M, Guaraldi MT, Mistry M, Kagan M, McDonald JL, Drew K, Radeke H, Azure M, Purohit A, Casebier DS, Robinson SP: BMS-747158-02: a novel PET myocardial perfusion imaging agent, *J Nucl Cardiol* 14(6):789–798, 2007, Epub 2007 Oct 22.

33. Nekolla SG, Reder S, Saraste A, et al: Evaluation of the novel myocardial perfusion PET tracer 18F-BMS-747158-02: comparison to 13N ammonia and validation with microspheres in a pig model, *Circulation* 2009, in press.

34. Patel AR, Epstein FH, Kramer CM: Evaluation of the microcirculation: advances in cardiac magnetic resonance perfusion imaging, *J Nucl Cardiol* 15(5):698–708, 2008, No abstract available.

35. Nandalur KR, Dwamena BA, Choudhri AF, Nandalur MR, Carlos RC: Diagnostic performance of stress cardiac magnetic resonance imaging in the detection of coronary artery disease: a meta-analysis, *J Am Coll Cardiol* 50(14):1343–1353, 2007, Epub 2007 Sep 17. Review.

36. Schwitter J, Wacker CM, van Rossum AC, Lombardi M, Al-Saadi N, Ahlstrom H, Dill T, Larsson HB, Flamm SD, Marquardt M, Johansson L: MR-IMPACT: comparison of perfusion-cardiac magnetic resonance with single-photon emission computed tomography for the detection of coronary artery disease in a multicentre, multivendor, randomized trial, *Eur Heart J* 29(4):480–489, 2008, Epub 2008 Jan 21.

37. Bodi V, Sanchis J, Lopez-Lereu MP, Nunez J, Mainar L, Monmeneu JV, Husser O, Dominguez E, Chorro FJ, Llacer A: Prognostic value of dipyridamole stress cardiovascular magnetic resonance imaging in patients with known or suspected coronary artery disease, *J Am Coll Cardiol* 50(12):1174–1179, 2007, Epub 2007 Sep 4.

38. Costa MA, Shoemaker S, Futamatsu H, Klassen C, Angiolillo DJ, Nguyen M, Siuciak A, Gilmore P, Zenni MM, Guzman L, Bass TA, Wilke N: Quantitative magnetic resonance perfusion imaging detects anatomic and physiologic coronary artery disease as measured by coronary angiography and fractional flow reserve, *J Am Coll Cardiol* 50(6):514–522, 2007, Epub 2007 Jul 23.

39. Lima JA, Judd RM, Bazille A, Schulman SP, Atalar E, Zerhouni EA: Regional heterogeneity of human myocardial infarcts demonstrated by contrast-enhanced MRI. Potential mechanisms, *Circulation* 92 (5):1117–1125, 1995.

40. Rochitte CE, Lima JA, Bluemke DA, Reeder SB, McVeigh ER, Furuta T, Becker LC, Melin JA: Magnitude and time course of microvascular obstruction and tissue injury after acute myocardial infarction, *Circulation* 98(10):1006–1014, 1998.

41. Petersen SE, Jerosch-Herold M, Hudsmith LE, Robson MD, Francis JM, Doll HA, Selvanayagam JB, Neubauer S, Watkins H: Evidence for microvascular dysfunction in hypertrophic cardiomyopathy: new insights from multiparametric magnetic resonance imaging, *Circulation* 115(18):2418–2425, 2007, Epub 2007 Apr 23.

42. Lanza GA, Buffon A, Sestito A, Natale L, Sgueglia GA, Galiuto L, Infusino F, Mariani L, Centola A, Crea F: Relation between stress-induced myocardial perfusion defects on cardiovascular magnetic resonance and coronary microvascular dysfunction in patients with cardiac syndrome X, *J Am Coll Cardiol* 51(4):466–472, 2008.

43. Cheng AS, Pegg TJ, Karamitsos TD, Searle N, Jerosch-Herold M, Choudhury RP, Banning AP, Neubauer S, Robson MD, Selvanayagam JB: Cardiovascular magnetic resonance perfusion imaging at 3-tesla for the detection of coronary artery disease: a comparison with 1.5-tesla, *J Am Coll Cardiol* 49(25):2440–2449, 2007, Epub 2007 Jun 11.

44. George RT, Jerosch-Herold M, Silva C, Kitagawa K, Bluemke DA, Lima JA, Lardo AC: Quantification of myocardial perfusion using

dynamic 64-detector computed tomography, *Invest Radiol* 42(12): 815–822, 2007.

45. George RT, Silva C, Cordeiro MA, DiPaula A, Thompson DR, McCarthy WF, Ichihara T, Lima JA, Lardo AC: Multidetector computed tomography myocardial perfusion imaging during adenosine stress, *J Am Coll Cardiol* 48(1):153–160, 2006, Epub 2006 Jun 21.

46. Nagao M, Matsuoka H, Kawakami H, Higashino H, Mochizuki T, Murase K, Uemura M: Quantification of myocardial perfusion by contrast-enhanced 64-MDCT: characterization of ischemic myocardium, *AJR Am J Roentgenol* 191(1):19–25, 2008.

47. Kido T, Kurata A, Higashino H, Inoue Y, Kanza RE, Okayama H, Higaki J, Murase K, Mochizuki T: Quantification of regional myocardial blood flow using first-pass multidetector-row computed tomography and adenosine triphosphate in coronary artery disease, *Circ J* 72 (7):1086–1091, 2008.

48. Salerno M, Beller GA: Non-invasive assessment of myocardial perfusion, *Circ Cardiovasc Imaging* 2009, in press.

49. Cury RC, Nieman K, Shapiro MD, Nasir K, Cury RC, Brady TJ: Comprehensive cardiac CT study: evaluation of coronary arteries, left ventricular function, and myocardial perfusion—is it possible? *J Nucl Cardiol* 14(2):229–243, 2007, Review.

50. Henneman MM, Schuijf JD, Dibbets-Schneider P, Stokkel MP, van der Geest RJ, van der Wall EE, Bax JJ: Comparison of multislice computed tomography to gated single-photon emission computed tomography for imaging of healed myocardial infarcts, *Am J Cardiol* 101 (2):144–148, 2008.

51. Kaul S: Myocardial contrast echocardiography: a 25-year retrospective, *Circulation* 118(3):291–308, 2008, No abstract available.

52. Lindner JR, Wei K: Contrast echocardiography, *Curr Probl Cardiol* 27 (11):454–519, 2002, Review. No abstract available.

53. Lepper W, Belcik T, Wei K, Lindner JR, Sklenar J, Kaul S: Myocardial contrast echocardiography, *Circulation* 109(25):3132–3135, 2004, Review. No abstract available.

54. Jeetley P, Hickman M, Kamp O, Lang RM, Thomas JD, Vannan MA, Vanoverschelde JL, van der Wouw PA, Senior R: Myocardial contrast echocardiography for the detection of coronary artery stenosis: a prospective multicenter study in comparison with single-photon emission computed tomography, *J Am Coll Cardiol* 47(1):141–145, 2006, Epub 2005 Dec 15.

55. Wei K: Contrast echocardiography: Fulfilling its promise, *ACC Curr J Rev* 27–32, 2005.

56. Wei K, Jayaweera AR, Firoozan S, Linka A, Skyba DM, Kaul S: Quantification of myocardial blood flow with ultrasound-induced destruction of microbubbles administered as a constant venous infusion, *Circulation* 97(5):473–483, 1998.

57. Bhatia VK, Senior R: Contrast echocardiography: evidence for clinical use, *J Am Soc Echocardiogr* 21(5):409–416, 2008.

Chapter 24

Cost-Effectiveness of Myocardial Perfusion Single-Photon Emission Computed Tomography

LESLEE J. SHAW

INTRODUCTION

Since peaking in the mid-1960s, reductions in mortality from coronary artery diseases have approached 50%.[1] Although a number of reasons have been put forth for this marked decline in death rates, a proportion of this reduction can be attributed to early and effective diagnostic testing techniques that result in improved outcomes for at-risk patients. Along with marked improvements in outcome, procedural utilization rates have skyrocketed. The current focus on the part of public and private health care payers is to contain "out of control" health care costs. Health care payers have reacted by focusing on programs to decrease reimbursement levels and to manage utilization of major growth procedures such as myocardial perfusion single-photon emission computed tomography (SPECT).[2] In fact, myocardial perfusion SPECT has been one of the largest growing procedures and is estimated to encumber approximately 2% of annual Medicare expenditures. To this end throughout the last few decades, there have been shifting foci between marked improvements in disease detection with medical advances in new technology and the reverberating excess expenditures associated with such developments. As a result, there has been a focus on developing rational approaches to containing health care costs and curbing unrestrained spending. The development of evidence-based medicine is an attempt to set guidelines for thresholds of evidence to justify the cost of a procedure. The bar has been set very high for diagnostic procedures where a test must now result in a net health improvement in clinical outcome (i.e., be effective). This is at the heart of cost-effectiveness analysis: striking a balance between spending and value.

For a diagnostic test in cardiology to be accepted and receive widespread utilization, using evidence-based standards, it must have a clear and demonstrated economic and clinical incremental value when compared with other modalities. Nuclear cardiology has a clear advantage with regard to setting higher standards of evidence, owing to the large (unparalleled) body of evidence from multicenter, observational series and randomized or controlled clinical trials from statistically powered, diverse patient populations. The current chapter will provide a synopsis of available evidence of gated myocardial perfusion SPECT, as well as review the guiding principles applied in the development of cost-effectiveness evidence.

HEALTH CARE COSTS FOR CARDIOVASCULAR DISEASE

In the United States, total health care costs for cardiovascular disease approached $450 billion in 2007.[3] In fact, lifetime costs for one symptomatic patient are reported at $1 million dollars.[4] Given that nearly 19 million patients have chronic stable angina, these costs of care are astronomical. It is then no wonder that the Medicare Panel Expenditure Survey ranked ischemic heart disease as the most expensive condition.[5] Recent estimates from the American College of Cardiology have noted that approximately 38% of all payments to cardiologists were for echocardiography and nuclear imaging.[6] Estimates from the 34th Bethesda Conference on atherosclerotic imaging noted an estimated 40 million noninvasive cardiac tests were performed during each of the past few years,[7] with total costs of over $1 billion in the year 2000.[3] For example, every year, a total of 6 million exercise electrocardiograms are billed. In the area of imaging, approximately 8.5 million nuclear scans are performed.[6] A report from the American College of Radiology reported annual growth rates for myocardial perfusion imaging exceeding 30% for cardiologists.[8] The largest growth sectors have been in the outpatient setting where reimbursement strategies have been more favorable. Given our aging population, as well as the dramatic increases in diabetes and obesity, it is estimated that there will be a continuing need for diagnostic imaging services to identify patients at risk for coronary artery disease (CAD). However, the challenge is to adequately service this growing population of at-risk patients with limited financial means within our current environment.

With the recent history of marked growth in nuclear cardiology, payers consider this test a "big target" for focusing cost-reduction efforts—in many cases, encouraging shifting to lower-cost procedures such as stress echocardiography. Thus the current review hopes to frame the utilization as supported by effective evidence to guide medical decision making, as well as to consider the advantages of a more noninvasive center approach to contain large health care costs associated with invasive coronary angiography. Similar to nuclear imaging, growth rates for cardiac catheterization have increased 300%+ with, on average, a third of catheterizations being considered inappropriate or not supported by accepted clinical indications.[9] From a clinical point of view, it is easy to envision that an overuse of coronary angiography can lead to higher rates and in some cases the unnecessary use of coronary revascularization procedures, defined as utilization that is not supported by evidence noting substantive improvements in outcome. Although SPECT imaging growth rates have been high, the cost savings resulting from decreased angiographic utilization, as will be illustrated later in this chapter, have been reportedly quite substantial. This is particularly true of patients with stable chest pain symptoms who are referred to diagnostic left heart catheterization.

Prior to discussing the available economic evidence, it will be helpful to define the calculation of cost-effectiveness and related standards for health policy decision making. An incremental cost-effectiveness ratio (ICER) requires not only necessary information on cost but also integrated evidence on diagnostic test accuracy and the ensuing therapeutic benefit of treatment.[10] Cost-effectiveness analyses are increasingly favored within health care systems where health care resources are increasingly finite; ICER is a tool to assist decision makers to assess and devise cost containment and value within their health care system. *ICER* is defined as an incremental or marginal cost-effectiveness ratio because it compares more than one test, therapy, or patient management approach. In general for cardiac imaging modalities, there are a number of published cost analyses.[7,11-26]

ICERs are increasingly being applied by larger health care systems and payers to develop systematic approaches to compare cardiac imaging modalities. Included in these approaches is the development of both clinical

and cost-effectiveness data. The development of both clinical outcome and economic data is consistent with our new standards of evidence-based medicine, where high-quality evidence is used to guide and support procedural utilization. For nuclear cardiology, a cost-effectiveness analysis can indicate how it compares to other tests or in what patient indications the results look favorable. Objectives of a cost-effectiveness analyses include the following:

1. To develop tools required to assess CAD diagnostic strategy costs and effectiveness for at-risk patients
2. To devise fair and equitable policy decisions based on the ICER results; with regard to this, should the ICER be low enough, a nuclear-drive strategy would be considered to achieve optimal economic value

A challenge with this reasoning is that for many comparisons, nuclear cardiology is a more expensive test. However, more expensive procedures can be cost-effective if they reduce induced costs or are substantially more effective. There are several scenarios in which nuclear cardiology may result in a favorable ICER. For the first case, if nuclear cardiology is less expensive and equally effective, then the result could be a favorable ICER. A favorable ICER could also result for nuclear cardiology testing even if it is initially more expensive but results in a reduction in downstream procedures with equally effective outcomes results. And finally, nuclear cardiology testing could be substantively more costly but also have a favorable ICER should it result in decidedly better outcome results. All of the above are simplified examples of how nuclear cardiology could be cost-effective; greater details of the methods for these types of analyses will be provided in the following discussions (Fig. 24-1).

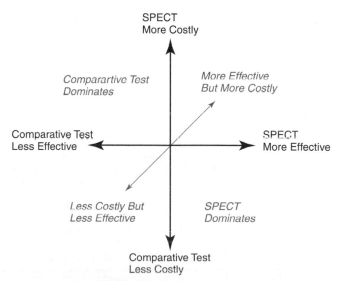

Figure 24-1 Simplistic view of cost-effectiveness plane comparing myocardial perfusion SPECT with other test modalities.

EVALUATING PROCEDURAL COST

It is important when discussing costs to differentiate between the actual test charge (which is regionally and locally based—mostly on payer contracts, insurance coverage, and other factors) and unit operating or production cost, with the difference being the test's contribution or profit margin. For much of this discussion, we will focus on the operating cost of a test with comparisons to similar evaluations for other imaging modalities. Because charges can vary widely, comparisons using it as a standard for economic evaluations can be misleading.

Although much has been made of the variability in imaging costs, it is helpful to examine data on the unit operating cost of a variety of cardiac diagnostic procedures.[7] There are two methods that can be applied to estimating cost: top-down and bottom-up. A top-down cost approach uses adjusted (technical and professional) charges and is calculated as the charge × the hospital-specific cost-charge ratio (set by the Center for Medicare and Medicaid Services). Recently, bottom-up costs have been employed and involve calculating both the fixed and variable labor costs (e.g., supplies, equipment, and labor costs). Using this type of calculation, procedural cost is predominately driven by laboratory volume, where high-volume laboratories have lower cost per test, achieving economies of scale with increasing volume. For SPECT imaging, cost is also influenced by noncardiac procedural volume. The use of quantitative scoring systems, such as calculating left ventricular ejection fraction, have lower labor inputs and are generally lower cost than systems utilizing greater labor components, especially those including physician labor. In large part, the use of quantitative scoring systems generally not only lowers initial costs but (because of improved reproducibility) also aids physician diagnostic confidence and the impact on induced posttest costs.[27]

For SPECT imaging, the cost of radioisotopes and pharmacologic stress agents is also included in the unit cost of a test. Recently, the commonly used technetium-99m sestamibi became generic, allowing for lower radioisotope costs to be realized. Factors that also influence test cost include labor and equipment necessary for laboratory standards or certification. A major component of the unit operating cost is equipment, where costs can vary widely from less than $1 million to up to $3 million for magnetic resonance, positron emission tomography, or multislice computed tomography scanners. Despite these high cost estimates, discounted prices and leasing agreements are common and reduce equipment prices substantially for most imaging modalities. The equipment space (e.g., cost at total square footage) and any necessary requirements (e.g., added concrete thickness for magnetic resonance imaging) for the equipment should be included in the equipment or fixed cost estimate. In the final step in calculating costs, estimates are then discounted and inflation-corrected to a given time period in order to establish a common metric for individual procedural estimates and for comparisons to other modalities.[28,29]

A review of current estimates for diagnostic procedures has been reported in several publications and is depicted in Figure 24-2.[7] Cost estimates should be viewed for all the modalities as "guesstimates," because there have been few attempts to calculate the true unit operating cost of each procedure. New imaging modalities in general have higher initial costs, but with greater experience and efficiency and equipment price reductions, cost estimates will decrease. Inexpensive tests include those that are "low tech" such as exercise electrocardiography. When integrating the available data, nuclear cardiology procedures appear to be in the midrange of diagnostic procedure cost estimates.

Adding Downstream Costs

Although rarely considered, the total cost of a procedure not only should include the upfront costs but should be

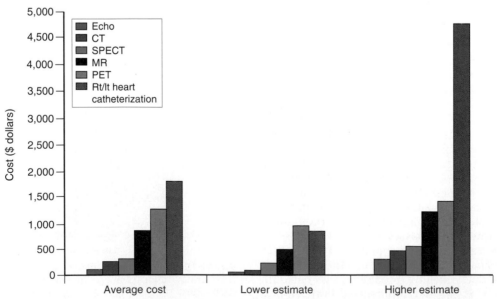

Figure 24-2 Average cost of common cardiac imaging procedures. Lt, left; Rt, right.

totaled throughout the episode of care (importantly, including induced costs). Drummond and Jefferson[30] have advised that any economic evaluation should consider the impact of test use on downstream resource consumption, including both additional procedure use and treatment costs. From a societal point of view, cost estimates should also consider those consumed by the patient, or indirect costs. By definition, *indirect costs* include travel time, out-of-pocket expenses, and days lost from work for both the patient and other caregivers. Downstream costs should also consider the induced costs of incidental findings, and this latter point will be a more critical cost component in vascular imaging. More recently, reports have been published on the radiation exposure associated with a number of cardiac imaging procedures. The associated cancer risk is also one component of cost that is rarely included but should be considered as a component of induced cost.[31]

Although precise delineation of induced costs may be difficult to enumerate, there is an expected proportional relationship between test results and expected costs of care.[32] That is, greater costs are expected for higher-risk test results (e.g., significant left ventricular dysfunction and multivessel or severely abnormal perfusion abnormalities), particularly in higher-likelihood patients. As expected, this latter population will require higher rates of coronary angiography, as well as revascularization procedures and (because of elevated, cumulative event rates) greater hospital admissions for acute coronary syndromes and lost life years as a result of premature death. Estimates of induced costs have revealed that the costs of downstream hospital and procedural care can be approximately 10- to 100-fold higher than the initial test cost itself.[32]

An easy method for estimating downstream care costs is to calculate a test's negative and positive disease rates, and this may be used to define cost waste induced by the procedure. True negative (lowest cost cohort) and positive tests result in effective resource consumption or costs as a result of their accurate identification or exclusion of disease. Of course, the economics of test misclassification can be affected by changes to the positivity threshold, the prevalence of disease in the population, and the length of follow-up for evaluating, in particular, false-negative results.[33] By definition, a false-positive test result is documented when a patient with abnormal SPECT results undergoes coronary angiography revealing normal or insignificant disease (Table 24-1). Of course, the defining of an intermediate stenosis that elicited a flow limitation may be wrongly termed a *false positive*. Yet it may be viewed as a false positive insofar as the abnormal nuclear finding failed to define revascularizable disease and, as such, from that perspective may be termed a *false positive*. This latter point suggests that the defining of a false positive should be used cautiously as a measure of cost inefficiency. Despite this, when downstream testing results in a lack of confirmatory findings, then the initial results misclassified the expected disease state in that patient. Repeated, redundant, and unnecessary testing contributes to high costs of care. Although false-positive results can be difficult to assess, many studies do not

Table 24-1 Cost Advantages Using Myocardial Perfusion Single-Photon Emission Computed Tomography

High sensitivity excludes disease more accurately and avoids the need for a secondary test if a less accurate primary test is used.

High sensitivity leads to fewer false-negative test results and avoids the cost of future events in patients with undiagnosed disease.

High specificity reduces the number of false-positive test results and consequent downstream testing.

Additional prognostic information avoids the need for further prognostic testing and focuses high-cost interventional care on patients with advanced disease with the most to gain in terms of improvement in clinical outcome.

allow a sufficient time period for follow-up to discern the rate of false-negative test results. A false-negative test result would be expected to occur when a patient with initially normal findings has an adverse event, or disease is confirmed at a later date. There are additional challenges with negative findings: They may change a patient's health-seeking behaviors, resulting in delays to treatment as well as litigation costs that are rarely considered in an economic analysis.[34] It is impossible to expect that any test would perfectly classify patients 100% of the time, and there are no standards for acceptability of false-negative and false-positive findings; however, a low rate of false-negative results is preferable (i.e., perhaps < 10%), because false-negative results are more costly and harmful to the patient.

DEFINING INCREMENTAL EFFECTIVENESS

In addition to delineating the costs of a diagnostic procedure, there are a variety of methods to define its effectiveness. There have been recent active discussions within health policy arenas as to what is the correct method to define the effectiveness of a diagnostic procedure. Historically, the diagnostic accuracy of a test has been the mainstay for gaining U.S. Food and Drug Administration (FDA) approval. More recently there has been an abundance of evidence on the prognostic accuracy of testing, including a large body of evidence on risk stratification with nuclear cardiology that is discussed in Chapters 15 and 16. A new standard of net improvement in health outcome has been introduced as a standard upon which to guide reimbursement. Where evidence for a given modality meets the criteria of net improvement in health outcome, then reimbursement should be favored for that given test or patient indication. In terms of defining what a net improvement in outcome means, patients must be "better off" after undergoing the diagnostic test when compared to no testing or an alternative modality. This type of examination of the effectiveness of a diagnostic test has to do with how the procedure is used to guide subsequent decisions on starting, stopping, or modifying therapies.[35]

Other positive improvements in health outcomes following a diagnostic test include:

1. Improvements in health status (e.g., symptoms, quality of life)
2. As a *gatekeeper* to invasive angiography or for medical therapy decisions
3. Improved fatal/morbid complications (e.g., life years saved) when compared to established modalities

We will discuss in detail how cost-effectiveness analyses are calculated, but it is important to note that several types of outcome measures may be applied. That is, one may see disease-specific cost-effectiveness analyses that incorporate diagnostic or prognostic outcomes. Or one may see the newer type of analyses that use costs related to changes in symptom burden or costs related to life years saved—all of which remain valid approaches to discerning different types of outcomes. However, it is likely that we will see the payer community rely more heavily on the more stringent approach of net improvement in outcome.

DEFINING INCREMENTAL COST-EFFECTIVENESS RATIO

For many clinicians, cost-effectiveness analysis can seem a bit obtuse; however, it is simply a ratio that reflects the amount of resources needed to change a patient's outcome. In other words, it is used to reflect the intensity of management in relation to any given outcome achieved. The aim of a cost-effectiveness analysis is to reflect or mirror clinical decision making where physicians make choices based on the information content and, generally, the invasive nature of the procedure (i.e., a surrogate for cost). A cost-effectiveness ratio (ICER) is most commonly expressed in cost per life year saved or, if adjusted by patient functional gain, in a modification as cost per quality-adjusted life year saved. For ICERs, cost per life year saved is rapidly becoming a common metric for comparisons to other medical interventions. A compendium of ICER data can be compiled in the form of a league table for comparisons to other medical and nonmedical procedures, therapies, and so forth.[32–57] Such comparisons may be more relevant to the health care policy analyst, but for the clinician, the link to an ICER for any given diagnostic test is best understood by a combination of factors that integrate accuracy, and resulting treatment efficacy and management intensity and timing. That is, a diagnostic test that is effective at identifying patients whose ensuing risk may be altered by aggressive therapeutic intervention will result in an aversion to more costly, end-stage care, thus resulting in cost-effective care for similar patients.

The theoretical approaches to adding value and improved cost-effectiveness with noninvasive testing are noted in Table 24-2. Tests that are ineffective result in redundant testing with rising cost-ineffective care. Simply stated, diagnostic tests that have high rates of false-negative and false-positive test results have

Table 24-2 Theoretical Approaches to Adding Value and Improved Cost-Effectiveness With Noninvasive Testing

Adding Value but Minimizing Cost Through Improved Test Accuracy Combination of Physiologic/Anatomic Assessment Adds to Cost Efficiency
For example, gated SPECT imaging, including evaluation of myocardial perfusion and global ventricular function
Containing Diagnostic Test Costs
For example, initial exercise electrocardiography followed by a cardiac imaging test (e.g., SPECT) in patients who have indeterminate or mildly positive ST-segment changes; lower overall evaluation costs, especially for patients with a normal resting 12-lead electrocardiogram
Tiered approach to testing, with a selective use of higher cost test for example, SPECT to those higher-risk patients
Lower Costs Tests Applied to Non-High-Risk
Selective coronary angiography in patients with SPECT ischemia
Using SPECT as a gatekeeper to conventional angiography, especially for patients with stable chest pain symptoms. The results of this strategy could be:
A reduction in procedural complications, hospital costs, and overall "workup" cost for a diagnostic catheterization; in-laboratory complications are $\sim$1%.

excessive cost waste and result in ICERs that are not economically attractive for the health and well-being of our society. High rates of false-positive tests lead to greater use of unnecessary coronary angiography, and high false-negative rates lead to higher rates of acute coronary syndromes in patients with initially negative results. This inefficiency leads to patient care that does not improve outcome and is cost inefficient.

An ICER is by definition a comparison, often called an *incremental or marginal cost-effectiveness ratio* because it compares more than one diagnostic test. Although an ICER is commonly defined as cost per life year saved, this ratio can be used to compare any difference in cost divided by a given delta outcome. Thus, the generic ICER equation is:

$$(\text{Test 1 Costs} - \text{Test 2 Costs})/(\text{Test 1 Outcomes} - \text{Test 2 Outcomes})$$

An incremental or marginal cost-effectiveness ratio includes a comparison of the differences in cost and effectiveness of more than one imaging modality. As previously stated, an ICER includes the calculation of upfront and downstream cost differences as well as near-term and/or long-term (i.e., life expectancy) outcome differences. Based on early work done on the evaluation of renal dialysis programs, the threshold for economic efficiency is set at less than $50,000 per life year saved (LYS), with many countries setting thresholds as low as less than $20,000 per LYS.[7,32–57] It does appear that the standards for an ICER are more appropriately designed for the evaluation of therapeutic regimens and, in some cases, screening programs.[7]

For SPECT imaging, a measure of an ICER is whether or not the test adds value in the form of either lowered cost or improved effectiveness in the management of patients. This economic benefit is more often achieved when one envisions patient care that does not include testing. That is, if a patient is not sent for a diagnostic procedure, then left untreated, the patient would present with more advanced if not unstable disease, resulting in substantially higher costs of care. Thus, a comparison to strategies of early detection and intervention results in an ICER that is economically attractive. The leverage point for this comparison is that SPECT imaging would offset the morbidity and perhaps premature mortality associated with a downstream presentation with more advanced coronary disease. The ultimate standard for the value of a test is that the downstream therapies (initiated based on SPECT abnormalities) result in an improvement in life expectancy as well as a higher quality of life and, for society, improved productivity. Although one can envision a favorable ICER when SPECT is compared to no testing, the real challenge arises when one compares SPECT to comparative modalities such as stress echocardiography. That is, most modalities will be favorable when compared to "doing nothing," but the real difficulties in driving health policy lie within the iterative comparison of SPECT as compared with other commonly applied diagnostic procedures; a review of available comparative evidence will be discussed later.

For clinicians, previous discussions on risk stratification have particular relevance and are the critical points for affecting cost-effective care for patients. That is, when a test risk stratifies, it also is a measure of the intensity of resources required to manage a given risk cohort and provides insight into the expected costs of care. There is a directly proportional relationship between risk and cost. Each event that is estimated in the many published reports should be equated to a given "high ticket" item in health care resource consumption (a myocardial infarction costs on average $14,000; chest pain hospitalization $\cong$ $6000, to name a few). In Chapters 15 and 16, there are reviews of the large body of evidence on risk stratification with SPECT imaging results. This compendium of data reveals that gated myocardial perfusion imaging is highly accurate for estimating major adverse cardiac events, including cardiac death and nonfatal myocardial infarction. This accuracy results in cost-effective care by streamlining the need for additional testing, resulting in more efficient care. In a recent review of the literature by Underwood and colleagues,[16] the rate of false-negative test results is minimal at around 12%, while the rate of false-positive results is around 26%. Opponents to SPECT imaging have been critical of this higher rate of false-positive results (i.e., diminished specificity). One should remember that flow limitations would be observed at subcritical lesions, and thus the calculation of diagnostic specificity using an obstructive lesion threshold of 70% or greater would be less valuable than understanding the ensuing prognosis associated with any given test abnormality. Accordingly, in many cases, diagnostic accuracy is not helpful in understanding the clinical or cost-effectiveness of a procedure. Risk stratification, however, has tremendous value in the course of everyday laboratory practice, in which the vast majority of patients undergoing SPECT imaging will have normal perfusion and function results, thus receiving posttest "low-cost" care. That is, the necessity for additional testing, in the setting of normal gated SPECT imaging, is minimal, and this information should be important to large health care payers and systems alike.

Mansley and McKenna[51] illustrate how one may design an ICER using five clear-cut steps:

1. Define the clinical or societal problem (i.e., analytical objectives), and include whether a societal or payer perspective is to be the focus of the analysis.
2. Define what is to be compared (e.g., stress echocardiography versus SPECT).
3. Define the outcome of interest (either near-term or long-term) in addition to data on the costs of care. (Although there has been a focus in the literature on comparing changes in life expectancy, there are minimal cardiac imaging data that estimate prognosis beyond 5 years. Therefore, these types of long-term models can be less reliable than those estimating ICER over a 2- to 5-year episode of care.)
4. Ensure that the amount of resources consumed mimics the time period for the outcome portion of this ratio, and be as "all inclusive" as possible (i.e., direct and indirect costs).
5. Attempt to consider and/or control for as many uncertainties and biases in any ICER, including the use of risk-adjustment techniques and sensitivity analyses.[51]

USE OF INTERMEDIATE OUTCOME MEASURES

A critical challenge of determining cost-effective testing is that the traditional definition includes examination of the incremental differences in cost per life year saved. As many clinicians involved in diagnostic testing understand, the use of any imaging modality does not directly impact patient survival but is used to identify risk. The ensuing risk is affected by the initiation of life-saving therapeutic intervention. An additional challenge with the use of cost-effective decision models is the lack of long-term data that may be used to estimate changes in life expectancy. Many individuals have advocated the use of intermediate outcome measures for diagnostic testing in order to emulate how clinicians utilize test content. This would include the derivation of economic models that determine the cost to identify or avert a major adverse cardiac event at 2 to 5 years after testing. As Hunink and Krestin recently described, outcome measures should reflect the physician's decision-making process.[52] In a review of the methods applied to establish cost-effectiveness of a diagnostic test, the link between diagnosis and end-stage care is often disparate or unrelated; most patients undergoing testing have nearly 2 decades of life years remaining.[53] From a practical standpoint, not all test abnormalities are acted on by the overseeing physicians. For example, one-third to two-thirds of patients with SPECT perfusion abnormalities are referred to coronary angiography, so the cost-effective models would be highly responsive and influenced by the intensity of posttest management, including both aggressive antiischemic and risk-factor modification therapies.

One of the major drawbacks for using an intermediate outcome measure is the lack of standardization or accepted metric (such as with cost per life year saved) upon which to derive comparisons across other health care choices. Nevertheless, there are several approaches that can be employed to discern whether ICER results are economically attractive societal health care choices. That is, the cost to avert a death or myocardial infarction should be less than the actual cost of these events, or in the range of $20,000 to $50,000 per patient. Another approach would be to examine the population benefit of this type of ICER calculation for a given cohort of 1000 patients. The resulting ranges would appear to be in the range of $250,000 to $500,000 (or under) to detect cardiac death or myocardial infarction.[32]

High-Risk Cost-Effectiveness Models

The concept of a high-risk cost-effectiveness model was introduced a number of years ago, and its utility appears to be highly relevant to the body of prognostic evidence with SPECT imaging.[53,54] A high-risk cost-effectiveness model is defined using the concept of proportional risk reduction as it is directly related to the underlying hazard in the population. That is, higher-risk patients receive a greater proportional therapeutic benefit from intervention. Using this reasoning, the more clinically beneficial the treatment, the more cost-effective care patterns will ensue. Or, in terms of imaging modalities, clinical effectiveness and cost-effectiveness generally parallel one another. For the clinician who struggles to find relevance in an ICER, this type of reasoning can be very helpful. Especially for nuclear cardiology procedures, the wealth and depth of evidence on risk assessment can become a template for understanding ICERs for SPECT. When SPECT is highly effective in any given patient cohort (intermediate-risk patients, stable chest pain patients, to name a few), one would also *expect* it to be cost-effective, since these two measures generally parallel one another. Clinicians should remember that clinical events are "big ticket" items that have direct cost implications, and it may be helpful to learn general ballpark estimates of major adverse events such as myocardial infarction (average cost = $14,000) or cardiac death (average societal cost = $10,000 per lost year of life).

ICERs have been evaluated using other imaging modalities, and the results reveal that economically attractive ratios can be achieved when identifying an optimal patient cohort, particularly where disease is prevalent[48] or for relevant age subsets.[55,56] For SPECT imaging, these results would yield attractive ICERs in intermediate high-risk patients (as compared to low-risk individuals) or in elderly (as compared with middle-aged) patients. This latter exercise also illustrates further

how we can extrapolate ICERs from our existing data on risk stratification. That is, for every prognostic series illustrating effective risk stratification, we can envision that this subset also derives a cost-effective benefit from testing. In a recent review of the prognostic value of SPECT imaging,[58] we noted that the differences in risk between low- and high-risk test results ranged from approximately 0.5% to 1.6% to 3% to 12% for suspected coronary disease to multivessel coronary disease patient subsets. ICERs would be favorable in patients with high-risk, multivessel disease cohorts (i.e., < $20,000 per life year saved [LYS]). These results would also be applicable to high-risk-disease equivalent patients such as diabetics or those with known cardiovascular disease (see Chapter 22). By comparison, in suspected disease subsets, cost-effective subsets (i.e., cohorts with an ICER < $50,000/LYS) of this population may include only those patients older than age 65 years or those with typical angina, to name a few.

ECONOMIC IMPACT OF NUCLEAR CARDIOLOGY AS A GATEKEEPER TO THE DIAGNOSTIC CATHETERIZATION LABORATORY

This section of the chapter will deal specifically with the available evidence on ICERs, as well as the simplistic comparison of marginal cost savings with SPECT imaging. Generally, the available economic data with SPECT imaging as compared with other diagnostic testing techniques—including exercise electrocardiography, echocardiography, and coronary angiography—evaluate costs as a result of a given management strategy resulting from the initial procedure. An example of how such an evaluation would be constructed is illustrated in Figure 24-3 and compares an echocardiographic versus SPECT imaging management approach. When evaluating the economic literature, one can see that there has been a growing use of more sophisticated ICER models over time. Older reports examined simple differences in test cost, but newer strategies employ models examining near-term and long-term ICERs.

Cost Minimization or Savings

One form of an ICER is a cost-savings model. When examining the calculation of an ICER, if the denominator is equivalent, then the economic advantages are leveraged based solely on cost differences (i.e., savings). Of course, this point is critical to most cost-savings models that consider resource consumption alone and fail to account for differences in patient outcome. Thus, a true cost-savings analysis should compare equivalent test choices that achieve similar outcomes. An example of this type of analysis was published from the Economics of Noninvasive Diagnosis (END) study group, in which 3-year rates of cardiac death or nonfatal myocardial infarction were statistically similar (Fig. 24-4).[15] This type of economic analysis is perhaps the most intuitive,

Care Path Diagram

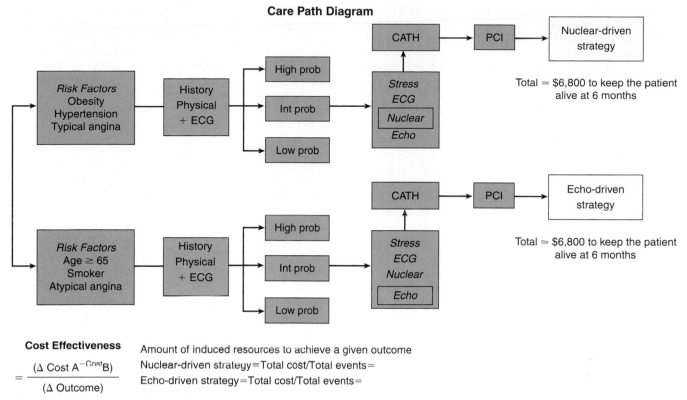

Cost Effectiveness

Amount of induced resources to achieve a given outcome

$$= \frac{(\Delta \text{ Cost A}^{-\text{Cost}}\text{B})}{(\Delta \text{ Outcome})}$$

Nuclear-driven strategy=Total cost/Total events=

Echo-driven strategy=Total cost/Total events=

Figure 24-3 Incremental cost-effectiveness ratio (ICER) of stress SPECT versus echocardiography in the evaluation of suspected ischemia in patients at intermediate pretest risk. CATH, catheterization; ECG, electrocardiogram; Echo, echocardiogram; Int, intermediate; PCI, percutaneous coronary intervention; Prob, probability.

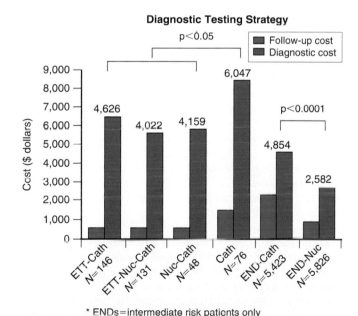

* ENDs=intermediate risk patients only

Figure 24-4 Two- to 3-year costs for varying diagnostic strategies: Economics of Myocardial Perfusion Imaging in Europe (EMPIRE) and Economics of Noninvasive Diagnosis (END) registries.

with the greatest potential for ease of understanding and assimilation of evidence into clinical practice. As a result, it is also one of the most commonly misapplied. That is, often the comparisons are based on cost only, without considering whether the two choices are equivalent or have similar diagnostic or prognostic accuracy. The term *cost savings* is also called *cost minimization* or *cost efficiency* because of the goal of achieving a streamlined pattern of care. An additional component to this type of analysis is that it also considers not only the upfront cost of a procedure but also the downstream use induced by the procedure itself.

Figure 24-2 explores the amount of resource consumption based on nuclear- and echocardiographic-driven diagnostic strategies. Using this example, patients with abnormal scans are referred for coronary angiography directly as a result of the SPECT results. Thus, including the cost of cardiac catheterization is a major component of calculating the costs of care. Although the added cost of coronary angiography was effective in identifying a patient with coronary disease in this illustration, *false-positive costs*, defined as an abnormal test but with normal coronaries, are considered cost waste in this diagnostic algorithm. Tests that are highly accurate also minimize cost waste, including a reduced false-positive rate. Therefore, the clinician evaluating not only cost evaluations but also diagnostic accuracy data may make inferences about cost waste by knowing the diagnostic specificity (= true negative/[true negative + false positive]) of a procedure. Since specificity gives us a false-positive rate, any laboratory can focus its daily laboratory practice of "cath correlations" on minimizing false positives, thus creating laboratory cost efficiency.

Furthermore, false-negative results are also a cost waste within this diagnostic construct. False-negative tests may be defined by calculating diagnostic sensitivity. However, a false negative is associated with a substantial economic burden to society, since it usually occurs when a patient presents downstream for additional testing or an acute coronary syndrome or death. In the latter case, average costs of this type of event are in the tens of thousands of dollars, with a great economic burden to society. To understand a false-negative rate, one must look beyond the near term and evaluate an adequate length of follow-up (e.g., 2 to 3 years). Although this is time-consuming for most laboratories, recent evidence from a community evaluation of prognosis with SPECT revealed that the overall false-negative rate is exceedingly low at less than 1%.[59] Using this type of analysis, most laboratories in the course of their quality evaluations may guesstimate their false-positive and false-negative or induced cost waste as well as their effective costs. The goal of this type of analysis would then be to optimize effective costs and minimize cost waste. This can be effective evidence to guide health care payer contracting.

One can then synthesize the published evidence about the cost savings of nuclear imaging based on several key publications from Cedars-Sinai Medical Center and from the Economics of Noninvasive Diagnosis multicenter study group.[15,60] One strategy that has been effective at realizing approximately 30% cost savings is that of limiting diagnostic catheterization to only those with inducible ischemia (i.e., conservative management or ischemia-guided care). This type of care is based on large bodies of evidence noting that the extent and severity of ischemia may be used to guide the proportional therapeutic benefit of risk reductions. For stable angina populations commonly referred to SPECT imaging, those indications for percutaneous coronary interventions noted in the recent stable angina guidelines include measures of the amount and severity of perfusion defects. Thus, by limiting referral to catheterization to only those with ischemia, a clinically effective paradigm is followed by a cost-efficient pattern of care. Cost savings are further realized for those patients with normal perfusion studies, inasmuch as intervention in this latter cohort is not associated with changes in outcome. Of course, this type of care is based on generalities that may not fit a given patient; other considerations such as exercise capacity and past medical history should also be considered in the management of stable chest-pain patients. However, this type of cost-efficient pathway can be used to guide a health care system that is both effective and cost efficient.

In more recent examples of cost savings, additional cost savings have been reported for patients who had an indeterminate exercise electrocardiogram. Due to effective risk stratification with SPECT imaging, cost efficiency can also be noted for patients with a normal resting 12-lead electrocardiogram. There are two large controlled clinical studies that have examined the cost implications of SPECT imaging when compared with other diagnostic approaches.[15,16] The smaller of the two studies, the Economics of Myocardial Perfusion Imaging in Europe (EMPIRE) study, compared stable chest-pain patients undergoing exercise electrocardiography, SPECT imaging, and direct coronary angiography (see Fig. 24-3). This study has value to extending prior results noted in the United States by the inclusion of four European countries with diverse health care and economic structures. The results of this study revealed that a noninvasive approach was decidedly cost efficient when compared with an invasive approach to care, at least for this cohort of patients with stable chest pain symptoms.

In the United States, the END study included a geographically diverse representation of multiple hospitals from within the United States and included 11,372 patients with Canadian Cardiovascular Society class II angina.[15] Patients enrolled in END were referred to direct coronary angiography or to initial SPECT imaging followed by selective catheterization in the setting of provocative ischemia. Figure 24-3 illustrates the diagnostic and follow-up costs of care for aggressively versus conservatively managed patients. These results revealed that over 3 years, there was an approximate 30% to 40% cost savings with initial SPECT imaging and a strategy of selective coronary angiography.

Both of these two large study results are consistent with prior modeling and observational datasets that support an economic advantage with the use of SPECT imaging in patients with stable chest-pain symptoms. If applied to a larger cohort of patients evaluated within a health care system, cost savings could be dramatic and approach several million dollars for every 1000 patients tested. The economic benefit of SPECT is based on the low catheterization rate required for patients with a normal perfusion scan. A number of reports have noted that only 1% to 3% of patients with normal perfusion results are referred to coronary angiography. Thus, the confirmation of normal SPECT findings can result in a marked reduction in costs of care and a reduced intensity of management. In the United Kingdom, the routine application of SPECT in this setting has been estimated to reduce costs by approximately £65,000 per year.[16]

At the heart of this research lies the concept of SPECT imaging as a gatekeeper to invasive coronary angiography. The above-mentioned research notes that gatekeeping can elicit substantive cost savings while maintaining equivalent patient outcomes. Recently, a review from the United Kingdom's National Institute of Clinical Excellence reported that when coronary angiography is used selectively following SPECT imaging, the resulting revascularization rates can be reduced by up to 50%, without a negative impact on outcomes.[61]

A recent report utilized this analytic method of identifying cost savings of SPECT compared with computed tomographic angiography (CTA).[62] This report compared 2313 patients who underwent CTA with 9252 patients referred to SPECT imaging. At 9 months of follow-up, the rates of worsening chest pain, myocardial infarction, or for any coronary disease hospitalization were similar for SPECT and CTA. However, dramatic cost differences were noted for both tests. That is, for patients with a history of coronary artery disease, CTA resulted in approximately $2500 higher costs of care.

This makes sense because of the importance of provocative ischemia in guiding therapeutic decision making in patients with a high likelihood for CAD and more prevalent revascularizable disease states. Conversely, in the low-risk patient with more atypical symptoms, the use of CTA resulted in cost savings of $603, largely driven by its high negative predictive accuracy. That is, the likelihood of significant CAD is very low when the CTA results do not reveal even minimal luminal irregularities. This report highlights the importance of pretest risk as a covariate in cost analysis. As shown in other reports, the extent and severity of regional myocardial perfusion provides important information that most prominently affects patients at higher risk, including those with known CAD.

There are also a number of reports focusing solely on the cost savings of SPECT imaging.[63] One area where the data are particularly strong for the utility of SPECT imaging is in the acute evaluation of chest pain.[63] In this setting, SPECT imaging has a high negative predictive value exceeding 95% and supported in the recent ACC/AHA guidelines by a class IA indication for patients with a nondiagnostic ECG and initially normal serum markers and enzymes.[64,65] Although SPECT imaging has been proposed as one of many strategies employed as a gatekeeper to hospitalization, the value of some form of testing lies in the nearly 3 million unnecessary hospitalizations accounting for some $5 to $8 billion dollars, as well as the approximately 5% of patients with acute coronary syndromes who are inappropriately sent home from the emergency department each year.[66–68] A review of this evidence was recently synthesized within the statement on cost-effectiveness published by the American Society of Nuclear Cardiology (ASNC),[63] in which the authors posit a nearly $800 cost savings when SPECT imaging is applied in the acute evaluation of chest pain in patients with indeterminate biomarkers. When compared to hospitalized patients, the use of SPECT imaging results in a lower rate of cardiac catheterization and shorter lengths of stay, both of which contribute to a positive yield in cost minimization. Moreover, the use of SPECT imaging to guide admissions results in a decrease in the rate of unnecessary hospitalizations by nearly 30% and a 6% reduction in inappropriate discharges. Perhaps the strongest piece of evidence was published from the ERASE trial noting that the use of SPECT imaging resulted in a 32% lower rate of admissions when compared to usual care.[69]

Several reports on the cost savings associated with predischarge use of SPECT imaging in patients with acute coronary syndromes have been published recently. The largest of these is from the Adenosine Sestamibi SPECT Postinfarction Evaluation (INSPIRE) Trial, where risk stratification based on quantitative estimates of ischemia resulted in substantial differences in cost (Table 24-3).[70] This report enrolled over 700 patients and noted that low-risk patients had average hospitalization costs of $5609 compared to high-risk patients, where the costs of care averaged $13,269 dollars ($P < 0.0001$). Much of the difference in cost had to do with a reduced length of stay for the low-risk patient with minimal ischemia. In fact, the average length of stay for low-risk patients

Table 24-3 Average In-Hospital Cost and Length of Stay in Postinfarction Patients Undergoing Myocardial Perfusion SPECT*

Estimated Hospital Costs (Not Charges)	
• Low risk	• $5609 ± $3632
• Intermediate risk	• $9967 ± $7344
• High risk (EF < 35%)	• $13,269 ± $6432
Average Length of Stay (Days)	
• Low risk	• 5.5 ± 2 days
• Intermediate risk	• 8.0 ± 5 days
• High risk (FF < 35%)	• 13.9 ± 13 days
Coronary Care Unit Length of Stay (Days)	
• Low risk	• 2.1 ± 1 day
• Intermediate risk	• 3.5 ± 3 days
• High risk (EF < 35%)	• 3.6 ± 2 days

*By extent of inducible ischemia, from low to high risk.[70]

was 5.5 days versus 13.9 days for high-risk patients ($P < 0.0001$), with high-risk patients remaining in the coronary care unit (CCU) an average of 2 additional days. The take-home message from the INSPIRE study was that low-risk patients with minimal ischemia can be safely discharged as soon as they are clinically stable. In fact, many of the low-risk patients spent little to no time in the CCU and were safely discharged within 3 days of admission. The majority of the aforementioned studies support the potential for significant cost savings as a result of using myocardial perfusion SPECT, with growing support of its utility postinfarction as an effective means of risk stratification and for identification of patients ready for early discharge.

Cost-Effectiveness of Myocardial Perfusion SPECT Compared to Other Diagnostic Procedures

There are a number of reports that have compared the marginal cost-effectiveness of stress myocardial perfusion SPECT with other modalities, notably stress echocardiography.[17–20] The majority of these reports have been decision models that have culled together pieces of data from related research, including test diagnostic accuracy and the effectiveness of revascularization in patients with CAD. The decision model is then formulated by including snippets of information from many diverse research reports. The problem with this type of analysis is that there are many assumptions about data inputs, and the selection of data is critical to devising the model and can heavily influence its results. It is for this reason that physicians should take care to scrutinize decision models, paying particular attention to the model inputs to evaluate their clinical relevance.

One recent report, however, evaluated a total of 4884 and 4637 patients undergoing exercise echocardiography and myocardial perfusion SPECT, respectively (Table 24-4).[71] The results reveal that for patients with

Table 24-4   Costs, Life Expectancy, and Incremental Cost-Effectiveness Ratio of Exercise Echocardiography Versus Myocardial Perfusion SPECT*

Median CAD Costs	Echocardiography	Myocardial Perfusion SPECT	P Value
Diagnostic	$294	$419	<0.0001
Annual hospitalization and event	$1647	$1604	<0.0001
Annual antiischemic drug therapy	$1101	$1272	<0.0001
Lifetime event and hospitalization	$42,644	$68,741	<0.0001
Median Life Expectancy (Years)			
No known coronary disease	20.2	23.6	<0.0001
Known coronary disease	18.3	19.4	<0.0001
Revascularization Within 90 Days			
No known coronary disease	2.2%	2.6%	0.18
Known coronary disease	3.7%	8.0%	<0.0001
Predicted Change in Life Expectancy with Revascularization (Years)			
No known coronary disease	2.0	1.6	<0.0001
Known coronary disease	1.8	3.0	<0.0001
Cost Effectiveness Calculation			
Echocardiography Versus SPECT Cost/Life Year Saved			
Intermediate Duke Treadmill Score	$39,506		
MPS Versus Echocardiography Cost/Life Year Saved			
Known coronary disease	$32,381		

*In patients with suspected and prior history of CAD undergoing exercise echocardiography (n = 4884) and exercise MPS (n = 4637).
CAD, coronary artery disease; MPS, myocardial perfusion scintigraphy; SPECT, single-photon emission computed tomography.

a high CAD likelihood, SPECT was decidedly more cost-effective than echocardiography. A number of patient subsets were included in this high-CAD-likelihood patient subset, notably the elderly, diabetics, patients with peripheral arterial disease, or those who are functionally impaired. The major driver for this cost-effectiveness advantage was the rapid referral of patients with abnormal myocardial perfusion results to coronary revascularization, with the result being a total of 3 additional years of life expectancy. Based on this, the resulting ICER was $32,381 for exercise SPECT versus echocardiography for the evaluation of stable chest pain. However, exercise echocardiography revealed a favorable ICER for lower-risk patients with a prior intermediate Duke Treadmill Score or indeterminate test results. In fact, the ICER was less than $20,000 for echocardiography compared to SPECT imaging when the estimated risk of cardiac death or nonfatal myocardial infarction was less than 2% per year (and largely included lower-risk patient cohorts). Once again, note the importance of pretest risk as guiding cost-effective test selection.

Based on a synthesis of results, initial test selection should be based on pretest likelihood of CAD. Using this reasoning, SPECT imaging is cost-effective when applied to higher-CAD-likelihood patients, including the elderly, patients with functional disability, diabetes, or peripheral arterial disease, and patients with a prior history of CAD. In general, this would include patients with an annual risk of CAD events of approximately 2% or

higher. Within this higher-likelihood population, SPECT imaging is decidedly more cost-effective when compared to both stress echocardiography and CTA.

American Society of Nuclear Cardiology Statement on Cost-Effectiveness of Nuclear Cardiology

The ASNC published a consensus statement on cost-effectiveness that may be helpful for readers to provide to local payers and as a tool for administrators to structure pathways of care that create efficiency and cost savings when using myocardial perfusion SPECT.[63] This ASNC statement highlighted several critical factors as strongly influencing downstream costs of care, including the greater accuracy of myocardial perfusion SPECT. A pattern of highly accurate testing can create cost efficiency or minimization of resources by reducing the need to layer testing; this pattern of cost efficiency has been reported for women and men with stable chest pain in diabetics, in the evaluation of acute chest pain in the emergency department, and for the predischarge evaluation following acute coronary syndrome. Each of these areas has been discussed in greater detail in prior parts of this chapter. For the interested laboratory, the creation of programs to ensure high-quality imaging will allow for pathways of care that create diagnostic efficiency. These programs should contain active quality assessment programs to assess near-term diagnostic or prognostic accuracy, including the assessment of referral patterns to coronary angiography for both low- and high-risk patients. The development of such programs can be important to payers and patients, ensuring that high-quality imaging is ensured within a given laboratory.

CONCLUSIONS

This chapter reveals that there is an increasingly large body of evidence on the economic value of SPECT imaging. Furthermore, the wealth of evidence on the diagnostic and prognostic value of nuclear cardiology has direct economic implications that may be inferred about the ensuing costs of care based on false-positive and false-negative test results. This evidence has been put forth largely in the past decade and has been widely accepted in this era focusing on cost containment. Evidence-based medicine standards are clearly met by the wealth and depth of data using SPECT imaging and provide a means to rationalize the use of nuclear imaging, even in the setting of a finite amount of health care resources.

As a result of this body of evidence, health care quality is ensured with SPECT imaging (when applied by supported research). Health care payer strategies that focus on near-term cost savings by using other imaging or nonimaging strategies will be shortsighted when compared with the data elucidating both the clinical and cost-effectiveness of myocardial perfusion SPECT. SPECT can add economic value to society by achieving an early, accurate diagnosis that results in improved patient outcome and reduced costs of care. Thus, SPECT imaging, if applied using evidence-based reasoning, can improve the allocation of resources and result in cost-effective care in the diagnosis and management of coronary disease. There is a particular advantage to the use of SPECT imaging for the evaluation of patients with known coronary disease that reveals its use is decidedly cost-effective when compared with other modalities, such as exercise echocardiography. The evidence with SPECT can be used to guide resource allocation and to leverage critical health care policy decisions that affect cohorts of patients commonly referred to nuclear laboratories.

REFERENCES

1. Benjamin EJ, Smith SC Jr, Cooper RS, et al: Task force #1: magnitude of the prevention problem: opportunities and challenges. 33rd Bethesda Conference, *J Am Coll Cardiol* 40:588–603, 2002.
2. http://www.rwjf.org/files/research/022008ib118final.pdf, Accessed March 15, 2008.
3. http://www.americanheart.org/presenter.jhtml?identifier=3018163., Accessed September 1, 2008.
4. Shaw LJ, Bairey Merz CN, Pepine CJ, Reis SE, Bittner V, Kip K, Kelsey SF, Olson M, Johnson BD, Mankad S, Sharaf BL, Rogers WJ, Pohost GM, Sopko G: for the WISE Investigators: The economic burden of angina in women with suspected ischemic heart disease: results from the National Institutes of Health–National Heart, Lung, and Blood Institute–Sponsored Women's Ischemia Syndrome Evaluation, *Circulation* 114:894–904, 2006.
5. http://www.meps.ahrq.gov/mepsweb/., Accessed March 15, 2008.
6. American College of Cardiology: Available at: www.acc.org/advocacy/advoc_issues/impactchart.htm. Accessed May 11, 2004.
7. Mark DB, Shaw LJ, Lauer MS, et al: Task force #5: is atherosclerotic imaging cost effective? From the 34th Bethesda Conference on Atherosclerotic Imaging, *J Am Coll Cardiol* 41:1906–1917, 2003.
8. Levin DC, Parker L, Intenzo CM, et al: Recent rapid increase in utilization of radionuclide myocardial perfusion imaging and related procedures: 1996–1998 practice patterns, *Radiology* 222:144–148, 2002.
9. Scanlon PJ, Faxon DP, Audet AM, et al: ACC/AHA Guidelines for coronary angiography: a report of the American College of Cardiology/American Heart Association Task Force on practice guidelines, *J Am Coll Cardiol* 33:1756–1824, 1999.
10. Goldman L, Garber AM, Grover SA, et al: 27th Bethesda Conference: matching the intensity of risk factor management with the hazard for CAD events. Task Force 6. Cost effectiveness of assessment and management of risk factors, *J Am Coll Cardiol* 27:1020–1030, 1996.
11. Underwood SR, Anagnostopoulos C, Cerqueira M, et al: Myocardial perfusion scintigraphy: the evidence. A consensus conference organised by the British Cardiac Society, the British Nuclear Cardiology Society and the British Nuclear Medicine Society, endorsed by the Royal College of Physicians of London and the Royal College of Radiologists, *Eur J Nuc Med Mol Imaging* 31:261–291, 2003.
12. Berry E, Kelly S, Hutton J, et al: A systematic literature review of spiral and electron beam computed tomography: with particular reference to clinical applications in hepatic lesions, pulmonary embolus and coronary artery disease, *Health Tech Assess* 3:1–118, 1999.
13. Berry E, Kelly S, Westwood ME, et al: The cost-effectiveness of magnetic resonance angiography for carotid artery stenosis and peripheral vascular disease: a systematic review, *Health Tech Assess* 6:1–155, 2002.
14. Rumberger JA, Behrenbeck T, Breen JF, et al: Coronary calcification by electron beam computed Tomography and obstructive coronary artery disease: a model for costs and effectiveness of diagnosis as compared with conventional cardiac testing methods, *J Am Coll Cardiol* 33:453–462, 1999.
15. Shaw LJ, Hachamovitch R, Berman DS, et al: The economic consequences of available diagnostic and prognostic strategies for the evaluation of stable angina patients: an observational assessment of the value of precatheterization ischemia. Economics of Noninvasive Diagnosis (END) Multicenter Study Group, *J Am Coll Cardiol* 33:661–669, 1999.
16. Underwood SR, Godman B, Salyani S, et al: Economics of myocardial perfusion imaging in Europe: the EMPIRE study, *Eur Heart J* 20:157–166, 1999.
17. Garber AM, Solomon NA: Cost-effectiveness of alternative test strategies for the diagnosis of coronary artery disease, *Ann Intern Med* 130:719–728, 1999.
18. Kuntz KM: Cost-effectiveness of diagnostic strategies for patients with chest pain, *Ann Intern Med* 130:709–718, 1999.
19. Marwick TH, Shaw LJ, Case C, et al: Clinical and economic impact of exercise electrocardiography and exercise echocardiography in clinical practice, *Eur Heart J* 24:1153–1163, 2003.
20. Lee DS, Jang MJ, Cheon GJ, et al: Comparison of the cost-effectiveness of stress myocardial perfusion SPECT and stress echocardiography in suspected coronary artery disease considering the prognostic value of false-negative results, *J Nucl Cardiol* 9:515–522, 2002.
21. Shaw LJ, Hachamovitch R, Eisenstein E, et al: Cost implications for implementing a selective preoperative risk screening approach for peripheral vascular surgery patients, *Am J Managed Care* 3:1817–1827, 1997.
22. Shaw LJ, Miller DD, Berman DS, et al: Clinical and economic outcomes assessment in nuclear cardiology, *Q J Nucl Med* 44:138–152, 2000.
23. Maddahi J, Ghambir SS: Cost-effective selection of patients for coronary angiography, *J Nucl Cardiol* 4:S141–S151, 1997.
24. Patterson RE, Eng C, Horowitz SF, et al: Bayesian comparison of cost-effectiveness of different clinical approaches to coronary artery disease, *J Am Coll Cardiol* 4:278–289, 1984.
25. Hunink MG, Kuntz KM, Fleischmann KE, et al: Noninvasive imaging for the diagnosis of coronary artery disease: focusing the development of new diagnostic technology, *Ann Intern Med* 131:673–680, 1999.
26. Sculpher M, Drummond M, Buxton M: The iterative use of economic evaluation as part of the process of health technology assessment, *J Health Serv Res* 2:26–30, 1997.
27. Callister TQ, Cooil B, Raya SP, et al: Coronary artery disease: improved reproducibility of calcium scoring with an electron-beam CT volumetric method, *Radiology* 208:807–814, 1998.
28. Smith DH, Hugh Gravelle H: The practice of discounting in economic evaluations of healthcare interventions, *Int J Tech Assess Health Care* 17:236–243, 2001.
29. Sheldon TA: Discounting in Health care decision-making: time for a change? *J Pub Health Med* 14:250–256, 1992.
30. Drummond MF, Jefferson TO: Guidelines for authors and peer reviewers of economic submissions to the BMJ. The BMJ Economic Evaluation Working Party, *BMJ* 313:275–283, 1996.
31. Einstein AJ, Henzlova MJ, Rajagopalan S: Estimating risk of cancer associated with radiation exposure from 64-slice computed tomography coronary angiography, *JAMA* 298(3)(Jul 18):317–323, 2007.
32. Shaw LJ, Raggi P, Berman DS, et al: Cost effectiveness of screening for cardiovascular disease with measures of coronary calcium, *Prog Cardiov Dis* 46:171–184, 2003.

33. Bell R, Petticrew M, Luengo S, et al: Screening for ovarian cancer: a systematic review, *Health Tech Assess* 2:1–84, 1998.

34. Petticrew MP, Sowden AJ, Lister-Sharp D, et al: False-negative results in screening programmes: systematic review of impact and implications, *Health Tech Assess* 4:1–60, 2000.

35. Mol: Characteristics of good diagnostic studies, *Semin Reprod Med* 21(1):17–25, 2003.

36. Shaw LJ, Eisenstein EL, Hachamovitch R, et al: A primer of biostatistic and economic methods for diagnostic and prognostic modeling in nuclear cardiology: Part II, *J Nucl Cardiol* 4(1 Pt 1):52–60, 1997.

37. Shaw LJ, Hachamovitch R, Papatheofanis FJ: *Outcomes and technology assessment in nuclear medicine*, Reston, VA, 1999, Society of Nuclear Medicine Press.

38. Mark D: Medical economics and health policy issues for interventional cardiology. In Topol E, editor: *Textbook of Interventional Cardiology*, ed 2, Philadelphia, 1993, WB Saunders.

39. Finkler S: *Cost accounting for health care organizations: concepts and applications*, Gaithersburg, MD, 1994, Aspen Publishers.

40. Laupacis A, Feeny D, Detsky AS, et al: How attractive does a new technology have to be to warrant adoption and utilization? Tentative guidelines for using clinical and economic evaluations, *CMAJ* 146:473–481, 1992.

41. Gold M: *Cost-effectiveness in Health and Medicine*, New York, NY, 1996, Oxford University Press.

42. Office of Technology Assessment: *The implications of cost-effectiveness analysis of medical technology, Chapters 1–4*, Washington, DC, 1980, U.S. Government Printing Office.

43. Doubilet P, Weinstein MC, McNeil BJ: Use and misuse of the term "cost effective" in medicine, *N Engl J Med* 314:253–256, 1986.

44. Garber AM, Phelps CE: Economic foundations of cost-effectiveness analysis, *J Health Econ* 16:1–31, 1997.

45. Siegel JE, Weinstein MC, Russell LB, et al: Recommendations for reporting cost-effectiveness analyses. Panel on Cost-Effectiveness in Health and Medicine, *JAMA* 276:1339–1341, 1996.

46. Weinstein MC, Siegel JE, Gold MR, et al: Recommendations of the Panel on Cost-effectiveness in Health and Medicine, *JAMA* 276:1253–1258, 1996.

47. Russell LB, Gold MR, Siegel JE, et al: The role of cost-effectiveness analysis in health and medicine. Panel on Cost-Effectiveness in Health and Medicine, *JAMA* 276:1172–1177, 1996.

48. Shaw LJ, Culler SD, Becker NR: Current evidence on cost effectiveness of noninvasive cardiac testing. Subsection E: analytic approaches to cost effectiveness and outcomes measurement in cardiovascular imaging. In Pohost G, O'Rourke R, Shah P, Berman D, editors: *Imaging in Cardiovascular Disease*, Philadelphia, 2000, Lippincott Williams & Wilkins, pp 479–500.

49. Petitti DB: *Meta-analysis, decision analysis, and cost-effectiveness analysis: Methods for quantitative synthesis in medicine*, New York, 1994, Oxford University Press.

50. Krumholz HM, Weintraub WS, Bradford WD, et al: The cost of prevention: can we afford it? Can we afford not to do it? *J Am Coll Cardiol* 40:603–605, 2002.

51. Mansley EC, McKenna MT: Importance of perspective in economic analyses of cancer screening decisions, *Lancet* 358:1169–1173, 2001.

52. Hunink MG, Krestin GP: Study design for concurrent development, assessment, and implementation of new diagnostic imaging technology, *Radiology* 222:604–614, 2002.

53. Mushlin AI, Ruchlin HS, Callahan MA: Cost effectiveness of diagnostic tests, *Lancet* 358:1353–1355, 2001.

54. Goldman L, Garber AM, Grover SA, et al: 27th Bethesda Conference: matching the intensity of risk factor management with the hazard for CAD events. Task Force 6. Cost effectiveness of assessment and management of risk factors, *J Am Coll Cardiol* 27:1020–1030, 1996.

55. Weinstein MC, Stason WB: Cost-effectiveness of interventions to prevent or treat coronary heart disease, *Annu Rev Public Health* 6:41–63, 1985.

56. Sonnenberg A, Delco F: Cost-effectiveness of a single colonoscopy in screening for colorectal cancer, *Arch Intern Med* 162:163–168, 2002.

57. Johnstone PA, Moore EM, Carrillo R, et al: Yield of mammography in selected patients age ≤30 years, *Cancer* 91:1075–1078, 2001.

58. Shaw LJ, Iskandrian AE: Prognostic value of stress gated SPECT in patients with known or suspected coronary artery disease, *J Nucl Cardiol* 11:171–185, 2004.

59. Thomas GS, Miyamoto MI, Morello AP III, et al: Technetium-99m based myocardial perfusion imaging predicts clinical outcome in the community outpatient setting: The Nuclear Utility in the Community ("NUC") Study, *J Am Coll Cardiol* 43:213–223, 2004.

60. Hachamovitch R, Berman DS, Shaw LJ, Kiat H, Cohen I, Cabico JA, Friedman J, Diamond GA: Incremental prognostic value of myocardial perfusion single photon emission computed tomography for the prediction of cardiac death: differential stratification for risk of cardiac death and myocardial infarction, *Circulation* 97:535–543, 1998.

61. Mowatt G, Brazzelli M, Gemmell H, Hillis GS, Metcalfe M, Vale L: Aberdeen Technology Assessment Group. Systematic review of the prognostic effectiveness of SPECT myocardial perfusion scintigraphy in patients with suspected or known coronary artery disease and following myocardial infarction, *Nucl Med Commun* 26:217–229, 2005.

62. Min JK, Shaw LJ, Berman DS: Cost-effective applications of cardiac computed tomography in coronary artery disease, *Expert Rev Cardiovasc Ther* 6(1):43–55, 2008.

63. DesPrez RD, Gillespie RL, Jaber WA, Noble GL, Soman P, Wolinsky DG, Williams KA, Shaw LJ: American Society of Nuclear Cardiology Information Statement on the Cost Effectiveness of Myocardial Perfusion Imaging, *J Nucl Cardiol* 12(6):750–759, 2005.

64. Heller GV, Stowers SA, Hendel RC, Herman SD, Daher E, Ahlberg AW, Baron JM, Mendes de Leon CF, Rizzo JA, Wackers FJ: Clinical value of acute rest technetium-99m tetrofosmin tomographic myocardial perfusion imaging in patients with acute chest pain and nondiagnostic electrocardiograms, *J Am Coll Cardiol* 31:1011–1017, 1998.

65. Klocke FJ, et al: ACC/AHA/ASNC guidelines for the clinical use of cardiac radionuclide imaging: executive summary, *Circulation* 108:1404–1418, 2003.

66. Fineberg HV, Scadden D, Goldman L: Care of patients with a low probability of acute myocardial infarction. Cost effectiveness of alternatives to coronary-care-unit admission, *N Engl J Med* 310:1301–1307, 1984.

67. Lee TH, Rouan GW, Weisberg MC, Brand DA, Acampora D, Stasiulewicz C, Walshon J, Terranova G, Gottlieb L, Goldstein-Wayne B, et al: Clinical characteristics and natural history of patients with acute myocardial infarction sent home from the emergency room, *Am J Cardiol* 60(4):219–224, 1987.

68. Pope JH, Aufderheide TP, Ruthazer R, Woolard RH, Feldman JA, Beshansky JR, Griffith JL, Selker HP: Missed diagnoses of acute cardiac ischemia in the emergency department, *N Engl J Med* 342(16):1163–1170, 2000.

69. Udelson JE, Beshansky JR, Ballin DS, Feldman JA, Griffith JL, Handler J, Heller GV, Hendel RC, Pope JH, Ruthazer R, Spiegler EJ, Woolard RH, Selker HP: Myocardial perfusion imaging for evaluation and triage of patients with suspected acute cardiac ischemia: a randomized controlled trial, *JAMA*. 288(21):2693–2700, 2002.

70. Mahmarian JJ, Shaw LJ, Filipchuk NG, Dakik HA, Iskander SS, Ruddy TD, Henzlova MJ, Keng F, Allam A, Pratt CM: INSPIRE Investigators. A multinational study to establish the value of early adenosine technetium-99m sestamibi myocardial perfusion imaging in identifying a low-risk group for early hospital discharge after acute myocardial infarction, *J Am Coll Cardiol* 48(12):2448–2457, 2006 Epub 2006 Nov 28.2006 Dec 19.

71. Shaw LJ, Marwick TH, Berman DS, Sawada S, Heller GV, Vasey C, Miller DD: Incremental cost effectiveness of exercise echocardiography versus SPECT imaging for the evaluation of stable chest pain, *Eur Heart J* 27(20):2448–2458, 2006, Epub 2006, Sep 26, 2006 Oct.

Chapter 25

Appropriate Use of Nuclear Cardiology

TODD D. MILLER AND RAYMOND J. GIBBONS

Spending on health care in the United States has been increasing at an alarming rate. Over the past 40 years, the annual increase in federal health care spending has outpaced the annual growth of the gross domestic product (GDP) by an average of 2.5%.[1] Currently, U.S. health care spending exceeds $2 trillion and accounts for 16% of the GDP.[2] The Congressional Budget Office projects that if current trends were to persist over the next 40 years, federal spending on Medicare and Medicaid (ignoring state spending on Medicaid) would approach 20% of the GDP (Fig. 25-1). To appreciate the significance of this projection, it is important to realize that total federal revenue over the past 60 years has ranged between 17.0% and 20.9% of the GDP and has never in the history of the United States exceeded 20.9%.[3] In other words, the projected federal spending on Medicare and Medicaid alone by the midpoint of this century would equal (as a percentage of the GDP) what has historically been spent on all components of the federal budget (social security, defense, education, interest on the national debt, agriculture, etc.).

Spending on cardiovascular diseases accounts for a substantial proportion of total health care spending. In 2007, the estimated direct and indirect costs for cardiovascular diseases were nearly $432 billion.[4] The rate of growth in cardiac imaging services has recently been especially steep. Stress imaging, which as defined by Medicare incorporates both stress single-photon emission computed tomography (SPECT) and stress echocardiography, grew at a rate of 6% per year between 1993 and 2001.[5] This rate of growth for stress imaging far exceeded the rate of growth in acute myocardial infarction, cardiac catheterizations, or coronary artery revascularization procedures during this time period (Fig. 25-2). Published data further demonstrate that the use of stress imaging is highly heterogenous across the country, with rates of imaging varying by more than 10-fold between different geographic regions (Fig. 25-3).[6]

In response to these concerns about the use of cardiovascular imaging, the American College of Cardiology Foundation (ACCF) initiated a process to address the appropriateness of different cardiovascular imaging procedures.[7] Examining the appropriateness of medical resource use is not a novel concept.[8-10] The American College of Radiology (ACR) published appropriateness criteria for radiologic imaging procedures in 1995.[11] The ACR criteria address a variety of imaging procedures across multiple medical and surgical disciplines. They have not been widely applied to the practice of clinical cardiology. The ACCF appropriateness criteria focus on single cardiovascular imaging procedures. In October 2005 the ACCF, in collaboration with the American Society of Nuclear Cardiology (ASNC), published the first set of appropriateness criteria, which addressed SPECT myocardial perfusion imaging (SPECT MPI).[12] Since then, appropriateness criteria have been published for cardiac computed tomography and cardiac magnetic resonance imaging,[13] transthoracic and transesophageal echocardiography,[14] stress echocardiography,[15] and coronary revascularization.[16]

The approach the ACCF has followed to examine the appropriateness of a cardiovascular imaging modality is based on a method originally developed by the RAND Corporation, in collaboration with researchers from the University of California, Los Angeles (UCLA), to examine the appropriateness of medical and surgical procedures.[17] Although the ACCF methodology is based on the RAND/UCLA approach, it is important to note that the RAND/UCLA method focuses on the therapeutic benefit of invasive procedures, whereas cardiovascular imaging has different goals. Another major difference relates to the number of clinical scenarios considered. The RAND/UCLA document addresses literally hundreds of clinical scenarios. The ACCF approach limits the number of situations to fewer, more broadly defined clinical scenarios where imaging is most commonly applied. The ACCF method follows the precedent set

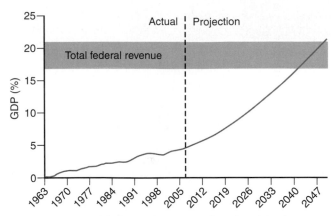

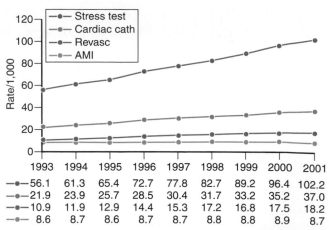

	1993	1994	1995	1996	1997	1998	1999	2000	2001
•	56.1	61.3	65.4	72.7	77.8	82.7	89.2	96.4	102.2
•	21.9	23.9	25.7	28.5	30.4	31.7	33.2	35.2	37.0
•	10.9	11.9	12.9	14.4	15.3	17.2	16.8	17.5	18.2
•	8.6	8.7	8.6	8.7	8.7	8.8	8.8	8.9	8.7

Figure 25-1 Federal spending on Medicaid and Medicare as a percent of GDP. Over the past 60 years, total federal revenue *(horizontal band)* has always been between 17% and 21% of the GDP. By 2040, spending on Medicaid and Medicare alone is projected to approximate 17% of the GDP. *(Reprinted from Orszag PR: Health care and the budget: Issues and challenges for reform. CBO Testimony before the Committee on the Budget, United States Senate, 2007.)*

Figure 25-2 Growth in Medicare stress imaging (which incorporates both SPECT and stress echocardiography) compared to cardiac catheterizations, revascularization procedures, and acute myocardial infarction between the years 1993 to 2001. The rate of growth of stress imaging far exceeded that of the other procedures or occurrence of myocardial infarction. *(Reprinted from Lucas FL, DeLorenzo MA, Siewers AE, et al: Temporal trends in the utilization of diagnostic testing and treatments for cardiovascular disease in the United State, Circulation 113:374–379, 2006.)*

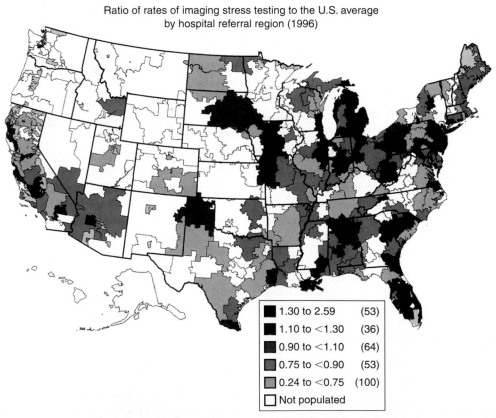

Figure 25-3 Dartmouth health care atlas map illustrating rates of stress imaging (both SPECT and stress echocardiography) studies in 1996 by Medicare referral regions compared to the national average. Regions in the darkest colors, concentrated primarily in selected locations in the Northeast, Southeast, Midwest, and Southwest, had rates far above the national average. *(Reprinted from Wennberg JE, Birkmeyer JD, Birkmeyer NJO, et al: The Dartmouth Atlas of Cardiovascular Health Care. Chicago: American Hospital Association Press, 1999.)*

by the ACR and uses the modified Delphi method to develop appropriateness criteria. With this approach, members of an expert panel assign ratings for imaging to various clinical indications, initially without any interaction with other panel members. The panel then meets to discuss the assigned ratings, and members again assign ratings after this panel interaction. The ACCF approach differs from the ACR approach by not trying to achieve consensus of panel members and by using fewer rounds of ratings.[7]

The definition of an appropriate imaging study selected by the ACCF is:[7]

"An appropriate imaging study is one in which the expected incremental information, combined with clinical judgment, exceeds the expected negative consequences* by a sufficiently wide margin for a specific indication that the procedure is generally considered acceptable care and a reasonable approach for the indication."

*Expected negative consequences include risks of the procedure (i.e., radiation or contrast exposure) and the downstream impact of poor test performance, such as delay in diagnosis (false negatives) or inappropriate diagnosis (false positives).

It is important to note that the "negative consequences" listed in this formal definition do not directly mention cost of the procedure. However, the ACCF methodology document does acknowledge the importance of cost: "Therefore, to identify the true risks of imaging, both inherent risks and downstream effects, including costs, must be considered. As such, if the imaging study provides little incremental information for an indication over standard clinical judgment and care, then cost considerations should contribute to deeming the procedure inappropriate."[7]

For each imaging modality being rated for appropriateness, the ACCF method follows 4 steps:
1. Develop list of specific clinical indications
2. Expert panel ratings
3. Expert panel meeting followed by re-ratings
4. Tabulation of appropriateness recommendations

The panelists assign a rating for each clinical indication using a 9-point scoring system. Following the second round of voting by panel members, scores are categorized as follows:

Median score 7 to 9: Appropriate test for that specific indication.
Median score 4 to 6: Uncertain or possibly appropriate test for that specific indication.
Median score 1 to 3: Inappropriate test for that indication.

It is important to distinguish between appropriateness criteria and clinical guidelines. ACCF/American Heart Association (AHA) guidelines are based on comprehensive reviews of the medical literature (evidence-based) and employ a level-of-evidence rating scheme to assign indications to diagnostic procedures and therapies. Conversely, the appropriateness criteria are based on consideration of benefit versus risk of performing the imaging modality. Panel members are encouraged to consider the published literature when assigning a rating for a given indication, but there is no requirement that the rating be based on the literature. The emphasis is on a less formal approach of whether it is "reasonable" to consider performing the imaging study.[7]

The technical panel for SPECT MPI appropriateness criteria was composed of 12 physicians, 58% of whom were specialists in nuclear cardiology. This panel rated 52 clinical indications for SPECT imaging. Most (49) of these indications addressed stress SPECT for detection or risk assessment of coronary artery disease, one indication addressed assessment of viability, and two indications addressed evaluation of ventricular function (Tables 25-1 through 25-9).[12] Of the 52 indications, 27 were rated appropriate, 12 uncertain, and 13 inappropriate.

In its initial document, the ACCF stated: "Both validation and evaluation of the proposed appropriateness ratings by modality are essential steps."[7] Since the ACCF appropriateness criteria ratings concept is only in its infancy, there are little published data that examines the application of the criteria in clinical practice.

We undertook a project to evaluate the appropriateness of stress SPECT MPI in our institution.[18] We retrospectively applied the criteria listed in the ACCF/ASNC document for stress SPECT MPI (see Tables 25-1 through 25-7) to 284 patients referred to our laboratory over a 2-week period between May 1 to 15, 2005. Since we were interested in studying the appropriateness of cardiovascular imaging in general terms, we also applied the same stress SPECT MPI criteria to 298 patients who underwent stress echocardiography at our institution during this same time period. For this initial project, we intentionally selected a timeframe before the publication of the ACCF appropriateness criteria for individual imaging techniques to establish a baseline for the use of stress imaging in our institution. Our goal in future projects will be to assess the impact of publication of the ACCF appropriateness criteria documents on our practice.

The major finding of our study was that 64% of stress SPECT MPI studies were appropriate, 11% were uncertain, and 14% were inappropriate. Eleven percent of the studies were unclassifiable. Results were similar for stress echocardiography (Fig. 25-4). The vast majority (88%) of inappropriate studies were performed for one of four indications: asymptomatic patients with low-risk Framingham score referred for screening for coronary artery disease and (indication #10 in Table 25-2 of the ACCF/ASNC SPECT MPI document); preoperative evaluation for intermediate-risk noncardiac surgery with normal exercise tolerance (indication #32 in Table 25-5); symptomatic patients with chest pain who had a low pretest probability for coronary artery disease and an interpretable ECG, and were able to exercise (indication #1 in Table 25-1); and preoperative evaluation for low-risk noncardiac surgery (indication #31 in Table 25-5).

Table 25-1 Detection of Coronary Artery Disease: Symptomatic

Indication	Appropriateness Criteria (Median Score)
Evaluation of Chest Pain Syndrome	
1. • Low pretest probability of CAD • ECG interpretable AND able to exercise	I (2.0)
2. • Low pretest probability of CAD • ECG uninterpretable OR unable to exercise	U* (6.5)
3. • Intermediate pretest probability of CAD • ECG interpretable AND able to exercise	A (7.0)
4. • Intermediate pretest probability of CAD • ECG uninterpretable OR unable to exercise	A (9.0)
5. • High pretest probability of CAD • ECG interpretable AND able to exercise	A (8.0)
6. • High pretest probability of CAD • ECG uninterpretable OR unable to exercise	A (9.0)
Acute Chest Pain (in Reference to Rest Perfusion Imaging)	
7. • Intermediate pretest probability of CAD • ECG—no ST elevation AND initial cardiac enzymes negative	A (9.0)
8. • High pretest probability of CAD • ECG—ST elevation	I (1.0)
New-Onset/Diagnosed Heart Failure With Chest Pain Syndrome	
9. • Intermediate pretest probability of CAD	A (8.0)

*Median scores of 3.5 and 6.5 were rounded to the middle (U).
A, appropriate; I, inappropriate; U, uncertain.

Table 25-2 Detection of Coronary Artery Disease: Asymptomatic (Without Chest Pain Syndrome)

Indication	Appropriateness Criteria (Median Score)
Asymptomatic	
10. • Low CAD risk (Framingham risk criteria)	I (1.0)
11. • Moderate CAD risk (Framingham)	U (5.5)
New-Onset or Diagnosed Heart Failure or LV Systolic Dysfunction Without Chest Pain Syndrome	
12. • Moderate CAD risk (Framingham) • No prior CAD evaluation AND no planned cardiac catheterization	A (7.5)
Valvular Heart Disease Without Chest Pain Syndrome	
13. • Moderate CAD risk (Framingham) • To help guide decision for invasive studies	U (5.5)
New-Onset Atrial Fibrillation	
14. • Low CAD risk (Framingham) • Part of the evaluation	U*(3.5)
15. • High CAD risk (Framingham) • Part of the evaluation	A (8.0)
Ventricular Tachycardia	
16. • Moderate to high CAD risk (Framingham)	A (9.0)

*Median scores of 3.5 and 6.5 are rounded to the middle (U).
A, appropriate; I, inappropriate; U, uncertain.

Table 25-3 Risk Assessment: General and Specific Patient Populations

Indication	Appropriateness Criteria (Median Score)
Asymptomatic	
17. • Low CAD risk (Framingham)	I (1.0)
18. • Moderate CAD risk (Framingham)	U (4.0)
19. • Moderate to high CAD risk (Framingham) • High-risk occupation (e.g., airline pilot)	A (8.0)
20. • High CAD risk (Framingham)	A (7.5)

A, appropriate; I, inappropriate; U, uncertain.

Performing this project highlighted many difficulties that arise related to the application of the ACCF appropriateness criteria to clinical databases.[18] The Mayo Clinic nuclear cardiology and stress echocardiography laboratories both have electronic databases. Because we had no previous experience applying the appropriate criteria to our databases, we first performed a pilot project applying these criteria to a single day of tests from both laboratories (50 patients). Five physicians and 2 experienced cardiovascular nurse abstractors independently attempted to apply the appropriateness criteria to these 50 patients. We discovered that a number of "assumptions" were necessary to apply the appropriateness criteria in a standardized manner. Some examples of these assumptions included assigning a hierarchical ranking to the appropriateness tables (since some patients met more than one test indication), assuming that certain surgical procedures not covered by the ACC/AHA preoperative guidelines would be low risk (e.g., endoscopic inguinal hernia repair), and interpreting the symptom of "dyspnea" as being equivalent to "atypical angina"

Table 25-4 Risk Assessment with Prior Test Results

Indication	Appropriateness Criteria (Median Score)
Asymptomatic OR Stable Symptoms	
Normal Prior SPECT MPI Study	
21. • Normal initial RNI study • High CAD risk (Framingham) • Annual SPECT MPI study	I (3.0)
22. • Normal initial RNI study • High CAD risk (Framingham) • Repeat SPECT MPI study after 2 years or greater	A (7.0)
Asymptomatic OR Stable Symptoms	
Abnormal Catheterization OR Prior SPECT MPI Study	
23. • Known CAD on catheterization OR prior SPECT MPI study in patients who have not had revascularization procedure • Asymptomatic OR stable symptoms • Less than 1 year to evaluate worsening disease	I (2.5)
24. • Known CAD on catheterization OR prior SPECT MPI study in patients who have not had revascularization procedure • Greater than or equal to 2 years to evaluate worsening disease	A (7.5)
Worsening Symptoms	
Abnormal Catheterization OR Prior SPECT MPI Study	
25. • Known CAD on catheterization OR prior SPECT MPI study	A (9.0)
Asymptomatic	
CT Coronary Angiography	
26. • Stenosis of unclear significance	U* (6.5)
Asymptomatic	
Prior Coronary Calcium Agatston Score	
27. • Agatston score greater than or equal to 400	A (7.5)
28. • Agatston score less than 100	I (1.5)
UA/NSTEMI, STEMI, or Chest Pain Syndrome	
Coronary Angiogram	
29. • Stenosis of unclear significance	A (9.0)
Duke Treadmill Score	
30. • Intermediate Duke Treadmill Score • Intermediate CAD risk (Framingham)	A (9.0)

*Median scores of 3.5 and 6.5 are rounded to the middle (U).
A, appropriate; I, inappropriate; U, uncertain.

Table 25-5 Risk Assessment: Preoperative Evaluation for Non-Cardiac Surgery

Indication	Appropriateness Criteria (Median Score)
Low-Risk Surgery	
31. • Preoperative evaluation for non-cardiac surgery risk assessment	I (1.0)
Intermediate-Risk Surgery	
32. • Minor to intermediate perioperative risk predictor • Normal exercise tolerance (greater than or equal to 4 METs)	I (3.0)
33. • Intermediate perioperative risk predictor OR • Poor exercise tolerance (less than 4 METs)	A (8.0)
High-Risk Surgery	
34. • Minor perioperative risk predictor • Normal exercise tolerance (greater than or equal to 4 METs)	U (4.0)
35. • Minor perioperative risk predictor • Poor exercise tolerance (less than 4 METs)	A (8.0)
36. • Asymptomatic up to 1 year post normal catheterization, noninvasive test, or previous revascularization	I (3.0)

A, appropriate; I, inappropriate; U, uncertain.

Table 25-6 Risk Assessment: Following Acute Coronary Syndrome

Indication	Appropriateness Criteria (Median Score)
STEMI—Hemodynamically Stable	
37. • Thrombolytic therapy administered • Not planning to undergo catheterization	A (8.0)
STEMI—Hemodynamically Unstable, Signs of Cardiogenic Shock, or Mechanical Complications	
38. • Thrombolytic therapy administered	I (1.0)
UA/NSTEMI—No Recurrent Ischemia OR No Signs of HF	
39. • Not planning to undergo early catheterization	A (8.5)
ACS Asymptomatic Post Revascularization (PCI or CABG)	
40. • Routine evaluation prior to hospital discharge	I (1.0)

A, appropriate; I, inappropriate; U, uncertain.

Table 25-7 Risk Assessment: Post-Revascularization (PCI or CABG)

Indication	Appropriateness Criteria (Median Score)
Symptomatic	
41. • Evaluation of chest pain syndrome	A (8.0)
Asymptomatic	
42. • Asymptomatic prior to previous revascularization • Less than 5 years after CABG	U (6.0)
43. • Symptomatic prior to previous revascularization • Less than 5 years after CABG	U (4.5)
44. • Asymptomatic prior to previous revascularization • Greater than or equal to 5 years after CABG	A (7.5)
45. • Symptomatic prior to previous revascularization • Greater than or equal to 5 years after CABG	A (7.5)
46. • Asymptomatic prior to previous revascularization • Less than 1 year after PCI	U* (6.5)
47. • Symptomatic prior to previous revascularization • Less than 1 year after PCI	I (3.0)
48. • Asymptomatic prior to previous revascularization • Greater than or equal to 2 years after PCI	U* (6.5)
49. • Symptomatic prior to previous revascularization • Greater than or equal to 2 years after PCI	U (5.5)

*Median scores of 3.5 and 6.5 are rounded to the middle (U).
A, appropriate; I, inappropriate; U, uncertain.

Table 25-8 Assessment of Viability/Ischemia

Indication	Appropriateness Criteria (Median Score)
Ischemic Cardiomyopathy	
Assessment of Viability/Ischemia (Includes SPECT Imaging for Wall Motion and Ventricular Function)	
50. • Known CAD on catheterization • Patient eligible for revascularization	A (8.5)

A, appropriate; I, inappropriate; U, uncertain.

Table 25-9 Evaluation of Ventricular Function

Indication	Appropriateness Criteria (Median Score)
Evaluation of Left Ventricular Function	
51. • Nondiagnostic echocardiogram	A (9.0)
Use of Potentially Cardiotoxic Therapy (e.g., doxorubicin)	
52. • Baseline and serial measurements	A (9.0)

A, appropriate; I, inappropriate; U, uncertain.

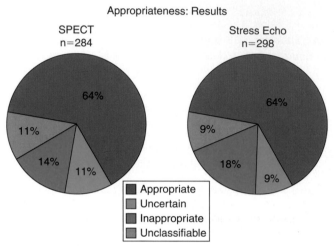

Appropriateness: Results

SPECT n=284 — 64%, 11%, 14%, 11%

Stress Echo n=298 — 64%, 9%, 18%, 9%

■ Appropriate
■ Uncertain
■ Inappropriate
■ Unclassifiable

Figure 25-4 Results of appropriateness criteria indication categories retrospectively assigned to 284 patients who underwent stress SPECT and 298 patients who underwent stress echocardiography over a 2-week period at the Mayo Clinic before the publication of the ACCF/ASNC appropriateness criteria document for SPECT MPI. Almost two-thirds of the studies were rated appropriate, but notably, 14% to 18% were rated inappropriate, and 9% to 11% of studies could not be classified. *(Reprinted from Gibbons RJ, Miller TD, Hodge DO, et al: Application of appropriateness criteria to stress single-photon emission computed tomography sestamibi studies and stress echocardiograms in an academic medical center, J Am Coll Cardiol 51:283–290, 2008.)*

for purposes of determining a patient's pretest probability of coronary artery disease. (The ACCF/ASNC SPECT MPI appropriateness criteria document indicates that an appropriateness rating can be assigned to patients being evaluated for dyspnea, but the published criteria for determining pretest probability of disease address only address chest pain and not dyspnea.) Once we completed the pilot project, the actual appropriateness ratings for the 284 SPECT MPI patients and the 298 stress echocardiography patients were assigned by the two experienced nurse abstractors, each blinded to the other's ratings and neither of whom was affiliated with either laboratory. Differences between the two nurses' ratings were resolved by consensus of two physicians. The overall level of agreement between the two nurses was only modest (kappa = 0.56). This finding illustrates the lack of consistency that is likely to occur when applying these ratings in clinical practice.

To date, the only other publication that addresses the application of the ACCF/ASNC SPECT MPI appropriateness criteria is a study from the University of Chicago nuclear cardiology laboratory involving 1209 patients who underwent stress SPECT MPI.[19] These authors found that a higher percentage (97%) of patients referred for SPECT MPI could be assigned to one of the indications in the ACCF/ASNC SPECT MPI document. In the patients who could be assigned to an indication, a higher percentage of patients were rated appropriate in this study compared to our study. The ratings results for the study by Mehta et al. were 80% appropriate, 7% uncertain, and 13% inappropriate. These authors also found that a small number (3) of similar indications accounted for the large majority (85%) of inappropriate tests: symptomatic patients with a low pretest probability of coronary artery disease, preoperative evaluation for low-risk surgery, and preoperative evaluation for intermediate-risk surgery with low to intermediate clinical predictors and normal exercise tolerance. Additional analyses undertaken by these authors included examination of the prevalence of normal SPECT MPI according to rating categories and the impact of the specialty of the ordering physician on rating categories. Predictably, the percentage of normal images was significantly smaller in the appropriate (45%) category versus the uncertain (53%) or inappropriate (68%) categories. Anesthesiologists were more likely to order SPECT MPI for inappropriate indications, compared to other physician specialties.

Differences in study methodology may explain some of the differences in results between the study by Mehta et al.[19] and our study.[18] The assignment of appropriateness category ratings by Mehta and colleagues was performed by a single individual affiliated with the University of Chicago nuclear cardiology laboratory. This individual understandably may have been biased toward rating studies as appropriate.[20] Additionally, the chart review in the Mehta et al. study was performed after the publication of the ACCF/ASNC SPECT MPI appropriateness criteria document. Conceivably, awareness of this document may have influenced test ordering at the University of Chicago.

These two studies[18,19] share common features, including application of retrospective chart review and similar practice settings (academic medical centers located in the Midwest). Use of SPECT MPI might be substantially different in private practice settings or in other geographic regions. Both the Rochester, Minnesota, and Chicago Medicare referral regions have reported rates of stress imaging that are far below those reported for multiple regions in Michigan, New Jersey, and Florida.[6] The results of these two studies should therefore not be interpreted to reflect the use of SPECT MPI on a national basis.

Currently there are only a limited number of studies that have applied appropriateness criteria to other imaging modalities.[21,22] Following our initial study,[18] we examined the application of the stress echocardiography appropriateness criteria[15] to the same 298 patients who underwent stress echocardiography in a subsequent study.[23] When stress SPECT MPI was applied to the stress echocardiography patients, 64% of studies were rated appropriate, 9% uncertain, 18% inappropriate, and 9% unclassifiable (see Fig. 25-4). Application of the stress echocardiography appropriateness criteria to the stress echocardiography patients resulted in significantly fewer studies (54%) rated as appropriate and more

studies (19%) rated as unclassifiable, with similar percentages rated as uncertain (8%) or inappropriate (19%) ($P < 0.001$ for overall difference compared to the ratings using the SPECT MPI criteria). These differences suggest that future revisions of appropriateness criteria documents for stress imaging should attempt to reduce the differences that currently exist in these criteria for the different imaging modalities.

The appropriateness criteria document for coronary revascularization[16] does not address the appropriate use of SPECT MPI but does require that the presence of ischemia or the presence of intermediate-risk or high-risk findings on noninvasive imaging be considered to assign a rating of appropriateness to many revascularization scenarios. For SPECT imaging specifically, intermediate-risk findings include mild to moderate resting left ventricular dysfunction (left ventricular ejection fraction 35% to 49%) or stress-induced moderate perfusion defect without left ventricular dilation or increased (thallium-201) lung uptake. There are several high-risk SPECT findings: severe resting left ventricular dysfunction (ejection fraction < 35%); severe exercise left ventricular dysfunction (exercise ejection fraction < 35%); stress-induced large perfusion defect (particularly if anterior); stress-induced multiple perfusion defects of moderate size; large fixed perfusion defect with left ventricular dilation or increased lung uptake; and stress-induced moderate perfusion defect with left ventricular dilation or increased lung uptake. Thus, the findings from SPECT MPI can play a major role in assigning a revascularization procedure to an appropriateness rating.

The ACCF appropriateness criteria initiative is intended to be a dynamic rather than a static process.[7] Once the appropriateness criteria documents are published, the ACCF anticipates that there will be many different groups applying these criteria to many different practices. The ACCF designed this process to include periodic reassessment of the individual documents, with revisions based on feedback from users. For instance, new indications may need to be added that were not addressed in the original document, and the rating category assigned to an individual indication may need to be altered based on experience or new published evidence. The ASNC Quality Assurance Committee has already published suggestions for revisions of the ACCF/ASNC SPECT MPI appropriateness criteria.[24]

Our laboratory has already published new evidence on the subject of screening for coronary artery disease in asymptomatic patients with new-onset atrial fibrillation.[25] The ACCF/ASNC criteria created separate indications for such patients based on clinical risk. Askew et al.[25] found that the distribution of summed stress scores in such patients was similar to asymptomatic patients without atrial fibrillation who were matched for age and gender (Fig. 25-5). There was no evidence that the identification of coronary artery disease was more likely in such patients. Moreover, clinical risk factors did not predict an increased prevalence of high-risk summed stress scores in such patients, as implied by the appropriateness ratings of "appropriate" for high-clinical-risk patients and "uncertain" for low-clinical-risk patients.

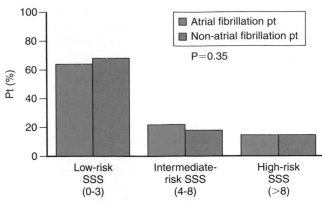

Figure 25-5 Percentages by summed stress score (SSS) categories for asymptomatic patients with atrial fibrillation matched to a cohort of patients without atrial fibrillation. There were no differences in SSS categories, suggesting that the presence of atrial fibrillation per se does not reflect a higher likelihood of coronary artery disease. *(Reprinted from Askew JW, Miller TD, Hodge DO, et al: The value of myocardial perfusion single-photon emission computed tomography in screening asymptomatic patients with atrial fibrillation for coronary artery disease, J Am Coll Cardiol 50:1080–1085, 2007.)*

Precisely how the ACCF appropriateness criteria documents[12–16] will be applied remains to be determined. The ACCF anticipates that clinicians, researchers, and payers will use these documents. A SPECT MPI appropriateness criteria decision support application has been developed to facilitate applying the criteria in the clinical setting. This tool can be downloaded from several different internet sites:

- WinCE: http://www.skyscape.com/download/reseller.asp? format=binary&os=win&device=ce&product=spectmpi
- Palm/Windows: http://www.skyscape.com/download/reseller.asp?format=binary&os=win&device=palm&product=spectmpi
- Palm/MAC: http://www.skyscape.com/download/reseller.asp?format=binary&os=mac&device=palm&product=spectmpi
- Windows Desktop: http://www.skyscape.com/download/reseller.asp?format=binary&os=win&device=pc&product=spectmpi

Clinicians can apply these documents to examine the appropriateness of test ordering in their institution. The ACCF hopes that indications rated as "uncertain" will stimulate research that will help assign these indications to a more certain rating category. Payers are expected to apply these documents to decide which imaging studies merit reimbursement. The ACCF has launched an initiative with United Health Care to test the appropriateness criteria at the point of service in 10 centers across the country to examine the impact on physician-ordering test patterns. A common goal between clinicians and payers should be to decrease and ultimately eliminate imaging studies being performed for inappropriate indications. Achievement of this goal will be an important step toward the goal of enhancing the efficiency of the health care system and containing escalating health care costs. Hopefully, they will be considered by the National Quality Forum during its ongoing project to develop "voluntary consensus standards for outpatient imaging efficiency."[26]

REFERENCES

1. Orszag PR: *Health care and the budget: issues and challenges for reform,* 2007, CBO Testimony before the Committee on the Budge United States Senate.
2. Orszag PR, Ellis P: The challenge of rising health care costs—a view from the Congressional Budget Office, *N Engl J Med* 357:1793–1795, 2007.
3. Gibbons RJ: Finding value in imaging: what is appropriate? *J Nucl Cardiol* 15:178–185, 2008.
4. Rosamond W, Flegal K, Friday G, et al: Heart disease and stroke statistics—2007 update: a report from the American Heart Association Statistics Committee and Stroke Statistics Subcommittee, *Circulation* 115:e69–e171, 2007.
5. Lucas FL, DeLorenzo MA, Siewers AE, et al: Temporal trends in the utilization of diagnostic testing and treatments for cardiovascular disease in the United States, *Circulation* 113:374–379, 2006.
6. Wennberg JE, Birkmeyer JD, Birkmeyer NJO, et al: *The Dartmouth Atlas of Cardiovascular Health Care,* Chicago, 1999, American Hospital Association Press.
7. Patel MR, Spertus JA, Brindis RG, et al: ACCF proposed method for evaluating the appropriateness of cardiovascular imaging, *J Am Coll Cardiol* 46:1606–1613, 2005.
8. Winslow CM, Solomon DH, Chassin MR, et al: The appropriateness of carotid endarterectomy, *N Engl J Med* 318:721–727, 1988.
9. Winslow CM, Kosecoff JB, Chassin M, et al: The appropriateness of performing coronary artery bypass surgery, *JAMA* 260:505–509, 1988.
10. Chassin MR, Kosecoff J, Park RE, et al: Does inappropriate use explain geographic variations in the use of health care services? A study of three procedures, *JAMA* 258:2533–2537, 1987.
11. American College of Radiology: *Appropriateness Criteria,* Reston, VA, 1995, American College of Radiology.
12. Brindis RG, Douglas PS, Hendel RC, et al: ACCF/ASNC appropriateness criteria for single-photon emission computed tomography myocardial perfusion imaging (SPECT MPI): a report of the American College of Cardiology Foundation Quality Strategic Directions Committee Appropriateness Criteria Working Group and the American Society of Nuclear Cardiology endorsed by the American Heart Association, *J Am Coll Cardiol* 46:1587–1605, 2005.
13. Hendel RC, Patel MR, Kramer CM, et al: ACCF/ACR/SCCT/SCMR/ASNC/NASCI/SCAI/SIR 2006 appropriateness criteria for cardiac computed tomography and cardiac magnetic resonance imaging: a report of the American College of Cardiology Foundation Quality Strategic Directions Committee Appropriateness Criteria Working Group, American College of Radiology, Society of Cardiovascular Computed Tomography, Society for Cardiovascular Magnetic Resonance, American Society of Nuclear Cardiology, North American Society for Cardiac Imaging, Society for Cardiovascular Angiography and Interventions, and Society of Interventional Radiology, *J Am Coll Cardiol* 48:1475–1497, 2006.
14. Douglas PS, Khandheria B, Stainback RF, et al: ACCF/ASE/ACEP/ASNC/SCAI/SCCT/SCMR 2007 appropriateness criteria for transthoracic and transesophageal echocardiography: a report of the American College of Cardiology Foundation Quality Strategic Directions Committee Appropriateness Criteria Working Group, American Society of Echocardiography, American College of Emergency Physicians, American Society of Nuclear Cardiology, Society for Cardiovascular Angiography and Interventions, Society of Cardiovascular Computed Tomography, and the Society for Cardiovascular Magnetic Resonance endorsed by the American College of Chest Physicians and the Society of Critical Care Medicine, *J Am Coll Cardiol* 50:187–204, 2007.
15. Douglas PS, Khandheria B, Stainback RF, et al: ACCF/ASE/ACEP/AHA/ASNC/SCAI/SCCT/SCMR 2008 appropriateness criteria for stress echocardiography, *J Am Coll Cardiol* 51:1127–1147, 2008.
16. Patel MR, Dehmer GJ, Hirshfeld JW, et al: ACCF/SCAI/STS/AATS/AHA/ASNC 2009 appropriateness criteria for coronary revascularization, *J Am Coll Cardiol* 53:530–553, 2009.
17. Fitch K, Bernstein SJ, Aguilar MS, et al: *The RAND/UCLA Appropriateness Method User's Manual,* Santa Monica, 2001, The RAND Corporation.
18. Gibbons RJ, Miller TD, Hodge DO, et al: Application of appropriateness criteria to stress single-photon emission computed tomography sestamibi studies and stress echocardiograms in an academic medical center, *J Am Coll Cardiol* 51:283–290, 2008.
19. Mehta R, Agarwal R, Chandra SW, et al: Evaluation of the ACCF/ASNC appropriateness criteria for SPECT myocardial perfusion imaging, *J Nucl Cardiol* 15:337–344, 2008.
20. Miller TD, Hendel RC: An appropriate challenge for the nuclear cardiology community, *J Nucl Cardiol* 15:305–307, 2008.
21. Ayyad AM, Cole J, Syed A, et al: Temporal trends in utilization of cardiac computed tomography, *J Cardiovasc Comput Tomogr* 3:16–21, 2009.
22. Ward RP, Mansour IN, Lemieux N, et al: Prospective evaluation of the clinical application of the American College of Cardiology Foundation/American Society of Echocardiography appropriateness criteria for

transthoracic echocardiography, *JACC Cardiovasc Imaging* 1:663–671, 2008.

23. McCully RB, Pellikka PA, Hodge DO, et al: Applicability of appropriateness criteria for stress imaging: Similarities and differences between stress echocardiography and single-photon emission computed tomography myocardial perfusion imaging (SPECT MPI) criteria, *Circ Cardiovasc Imaging* 2:213–218, 2009.

24. Ward RP, Al-Mallah MH, Grossman GB, et al: American Society of Nuclear Cardiology review of the ACCF/ASNC appropriateness criteria for single-photon emission computed tomography myocardial perfusion imaging (SPECT MPI), *J Nucl Cardiol* 14:e26–e38, 2007.

25. Askew JW, Miller TD, Hodge DO, et al: The value of myocardial perfusion single-photon emission computed tomography in screening asymptomatic patients with atrial fibrillation for coronary artery disease, *J Am Coll Cardiol* 50:1080–1085, 2007.

26. http://www.qualityforum.org/projects/ongoing. Last accessed April 26, 2008.

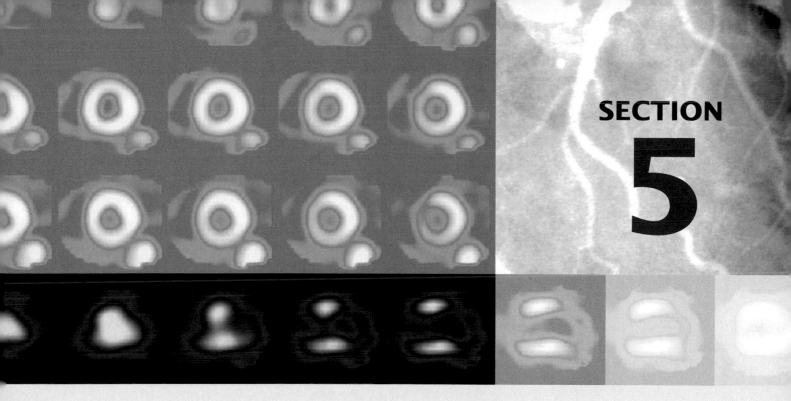

Disease/Gender-Specific Issues

Chapter 26

Imaging in Women

DONNA M. POLK, LAURA FORD-MUKKAMALA AND GARY V. HELLER

INTRODUCTION

Despite recent declines in the rates of cardiovascular deaths in women, cardiovascular disease (CVD) is the leading cause of mortality in women.[1] In the United States, more than 500,000 women each year will die of CVD, mostly coronary artery disease (CAD), more than in men (Fig. 26-1).[1] This is not just a disease of aging women. Ischemic heart disease is the number one killer of women at all ages, and the mortality for younger women is greater than for men. Women younger than age 75 have higher in hospital mortality post myocardial infarction (MI), and until the age of 60 have higher 2-year post-MI mortality.[2,3] There is a gap between these staggering statistics and a woman's perception of her own health risk. With campaigns aimed at increasing awareness of the risk of heart disease in women, the recognition of heart disease as a women's issue has improved, but in an American Heart Association (AHA) survey, only 13% of women identified CVD as their own greatest risk.[4] Only 38% of these women reported that they had had a discussion with their physician about their risk for CVD, thus providing an opportunity for education and assessment.[4]

Women often experience typical symptoms of CAD, but there are gender differences in both how women present with acute coronary syndromes and the symptoms they report. Despite the fact that women present more commonly with unstable angina than with ST elevation MI, they have a higher mortality than men.[5-9] Women appear to have less plaque rupture leading to ST elevation MI, and more plaque erosion resulting in unstable angina. In autopsy studies, women have less evidence of obstructive disease until the 7th decade of life.[10] Two-thirds of women have fatal MI without recognized prodromal symptoms as their initial presentation of CAD.[1] There is evidence that there are gender differences in pain perception, and this may contribute to the lack of specificity of typical anginal symptoms in women.[11,12] Contributing to the challenge in diagnosing CAD in women is the variability in the reporting of chest pain as the predominant symptom in women who present with CAD. In one study, Milner et al. reviewed 550 individuals (41% women) who had

evidence of ischemia or MI and found that both men and women reported chest pain with equal frequency.[13] Women, however, were more likely to report an increased number of symptoms that were atypical, such as mid back pain, nausea, vomiting, dyspnea, palpitations, and indigestion. This increased symptomatology likely contributes to the difficulty in obtaining an accurate diagnosis of CAD in women. Other studies support the higher frequency of atypical symptoms and less chest pain prior to presentation as well as at the time of diagnosis. Women were more likely to describe back pain, jaw pain, rest pain, pain related to mental stress, and pain that awoke them from sleep.[14-16] In a recent study, 515 women were surveyed 4 to 6 months post MI, and 43% did not describe any chest discomfort at the time of their MI.[17] They did, however, report atypical prodromal symptoms, including unusual fatigue, sleep disturbance, and shortness of breath during the month before their MI, with only a minority reporting chest discomfort (29.7%).[17] This variation in presentation and symptomatology has contributed to the difficulty in diagnosing heart disease in women and missed opportunities to diagnose and treat women with CAD.

Traditional risk factors for CAD are similar in men and women, but certain risk factors such as dyslipidemia and the presence of diabetes play a more important role in women. Elevated LDL levels play a central role in the development of CAD in both men and women, as evidenced by the linear relationship between LDL levels and risk for CAD. This is particularly true in women younger than 65 years of age.[18-20] For women, the risk associated with elevated triglycerides has been shown to be an independent predictor of risk for CAD.[21] Additionally, low HDL levels in women convey a greater risk than in men. For every 1 mg/dL increase in HDL, the risk of CAD decreases 3% in women, compared to 2% in men.[22] Notably, the risk for death from CAD was more than two times higher in women with HDL levels below 50 mg/dL compared to those with levels above 60 mg/dL.[18] Postmenopausal lipid levels are more atherogenic, with higher LDL and triglyceride levels and lower HDL levels.[23,24]

Although diabetes has a prevalence of 5% to 10% in both men and women, the risk for CVD is markedly

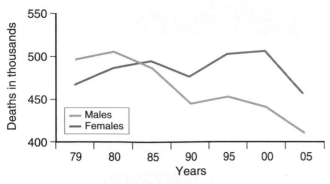

Figure 26-1 Cardiovascular disease mortality trends for males and females, United States (1979–2005). *(From NCHS and NHLBI.)*

higher in women. In a 20-year follow-up of the Framingham data, nondiabetic women had half the mortality rate of men.[25] Those *with* diabetes had death rates equal to men, a disproportionate increase in mortality.

Metabolic syndrome, characterized by central obesity, hypertension, impaired glucose tolerance, low HDL-C, and elevated triglycerides affects almost a quarter of U.S. women.[26] This dysmetabolic state increases the risk for the development of atherosclerosis and subsequent cardiovascular events.[27] In women with suspected ischemia, Marroquin and investigators for the Women's Ischemia Syndrome Evaluation (WISE) showed that there was a greater burden of atherosclerotic disease in those with metabolic syndrome compared to normal-metabolic women with angiographic evidence of disease (Fig. 26-2).[27] This evidence illustrates the increased risk associated with the dysmetabolic state and alerts us to focus on preventive strategies in women at risk.

While public awareness regarding the detrimental effects of tobacco appears to be increasing, the Surgeon General reported in 2001 that the overall rate of cigarette use in women is on the rise, particularly in younger, less educated women.[28] The Nurses' Health Study showed increased cardiovascular mortality with cigarette use, which declined after 10 years with smoking cessation.[29,30] Age-adjusted mortality rates were substantially increased in women with diabetes who also smoked. In comparison to nonsmokers, the relative risk (RR) of smokers of 1 to 14 cigarettes a day was 0.92.[29] This risk increased in a dose-dependent manner to an RR of 1.95 for those with a history of over 50 pack-years.[29] For diabetic patients who smoked more than 15 cigarettes a day, the RR of a cardiovascular event was 7.67.[30]

Because CVD is the leading cause of mortality in women, physicians need to be aware of the potential gender differences in the presentation, assessment, and treatment of cardiovascular risk and disease in women. The diagnosis of heart disease can be challenging in women; it is clear that noninvasive evaluation is effective for both diagnosis and prognostication. Detection and aggressive treatment of cardiovascular risk factors and disease are likely the most cost-effective way to reduce the heart disease epidemic in women.

DIAGNOSING CORONARY ARTERY DISEASE IN WOMEN

Diagnosis of CAD can be challenging in women, given the lower prevalence of obstructive disease, greater symptomatology, and lower functional capacity. Establishing the pretest likelihood of disease in a women is

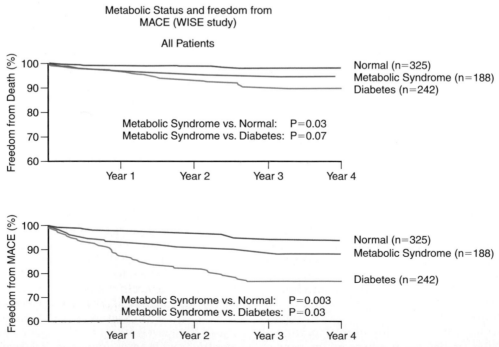

Figure 26-2 Event-free survival by metabolic status. *(From Marroquin OC, Kip KE, Kelley DE, et al., for the Women's Ischemia Syndrome Evaluation Investigators: Metabolic syndrome modifies the cardiovascular risk associated with angiographic coronary artery disease in women: A report from the Women's Ischemia Syndrome Evaluation, Circulation 109:714–721, 2004.)*

Table 26-1 The Effect of Age and the Presence of Symptoms on the Probability of Underlying Coronary Artery Disease in Men and Women

Age (Yr)	NONANGINAL CHEST PAIN		ATYPICAL ANGINA		TYPICAL ANGINA	
	Men	**Women**	**Men**	**Women**	**Men**	**Women**
30–39	5.7 ± 0.8	0.8 ± 0.3	21.8 ± 2.4	4.2 ± 1.3	69.7 ± 3.2	25.8 ± 6.6
40–49	14.1 ± 1.3	2.8 ± 0.7	46.1 ± 1.3	13.3 ± 2.9	87.3 ± 1.0	35.2 ± 6.5
50–59	21.5 ± 1.7	8.4 ± 1.9	58.9 ± 1.5	32.4 ± 3.0	92.3 ± 0.6	79.4 ± 2.4
60–69	21.1 ± 1.9	18.6 ± 1.9	67.1 ± 1.3	54.4 ± 2.4	94.3 ± 0.4	90.6 ± 1.0

key in the diagnosis of CAD, balancing the probability of false positives when the disease prevalence is low with the need to avoid unnecessary additional and/or invasive testing. Diamond and Forrester analyzed the pretest probability of CAD as well as sensitivity and specificity in patients undergoing exercise electrocardiography.[31] The prevalence of coronary disease by angiography was stratified into asymptomatic, nonanginal, atypical, and typical angina categories. Table 26-1 demonstrates interaction of gender and age with type of symptoms. Using this type of strategy can help further refine the likelihood of disease and hence direct

the most appropriate testing, such as cardiac catheterization for high-risk individuals and exercise tolerance testing for low-risk individuals. In the WISE study, this strategy was found to overestimate the degree of obstructive disease (Fig. 26-3).[32]

There is growing recognition that women can have anginal symptoms, evidence of ischemia by exercise or noninvasive testing, but no evidence of obstructive disease at the time of cardiac catheterization. In the WISE study, women who had evidence of ischemia on phosphorus-31 nuclear magnetic resonance spectroscopy stress testing and no evidence of obstructive CAD

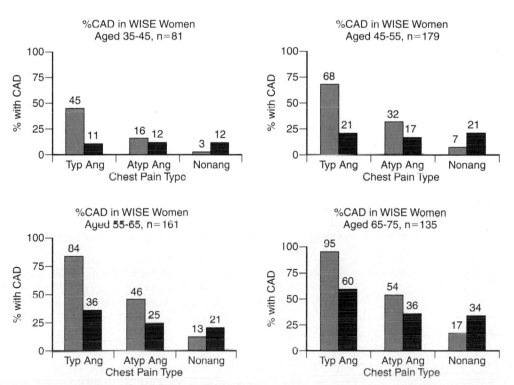

From the National Heart, Lung, and Blood Institute Women's Ischemia Syndrome Evaluation (WISE), the Diamond probability of coronary artery disease (CAD) as compared with observed coronary disease prevalence in symptomatic women ages 35 to 45, 46 to 55, 56 to 65, and 66 to 75 years

Figure 26-3 Diamond probability of coronary artery disease compared with observed coronary disease prevalence in symptomatic women in WISE study. *(From Shaw LJ, Bairey Merz CN, Pepine CJ, et al. Insights from the NHLBI sponsored Women's Ischemia Syndrome Evaluation (WISE) study. Part I: Gender differences in traditional and novel risk factors, symptom evaluation, and gender-optimized diagnostic strategies. J Am Coll Cardiol 47:S4–S20, 2006.)*

had higher rates of hospitalization for anginal symptoms, repeat catheterization, and overall costs.[32] Additional information from the WISE study showed that coronary microvascular dysfunction is seen in almost half of women with chest pain and nonobstructive disease.[33] This group of women present a challenge in both diagnosis and treatment.

Exercise Tolerance Testing

In symptomatic women in whom the presence of CAD is uncertain, exercise tolerance testing (ETT) is the simplest and least expensive testing modality. In certain populations, such as women with a low likelihood of CAD and low disease prevalence, this test is appropriate and is supported by current guidelines. In this group, a negative exercise electrocardiographic response with normal hemodynamics has been associated with a high negative predictive value.[34]

A major limitation of ETT is its compromised diagnostic accuracy (Table 26-2). A meta-analysis reported by Kwok and colleagues reported 15 studies with a sensitivity of 61% (range, 46% to 79%) and specificity of 69% (range, 51% to 86%).[35] These testing results suggest a limited value of ETT alone in the appropriate diagnosis of CAD in women. Additionally, the increased age in women on presentation is concomitant with functional impairment. This results in reduced exercise capacity and inability to complete a diagnostic stress test. Other factors contribute to ETT being suboptimal: resting ST-T wave changes in hypertensive women, lower electrocardiogram (ECG) voltage, and hormonal factors.[36-41] For example, endogenous estrogen has a digoxin-like effect, resulting in a false-positive ECG response, particularly midcycle when estrogen levels are highest.[42] In an effort to determine the most cost-effective way to identify women at high risk for CVD, the What is the Optimal Method for Ischemia Evaluation in Women (WOMEN) Study is being conducted with intermediate- and high-risk women with chest pain or equivalent symptoms suggestive of ischemic heart disease. The study's objective is to determine whether exercise ECG has the same negative predictive value for risk detection as gated myocardial perfusion single-photon emission computed tomography (SPECT) in women.[43] Currently, use of the Framingham Risk Score (FRS) to predict the presence of disease may underestimate the degree of atherosclerosis. In the Multi-Ethnic Study of Atherosclerosis (MESA), 32% of women classified as low risk by FRS had evidence of coronary artery calcium indicative of atherosclerotic disease.[44] These women also had higher rates of coronary artery disease and cardiovascular events.

Women with diabetes are of particular concern. It has been recognized that such patients are at heightened risk for premature as well as accelerated atherosclerosis, MI, and cardiac death.[1] It has also been reported that ECG is less reliable in diabetic patients,[45] so in diabetic women, ETT alone may be particularly misleading (see Chapter 22).

Despite these limitations, if exercise testing is to be used in women, interpretation of the test should include factors in addition to ST-T segment depression.[46,47] This should include parameters such as changes in ST/heart rate and the Duke Treadmill Score. Despite the described limitations, it should be also noted that the American Heart Association/American College of Cardiology (AHA/ACC) Guidelines recommend exercise testing in women with intermediate likelihood of CAD.[48] Generally, optimal diagnostic stress testing is assumed when a patient achieves 85% or greater of predicted maximal heart rate. However, in deconditioned women, a hyperexaggerated response may yield a rapid and marked increase in heart rate. The test should be continued, and if a female patient cannot achieve at least 5 metabolic equivalents (METs) of exercise, they should be considered a candidate for pharmacologic myocardial perfusion imaging.[38] Women with lower functional capacity have been found to have higher prevalence of cardiovascular risk factors, angiographic evidence of CAD, and adverse events compared to those with higher functional capacity.[49] Functional capacity is associated with better prognostic value than electrocardiographic evidence of ischemia.[50] Exercise capacity is an important predictor of cardiovascular outcome in women, and unless functional capacity is significantly limited, all stress testing should be done with exercise (Fig. 26-4).[38]

Table 26-2 Sensitivity and Specificity of Exercise Tolerance Testing in the Diagnosis of Coronary Artery Disease

| Study, Year | ANGIOGRAPHIC END POINT | | | | |
	Women (n)	Men (n)	Stenosis (%)	Sensitivity (%)	Specificity (%)
Detry et al., 1979*	47	231	≥50%	80 in women/87 in men	63 in women/74 in men
Weiner et al., 1979	580	1465	≥70 or ≥50 LM	76 in women/80 in men	64 in women/74 in men
Barolsky et al., 1979	92	85	≥75	60 in women/65 in men	68 in women/89 in men
Friedman et al., 1982	60	NA	≥70	32	41
Guiteras et al., 1982	112	NA	≥70	79	66
Hung et al., 1984	92	NA	≥70 or ≥50 LM	73	59
Morise et al., 1995	284	504	≥50	47 in women/56 in men	73 in women/81 in men
Miller et al., 2001	205	838	≥70 or ≥50 LM	53 in women/63 in men	69 in women/74 in men

*Included patients with and without history of myocardial infarction. All other studies cited excluded patients with history of myocardial infarction.
LM, left main coronary stenosis; NA, not applicable.

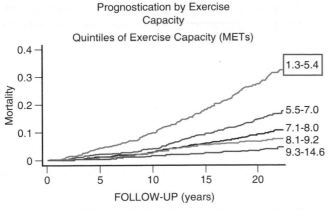

Prognostication by Exercise
Capacity
Quintiles of Exercise Capacity (METs)

Figure 26-4 Prognostication by exercise capacity. *(From Mora S, Redberg R, Cui Y, et al: Ability of exercise testing to predict cardiovascular and all-cause death in asymptomatic women: A 20-year follow-up of the Lipid Research Clinics Prevalence Study, JAMA 290:1600–1607, 2003.)*

Stress Myocardial Perfusion Imaging in Women

Stress myocardial perfusion imaging (MPI) was first developed to offset the limitations of ETT in the accurate diagnosis and location of CAD in patients. Using exercise as the stress modality, radionuclide perfusion imaging with thallium (Tl)-201 has been shown to have on average a sensitivity of 83% and specificity of 88% using planar imaging.[51] This represents approximately 20% to 25%, improvement in diagnostic accuracy in comparison to ETT alone. However, a considerable number of laboratories are now using SPECT and technetium (Tc)-99m-based imaging agents. SPECT imaging studies have been shown to be more accurate than planar imaging in the diagnosis of CAD and in separating single-vessel from multivessel disease.[51]

Of considerable importance, Stratman and colleagues demonstrated for all levels of exercise that Tc-99m-sestamibi SPECT imaging was significantly more sensitive in the detection of CAD than ECG with exercise data alone.[52] Several studies have noted improved diagnosis of multivessel disease in comparison with planar methods. Unfortunately, few studies are available in women alone.

Pharmacologic Myocardial Perfusion Imaging (See Chapter 15)

An important advantage of MPI is the ability to assess patients unable to complete adequate exercise. For such patients unable to achieve 85% maximally predicted heart rate, the diagnostic utility of the exercise ECG falls precipitously.[53–54] In such circumstances, MPI with pharmacologic stress provides an important and diagnostically useful alternative (see Chapter 14).

It has been estimated that 35% to 40% of all stress MPI is performed with pharmacologic stress. The most common pharmacologic type is that of vasodilator stress with either dipyridamole or adenosine. Pharmacologic vasodilator stress MPI has been shown to be comparable between dipyridamole and adenosine using either

planar or SPECT imaging.[55] Similar results have been reported with Tc-99m imaging agents.[56]

For women, Amanullah and colleagues found high sensitivity and moderate specificity ranges with adenosine in women despite their symptom complex. The sensitivity and specificity in nonanginal versus anginal symptoms was 93% and 69% versus 92% and 83%, respectively.[56] They then compared sensitivity and specificity with respect to pretest probability of CAD. The sensitivity ranged from 82% and increased to 95% with a high-likelihood status. Given the fact that woman's symptoms are more difficult to decipher clinically, these data support the use of adenosine MPI in evaluating symptomatic patients for CAD. Studies using another vasodilator, dipyridamole, have shown a sensitivity of 87% in women for detecting single-vessel disease.[55] A retrospective review of women and men who underwent dipyridamole with ^{99m}Tc-sestamibi and cardiac catheterization surprisingly demonstrated an improved sensitivity for detecting left anterior descending (LAD) disease in women compared to men.[57] These findings suggest the diagnostic accuracy of pharmacologic stress MPI is high regardless of the agent and should be used in women unable to exercise.

Dobutamine is an alternative for women with contraindications to vasodilator stress (reactive airway disease). This agent depends on a chronotropic response, and data suggest a similar accuracy to vasodilators. However, as with exercise, the accuracy of dobutamine is heart-rate dependent.[58] In general, then, both exercise and pharmacologic stress are superior to exercise ECG alone. In a review of the literature, Leppo found the diagnostic accuracy, including dobutamine, to be equivalent.[59]

GENDER-RELATED CHALLENGES IN THE DIAGNOSIS OF CORONARY ARTERY DISEASE

The previous section laid the groundwork for diagnostic accuracy of stress MPI. Unfortunately, over 75% of patients enrolled in these studies were men. Studies in a female population alone are less available but indicate a similar accuracy with a few notable exceptions.

Overall, accuracy with exercise MPI in women appears to be similar to that in men.[37,38] However, the identification of single-vessel CAD in women may be lower than in men.[60] Reasons for this are not clear, although the difference may relate to heart size. Hansen and colleagues analyzed men and women who underwent exercise ^{201}Tl stress tests.[60] Women were statistically more likely to have smaller chamber sizes. When chamber volumes were compared, larger chamber sizes correlated with better diagnostic accuracy (Fig. 26-5). When men and women with smaller chamber sizes were compared, diagnostic accuracy was similar but less than in those with larger chambers (Figs. 26-6 and 26-7). Whether there is a true gender difference within the smaller heart subset is unclear, owing to fewer numbers of men with small hearts. Speculation by the authors was made regarding

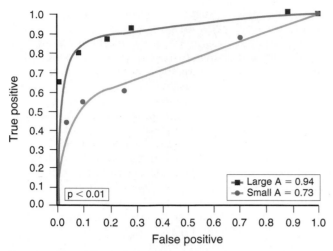

Figure 26-5 Effect of chamber size on diagnostic accuracy: ROC analysis of large versus small chamber demonstrating reduced accuracy with small hearts. ROC, receiver operating characteristic. *(From Hansen CL, Crabbe D, Rubin S: Lower diagnostic accuracy of thallium-201 SPECT myocardial perfusion imaging in women: An effect of smaller chamber size, J Am Coll Cardiol 28:1214–1219, 1996.)*

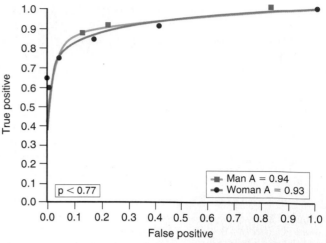

Figure 26-7 Effect of chamber size and gender on diagnostic accuracy. When men and women with large chamber size are compared, there is no statistical difference in accuracy. *(From Hansen CL, Crabbe D, Rubin S: Lower diagnostic accuracy of thallium-201 SPECT myocardial perfusion imaging in women: An effect of smaller chamber size, J Am Coll Cardiol 28:1214–1219, 1996.)*

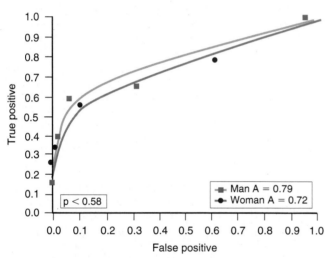

Figure 26-6 Effect of chamber size and gender on diagnostic accuracy. When men and women with small chamber size are compared, there is no statistical difference in accuracy. *(From Hansen CL, Crabbe D, Rubin S: Lower diagnostic accuracy of thallium-201 SPECT myocardial perfusion imaging in women: An effect of smaller chamber size, J Am Coll Cardiol 28:1214–1219, 1996.)*

the oversight of a lesion in a smaller heart, inasmuch as it may be less likely to be visualized in a small heart compared to a large heart. Thus, heart size may be a factor in diagnostic accuracy and appears to be an issue more frequently in women. Regardless of this limitation, data have shown a higher accuracy of exercise MPI for single-vessel disease over exercise alone.[37]

Attenuation artifact is a critical issue in the accurate diagnosis of CAD in patients, especially women. It is well recognized that attenuation artifact in nuclear cardiology procedures is commonplace, affecting overall accuracy and primary specificity. Common areas of attenuation artifact are in the anterior and inferior walls

(see Chapter 5). Attenuation artifact is often observed equally in stress and rest images, but reversible attenuation is also possible. For women, attenuation artifact is of considerable importance because it can commonly occur in the anterior wall from breast, as well as the inferior wall for multiple reasons, including pharmacologic stress (liver). Prior to the past several years, this resulted in reduced specificity, even in comparison with stress echocardiography.[35]

A meta-analysis compared exercise-ECG stress MPI and stress echo in 21 studies involving 4113 women.[35] While stress MPI was clearly superior to ETT alone, a reduced specificity in relation to stress echocardiography was suggested. Of importance, the perfusion studies included in the analysis were antiquated, not incorporating modern approaches to resolve attenuation artifact. It does point out the necessity of resolving attenuation artifact using appropriate and often newer techniques.

Solutions to attenuation artifact have centered on three approaches: prone imaging, ECG-gated SPECT imaging, and attenuation correction. The first, prone imaging, requires acquisition of SPECT perfusion data while the patient is in a prone position, and data are compared to supine imaging. The assumption is that inferior attenuation from diaphragm will be noted in the supine position "normalized" by prone imaging. Recent documentation supports this claim,[61] although it is unclear whether this can be applied to attenuation artifact from other sources such as liver or breast. It is theoretically valuable for both fixed or reversible attenuation artifacts in the inferior wall. It is also not clear how often an incomplete solution results from prone imaging.

ECG-gated SPECT imaging has also been used to distinguish attenuation artifact from CAD. Applied to fixed defects only, it is assumed that if wall motion is normal in the area of the perfusion abnormality, the perfusion abnormality is due to attenuation artifact. Conversely, if wall motion is abnormal, this is consistent with CAD, either stunned myocardium or prior MI. Taillefer and colleagues demonstrated the improved specificity in diagnosing coronary disease in women, utilizing gating to help differentiate attenuation from stunned or scarred myocardium.[40] In addition, two other studies involving 170 patients have confirmed the value of this technique in women.[34,52] In the study by Taillefer et al., the specificity of gated SPECT imaging was 92%, compared with 67% with nongated thallium studies in the same patients.[40] These results were both higher than the confidence intervals in regard to the specificity in the previously mentioned meta-analysis. This supports the enhanced diagnostic accuracy of gated SPECT imaging in women (Fig. 26-8).

A more recent approach to attenuation artifact uses attenuation correction with transmission line sources (usually gadolinium-100; see Chapters 6 and 7). This solution differs from ECG-gated SPECT in that both fixed and reversible attenuation artifact can be evaluated. Recent data from Bateman et al. and Links et al. demonstrated improved specificity in comparison with ECG-gated SPECT imaging in both genders.[62,63] Bateman reported an improved specificity for both genders and an improved normalcy rate in women.[63]

In summary, the use of stress MPI for the diagnosis of CAD in women is very important and provides substantially higher accuracy than ETT alone.[64] Using pharmacologic stress in appropriate patients is of considerable value in women, given the fact that CAD is more prevalent in a population less likely to complete adequate

exercise protocols. One limitation in comparison to men may be the ability to identify single-vessel disease in women, although further studies are necessary. Finally, attenuation artifact is a very important issue, and such solutions as ECG-gated SPECT imaging or attenuation correction are extremely important to use when assessing female patients. A very useful algorithm for the evaluation of women with suspected or known coronary disease is illustrated in Figure 26-9.[38]

RISK STRATIFICATION IN WOMEN (See Chapter 16)

The previous sections presented evidence that stress MPI, particularly with modern techniques like ECG-gated SPECT imaging and attenuation correction, can provide high diagnostic accuracy. Of equal importance is the ability to categorize a patient's risk of cardiac events such as nonfatal MI or cardiac death. MPI results have been shown in multiple investigations including over 22,000 patients to provide a powerful role in risk stratification (see Chapters 15 and 16). Data suggest that patients with normal stress MPI, particularly with exercise as the stress, have a low risk of cardiac events.[65,66] This risk is essentially the same as a normal population. Conversely, patients with abnormal studies[65] have a 12-fold higher annualized risk of a cardiac event[69] based on a review of 14 studies (Fig. 26-10). The general concept proposed is the size and severity of the perfusion abnormality is also related to risk of coronary events (Figs. 26-11 and 26-12).[67-70] Cardiac survival is also predicted by the number of ischemic vascular territories (Fig. 26-13).[70,72] These findings may help direct therapies. For example, those with normal studies most likely do not need further testing unless symptoms continue. Patients with low-risk images (one-vessel or mild perfusion abnormalities) may be adequately treated with aggressive medical therapies. An analysis by O'Keefe and colleagues supports this position, demonstrating excellent outcomes in patients with low-risk scans being treated solely with medical approaches.[73] Finally, patients with large or severe abnormalities are candidates for both revascularization and aggressive medical therapies.

The prognostic value of stress MPI has also been accumulating for women. Data in over 8000 women suggest the cardiac event rate in patients with normal stress myocardial perfusion results is less than 1%.[71,74-80] This low event rate has been found even in patients in whom a high pretest likelihood of CAD is present. Similarly, the revascularization in women with a normal perfusion study was very low. Similar to the general population, the size and severity of the perfusion abnormality also is associated with an increase in the higher cardiac event rate.[71,74-80] This appears to be true even in patients with a high pretest likelihood. As the extent of the perfusion abnormality increases, the rates for both MI and cardiac death increase four to sixfold. In women, both the size of the defect (summed stress score [SSS] > 22) and ejection fraction (EF) (<52%) are predictive of cardiac death, MI, or ventricular fibrillation (see Fig. 26-13).[81] An SSS of higher than 14 was predictive of all cardiac events,

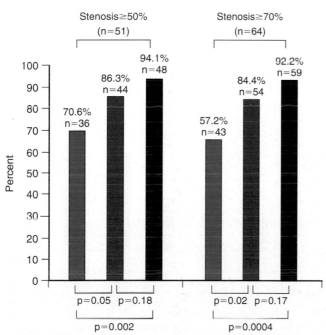

Figure 26-8 Specificity of Tl-201, Tc-99m-sestamibi perfusion, and gated SPECT studies for both patients without coronary artery disease and normal volunteers. Tc, thallium; Tl, thallium. *(From Taillefer R, DePuey EG, Udelson JE, et al: Comparative diagnostic accuracy of Tl-201 and Tc-99m sestamibi SPECT imaging [perfusion and ECG-gated SPECT] in detecting coronary artery disease in women, J Am Coll Cardiol 29:69-77, 1997.)*

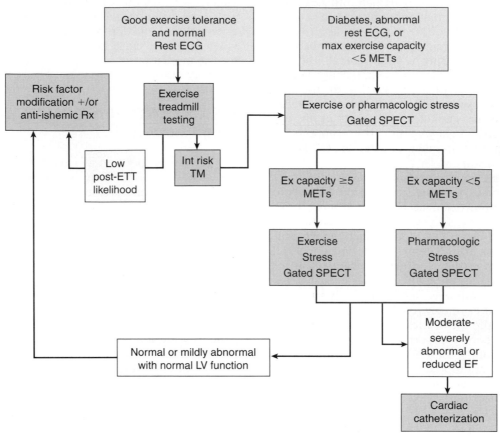

Intermediate–High Likelihood Women with Atypical or Typical Chest Pain Symptoms, Dyspnea, or Reduced Activities of Daily Living

Figure 26-9 Recommended algorithm for the evaluation of women with suspected or known coronary disease. *(From Mieres JH, Shaw LJ, Hendel RC, et al: A report of the American Society of Nuclear Cardiology Task Force on Women and Heart Disease [writing group on perfusion imaging in women], J Nucl Cardiol 10:95–101, 2003. Reprinted with permission from the American Society of Nuclear Cardiology.)*

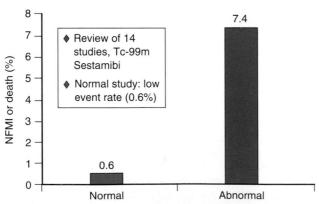

Figure 26-10 Prognostic significance of a normal study. *(From Iskander S, Iskandrian AE: Risk assessment using single-photon emission computed tomographic technetium-99m sestamibi imaging, J Am Coll Cardiol 32:57–62, 1998.)*

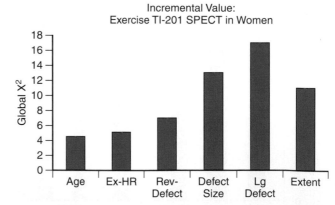

Figure 26-11 Incremental value of exercise thallium-201 SPECT in women. *(From Pancholy SB, Fattah AA, Kamal AM, et al: Independent and incremental prognostic value of exercise thallium single-photon emission computed tomographic imaging in women, J Nucl Cardiol 2(2 Pt 1):110–116, 1995.)*

including revascularization, in a series of 453 consecutive female patients. Additional data from nearly 900 patients referred for SPECT further support the prognostic role of EF in women, with high event rates occurring in those with lower EFs.[82] Women with hard events had larger end-systolic volume index (63 versus 35 mL/m^2) and end-diastolic volume index (106 versus 76 mL/m^2) compared to men, as well as lower EFs (<44%).[82]

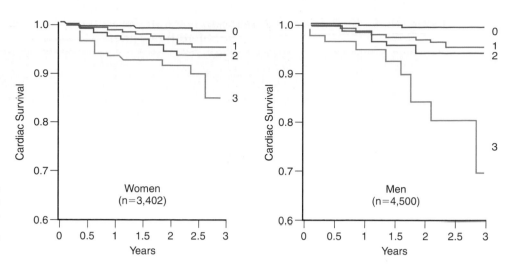

Figure 26-12 Cardiac survival by number of SPECT vascular territories with ischemia in women and men. *(From Marwick TH, Shaw LJ, Lauer MS, et al: The noninvasive prediction of cardiac mortality in men and women with known or suspected coronary artery disease. Economics of Noninvasive Diagnosis (END) Study Group, Am J Med 106:172–178, 1999.)*

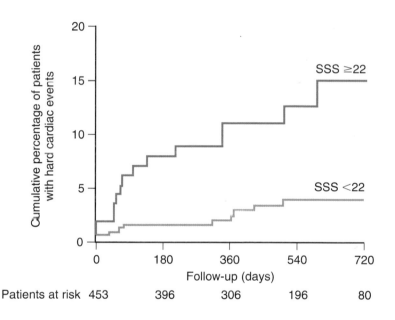

Figure 26-13 Relationship between extent of ischemia and cardiac events. *(From Ladenheim ML, Pollock BH, Rozanski A, et al: Extent and severity of myocardial hypoperfusion as predictors of prognosis in patients with suspected coronary artery disease, J Am Coll Cardiol 7:464–471, 1986.)*

Referral for catheterization appears to have shifted more recently and appears to be based on imaging results rather than solely upon the gender of the patient.[79]

Clinical factors have been found to also be important predictors of cardiac events. However, in the setting of risk factors, the severity and extent of the perfusion abnormality still independently predict cardiac events. Incremental chi-square analysis has demonstrated a significantly greater ability to predict coronary events, even in the presence of clinical rest or ECG stress data.

Women with diabetes mellitus constitute a very high-risk population, even in comparison to men with the same disorder.[83–85] Several studies have now demonstrated the prognostic value of SPECT MPI (Fig. 26-14).[73,86,87] Given the severity of perfusion abnormality, the presence of diabetes mellitus was associated with a significantly higher event rate when compared with men (Table 26-3 and Fig. 26-15).[87] In this multivariable analysis, gender was no longer an independent predictor of coronary events,

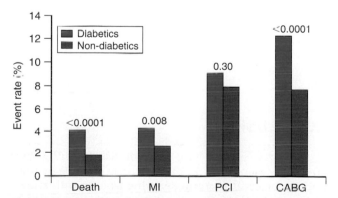

Figure 26-14 Outcomes of cardiac death, MI, PCI, and CABG in diabetics versus nondiabetics. CABG, coronary artery bypass graft; MI, myocardial infarction; PCI, percutaneous coronary intervention. *(From Giri S, Shaw LJ, Murthy DK, et al: Impact of diabetes on the risk stratification using stress single-photon emission computed tomography myocardial perfusion imaging in patients with symptoms suggestive of coronary artery disease, Circulation 105:32–40, 2002.)*

Table 26-3 Kaplan-Meier 3-Year Survival Rate for Patients With and Without Diabetes Stratified by Gender*

| | DEATH | | | DEATH | | |
Group	0-Vessel Ischemia	1-Vessel Ischemia	≥2-Vessel Ischemia	0-Vessel Ischemia	1-Vessel Ischemia	≥2-Vessel Ischemia
Diabetic men	93.75	93.0	91.25	96.26	77.0	79.0
Nondiabetic men	99.0	86.5	95.0	93.75	88.0	85.0
Diabetic women	99.0	88.0[†]	81.25[†]	96.50	72.50[†]	60.00[†]
Nondiabetic women	98.75	97.50	97.0	95.50	85.00	77.50

*Demonstrating lowest survival rates for diabetic women for any given extent of myocardial ischemia. Extent of ischemia was determined by the number of vascular territories (0, 1, or ≥ 2 vessel) involved in the reversible perfusion defect.
†$P < 0.05$.

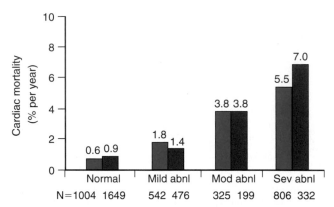

Figure 26-15 Annual rates of cardiac death in women and men as a function of myocardial perfusion single-photon emission computed tomography results. *(From Berman DS, Kang X, Hayes SW, et al: Adenosine myocardial perfusion single-photon emission computed tomography in women compared with men: Impact of diabetes mellitus on incremental prognostic value and effect on patient management, J Am Coll Cardiol 41:1125–1133, 2003.)*

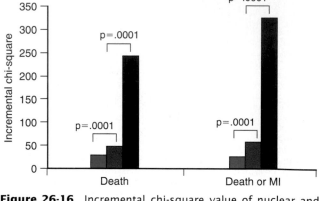

Figure 26-16 Incremental chi-square value of nuclear and clinical variables in the prediction of cardiac death or cardiac death/myocardial infarction in diabetic patients. *(From Giri S, Shaw LJ, Murthy DK, et al: Impact of diabetes on the risk stratification using stress single-photon emission computed tomography myocardial perfusion imaging in patients with symptoms suggestive of coronary artery disease, Circulation 105:32–40, 2002.)*

whereas severity of the perfusion abnormality was. In addition to the clinical risk assessment and the presence of diabetes mellitus, the addition of nuclear imaging added significantly to risk stratification (Fig. 26-16). Beyond the presence or absence of diabetes mellitus, the type of diabetes also played a role in the overall prognosis (Fig. 26-17).[86]

CONCLUSIONS

In summary, women face a major risk for CVD; over 50% of women die from this disorder. The role of stress MPI has been discussed in assessing women with known or suspected CAD. Previous limitations with regard to attenuation artifact have now been conquered with the use of ECG-gated SPECT imaging and attenuation correction. The role of risk stratification in women has now been elucidated. These data suggest that stress MPI is an effective tool in the evaluation of women with known or suspected CAD.

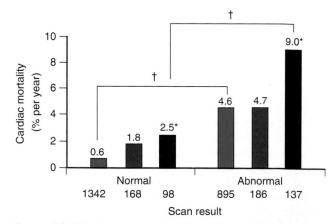

Figure 26-17 Cardiac mortality in patients without diabetes mellitus, with non-insulin-dependent diabetes mellitus, and with insulin-dependent diabetes mellitus. *(From Berman DS, Kang X, Hayes SW, et al: Adenosine myocardial perfusion single-photon emission computed tomography in women compared with men: Impact of diabetes mellitus on incremental prognostic value and effect on patient management, J Am Coll Cardiol 41:1125–1133, 2003.)*

REFERENCES

1. American Heart Association and National Center on Health Statistics: *Heart Disease and Stroke Statistics–2004 Update*, Dallas, TX, 2004, National Heart, Lung and Blood Institute.
2. Vaccarino V, Krumholz HM, Yarzebski J, Gore JM, Goldberg RJ: Sex differences in 2-year mortality after hospital discharge for myocardial infarction, *Ann Intern Med* 134:173–181.
3. Robinson K, Conroy RM, Mulcahy R, Hickey N: The 15-year prognosis of a first acute coronary episode in women, *Eur Heart J* 13:67–69, 1992.
4. Mosca L, Ferris A, Fabunmi R, Robertson RM: Tracking women's awareness of heart disease: An American Heart Association National Study, *Circulation* 190:573–579, 2004.
5. Lerner DJ, Kannel WB: Patterns of coronary artery disease morbidity and mortality in the sexes: a 26-year follow-up of the Framingham population, *Am Heart J* 111:383–390, 1986.
6. Hochman JS, McCabe CH, Stone PH, et al: Outcome and profile of women and men presenting with acute coronary syndromes: A report from TIMI IIIB, *J Am Coll Cardiol* 30:141–148, 1997.
7. Hochman JS, Tamis JE, Thompson TD, et al: Sex, clinical presentation and outcome in patients with acute coronary syndromes, *N Engl J Med* 341:226–232[1], 1999.
8. Marrugat J, Sala J, Malia R, et al: Mortality differences between men and women following first myocardial infarction, *JAMA* 2801:1405–1409, 1998.
9. Chang WC, Kaul P, Westerhout CM, et al: Impact of sex on long-term mortality from acute myocardial infarction vs unstable angina, *Arch Intern Med* 163:2476–2484, 2003.
10. Shaw LJ, Shaw RE, Radford M, et al: for the ACC-National Cardiovascular Data Registry: Sex and ethnic differences in the prevalence of significant and severe coronary artery disease in the ACC-National Cardiovascular Data Registry, *Circulation* 110: SIII800, 2004.
11. Rollman GB, Lauterbacher S, Jones KS: Sex and gender differences in responses to experimentally induced pain in humans. In Fillingham RB, editor: *Sex, Gender and Pain*, vol 17, Seattle, 2001, International Association for the Study of Pain.
12. Sheps DS, McMahon RP, Light KC, et al: Low hot pain threshold predicts shorter time to exercise-induced angina: results from the psychophysiological investigations of myocardial ischemia (PIMI) study, *J Am Coll Cardiol* 33:1855–1862, 1999.
13. Milner KA, Funk M, Richards S, Wilmes RM, Vaccarino V, Krumholz HM: Gender differences in symptom presentation associated with coronary heart disease, *Am J Cardiol* 84:396–399, 1999.
14. Culic V, Eterovic D, Dinko M, Rumboldt Z, Izet H: Gender differences in triggering of acute myocardial infarction, *Am J Cardiol* 85:753–756, 2000.
15. Goldberg RJ, O'Donnell C, Yarzebski J, Bigelow C, Savageau J, Gore JM: Sex differences in symptom presentation associated with acute myocardial infarction: A population-based perspective, *Am Heart J* 136:189–195, 1998.
16. Kudenchuk PJ, Maynard C, Martin JS, Wirkus M, Weaver WD: Comparison of presentation, treatment and outcomes of acute myocardial infarction in men versus women (the Myocardial Infarction Triage and Intervention Registry), *Am J Cardiol* 78:9–14, 1996.
17. McSweeney JC, Cody M, O'Sullivan P, Elberson K, Moser DK, Garvin BJ: Women's early warning symptoms of acute myocardial infarction, *Circulation* 108:2619–2623, 2004.
18. Manolio TA, Pearson TA, Wenger NK, Barrett-Connor E, Payne GH, Harlan WH: Cholesterol and heart disease in older persons and women: Review of an NHLBI workshop, *Ann Epidemiol* 2:161–176, 1992.
19. Stamier J, Wentworth D, Neaton JD: for the MRFIT Research Group: Is relationship between serum cholesterol and risk for premature death from coronary heart disease continuous and graded? Findings in 356,222 primary screenees of the Multiple Risk Factor Intervention Trial (MRFIT), *JAMA* 256:2823–2828, 1986.
20. Gordon T, Castelli WP, Hjortland MC, Kannel WB, Dawber TR: High density lipoprotein as a protective factor against coronary heart disease. The Framingham Study, *Am J Med* 62:707–714, 1977.
21. Castelli WP: Cholesterol and lipids in the risk of coronary artery disease- the Framingham Heart Study, *Can J Cardiol* 4:5A–10A, 1988.
22. Gordon DJ, Probstfield JL, Barrison RJ, et al: High-density lipoprotein cholesterol and cardiovascular disease in men and women. Four prospective American studies, *Circulation* 79:8–15, 1989.
23. Stevenson JC, Crook D, Godsland IF: Influence of age and menopause on serum lipids and lipoproteins in healthy women, *Atherosclerosis* 98:83–90, 1993.
24. Jenner JL, Ordovas JM, Lamon-Fava S, et al: Effects f age, sex and menopausal status on plasma lipoprotein(a) levels. The Framingham Offspring Study, *Circulation* 87:1135–1141, 1993.
25. Hu FB, Stampfer MJ, Solomon CG, et al: The impact of diabetes mellitus on mortality from all causes and coronary heart disease in women, *Arch Intern Med* 161:1717–1723, 2001.
26. Ford ES, Giles WH, Dietz Wh: Prevalence of the metabolic syndrome among US adults: findings from the third National Health and Nutrition Examination Survey, *JAMA* 287:356–359, 2002.
27. Marroquin OC, Kip KE, Kelley DE, et al: for the Women's Ischemia Syndrome Evaluation Investigators: Metabolic syndrome modifies the cardiovascular risk associated with angiographic coronary artery disease in women: A report from the Women's Ischemia Syndrome Evaluation, *Circulation* 109:714–721, 2004.
28. *Survey by ADA and AHA*, 2001.
29. Al Delaimy WK, Willett WC, Manson JE, et al: Smoking and mortality among women with type 2 diabetes: The Nurses' Health Study cohort, *Diabetes Care* 24(12):2043–2048, 2001.
30. Al Delaimy WK, Manson JE, Solomon CG, et al: Smoking and risk of coronary heart disease among women with type 2 diabetes mellitus, *Arch Intern Med* 162(3):273–279, 2002.
31. Diamond GA, Forrester JS: Analysis of probability as an aid in the clinical diagnosis of coronary-artery disease, *N Engl J Med* 300(24): 1350–1358, 1979.
32. Shaw LJ, Bairey Merz CN, Pepine CJ, et al: Insights from the NHLBI-sponsored Women's Ischemia Syndrome Evaluation (WISE) study. Part I: Gender differences in traditional and novel risk factors, symptom evaluation, and gender-optimized diagnostic strategies, *J Am Coll Cardiol* 47:S4–S20, 2006.
33. Reis SE, Holubkov R, Conrad Smith AJ, et al: Coronary microvascular dysfunction in women is highly prevalent in women with chest pain in the absence of coronary artery disease: results from the NHLBI WISE study, *Am Heart J* 141:735–741, 2001.
34. Santana-Boado C, Candell-Riera J, Castell-Conesa J, et al: Diagnostic accuracy of technetium-99m-MIBI myocardial SPECT in women and men [commentary], *J Nucl Med* 39(5):751–755, 1998.
35. Kwok Y, Kim C, Grady D, et al: Meta-analysis of exercise testing to detect coronary artery disease in women [commentary], *Am J Cardiol* 83(5):660–666, 1999.
36. Arruda-Olson AM, Juracan EM, Mahoney DW, et al: Prognostic value of exercise echocardiography in 5,798 patients: Is there a gender difference? *J Am Coll Cardiol* 39(4):625–631, 2002.
37. Friedman TD, Greene AC, Iskandrian AS, et al: Exercise thallium-201 myocardial scintigraphy in women: Correlation with coronary arteriography, *Am J Cardiol* 49(7):1632–1637, 1982.
38. Mieres JH, Shaw LJ, Hendel RC, et al: A report of the American Society of Nuclear Cardiology Task Force on Women and Heart Disease (writing group on perfusion imaging in women), *J Nucl Cardiol* 10(1): 95–101, 2003.
39. Schmermund A, Erbel R, Silber S: Age and gender distribution of coronary artery calcium measured by four-slice computed tomography in 2,030 persons with no symptoms of coronary artery disease, *Am J Cardiol* 90(2):168–173, 2002.
40. Taillefer R, DePuey EG, Udelson JE, et al: Comparative diagnostic accuracy of Tl-201 and Tc-99m sestamibi SPECT imaging (perfusion and ECG-gated SPECT) in detecting coronary artery disease in women, *J Am Coll Cardiol* 29(1):69–77, 1997.
41. White MP: Pharmacologic stress testing: Understanding the options, *J Nucl Cardiol* 6(6):672–675, 1999.
42. Morise AP, Dalal JN, Duval RD: Value of a simple measure of estrogen status for improving the diagnosis of coronary artery disease in women, *Am J Med* 94(5):491–496, 1993.
43. Mieres JH, Shaw LJ, Hendel RC, et al: The WOMEN Study: What is the Optimal Method for Ischemia Evaluation in WomeN? A multi-center, prospective, randomized study to establish the optimal method for detection of coronary artery disease (CAD) risk in women at an intermediate-high pretest likelihood of CAD: study design, *J Nucl Cardiol* 16:105–112, 2009.
44. Lakoski SG, Greenland P, Wong ND, et al: Coronary artery calcium scores and risk for cardiovascular events in women classified as "low risk" based on Framingham risk score. The Multi-Ethnic Study of Atherosclerosis (MESA), *Arch Intern Med* 167(22):2437–2442, 2007.
45. Nesto RW, Phillips RT, Kett KG, et al: Angina and exertional myocardial ischemia in diabetic and nondiabetic patients: assessment by exercise thallium scintigraphy [erratum appears in Ann Intern Med 108 (4):646, 1988], *Ann Intern Med* 108(2).170–175, 1988.
46. Alexander KP, Shaw LJ, Shaw LK, et al: Value of exercise treadmill testing in women [erratum appears in J Am Coll Cardiol 1999 Jan;33 (1):289], *J Am Coll Cardiol* 32(6):1657–1664, 1998.
47. Okin PM, Kligfield P: Gender-specific criteria and performance of the exercise electrocardiogram, *Circulation* 92(5):1209–1216, 1995.
48. Gibbons RJ, Balady GJ, Bricker JT, et al: ACC/AHA 2002 guideline update for exercise testing: summary article. A report of the American College of Cardiology/American Heart Association Task Force on Practice Guidelines (Committee to Update the 1997 Exercise Testing Guidelines), *J Am Coll Cardiol* 40(8):1531–1540, 2002.
49. Wessel TR, ARant CV, Olson MB, et al: Relationship of physical fitness vs body mass index with coronary artery disease and cardiovascular events in women, *JAMA* 292:1179–1187, 2004.

50. Gulati M, Pandy DK, Arnsdorf MF, et al: Exercise capacity and the risk of death in women: the St. James Women Take Heart Project, *Circulation* 108:1554–1559, 2003.

51. Goodgold HM, Rehder JG, Samuels LD, et al: Improved interpretation of exercise Tl-201 myocardial perfusion scintigraphy in women: Characterization of breast attenuation artifacts, *Radiology* 165(2):361–366, 1987.

52. Stratmann HG, Williams GA, Wittry MD, et al: Exercise technetium-99m sestamibi tomography for cardiac risk stratification of patients with stable chest pain, *Circulation* 89(2):615–622, 1994.

53. Heller GV, Ahmed I, Tilkemeier PL, et al: Comparison of chest pain, electrocardiographic changes, and thallium-201 scintigraphy during varying exercise intensities in men with stable angina pectoris, *Am J Cardiol* 68:569–574, 1999.

54. Heller GV, Ahmed I, Tilkemeier PL, et al: Influence of exercise intensity upon the presence, distribution and size of thallium-201 defect, *Am Heart J* 123:909–916, 1992.

55. Navare SM, Kapetanopoulos A, Heller GV: Pharmacologic radionuclide myocardial perfusion imaging, *Curr Cardiol Rep* 5(1):16–24, 2003.

56. Amanullah AM, Kiat H, Friedman JD, et al: Adenosine technetium-99m sestamibi myocardial perfusion SPECT in women: Diagnostic efficacy in detection of coronary artery disease, *J Am Coll Cardiol* 27 (4):803–809, 1996.

57. Travin MI, Katz MS, Moulton AW, et al: Accuracy of dipyridamole SPECT imaging in identifying individual coronary stenoses and multivessel disease in women versus men, *J Nucl Cardiol* 7(3):213–220, 2000.

58. Shehata AR, Gillam LD, Mascitelli VA, et al: Impact of acute propranolol administration on dobutamine-induced myocardial ischemia as evaluated by myocardial profusion imaging and echocardiography, *Am J Cardiol* 80:268–272, 1997.

59. Leppo JA: Comparison of pharmacologic steroagents, *J Nucl Cardiol* 3(6 Pt 2):522–526, 1996.

60. Hansen CL, Crabbe D, Rubin S: Lower diagnostic accuracy of thallium-201 SPECT myocardial perfusion imaging in women: An effect of smaller chamber size, *J Am Coll Cardiol* 28(5):1214–1219, 1996.

61. Hayes SW, De Lorenzo A, Hachamovitch R, et al: Prognostic implications of combined prone and supine acquisitions in patients with equivocal or abnormal supine myocardial perfusion SPECT, *J Nucl Med* 44:1633–1640, 2003.

62. Bateman TM, Heller GV, Johnson LL, et al: Does attenuation correction add value to non-attenuation corrected ECG-gated technetium-99m sestamibi SPECT? [abstract], *J Nucl Cardiol* 10:S91, 2003.

63. Links JM, DePuey EG, Taillefer R, et al: Attenuation correction and gating synergistically improve the diagnostic accuracy of myocardial perfusion SPECT, *J Nucl Cardiol* 9(2):183–187, 2002.

64. Iskandrian AE, Heo J, Nallamothu N: Detection of coronary artery disease in women with use of stress single-photon emission computed tomography myocardial perfusion imaging, *J Nucl Cardiol* 4(4):329–335, 1997.

65. Iskander S, Iskandrian AE: Risk assessment using single-photon emission computed tomographic technetium-99m sestamibi imaging, *J Am Coll Cardiol* 32(1):57–62, 1998.

66. Gibbons RJ, Hodge DO, Berman DS, et al: Long-term outcome of patients with intermediate-risk exercise electrocardiograms who do not have myocardial perfusion defects on radionuclide imaging, *Circulation* 100(21):2140–2145, 1999.

67. Heller GV, Herman SD, Travin MI, et al: Independent prognostic value of intravenous dipyridamole with technetium-99m sestamibi tomographic imaging in predicting cardiac events and cardiac-related hospital admissions, *J Am Coll Cardiol* 26(5):1202–1208, 1995.

68. Galassi AR, Azzarelli S, Tomaselli A, et al: Incremental prognostic value of technetium-99m-tetrofosmin exercise myocardial perfusion imaging for predicting outcomes in patients with suspected or known coronary artery disease, *Am J Cardiol* 88(2):101–106, 2001.

69. Vanzetto G, Ormezzano O, Fagret D, et al: Long-term additive prognostic value of thallium-201 myocardial perfusion imaging over clinical and exercise stress test in low to intermediate risk patients: Study in 1137 patients with 6-year follow-up, *Circulation* 100(14):1521–1527, 1999.

70. Ladenheim ML, Pollock BH, Rozanski A, et al: Extent and severity of myocardial hypoperfusion as predictors of prognosis in patients with suspected coronary artery disease, *J Am Coll Cardiol* 7(3):464–471, 1986.

71. Pancholy SB, Fattah AA, Kamal AM, et al: Independent and incremental prognostic value of exercise thallium single-photon emission computed tomographic imaging in women, *J Nucl Cardiol* 2(2 Pt 1):110–116, 1995.

72. Marwick TH, Shaw LJ, Lauer MS, et al: The noninvasive prediction of cardiac mortality in men and women with known or suspected coronary artery disease. Economics of Noninvasive Diagnosis (END) Study Group, *Am J Med* 106(2):172–178, 1999.

73. O'Keefe JH Jr, Bateman TM, Ligon RW, et al: Outcome of medical versus invasive treatment strategies for non-high-risk ischemic heart disease [commentary], *J Nucl Cardiol* 5(1):28–33, 1998.

74. Cacciabaudo JM, Hachamovitch R: Stress myocardial perfusion SPECT in women: Is it the cornerstone of the noninvasive evaluation? [commentary], *J Nucl Med* 39(5):756–759, 1998.

75. Hachamovitch R, Berman DS, Kiat H, et al: Effective risk stratification using exercise myocardial perfusion SPECT in women: Gender-related differences in prognostic nuclear testing, *J Am Coll Cardiol* 28(1):34–44, 1996.

76. Machecourt J, Longere P, Fagret D, et al: Prognostic value of thallium-201 single-photon emission computed tomographic myocardial perfusion imaging according to extent of myocardial defect. Study in 1,926 patients with follow-up at 33 months, *J Am Coll Cardiol* 23(5):1096–1106, 1994.

77. Stratmann HG, Tamesis BR, Younis LT, et al: Prognostic value of dipyridamole technetium-99m sestamibi myocardial tomography in patients with stable chest pain who are unable to exercise, *Am J Cardiol* 73(9):647–652, 1994.

78. Amanullah AM, Kiat H, Hachamovitch R, et al: Impact of myocardial perfusion single-photon emission computed tomography on referral to catheterization of the very elderly. Is there evidence of gender-related referral bias, *J Am Coll Cardiol* 28(3):680–686, 1996.

79. Travin MI, Duca MD, Kline GM, et al: Relation of gender to physician use of test results and to the prognostic value of stress technetium 99m sestamibi myocardial single-photon emission computed tomography scintigraphy, *Am Heart J* 134(1):73–82, 1997.

80. Barrett-Connor EL, Cohn BA, Wingard DL, et al: Why is diabetes mellitus a stronger risk factor for fatal ischemic heart disease in women than in men? The Rancho Bernardo Study. [erratum appears in JAMA 1991 Jun 26;265(24):3249], *JAMA* 265(5):627–631, 1991.

81. America YG, Bax JJ, Boersma E, et al: The additive prognostic value of perfusion and functional data assessed by quantitative gated SPECT in women, *J Nucl Cardiol* 16:10–19, 2009.

82. Wexler O, Yoder SR, Elder JL, et al: Effect of gender on cardiovascular risk stratification with ECG gated SPECT left ventricular volume indices and ejection fraction, *J Nucl Cardiol* 16:28–37, 2009.

83. Heyden S, Heiss G, Bartel AG, et al: Sex differences in coronary mortality among diabetics in Evans County, Georgia, *J Chron Dis* 33(5):265–273, 1980. Kannel WB, McGee DL: Diabetes and glucose tolerance as risk factors for cardiovascular disease: The Framingham study, *Diabetes Care* 2(2):120–126, 1979.

84. Pan WH, Cedres LB, Liu K, et al: Relationship of clinical diabetes and asymptomatic hyperglycemia to risk of coronary heart disease mortality in men and women, *Am J Epidemiol* 123(3):504–516, 1986.

85. Giri S, Shaw LJ, Murthy DR, et al: Impact of diabetes on the risk stratification using stress single-photon emission computed tomography myocardial perfusion imaging in patients with symptoms suggestive of coronary artery disease, *Circulation* 105(1):32–40, 2002.

86. Berman DS, Kang X, Hayes SW, et al: Adenosine myocardial perfusion single-photon emission computed tomography in women compared with men. Impact of diabetes mellitus on incremental prognostic value and effect on patient management, *J Am Coll Cardiol* 41(7):1125–1133, 2003.

87. Mora S, Redberg R, Cui Y, et al: Ability of exercise testing to predict cardiovascular and all-cause death in asymptomatic women: A 20 year follow-up of the Lipid Research Clinics Prevalence Study, *JAMA* 290:1600–1607, 2003.

Imaging for Preoperative Risk Stratification

SETH T. DAHLBERG AND JEFFREY A. LEPPO

INTRODUCTION

The evaluation of preoperative cardiac risk in patients undergoing noncardiac surgery has been a challenging and important topic over the past 25 years. The incidence of perioperative cardiac mortality has declined in recent years, but the prevalence of both coronary artery disease (CAD) and noncardiac surgical procedures in the United States[1,2] is predicted to significantly increase over the next 30 years. Therefore, preoperative evaluation for cardiac risk will continue to be an important issue for surgeons, cardiologists, and medical consultants.[2-6]

This chapter will review the use of nuclear cardiology myocardial perfusion imaging (MPI) for preoperative and long-term risk stratification, including recommendations from the recently revised 2007 Guidelines on Perioperative Cardiovascular Evaluation and Care for Noncardiac Surgery[2] for which patients benefit from preoperative imaging. The recommendations for preoperative risk assessment in the current Guidelines are also included in the recent American College of Cardiology/American Heart Association SPECT (single-photon emission computed tomography) Appropriateness criteria.[7] Although controlled prospective randomized clinical trials are lacking, there are many retrospective reports and a few meta-analyses that demonstrate the utility of MPI in this evaluation process. We will focus on the evaluation of ischemia and left ventricular (LV) function, both of which have been shown to have significant prognostic utility for cardiac events such as myocardial infarction (MI) or cardiac death[8] in patients with CAD. The issues of perioperative medical therapy and revascularization will also be reviewed.

The 2007 revised Guidelines divide preoperative clinical cardiac risk assessment into five steps.[2] Overall clinical risk is determined by individual patient risk factors, the risk of the surgical procedure, and the patient's functional capacity. This initial clinical evaluation can determine which patients may warrant further risk stratification with stress MPI.

STEP ONE: DETERMINE THE URGENCY OF THE SURGERY

Evaluation of patients who must undergo emergency surgery is generally limited to identifying and managing active cardiac conditions. However, after surgical recovery, it may be helpful to complete a more thorough evaluation, including stress MPI when appropriate, in those patients with significant cardiac problems. While this may not impact immediate perioperative treatment, such an evaluation can assist in long-term cardiac management. Communication with the referring primary care physician and cardiologist is an important aspect of this evaluation.

STEP TWO: EVALUATE AND TREAT ACTIVE CARDIAC CONDITIONS

The next step is to identify and treat active cardiac conditions, including acute coronary syndrome, recent MI, decompensated congestive heart failure (CHF), significant arrhythmia, and severe valvular heart disease. These conditions will often lead to delay or cancellation of elective surgery and may warrant cardiac catheterization. If bleeding, stroke, or renal disease increase the risk of coronary angiography, MPI can be a useful strategy for risk stratification after initial treatment. When percutaneous coronary intervention (PCI) is indicated, the timing of the noncardiac surgery with its associated risk of perioperative stent thrombosis will affect the choice of balloon angioplasty or bare metal or drug-eluting stent.

Table 27-1 Risk associated with Various Types of Surgery[2]

High Surgical Risk:
Aortic and other major vascular surgery
Peripheral vascular surgery
Intermediate Surgical Risk:
Carotid endarterectomy
Head and neck surgery
Intraperitoneal and intrathoracic surgery
Orthopedic surgery
Prostate surgery
Low Surgical Risk:
Endoscopic procedures
Superficial procedures
Cataract surgery
Breast surgery
Ambulatory surgery

STEP THREE: DETERMINE WHETHER THE PLANNED PROCEDURE IS LOW-RISK SURGERY

The type of surgery has an important impact on perioperative risk. In Table 27-1,[2] the major types of surgical procedures are divided into high-, intermediate-, and low-risk groups. High-risk surgery, with a combined perioperative MI/cardiac death rate greater than 5%, includes major vascular, aortic, and peripheral vascular surgery that often warrants preoperative assessment with MPI. Intermediate-risk surgery includes intrathoracic, intraperitoneal, orthopedic, prostate, and head/neck surgery. Low-risk surgery includes superficial, endoscopic, breast, cataract, and ambulatory surgery. An important change in the 2007 Guidelines is the recognition that preoperative MPI rarely changes management of patients undergoing low-risk surgery, even in patients with clinical risk factors and poor functional capacity. Therefore, low-risk procedures can generally be performed without additional preoperative imaging.

STEP FOUR: ASSESS FUNCTIONAL CAPACITY

A key factor in the Guidelines for predicting perioperative cardiac risk is the patient's functional capacity, which can be estimated from a careful history of daily activity or determined with exercise stress testing. The Duke Activity Status Index[9] can be used to approximate the metabolic equivalents (METs) for many daily activities. If the patient can exceed 4 METs with daily activity without symptoms (climbs one to two flights of stairs, performs own housework, or exercises regularly), then that patient will typically have sufficient cardiovascular reserve to tolerate the stress of surgery. The 2007 revised Guidelines recognize

that stress MPI is unlikely to alter management in asymptomatic patients with good functional capacity. In contrast, symptomatic patients or those with very limited functional capacity may have poor cardiovascular reserve, with worse perioperative and long-term outcomes after noncardiac surgery.

STEP FIVE: ASSESS CLINICAL RISK IN SYMPTOMATIC PATIENTS OR PATIENTS WITH POOR/UNKNOWN FUNCTIONAL CAPACITY

Although the clinical question that is often posed to the medical or cardiac consultant is whether or not to "clear" the patient for noncardiac surgery, the Guidelines[2] suggest an overall conservative approach to the use of expensive tests and interventions. The real challenge is in symptomatic or mildly symptomatic patients who are being evaluated for elective surgical procedures. A detailed medical history, physical examination, and electrocardiogram (ECG) should include information about angina, prior MI, CHF, symptomatic arrhythmia, diabetes, peripheral vascular disease, and prior history of coronary angiography or revascularization procedures. Even in the presence of known CAD, the risk of perioperative death or MI is less than 1% in patients who have undergone revascularization within the previous 4 years.[10] It is also reasonable to proceed to surgery if the patient has had a recent coronary angiogram or stress test that reveals favorable results with no change in clinical symptoms. However, the presence of cardiac symptoms or prior cardiovascular disease, as already noted, should alert the consulting physician to consider further noninvasive testing. This decision to consider further testing such as stress MPI in patients with poor functional capacity can be made based on clinical risk factors and surgical risk.

Clinical Risk Score

Since the initial report by Goldman et al.[11] demonstrated the utility of a clinical risk score for prediction of perioperative risk, several authors have published similar clinical risk scores based on the presence of clinical cardiovascular disease, diabetes mellitus (DM), renal disease, or other medical comorbidities.[11-13] The 2007 Guidelines incorporate the Revised Clinical Risk Index developed by Lee et al.[13]

Lee et al.[13] evaluated a total of 4315 patients undergoing elective noncardiac surgery. They derived a simple clinical index of six factors that could predict perioperative cardiac events: The presence of high-risk surgery, a history of CAD, history of CHF, history of cerebrovascular disease, diabetes treated with insulin, and a serum creatinine above 2 mg/dL constitute a useful index for risk assessment. In a validation population, the authors noted that when zero to one of these six factors was present (74% of all patients), the postoperative cardiac event rate was less than 1%. In contrast, the event rate in patients with any two factors was 7% (18% of all patients), and in those patients with three or more factors (8% of all patients), the event rate was 11%. Therefore, the Revised Clinical Risk Index classified three-quarters of the patients as low risk. A decision to consider further testing such as stress MPI can be made based on the presence of the five clinical risk factors together with surgical risk (the sixth risk factor).

Surgical Risk

In addition to the patient's clinical cardiac risk, the risk of the planned surgery (see Table 27-1) should be considered in the decision for preoperative MPI testing. As discussed, current Guidelines now recommend proceeding directly to low-risk surgery without preoperative imaging. High-risk vascular surgery or intermediate-risk surgery often warrants preoperative assessment with MPI when the patient's clinical risk is increased and functional capacity is poor.

Vascular Surgery

Assessment of cardiac risk is of particular importance prior to elective peripheral vascular surgery, owing to the high prevalence (~60%) of coexisting coronary artery disease.[14,15] The incidence of nonfatal MI or cardiac death in this population is summarized in Table 27-2. These data show that although vascular procedures are considered high-risk surgery, the perioperative cardiac death rate

Table 27-2 Perioperative Cardiac Events in Vascular Surgery (n ≥ 100 patients)

Vascular Surgery	No. Patients	INCIDENCE OF	
		NFMI (%)	CV Death (%)
Young '77[73] 1958–68	75	12.5	8.0
1968–76	143	12.5	8.0
Hertzer '81[74] Aortic	343	N/A	6.1
Peripheral	273	N/A	3.3
Cutler '87[75]	116	7.8	0
Raby '89[76]	176	2.3	0.6
Eagle '89[26]	200	4.5	3.0
Younis '90[77]	111	3.6	3.6
Hendel '92[60]	327	6.7	2.1
Taylor '91[78]	491	3.5	0.8
Kresowik '93[79]	170	2.4	0.6
McFalls '93[80]	116	17.0	1.7
Baron '94[81]	457	4.8	2.2
Bry '94[82]	237	5.9	1.3
Seeger '94[83]	172 (no test)	1.1	0.6
	146 (test)	3.4	0.7
Fleisher '95[84]	109	3.7	0.9

CV, cardiovascular; NFMI, nonfatal myocardial infarction; N/A, not applicable; No., number.

for vascular surgery has fallen to less than 2% as a result of improved preoperative assessment and perioperative management. However, these data also show that although the rate of nonfatal perioperative MI has also decreased, it remains two- to threefold higher than perioperative cardiac death. Therefore, it appears that while preoperative assessment and perioperative management have resulted in a lower perioperative death rate, the ability to predict and prevent perioperative MI is more difficult. The observation that nonfatal perioperative MI is a powerful predictor of late cardiac events[16–18] suggests the need to combine preoperative risk assessment with longer-term coronary management.

Transplant Surgery

The question of routine screening for all patients undergoing renal transplantation is primarily an issue of long-term cardiac prognosis. There is little immediate risk in performing transplant surgery, but it is clear that cardiac morbidity and mortality can have a significant impact on long-term postoperative survival. This seems to be especially true for patients with diabetes[19] and can result in a policy of routine noninvasive stress imaging or coronary angiography in many patients before transplantation. Heston et al.[20] have shown that an "expert system" using clinical risk predictors and thallium stress testing achieved an overall accuracy of 89% in predicting 4-year cardiac mortality among 189 renal transplant candidates. Other studies[21,22] show that if there are no clinical risk predictors, such as a history of CHF, angina, insulin-dependent diabetes, age older than 50 years, or an abnormal ECG (excluding LV hypertrophy), no further cardiac evaluation is needed prior to renal transplantation.

In patients being evaluated for cardiac risk prior to liver transplantation, there has been little published experience. A study from Kryzhanovski and Beller[23] suggests that perioperative cardiac risk is too low to warrant routine stress MPI or radionuclide angiography prior to liver transplantation. There were no cardiac events in 63 liver transplant procedures, and only one patient had a high-risk scan. Therefore, cardiac evaluations should be used in this patient subgroup only when there is clear evidence of coronary disease or when clinical risk factors are present.

THE DECISION TO OBTAIN PREOPERATIVE TESTING: A SHORTCUT APPROACH

After initial clinical assessment, a large group of patients with good functional capacity or those undergoing low-risk surgery can proceed to surgery without further testing. However, there remains a group of patients with clinical evidence of cardiovascular disease and poor functional capacity whose risk is uncertain or increased. Table 27-3 presents a shortcut approach to a large number of patients in whom the decision to recommend testing prior to surgery can be difficult. Basically, if

Table 27-3 Preoperative Risk: Shortcut Approach

Consider preoperative noninvasive testing when all three factors are present:
1. Clinical risk factors are present (ischemic heart disease, congestive heart failure, diabetes mellitus, renal insufficiency, cerebrovascular disease)
2. Symptomatic (angina, dyspnea) or poor/unknown functional capacity (<4 METs)
3. Intermediate or high surgical risk (aortic or other major vascular surgery, peripheral vascular surgery, intraperitoneal or intrathoracic surgery, carotid endarterectomy, head and neck surgery, orthopedic surgery, prostate surgery).

all of the three listed factors are true, then the Guidelines suggest that noninvasive cardiac testing can be considered as part of the preoperative evaluation.

RISK ASSESSMENT WITH PREOPERATIVE STRESS IMAGING

For patients with clinical risk factors undergoing intermediate- to high-risk surgery, MPI is appropriate for further risk stratification. MPI effectively separates patients into a lower-risk group that can safely proceed to surgery and a higher-risk group that warrants intensive perioperative medical management and sometimes revascularization.

The utility of vasodilator (dipyridamole or adenosine) MPI imaging in more than 3000 patients is summarized in Table 27-4. In the upper section, all studies involved vascular surgery, and the incidence of thallium redistribution was 42%. The overall positive predictive accuracy of a reversible perfusion defect (ischemia) for prediction of perioperative MI or cardiac death is 12%. In the vascular surgery population, in which the prevalence of CAD is 60% to 70%, 38% (930/2417) of the patients have a normal stress perfusion scan. The average negative predictive accuracy is 99%, which indicates that a normal stress perfusion study is a powerful prognostic indicator.

The lower section of Table 27-4 summarizes similar results for patients with nonvascular surgery. Most patients in this section were studied because of increased clinical risk of CAD, and the overall event rate of 6% was similar to the vascular surgery group. It is interesting to note that although the incidence of thallium redistribution was somewhat lower, the positive and negative predictive values are similar to those noted in the vascular surgery group.

Table 27-4 Pharmacologic Perfusion Imaging for Preoperative Assessment of Cardiac Risk

Author	Thallium Redist (%)	Periop Events MI/Dead (%)	Ischemia Pos. Pred (%)	Normal Scan Neg. Pred (%)
Vascular Surgery Only				
Boucher '85[85]	33	6	19	100
Cutler '87[75]	47	10	20	100
Fletcher '88[86]	22	4	37	100
Sachs '88[87]	31	4	14	100
Eagle '89[26]	41	8	16	98
Younis '90[77]	36	7	15	100
Mangano '91[88]	37	5	5	95
Lette '92[31]	45	8	17	99
Hendel '92[60]	51	9	14	99
Kresowik '93[79]	39	3	4	98
Baron '94[81]	35	5	4	96
Bry '94[82]	46	7	11	100
Koutelou '95[89]	44	3	6	100
Marshall '95[90]	47	10	16	97
Total (weighted avg)	42	7	12	99
2417 Total patients				
Other Surgery				
Coley '92[91]	36	4	11	99
Shaw '92[92]	47	10	21	100
Brown '93[30]	33	5	13	99
Younis '94[93]	31	9	18	98
Stratmann '96[94]	29	4	6	99
Van Damme '97[95]	34	2	N/A	N/A
Total (weighted avg)	33	6	13	99
923 Total patients				

Shaw et al. reviewed the utility of preoperative noninvasive testing in a large meta-analysis.[24] These authors reviewed stress imaging studies from 1985 to 1994 in which either dipyridamole thallium (n = 1994) or dobutamine echocardiography (n = 455) was used for perioperative risk stratification. Reversible perfusion defects were noted in 26% of patients, and perioperative nonfatal MI or cardiovascular death occurred in 9% of these cases. In contrast, 430 (22%) patients had normal perfusion scans with an event rate of 1.4%. Similar prognostic utility was noted in the dobutamine echocardiography studies. New wall-motion abnormalities during dobutamine-induced stress were noted in 39% of the patients, and 11% of these patients had a major cardiac event. In the 270 (61%) patients without new regional wall-motion abnormalities, the event rate was 0.4%. The authors of this meta-analysis concluded that (1) reversible perfusion defects have significant positive predictive accuracy, but the overall accuracy depends on the prevalence of CAD and clinical risk factors; (2) dobutamine-induced wall-motion abnormalities predict adverse outcomes, but the relatively small population size yields wider confidence limits; (3) the use of semiquantitative image analysis for MPI should improve its prognostic utility; and (4) fixed defects predict long-term cardiac events with an accuracy equal to reversible defects for perioperative events.

The issue of a possible gender difference in perioperative risk stratification was studied by Hendel et al.[25] This study of 567 vascular surgery patients showed that, overall, perioperative and long-term cardiac events were similar for both men and women. Clinical predictors of cardiac risk were less useful in women versus men. ECG ST-segment depression with dipyridamole infusion predicted increased perioperative risk for men but not for women. An important finding was that multivariate analysis showed thallium redistribution to be an independent predictor of risk for both men and women.

Several authors have evaluated the use of clinical risk factors to identify the intermediate, risk patients who most benefit from preoperative stress MPI. Eagle et al.[26] evaluated the utility of preoperative dipyridamole thallium MPI in 200 patients undergoing vascular surgery. In the 32% of patients at low clinical risk, with no DM or clinical risk factors for CAD, the perioperative rate of cardiac death, perioperative MI, pulmonary edema, or unstable angina was 3.1%. Thallium redistribution stratified the 54% of patients at intermediate risk (one or two risk factors) into a low-risk group with a perioperative event rate equal to that for patients with no risk factors and a high-risk group with a perioperative event rate of 30%. Therefore, these data support the current recommendation to reserve preoperative stress MPI for patients with clinical risk factors.

L'Italien et al. showed similar results in a multicenter analysis of over 1081 patients undergoing vascular surgery.[27] In this study, clinically low-risk patients with a 3% perioperative event rate and high-risk patients with a 19% event rate were not more accurately risk stratified by preoperative dipyridamole thallium MPI. However, clinical assessment classified 51% of the patients as being at intermediate surgical risk, and stress thallium MPI effectively separated more than 80% of these intermediate-risk patients into low-risk or high-risk groups.

In a prospective clinical trial of patients undergoing abdominal aortic surgery, Vanzetto et al.[28] identified patients at increased clinical risk based on the presence of two or more of the following predictors: age older than 70 years; history of MI, angina, CHF, DM, hypertension with LV hypertrophy; or a resting ECG that shows Q waves or ST-segment ischemia. Of 457 patients, 69% were classified as low risk and underwent surgery without preoperative stress testing. There was a 4% event rate in patients with one risk factor and a rate of approximately 2% in patients without any CAD risk predictors. One hundred forty-seven (32%) of the patients were classified as increased risk, and subsequently, 134 of these 147 patients underwent surgery after dipyridamole SPECT thallium scans. On the basis of these clinical criteria alone, 9% of the higher-risk patients had cardiac events. The perioperative rate of cardiac death or MI was 13% in patients with abnormal perfusion scans, compared to 1.9% in those with normal MPI. It is also important to add that Vanzetto et al.[28] performed a multivariate analysis that showed that the number of ischemic segments was the single best predictor of perioperative events.

In another study of preoperative cardiac risk assessment, Bartels et al.[29] evaluated a strategy that emulated the ACC/AHA recommendations for cardiac risk. Clinical risk classifications were assigned to 201 patients who were to undergo major vascular surgery. Approximately 10% of the patients were defined as high risk based on the presence of major clinical predictors of cardiac risk, 40% at intermediate risk, and the remaining 50% at low risk. All the low-risk patients and the intermediate-risk patients (52%) with a functional capacity of greater than 5 METs based on a questionnaire (Duke Activity Status Index)[9] proceeded directly to major aortic surgery without further testing. The remaining intermediate-risk patients (48%) who had a functional capacity of less than 5 METs on the questionnaire underwent noninvasive testing (40%) or intensified medical care (60%) before surgery. In the high-risk group, approximately half underwent noninvasive testing, and the other half received intensified medical treatment. Subsequently, five (6%) intermediate risk and two (9%) high-risk patients underwent preoperative coronary angiography, resulting in one coronary bypass procedure and two cancellations of further elective surgery. Cardiac events occurred in 5% of the high-risk group and in 9% of the intermediate-risk group patients. The low-risk group had an event rate of 2%.

Patients with a mildly abnormal preoperative MPI study can generally undergo surgery with medical treatment for coronary disease. However, when preoperative stress MPI indicates very high risk of a perioperative cardiac complication, the Guidelines recommend evaluation with coronary angiography. Identification of patients at the highest cardiac risk with stress MPI is based on detection of a large area of multivessel ischemia together with markers of LV dysfunction such as LV dilation, increased thallium lung uptake, and reduced left ventricular ejection fraction (LVEF). Brown et al.[30] showed that ischemic defect size detected with dipyridamole thallium MPI correlated with surgical risk. A large reversible scan defect and DM identified patients at highest risk for perioperative cardiac events. Lette et al.[31] also found that large perfusion defects in multiple coronary territories or transient LV dilation with dipyridamole identified high-risk patients with a 52% incidence of perioperative cardiac death or MI. In contrast, the 63% of the patients with normal MPI or small apical scan defects and normal LV cavity size had a perioperative event rate of only 1.3%. In the study of SPECT thallium MPI prior to aortic aneurysm surgery discussed earlier, Vanzetto et al.[28] showed that the best multivariate predictor of perioperative cardiac death or MI was the number of ischemic segments detected by dipyridamole SPECT MPI. A classification of perioperative risk based on MPI results is shown in Table 27-5, with specific patient examples shown in Figures 27-1 and 27-2.

In summary, clinical risk assessment can identify a large group of patients at low risk who can safely undergo noncardiac surgery. Higher-risk patients can be further risk stratified with preoperative stress MPI. When MPI shows multivessel ischemia and LV dysfunction indicating very high risk, one needs to reassess the need for surgery or consider canceling the procedure, ensure intensive medical therapy, and consider coronary angiography and revascularization.

Table 27-5   Prognostic Gradient of Nuclear Stress Nuclear Perfusion Imaging

Very Low Risk:
Normal stress perfusion study with normal LVEF
Low Risk:
Stress-induced or fixed perfusion defects of small size with normal LVEF
Intermediate Risk:
Stress-induced or fixed perfusion defects of moderate size without LV dilation or increased thallium-201 lung uptake
Mildly to moderately depressed resting LVEF 35%-49%
High Risk:
Large stress-induced perfusion defect (particularly if anterior)
Multiple stress-induced perfusion defects of moderate size
Large, fixed perfusion defect with LV dilation or increased thallium-201 lung uptake
Moderate stress-induced perfusion defect with LV dilation, increased thallium-201 lung uptake, or diabetes mellitus
Severely depressed LVEF < 35%

LVEF, left ventricular ejection fraction; LV, left ventricular.
Based in part on summary recommendations from International Nuclear Cardiology Retreat[96] and ACC/AHA 2007 Guidelines for the Management of Patients With Unstable Angina/Non-ST-Elevation Myocardial Infarction.[97]

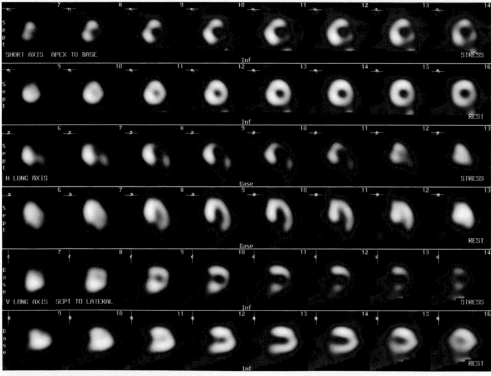

Figure 27-1   GR, 76-year-old female who is preop for a vascular left foot ulcer. She has no angina, dyspnea, CHF, or history of CAD but has limited activity due to peripheral vascular disease. Given the combination of low functional capacity, diabetes, and major vascular surgery, a dipyridamole thallium scan was performed. The scan shows a large area of ischemia with reversible cavity dilation and LVEF of 50%, with mild anterior and posterolateral wall hypokinesis. At coronary angiography, she was noted to have three-vessel disease and a left main stenosis. She underwent a three-vessel CABG and then had an aortobifemoral bypass, with no cardiac events. This case illustrates the utility of stress perfusion imaging in patients with clinical risk factors and poor exercise tolerance, even if they are asymptomatic for CAD. CABG, coronary artery bypass graft; CAD, coronary artery disease; CHF, congestive heart failure; LVEF, left ventricular ejection fraction.

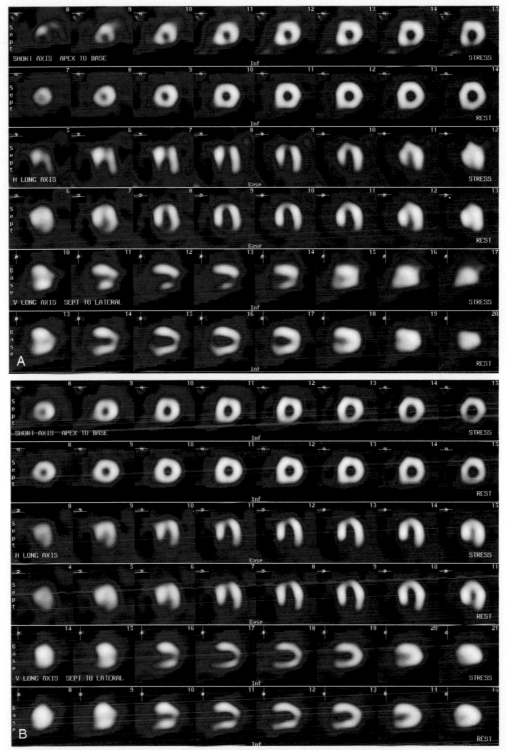

Figure 27-2 ME-CAD1(**A**) & CAD2(**B**) are from a 61-year-old male with a past MI and CABG 11 years ago. Presently he has no angina or CHF, but he has a history of peripheral vascular disease and is status-post aortobi-iliac bypass and right above-the-knee amputation. He can climb two flights of stairs with a leg prosthesis and is active walking, with no cardiac symptoms. The first scan (**A**) shows a moderate area of ischemia and small infarct, with LVEF of 47% with inferoapical hypokinesis. His medical therapy was reemphasized to him and adjusted to include: aspirin, atorvastatin, niacin, atenolol, and also isosorbide for atypical neck burning. A repeat scan (**B**) 6 months later for atypical symptoms and preop for carotid surgery showed less ischemia on this medical therapy, and the LVEF was 48% with no focal wall-motion abnormalities. This case illustrates that medical therapy without cardiac catheterization can be a good choice in patients with good exercise capacity, despite an initial scan with moderate risk. CABG, coronary artery bypass graft; CHF, congestive heart failure; LVEF, left ventricular ejection fraction; MI, myocardial infarction.

PERIOPERATIVE MEDICAL TREATMENT

For patients found to be at increased perioperative risk, medical therapy should be considered. While Mangano et al.[32] showed no reduction in perioperative risk with atenolol treatment, Poldermans et al.[33] found a marked reduction in risk with bisoprolol treatment. Recent studies of perioperative β-blockade in diabetic[34] and vascular surgery[35] patients have shown no clear benefit. The multicenter Perioperative Ischemic Evaluation (POISE) Trial[36] showed conflicting results. Perioperative metoprolol treatment resulted in an overall reduction in perioperative cardiac events (driven primarily by a reduction in MI) but significantly increased perioperative stroke and death. Recommendations for the use of perioperative β-blockers range from the view of no clear benefit[37–39] to the view that all vascular surgery patients should receive β-blockers and omit preoperative stress imaging.[40] Two recent meta-analyses also showed contradictory results about the benefit of perioperative β-blockade.[41,42] Further research on the role of perioperative β-blockade is warranted, but the 2006 ACC/AHA focused update on perioperative β-blocker therapy[43] recommends perioperative β-blockers for most patients undergoing vascular surgery and for other surgical patients with CAD or multiple cardiac risk factors.

The benefit of perioperative statin therapy has been addressed in two studies. A case-control study found significantly lower mortality in vascular surgery patients who were treated with perioperative statins.[44] A randomized trial of atorvastatin in vascular surgery patients showed an early and sustained reduction in postoperative mortality.[45]

CORONARY ANGIOGRAPHY AND REVASCULARIZATION

The Guidelines note that coronary angiography is often performed for evaluation of severe angina, recent MI, or for high-risk noninvasive stress imaging.

The indications for coronary artery bypass graft (CABG) are essentially identical to those for most patients with CAD. For most patients, CABG is rarely indicated to "get them through" noncardiac surgery, but it should be considered in appropriate patients to improve long-term prognosis.

PCI has not been clearly shown to reduce perioperative mortality. There is a high cardiac risk if noncardiac surgery is performed within 4 to 6 weeks after bare metal stenting and concern about risk within 12 months after treatment with a drug-eluting stent.[46–48] While balloon angioplasty is sometimes considered as an alternative to avoid the risk of stent thrombosis, perioperative risk early after angioplasty may be similar to that with a coronary stent.[49] The Guidelines recommend delaying elective noncardiac surgery for at least 14 days after balloon angioplasty, 30 to 45 days after bare metal stenting, and 365 days after a drug-eluting stent (Fig. 27-3).[2]

The Coronary Artery Revascularization Prophylaxis (CARP) trial showed no benefit of revascularization over optimal medical management in most patients undergoing noncardiac vascular surgery (Fig. 27-4)[50] when the highest-risk patients with left main CAD or severe LV dysfunction were excluded. Although there is some uncertainty about the subgroup of patients with multiple clinical risk factors and a large area of ischemia detected with preoperative imaging,[50,51] most patients at increased cardiac risk should be managed with

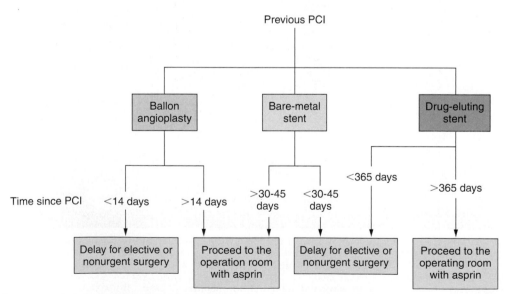

Figure 27-3 Recommended timing of noncardiac surgery after prior percutaneous coronary intervention (PCI). Reproduced, with permission, from Fleisher et al.[2] *(From Fleisher LA, Beckman JA, Brown KA, et al: ACC/AHA 2007 guidelines on perioperative cardiovascular evaluation and care for noncardiac surgery: A report of the American College of Cardiology/ American Heart Association Task Force on Practice Guidelines [Writing Committee to Revise the 2002 Guidelines on Perioperative Cardiovascular Evaluation for Noncardiac Surgery] developed in collaboration with the American Society of Echocardiography, American Society of Nuclear Cardiology, Heart Rhythm Society, Society of Cardiovascular Anesthesiologists, Society for Cardiovascular Angiography and Interventions, Society for Vascular Medicine and Biology, and Society for Vascular Surgery [erratum appears in J Am Coll Cardiol 50:e242, 2007], J Am Coll Cardiol 50:e159-e241, 2007.)*

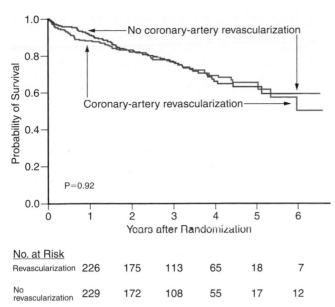

Figure 27-4 Survival of patients undergoing vascular surgery in the Coronary Artery Revascularization Prophylaxis (CARP) trial.[50] There was no significant difference in survival with or without preoperative revascularization. Reproduced, with permission, from McFalls et al.[50] Copyright © 2004 *Massachusetts Medical Society. All rights reserved.*

appropriate medical therapy, with coronary angiography and revascularization reserved for the highest-risk patients who will benefit from improvement in long-term prognosis.

LONG-TERM PROGNOSIS AFTER NONCARDIAC SURGERY

When performing a preoperative consultation for cardiac risk, assessment and management of long-term prognosis may be even more important than short-term

perioperative cardiac risk, particularly in vascular surgery patients. Table 27-6 summarizes late cardiac events that occurred in a population dominated by vascular surgery procedures. It appears that long-term cardiac mortality has been decreasing over the past decade, as noted previously in Table 27-2 for perioperative events, but CAD still correlates with a worse long-term prognosis. Cardiac risk factors should be appropriately treated (hypertension, diabetes, hyperlipidemia, smoking, ischemia, heart failure). This evaluation and recommendations should be communicated to the patient and the primary care physician so that it becomes part of long-term medical care. This is especially important for any patient who sustains a severe ischemic episode, heart failure, or nonfatal MI in the perioperative period, since all of these events carry high risk for future cardiac events over the next 2 to 4 years.[52]

In a review of the vascular surgery literature from 1975 through 1987, Hertzer[53] noted that late mortality in patients with aortic aneurysms was 44% in those with probable CAD versus 22% in those without CAD. This review also noted increased long-term mortality among patients having infrainguinal or carotid surgery based on the presence of symptomatic CAD. L'Italien et al.[54] also showed that patients undergoing infrainguinal or carotid surgery had significantly lower cumulative survival compared with aortic surgery patients. However, after adjustment for cardiac risk factors, the differences in long-term cardiac event rates for the specific surgical procedures were significantly reduced. Multivariate analysis showed that a history of angina or CHF, DM, fixed dipyridamole thallium defects, and perioperative MI were the best predictors of long-term events. In contrast, survival in patients without any CAD risk factors was above 95% in all three surgical groups. Therefore, these authors concluded that cardiac status, DM, and MPI results were critical predictors for long-term prognosis, whereas the specific type of vascular surgery was less important.

Table 27-6 Cardiac Event Rate in Long-Term Postoperative Follow-Up

Author	Avg FU Years	# Pts	NFMI	CV Death
Hertzer '80[74]	6–7	286	N/A	22.0%
Hertzer '81[98]	7–8	256	N/A	22.0%
Roger '89[99]	8	75 no CAD	12.0%	12.0%
		47 CAD	28.0%	38.0%
Hertzer '87[100]	4.6	228	N/A	6.1%
Younis '90[77]	1.5	127	—12%—*	
Lette '92[59]	1.3	355	5.4%	6.8%
Mangano '92[52]	2	444	2.5%	5.4%
Seeger '94[83]	2.8	171 no test	N/A	1.2%
		144 test	N/A	3.6%
Hendel '95[25]	4.2	556	5.0%	7.7%
Fleisher '95[84]	1.4	108	6.5%	3.7%
Poldermans '97[101]	1.6	316	3.5%	3.5%

*Combined rate of NFMI and CV death.

Avg FU, average follow-up; CV death, cardiac death; N/A, not applicable; NFMI, nonfatal myocardial infarction; # Pts, number patients in each study.

UTILIZING PREOPERATIVE TESTING FOR LONG-TERM PROGNOSIS

There is evidence that both the data collected and the process of evaluation and subsequent workup or intervention (medical or surgical) have resulted in better outcomes and predictions. A recent review of a national Medicare population sample identified a cohort of patients (n = 6895) who underwent elective vascular surgery during a 17-month period in 1991 and 1992. The authors noted a relatively high mortality (14%) at 1 year of follow-up. However, in those patients undergoing preoperative stress testing with or without coronary bypass surgery, the mortality rate was lower (<6%).[55] In another follow-up study of peripheral vascular surgery patients (n = 343) for a mean of 40 months, cardiac events were significantly more frequent in those who had an LVEF of less than 35% or ischemia on dipyridamole-thallium imaging.[56] Other studies[31,57] also confirm the value of semiquantitative analysis of MPI when using these types of preoperative tests to predict future cardiac events. All these studies have the ability to combine an assessment of myocardial ischemia and left ventricular function into a more useful clinical index.

Table 27-7 shows the long-term survival after aortic vascular surgery in different patient studies using various clinical parameters that have demonstrated significant preoperative prognostic utility. The clinical risk index[58] can be divided into low, intermediate, and high-risk groups, and there is a significant survival difference between low- and high-risk patients. As expected, the mortality is elevated in the high-risk group, but the low-risk patients have 22% mortality over 5 years. This is the same group of patients who are often sent directly to elective surgery without cardiac testing and typically have low (~2%) perioperative event rates. It is possible that assessment of functional capacity or use of stress MPI could identify some patients at higher long-term risk, even in this lower-risk group. Intermediate-risk patients also have a fairly high (>50%) mortality over the 5-year follow-up period and may warrant further investigation.

LVEF is another powerful predictor of survival in patients with CAD. Although early studies of MPI utilized indirect measurements of LV function, such as increased LV size[31,57,59] and extent of fixed defects,[24,60] it is now routine to measure LVEF with gated SPECT imaging.[61,62] In Table 27-7, Kazmers et al.[63] show that 3-year survival is significantly better in patients with an LVEF above 35% than in those with lower LVEF. However, even patients with preserved LVEF have a mortality of approximately 6% per year. Therefore, having an LVEF above 35% does not necessarily ensure an excellent event-free survival.

The long-term prognostic power of multivessel CAD has been demonstrated by Hertzer.[53] In Table 27-7, a summary of data collected after vascular surgery is shown. These investigators noted that patients with two- or three-vessel CAD had a 5-year event-free survival of only 22%. In contrast, those patients with only single-vessel CAD or normal coronary angiograms had a survival of 85%. Although this identifies a relatively low-risk group with a 3% per year cardiac event rate, MPI can also identify these low-risk patients without the need for routine coronary angiography.

A study of long-term prognosis by Cutler et al.[64] is presented in Table 27-7. The authors report a very low event rate of less than 1% per year in vascular patients who had a normal stress MPI scan. In contrast, fixed perfusion defects identified patients at higher long-term risk. In a subsequent study,[57] Emlein et al. reported that the extent of LV cavity dilation was the most important factor in predicting cardiac death among patients with abnormal MPI scans. These studies clearly show that patients with a normal MPI scan have a very low risk of long-term cardiac events, similar to the data in Table 27-3 that show a high negative predictive value of a normal MPI scan for perioperative events. Therefore, pharmacologic stress MPI can be used to assess appropriate patient populations for both perioperative and long-term events by use of slightly different predictors.

In a study of long-term prognosis of peripheral vascular surgery patients (n = 343) for a mean of 40 months, cardiac events were significantly more frequent in those who had an LVEF of below 35% or ischemia on dipyridamole thallium MPI.[56] Other studies[57,65] also confirm the value of semiquantitative analysis of MPI to predict long-term cardiac events. These studies combine an

Table 27-7 Prediction of Long-Term Survival After Aortic Reconstruction

	CUMULATIVE SURVIVAL			
	1 Yr (%)	2 Yr (%)	3 Yr (%)	5 Yr (%)
Screening Test				
White et al., 1988[58]				
Goldman risk index[11] (clinical)				
I (low)	98	90	84	78
II/III (intermediate)	84	78	66	46
IV (high)	55	40	30	18
Kazmers et al., 1988[63]				
Radionuclide ventriculogram				
≥35% LVEF	90	82	82	—
<35% LVEF	56	56	37	—
Hertzer 1987[53]				
CAD by angiography				
≤single vessel	97	95	92	85
≥double vessel	83	74	53	22
Cutler et al., 1992[64]				
Dipyridamole thallium-201 scan				
Normal scan	99	97	97	97
Fixed defect	88	79	69	55

CAD, coronary artery disease; LVEF, left ventricular ejection fraction.

assessment of myocardial ischemia and LV function into a more accurate prognostic index.

Therefore, pharmacologic stress MPI can be used to assess both perioperative and long-term risk by means of slightly different predictors. The extent of reversible perfusion defects predicts short-term perioperative events, which typically involve nonfatal MI, whereas large LV cavity size, reduced LVEF, and fixed perfusion defects predict long-term events, which usually involve cardiac death.

When vascular or other surgical patients are identified at high long-term risk for cardiac events, medical therapy for coronary disease and appropriate use of revascularization using standard guidelines should be considered. Despite their increased operative mortality with CABG,[66] patients with peripheral vascular disease derive equal or greater long-term survival benefit from revascularization. The European Coronary Surgery Study Group showed that in patients with peripheral vascular disease and multivessel CAD, the 5-year survival of 66% was significantly improved to 89% with CABG.[67] An analysis of data from the Coronary Artery Surgery Study registry by Rihal et al.[68] of patients with combined coronary and peripheral arterial disease showed a significant survival benefit of CABG for patients with three-vessel CAD. The benefit was greatest for patients with reduced LVEF. Landesberg et al.[69,70] showed that long-term survival in vascular surgery patients with moderate to severe ischemia detected by stress MPI, long-term survival was significantly improved by revascularization. These authors noted that patients with moderate to severe ischemia who were selected for revascularization had a 5-year survival (74%) similar to that patients with only mild or no perfusion defects. In contrast, those patients with moderate to severe defects who did not undergo revascularization had a 53% 5-year survival.[70] Patients with reduced LVEF appeared to derive the greatest benefit.

CONCLUSION: USE OF GUIDELINES FOR COST-EFFECTIVE RISK ASSESSMENT

This review of perioperative cardiac risk stratification shows that a large group of patients can safely proceed to surgery after assessment of clinical and surgical risk. The ACC/AHA Guidelines recommend perioperative treatment with β-blockers for most patients undergoing vascular surgery and many others with CAD or clinical risk factors. Patients at higher clinical risk with poor functional capacity, particularly those undergoing vascular surgery, often warrant further risk assessment with MPI and sometimes coronary angiography.

Data from Almanaseer et al.[71] and Froelich et al.[72] show that adherence to the Guidelines significantly reduced preoperative stress imaging, perioperative length of stay and cost, and increased use of perioperative β-blockers while maintaining a low rate of perioperative cardiac death and MI.

REFERENCES

1. Rosamond W, Flegal K, Furie K, et al: Heart disease and stroke statistics 2008 update: a report from the American Heart Association Statistics Committee and Stroke Statistics Subcommittee, *Circulation* 117(4):e25–e146, 2008.
2. Fleisher LA, Beckman JA, Brown KA, et al: ACC/AHA 2007 guidelines on perioperative cardiovascular evaluation and care for noncardiac surgery: a report of the American College of Cardiology/American Heart Association Task Force on Practice Guidelines (Writing Committee to Revise the 2002 Guidelines on Perioperative Cardiovascular Evaluation for Noncardiac Surgery) developed in collaboration with the American Society of Echocardiography, American Society of Nuclear Cardiology, Heart Rhythm Society, Society of Cardiovascular Anesthesiologists, Society for Cardiovascular Angiography and Interventions, Society for Vascular Medicine and Biology, and Society for Vascular Surgery [erratum appears in *J Am Coll Cardiol* 50(17):e242, 2007], *J Am Coll Cardiol* 50(17):e159–e241, 2007.
3. Mangano DT, Goldman L: Preoperative assessment of patients with known or suspected coronary disease, *N Engl J Med* 333(26):1750–1756, 1995.
4. Fleisher LA, Eagle KA: Clinical practice. Lowering cardiac risk in noncardiac surgery, *N Engl J Med* 345(23):1677–1682, 2001.
5. Poldermans D, Hoeks SE, Feringa HH: Pre-operative risk assessment and risk reduction before surgery, *J Am Coll Cardiol* 51(20):1913–1924, 2008.
6. Hoeks SE, Schouten O, van d V, Poldermans D: Preoperative cardiac testing before major vascular surgery, *J Nucl Cardiol* 14(6):885–891, 2007.
7. Brindis RG, Douglas PS, Hendel RC, et al: ACCF/ASNC appropriateness criteria for single-photon emission computed tomography myocardial perfusion imaging (SPECT MPI): a report of the American College of Cardiology Foundation Quality Strategic Directions Committee Appropriateness Criteria Working Group and the American Society of Nuclear Cardiology endorsed by the American Heart Association, *J Am Coll Cardiol* 46(8):1587–1605, 2005.
8. Califf RM, Armstrong PW, Carver JR, D'Agostino RB, Strauss WE: Task force 5: Stratification of patients into high, medium and low risk subgroups for purposes of risk factor management, *J Am Coll Cardiol* 27:1007–1019, 1996.
9. Hlatky MA, Boineau RE, Higginbotham MB, et al: A brief self-administered questionnaire to determine functional capacity (the Duke Activity Status Index), *Am J Cardiol* 64:651–654, 1989.
10. Hassan SA, Hlatky MA, Boothroyd DB, et al: Outcomes of noncardiac surgery after coronary bypass surgery or coronary angioplasty in the Bypass Angioplasty Revascularization Investigation (BARI) [commentary], *Am J Med* 110(4):260–266, 2001.
11. Goldman L, Caldera DL, Nussbaum SR, et al: Multifactorial index of cardiac risk in noncardiac surgical procedures, *N Engl J Med* 297:845–850, 1977.
12. Detsky AS, Abrams HB, Forbath N, Scott JG, Hilliard JR: Cardiac assessment for patients undergoing noncardiac surgery: A multifactorial clinical risk index, *Arch Intern Med* 146:2131–2134, 1986.
13. Lee TH, Marcantonio ER, Mangione CM, et al: Derivation and prospective validation of a simple index for prediction of cardiac risk of major noncardiac surgery, *Circulation* 100(10):1043–1049, 1999.
14. Gersh BJ, Rihal CS, Rooke TW, Ballard DJ: Evaluation and management of patients with both peripheral vascular and coronary artery disease, *J Am Coll Cardiol* 18:203–214, 1991.
15. Hertzer NR, Beven EG, Young JR, et al: Coronary artery disease in peripheral vascular patients: A classification of 1000 coronary angiograms and results of surgical management, *Ann Surg* 199:223–233, 1984.
16. Hollenberg M, Mangano DT, Browner WS, London MJ, Tubau JF, Tateo IM: Predictors of postoperative myocardial ischemia in patients undergoing noncardiac surgery. The Study of Perioperative Ischemia Research Group, *JAMA* 268(2):205–209, 1992.
17. Mangano DT, Browner WS, Hollenberg M, Li J, Tateo IM: Long-term cardiac prognosis following noncardiac surgery. The Study of Perioperative Ischemia Research Group, *JAMA* 268(2):233–239, 1992.
18. Kertai MD, Boersma E, Klein J, van UH, Bax JJ, Poldermans D: Long-term prognostic value of asymptomatic cardiac troponin T elevations in patients after major vascular surgery, *Eur J Vasc Endovasc Surg* 28(1):59–66, 2004.
19. Weinrauch LA, D'Elia JA, Healy RW, et al: Asymptomatic coronary artery disease: Angiography in diabetic patients before renal transplantation: Relations of findings to postoperative survival, *Ann Intern Med* 88:346–348, 1978.
20. Heston TF, Norman DJ, Barry JM, Bennett WM, Wilson RA: Cardiac risk stratification in renal transplantation using a form of artificial intelligence, *Am J Cardiol* 79:415–417, 1997.
21. Iqbal A, Gibbons RJ, McGoon MD, Steinoff S, Frohnert PT, Velosa JA: Noninvasive assessment of cardiac risk in insulin-dependent diabetic patient being evaluated for pancreatic transplantation using

thallium-201 myocardial perfusion scintigraphy, *Transplant Proc* 23:1690–1691, 1991.

22. Le A, Wilson R, Douek K, et al: Prospective risk stratification in renal transplant candidates for cardiac death, *Am J Kidney Dis* 24:65–71, 1994.
23. Kryzhanovski VA, Beller GA: Usefulness of preoperative noninvasive radionuclide testing for detecting coronary artery disease in candidates for liver transplantation, *Am J Cardiol* 79(7):986–988, 1997.
24. Shaw LJ, Eagle KA, Gersh BJ, Miller DD: Meta-analysis of intravenous dipyridamole-thallium-201 imaging (1985 to 1994) and dobutamine echocardiography (1991 to 1994) for risk stratification before vascular surgery, *J Am Coll Cardiol* 27(4):787–798, 1996.
25. Hendel RC, Chen MH, L'Italien GJ, et al: Sex differences in perioperative and long-term cardiac event-free survival in vascular surgery patients: An analysis of clinical and scintigraphic variables, *Circulation* 91:1044–1051, 1995.
26. Eagle KA, Coley CM, Newell JB, et al: Combining clinical and thallium data optimizes preoperative assessment of cardiac risk before major vascular surgery, *Ann Intern Med* 110:859–866, 1989.
27. L'Italien GJ, Paul SD, Hendel RC, et al: Development and validation of a Bayesian model for perioperative cardiac risk assessment in a cohort of 1,081 vascular surgical candidates, *J Am Coll Cardiol* 27(4):779–786, 1996.
28. Vanzetto G, Machecourt J, Blendea D, et al: Additive value of thallium single-photon emission computer tomography myocardial imaging for prediction of perioperative events in clinically selected high cardiac risk patients having abdominal aortic surgery, *Am J Cardiol* 77: 143–148, 1996.
29. Bartels C, Bechtel JFM, Hossmann V, Horsch S: Cardiac risk stratification for high-risk vascular surgery, *Circulation* 95:2473–2475, 1997.
30. Brown KA, Rowen M: Extent of jeopardized viable myocardium determined by myocardial perfusion imaging best predicts perioperative cardiac events in patients undergoing noncardiac surgery, *J Am Coll Cardiol* 21:325–330, 1993.
31. Lette J, Waters D, Cerino M, Picard M, Champagne P, Lapointe J: Preoperative coronary artery disease risk stratification based on dipyridamole imaging and a simple three-step, three-segment model for patients undergoing noncardiac vascular surgery or major general surgery, *Am J Cardiol* 69:1553–1558, 1992.
32. Mangano DT, Layug EL, Wallace A, Tateo I: Effect of atenolol on mortality and cardiovascular morbidity after noncardiac surgery, *N Engl J Med* 335:1713–1720, 1996.
33. Poldermans D, Boersma E, Bax JJ, et al: The effect of bisoprolol on perioperative mortality and myocardial infarction in high-risk patients undergoing vascular surgery. Dutch Echocardiographic Cardiac Risk Evaluation Applying Stress Echocardiography Study Group, *N Engl J Med* 341(24):1789–1794, 1999.
34. Juul AB, Wetterslev J, Gluud C, et al: Effect of perioperative beta blockade in patients with diabetes undergoing major non-cardiac surgery: randomised placebo controlled, blinded multicentre trial, *BMJ* 332 (7556):1482, 2006.
35. Yang H, Raymer K, Butler R, Parlow J, Roberts R: The effects of perioperative beta-blockade: results of the Metoprolol after Vascular Surgery (MaVS) study, a randomized controlled trial, *Am Heart J* 152(5): 983–990, 2006.
36. POISE Study Group: Devereaux PJ, Yang H, et al: Effects of extended-release metoprolol succinate in patients undergoing non-cardiac surgery (POISE trial): a randomised controlled trial, *Lancet* 371 (9627):1839–1847, 2008.
37. Devereaux PJ, Yusuf S, Yang H, Choi PT, Guyatt GH: Are the recommendations to use perioperative beta-blocker therapy in patients undergoing noncardiac surgery based on reliable evidence? *CMAJ* 171(3):245–247, 2004.
38. Devereaux PJ, Leslie K, Yang H: The effect of perioperative beta-blockers on patients undergoing noncardiac surgery: Is the answer in, *Can J Anaesth* 51(8):749–755, 2004.
39. Devereaux PJ, Beattie WS, Choi PT, et al: How strong is the evidence for the use of perioperative beta blockers in non-cardiac surgery? Systematic review and meta-analysis of randomised controlled trials, *BMJ* 331(7512):313–321, 2005.
40. Poldermans D, Bax JJ, Schouten O, et al: Should major vascular surgery be delayed because of preoperative cardiac testing in intermediate-risk patients receiving beta-blocker therapy with tight heart rate control? *J Am Coll Cardiol* 48(5):964–969, 2006.
41. Schouten O, Shaw LJ, Boersma E, et al: A meta-analysis of safety and effectiveness of perioperative beta-blocker use for the prevention of cardiac events in different types of noncardiac surgery, *Coron Artery Dis* 17(2):173–179, 2006.
42. Bangalore S, Wetterslev J, Pranesh S, Sawhney S, Gluud C, Messerli FH: Perioperative beta blockers in patients having non-cardiac surgery: a meta-analysis [commentary], *Lancet* 372(9654):1962–1976, 2008.
43. Fleisher LA, Beckman JA, Brown KA, et al: ACC/AHA 2006 guideline update on perioperative cardiovascular evaluation for noncardiac surgery: focused update on perioperative beta-blocker therapy: a report of the American College of Cardiology/American Heart Association Task Force on Practice Guidelines (Writing Committee to Update the 2002 Guidelines on Perioperative Cardiovascular Evaluation for Noncardiac Surgery) developed in collaboration with the American Society of Echocardiography, American Society of Nuclear Cardiology, Heart Rhythm Society, Society of Cardiovascular Anesthesiologists, Society for Cardiovascular Angiography and Interventions, and Society for Vascular Medicine and Biology, *J Am Coll Cardiol* 47(11):2343–2355, 2006.

44. Poldermans D, Bax JJ, Kertai MD, et al: Statins are associated with a reduced incidence of perioperative mortality in patients undergoing major noncardiac vascular surgery, *Circulation* 107(14):1848–1851, 2003.
45. Durazzo AE, Machado FS, Ikeoka DT, et al: Reduction in cardiovascular events after vascular surgery with atorvastatin: a randomized trial, *J Vasc Surg* 39(5):967–975, 2004.
46. Kaluza GL, Joseph J, Lee JR, Raizner ME, Raizner AE: Catastrophic outcomes of noncardiac surgery soon after coronary stenting, *J Am Coll Cardiol* 35(5):1288–1294, 2000.
47. Wilson SH, Fasseas P, Orford JL, et al: Clinical outcome of patients undergoing non-cardiac surgery in the two months following coronary stenting, *J Am Coll Cardiol* 42(2):234–240, 2003.
48. Compton PA, Zankar AA, Adesanya AO, Banerjee S, Brilakis ES: Risk of noncardiac surgery after coronary drug-eluting stent implantation, *Am J Cardiol* 98(9):1212–1213, 2006.
49. Leibowitz D, Cohen M, Planer D, et al: Comparison of cardiovascular risk of noncardiac surgery following coronary angioplasty with versus without stenting, *Am J Cardiol* 97(8):1188–1191, 2006.
50. McFalls EO, Ward HB, Moritz TE, et al: Coronary-artery revascularization before elective major vascular surgery, *N Engl J Med* 351(27): 2795–2804, 2004.
51. Boersma E, Poldermans D, Bax JJ, et al: Predictors of cardiac events after major vascular surgery: Role of clinical characteristics, dobutamine echocardiography, and beta-blocker therapy, *JAMA* 285(14): 1865–1873, 2001.
52. Mangano DT, Browner WS, Hollenberg M, Li J, Tateo IM: Long-term cardiac prognosis following noncardiac surgery, *JAMA* 268:233–239, 1992.
53. Hertzer NR: Basic data concerning associated coronary artery disease in peripheral vascular disease, *Ann Vasc Surg* 1:616–620, 1987.
54. L'Italien GJ, Cambria RP, Cutler BS, et al: Comparative early and late cardiac morbidity among patients requiring different vascular surgery procedures, *J Vasc Surg* 21:935–944, 1995.
55. Fleisher LA, Eagle KA, Shaffer T, Anderson GF: Perioperative- and long-term mortality rates after major vascular surgery: the relationship to preoperative testing in the Medicare population, *Anesth Analg* 89 (4):849–855, 1999.
56. Schueppert MT, Kresowik TF, Corry DC, et al: Selection of patients for cardiac evaluation before peripheral vascular operations, *J Vasc Surg* 23 (5):802–808, 1996.
57. Emlein G, Villegas B, Dahlberg S, Leppo J: Left ventricular cavity size determined by preoperative dipyridamole thallium scintigraphy as a predictor of late cardiac events in vascular surgery patients, *Am Heart J* 131:907–914, 1996.
58. White GH, Advani SM, Williams RA, Wilson SE: Cardiac risk index as a predictor of long-term survival after repair of abdominal aortic aneurysm, *Am J Surg* 156:103–107, 1988.
59. Lette J, Waters D, Champagne P, Picard M, Cerino M, Lapointe J: Prognostic implications of a negative dipyridamole-thallium scan: Results in 360 patients, *Am J Med* 92:615–620, 1992.
60. Hendel RC, Whitfield SS, Villegas BJ, Cutler BS, Leppo JA: Prediction of late cardiac events by dipyridamole thallium imaging in patients undergoing elective vascular surgery, *Am J Cardiol* 70:1243–1249, 1992.
61. Garcia EV, Bacharach SL, Mahmarian JJ, et al: Imaging guidelines for nuclear cardiology procedures. Part 1. *J Nucl Cardiol* 3:G1–G46, 1996.
62. Sharir T, Germano G, Kavanagh PB, et al: Incremental prognostic value of post-stress left ventricular ejection fraction and volume by gated myocardial perfusion single photon emission computed tomography, *Circulation* 100(10):1035–1042, 1999.
63. Kazmers A, Cerqueira MD, Zierler RE: Perioperative and late outcome in patients with left ventricular ejection fraction of 35% or less who require major vascular surgery, *J Vasc Surg* 8:307–315, 1988.
64. Cutler BS, Hendel RC, Leppo JA: Dipyridamole-thallium scintigraphy predicts perioperative and long-term survival after major vascular surgery, *J Vasc Surg* 15:972–981, 1992.
65. Lette J, Waters D, Bernier H, et al: Perioperative and long-term cardiac risk assessment, *Ann Surg* 216:192–204, 1991.
66. Mullany CJ, Darling GE, Pluth JR, et al: Early and late results after isolated coronary artery bypass surgery in 159 patients aged 80 years and older, *Circulation* 82(Suppl IV):IV-229–IV-236, 1990.
67. European Coronary Surgery Study Group: Long-term results of prospective randomised study of coronary artery bypass surgery in stable angina pectoris, *Lancet* 2(8309):1173–1180, 1982.
68. Rihal CS, Eagle KA, Mickel MC, Foster ED, Sopko G, Gersh BJ: Surgical therapy for coronary artery disease among patients with combined

coronary artery and peripheral vascular disease, *Circulation* 91(1): 46–53, 1995.

69. Landesberg G, Wolf Y, Schechter D, et al: Preoperative thallium scanning, selective coronary revascularization, and long-term survival after carotid endarterectomy, *Stroke* 29(12):2541–2548, 1998.

70. Landesberg G, Mosseri M, Wolf YG, et al: Preoperative thallium scanning, selective coronary revascularization, and long-term survival after major vascular surgery, *Circulation* 108(2):177–183, 2003.

71. Almanaseer Y, Mukherjee D, Kline-Rogers EM, et al: Implementation of the ACC/AHA guidelines for preoperative cardiac risk assessment in a general medicine preoperative clinic: improving efficiency and preserving outcomes, *Cardiology* 103(1):24–29, 2005.

72. Froehlich JB, Karavite D, Russman PL, et al: American College of Cardiology/American Heart Association preoperative assessment guidelines reduce resource utilization before aortic surgery, *J Vasc Surg* 36(4):758–763, 2002.

73. Young AE, Sandberg GW, Couch NP: The reduction of mortality of abdominal aortic aneurysm resection, *Am J Surg* 134:585–590, 1977.

74. Hertzer NR: Fatal myocardial infarction following abdominal aortic aneurysm resection: Three hundred forty-three patients followed 6–11 years postoperatively, *Ann Surg* 192:667–673, 1980.

75. Cutler BS, Leppo JA: Dipyridamole thallium 201 scintigraphy to detect coronary artery disease before abdominal aortic surgery, *J Vasc Surg* 5:91–100, 1987.

76. Raby KE, Goldman L, Creager MA, et al: Correlation between preoperative ischemia and major cardiac events after peripheral vascular surgery, *N Engl J Med* 321:1296–1300, 1989.

77. Younis LT, Aguirre F, Byers S, et al: Perioperative and long-term prognostic value of intravenous dipyridamole thallium scintigraphy in patients with peripheral vascular disease, *Am Heart J* 119:1287–1292, 1990.

78. Taylor LM Jr., Yeager RA, Moneta GL, McConnell DB, Porter JM: The incidence of perioperative myocardial infarction in general vascular surgery, *J Vasc Surg* 15:52–61, 1991.

79. Kresowik TF, Bower TR, Garner SA, et al: Dipyridamole thallium imaging in patients being considered for vascular procedures, *Arch Surg* 128:299–302, 1993.

80. McFalls EO, Doliszny KM, Grund F, Chute E, Chesler E: Angina and persistent exercise thallium defects: Independent risk factors in elective vascular surgery, *J Am Coll Cardiol* 21:1347–1352, 1993.

81. Baron JF, Mundler O, Bertrand M, et al: Dipyridamole-thallium scintigraphy and gated radionuclide angiography to assess cardiac risk before abdominal aortic surgery, *N Engl J Med* 330:663–669, 1994.

82. Bry JDL, Belkin M, O'Donnell TF Jr: An assessment of the positive predictive value and cost-effectiveness of dipyridamole myocardial scintigraphy in patients undergoing vascular surgery, *J Vasc Surg* 19:112–124, 1994.

83. Seeger JM, Rosenthal GR, Self SB, Flynn TC, Limacher MC, Harward TRS: Does routine stress-thallium cardiac scanning reduce postoperative cardiac complications? *Ann Surg* 219:654–663, 1994.

84. Fleisher LA, Rosenbaum SH, Nelson AH, Jain D, Wackers FJTh, Zaret BL: Preoperative dipyridamole thallium imaging and ambulatory electrocardiographic monitoring as a predictor of perioperative cardiac events and long term outcome, *Anesthesiology* 83:906–917, 1995.

85. Boucher CA, Brewster DC, Darling C, Okada R, Strauss HW, Pohost GM: Determination of cardiac risk by dipyridamole-thallium imaging before peripheral vascular surgery, *N Engl J Med* 312:389–394, 1985.

86. Fletcher JP, Antico VF, Gruenewald S, Kershaw LZ: Dipyridamole-thallium scan for screening of coronary artery disease prior to vascular surgery, *J Cardiovasc Surg* 29:666–669, 1988.

87. Sachs RN, Tellier P, Larmignat P, et al: Assessment by dipyridamole-thallium-201 myocardial scintigraphy of coronary risk before peripheral vascular surgery, *Surgery* 103:584–587, 1988.

88. Mangano DT, London MJ, Tubau JF, et al: Dipyridamole thallium-201 scintigraphy as a preoperative screening test: A reexamination of its predictive potential, *Circulation* 84:493–502, 1991.

89. Koutelou MG, Asimacopoulos PJ, Mahmarian JJ, Kimball KT, Verani MS: Preoperative risk stratification by adenosine thallium 201 single-photon emission computed tomography in patients undergoing vascular surgery, *J Nucl Med* 2:389–394, 1995.

90. Marshall ES, Raichlen JS, Forman S, Heyrich GP, Keen WD, Weitz HH: *Adenosine* radionuclide perfusion imaging in the preoperative evaluation of patients undergoing peripheral vascular surgery, *Am J Cardiol* 76:817–821, 1995.

91. Coley CM, Field TS, Abraham SA, Boucher CA, Eagle KA: Usefulness of dipyridamole-thallium scanning for preoperative evaluation of cardiac risk for nonvascular surgery, *Am J Cardiol* 69:1280–1285, 1992.

92. Shaw L, Miller DD, Kong BA, et al: Determination of perioperative cardiac risk by adenosine thallium-201 myocardial imaging, *Am Heart J* 124:861–869, 1992.

93. Younis L, Stratmann H, Takase B, Byers S, Chaitman BR, Miller DD: Preoperative clinical assessment and dipyridamole thallium-201 scintigraphy for prediction and prevention of cardiac events in patients having major noncardiovascular surgery and known or suspected coronary artery disease, *Am J Cardiol* 74:311–317, 1994.

94. Stratmann HG, Younis LT, Wittry MD, Amato M, Mark AL, Miller DD: Dipyridamole technetium-99m sestamibi myocardial tomography for preoperative cardiac risk stratification before major or minor nonvascular surgery, *Am Heart J* 132:536–541, 1996.

95. Van Damme H, Pierard L, Rigo PLR: Cardiac risk assessment before vascular surgery: a prospective study comparing clinical evaluation, dobutamine stress echocardiography, and dobutamine Tc-99m sestamibi tomoscintigraphy, *J Cardiovasc Surg* 5:54–64, 1997.

96. Beller GA, Brown KA, Hendel RC, Shaw LJ, Williams KA: Unresolved issues in risk stratification: Chronic coronary artery disease including preoperative testing, *J Nucl Cardiol* 4:92–95, 1997.

97. Anderson JL, Adams CD, Antman EM, et al: ACC/AHA 2007 guidelines for the management of patients with unstable angina/non ST-elevation myocardial infarction: a report of the American College of Cardiology/American Heart Association Task Force on Practice Guidelines (Writing Committee to Revise the 2002 Guidelines for the Management of Patients With Unstable Angina/Non ST-Elevation Myocardial Infarction): developed in collaboration with the American College of Emergency Physicians, the Society for Cardiovascular Angiography and Interventions, and the Society of Thoracic Surgeons: endorsed by the American Association of Cardiovascular and Pulmonary Rehabilitation and the Society for Academic Emergency Medicine, *Circulation* 116(7):e148–e304, 2007.

98. Hertzer NR: Fatal myocardial infarction following lower extremity revascularization: Two hundred seventy-three patients followed six to eleven postoperative years, *Ann Surg* 193:492–498, 1981.

99. Roger VL, Ballard DJ, Hallett JW Jr, Osmundson PJ, Puetz PA, Gersh BJ: Influence of coronary artery disease on morbidity and mortality after abdominal aortic aneurysmectomy: A population-based study, 1971–1987, *J Am Coll Cardiol* 14:1245–1252, 1989.

100. Hertzer NR, Young JR, Beven EG, et al: Late results of coronary bypass in patients with infrarenal aortic aneurysms: The Cleveland Clinic study, *Ann Surg* 205:360–367, 1987.

101. Poldermans D, Arnese M, Fioretti PM, et al: Sustained prognostic value of dobutamine stress echocardiography for late cardiac events after major noncardiac vascular surgery, *Circulation* 95(1):53–58, 1997.

Chapter 28

Nuclear Imaging in Revascularized Patients with Coronary Artery Disease

KENNETH A. BROWN AND JANUSZ K. KIKUT

....

BACKGROUND

Mechanical coronary revascularization with coronary artery bypass graft (CABG) surgery and percutaneous coronary intervention (PCI) have become important established techniques for treating selected patients with coronary artery disease (CAD). Optimal outcome of the invasive therapy is limited by several factors, including inability to establish complete revascularization in patients with diffuse disease, the finite patency rates, particularly for saphenous vein grafts, the development of in-stent restenosis, and progressive native CAD in nonrevascularized coronary vessels over time. With an established ability to identify myocardium at risk and hence prognostic value and an ability to localize ischemic myocardium to specific coronary territories, nuclear cardiac imaging can play an important role in evaluating revascularized CAD patients. Nuclear cardiac imaging can assess short- and long-term cardiac risk, predict restenosis in patients undergoing PCI, and identify new areas of myocardium at risk remote to prior revascularization.

Single-photon emission tomography (SPECT) continues to be the mainstay of scintigraphy. Many technical improvements have been made over last decade, allowing shortening of acquisition protocols and attenuation correction. Hybrid SPECT/CT and positron emission tomography PET/CT systems have grown throughout the United States, opening an opportunity for more accurate noninvasive myocardial perfusion imaging[1] PET unlike standard SPECT allows assessment of true coronary flow reserve.[1] However, vasodilator stress nitrogen (N)-13-ammonia or oxygen (O)-15-water requires on-site isotope production and additional capital investment for a cyclotron that may be prohibitively expensive for most PET centers. Rubidium-82 PET imaging is a more practical and financially feasible alternative to SPECT imaging,

with advantages of higher image quality and shorter patient time commitment.[2]

EVALUATION AFTER CORONARY ARTERY BYPASS GRAFT

Abnormalities observed on stress nuclear myocardial perfusion imaging (MPI) in patients who have undergone CABG will reflect a complex constellation of underlying pathophysiology that involves variable time courses. Early after CABG, abnormal perfusion may be related to early graft closure, which occurs in 12% to 20% within the first year.[3] However, it may also reflect myocardium supplied by diseased vessels that were technically unable to be grafted due to anatomic limitations. Alternatively, early MPI ischemia may be the result of coronary lesions proximal to patent grafts that compromise retrograde flow. When this involves the left anterior descending (LAD), a pattern of basal ischemia involving the anterior and lateral walls may be seen. Therefore, analysis and interpretation of MPI in revascularized patients should be done with knowledge of the coronary anatomy and operative results on hand.

Late after CABG, MPI abnormalities can reflect development of intercurrent venous graft closure, which is 2% to 4% per graft per year for years 1 through 5 and reaches 50% by 5 years.[3] Late ischemia on MPI can also reflect progression of native CAD.

Detection of Graft Disease

Several studies have evaluated the ability of nuclear MPI to detect graft disease, although their value is limited by relativity small sample size and older planar technology.[4,5] Combining these studies, the sensitivity for detecting occluded grafts was 19/22 (86%) grafts, with a specificity of 56/64 (88%). MPI SPECT imaging has shown similar results. In a series of 109 patients undergoing adenosine SPECT MPI nearly 7 years after CABG, the sensitivity of detecting graft disease was 96%. The specificity was only 61%, but the large majority of "false positives" were explained by significant lesions in non-revascularized native CAD or prior myocardial infarction with fixed defects.[6] Sensitivity of 80% to 84% with specificity of 80% to 90% has been reported in several smaller studies.[7,8] Localization of graft-site occlusion using stress nuclear MPI is quite accurate, with individual coronary territory sensitivities of 92%, 82%, and 75%, respectively, for the LAD, right coronary (RCA), and left circumflex (LCX).[8] The corresponding specificities were 91%, 90%, and 75%. The lower accuracy for the LCX territory is consistent with MPI data for native CAD and probably reflects the smaller myocardial territory and overlapping distributions with both RCA and LAD.

Anatomy Versus Physiology Considerations

Because stress nuclear MPI will reflect the hemodynamic significance of a coronary or graft lesion that may not correspond to conventional paradigms of angiographically significant lesions, descriptions of sensitivity and specificity for stress MPI based on such anatomic standards is limited. For example, Salm and colleagues found that 50% of grafts with a greater than 50% diameter stenosis had normal perfusion.[9] However, when graft lesions were assessed hemodynamically by Doppler coronary flow reserve, all of the grafts with depressed flow reserve had abnormal stress MPI, and 79% of grafts with normal flow reserve had normal MPI. Similar findings were reported by the same group using coronary flow reserve measured by cardiac MRI.[10] Zafir and colleagues identified that in patients with left internal mammary artery (LIMA) to LAD anastomosis, myocardial ischemia by MPI can occur without angiographic luminal stenosis, concluding that flow-limiting factors like mismatch between LAD and LIMA diameters at the anastomosis take place.[11]

Prognostic Implications of Stress Nuclear MPI after CABG

Because revascularization, even when "complete," reflects a moment in time in a disease process that is inevitably progressive, over time patients remain vulnerable for early and late graft closure and development or worsening of native coronary lesions. Not only can stress nuclear MPI detect the presence of such progressive disease, but more important, it can quantitate the risk of hard cardiac events, including cardiac death and future myocardial infarction (MI).

Assessment Early After CABG (2 to 3 Years)

Miller and colleagues evaluated the prognostic value of stress thallium-201 MPI SPECT performed within 2 years of CABG (mean, 11 months) and followed for 5.8

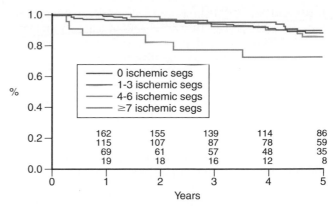

Figure 28-1 Kaplan-Meier curves for survival free of cardiac death or MI for the study group separated on the basis of the size of ischemic defect ($P = 0.007$). Influence of extent of ischemia on outcome seems to have threshold effect at ≥ 7 segments. MI, myocardial infarction; segs, segments. *(From Miller TD, Christian TF, Hodge DO, et al: Prognostic value of exercise thallium-201 imaging performed within 2 years of coronary artery bypass graft surgery, J Am Coll Cardiol 31:848–854, 1988.)*

years.[12] They found that the only significant multivariate predictors of cardiac death or MI were the exercise angina score and the number of abnormal segments on stress MPI, which reflects the extent of ischemia plus scar. Five-year event-free survival was 93% without angina and either normal MPI or a small postexercise perfusion defect (less than 3 abnormal segments of 14 total segments), compared to 71% for patients with angina and a moderate to large defect and 83% for patients with either of these adverse prognostic factors. Looking at the prognostic impact of reversible defects, indicating jeopardized viable myocardium, there was a threshold effect where patients with more than 7 ischemic segments had a worse outcome (72% 5-year death/ MI event-free rate) compared to patients with 0 to 6 reversible segments (85% to 89% 5-year event-free survival) (Fig. 28-1). Importantly, patients with normal MPI had a 5-year death/MI free rate of 92%, yielding an annual event rate of 1.6% per year. An interesting finding in this study was that ischemia proximal to bypass anastomosis was not associated with adverse outcome.

In a series of 75 patients undergoing stress MPI a mean of 38 months after CABG, the best predictor of cardiac events was the summed reversibility score (SRS), reflecting the extent of jeopardized viable myocardium.[13] This variable added significant incremental prognostic value to clinical and exercise data and nearly doubled the chi-square of the predictive model. A meta-analysis of functional testing for graft stenosis or progression of native disease showed superior sensitivity for stress MPI compared to exercise treadmill testing (ETT) (68% versus 45%), with similar specificity (84% versus 82%, respectively).[14]

Assessment Late After CABG (Beyond 5 Years)

Several studies have consistently shown that stress MPI performed late after CABG predicts future cardiac death and MI.[15–20] Palmas and colleagues evaluated 294 patients undergoing stress ^{201}Tl MPI at least 5 years after CABG.[16] They found that the SRS reflecting jeopardized viable myocardium was significantly related to future death or MI and had significant incremental predictive value to clinical and exercise data, doubling the predictive model chi-square. Stress nuclear MPI data in patients 5 years after CABG have also been shown to add significant prognostic value to angiographic data, doubling the predictive model chi-square for cardiac death/MI when added to clinical, exercise, and angiographic data.[17] Significant multivariate predictors of cardiac death or MI included the extent of the perfusion defect, multivessel perfusion defects, and increased ^{201}Tl lung uptake. Zellweger and colleagues also found that the extent of reversible defects in patients undergoing stress MPI more than 5 years after CABG was a significant multivariate predictor of cardiac death.[18]

Even in asymptomatic patients presenting 6 to 7 years out from their CABG, stress nuclear MPI is a powerful predictor of death or MI.[19] Reversible perfusion defects and exercise capacity were multivariate predictors of death or MI when clinical factors were adjusted. The presence of any reversible defect was associated with a 13% death/MI rate over 3 years, compared to 7% without reversible defect ($P = 0.004$) (Fig. 28-2), with separation in risk appearing to grow over additional time.

Interestingly, there was an inverse relationship between the time elapsed since CABG and the predictive value of a reversible defect. The relative risk associated with reversible defect for death/MI was 4.12 ($P = 0.02$) when performed 3 years after CABG, compared to 3.42 ($P = 0.01$) 3 to 6 years after CABG, 1.91 ($P = $ NS) 6 to 9 years after CABG, and 0.66 ($P = $ NS) more then 9 years after CABG. This suggests that stress MPI is detecting accelerated vein graft disease rather than progressive native disease. Finally, the authors evaluated the economic impact of evaluating this asymptomatic cohort and found that the costs of identifying patients at risk for the important cardiac events of death or MI were reasonable at approximately $1000 in 1998 dollars.

EVALUATION AFTER PERCUTANEOUS CORONARY INTERVENTION

Stress nuclear MPI can play an important role in evaluating patients with prior PCI who present with chest pain. Stress MPI can distinguish restenosis from other unrevascularized native CAD because of its abilities to locate ischemia to specific coronary artery territories. It also may be valuable in screening patients with recent PCI for development of occult restenosis. Accuracy of MPI and implications of the results differ with time after PCI. Three distinct time frames after PCI are discussed.

Early After PCI

There is little role for performing screening MPI before 6 weeks, because generally the restenosis phenomenon does not begin to occur before this time. Nevertheless, in patients presenting with chest pain, stress MPI may be helpful in ruling out ischemia as a basis even in this time frame, although interpretation of images requires an understanding of the impact of coronary intervention on coronary responsiveness to hyperemic stimuli. In the days of balloon angioplasty without stent placement, the initial vascular response to reduction of diameter narrowing with mechanical plaque rupture was variable. Several studies showed that perfusion defects on stress MPI early after angioplasty predicted development of restenosis.[20–23] Furthermore, even in arteries that do not show restenosis early, perfusion defect on stress MPI can be seen at a mean 9 days after angioplasty and progressively resolves on serial imaging at 3 and 7 months after angioplasty.[24] Similar findings have been described for coronary stenting, despite generally more satisfactory initial angiographic results.[25–28] The initial perfusion defect may reflect residual vessel obstruction, regional microvascular distal dysfunction in the territory of the dilated artery, angiographically unapparent dissections, or new accumulations of focally extruded plaque. The initial perfusion defect and diminished coronary flow reserve may also reflect endothelial dysfunction and medial injury without coronary stenosis that resolves with time.[29–31] These factors contribute to decreased specificity of MPI early after PCI, which substantially impairs the clinical utility of stress MPI in this time frame.

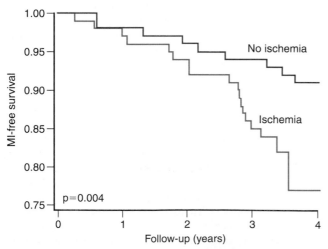

Figure 28-2 Kaplan-Meier plot associating reversible thallium defects with MI-free survival in asymptomatic patients late after coronary artery bypass surgery. Patients with ischemia had a significantly worse outcome than patients without ischemia. *(From Lauer MS, Lytle B, Pashkow F, et al: Prediction of death and myocardial infarction by screening with exercise-thallium testing after coronary-artery-bypass grafting, Lancet 351:615–622, 1998.)*

3 to 6 Months After PCI

This time frame represents the general period during which the restenosis phenomenon becomes completed. A large body of literature has evaluated the role of stress nuclear MPI in this clinical setting. It supports the use of stress MPI for detecting the presence of silent or symptomatic restenosis and documents its incremental prognostic value compared to treadmill testing and angiography, its cost-effectiveness, and its overall ability to predict cardiac events and guide management decisions.[32–41]

In a series of 116 patients 6 months out from angioplasty, stress nuclear MPI and treadmill testing were compared for predicting restenosis.[42] SPECT MPI had superior sensitivity (93% versus 52%), specificity (77% versus 64%), and accuracy (86% versus 57%) compared to treadmill testing. In addition, MPI was able to correctly identify the culprit vessel with 86% accuracy. Importantly, many patients with angiographic restenosis are asymptomatic, and the accuracy of stress MPI is not affected by manifestation of the symptoms. Hecht and colleagues reported that in their series of 116 patients, angiographic restenosis occurred in 61% of symptomatic and 59% of asymptomatic patients.[43] The ability of stress MPI to detect restenosis was similar: 96% and 91% sensitivity for asymptomatic and symptomatic patients, respectively, with 75% and 77% specificity, respectively. The sensitivity of stress EKG was substantially lower, 40% and 59%, respectively for silent and symptomatic patients. A series by Marie et al. confirmed that asymptomatic restenosis is common but well detected by stress MPI. Silent and symptomatic restenosis occurred at equal rates, and stress nuclear MPI detected 100% of the lesions, whereas stress ECG detected only 25%.[44] Numerous other studies, including a meta-analysis of publications between 1975 and 2000, have showed sensitivity of 80% to 90% for detecting restenosis, compared to 40% to 50% for treadmill exercise testing.[45–47]

Late After PCI

During the late time period after PCI, progression of disease in untreated vessel segments is more prevalent than restenosis.[48–52] Beyond simply detecting the presence or absence of restenosis after PCI, stress nuclear MPI performed outside the window of restenosis has the ability to predict major cardiac events, including death or MI. In a series of 211 patients undergoing stress ^{201}Tl MPI 1 to 3 years after balloon angioplasties, future cardiac death or MI was best predicted by the summed stress score, which will reflect the extent of ischemia plus scar.[53] The Duke Treadmill Score was not a significant predictor of outcome. In a series of 206 patients undergoing stress nuclear MPI 12 to 18 months after PCI (139 with stenting), the summed difference score (SDS) reflecting ischemia was the best predictor of death or MI.[54] Death or MI occurred in 36% patients with reversible defects compared to only 5% without reversible defects. Importantly, of the 124 asymptomatic patients, 24 (19%) had ischemia on MPI, of whom 8/24 (33%) died or developed MI.[54] In a larger series of 356 patients who had stress nuclear MPI 6 months after PCI stenting, 23% of patients had evocable target vessel ischemia by MPI that was clinically silent in 62% of cases.[55] Risk of cardiac events was directly proportionally related to the extent of

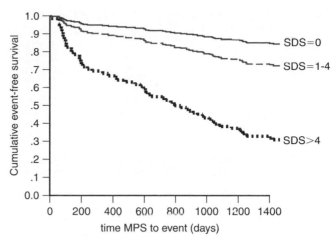

Figure 28-3 Cardiac risk in patients late after PCI is directly related to extent of jeopardized viable myocardium reflected in summed difference scores (SDS). MPS, myocardial perfusion single-photon emission computed tomography; PCI, percutaneous coronary intervention. *(From Zellweger MJ, Weinbacher M, Zutter AW, et al: Long-term outcome of patients with silent versus symptomatic ischemia six months after percutaneous coronary intervention and stenting, J Am Coll Cardiol 42: 33–40, 2003.)*

reversible defects manifested by the SDS: As SDS increased from 0, 1 to 4, and greater than 4, the cardiac event rates were 17%, 29%, and 69%, respectively (Fig. 28-3). Thus, absence of symptoms in this cohort was not a marker of low risk, and stress MPI was able to identify the high-risk subgroup. Similarly, in another study of 318 post-PCI patients, multivariate analysis showed the summed stress score to be the best independent predictor for hard cardiac events and the SDS the strongest independent predictor of soft cardiac events.[56] In the cohort, outcome was also not related to symptomatic status.[56] Target vessel ischemia appears to be less common with drug-eluting stents, but late cardiac events are still predicted by stress nuclear MPI. In a series of 476 patients who underwent stress nuclear MPI at 6 months after PCI (66% drug-eluting stents [DES], 34% bare metal stents [BMS]), target vessel ischemia was seen in 10% of BMS compared to 5% of DES ($P = 0.045$).[57] Most patients (68%) with target vessel ischemia were asymptomatic. Target vessel ischemia was associated with a greater then fivefold increased risk of major adverse cardiac events (MACE) (Fig. 28-4). Furthermore, the risk of cardiac events was directly related to extent of jeopardized viable myocardium reflected in the SDS (Fig. 28-5). The increased risk of MACE with target vessel ischemia persisted even if events occurring within 2 months of the MPI (which might have included revascularization events induced by the positive MPI results) were excluded (28% MACE with target vessel ischemia compared to only 5% without; $P < 0.0001$). Importantly, target vessel ischemia did not predict events related to late stent thrombosis, suggesting that such events are related to a different pathophysiology than intima hyperplasia.

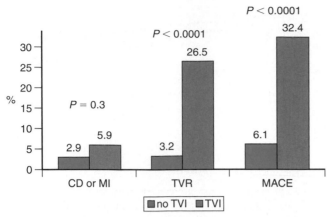

Figure 28-4 In patients late after PCI, target vessel ischemia (TVI) seen on stress nuclear MPI was associated with a fivefold increase in overall risk of major adverse cardiac events (MACE). MPI, myocardial perfusion imaging; PCI, percutaneous coronary intervention. *(From Zellweger MJ, Kaiser C, Brunner-LaRocca HP, et al: Value and limitations of target-vessel ischemia in predicting late clinical events after drug-eluting stent implantation, J Nucl Med 49:550–556, 2008.)*

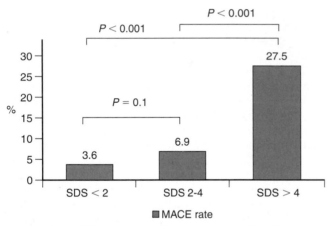

Figure 28-5 The risk of cardiac events was directly proportional to the extent of jeopardized viable myocardium manifested as summed difference scores (SDS) on stress MPI. *(From Zellweger MJ, Kaiser C, Brunner-LaRocca HP, et al: Value and limitations of target-vessel ischemia in predicting late clinical events after drug-eluting stent implantation, J Nucl Med 49:550–556, 2008.)*

Time Dependency of Risk

Although normal stress MPI performed late after PCI generally predicts a low cardiac event rate, the event rate is time dependent and also influenced by clinical risk factors. Prior studies have showed that in patients with CAD but normal MPI results, the risk of hard cardiac events increases with time.[58] In a series of 396 patients undergoing stress MPI 12 to 18 months after PCI, Acampa and colleagues found, over a 31-month follow-up, that clinical likelihood of ischemia and MPI SPECT ischemia were independent significant predictors of cardiac death or MI.[59] Importantly, they found that cardiac risk accelerated with time for both patients with and without MPI ischemia, and this risk was also influenced by clinical likelihood of ischemia (Fig. 28-6). Patients

with MPI ischemia and a high clinical likelihood of ischemia exceeded a calculated 2% annual death/MI rate by 10 months after imaging, while it took patients 30 months to reach that threshold if they had a low clinical likelihood of ischemia. Conversely, in patients without MPI ischemia and low clinical likelihood of ischemia, the annual risk of death/MI remained less than 2% throughout the follow-up. Patients without MPI ischemia but an intermediate-high clinical likelihood of ischemia exceeded 2% annual risk of death/MI by 20 months.

NOVEL REVASCULARIZATION METHODS AND RESEARCH TRENDS

Despite technical improvements of PCI and CABG procedures, there are a substantial number of patients with advanced coronary disease who are not suitable candidates for standard mechanical revascularization. Alternative medical and interventional revascularization treatments are being developed that may be suitable for these refractory patients. These include transmyocardial laser revascularization, percutaneous laser revascularization, and medical induction of angiogenesis. Nuclear myocardial scintigraphy may play an important role as an objective measure of efficiency of these alternative revascularization methods.

Transmyocardial laser revascularization (TMLR) is a surgical technique performed through a left thoracotomy or thoracoscopically, that uses a laser to bore transmural channels from the epicardial to the endocardial surfaces through the left ventricular myocardium in an attempt to improve local perfusion to ischemic myocardial territories not being reached by diseased arteries. TMLR has demonstrated improvement of symptoms in patients with refractory angina.[60,61] The basis of the beneficial effect of the procedure is unclear. Although it has been proposed that the clinical benefit could be related to creation of new intramuscular oxygen delivery channels, several studies have shown modest to no myocardial perfusion improvement by SPECT or quantitative PET.[62-65] Others have attributed the decrease in anginal symptoms to a decrease in sympathetic innervation after TMLR rather than improvement in myocardial perfusion.[66] Interestingly, myocardial sympathetic denervation has been documented by I-123 metaiodobenzylguanidine (MIBG) imaging in patients undergoing TMLR, and the duration of denervation corresponds to the duration of reduced anginal symptoms after TMLR.[67] Further data are required to determine whether MIBG SPECT has a role for following patients after TMLR treatment.

Percutaneous transmyocardial laser revascularization (PTMR) is a catheter-based technique of laser revascularization for refractory angina in no-option patients.[72] However, similar to TMLR, a reduction in anginal score does not correspond to an improvement in myocardial perfusion,[72] suggesting that any beneficial effect of PTMR is also not based on increased myocardial perfusion through the bored channels. Furthermore, initial

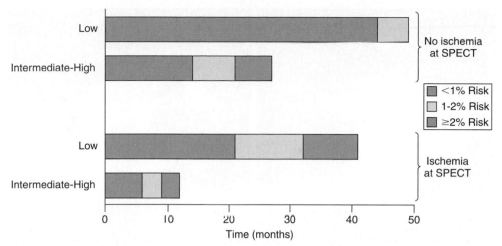

Figure 28-6   The acceleration of cardiac risk following stress MPI performed late after PCI depends on two factors: presence of ischemia seen on MPI and clinical indices of risk. Patients with MPI ischemia and an intermediate-high clinical risk exceed an annual death/MI rate of 2% within only 10 months, whereas those with ischemia but low clinical risk took 30 months to reach that threshold. In patients without MPI ischemia but an intermediate-high clinical risk, the 2% annual death/MI rate was reached at 20 months. Those without ischemia and with low clinical risk never reached that threshold. MI, myocardial infarction; MPI, myocardial perfusion imaging; PCI, percutaneous coronary intervention. *(From Acampa W, Evangelista L, Petretta M, et al: Usefulness of stress cardiac single-photon emission computed tomographic imaging late after percutaneous coronary intervention for assessing cardiac events and time of such events, Am J Cardiol 100:436–441, 2007.)*

promising results of PTMR[68] could not be reproduced in a subsequent randomized trial.[69]

Medical induction of angiogenesis: Over a decade of research in coronary angiogenesis[70] has led to developments of exciting methods in nonsurgical coronary revascularization, allowing more effective and targeted induction of angiogenesis. MPI has been shown to be useful as a surrogate of treatment efficacy in this cohort. Intracoronary administration of adenoviral particles containing gene-encoding fibroblast growth factor Ad5FGF-4 resulted in reduction of ischemic defect size by SPECT adenosine MPI.[71] Vascular endothelial growth factor (VEGF) gene transfer using adenoviral vector administered after PTCA and stenting showed no measurable benefit in restenosis rate at 6 months but showed improvement in myocardial perfusion by exercise MPI.[72] Intracoronary administration of these vectors may be intrinsically limited in reaching the target myocardium in no-option patients with severely diseased or occluded vessels. Therefore, transendocardial stereotactic injection systems have been developed to deliver angiogenesis factors directly to ischemic viable myocardium.[73] Stress nuclear MPI has been used then to determine objective response to treatment. Tio and colleagues compared treatment of end-stage CAD with transendocardial-delivered VEGF (using electrical and mechanical data to define ischemic viable segments) to PTLR[74] in a randomized trial.[73] PET imaging showed an improvement in extent of ischemia only in the VEGF-treated group. Gyongyosi and colleagues took a different approach and instead used the results of stress nuclear MPI SPECT as a navigational map to define segments of ischemic viable myocardium, based on the location or reversible defects, that were suitable for transendocardial injections of VEGF (Fig. 28-7).[75]

Patients were randomized to active agent or placebo injections. The target area of SPECT reversibility was substantially and significantly reduced in the VEGF group compared to placebo (*P* < 0.01) (Fig. 28-8). Direct endocardial implantation of bone marrow cells has also been used to attempt to improve myocardial perfusion in end-stage CAD. Tse and colleagues compared perfusion and clinical symptom response to endocardial injections of bone marrow cells versus PTMR.[76] Selection of sites for endocardial injections was guided by SPECT MPI and electromechanical mapping, whereas PTMR was guided by electromechanical mapping alone. Although there was significant improvement in quality of life scores in both groups, only the bone marrow injection group showed improvement in extent of jeopardized viable myocardium reflected in reversibility score (Fig. 28-9) at 6 months. Ongoing research in this area will further define the long-term benefit of these novel approaches to revascularization as well as the utility of stress MPI for mapping vulnerable areas and determining the success of revascularization.

Gene transfection is another promising technology of medical myocardial revascularization.[77] Ongoing investigations are addressing the appropriate choice of the therapeutic gene type, its structure and form, vector for delivery, method of selective delivery to target tissue, and preferable controllable gene expression.[74,78] Molecular imaging probes may be helpful in monitoring the gene expression at the cellular level. Combining traditional scintigraphic technologies with precise anatomic information from CT in hybrid technologies like SPECT/CT and PET/CT may result in a potent imaging tool for translational research,[79] but much more research will be required to define the role of radionuclide imaging in this setting.

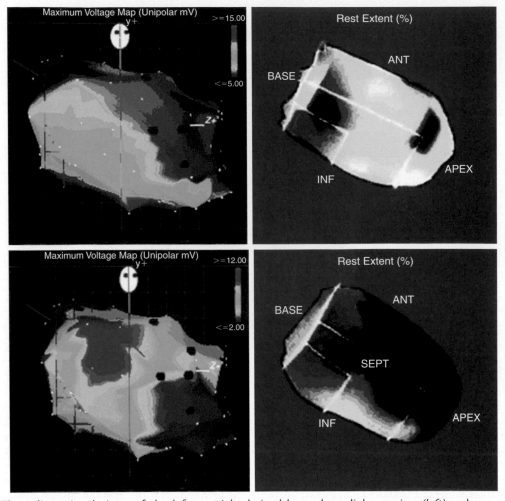

Figure 28-7 Three-dimensional views of the left ventricle derived by endocardial mapping *(left)* and myocardial perfusion scintigraphy derived by SPECT *(right)*. Decreased unipolar voltage (as index of viability) *(upper left)* and local linear shortening (index of rest local wall motion) *(bottom left)* in the anterior/anterolateral wall are shown, with the locations of the intramyocardial injections of phVEGF-A165 *(brown points)*. Small perfusion abnormality at rest SPECT (index of resting myocardial perfusion) *(upper right)* and large perfusion defect at stress SPECT (index of stress-induced perfusion abnormality) *(bottom right)* in the anterior wall in a patient with three-vessel disease and no previous myocardial infarction are shown. The transendocardial-treated area does not completely cover the scintigraphic ischemic area. The injection area at the endocardial map was approximated from the location of stress-induced ischemia at SPECT. SPECT, single-photon emission computed tomography; VEGF, vascular endothelial growth factor. *(From Gyongyosi M, Khorsand A, Zamini S, et al: NOGA-guided analysis of regional myocardial perfusion abnormalities treated with intramyocardial injections of plasmid encoding vascular endothelial growth factor A-165 in patients with chronic myocardial ischemia: Subanalysis of the EUROINJECT-ONE Multicenter Double-Blind Randomized Study, Circulation 112:I-157–I-165, 2005.)*

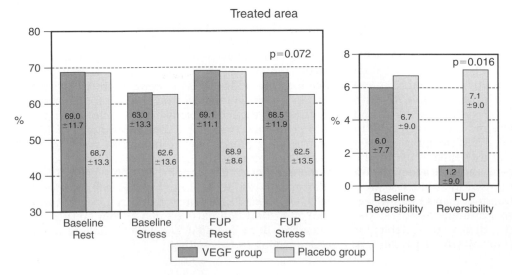

Figure 28-8 Reduction of MPI reversibility following transendocardial introduction of VEGF compared to placebo in end-stage CAD on follow-up imaging (FUP). CAD, coronary artery disease; MPI, myocardial perfusion imaging; VEGF, vascular endothelial growth factor. *(From Gyongyosi M, Khorsand A, Zamini S, et al: NOGA-guided analysis of regional myocardial perfusion abnormalities treated with intramyocardial injections of plasmid encoding vascular endothelial growth factor A-165 in patients with chronic myocardial ischemia: Subanalysis of the EUROINJECT-ONE Multicenter Double-Blind Randomized Study, Circulation 112:I-157–I-165, 2005.)*

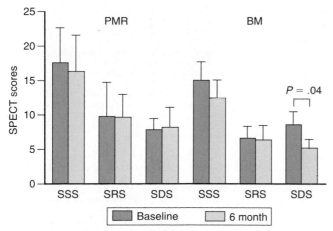

Figure 28-9 Improvement of stress MPI ischemia reflected in serial summed difference score (SDS) performed 6 months following transendocardial injection of bone marrow cells (BM) or percutaneous laser revascularization (PMR). Only the cohort receiving bone marrow cells showed an improvement in extent of ischemic myocardium. *(From Tse HF, Thambar S, KwongYL, et al: Comparative evaluation of long-term clinical efficacy with catheter-based percutaneous intramyocardial autologous bone marrow cell implantation versus laser myocardial revascularization in patients with severe coronary artery disease, Am Heart J 154:982e.1–1982.e6, 2007.)*

SUMMARY

Nuclear imaging is a valuable tool to evaluate patients with CAD who have undergone coronary revascularization. It can detect bypass graft disease and restenosis following PCI and define short-term and long-term prognosis in both cohorts. Furthermore, nuclear imaging may develop into a critical tool in assessing patients undergoing more novel approaches to revascularization.

REFERENCES

1. Raymondo I, et al: A prospective comparison of rubidium-82 and thallium-201 SPECT myocardial perfusion imaging utilizing a single dipyridamole stress in the diagnosis of coronary artery disease, *J Nucl Med* 21:1899–1905, 1990.
2. Katsuya Y, et al: Coronary flow and flow reserve by PET simplified for clinical applications using rubidium-82 or nitrogen-13-ammonia, *J Nucl Med* 37:1701–1712, 1996.
3. Grondin CN, et al: Coronary artery bypass grafting with saphenous vein, *Circulation* 79(Suppl I):24, 1989.
4. Pfisterer M, Emmenegger H, Schmitt HE, Muller-Brand J, Hasse J, Gradel E, Laver MB, Burckhardt D, Burkart F: Accuracy of serial myocardial perfusion scintigraphy with thallium-201 for prediction of graft patency early and late after coronary artery bypass surgery. A controlled prospective study, *Circulation* 66(5):1017–1024, 1982.
5. Ritchie JL, Narahara KA, Trobaugh GB, Williams DL, Hamilton GW: Thallium-201 myocardial imaging before and after coronary revascularization. Assessment of regional myocardial blood flow and graft patency, *Circulation* 56:830–836, 1977.
6. Khoury AF, Rivera JM, Mahmarian JJ, Verani MS: Adenosine thallium-201 tomography in evaluation of graft patency late after coronary artery bypass graft surgery, *J Am Coll Cardiol* 29:1290–1295, 1997.
7. Lakkis NM, Mahmarian JJ, Verani MS: Exercise thallium-201 single photon emission computed tomography for evaluation of coronary artery bypass graft patency, *Am J Cardiol* 76:107–111, 1995.
8. Elhendy A, et al: Dobutamine-atropine stress myocardial perfusion SPECT imaging in the diagnosis of graft stenosis after coronary bypass grafting, *J Nucl Cardiol* 5:491–497, 1998.
9. Salm LP, Bax JJ, Jukema JW, Langerak SE, Vliegen HW, Steendijk P, Lamb HJ, de Roos A, van der Wall EE: *J Nucl Cardiol* 12:545–552, 2005.
10. Salm LP, Bax JJ, Vliegen HW, Langerak SE, Dibbets P, Jukema JW, Lamb HJ, Pauwels EK, de roos A, van der Wall EE: Functional significance of stenoses in coronary artery bypass grafts. Evaluation by single-photon emission tomography perfusion imaging, cardiovascular magnetic resonance, and angiography, *J Am Coll Cardiol* 44:1877–1882, 2004.
11. Zafrir N, et al: Discrepancy between myocardial ischemia and luminal stenosis in patients with left internal mammary artery grafting to left anterior descending coronary, *J Nucl Cardiol* 10:663–668, 2003.
12. Miller TD, Christian TF, Hodge DO, Mullan BP, Gibbons RJ: Prognostic value of exercise thallium-201 imaging performed within 2 years of coronary artery bypass graft surgery, *J Am Coll Cardiol* 31:848–854, 1988.
13. Desideri A, et al: Exercise technetium-99m sestamibi single-photon emission tomography late after coronary artery bypass surgery: Long term follow-up, *Clin Cardiol* 20:779, 1997.
14. Chin AS, et al: Functional testing after coronary artery bypass graft surgery: a meta analysis, *Can J Cardiol* 19(7):802–808, 2003.
15. Sales dos Santos MM, et al: Prognostic value of technetium-99m labeled single photon emission computerized tomography in the follow-up of patients after their first myocardial revascularization surgery, *Arq Bras Cardiol* 80:25–30, 2003.
16. Palmas W, Bingham S, Diamond GA, Denton TA, Kiat H, Friedman JD, Scarlata D, Maddahi J, Cohen I, Berman D: Incremental prognostic value of exercise thallium-201 myocardial single-photon emission computed tomography late after coronary artery bypass surgery, *J Am Coll Cardiol* 25:403–409, 1995.
17. Nallamothu N, Johnson JH, Bagheri B, Heo J, Iskandrian AE: Utility of stress single-photon emission computed tomography (SPECT) perfusion imaging in predicting outcome after coronary artery bypass grafting, *Am J Cardiol* 80:1517–1521, 1997.
18. Zellweger MJ, Lewin HC, Lai S, Dubois EA, Friedman JD, Germano G, Kang X, Sharir T, Berman DS: When to stress patients after coronary artery bypass surgery, *J Am Coll Cardiol* 37:144–152, 2001.
19. Lauer MS, Lytle B, Pashkow F, Snader CE, Marwick TH: Prediction of death and myocardial infarction by screening with exercise-thallium testing after coronary-artery-bypass grafting, *Lancet* 351:615–622, 1998.
20. Cubukcu AA, Sivananthan UM, Thorley PJ, Verma SP, Sheard K, Williams GJ, Rees MR: Value of thallium-201 studies to assess coronary stent patency and to detect restenosis, *Am J Noninvas Cardiol* 8:225–229, 1994.
21. Wijns W, Serruys PW, Simoons ML, van den Brand M, De Feijter PJ, Reiber JH, Hugenholtz PG: Predictive value of early maximal exercise test and thallium scintigraphy after successful percutaneous transluminal coronary angioplasty, *Br Heart J* 53:194–200, 1985.
22. Breisblatt WM, Weiland F, Spaccavento LJ: Stress thallium-201 imaging after coronary angioplasty predicts restenosis and recurrent symptoms, *J Am Coll Cardiol* 12:1199–12204, 1988.
23. Wijns W, Serruys PW, Reiber JHC, de Feyter PJ, den Brand M, Simoons ML, Hugenholtz PG, Tijssen JGP: Early detection of restenosis after successful percutaneous transluminal coronary angioplasty by exercise-redistribution thallium scintigraphy, *Am J Cardiol* 55:357–361, 1985.
24. Manyari DE, Knudtson M, Kloiber R, Roth D: Sequential thallium-201 myocardial perfusion studies after successful percutaneous transluminal coronary artery angioplasty: delayed resolution of exercise-induced scintigraphic abnormalities, *Circulation* 77:86–95, 1988.
25. Rodes-Cabau J, et al: Frequency of Clinical significance of myocardial ischemia detected early after coronary stent implantation, *J Nucl Med* 42:1768–1772, 2001.
26. Nagaoka H, et al: Redistribution in thalium-201 imaging soon after successful coronary stenting: tomographic evaluation during coronary hyperemia induced by adenosine, *Jpn Circ J* 62:160–166, 1998.
27. Bachmann R, et al: Dipyridamole scintigraphy and intravascular ultrasound after successful coronary intervention, *J Nucl Med* 38:553–558, 1997.
28. Versafil F, et al: Differences of regional coronary flow reserve by adenosine thallium-201 scintigraphy early and six months after successful percutaneous transluminal coronary angioplasty or stent implantation, *Am J Cardiol* 78:1097–11102, 1996.
29. DePuey EG: Myocardial perfusion imaging with thallium-201 to evaluate patients before and after percutaneous transluminal coronary angioplasty, *Circulation* 84:159–165, 1991.
30. Wilson RF, et al: The effect of coronary angioplasty on coronary flow reserve, *Circulation* 77:873–885, 1988.
31. Uren NG, et al: Delayed recovery of resistive vessel function after coronary angioplasty, *J Am Coll Cardiol* 21:612–621, 1993.
32. Mishra J, Iskandrian AE: Stress myocardial perfusion imaging after coronary angioplasty, *Am J Cardiol* 81:766, 1998.
33. Alzaraki P, Krawczynska EG: Thallium imaging in management of post-revascularization patients, *Q J Nucl Med* 40:85, 1996.
34. Miller DD, Verani MS: Current status of myocardial perfusion imaging after percutaneous transluminal coronary angioplasty, *J Am Coll Cardiol* 24:260, 1994.

35. Miller DD, Liu P, Strauss HW, et al: Prognostic value of computer-quantitated exercise thallium imaging early after percutaneous transluminal coronary angioplasty, *J Am Coll Cardiol* 10:275, 1987.

36. Rosin DR, Van Raden MJ, Mincemoyer RM, et al: Exercise electrocardiographic and functional responses after percutaneous transluminal coronary angioplasty, *Am J Cardiol* 53:36C, 1984.

37. Herzel HO, Nuesch K, Gruentzig AR, et al: Short and long-term changes in myocardial perfusion after percutaneous transluminal coronary angioplasty assessed with thallium-201 exercise scintigraphy, *Circulation* 63:1001, 1981.

38. Scoll JM, Chaitman BR, David PR, et al: Exercise electrocardiography and myocardial scintigraphy in the serial evaluation of the results of percutaneous transluminal coronary angioplasty, *Circulation* 66:380, 1982.

39. Cottin Y, Rezaizadeh K, Touzery C, et al: Long-term prognostic value of ^{201}Tl single-photon emission computed tomographic myocardial perfusion imaging after coronary stenting, *Am Heart J* 141:999–1006, 2001.

40. Kaminek M, et al: Prognostic value of myocardial perfusion tomographic imaging in patients after percutaneous transluminal coronary angioplasty, *Clin Nucl Med* 25:775–778, 2000.

41. Zhang XL, et al: 99mTc-MIBI stress-rest SPECT imaging for evaluation of outcome after percutaneous transluminal coronary angioplasty, *Chin J Nucl Med* 20:97–100, 2000.

42. Hecht HS, Shaw R, Buce RT, et al: Usefulness of tomographic thallium-201 imaging for detection of restenosis after percutaneous transluminal coronary angioplasty, *Am J Cardiol* 6:1314, 1990.

43. Hecht HS, Shaw RE, Chin HL, et al: Silent ischemia after coronary angioplasty: Evaluation of restenosis and extent of ischemia in asymptomatic patients by tomographic thallium-201 exercise imaging and comparison with symptomatic patients, *J Am Coll Cardiol* 17:670, 1991.

44. Marie PY, Danchin N, Karcher G, et al: Usefulness of exercise SPECT thallium to detect asymptomatic restenosis in patients who had angina before coronary angioplasty, *Am Heart J* 126:571, 1993.

45. Georoulias P, Demakopoulos N, Kontos A, et al: Tc-99m tetrofosmin myocardial perfusion imaging before and six months after percutaneous transluminal coronary angioplasty, *Clin Nucl Med* 23:678, 1998.

46. Milan E, Zoccarto O, Terzi A, et al: Technetium-99m Sestamibi SPECT to detect restenosis after successful percutaneous coronary angioplasty, *J Nucl Med* 37:1300, 1996.

47. Garzon PP, Eisnberg MJ: Functional testing for the detection of restenosis after percutaneous transluminal coronary angioplasty: a meta-analysis, *Can J Cardiol* 17:41, 2001.

48. Suresh CG, et al: Late symptom recurrence after successful coronary angioplasty: angiographic outcome, *Int J Cardiol* 42:257–262, 1993.

49. Fleisch M, et al: Management and outcome of stents in 1998, *Cardiol Rev* 7:215–218, 1999.

50. Kober G, et al: Results of repeat angiography up to eight years following percutaneous transluminal angioplasty, *Eur Hear J* 10(Suppl G):49–53, 1989.

51. Kober G, et al: Results of repeat angiography up to eight years following percutaneous transluminal angioplasty, *Eur Heart J* 10(Suppl G):49–53, 1989.

52. Serruys PW, Luijten HE, Beatt KJ, et al: Incidence of restenosis after successful coronary angioplasty: A time-related phenomenon. A quantitative angiographic study in 342 consecutive patients at 1, 2, 3, and 4 months, *Circulation* 77:361–371, 1988.

53. Ho KT, Miller TD, Holmes DR, et al: Long-term prognostic of Duke Treadmill Score and exercise thallium-201 imaging performed one to three years after percutaneous transluminal coronary angioplasty, *Am J Cardiol* 84:1323, 1999.

54. Acampa W, Petretta M, Florimonte L, et al: Prognostic value of exercise cardiac tomography performed late after percutaneous coronary intervention in symptomatic and symptom free patient, *Am J Cardiol* 91:259–263, 2003.

55. Zellweger MJ, Weinbacher M, Zutter AW, et al: Long-term outcome of patients with silent versus symptomatic ischemia six months after percutaneous coronary intervention and stenting, *J Am Coll Cardiol* 42:33–40, 2003.

56. Zhang X, et al: Long-term prognostic value of exercise 99mTc-MIBI SPET myocardial perfusion imaging in patients after percutaneous coronary intervention, *Eur J Nucl Med Mol Imaging* 31:655–662, 2004.

57. Zellweger MJ, Kaiser C, Brunner-LaRocca HP, Buser PT, Osswald S, Weiss P, Mueller-Brand J, Pfisterer ME: Value and limitations of target-vessel ischemia in predicting late clinical events after drug-eluting stent implantation, *J Nucl Med* 49:550–556, 2008.

58. Hachamovitch R, et al: Determinants of risk and its temporal variation in patients with normal stress myocardial perfusion scans: what is the warranty period of a normal scan? *J Am Coll Cardiol* 41:1329–1340, 2003.

59. Acampa W, et al: Usefulness of stress cardiac single-photon emission computed tomographic imaging late after percutaneous coronary intervention for assessing cardiac events and time of such events, *Am J Cardiol* 100:436–441, 2007.

60. Spertus JA, Jones PG, Coen M, et al: Transmyocardial CO$_2$ laser revascularization improves symptoms, function and quality of life: 12 month results from a randomized controlled trial, *Am J Med* 111:341, 2001.

61. Horvath KA, Aranki SF, Chn LH, et al: Sustained angina relief 5 years after transmyocardial laser revascularization with a CO$_2$ laser, *Circulation* 104:181, 2001.

62. Cooley DA, Frazier OH, Kadipasaoglu KA, et al: Transmyocardial laser revascularization: clinical experience with twelve months follow-up, *J Thorac Cardiovasc Surg* 111:791–799, 1996.

63. Rimoldi O, Burns SM, Rosen SD, et al: Measurements of myocardial blood flow with positron emission tomography before and after transmyocardial laser revascularization, *Circulation* 100:II 134, 1999.

64. Horvath KA, Cohn LH, Cooley DA, et al: Transmyocardial laser revascularization: results of a multicenter trial with transmyocardial laser revascularization used as sole therapy for end-stage coronary artery disease, *J Thorac Cardiovasc Surg* 113:645–653, 1997.

65. Holmstrom M, et al: Wall motion and perfusion analysis of transmyocardial laser revascularization, *Scand Cardiovasc J* 37(2):91–97, 2003.

66. Al-Sheikh T, Allen KB, Straka SP, et al: Cardiac sympathetic denervation after transmyocardial laser revascularization, *Circulation* 100:135, 1999.

67. Teresinska, et al: Changes in cardiac adrenergic nervous system after transmyocardial laser revascularization assessed by I-123 MIBG SPECT, *Kardiol Pol* 60:15–20, 2004.

68. Oesterle SN, Sanborn TA, Ali N, et al: Percutaneous transmyocardial laser revascularization for severe angina: The PACIFIC randomized trial. Potential Class Improvement From Intramyocardial Channels, *Lancet* 356(9243):1705–1710, 2000.

69. Liao L, Sarria-Santamera A, Matchar DB, et al: Meta-analysis of survival and relief of angina pectoris after transmyocardial revascularization, *Am J Cardiol* 95(10):1243–1245, 2005.

70. Lazarous DF, Shou M, Scheinowitch M, et al: Comparative effects of basic fibroblast growth factor and vascular endothelial growth factor on coronary collateral development and the arterial response to injury, *Circulation* 94:1074–1082, 1996.

71. Grines C, Watkins M, Mahmarian J, et al: A randomized, double-blind, placebo-controlled trial of Ad5FGF-4 gene therapy and its effect on myocardial perfusion in patients with stable angina, *J Am Coll Cardiol* 42:1339–1347, 2003.

72. Hedman M, Hartikainen J, Syvanne M, et al: Safety and feasibility of catheter-based local intracoronary vascular endothelial growth factor gene transfer in the prevention of postangioplasty and in-stent restenosis and in the treatment of chronic myocardial ischemia, *Circulation* 2003:107, 2677.

73. Tio RA, et al: PET for evaluation of differential myocardial perfusion dynamics after VEGF gene therapy and laser therapy in end-stage coronary artery disease, *J Nucl Med* 45(9):1437–1443, 2004.

74. Gaffney MM, Hynes SO, Barry F, O'Brien T: Cardiovascular gene therapy: current status and therapeutic potential, *Br J Pharmacol* 152:175–188, 2007.

75. Gyongyosi M, Khorsand A, Zamini S, et al: NOGA-guided analysis of regional myocardial perfusion abnormalities treated with intramyocardial injections of plasmid encoding vascular endothelial growth factor A-165 in patients with chronic myocardial ischemia: Subanalysis of the EUROINJECT-ONE Multicenter Double-Blind Randomized Study, *Circulation* 112:I–157–I–165, 2005.

76. Tse HF, et al: Comparative evaluation of long-term clinical efficacy with catheter-based percutaneous intramyocardial autologous bone marrow cell implantation versus laser myocardial revascularization in patients with severe coronary artery disease, *Am Heart J* 14(982e):1–1982.e6, 2007.

77. Hedman M, Turunen MP, Ylä-Herttuala S: New technologies in cardiovascular research: Gene therapy. In Pasterkamp G, de Kleijn D, editors: *Cardiovascular Research: New Technologies, Methods, and Applications*, New York, 2005, Springer, pp 89–98.

78. Rissanen TT, Ylä-Herttuala S: Current status of cardiovascular gene therapy, *Mol Ther* 15:1233–1247, 2007.

79. Jaffer FA: Seeing within. Molecular imaging of the cardiovascular system, *Circ Res* 94:433–445, 2004.

Chapter 29

Stress Myocardial Perfusion Imaging in Patients with Diabetes Mellitus

FRANS J.TH. WACKERS AND JEROEN J. BAX

INTRODUCTION

In 2005, the Centers for Disease Control and Prevention (CDC) estimated that there were approximately 21 million people with diabetes mellitus in the United States: 15 million with diagnosed diabetes mellitus and 6 million with undiagnosed diabetes. Greater than 95% of these individuals have type 2 diabetes.[1] The number of patients with diabetes mellitus increases every year by 5%, adding approximately 1.5 million new cases annually. Compared to the nondiabetic population, patients with diabetes mellitus have an increased risk of developing cardiovascular disease and an increased risk for death from myocardial infarction or congestive heart failure. Although in the general population, the overall age-adjusted mortality from cardiovascular diseases decreased by 30% between 1990 and 2000, the mortality rate in patients with diabetes mellitus has increased by approximately the same amount (Fig. 29-1). Importantly, 80% of the mortality among diabetics can be attributed to cardiovascular causes. Because of these alarming statistics, the American Diabetes Association; the National Heart, Lung and Blood Institute; the Juvenile Diabetes Foundation International; the National Institute of Diabetes and Digestive and Kidney Diseases; and the American Heart Association issued a joint statement in 1999 indicating the importance of diabetes mellitus as a major risk factor for cardiovascular disease.[2]

EARLY DETECTION OF CORONARY ARTERY DISEASE IN DIABETES MELLITUS

To maximize the effect of appropriate treatment of cardiovascular disease, it is important that diabetic patients at risk of developing or who have already developed coronary artery disease (CAD) are identified as early as possible.

A major hurdle toward this goal is that CAD in patients with diabetes is frequently silent; when clinically manifest, it is often in an advanced stage. Twenty-five percent of patients with diabetes mellitus in the Framingham Study had electrocardiographic evidence of prior unrecognized infarction, and half of these individuals were asymptomatic.[3–5] Less than a third of diabetic patients with exercise-induced ischemia on myocardial perfusion imaging (MPI) had angina during exertion, compared to more than two-thirds of nondiabetic patients. In 1998, the American Diabetes Association published a consensus statement on diagnostic testing for CAD in people with diabetes mellitus.[6] It was recommended that asymptomatic diabetic patients with two or more risk factors for CAD in addition to diabetes mellitus should have exercise stress testing. The consensus statement further recommended exercise electrocardiography (ECG) as the first diagnostic test. These recommendations were based on the clinical judgment of a panel of experts rather than on published scientific data in truly asymptomatic patients. At the time of the consensus statement, it was evident that a substantial gap existed in the knowledge about the prevalence of silent ischemia, how to detect preclinical CAD, and how to manage asymptomatic patients with diabetes in whom silent ischemia was demonstrated. In subsequent years, a number of studies have demonstrated unequivocally that the presence or absence of traditional risk factors for CAD in patients with diabetes are not helpful for predicting silent myocardial ischemia. Therefore, other clinical and diagnostic algorithms need to be explored for identifying diabetic patients at increased cardiovascular risk.

Stress Modality

In the general population, the preferred stress modality for detecting myocardial ischemia is physical exercise on a treadmill or bicycle. However, many diabetic

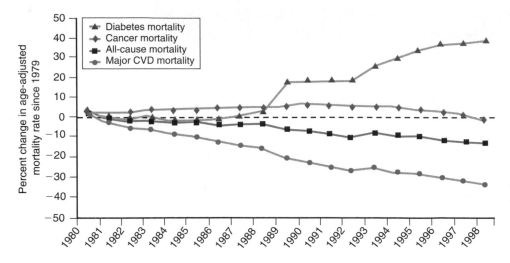

Figure 29-1 Change in age-adjusted mortality rates over the previous decades. In contrast to the decrease in major cardiovascular disease (CVD) mortality, the mortality from diabetes has increased. *(From Centers for Disease Control and Prevention Mortality Database.)*

patients have diminished exercise ability because of obesity, deconditioning, peripheral neuropathy, or peripheral vascular disease. Several studies have observed that about a third to half of diabetic patients were unable to achieve adequate exercise levels for diagnostic testing.[7] Therefore, pharmacologic stress may be the more appropriate stress modality in many patients with diabetes. Stress MPI has been shown to have comparable sensitivity and specificity in nondiabetics and diabetic patients for detecting CAD (Fig. 29-2).[8] Moreover, the incremental prognostic value of pharmacologic MPI was similar to that using physical exercise (Fig. 29-3).[9,10]

Prevalence of Silent Myocardial Ischemia

Screening for CAD is a controversial issue in clinical cardiology. To avoid an unacceptably large number of false-

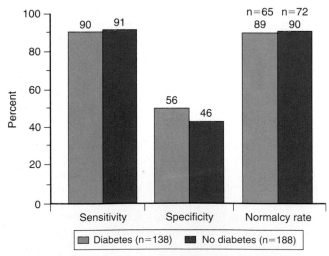

Figure 29-2 Comparative sensitivity and specificity for detecting coronary artery disease (stenosis > 70%) and normalcy rate in patients with and without diabetes. There is no significant difference for each comparison. *(Modified from Kang X, Berman DS, Lewin H, et al: Comparative ability of myocardial perfusion single-photon emission computed tomography to detect coronary artery disease in patients with and without diabetes mellitus, Am Heart J 137:949–957, 1999.)*

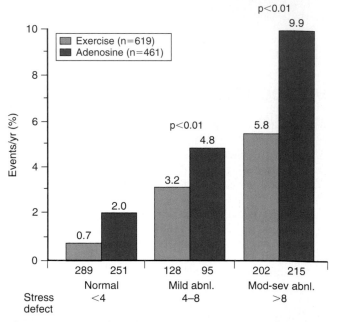

Figure 29-3 Hard cardiac event rates (death and nonfatal myocardial infarction) in relation to the extent and severity of myocardial perfusion abnormality in patients with diabetes who had exercise stress and adenosine vasodilation. With both exercise and adenosine, event rates increased with increasing stress defect size. *(Modified from Kang X, Berman DS, Lewin HC, et al: Incremental prognostic value of myocardial perfusion single-photon emission computed tomography in patients with diabetes mellitus, Am Heart J 138:1025–1032, 1999.)*

positive test results, the prevalence of the disease for which screening is to be performed must be at least intermediate. The true prevalence of silent myocardial ischemia in asymptomatic patients with diabetes was until recently unknown because most estimates were based on retrospective database analyses. The results of the prospective Detection of Ischemia in Asymptomatic Diabetics (DIAD) study made very clear that indeed most previous studies were significantly biased owing to patient selection. Retrospective database analyses may not be accurate because patients were most likely referred for stress testing to investigate symptoms suspected to be due to CAD. The available published information consisted of three types of analyses: retrospective analysis of large, combined nuclear cardiology databases, retrospective analysis of single laboratory databases, and prospective epidemiologic studies. In two large retrospective database studies, the prevalence of abnormal myocardial perfusion images ranged from 41% to 58%.[8,11,12] Detailed information on patients' symptoms was not available, and it was unclear how many patients were truly asymptomatic. In other retrospective analyses of apparently asymptomatic patients with diabetes, 26% to 59% had abnormal stress myocardial perfusion images.[13-16] These patients were referred for risk assessment before general surgery or because of the presence of multiple risk factors for CAD. Several prospective studies have been performed in Europe in asymptomatic patients with diabetes. The observed prevalence of ischemia in these studies varied as well. Whereas Janand-Delenne and colleagues[17] reported a prevalence of silent myocardial ischemia of 18.4%, Gazzaruso and colleagues[18] and the Italian MiSAD group[19] reported a prevalence of 8.6% and 6.4%, respectively. In the latter studies, characteristically, exercise electrocardiography was the first stress test, and MPI was only performed if exercise electrocardiography was positive or equivocal. Because of the known low sensitivity of exercise electrocardiography, a substantial number of patients may have been missed in these studies.

The prospective multicenter DIAD study[20] published in 2004 shed a different light on the practical problem of silent myocardial ischemia in asymptomatic patients with diabetes. It is important to consider the entry criteria for the DIAD study. All patients enrolled in the study had type 2 diabetes mellitus, were 50 to 75 years of age, had no symptoms suggesting CAD (including a negative Rose questionnaire for angina or chest discomfort), had a normal resting electrocardiogram, and had no prior cardiac stress testing. In addition to carefully ruling out symptoms of angina and anginal equivalents, the requirement of a normal rest ECG is an important characteristic of this study. Well over 1100 patients were recruited and randomized to either screening for CAD with adenosine technetium ^{99m}Tc sestamibi gated single-photon emission computed tomography (SPECT) imaging or no screening. The prevalence of *silent myocardial ischemia*, defined as regional myocardial perfusion abnormalities on imaging or ischemic ECG changes during adenosine infusion, was lower in the DIAD study than previously suggested in the literature. Although 22% of asymptomatic subjects had abnormal screening test results, in only 6% of participants were the myocardial perfusion abnormalities severe.[20] Thus, 1 out of every 5 asymptomatic patients with diabetes may have silent CAD, and 1 of 16 may have markedly abnormal screening results. In a recent French study, similar to the DIAD study in design, age appeared to be an important factor for the occurrence of silent ischemia. Whereas asymptomatic patients with diabetes younger than 60 years had a prevalence of about 30%, patients older than 60 years had a prevalence of 43%.[21]

Endothelial Dysfunction

Many patients with diabetes mellitus have evidence for endothelial dysfunction.[22,23] Persistent hyperglycemia may be in part responsible for impaired endothelial-dependent vasodilation. Oxidative stress and hyperproduction of superoxide are common in diabetes and might cause impaired endothelial nitric oxide synthesis. In addition, the insulin-resistant state itself may blunt nitric oxide–mediated vasodilation. Impaired regional coronary flow reserve has been observed in patients with diabetes mellitus, in particular in conjunction with cardiac autonomic dysfunction. The presence of microvascular endothelial dysfunction is of relevance for MPI. Regional myocardial perfusion abnormalities may occur in the absence of significant epicardial CAD.[24] Whether such myocardial perfusion abnormalities have the same prognostic implications as those associated with epicardial CAD is as yet unclear. Emmett et al.[25] reported that transient ischemic left ventricular dilation (TID) on SPECT imaging was strongly associated with diabetes mellitus and left ventricular hypertrophy, rather than with the amount of ischemia or severity of CAD. Thus, microvascular disease and endothelial dysfunction may play an important role in the etiology of TID.

ABNORMAL MYOCARDIAL PERFUSION IMAGING IN PATIENTS WITH SUSPECTED OR KNOWN CORONARY ARTERY DISEASE (See Chapter 16)

Observations in selected patient populations suggest that SPECT myocardial perfusion abnormalities in patients with diabetes mellitus carry a significantly worse prognosis than similar abnormalities in patients without diabetes mellitus. The most extensive retrospective five-center database analysis published thus far involved 4755 patients, of whom 929 had diabetes mellitus.[11] More patients with diabetes were unable to exercise adequately and had vasodilator stress. Abnormal SPECT MPI was an independent predictor of cardiac death and nonfatal myocardial infarction in both nondiabetic patients and diabetic patients. However, in spite of higher revascularization rate, patients with diabetes had an almost two times higher cardiac event rate than nondiabetic patients. Unadjusted cardiac survival rate was lower for diabetic patients but became comparable to that in nondiabetic patients after adjustment for pretest clinical risk and severity of MPI abnormalities. An important observation was that diabetic women had a significantly worse outcome for any given extent of myocardial ischemia on SPECT imaging (Fig. 29-4).[11,26] Another study that evaluated specifically the value of adenosine stress SPECT MPI in women confirmed the preceding observations.[10] Although men and women without diabetes mellitus had similar outcomes for any given MPI abnormality, women with diabetes mellitus had significantly higher cardiac mortality. Furthermore, insulin-dependent patients were at higher risk than non-insulin-dependent diabetic patients (Fig. 29-5).[10]

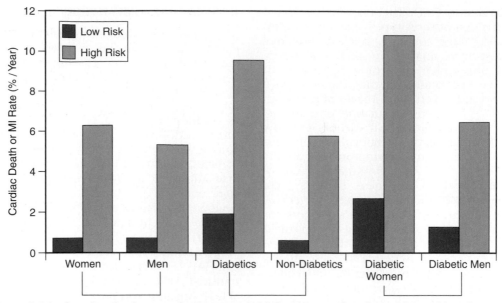

Figure 29-4 Annual risk of cardiac death or nonfatal myocardial infarction as a function of the results of stress SPECT imaging based on meta-analysis of 39 peer-reviewed publications. The annual risk for patients with normal SPECT imaging (low risk) is substantially higher in patients with diabetes, particularly diabetic women, than in nondiabetic patients. Similarly, diabetic patients with moderate to severely abnormal SPECT images, particularly women, are at higher annual risk for hard cardiac events than nondiabetic patients. *(From Shaw LJ, Iskandrian AE: Prognostic value of gated myocardial perfusion SPECT, J Nucl Cardiol 11:171–185, 2004.)*

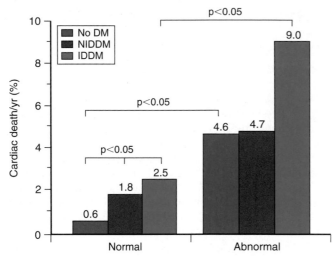

Figure 29-5 Cardiac mortality in patients with normal and abnormal stress myocardial perfusion SPECT images, in patients with no diabetes mellitus (DM), with non-insulin-dependent diabetes mellitus (NIDDM), and with insulin-dependent diabetes. Patients with insulin-dependent diabetes and normal and abnormal stress SPECT images had significantly higher mortality than patients without diabetes. *(Modified from Berman DS, Kang X, Hayes SW, et al: Adenosine myocardial perfusion single-photon emission computed tomography in women compared to men. Impact of diabetes mellitus on incremental prognostic value and effect on patient management, J Am Coll Cardiol 41:1125–1133, 2003.)*

Not unexpectedly, many asymptomatic patients with diabetes mellitus who are screened have entirely normal stress myocardial perfusion images. In the general population, patients with normal exercise myocardial perfusion images have an excellent prognosis with a low hard cardiac event rate of less than 1% per year.[27]

However, in patients with diabetes mellitus, this expectation appeared invalid. In a retrospective database analysis, Giri and colleagues[11] observed that even though the prognosis in patients with diabetes mellitus and normal stress perfusion images was significantly better than that of patients with diabetes and perfusion abnormalities, their prognosis was worse compared to patients without diabetes mellitus (Fig. 29-6). Outcome was even worse in insulin-dependent patients with normal perfusion images (see Fig. 29-4).[10] Thus, the "warranty period" of normal stress perfusion images in patients with diabetes mellitus is apparently limited. Hachamovitch and colleagues[28] subsequently demonstrated that the prognostic value of normal stress perfusion images must be viewed in the clinical context and is less favorable in the elderly, patients with known CAD, those who require pharmacologic testing, and, in particular those with diabetes.

In the recently completed DIAD study, 1123 patients without symptoms or clinical signs of CAD were followed prospectively for 5 years.[29] Unexpectedly, the outcome in these patients was considerably more favorable than anticipated. This illustrates (again) that retrospective database analyses may have significant limitations. The cumulative 5-year hard cardiac event rate (cardiac death or nonfatal myocardial infarction) in DIAD was only 2.9%, or less than 1% per year.[29] Moreover, cardiac event rate was not different in patients randomized to screening or no screening (Fig. 29-7). A relatively small and equal number of patients in both groups had coronary revascularization, so this does not explain the favorable outcome. In the DIAD study, the only intervention consisted of systematic screening with adenosine stress SPECT imaging in one group of the participants. The other group had no intervention but

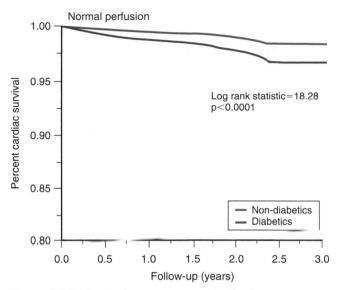

Figure 29-6 Survival curves comparing the 3-year outcome in patients with normal stress myocardial perfusion SPECT images, with and without diabetes mellitus. After 2 years of follow-up, patients with diabetes had a higher incidence of cardiac events than patients without diabetes. *(From Giri S, Shaw LJ, Murthy DR, et al: Impact of diabetes on the risk stratification using stress single-photon emission computed tomography myocardial perfusion imaging in patients with symptoms suggestive of coronary artery disease, Circulation 105:32–40, 2002.)*

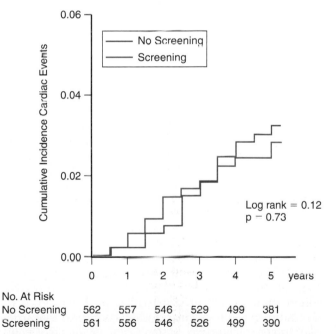

No. At Risk

No Screening	562	557	546	529	499	381
Screening	561	556	546	526	499	390

Figure 29-7 Cumulative incidence of cardiac events (cardiac death or nonfatal myocardial infarction) in participants in the DIAD study. Patients with type 2 diabetes mellitus without symptomatic or previously diagnosed coronary artery disease were randomized to screening with stress myocardial perfusion imaging or no screening. *(From Young LH, Wackers FJTh, Chyun DA, et al: Cardiac outcomes after screening for asymptomatic coronary artery disease in patients with type 2 diabetes: The DIAD study: A randomized controlled clinical trial, JAMA 301:1547–1555, 2009.)*

regular follow-up. Screened participants with normal stress images or small myocardial perfusion defects had a very low cardiac event rate (0.4% per year), whereas participants with moderate to large myocardial perfusion defects had a significantly higher cardiac event rate (2.4% per year) (Fig. 29-8). Subsequent clinical management in both groups was entirely at the discretion of the patients' medical providers, and one can argue therefore that DIAD reflects "real world" contemporary clinical care. Importantly, during the course of the study, the majority of DIAD patients were aggressively treated with antiischemic medications (statins, angiotensin-converting enzyme [ACE] inhibitors, aspirin). Thus it appears that patients with type 2 diabetes mellitus without symptoms or signs of CAD fare very well on contemporary and aggressive primary cardiac preventive treatment.[29]

CLINICAL PREDICTORS OF SILENT MYOCARDIAL ISCHEMIA

Because of the relatively low prevalence of silent ischemia in asymptomatic patients with diabetes, and because of the large number of asymptomatic diabetic patients potentially to be screened, investigators have tried to derive simple and inexpensive clinical markers that would identify a subgroup of patients at higher risk. A number of predictors for the presence of silent CAD have been suggested in various studies: retinal vasculopathy,[17] micro/macro albuminuria,[30] C-reactive protein, hemoglobin A_{1c}, duration of diabetes, body mass index (BMI), peripheral neuropathy, lipoprotein (a),[18] traditional risk factors for CAD,[2,17] peripheral arterial disease, rest electrocardiogram,[19] and cardiac autonomic dysfunction.[20,31-35] Many of these variables either have too high a prevalence in the diabetic population to be practically useful, or their statistical association with ischemia has been inconsistent in various published studies. In recent years, a number of studies confirmed that conventional risk factors for CAD were not predictive of stress-inducible ischemia.[20,36] The DIAD study showed that male gender, duration of diabetes, and the presence of cardiac autonomic dysfunction were strong predictors of inducible ischemia.[20] Although the statistical association of cardiac autonomic dysfunction and myocardial ischemia was strong, the positive predictive value was low.

The anatomic substrate of cardiac autonomic dysfunction has been visualized by positron emission tomography with C-11 hydroxyephedrine. In patients with diabetes, myocardial uptake of hydroxyephedrine often was heterogeneous, consistent with regional sympathetic denervation, and was associated with diminished coronary flow reserve due to endothelial dysfunction.[37,38] In addition, increased in vitro platelet activation[39] has been reported in conjunction with cardiac autonomic dysfunction in patients with type 1 diabetes mellitus, potentially explaining the association with impaired myocardial perfusion. It is as yet unclear whether there is a causal relationship between the presence of cardiac autonomic dysfunction and coronary vasculopathy or whether it is merely an epiphenomenon. Valensi et al.[40] observed in a large multicenter study that about 25% of patients with

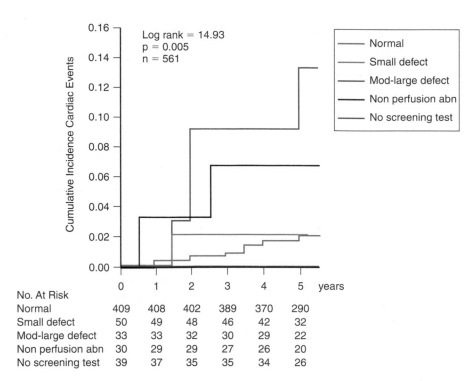

Figure 29-8 Cumulative incidence of cardiac events (cardiac death or nonfatal myocardial infarction) according to the results of screening in the DIAD study. Participants with moderate to large stress myocardial perfusion defects had significantly worse outcome than those with normal screening images or small perfusion defects. *(From Young LH, Wackers FJTh, Chyun DA, et al: Cardiac outcomes after screening for asymptomatic coronary artery disease in patients with type 2 diabetes: The DIAD study: A randomized controlled clinical trial, JAMA 301:1547–1555, 2009.)*

type 1 and type 2 diabetes have evidence of cardiac autonomic dysfunction. Although clinical testing for cardiac autonomic dysfunction has recently become easier, more standardized, and more reproducible by the development of automated portable devices, it is not a routine test in most outpatient clinics. Another relatively simple method to recognize cardiac autonomic dysfunction may be to assess heart rate response to vasodilator stress testing with adenosine. The normal increase of heart rate that may be observed in response to coronary vasodilation is significantly blunted in patients with diabetes, compared to nondiabetic patients.[41] However, in individual patients, the threshold of an abnormal response associated with increased cardiac risk is not yet defined.

MULTIMODALITY APPROACH FOR DETECTION OF CAD IN DIABETES MELLITUS (See Chapter 20)

Another potentially attractive and perhaps cost-effective first step in the screening of asymptomatic patients with diabetes may be the assessment of coronary artery calcium by x-ray computed tomography.[42–44] The degree of calcification, expressed as the coronary artery calcium (CAC) score, is a measure of atherosclerotic plaque burden.[45] In the general population, patients with high levels of coronary artery calcium have a high incidence of abnormal stress myocardial perfusion images, whereas in the absence of significant calcium deposits, this incidence is low.[46] In selected populations, high CAC scores have been shown to be associated with higher future cardiac event rates.[47–49] In a study of self-referred low- to intermediate-risk asymptomatic patients, calcium scoring

appeared to be an independent predictor for hard and soft cardiac events, in addition to conventional risk factors.[49] A number of recent studies explored the prognostic value of coronary artery calcium in the diabetic population.[50–54] In a retrospective analysis of a largely self-referred population of asymptomatic subjects, subjects with metabolic syndrome or diabetes had a significantly higher likelihood of having significant coronary artery calcium on electron beam computed tomography (EBCT) compared to subjects with neither.[52] In comparison to nondiabetic patients, patients with CAC scores above 100 Agatston units (Au) and metabolic syndrome or diabetes had a higher likelihood of inducible ischemia.[53] Anand et al.[54] prospectively studied asymptomatic patients with diabetes mellitus using a stepwise diagnostic approach: After initial EBCT coronary calcium scoring, patients with a calcium score over 100 Au had stress MPI. With increasing calcium burden, the number of patients with abnormal SPECT increased substantially; 60% of patients with CAC scores above 400 Au had abnormal stress SPECT (Fig. 29-9). In addition, significant coronary artery calcification (>400 Au) was associated with adverse outcome in these asymptomatic patients with diabetes (Fig. 29-10). The recent PREDICT study, a prospective cohort study of 589 patients with type 2 diabetes with no history of cardiovascular disease, confirmed that coronary artery calcium was a significant predictor of combined hard and soft cardiac events.[55]

Although the presence of calcium in coronary arteries must be considered pathologic, it does not necessarily imply that significant obstructive CAD is present. In fact, the specificity of coronary calcium for significant angiographic coronary artery stenoses is in the 60% to 70% range. Neither does the absence of calcium guarantee absence of obstructive CAD.

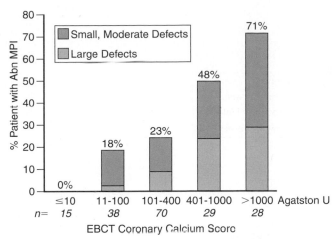

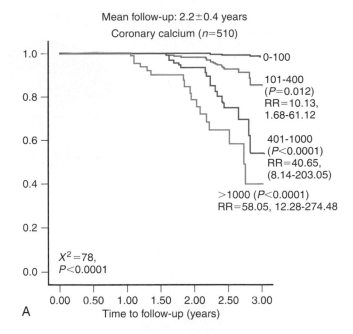

Figure 29-9 Abnormal myocardial perfusion imaging (MPI) and coronary artery calcium detected by electron beam computed tomography (EBCT) in 180 asymptomatic patients with type 2 diabetes mellitus. With increasing coronary artery calcium score, the overall percentage of patients with abnormal MPI increases. Large defects are more frequent when the calcium score is above 400 Agatston units. *(Modified from Anand DV, Lim E, Hopkins D, et al: Risk stratification in uncomplicated type 2 diabetes: Prospective evaluation of the combined use of coronary artery calcium imaging and selective myocardial perfusion scintigraphy, Eur Heart J 27:713–721, 2006.)*

A recent study by Scholte et al.[56] explored prospectively the interrelationship of SPECT stress myocardial perfusion abnormalities, significant coronary artery calcium, and significant coronary artery stenoses on non-invasive CT angiography in the same asymptomatic patients with diabetes mellitus. Anatomic evidence of CAD (coronary calcium and luminal stenoses) occurred more frequently than functional evidence of CAD by stress SPECT imaging. Clinically significant manifestations of CAD by any of the three technologies occurred in about one-quarter to one-fifth of patients, either alone or in combination (Fig. 29-11). At the present time, the comparative prognostic significance of these different manifestations of CAD is still unclear and needs to be clarified by long-term follow-up.

TREATMENT OF SILENT MYOCARDIAL ISCHEMIA IN PATIENTS WITH DIABETES

Once silent myocardial ischemia has been detected in asymptomatic patients with diabetes, a dilemma presents itself: how to treat these patients. Is outcome in these asymptomatic patients sufficiently poor to justify major interventions such as revascularization? A retrospective database study suggested a significantly worse outcome in diabetic patients with evidence of inducible ischemia, particularly if the presenting symptom was shortness of breath.[14] However, preliminary follow-up data of the DIAD study suggest that the overall 5-year prognosis of initially asymptomatic patients is very favorable, even in patients with mild inducible ischemia.[29] Patients with severe myocardial perfusion

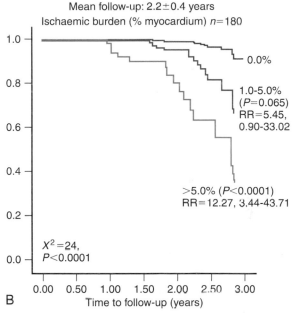

Figure 29-10 Event-free survival during an average follow-up of 2.2 ± 0.4 years by a Cox proportional hazard model. Survival curves according to the extent of coronary calcification (**A**) and SPECT myocardial perfusion abnormalities (**B**) are shown. Relative risk ratios (RR), confidence intervals, and *P* values are shown for each coronary calcium and ischemia on SPECT imaging category. *(From Anand DV, Lim E, Hopkins D, et al: Risk stratification in uncomplicated type 2 diabetes: Prospective evaluation of the combined use of coronary artery calcium imaging and selective myocardial perfusion scintigraphy, Eur Heart J 27:713–721, 2006.)*

abnormalities and ischemia ECG during adenosine infusion have a significantly poorer prognosis, however (see Fig. 29-8).[29] The ongoing BARI-2D trial can be expected to provide new insights in how to treat these patients.[57] The only data available at present are those from a non-randomized retrospective study that evaluated outcome after revascularization of asymptomatic patients with

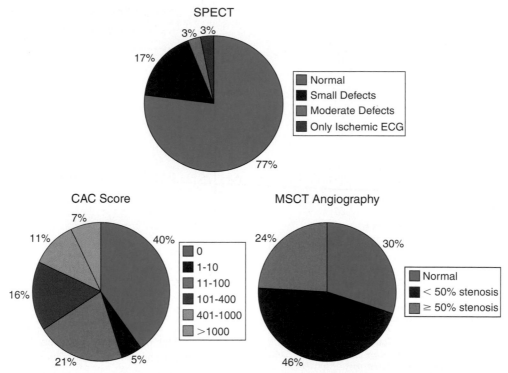

Figure 29-11 Distribution (%) of diagnostic findings on stress single-photon emission computed tomography (SPECT), coronary artery calcium (CAC) score, and multislice computed tomography (MSCT) angiography in 100 asymptomatic patients with type 2 diabetes mellitus. *(Modified from Scholte AJHA, et al: Different manifestations of coronary artery disease by stress myocardial perfusion imaging, coronary calcium scoring, and multislice CT coronary angiography in asymptomatic patients with type 2 diabetes mellitus, J Nucl Cardiol 15:503–509, 2008.)*

diabetes with inducible silent ischemia on SPECT imaging.[58] Only patients who had severe stress myocardial perfusion abnormalities had improved outcome after coronary bypass surgery, but not after coronary angioplasty. Patients who had mild inducible myocardial ischemia had no difference in outcome when treated medically or when treated by revascularization.

Interestingly, repeat stress SPECT imaging after 3 years in the DIAD study showed unexpected resolution of inducible myocardial ischemia in a significant number of patients. This appeared to be most likely due to optimized medical treatment with aspirin, statins, and ACE inhibitors.[59]

For patients with diabetes mellitus, the stakes are too high to wait for the first obvious clinical manifestation of CAD. When symptoms occur, it may already be too late for many patients because of the advanced stage of CAD. Screening of selected subgroups of asymptomatic patients with diabetes is probably justified. However, as the results of the DIAD study suggested,[29] careful clinical observation and appropriately timed stress radionuclide MPI, alone or in conjunction with other diagnostic tests, can play important roles in early detection of CAD in patients with diabetes mellitus.

REFERENCES

1. Centers for Disease Control and Prevention mortality database: Available at: www.cdc.gov.
2. Diabetes mellitus: A major risk factor for cardiovascular disease. A joint editorial statement by the American Diabetes Association; the National Heart, Lung, and Blood Institute; the Juvenile Diabetes Foundation International; the National Institute of Diabetes and Digestive and Kidney Diseases; and the American Heart Association, *Circulation* 100:1132–1133, 1999.
3. Nesto RW: Screening for asymptomatic coronary artery disease in diabetes [editorial; comment], *Diabetes Care* 22(9):1393–1395, 1999.
4. Boland LL, Folsom AR, Sorlie PD, et al: Occurrence of unrecognized myocardial infarction in subjects aged 45 to 65 years (The ARIC Study), *Am J Cardiol* 90:927–931, 2002.
5. Naka M, Hiramatsu K, Aizawa T, et al: Silent myocardial ischemia in patients with non-insulin-dependent diabetes mellitus as judged by treadmill exercise testing and coronary angiography, *Am Heart J* 123:46–52, 1992.
6. ADA consensus statement American Diabetes Association: Consensus development conference on the diagnosis of coronary heart disease in people with diabetes, *Diabetes Care* 21:1551–1559, 1998.
7. Vanzetto G, Halimi S: Hammoud, et al: Prediction of cardiovascular events in clinically selected high-risk NIDDM patients. Prognostic value of exercise stress test and thallium-201 single-photon emission computed tomography, *Diabetes Care* 22:19–26, 1999.
8. Kang X, Berman DS, Lewin H, et al: Comparative ability of myocardial perfusion single-photon emission computed tomography to detect coronary artery disease in patients with and without diabetes mellitus, *Am Heart J* 137:949–957, 1999.
9. Kang X, Berman DS, Lewin HC, et al: Incremental prognostic value of myocardial perfusion single photon emission computed tomography in patients with diabetes mellitus, *Am Heart J* 138:1025–1032, 1999.
10. Berman DS, Kang X, Hayes SW, et al: Adenosine myocardial perfusion single-photon emission computed tomography in women compared to men. Impact of diabetes mellitus on incremental prognostic value and effect on patient management, *J Am Coll Cardiol* 41:1125–1133, 2003.
11. Giri S, Shaw LJ, Murthy DR, et al: Impact of diabetes on the risk stratification using stress single-photon emission computed tomography myocardial perfusion imaging in patients with symptoms suggestive of coronary artery disease, *Circulation* 105:32–40, 2002.
12. Rajagopalan N, Miller TD, Hodge DO, Frye RL, Gibbons RJ: Identifying high-risk asymptomatic diabetic patients who are candidates for screening stress single-photon emission computed tomography imaging, *J Am Coll Cardiol* 45:43–49, 2005.
13. DeLorenzo A, Lima R, Siqueira-Filho AG, et al: Prevalence and prognostic value of perfusion defects detected by stress technetium-99m sestamibi myocardial perfusion single-photon emission computed

tomography in asymptomatic patients with diabetes mellitus and no known coronary artery disease, *Am J Cardiol* 90:827–832, 2002.

14. Zellweger MJ, Hachamovitch R, Kang X, Hayes SW, Friedman JD, Germano G, Pfisterer ME, Berman DS: Prognostic relevance of symptoms versus objective evidence of coronary artery disease in diabetic patients, *Eur Heart J* 25:543–550, 2004.

15. Prior JO, Monbaron D, Koehli M, Calcagni ML, Ruiz J, Bischof Delaloye A: Prevalence of asymptomatic and silent stress-induced perfusion defects in diabetic patients with suspected coronary artery disease referred for myocardial perfusion scintigraphy, *Eur J Nucl Med Mol Imaging* 32:60–69, 2005.

16. Miller TD, Rajagopalan N, Hodge DO, Frye RL, Gibbons RJ: Yield of stress single-photon emission computed tomography in asymptomatic patients with diabetes, *Am Heart J* 147:890–896, 2004.

17. Janand-Delenne B, Savin B, Habib G, et al: Silent myocardial ischemia in patients with diabetes, *Diabetes Care* 22:1396–1400, 1999.

18. Gazzaruso C, De Amici E, Garzaniti A, et al: Assessment of asymptomatic coronary artery disease in apparently uncomplicated type 2 diabetic patients, *Diabetes Care* 25:1418–1424, 2002.

19. Milan Study on Atherosclerosis and Diabetes Group: Prevalence of unrecognized silent myocardial ischemia and its association with atherosclerotic factors in noninsulin-dependent diabetes mellitus, *Am J Cardiol* 79:134–139, 1997.

20. Wackers FJTh, Young LH, Inzucchi SE, et al: Detection of silent myocardial ischemia in asymptomatic diabetic subjects-The DIAD study, *Diabetes Care* 27:1954–1961, 2004.

21. Valensi P, Paries J, Brulport-Cerisier V, et al: Predictive value of silent myocardial ischemia for cardiac events in diabetic patients, *Diabetes Care* 28:2722–2727, 2005.

22. Williams SB, Cusco JA, Roddy MA, et al: Impaired nitric oxide-mediated vasodilation in patients with non-insulin-dependent diabetes mellitus, *J Am Coll Cardiol* 27:567–574, 1996.

23. Hogykian RV, Galecki AT, Pitt B, et al: Specific impairment of endothelium-dependent vasodilation in subjects with type 2 diabetes, *J Clin Endocrinol Metab* 83:1946–1952, 1998.

24. Hasdai D, Gibbons RJ, Holmes DR, et al: Coronary endothelial dysfunction in humans is associated with myocardial perfusion defects, *Circulation* 96:3390–3395, 1997.

25. Emmett L, Van Gaal WJ, Magee M, Bass S, Ali O, Freedman B, Van der Wall H, Kritharides L: Prospective evaluation of the impact of diabetes and left ventricular hypertrophy on the relationship between ischemia and transient ischemic dilation of the left ventricle on single-day adenosine Tc-99m myocardial perfusion imaging, *J Nucl Cardiol* 15:638–643, 2008.

26. Shaw LJ, Iskandrian AE: Prognostic value of gated myocardial perfusion SPECT, *J Nucl Cardiol* 11:171–185, 2004.

27. ASNC statement: Bateman T: Clinical relevance of a normal myocardial perfusion scintigraphy study, *J Nucl Cardiol* 4:172–173, 1996.

28. Hachamovitch R, Hayes S, Friedman JD, et al: Determinants of risk and its temporal variation in patients with normal stress myocardial perfusion scans. What is the warranty period of a normal scan, *J Am Coll Cardiol* 41:1329–1340, 2003.

29. Young LH, Wackers FJTh, Chyun DA, et al: Cardiac outcomes after screening for asymptomatic coronary artery disease in patients with type 2 diabetes: The DIAD study: A randomized controlled clinical trial, *JAMA* 301:1547–1555, 2009.

30. Rutter MK, McComb JM, Brady S, et al: Silent myocardial ischemia and microalbuminuria in asymptomatic subjects with non-insulin-dependent diabetes mellitus, *Am J Cardiol* 83:27–31, 1999.

31. Langer A, Freeman MR, Josse RG, et al: Detection of silent myocardial ischemia in diabetes mellitus, *Am J Cardiol* 67:1073–1078, 1992.

32. Ziegler D: Cardiovascular autonomic neuropathy: clinical manifestations and measurement, *Diabetes Rev* 7:342, 1999.

33. Seshadri N, Acharya N, Lauer M: Association of diabetes mellitus with abnormal heart rate recovery in patients without known coronary artery disease, *Am J Cardiol* 91:108–111, 2003.

34. Lee K, Jang H, Kim Y, et al: Prognostic value of cardiac autonomic neuropathy independent and incremental to perfusion defects in patients with diabetes and suspected coronary artery disease, *Am J Cardiol* 92:1458–1461, 2003.

35. Marchant B, Umachandran V, Stevenson R, et al: Silent myocardial ischemia: Role of subclinical neuropathy in patients with and without diabetes, *J Am Coll Cardiol* 22:1433–1437, 1993.

36. Scognamiglio R, Negut C, Ramondo A, Tiengo A, Avogaro A: Detection of coronary artery disease in asymptomatic patients with type 2 diabetes mellitus, *J Am Coll Cardiol* 47:65–71, 2006.

37. Allman KC, Stevens MJ, Wieland DM, et al: Noninvasive assessment of cardiac diabetic neuropathy by carbon-11 hydroxyephedrine and positron emission tomography, *J Am Coll Cardiol* 22:1425–1432, 1993.

38. Stevens MJ, Dayanikli F, Raffel DM, et al: Scintigraphic assessment of regionalized defects in myocardial sympathetic innervation and blood flow regulation in diabetic patients with autonomic neuropathy, *J Am Coll Cardiol* 31:1575–1584, 1998.

39. Rauch U, Ziegler D, Piolot R, et al: Platelet activation in diabetic cardiovascular autonomic neuropathy, *Diabetes Med* 16:848–852, 1999.

40. Valensi P, Paries J, Attali JR: and the French Group for Research and Study of Diabetes Neuropathy: Cardiac autonomic neuropathy in diabetic patients: influence of diabetes duration, obesity, and microangiopathic complications: The French multicenter study, *Metabolism* 52:815–820, 2003.

41. Bravo PE, Hage FG, Woodham RM, Heo J, Iskandrian AE: Heart rate response to adenosine in patients with diabetes mellitus and normal myocardial perfusion imaging, *Am J Cardiol* 102:1103–1106, 2008.

42. Agatston AS, Janowitz WR, Hildner FJ, et al: Quantification of coronary artery calcium using ultrafast computed tomography, *J Am Coll Cardiol* 15:827–832, 1990.

43. Achenbach S, Moshage W, Ropers D, et al: Value of electron-beam computed tomography for the noninvasive detection of high-grade coronary artery stenoses and occlusions, *N Engl J Med* 339:1964–1971, 1998.

44. Budoff MJ, Diamond GA, Raggi P, et al: Continuous probabilistic prediction of angiographically significant coronary artery disease using electron beam tomography, *Circulation* 105:1791–1796, 2002.

45. Rumberger J, Simons DB, Fitzpatrick LA, et al: Coronary artery calcium areas by electron-beam computed tomography and coronary atherosclerotic plaque area: A histopathologic correlative study, *Circulation* 92:2157–2162, 1995.

46. Berman DS, Wong ND, Gransar H, et al: Relationship between stress myocardial perfusion SPECT and the extent of subclinical atherosclerosis assessed by CT coronary calcium, *Circulation* 108(Suppl 4):634, 2003.

47. Arad Y, Spadaro LA, Goodman K, et al: Predictive value of electron beam computed tomography of the coronary arteries: 19-month follow-up of 1173 asymptomatic subjects, *J Am Coll Cardiol* 36:1253–1260, 2000.

48. Raggi P, Callister TQ, Cooil B, et al: Identification of patients at increased risk of first unheralded acute myocardial infarction by electron-beam computed tomography, *Circulation* 101:850–855, 2000.

49. Kondos GT, Hoff JA, Sevrukov A, et al: Electron-beam tomography coronary artery calcium and cardiac events: A 37-month follow-up of 5635 initially asymptomatic low- to intermediate-risk adults, *Circulation* 107:2571–2576, 2003.

50. Starkman HS, Cable G, Hala V, et al: Delineation of prevalence and risk factors for early coronary artery disease by electron beam computed tomography in young adults with type 1 diabetes, *Diabetes Care* 26:433–436, 2003.

51. Wolfe ML, Gefter NI, Warren G, et al: Coronary artery calcification at electron beam computed tomography is increased in asymptomatic type 2 diabetics independent of traditional risk factors, *J Cardiovasc Risk* 9:369–376, 2002.

52. Wong ND, Sciammarella MG, Polk D, et al: The metabolic syndrome, diabetes, and subclinical atherosclerosis assessed by coronary calcium, *J Am Coll Cardiol* 41:1547–1553, 2003.

53. Wong ND, Rozanski A, Gransar H, Miranda-Peats R, Kang X, Hayes S, Shaw L, Friedman J, Polk D, Berman DS: Metabolic syndrome and diabetes are associated with an increased likelihood of inducible ischemia among patients with subclinical atherosclerosis, *Diabetes Care* 28:1445–1450, 2005.

54. Anand DV, Lim E, Hopkins D, Corder R, Shaw LJ, Sharp P, Lipkin D, Lahiri A: Risk stratification in uncomplicated type 2 diabetes: prospective evaluation of the combined use of coronary calcium imaging and selective myocardial perfusion scintigraphy, *Eur Heart J* 27:713–721, 2006.

55. Elkeles RS, Godsland IF, Feher MD, Rubens MB, Roughton M, Nugara F, Humphries SF, Richmond W, Flather MD: for the PREDICT study group. Coronary calcium measurement improves prediction of cardiovascular events in asymptomatic patients with type 2 diabetes: the PREDICT study, *Eur Heart J* 29:2244–2251, 2008.

56. Scholte AJHA, Schuijf JD, Kharagjitsingh AV, Dibbets-Schneider P, Stokkel MP, Jukema JW, vander Wall EE, Bax JJ, Wackers FJTH: Different manifestations of coronary artery disease by stress SPECT myocardial perfusion imaging, coronary calcium scoring, and multislice CT coronary angiography in asymptomatic patients with type 2 diabetes mellitus, *J Nucl Cardiol* 15:503–509, 2008.

57. Sobel BE, Frye R, Detre KM: Burgeoning dilemmas in the management of diabetes and cardiovascular disease. Rationale for the Bypass Angioplasty Revascularization Investigation 2 Diabetes (BARI 2D) trial, *Circulation* 107:636–642, 2003.

58. Sorajja P, Chareonthaitawee P, Rajagopalan N, Miller TD, Frye RL, Hodge DO, Gibbons RJ: Improved survival in asymptomatic diabetic patients with high-risk SPECT imaging treated with coronary bypass grafting, *Circulation* 112(Suppl I):I-311–I-316, 2005.

59. Wackers FJTh, Chyun DA, Young LH, et al: Resolution of asymptomatic myocardial ischemia in patients with type 2 diabetes in the Detection of Ischemia in Asymptomatic Diabetics (DIAD) study, *Diabetes Care* 30:2892–2898, 2007.

Chapter 30

Radionuclide Imaging in Heart Failure

PREM SOMAN

INTRODUCTION

The epidemic of heart failure affects 5 million people in the United States, with 500,000 new diagnoses made every year.[1] Physicians treating heart failure seek answers to several important clinical questions that impact on management:

1. What is the etiology of heart failure?
2. Among patients with ischemic left ventricular (LV) dysfunction, who will benefit from coronary revascularization?
3. Is left ventricular systolic function impaired, and if so, to what degree?
4. Will the patient benefit from an implantable cardioverter defibrillator (ICD) or cardiac resynchronization therapy (CRT)?

This chapter will review the application of radionuclide imaging tests to address these questions and the ongoing investigations into potential new applications of radionuclide imaging in heart failure patients.

ESTABLISHED USES OF RADIONUCLIDE IMAGING IN HEART FAILURE

Determining Heart Failure Etiology

Data from epidemiologic studies and clinical trials suggest that 60% to 70% of patients with heart failure have coronary artery disease (CAD). These data underscore the fact that CAD has now overtaken hypertension as the most common cause of heart failure. In a review of 13 randomized, multicenter clinical trials of patients with established heart failure reported in the *New England Journal of Medicine*, Gheorghiade and Bonow reported that 68% of patients had CAD.[2] It is likely that these data underestimate the true prevalence of CAD in heart failure, since patients presenting with LV dysfunction due to acute MI were generally excluded from these

trials. It is also important to note that the majority of these reports pertained to patients with chronic heart failure. However, adjudicating etiology is most relevant in patients with new-onset heart failure in whom the detection of significant CAD has important therapeutic and prognostic implications.[3]

More important, in these clinical trials, an "ischemic" etiology of heart failure was generally attributed to patients with *any* significant epicardial CAD (usually defined as = 50% diameter stenosis). However, in patients with heart failure and limited-extent CAD (e.g., single-vessel disease) and severe LV dysfunction, the underlying pathophysiology is unlikely to be ischemic LV dysfunction but rather cardiomyopathy of other etiologies coexisting with minor CAD. This distinction between heart failure patients with LV dysfunction resulting from extensive CAD and those with nonischemic LV dysfunction coexisting with limited-extent CAD is prognostically important, as was demonstrated by Felker and colleagues, who followed up 1921 symptomatic heart failure patients enrolled in the Duke database.[4] Patients were categorized as having ischemic and nonischemic cardiomyopathy based on two separate definitions. In the traditional definition, heart failure patients with any epicardial CAD equal to 75% were classified as having ischemic cardiomyopathy. In the modified definition, an ischemic etiology was attributed only to patients with extensive CAD, defined as significant left main or proximal left anterior descending coronary artery stenosis, three-vessel disease, or single-vessel disease with prior MI or coronary revascularization, that is, patients with extensive CAD more likely to be etiologically related to heart failure. Therefore, in the modified definition, heart failure patients with single-vessel disease without prior MI or coronary revascularization were categorized as having nonischemic cardiomyopathy. At the end of a median follow-up period of 3.1 years (interquartile range 1.0 to 6.2 years), the authors reported that the modified definition of ischemic cardiomyopathy was a more powerful discriminator of prognosis, and

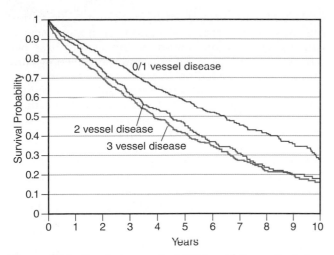

Figure 30-1 Survival curves for 1921 heart failure patients from the Duke database, adjusted for age, ejection fraction, gender, NYHA class, diabetes mellitus, and valvular disease. When patients were categorized based on the number of obstructed coronary arteries, the prognosis of patients with single-vessel disease was identical to that of patients with unobstructed coronary arteries. *(From Felker GM, Shaw LK, O'Connor CM: A standardized definition of ischemic cardiomyopathy for use in clinical research, J Am Coll Cardiol 39:210–218, 2002.)*

Table 30-1 Clinical Studies of Myocardial Perfusion Imaging in Chronic Heart Failure

Author	Technique	PREDICTIVE VALUE (%)	
		Negative	Positive
Bulkley (1977)	Tl-201	100	72
Dunn (1982)	Tl-201	100	40
Saltissi (1981)	Tl-201	100	65
Eichorn (1988)	Tl-201	100	71
Tauberg (1993)	Tl-201	100	61
Chikamori (1992)	Tl-201	100	65

Tl, thallium.
Adapted from Udelson JE, Shafer CD, Carrio I: Radionuclide imaging in heart failure: Assessing etiology and outcomes and implications for management, J Nucl Cardiol 9:40S–52S, 2002.

the prognosis of heart failure patients with single-vessel CAD without prior MI or coronary revascularization was identical to that of heart failure patients without CAD (Fig. 30-1). This important observation indicates that the standard definition of ischemic cardiomyopathy applied to most heart failure studies ($\geq$50% diameter stenosis in any coronary artery) may be inadequate for the characterization of heart failure etiology and risk, since it does not enable a distinction between extensive CAD that is likely to be the etiology of heart failure and limited-extent CAD coexisting with heart failure of other etiologies. Making this distinction is a critical step in the evaluation of heart failure patients, since the presence of extensive CAD implies potential benefit from coronary revascularization.[5]

Current practice guidelines mandate coronary angiography in heart failure patients with angina.[6] However, up to 60% of patients with ischemic LV dysfunction do not have angina,[7] and the guidelines do not offer firm recommendations for the optimal initial evaluation strategy of these patients.[6,8] Given this lack of a unified approach and the potential adverse consequences of not identifying extensive CAD, most heart failure patients are likely to undergo at least one coronary angiogram to exclude CAD, especially after the initial onset of symptoms. Many patients end up having repeat coronary angiograms when clinical symptoms worsen or left ventricular ejection fraction (LVEF) deteriorates.

The role of myocardial perfusion imaging (MPI) to diagnose CAD noninvasively in patients with heart failure has been investigated.[9] Many of these studies predated contemporary MPI methodology, for example, using nongated, planar thallium-(^{201}Tl) scintigraphy, and yet showed a near-perfect sensitivity and negative predictive value (NPV) (Table 30-1). A more recent study using gated technetium-99m (^{99m}Tc) sestamibi single-

photon emission computed tomographic (SPECT) MPI incorporating information on both perfusion and regional LV function demonstrated a high sensitivity of 94% but specificity of only 32%.[10] Thus, these studies performed in patients with *chronic* heart failure suggest that MPI may be used to exclude significant CAD in heart failure patients with a high degree of accuracy, but because of the poor specificity of the technique, many heart failure patients without CAD will undergo coronary angiography based on falsely positive MPI results.

The Investigation of Myocardial Gated SPECT Imaging as Initial Strategy (IMAGING) in Heart Failure study prospectively explored the role of MPI in 201 patients presenting with *new-onset* heart failure, recruited from 14 hospitals in the United States and United Kingdom.[11] Patients underwent exercise or pharmacologic stress MPI with ^{99m}Tc sestamibi gated SPECT imaging during or within 2 weeks of the index hospitalization for heart failure. The diagnosis of heart failure was based on the Framingham criteria.[12] A subset of patients (37%) underwent coronary angiography based on clinical indications, and the performance characteristics of MPI for CAD diagnosis were derived from this angiographic cohort. A positive MPI was defined by a summed stress score greater than 3 (the sum of the individual segmental perfusion scores on stress MPI, using a 17-segment LV model and a 5-point semiquantitative perfusion score ranging from 0 = normal to 4 = absent perfusion), as validated previously.[13] For the diagnosis of *any* angiographic CAD (= 70% diameter stenosis, prevalence 51%), the sensitivity, specificity, positive predictive value (PPV), and NPV of MPI were 82%, 57%, 67%, and 75%, respectively. For the diagnosis of more extensive CAD, indicating the presence of ischemic LV dysfunction (= 70% stenosis in the left main or proximal left anterior descending coronary artery, = 70% stenosis in two or more major epicardial coronary arteries, or any stenosis = 70% with prior MI or coronary revascularization, prevalence 36%), the corresponding values were 96%, 56%, 55%, and 95%, respectively (Table 30-2). Thus, the principal finding of this study in patients with *new-onset* heart failure was concordant with prior studies

Table 30-2 Performance Characteristics of Gated SPECT ^{99m}Tc Sestamibi for CAD Diagnosis in Patients with New-Onset Heart Failure from the IMAGING in Heart Failure Study[103]

CAD definition	Any CAD: ≥70% stenosis in any coronary artery	Extensive CAD: stenosis ≥ 70% in the LM or proximal LAD, ≥ 70% in ≥ two major epicardial coronary arteries, or any stenosis ≥ 70% with a prior MI or coronary revascularization
CAD prevalence by angiography	51% (n = 38)	36% (n = 27)
Sensitivity % (95% CI)	82 (66-92)	96 (81-99)
Specificity % (95% CI)	57 (40-72)	56 (41-71)
PPV %	67	55
NPV %	75	96

Criteria for positive SPECT was summed stress score > 3.
CAD, coronary artery disease; LAD, left anterior descending coronary artery; LM, left main coronary artery; MPI, myocardial perfusion imaging; NPV, negative predictive value; PPV, positive predictive value; SPECT, single-photon emission computed tomography; Tc, technetium.
From Soman P, Lahiri A, Mieres JH, et al: Etiology and pathophysiology of new-onset heart failure: Evaluation by myocardial perfusion imaging, J Nucl Cardiol 16:82-91, 2009.

in patients with established heart failure in that MPI has a high NPV for excluding an ischemic etiology for LV dysfunction. Several limitations of this study should be noted. Although prospective and the first study to explore MPI in patients with new-onset heart failure, this was an observational cohort of nonconsecutive patients. Furthermore, coronary angiography was performed in only 37% of patients and was driven by clinical indications, including in some cases, the results of the MPI. Therefore the results were subject to verification bias, which is known to falsely lower specificity and overestimate sensitivity. Selection bias may have also been operative in patients with new-onset heart failure and known CAD, who are sometimes referred directly for coronary angiography. Thus, the applicability of these results to all patients with new-onset heart failure needs further confirmation. Nevertheless, this study in patients with new-onset heart failure, and prior studies in patients with chronic disease, indicate that heart failure patients with a normal MPI are highly unlikely to have significant, etiologically related CAD. Using MPI as an early investigative strategy might avoid the routine use of coronary angiography in some patients. Figure 30-2 shows characteristic patterns of perfusion and function in heart failure patients. Patients with cardiomyopathy of nonischemic etiologies generally have normal or near-normal perfusion. In these patients, coronary angiography can be safely avoided.

The predominant cause of false-positive MI is soft-tissue attenuation, although pathophysiologic phenomena such as myocardial fibrosis and endothelial dysfunction produce abnormal MPI in some patients with unobstructed epicardial coronary arteries.[14,15] Although quantitative attenuation-correction techniques have been shown in clinical trials to improve diagnostic specificity of SPECT MPI, this approach has not been tested specifically in patients with heart failure.[16] Given the propensity of attenuation artifacts in patients with a dilated LV, attenuation correction is likely to favorably impact specificity in this population. Figure 30-3 shows

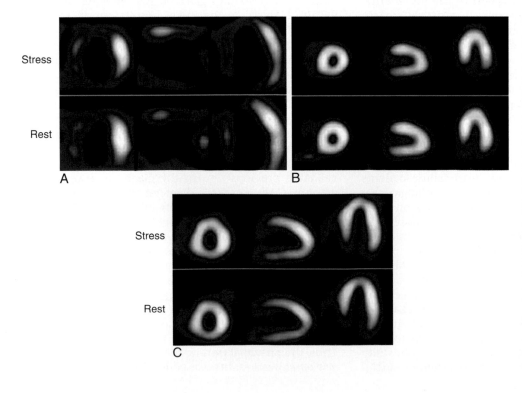

Figure 30-2 Categorization of heart failure (HF) etiology using technetium-99m sestamibi myocardial perfusion imaging. **A,** Left ventricular (LV) dilation (abnormal LV systolic function by gated SPECT not shown) with large, fixed perfusion defects in the septum, anterior wall, apex, and inferior wall, suggestive of CAD-related ("ischemic") cardiomyopathy. **B,** Normal stress/rest perfusion and LV size (normal LVEF on gated SPECT not shown) indicative of HF likely related to diastolic mechanisms. **C,** LV dilation (with abnormal LV systolic function on gated SPECT, not shown) and normal perfusion suggestive of non-CAD related ("nonischemic") cardiomyopathy. CAD, coronary artery disease; LVEF, left ventricular ejection fraction; SPECT, single-photon emission computed tomography. *(From Soman P, Lahiri A, Mieres JH, et al: Etiology and pathophysiology of new-onset heart failure: Evaluation by myocardial perfusion imaging, J Nucl Cardiol 16:82–91, 2009.)*

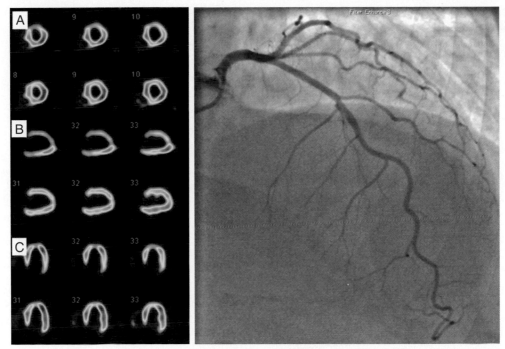

Figure 30-3 Use of gadolinium-153 transmission scan attenuation correction to improve diagnostic accuracy of myocardial perfusion imaging. *Left*, short-axis (**A**), horizontal long-axis (**B**) and vertical long-axis (**C**) images from the stress technetium-99m sestamibi myocardial perfusion (images) (of) a patient presenting with heart failure. In each of these sections, the *upper and lower rows* show uncorrected and attenuation-corrected images, respectively. While there appears to be a perfusion abnormality involving the apex and anterior wall, suggesting ischemia in the left anterior descending (LAD) coronary artery territory on the uncorrected images, the attenuation-corrected images show substantial resolution of this defect, indicating that this is an attenuation artifact, most likely due to breast tissue in this female patient. *Right*, coronary angiography demonstrating a normal LAD coronary artery.

the gated SPECT images from a patient in whom the attenuation correction formed using a gadolinium-153 transmission scan was useful in correctly identified non-ischemic LV dysfunction.

With the advent of cardiac CT, small, single-center studies have explored the utility of coronary calcium scoring and CT coronary angiography for the diagnosis of CAD in heart failure patients.[17,18] Like MPI, coronary calcium scoring and CT coronary angiography have good NPV for this application. In the future, combined SPECT/CT imaging may improve diagnostic accuracy.

Measuring Left Ventricular (Dys)Function (See Chapters 12 and 13)

Radionuclide techniques are well validated and widely applied for the assessment of LV function. While radionuclide ventriculography (RVG) was the traditional radionuclide technique used to determine LV systolic and diastolic function, this method has been largely supplanted by gated SPECT imaging, which is extensively used for myocardial perfusion assessment and provides simultaneous information on LV systolic function. Sixteen-frame ECG gating provides an accurate assessment of LV systolic function, but it may not provide a sufficiently high-fidelity time-volume curve for diastolic function assessment (Fig. 30-4).[19] Assessment of diastolic function can be performed with 32- or 64-frame gating, which can be impractical for routine MPI because of the long scanning time required for collection of adequate counts.[19,20]

Assessment of ejection fraction by gated SPECT imaging has been validated against other established imaging modalities, including echocardiography, radionuclide ventriculography, and newer techniques with high spatial resolution, such as magnetic resonance imaging, with excellent correlation.[20] However, it must be noted that the normal limits of ejection fraction vary depending on the modality used.[21,22] This intermodality variability is exaggerated in patients with LV systolic dysfunction,[22] an observation that has been overlooked even in the design of major clinical trials requiring precise measurement of LV function, such as the implantable cardioverter-defibrillator trials in heart failure patients. While these trials recruited patients based on specific ejection fraction criteria, a modality of ejection fraction measurement was usually not specified.[23,24] Normal limits also vary based on gated SPECT methodology, with 8-frame gating resulting in lower ejection fraction values that correlate less well with RVG compared to 16-frame gating[19,25] and with the software used for quantification of ejection fraction and volumes (see Fig. 30-4).[26] In some laboratories including the author's, the lower limit of normality for ejection fraction measurement by gated SPECT is set variably depending on the frame rate used for gating (45% and 50% for 8-frame and 16-frame gating, respectively). Compared to two-dimensional echocardiography, which is also widely used for assessment of LV systolic function, a significant advantage of gated SPECT estimation of LV systolic function is its fully automated application, resulting in high

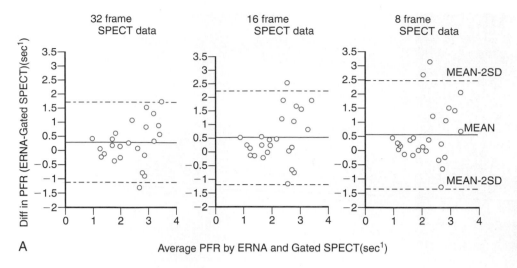

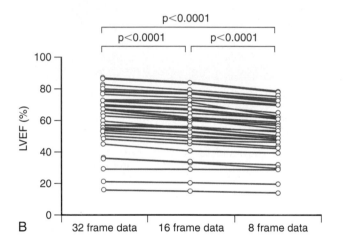

Figure 30-4 **A,** Comparison of left ventricular peak filling rate (PFR) in 48 patients obtained by 8-, 16-, and 32-frame gated SPECT imaging and equilibrium radionuclide angiography (ERNA). The Bland-Altman plots show better agreement between the techniques when gated SPECT is performed with higher frame rates. **B,** Comparison of left ventricular ejection fraction obtained by 32-, 16-, and 8-frame gated SPECT MPI. The higher frame rates produced higher values of ejection fraction. MPI, myocardial perfusion imaging; SPECT, single-photon emission computed tomography. *(From Kumita S, Cho K, Nakajo H, et al: Assessment of left ventricular diastolic function with electrocardiography-gated myocardial perfusion SPECT: Comparison with multigated equilibrium radionuclide angiography, J Nucl Cardiol 8:568–574, 2001.)*

reproducibility. Studies indicate that the variability in serial estimations of LV ejection fraction from gated rest ^{99m}Tc SPECT scans is approximately ±5% (Fig. 30-5).[27,28] Serial gated SPECT imaging can be effectively used to assess changes in perfusion and function following therapeutic interventions (Fig. 30-6A and B).

Predicting Benefit from Coronary Revascularization: Assessment of Myocardial Viability (See Chapters 37 and 38)

In patients with ischemic LV dysfunction, the assessment of myocardial viability is a critical step in management planning. On one hand, patients with severe LV

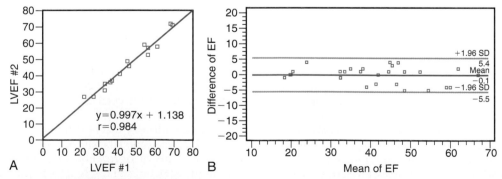

Figure 30-5 Reproducibility of left ventricular ejection fraction (LVEF) on serial resting gated SPECT imaging. **A,** Data from Johnson et al.[27] on 15 patients who underwent serial rest thallium-201 imaging. LVEF obtained from the first and second studies are plotted on the *x-* and *y-*axes, respectively. The regression line is not significantly different from the line of identity, indicating close correlation between the two measurements. **B,** Data from Hyun et al.[28] on 26 patients, showing that the 2-SD limits of difference in two serial measurements of LVEF by technetium-99m gated SPECT imaging assessed by Bland-Altman plotting was ± 5.5%. In this study, the variability between serial gated SPECT thallium-201 imaging was higher.

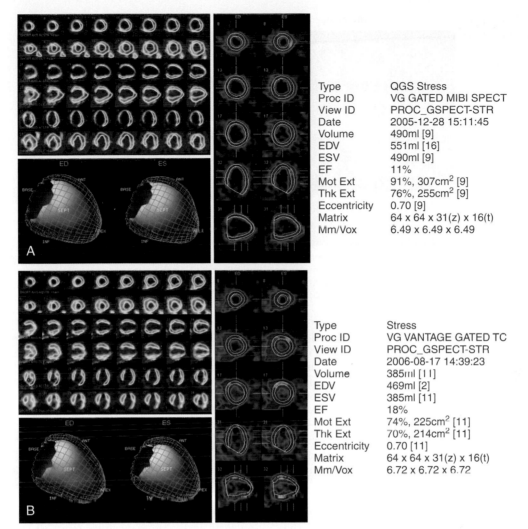

Type	QGS Stress
Proc ID	VG GATED MIBI SPECT
View ID	PROC_GSPECT-STR
Date	2005-12-28 15:11:45
Volume	490ml [9]
EDV	551ml [16]
ESV	490ml [9]
EF	11%
Mot Ext	91%, 307cm^2 [9]
Thk Ext	76%, 255cm^2 [9]
Eccentricity	0.70 [9]
Matrix	64 x 64 x 31(z) x 16(t)
Mm/Vox	6.49 x 6.49 x 6.49

Type	Stress
Proc ID	VG VANTAGE GATED TC
View ID	PROC_GSPECT-STR
Date	2006-08-17 14:39:23
Volume	385ml [11]
EDV	469ml [2]
ESV	385ml [11]
EF	18%
Mot Ext	74%, 225cm^2 [11]
Thk Ext	70%, 214cm^2 [11]
Eccentricity	0.70 [11]
Matrix	64 x 64 x 31(z) x 16(t)
Mm/Vox	6.72 x 6.72 x 6.72

Figure 30-6   Utility of serial myocardial perfusion imaging to monitor changes in left ventricular perfusion and function following therapeutic intervention. **A,** The perfusion images *(left upper panel)* show a reversible perfusion defect in the left anterior descending coronary territory (apex, anterior wall, and septum). Functional information is shown on the three-dimensional surface-rendered images *(bottom left panel)* and on representative short-axis, vertical long-axis, and horizontal long-axis slices, with epicardial and endocardial border contouring *(middle panel)*. Quantitative values generated by the automated algorithm are shown in the *right panel*. In this patient, the left ventricular end-diastolic and end-systolic volumes were markedly increased, with a severe reduction in ejection fraction. **B,** The corresponding images 7 months after revascularization of a mid-LAD stenosis. The perfusion images now show an apical infarction, with improved perfusion in the anterior wall and septum. There was some reduction in LV volumes and a small improvement in ejection fraction, which, however, still remains severely depressed. LAD, left anterior descending coronary artery; LV, left ventricular.

systolic dysfunction undergoing coronary bypass grafting are at high risk for perioperative mortality.[29] On the other, the presence of significant amounts of residual myocardial viability portends the potential for improvement in symptoms,[30–32] regional LV function,[33,34] global LV function,[35,36] and prognosis[5,37] following coronary revascularization. It is important to note that while the use of functional recovery is a convenient standard for viability studies, it may not capture the full benefit of revascularization, which may confer other important benefits such as attenuation of progressive remodeling and prevention of arrhythmia independently of functional recovery.[38–40] LV function may also continue to improve for several months following revascularization, so a single assessment, if not timed appropriately, may underestimate the full extent of functional recovery.[39]

Finally, resting regional function is primarily determined by endocardial thickening, which is unlikely to improve in patients who have suffered a subendocardial MI despite preserved myocardial viability.[41–43] A more important criterion for assessing the usefulness of noninvasive viability testing should be whether it can drive therapeutic decisions that ultimately improve patient outcome. While the field of viability testing is somewhat limited by the lack of randomized control studies, a meta-analysis by Allman and colleagues[5] of 24 studies of viability testing with MPI or dobutamine echocardiography that reported on survival after coronary revascularization provides important insights. In patients with predominantly viable myocardium, follow-up on medical therapy was associated with a 16% annual mortality. Similar patients who were revascularized experienced an annual

Patient A   Patient B

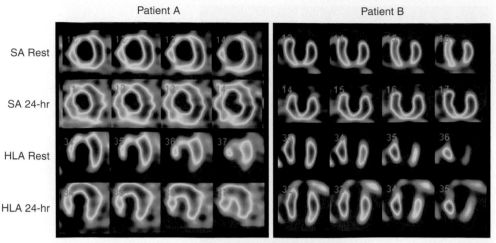

Figure 30-7 Examples of rest 24-hour redistribution thallium-^{201}Tl images for viability assessment. In Patient **A**, the presence of significant residual myocardial viability is indicated by "redistribution" of ^{201}Tl in the apex, septum, and anterior wall. In Patient **B**, the large perfusion defect involving the apex and anterior wall show no significant redistribution of Tl-201, suggesting the absence of viable myocardium. SA, short axis, HLA, horizontal long axis.

mortality of only 3.2%—that is, an 80% reduction in mortality. In contrast, the choice of medical therapy or revascularization had no significant impact on annual mortality (7.7% versus 6.2%, respectively) in patients with predominantly nonviable myocardium. Despite the known limitations of pooling data from observational cohort studies, which can bring into play selection biases that cannot be evaluated when meta-analyzing published literature, these data provide a strong signal that the presence of residual myocardial viability in patients with LV systolic dysfunction is a marker of very high risk without revascularization.

Clinical studies suggest that residual myocardial viability is prevalent among patients with ischemic LV dysfunction.[44,45] For example, in the CHRISTMAS trial of 489 patients with chronic heart failure due to ischemic LV dysfunction (LVEF 29 ± 11%), 79% had viable myocardium demonstrated by [99mTc] sestamibi SPECT imaging.[45] It must be noted that viability exists as a continuum, ranging from patients with extensive scar tissue and minimal residual viability, to those with minimal scar tissue and predominantly viable but dysfunctional myocardium due to varying combinations of hibernating and repetitive stunning.[46,47] Patient outcome is dependent on not only the presence but also the extent of viability, and a critical threshold mass of viable myocardium may be necessary for functional recovery and prognostic benefit to occur from revascularization.[48] Therefore, while several clinical and laboratory parameters, including anginal symptoms, absence of Q waves on the electrocardiogram, and absence of thinning and akinesis on echocardiography, indicate the presence of *some* viability, a systematic assessment of the *degree and extent* of viability is often indicated for management planning and prognostication. Techniques used for viability assessment are based on the demonstration of preserved myocyte metabolism (F-18 fluorodeoxyglucose positron emission tomography [PET]), cellular integrity (SPECT with ^{201}Tl or [99mTc] ligands), contractile reserve (dobutamine echocardiography), microvascular integrity

(myocardial contrast echocardiography), or the absence of scar tissue (gadolinium-enhanced cardiac magnetic resonance [CMR] imaging). The use of PET and SPECT for viability assessment is backed by a substantial literature, with SPECT having the advantages of wider availability and relative ease of use, and PET having a slightly higher overall accuracy.[33] The property of redistribution confers an advantage to ^{201}Tl compared with [99mTc] agents for viability assessment in dysfunctional myocardial segments supplied by a critically stenosed coronary artery. Here the continued uptake of ^{201}Tl over time results in higher tracer uptake on the delayed compared to early scan, thus signaling the presence of viable myocardium (Fig. 30-7).[49,50] However, when used with nitrate enhancement and quantitative interpretation, [99mTc]-sestamibi SPECT has comparable accuracy for viability assessment.[51,52] When compared with other imaging modalities for viability assessment, radionuclide techniques have comparable predictive accuracy for functional recovery.[33] Comparative studies also indicate that slight differences in sensitivity and specificity among these modalities may not impact on management decision making in a clinically meaningful way.[53] Furthermore, other information that can be derived from PET and SPECT imaging, such as the degree of remodeling, may interact with the amount of residual viability to determine outcome after revascularization.[54]

EVOLVING APPLICATIONS OF RADIONUCLIDE TECHNIQUES IN HEART FAILURE

Targeted Molecular Imaging and Imaging Myocardial Metabolism (See Chapters 40 and 41)

The most recent American College of Cardiology/American Heart Association guidelines for the diagnosis and management of heart failure includes a preclinical class (stage A) consisting of patients with conditions that are associated with a high likelihood of the development of heart failure.[6] It is established that molecular mechanisms mediating heart failure are already operative at this stage,[55] and imaging these mechanisms may facilitate the important goals of enhancing our understanding of heart failure pathophysiology and testing early therapy to halt disease progression. Molecular and metabolic imaging at later stages in the evolution of heart failure helps identify specific processes that may predominate in individual patients or patient groups and explain the heterogeneity in response to therapy (e.g., β-blockers). Such an approach may in future facilitate personalized medicine for heart failure. Both SPECT- and PET-based imaging can be potentially applied to a wide array of molecular targets. PET has the advantage of better spatial resolution and quantification.[56] The areas of heart failure where there are substantial ongoing research efforts directed to the application of molecular and metabolic imaging are (1) the imaging of cellular mechanisms underlying heart failure and (2) imaging of regenerative cell therapy.

Imaging Cellular Mechanisms in Heart Failure

Apoptosis: The imaging of programmed cell death (apoptosis) is one area where a substantial amount of animal work has already led to encouraging preliminary clinical data. The current approach uses radiolabeled annexin-V, a phosphatidyl-binding protein, to target phosphatidylserine, which is an intracellular cell-membrane phospholipid that is translocated to the cell surface during apoptosis. Small clinical studies using ^{99m}Tc annexin-V SPECT imaging have successfully imaged apoptosis in humans.[57] Potential applications in heart failure include imaging myocarditis, chemotherapy-induced cardiomyopathy, and cardiac transplant rejection.[58]

Renin-Angiotensin System (RAS): ^{18}F-Captopril and ^{18}F-lisinopril have been used to image the activity of the angiotensin-converting enzyme (ACE), which is increased in heart failure and modulates fibrosis, inflammation, and apoptosis through angiotensin II. Many of the effects of the RAS are paracrine, by components produced locally in the heart, and ^{18}F-lisinopril may have an advantage in that it has a higher affinity for tissue-bound ACE than ^{18}F-captopril.[55] An ^{99m}Tc-labeled angiotensin II type I receptor ligand is also being studied.[55]

Myocardial Sympathetic Neuronal Activity: The heart is richly supplied with sympathetic nerves that are intricately involved in the control of heart rate and contractility. Sympathetic dysregulation is a prominent component of the pathophysiology of heart failure and has established prognostic significance.[59,60] The use of ^{123}I-metaiodobenzylguanidine (MIBG) for scintigraphic imaging of the myocardium was first reported by Wieland and colleagues in 1981.[61] MIBG is an analogue of norepinephrine with identical mechanisms of uptake, storage, and release. However, unlike norepinephrine, it is retained in the sympathetic nerve endings unbound and largely unmetabolized, and it is therefore useful for scintigraphic imaging.[62] Current protocols used for MIBG imaging are designed to obtain comprehensive information about the functional activation state and anatomic distribution of the myocardial sympathetic innervation. Early (15-minute) and late (4-hour) anterior planar and SPECT imaging are performed. The MIBG uptake of the myocardium is represented as the heart-to-mediastinum (H/M) ratio on planar imaging. The H/M ratio on the early planar image is a reflection of the degree of uptake of MIBG by the myocardial sympathetic neurons. The H/M ratio on the delayed images is a reflection of the washout rate of MIBG, calculated as the difference in the background-subtracted (heart counts − mediastinum counts) myocardial counts between the early and late planar images, expressed as a percentage of the counts in the early image (Fig. 30-8). The washout rate is

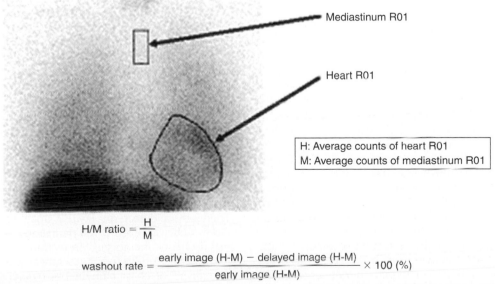

$$H/M \text{ ratio} = \frac{H}{M}$$

H: Average counts of heart R01
M: Average counts of mediastinum R01

$$\text{washout rate} = \frac{\text{early image (H-M)} - \text{delayed image (H-M)}}{\text{early image (H-M)}} \times 100 \ (\%)$$

Figure 30-8 Method of calculating the heart-to-mediastinum (H/M) ratio and washout rate on MIBG planar images. *(From Yamashina S, Yamazaki JI: Neuronal imaging using SPECT, Eur J Nucl Med Mol Imaging 34:939–950, 2007.)*

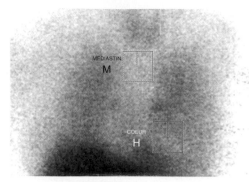

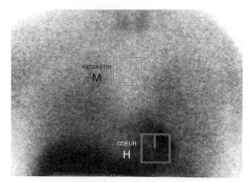

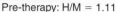

Pre-therapy: H/M = 1.11   Post-therapy: H/M = 1.62

Figure 30-9 Serial planar imaging with ^{123}I-MIBG showing improvement in the heart-to-mediastinum (H/M) ratio with heart failure therapy. *(From Agostini D, Belin A, Amar MH, et al: Improvement of cardiac neuronal function after carvedilol treatment in dilated cardiomyopathy: A ^{123}I-MIBG scintigraphic study, J Nucl Med 41:845–851, 2000.)*

an index of the state of activation of the myocardial sympathetic neurons. A high washout rate (and thus, a lower H/M ratio on the delayed image) is indicative of down-regulation of the myocardial sympathetic neurons, commonly seen in patients with heart failure. The degree of reduction in the H/M ratio is proportional to the degree of heart failure, varies directly with changes in LV systolic function (Fig. 30-9),[62] and therefore can be used to follow response to therapy. Attempts to predict response to therapy, however, have produced mixed results.[62] The H/M ratio and washout rate have been established as strong predictors of prognosis in heart failure, and in one study by Merlet et al., surpassed LV ejection fraction in this regard.[63] An improvement in MIBG uptake with therapy has also been associated with a favorable prognosis in heart failure patients.[64]

The SPECT image enables determination of regional differences in MIBG uptake. The sympathetic neurons are exquisitely sensitive to myocardial ischemia, and the resultant regional sympathetic dysfunction persists after ischemia resolution. As a result, after an ischemic insult, regional abnormalities in MIBG uptake extend beyond the boundaries of the perfusion defect on ^{201}Tl or ^{99m}Tc scintigraphy and persist longer. This phenomenon has potential utility for more accurate identification of the extent of myocardium at risk in acute coronary syndromes.

MIBG scintigraphy is the subject of several phase III clinical trials currently ongoing in the United States, with the objective of establishing this imaging agent as a powerful prognostic indicator in heart failure that may help individualize pharmacotherapy and identify patients who will benefit from invasive device therapy such as ICD or cardiac resynchronization therapy.

Imaging Myocardial Metabolism: Ischemia shifts myocardial metabolism from long-chain fatty acids, which is the predominant substrate under aerobic conditions, to glucose.[65] This finding prompted the investigation of several radionuclide-labeled fatty acid compounds for use in myocardial imaging. The uptake and washout kinetics of these agents are reflective of distinct pathways of myocardial fatty acid metabolism that are altered in acute ischemia, chronic ischemia, and the different states of dysfunctional but viable myocardium. Initial studies used C-11 palmitate and PET imaging,

with encouraging results.[66,67] Subsequent efforts were directed at adapting these tracers and protocols for the more widely available SPECT cameras and obviating the need for cyclotron production, resulting in the introduction of I-123-labeled agents.

^{123}I-Iodophenylpentadecanoic acid (IPPA) is a straight-chain fatty acid that is taken up by the myocardium in proportion to regional perfusion. Under nonischemic conditions, this tracer is rapidly metabolized and released, resulting in rapid washout kinetics.[68] Suppressed metabolism in the presence of ischemia results in longer myocardial retention and a "redistribution" pattern on serial imaging.[69] Qualitative and semiquantitative analysis of IPPA uptake and washout have been used in various clinical trials to successfully diagnose coronary stenosis,[68] detect myocardial ischemia,[70] determine myocardial viability,[71–73] and predict recovery of regional LV dysfunction following revascularization.[74] One study, for example, demonstrated superiority of this agent over rest-redistribution ^{201}Tl imaging for viability detection.[73] However, the rapid dynamics of straight-chain fatty acid uptake and metabolism is a critical problem for SPECT imaging.

Methyl-branching of the fatty acid chain protects against beta oxidation and considerably slows down washout from the myocardium (metabolic trapping).[75] Of the methyl-branched fatty acid tracers, ^{123}I-(p-iodophenyl)-3-(R,S)-methylpentadecanoic acid (BMIPP)[76] has been extensively studied in Japan and Europe and more recently in the United States. Excellent-quality images with high heart-to-background ratios can be obtained 15 to 30 minutes after tracer administration.[77] Because of the metabolic modulation, however, separate imaging with ^{201}Tl or one of the ^{99m}Tc ligands is required for perfusion assessment.

The clinical utility of BMIPP imaging stems from the fact that abnormalities of fatty acid metabolism resulting from transient ischemia persist for prolonged periods.[77,78] Therefore, a defect on BMIPP imaging is indicative of recent ischemia, even when perfusion has returned to normal (ischemic memory).[78] Detection of ischemic memory has potential utility in many clinical situations, including assessment of chest pain in the emergency department, diagnosis of CAD without stress testing, and diagnosis of vasospastic angina. There is also potential utility for risk stratification of patients with high likelihood of CAD.[79] In dysfunctional myocardium, a disproportionately greater decrease in BMIPP compared to a perfusion trace uptake likely represents recurrent ischemia with stunning and has been shown to correlate with preserved inotropic reserve,[80] histologic evidence of viability,[81] and postrevascularization recovery of function.[80,82,83] On the other hand, a concordant severe reduction in both BMIPP uptake and perfusion indicates scar tissue.

Monitoring Regenerative Cell Therapy: Regenerative cell therapy using embryonic stem cells, bone marrow–derived stem cells, and endothelial progenitor cells is being investigated for heart failure. Such therapy, delivered by intracoronary, intramyocardial, or systemic venous injection, requires monitoring of the homing, engraftment, and survival of the injected cells. In addition to providing information on these aspects, radionuclide imaging has the advantage of being able to assess myocardial remodeling, regional myocardial perfusion and viability, and regional and global function, which can be used as measures of outcome in regenerative therapy. Two approaches have been used. *Direct radiolabeling of cells* enables monitoring of homing and engraftment. [111]Indium oxine and ^{99m}Tc exametazime labeling have been used for SPECT imaging[84] and F-18 fluorodeoxyglucose for PET imaging.[85] X-ray CT can be used conjointly to enable localization.[86] Disadvantages of this approach include persistence of radioactivity despite cell death, which may provide unreliable information regarding cell survival, and the fact that the duration of monitoring is limited by radioactive decay of the label.[87] *Reporter gene imaging* overcomes some of these limitations of direct radiolabeling. In this process, a reporter gene that encodes for a protein product is transferred to regenerative cells in vitro before they are applied therapeutically. After engraftment, the cells produce the protein product, which is then detected by the intravenous injection of highly specific radiolabeled reporter probes, followed by imaging. This method ensures that the imaging signals detected are from viable cells capable of expressing the reporter gene. Furthermore, repeated imaging can be performed to monitor cell survival and activity.[87]

Assessing LV Remodeling: Shape Indices

The cellular and interstitial changes that underlie the phenomenon of LV remodeling are accompanied by a transformation of the normally ellipsoid LV into a more spherical structure. The degree of remodeling can be assessed by calculating a *sphericity index*, defined as the ratio of the largest long-axis and short-axis diameters of the LV,[88] which has established utility in predicting response to therapy and prognosis in heart failure.[38,88–90] The sphericity index has generally been calculated based on echocardiographic measurements, but Fukuchi and colleagues manually determined the sphericity index on gated SPECT imaging as the ratio of the LV long-axis diameter to the LV vertical diameter on the end-diastolic vertical long-axis frame (Fig. 30-10).[91] In 38 patients with idiopathic dilated cardiomyopathy treated with β-adrenergic blockers, the sphericity index at baseline identified patients who responded to therapy (defined as = 10% increase in EF at a mean follow-up of 4 months). The mean sphericity index was 1.77 ± 0.26 versus 1.52 ± 0.15 in responders and nonresponders, respectively; $P < 0.05$. The only other parameter predictive of response was the presence of myocardial perfusion defects in these patients with idiopathic dilated cardiomyopathy, presumably indicative of myocardial

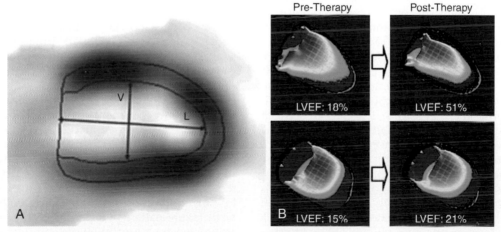

Figure 30-10 **A,** Assessment of left ventricular (LV) geometry using gated SPECT. The sphericity index was manually calculated as the ratio of the LV long-axis diameter (L) to the LV vertical diameter (V) on the end-diastolic vertical long axis frame. **B,** Representative three-dimensional displays of end-diastolic *(grid)* and end-systolic *(solid)* surfaces from gated SPECT imaging to show the effect of LV remodeling on response to β-adrenergic blocker therapy in heart failure. The pretherapy images in the *top row* show preservation of the elliptical shape of the LV, and the posttherapy images show significant improvement in LV ejection fraction (EF) after 4 months of therapy. The pretherapy images in the *bottom row* show a spherical LV, indicative of extensive remodeling, and the posttherapy images show a much smaller increase in EF with therapy. *(From Fukuchi K, Yasumura Y, Kiso K, et al: Gated myocardial SPECT to predict response to β-blocker therapy in patients with idiopathic dilated cardiomyopathy. J Nucl Med 45:527–531, 2004.)*

fibrosis.[91] Abidov and colleagues[92] recently reported an automated algorithm on gated SPECT MPI to define LV geometry. Taking advantage of the true three-dimensional nature of SPECT data and the completely operator-independent execution of the QGS program (Cedars-Sinai Medical Center, Los Angeles, CA), they developed an algorithm for the calculation of an *LV shape index* (LVSI), defined as the ratio of the maximum three-dimensional short- and long-axis dimensions of the left ventricle in systole, LVSIs, and diastole, LVSId. Normal limits were determined from 186 consecutive patients with = 5 likelihood of CAD *and* normal MPI, and then applied prospectively in 93 hospitalized patients, of whom 25 had a discharge diagnosis of worsening heart failure. Repeatability was tested in a group of 52 patients who had sequential MPI within 60 days of each other, without clinical events in between. The LVSI was significantly different in the CHF group compared to normal subjects and also the non-CHF group; it was superior to all conventional variables, including LVEF, for predicting CHF hospitalizations. A cutoff LVSIs of 0.54 had a sensitivity of 68% and specificity of 95% for predicting CHF hospitalizations, and a normalcy rate of 99% in the control population. LVSIs and LVSId had good reproducibility on serial measurement (R^2 = 0.8497 and 0.8233, respectively). Gated SPECT imaging offers a widely available and reproducible method to determine LV geometry, which is an indicator of the degree of remodeling and has potential utility for the prediction of functional recovery and prognosis following therapeutic interventions in patients with LV systolic dysfunction.

Assessment of LV Mechanical (Dys)Synchrony

Cardiac resynchronization therapy (CRT) has been shown to improve symptoms and prognosis in selected patients with LV systolic dysfunction (EF = 35%), severe symptoms (NYHA class III or IV), and evidence of mechanical dyssynchrony (QRS duration = 120 ms on the surface electrocardiogram).[93,94] Much effort has been directed toward optimizing patient selection for this invasive and costly therapy. Using the conventional criteria listed above, less than two-thirds of patients who undergo CRT derive symptomatic benefit from it. This disparity is most likely due to a dissociation between mechanical synchrony and the QRS duration in some patients.[95] Echocardiography-derived indices of dyssynchrony using tissue Doppler imaging and speckle tracking have been used to improve detection of mechanical dyssynchrony and response to CRT, and encouraging results were obtained in individual studies, including studies in patients with LV systolic dysfunction and narrow QRS complexes.[95] However, the poor reproducibility of echo-based assessments is a significant limitation to the widespread application of this approach, as was demonstrated in the recent multicenter Predictors of Response to Cardiac Resynchronization Therapy (PROSPECT) trial.[96]

Phase analysis of radionuclide images of the heart is well suited for the assessment of ventricular synchrony (Fig. 30-11). This has hitherto been performed on

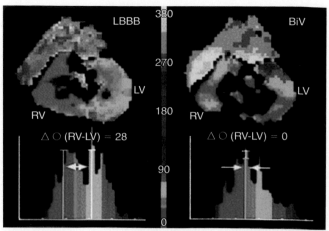

Figure 30-11 Phase analysis of radionuclide ventriculography showing the effect of biventricular pacing (BiV) on a patient with dilated cardiomyopathy and left bundle branch block (LBBB). The contraction sequence is represented *from early to late* in green, azure, navy, violet, orange, and yellow. The histograms illustrate dispersion of phase angles during ventricular ejection, plotted as phase angle (*x*-axis) versus number of pixels (*y*-axis). *Vertical bars* represent the arithmetic mean phase angle, Ø, computed for right ventricular (RV) and left ventricular (LV) blood pools. *Left*, Dyssynchronous RV and LV phase pattern in sinus rhythm. The bulk of the RV *(green)* contracts before onset of LV contraction *(azure)*. Histogram illustrates bimodal distribution of phase angles for the RV and LV, with a difference in mean phase between the RV and LV (ΔØ) of 28 degrees. *Right*, During BiV, ventricular activation originates simultaneously at the LV and RV apices *(green)*, followed by RV outflow tract *(azure)* and LV base *(azure, navy)*. A more symmetrical RV and LV phase pattern is observed with restoration of early septal contraction *(green)*. Histogram illustrates a decrease in ΔØ to 0 degrees, representing a 28-degree correction of baseline interventricular dyssynchrony. *(From Kerwin WF, Botvinick EH, O'Connell JW, et al: Ventricular contraction abnormalities in dilated cardiomyopathy: Effect of biventricular pacing to correct interventricular dyssynchrony, J Am Coll Cardiol 35:1221–1227, 2000.)*

radionuclide ventriculography, from which an indirect assessment of regional LV function is obtained by measuring changes in regional (counts) within the LV blood pool (indicative of regional shifts in blood volume related to regional wall motion).[97] Phase analysis on gated-SPECT imaging has recently been investigated as a modality to assess the synchrony of LV mechanical contraction.[98] Preliminary studies indicate ability to distinguish between patients with normal conduction and LV systolic function from those with LV systolic dysfunction, left bundle branch block, right bundle branch block, or right ventricular pacing.[99] Small studies also suggest that baseline phase analysis variables can predict response to CRT.[100] Advantages of gated SPECT imaging for this application are its existing widespread use in heart failure patients for perfusion imaging, completely automated function involving minimal operator input (resulting in excellent reproducibility), and the ability to simultaneously generate information on scar burden, viability, and remodeling, all of which may have important bearing on response to CRT. Phase analysis is based on the linear relationship between LV regional myocardial thickening and change in regional counts (brightening) between diastole and systole due to the partial volume effect.[101] This change in regional counts can be used to determine the onset of thickening (mechanical contraction) in each region of the LV myocardium. A phase analysis is performed by applying Fourier transformation to the count variation over time in each myocardial voxel, thus generating a three-dimensional phase distribution. This phase distribution is displayed as a function of the R-R interval, so that the percentage of LV myocardium initiating mechanical contraction (thickening) at any point in the cardiac cycle can be determined.[98] This information is used to determine how homogeneous or heterogeneous the onset of mechanical contraction (synchrony or dyssynchrony) is across the LV myocardium. The phase analysis tool is implemented in the Emory Cardiac Toolbox and described in the recent publication by Chen and colleagues.[98] As shown in Figure 30-12, the phase analysis is represented as polar maps and phase histograms. The coordinates for the histogram are the cardiac cycle on the x-axis (the R-R interval divided into 360 degrees, which can be converted to milliseconds if the heart rate is known) and percentage of the myocardium initiating mechanical contraction during any gating frame on the y-axis. With coordinated ventricular contraction, most myocardial segments have nearly the same phase, resulting in a uniform phase image and a narrow and highly peaked phase histogram. The following previously validated indices with known normal limits are measured to quantify LV dyssynchrony:

1. *Peak phase (degrees)* is the most frequent phase and represents the time in the cardiac cycle during which the largest extent of LV myocardium is initiating contraction.
2. *Phase standard deviation (SD)* is SD of phase distribution in degrees. Lower values indicate more synchronous LV contraction.
3. *Phase histogram bandwidth* represents the range of degrees of the cardiac cycle during which 95% of the myocardium is initiating contraction. A smaller dispersion of the histogram reflects more synchronous LV contraction.

CONCLUSION

Radionuclide imaging techniques can be used to evaluate several aspects of the heart failure syndrome and provide clinically meaningful data that can be applied effectively to patient care. Established applications include the determination of heart failure etiology, measurement of LV function, assessment of myocardial remodeling, and the optimal selection of patients for coronary revascularization. The major strengths of the modality include wide availability and completely automated quantitation of perfusion and function, resulting in excellent reproducibility. Encouraging preliminary results indicate that it could be useful for the assessment of myocardial dyssynchrony. There is extensive ongoing clinical and translational research related to the use of radionuclide tracers for molecular and metabolic imaging. Thus, in the future, the applicability of radionuclide imaging to heart failure patients is likely be expanded even further.

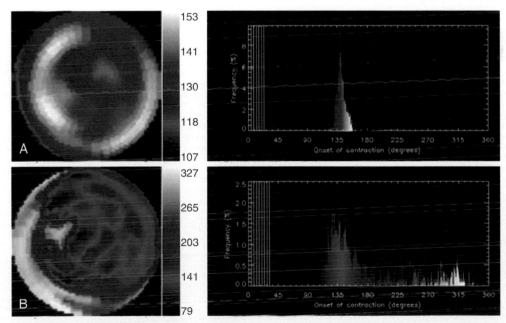

Figure 30-12 Assessment of left ventricular (LV) mechanical synchrony by gated SPECT. Results are presented on a polar map *(left panels)* and as a phase histogram *(right panels)* on which the x-axis represents the timing of one cardiac cycle (R-R interval), and the y-axis represents the percentage of myocardium initiating mechanical contraction during any particular phase of the cardiac cycle. A uniform phase polar map and a narrow and high peaked phase histogram are characteristic of patients with synchronous LV contraction **(A)**, whereas a heterogeneous polar map and a widely dispersed histogram indicate mechanical dyssynchrony **(B)**. *(From Chen J, Henneman MM, Trimble MA, et al: Assessment of left ventricular mechanical dyssynchrony by phase analysis of ECG-gated SPECT myocardial perfusion imaging, J Nucl Cardiol 15:127–136, 2008.)*

REFERENCES

1. Rosamond W, Flegal K, Friday G, Furie K, Go A, Greenlund K, Haase N, Ho M, Howard V, Kissela B, Kittner S, Lloyd-Jones D, McDermott M, Meigs J, Moy C, Nichol G, O'Donnell CJ, Roger V, Rumsfeld J, Sorlie P, Steinberger J, Thom T, Wasserthiel-Smoller S, Hong Y: for the American Heart Association Statistics Committee and Stroke Statistics Subcommittee. Heart Disease and Stroke Statistics–2007 Update: A Report From the American Heart Association Statistics Committee and Stroke Statistics Subcommittee, *Circulation* 115:e69–e171, 2007.
2. Gheorghiade M, Bonow RO: Chronic heart failure in the United States: a manifestation of coronary artery disease, *Circulation* 97:282–289, 1998.
3. Velagaleti RS, Vasan RS: Heart failure in the twenty-first century: is it a coronary artery disease or hypertension problem? *Cardiol Clin* 25:487–495, 2007.
4. Felker GM, Shaw LK, O'Connor CM: A standardized definition of ischemic cardiomyopathy for use in clinical research, *J Am Coll Cardiol* 39:210–218, 2002.
5. Allman KC, Shaw LJ, Hachamovitch R, Udelson JE: Myocardial viability testing and impact of revascularization on prognosis in patients with coronary artery disease and left ventricular dysfunction: a meta-analysis, *J Am Coll Cardiol* 39:1151–1158, 2002.
6. Hunt SA, Abraham WT, Chin MH, Feldman AM, Francis GS, Ganiats TG, Jessup M, Konstam MA, Mancini DM, Michl K, Oates JA, Rahko PS, Silver MA, Stevenson LW, Yancy CW, Antman EM, Smith SC Jr, Adams CD, Anderson JL, Faxon DP, Fuster V, Halperin JL, Hiratzka LF, Hunt SA, Jacobs AK, Nishimura R, Ornato JP, Page RL, Riegel B: ACC/AHA 2005 Guideline update for the diagnosis and management of chronic heart failure in the adult—Summary article: A report of the American College of Cardiology/American Heart Association Task Force on Practice Guidelines (Writing Committee to Update the 2001 Guidelines for the Evaluation and Management of Heart Failure): Developed in collaboration with the American College of Chest Physicians and the International Society for Heart and Lung Transplantation: Endorsed by the Heart Rhythm Society, *Circulation* 112:1825–1852, 2005.
7. Poole-Wilson PA, Swedberg K, Cleland JG, Di L, Hanrath P, Komajda M, Lubsen J, Lutiger B, Metra M, Remme WJ, Torp-Pedersen C, Scherhag A, Skene A, Carvedilol O: Comparison of carvedilol and metoprolol on clinical outcomes in patients with chronic heart failure in the Carvedilol Or Metoprolol European Trial (COMET): randomised controlled trial, *Lancet* 362:7–13, 2003.
8. Klocke FJ, Baird MG, Lorell BH, Bateman TM, Messer JV, Berman DS, O'Gara PT, Carabello BA, Russell ROJ, Cerqueira MD, St J, DeMaria AN, Udelson JE, Kennedy JW, Verani MS, Williams KA, Antman EM, Smith SCJ, Alpert JS, Gregoratos G, Anderson JL, Hiratzka LF, Faxon DP, Hunt SA, Fuster V, Jacobs AK, Gibbons RJ, Russell RO, American C, American H, American S: ACC/AHA/ASNC guidelines for the clinical use of cardiac radionuclide imaging—Executive summary: A report of the American College of Cardiology/American Heart Association Task Force on Practice Guidelines (ACC/AHA/ASNC Committee to Revise the 1995 Guidelines for the Clinical Use of Cardiac Radionuclide Imaging), *Circulation* 108:1404–1418, 2003.
9. Udelson JE, Shafer CD, Carrio I: Radionuclide imaging in heart failure: assessing etiology and outcomes and implications for management, *J Nucl Cardiol* 9:40S–52S, 2002.
10. Danias PG, Papaioannou GI, Ahlberg AW, O'Sullivan DM, Mann A, Boden WE, Heller GV: Usefulness of electrocardiographic-gated stress technetium-99m sestamibi single-photon emission computed tomography to differentiate ischemic from nonischemic cardiomyopathy, *Am J Cardiol* 94:14–19, 2004.
11. Soman P, Lahiri A, Mieres JH, Calnon DA, Wolinsky D, Beller GA, Sias T, Burnham K, Conway L, McCullough PA, Daher E, Walsh MN, Wight J, Heller GV, Udelson JE: Etiology and pathophysiology of new-onset heart failure: Evaluation by myocardial perfusion imaging, *J Nucl Cardiol* 16:82–91, 2009.
12. Di B, Pozzi C, Cavallini MC, Innocenti F, Baldereschi G, De A, Antonini E, Pini R, Masotti G, Marchionni N: The diagnosis of heart failure in the community. Comparative validation of four sets of criteria in unselected older adults: the ICARe Dicomano Study, *J Am Coll Cardiol* 44:1601–1608, 2004.
13. Hachamovitch R, Hayes SW, Friedman JD, Cohen I, Berman DS: Comparison of the short-term survival benefit associated with revascularization compared with medical therapy in patients with no prior coronary artery disease undergoing stress myocardial perfusion single-photon emission computed tomography, *Circulation* 107:2900–2907, 2003.
14. Doi YL, Chikamori T, Tukata J, Yonezawa Y, Poloniecki JD, Ozawa T, McKenna WJ: Prognostic value of thallium-201 perfusion defects in idiopathic dilated cardiomyopathy, *Am J Cardiol* 67:188–193, 1991.
15. Soman P, Dave DM, Udelson JE, Han H, Ouda HZ, Patel AR, Karas RH, Kuvin JT: Vascular endothelial dysfunction is associated with reversible myocardial perfusion defects in the absence of obstructive coronary artery disease, *J Nucl Cardiol* 13:756–760, 2006.
16. Heller GV, Links J, Bateman TM, Ziffer JA, Ficaro E, Cohen MC, Hendel RC: American Society of Nuclear Cardiology and Society of Nuclear Medicine joint position statement: Attenuation correction of myocardial perfusion SPECT scintigraphy, *J Nucl Cardiol* 11:229–230, 2004.
17. Budoff MJ, Jacob B, Rasouli ML, Yu D, Chang RS, Shavelle DM: Comparison of electron beam computed tomography and technetium stress testing in differentiating cause of dilated versus ischemic cardiomyopathy, *J Comput Assist Tomogr* 29:699–703, 2005.
18. Andreini D, Pontone G, Pepi M, Ballerini G, Bartorelli AL, Magini A, Quaglia C, Nobili E, Agostoni P: Diagnostic accuracy of multidetector computed tomography coronary angiography in patients with dilated cardiomyopathy, *J Am Coll Cardiol* 49:2044–2050, 2007.
19. Kumita S, Cho K, Nakajo H, Toba M, Uwamori M, Mizumura S, Kumazaki T, Sano J, Sakai S, Munakata K: Assessment of left ventricular diastolic function with electrocardiography-gated myocardial perfusion SPECT: Comparison with multigated equilibrium radionuclide angiography, *J Nucl Cardiol* 8:568–574, 2001.
20. Germano G, Kavanagh PB, Slomka PJ, Van Kriekinge SD, Pollard G, Berman DS: Quantitation in gated perfusion SPECT imaging: The Cedars-Sinai approach, *J Nucl Cardiol* 14:433–454, 2007.
21. Rozanski A, Nichols K, Yao SS, Malhotra S, Cohen R, DePuey EG: Development and application of normal limits for left ventricular ejection fraction and volume measurements from 99mTc-sestamibi myocardial perfusion gates SPECT, *J Nucl Med* 41:1445–1450, 2000.
22. Bellenger NG, Burgess MI, Ray SG, Lahiri A, Coats AJS, Cleland JGF, Pennell DJ: Comparison of left ventricular ejection fraction and volumes in heart failure by echocardiography, radionuclide ventriculography and cardiovascular magnetic resonance. Are they interchangeable? *Eur Heart J* 21:1387–1396, 2000.
23. Moss AJ, Zareba W, Hall WJ, Klein H, Wilber DJ, Cannom DS, Daubert JP, Higgins SL, Brown MW, Andrews ML: the Multicenter Automatic Defibrillator Implantation Trial II Investigators: Prophylactic implantation of a defibrillator in patients with myocardial infarction and reduced ejection fraction, *N Engl J Med* 346:877–883, 2002.
24. Bigger JT: The Coronary Artery Bypass Graft (CABG) Patch Trial Investigators: Prophylactic use of implanted cardiac defibrillators in patients at high risk for ventricular arrhythmias after coronary-artery bypass graft surgery, *N Engl J Med* 337:1569–1575, 1997.
25. Manrique A, Koning R, Cribier A, et al: Effect of temporal sampling on evaluation of left ventricular ejection fraction by means of thallium-201 gated SPET: comparison of 16- and 8-interval gating, with reference to equilibrium radionuclide angiography, *Eur J Nucl Med Mol Imaging* 27:694–699, 2000.
26. Nakajima K, Higuchi T, Taki J, Kawano M, Tonami N: Accuracy of ventricular volume and ejection fraction measured by gated myocardial SPECT: Comparison of 4 software programs, *J Nucl Med* 42:1571–1578, 2001.
27. Johnson LL, Verdesca SA, Aude WY, Xavier RC, Nott LT, Campanella MW, Germano G: Postischemic stunning can affect left ventricular ejection fraction and regional wall motion on post-stress gated sestamibi tomograms, *J Am Coll Cardiol* 30:1641–1648, 1997.
28. Hyun IY, Kwan J, Park KS, Lee WH: Reproducibility of Tl-201 and Tc-99m sestamibi gated myocardial perfusion SPECT measurement of myocardial function, *J Nucl Cardiol* 8:182–187, 2001.
29. Muhlbaier LH, Pryor DB, Rankin JS, Smith LR, Mark DB, Jones RH, Glower DD, Harrell FEJ, Lee KL, Califf RM, et al: Observational comparison of event-free survival with medical and surgical therapy in patients with coronary artery disease. 20 years of follow-up, *Circulation* 86:II198–II204, 1992.
30. Di Carli MF, Asgarzadie F, Schelbert HR, Brunken RC, Laks H, Phelps ME, Maddahi J: Quantitative relation between myocardial viability and improvement in heart failure symptoms after revascularization in patients with ischemic cardiomyopathy, *Circulation* 92:3436–3444, 1995.
31. Marwick TH, Zuchowski C, Lauer MS, Secknus MA, Williams Lytle BW: Functional status and quality of life in patients with heart failure undergoing coronary bypass surgery after assessment of myocardial viability, *J Am Coll Cardiol* 33:750–758, 1999.
32. Bax JJ, Poldermans D, Elhendy A, Cornel JH, Boersma E, Rambaldi R, Roelandt JR, Fioretti PM: Improvement of left ventricular ejection fraction, heart failure symptoms and prognosis after revascularization in patients with chronic coronary artery disease and viable myocardium detected by dobutamine stress echocardiography, *J Am Coll Cardiol* 34:163–169, 1999.
33. Bax JJ, Wijns W, Cornel JH, Visser FC, Boersma E, Fioretti PM: Accuracy of currently available techniques for prediction of functional recovery after revascularization in patients with left ventricular dysfunction due to chronic coronary artery disease: comparison of pooled data, *J Am Coll Cardiol* 30:1451–1460, 1997.
34. Kim RJ, Wu E, Rafael A, Chen EL, Parker MA, Simonetti O, Klocke FJ, Bonow RO, Judd RM: The use of contrast-enhanced magnetic resonance imaging to identify reversible myocardial dysfunction, *N Engl J Med* 343:1445–1453, 2000.
35. Meluzin J, Cigarroa CG, Brickner ME, Cerny J, Spinarova L, Frelich M, Stetka F, Groch L, Grayburn PA: Dobutamine echocardiography in

predicting improvement in global left ventricular systolic function after coronary bypass or angioplasty in patients with healed myocardial infarcts, *Am J Cardiol* 76:877–880, 1995.

36. Senior R, Kaul S, Raval U, Lahiri A: Impact of revascularization and myocardial viability determined by nitrate-enhanced Tc-99m sestamibi and Tl-201 imaging on mortality and functional outcome in ischemic cardiomyopathy, *J Nucl Cardiol* 9:454–462, 2002.

37. Pagley PR, Beller GA, Watson DD, Gimple LW, Ragosta M: Improved outcome after coronary bypass surgery in patients with ischemic cardiomyopathy and residual myocardial viability, *Circulation* 96:793–800, 1997.

38. Senior R, Lahiri A, Kaul S: Effect of revascularization on left ventricular remodeling in patients with heart failure from severe chronic ischemic left ventricular dysfunction, *Am J Cardiol* 88:624–629, 2001.

39. Bonow RO: Identification of viable myocardium, *Circulation* 94:2674–2680, 1996.

40. Samady H, Elefteriades JA, Abbott BG, Mattera JA, McPherson CA, Wackers FJ: Failure to improve left ventricular function after coronary revascularization for ischemic cardiomyopathy is not associated with worse outcome, *Circulation* 100:1298–1304, 1999.

41. Myers JH, Stirling MC, Choy M, Buda AJ, Gallagher KP: Direct measurement of inner and outer wall thickening dynamics with epicardial echocardiography, *Circulation* 74:164–172, 1986.

42. Lieberman AN, Weiss JL, Jugdutt BI, Becker LC, Bulkley BH, Garrison JG, Hutchins GM, Kallman CA, Weisfeldt ML: Two-dimensional echocardiography and infarct size: relationship of regional wall motion and thickening to the extent of myocardial infarction in the dog, *Circulation* 63:739–746, 1981.

43. Kaul S: There may be more to myocardial viability than meets the eye, *Circulation* 92:2790–2793, 1995.

44. Auerbach MA, Schoder H, Hoh C, Gambhir SS, Yaghoubi S, Sayre JW, Silverman D, Phelps ME, Schelbert HR, Czernin J: Prevalence of myocardial viability as detected by positron emission tomography in patients with ischemic cardiomyopathy, *Circulation* 99:2921–2926, 1999.

45. Cleland JG, Pennell DJ, Ray SG, Coats AJ, Macfarlane PW, Murray GD, Mule JD, Vered Z, Lahiri A: Carvedilol hm. Myocardial viability as a determinant of the ejection fraction response to carvedilol in patients with heart failure (CHRISTMAS trial): randomised controlled trial, *Lancet* 362:14–21, 2003.

46. Camici PG, Wijns W, Borgers M, De S, Ferrari R, Knuuti J, Lammertsma AA, Liedtke AJ, Paternostro G, Vatner SF: Pathophysiological mechanisms of chronic reversible left ventricular dysfunction due to coronary artery disease (hibernating myocardium), *Circulation* 96:3205–3214, 1997.

47. Wijns W, Vatner SF, Camici PG: Hibernating myocardium, *N Engl J Med* 339:173–181, 1998.

48. Ragosta M, Beller GA, Watson DD, Kaul S, Gimple LW: Quantitative planar rest-redistribution ^{201}Tl imaging in detection of myocardial viability and prediction of improvement in left ventricular function after coronary bypass surgery in patients with severely depressed left ventricular function, *Circulation* 87:1630–1641, 1993.

49. Pohost GM, Zir LM, Moore RH, McKusick KA, Guiney TE, Beller GA: Differentiation of transiently ischemic from infarcted myocardium by serial imaging after a single dose of thallium-201, *Circulation* 55:294–302, 1977.

50. Bonow RO, Dilsizian V: Thallium-201 and technetium-99m-sestamibi for assessing viable myocardium, *J Nucl Med* 33:815–818, 1992.

51. Udelson JE, Coleman PS, Metherall J, Pandian NG, Gomez AR, Griffith JL, Shea NL, Oates E, Konstam MA: Predicting recovery of severe regional ventricular dysfunction. Comparison of resting scintigraphy with 201Tl and 99mTc-sestamibi, *Circulation* 89:2552–2561, 1994.

52. Sciagra R, Bisi G, Santoro GM, Zerauschek F, Sestini S, Pedenovi P, Pappagallo R, Fazzini PF: Comparison of baseline-nitrate technetium-99m sestamibi with rest-redistribution thallium-201 tomography in detecting viable hibernating myocardium and predicting postrevascularization recovery, *J Am Coll Cardiol* 30:384–391, 1997.

53. Siebelink HM, Blanksma PK, Crijns HJ, Bax JJ, van B, Kingma T, Piers DA, Pruim J, Jager PL, Vaalburg W: Van d. No difference in cardiac event-free survival between positron emission tomography-guided and single-photon emission computed tomography-guided patient management: a prospective, randomized comparison of patients with suspicion of jeopardized myocardium, *J Am Coll Cardiol* 37:81–88, 2001.

54. Schinkel AF, Poldermans D, Rizzello V, Vanoverschelde JL, Elhendy A, Boersma E, Roelandt JR, Bax JJ: Why do patients with ischemic cardiomyopathy and a substantial amount of viable myocardium not always recover in function after revascularization? *J Thorac Cardiovasc Surg* 127:385–390, 2004.

55. Shirani J, Narula J, Eckelman WC, Narula N, Dilsizian V: Early imaging in heart failure: Exploring novel molecular targets, *J Nucl Cardiol* 14:100–110, 2007.

56. Shirani J, Dilsizian V: Molecular imaging in heart failure, *Curr Opin Biotechnol* 18:65–72, 2007.

57. Thimister PW, Hofstra L, Liem IH, Boersma HH, Kemerink G, Reutelingsperger CP, Heidendal GA: In vivo detection of cell death in the area at risk in acute myocardial infarction, *J Nucl Med* 44:391–396, 2003.

58. Korngold EC, Jaffer FA, Weissleder R, Sosnovik DE: Noninvasive imaging of apoptosis in cardiovascular disease, *Heart Fail Rev* 13:163–173, 2008.

59. Ferrari R, Ceconi C, Curello S, Visioli O: The neuroendocrine and sympathetic nervous system in congestive heart failure, *Eur Heart J* 19:F45–F51, 1998.

60. Schrier RW, Abraham WT: Hormones and hemodynamics in heart failure, *N Engl J Med* 341:577–585, 1999.

61. Wieland DM, Brown LE, Rogers WL, Worthington KC, Wu JL, Clinthorne NH, Otto CA, Swanson DP, Beierwaltes WH: Myocardial imaging with a radioiodinated norepinephrine storage analog, *J Nucl Med* 22:22–31, 1981.

62. Yamashina S, Yamazaki J: Neuronal imaging using SPECT, *Eur J Nucl Med Mol Imaging* 34:939–950, 2007.

63. Valette H, Bourguignon MH, Le Guludec D, Merlet P, Dove PJ, Kiger JP, Slama M, Motte G, Raynaud C, Syrota A: ECG gated thallium 201 myocardial images: value in detecting multivessel disease in patients on anti anginal therapy 1–3 months after myocardial infarction, *Eur J Nucl Med* 13:551–556, 1988.

64. Fujimoto S, Inoue A, Hisatake S, Yamashina S, Yamashina H, Nakano H, Yamazaki J: Usefulness of meta-iodobenzylguanidine myocardial scintigraphy for predicting cardiac events in patients with dilated cardiomyopathy who receive long-term beta blocker treatment, *Nucl Med Commun* 26:97–102, 2005.

65. Neely JR, Rovetto MJ, Oram JF: Myocardial utilization of carbohydrate and lipids, *Prog Cardiovasc Dis* 15:289–329, 1972.

66. Goldstein RA, Klein MS, Welch MJ, Sobel BE: External assessment of myocardial metabolism with C-11 palmitate in vivo, *J Nucl Med* 21:342–348, 1980.

67. Schon HR, Schelbert HR, Robinson G, Najafi A, Huang SC, Hansen H, Barrio J, Kuhl DE, Phelps ME: C-11 labeled palmitic acid for the noninvasive evaluation of regional myocardial fatty acid metabolism with positron-computed tomography. I. Kinetics of C- 11 palmitic acid in normal myocardium, *Am Heart J* 103:532–547, 1982.

68. Reske SN, Biersack HJ, Lackner K, Machulla HJ, Knopp R, Hahn N, Winkler C: Assessment of regional myocardial uptake and metabolism of omega-(p-123I-phenyl) pentadecanoic acid with serial single-photon emission tomography, *Nuklearmedizin* 21:249–253, 1982.

69. Yang JY, Ruiz M, Calnon DA, Watson DD, Beller GA, Glover DK: Assessment of myocardial viability using ^{123}I-labeled iodophenylpentadecanoic acid at sustained low flow or after acute infarction and reperfusion, *J Nucl Med* 40:821–828, 1999.

70. Caldwell JH, Martin GV, Link JM, Krohn KA, Bassingthwaighte JB: Iodophenylpentadecanoic acid-myocardial blood flow relationship during maximal exercise with coronary occlusion, *J Nucl Med* 31:99–105, 1990.

71. Murray G, Schad N, Ladd W, Allie D, vander Z, Avet P, Rockett J: Metabolic cardiac imaging in severe coronary disease: assessment of viability with iodine-123-iodophenylpentadecanoic acid and multicrystal gamma camera, and correlation with biopsy, *J Nucl Med* 33:1269–1277, 1992.

72. Hansen CL, Heo J, Oliner C, Van D, Iskandrian AS: Prediction of improvement in left ventricular function with iodine-123-IPPA after coronary revascularization, *J Nucl Med* 36:1987–1993, 1995.

73. Iskandrian AS, Powers J, Cave V, Wasserleben V, Cassell D, Heo J: Assessment of myocardial viability by dynamic tomographic iodine 123 iodophenylpentadecanoic acid imaging: comparison with rest-redistribution thallium 201 imaging, *J Nucl Cardiol* 2:101–109, 1995.

74. Verani MS, Taillefer R, Iskandrian AE, Mahmarian JJ, He ZX, Orlandi C: ^{123}I-IPPA SPECT for the prediction of enhanced left ventricular function after coronary bypass graft surgery. Multicenter IPPA Viability Trial Investigators. ^{123}I-iodophenylpentadecanoic acid, *J Nucl Med* 41:1299–1307, 2000.

75. Tamaki N, Tadamura E, Kawamoto M, Magata Y, Yonekura Y, Fujibayashi Y, Nohara R, Sasayama S, Konishi J: Decreased uptake of iodinated branched fatty acid analog indicates metabolic alterations in ischemic myocardium, *J Nucl Med* 36:1974–1980, 1995.

76. Knapp FFJ, Goodman MM, Callahan AP, Kirsch G: Radioiodinated 15-(p-iodophenyl)-3,3-dimethylpentadecanoic acid: a useful new agent to evaluate myocardial fatty acid uptake, *J Nucl Med* 27:521–531, 1986.

77. Tamaki N, Kawamoto M, Yonekura Y, Fujibayashi Y, Takahashi N, Konishi J, Nohara R, Kambara H, Kawai C, Ikekubo K, et al: Regional metabolic abnormality in relation to perfusion and wall motion in patients with myocardial infarction: assessment with emission tomography using an iodinated branched fatty acid analog, *J Nucl Med* 33:659–667, 1992.

78. Dilsizian V, Bateman TM, Bergmann SR, Des P, Magram MY, Goodbody AE, Babich JW, Udelson JE: Metabolic imaging with β-methyl-p-iodophenyl-pentadecanoic acid identifies ischemic memory after demand ischemia, *Circulation* 112:2169–2174, 2005.

79. Nishimura M, Tsukamoto K, Hasebe N, Tamaki N, Kikuchi K, Ono T: Prediction of cardiac death in hemodialysis patients by myocardial fatty acid imaging, *J Am Coll Cardiol* 51:139–145, 2008.

80. Hambye AS, Vaerenberg MM, Dobbeleir AA, Van d, Franken PR: Abnormal BMIPP uptake in chronically dysfunctional myocardial segments: correlation with contractile response to low-dose dobutamine, *J Nucl Med* 39:1845–1850, 1998.

81. Kudoh T, Tadamura E, Tamaki N, Hattori N, Inubushi M, Kubo S, Magata Y, Nishimura K, Matsuda K, Konishi J: Iodinated free fatty acid and 201T1 uptake in chronically hypoperfused myocardium: histologic correlation study, *J Nucl Med* 41:293–296, 2000.

82. Ito T, Tanouchi J, Kato J, Morioka T, Nishino M, Iwai K, Tanahashi H, Yamada Y, Hori M, Kamada T: Recovery of impaired left ventricular function in patients with acute myocardial infarction is predicted by the discordance in defect size on ^{123}I-BMIPP and ^{201}Tl SPECT images, *Eur J Nucl Med* 23:917–923, 1996.

83. Naruse H, Arii T, Kondo T, Morita M, Ohyanagi M, Iwasaki T, Fukuchi M: Clinical usefulness of iodine 123-labeled fatty acid imaging in patients with acute myocardial infarction, *J Nucl Cardiol* 5:275–284, 1998.

84. Barbash IM, Chouraqui P, Baron J, Feinberg MS, Etzion S, Tessone A, Miller L, Guetta E, Zipori D, Kedes LH, Kloner RA, Leor J: Systemic delivery of bone marrow-derived mesenchymal stem cells to the infarcted myocardium: Feasibility, cell migration, and body distribution, *Circulation* 108:863–868, 2003.

85. Hofmann M, Wollert KC, Meyer GP, Menke A, Arseniev L, Hertenstein B, Ganser A, Knapp WH, Drexler H: Monitoring of bone marrow cell homing into the infarcted human myocardium, *Circulation* 111:2198–2202, 2005.

86. Kraitchman DL, Tatsumi M, Gilson WD, Ishimori T, Kedziorek D, Walczak P, Segars WP, Chen H, Fritzges D, Izbudak I, Young RG, Marcelino M, Pittenger MF, Solaiyappan M, Boston RC, Tsui BMW, Wahl RL, Bulte JWM: Dynamic imaging of allogeneic mesenchymal stem cells trafficking to myocardial Infarction, *Circulation* 112:1451–1461, 2005.

87. Bengel F: Nuclear imaging in cardiac cell therapy, *Heart Fail Rev* 11:325–332, 2006.

88. Douglas PS, Morrow R, Ioli A, Reichek N: Left ventricular shape, afterload and survival in idiopathic dilated cardiomyopathy, *J Am Coll Cardiol* 13:311–315, 1989.

89. Lowes BD, Gill EA, Abraham WT, Larrain JR, Robertson AD, Bristow MR, Gilbert EM: Effects of carvedilol on left ventricular mass, chamber geometry, and mitral regurgitation in chronic heart failure, *Am J Cardiol* 83:1201–1205, 1999.

90. Hall SA, Cigarroa CG, Marcoux L, Risser RC, Grayburn PA, Eichhorn EJ: Time course of improvement in left ventricular function, mass and geometry in patients with congestive heart failure treated with β-adrenergic blockade, *J Am Coll Cardiol* 25:1154–1161, 1995.

91. Fukuchi K, Yasumura Y, Kiso K, Hayashida K, Miyatake K, Ishida Y: Gated myocardial SPECT to predict response to β-blocker therapy in patients with idiopathic dilated cardiomyopathy, *J Nucl Med* 45:527–531, 2004.

92. Abidov A, Slomka PJ, Nishina H, et al: Left ventricular shape index assessed by gated stress myocardial perfusion SPECT: Initial description of a new variable, *J Nucl Cardiol* 13:652–659, 2006.

93. Bristow MR, Saxon LA, Boehmer J, Krueger S, Kass DA, De Marco T, Carson P, DiCarlo L, DeMets D, White BG, DeVries DW, Feldman AM: Comparison of Medical Therapy, Pacing, and Defibrillation in Heart Failure (COMPANION) Investigators. Cardiac-resynchronization therapy with or without an implantable defibrillator in advanced chronic heart failure, *N Engl J Med* 350:2140–2150, 2004.

94. Cleland JGF, Daubert JC, Erdmann E, Freemantle N, Gras D, Kappenberger L, Tavazzi L: For the Cardiac Resynchronization-Heart Failure (Care-HF) Study Investigators. The effect of cardiac resynchronization on morbidity and mortality in heart failure, *N Engl J Med* 352:1539–1549, 2005.

95. Gorcsan J: Role of echocardiography to determine candidacy for cardiac resynchronization therapy, *Curr Opin Cardiol* 23:16–22, 2008.

96. Chung ES, Leon AR, Tavazzi L, Sun JP, Nihoyannopoulos P, Merlino J, Abraham WT, Ghio S, Leclercq C, Bax JJ, Yu CM, Gorcsan J, St J, De S, Murillo J: Results of the Predictors of Response to CRT (PROSPECT) trial, *Circulation* 117:2608–2616, 2008.

97. Kerwin WF, Botvinick EH, O'Connell JW, Merrick SH, DeMarco T, Chatterjee K, Scheibly K, Saxon LA: Ventricular contraction abnormalities in dilated cardiomyopathy: effect of biventricular pacing to correct interventricular dyssynchrony, *J Am Coll Cardiol* 35:1221–1227, 2000.

98. Chen J, Henneman MM, Trimble MA, Bax JJ, Borges-Neto S, Iskandrian AE, Nichols KJ, Garcia EV: Assessment of left ventricular mechanical dyssynchrony by phase analysis of ECG-gated SPECT myocardial perfusion imaging, *J Nucl Cardiol* 15:127–136, 2008.

99. Trimble MA, Borges-Neto S, Smallheiser S, Chen J, Honeycutt EF, Shaw LK, Heo J, Pagnanelli RA, Tauxe EL, Garcia EV, Esteves F, Seghatol-Eslami F, Kay GN, Iskandrian AE: Evaluation of left ventricular mechanical dyssynchrony as determined by phase analysis of ECG-gated SPECT myocardial perfusion imaging in patients with left ventricular dysfunction and conduction disturbances, *J Nucl Cardiol* 14:298–307, 2007.

100. Henneman MM, Chen J, Dibbets-Schneider P, Stokkel MP, Bleeker GB, Ypenburg C, van der Wall EE, Schalij MJ, Garcia EV, Bax JJ: Can LV dyssynchrony as assessed with phase analysis on gated myocardial perfusion SPECT predict response to CRT? *J Nucl Med* 48:1104–1111, 2007.

101. Marcassa C, Marzullo P, Parodi O, Sambuceti G, L'Abbate A: A new method for noninvasive quantitation of segmental myocardial wall thickening using technetium-99m 2-methoxy-isobutyl-isonitrile scintigraphy—results in normal subjects, *J Nucl Med* 31:173–177, 1990.

Chapter 31

Imaging in Patients Receiving Cardiotoxic Chemotherapy

BARRY L. ZARET

INTRODUCTION

Of the many chemotherapeutic agents used in the treatment of malignancies, the anthracycline doxorubicin is well established for its therapeutic efficacy, despite its potential cardiotoxicity. Doxorubicin (Adriamycin) has been available for more than 30 years.[1,2] Although a number of other anthracycline derivatives are available, doxorubicin is the most extensively used agent. Currently, it is used widely in the treatment of breast and gynecologic malignancies, lymphoma, and lung cancer. The cardiotoxicity associated with doxorubicin can be both acute and chronic.[3] Acute cardiotoxicity is transient and without permanent consequences. It involves hypotension, pericarditis, tachycardia, or other arrhythmias. Chronic cardiotoxicity is of greater concern because it can cause progressive left ventricular dysfunction leading to clinical congestive heart failure, which in its most severe form can be fatal.

Some of the earliest clinical paradigms for nuclear cardiology techniques for monitoring and assessing therapeutic efficacy involved doxorubicin and its cardiotoxicity. Remarkably, techniques first reported in the late 1970s continue to be relevant.[4] This chapter focuses on nuclear cardiology approaches to following patients receiving potentially cardiotoxic chemotherapy. It focuses on global left ventricular function monitoring, which is the most widely used clinical approach, and also discusses alternative nuclear and nonnuclear monitoring strategies.

MECHANISMS OF CARDIOTOXICITY

The most commonly accepted view of the mechanism of doxorubicin cardiotoxicity involves a combination of oxidative stress, or free radical production by the metabolites of doxorubicin, coupled with sensitivity of the myocardium to the cytotoxic effects of oxidative stress.[5,6] Generated free radicals are usually toxic, reacting with a number of cell constituents and leading to lipid peroxidation, depletion of specific peptides, and damage to nucleic acids. In addition, mammalian myocardium, in contrast to other organs, is relatively deficient in enzymatic free radical scavengers that can potentially reverse the process. Doxorubicin metabolites also may have direct effects on these enzymes. In addition, doxorubicin can bind to cellular ionic iron, resulting in a complex that is highly toxic to intracellular proteins and membrane lipids.[7]

Alternative mechanisms involve calcium overload, release of vasoactive amines, decrease in cardiac muscle protein gene expression, and induction of apoptosis.[8–12]

PATHOLOGY

The myocardial damage associated with doxorubicin toxicity involves myofibrolysis, cytoplasmic vacuolization as a result of ballooning of sarcoplasmic reticulum, and degeneration of nuclei and mitochondria.[13] Such changes ultimately result in substantial fibrosis. Minor grades of change are usually seen, even after lower doses. Higher grades are associated with impending congestive heart failure.[14] A grading system for evaluating histopathologic changes based on the findings of endomyocardial biopsy has been described (Table 31-1). Intrinsic relationships between the severity of histopathologic abnormality and the degree of left ventricular dysfunction are poor. Even though there is an approximate linear relationship between histopathologic changes and cumulative dose, there is such marked variation that specific relationships cannot be readily established in individual patients.[15] Further, sampling of biopsy

Table 31-1 Histopathologic Grading of Doxorubicin Cardiotoxicity

Grade 0	No abnormality
Grade 1	Minimal number of cells (<5% of total cells in each block) with early changes (early myofibrillar loss or distended sarcoplasmic reticulum)
Grade 1.5	Small groups of cells involved (5%-15% of total number), some of which have definite changes (marked myofibrillar loss or cytoplasmic vacuolization)
Grade 2	Groups of cells involved 16%-25% of total number, some of which have definite changes (marked myofibrillar loss or cytoplasmic vacuolization)
Grade 2.5	Groups of cells involved 26%-35% of total number, some of which have definite changes (marked myofibrillar loss or cytoplasmic vacuolization)
Grade 3	Diffuse cell damage (>35% of total number of cells) with marked changes (total loss of contractile elements, loss of organelles, mitochondrial and nuclear degeneration)

Adapted from Billingham ME, Mason JW, Bristow MR, Daniels JR: Anthracycline cardiomyopathy monitored by morphologic changes, Cancer Treat Rep 62:865–872, 1978.

material, because of the small sample size, may lead to inadequate identification of a more severe problem. On the other hand, the reverse can occur, and the degree of dysfunction can be overestimated based on a sampling error as a result of the nonuniform pathologic process.

INCIDENCE OF CARDIOTOXICITY

Although the severity and occurrence of clinical cardiotoxicity are dose dependent, there is considerable variability in individual susceptibility. As a result, some patients may experience substantial left ventricular dysfunction at relatively lower doses, whereas others may tolerate high cumulative doses with minimal if any effects. Usually, doses of more than 450 to 500 mg/m² result in increased occurrence of cardiotoxicity. Older studies reported an incidence of heart failure of approximately 2% at a cumulative dose of 300 mg/m² or less and 7% at a dose of 550 mg/m². The incidence rose to more than 20% at a cumulative dose of more than 700 mg/m².[16,17] No specific genetic or biochemical markers to predict susceptibility have been identified. However, retrospective analysis shows that certain clinical risk factors are associated with a predilection for doxorubicin cardiotoxicity, including antecedent cardiac disease, age, mediastinal radiation, concomitant cyclophosphamide therapy, concomitant paclitaxel therapy, and, more recently, concomitant therapy with monoclonal antibody against epidermal growth factor (HER2).[3]

CLINICAL COURSE

Left ventricular dysfunction may occur without identifiable cardiac symptoms before clinical congestive heart failure develops. Left ventricular dysfunction induced by doxorubicin is usually irreversible. However, in a significant number of patients, improvement (and even normalization) has occurred after discontinuation of doxorubicin therapy or institution of appropriate therapy for congestive heart failure.[18–20] If treatment with doxorubicin is continued after asymptomatic left ventricular dysfunction occurs, a progressive and rapid decline in ventricular performance leading to the clinical manifestation of congestive heart failure is likely.[20] It is unusual for patients who have completed a course of doxorubicin chemotherapy to have ventricular dysfunction and heart failure after discontinuation of therapy.[11] However, this phenomenon is seen in a relatively small proportion of patients.

MONITORING FOR CARDIOTOXICITY

Radionuclide angiocardiography, initially by first-pass techniques and more recently by equilibrium techniques, remains the standard for assessing potential cardiotoxicity (see Chapter 12).[19] Neither clinical examination nor electrocardiography or more standard clinical laboratory evaluation is efficacious in this regard. The use of radionuclide angiocardiography for measuring left ventricular ejection fraction as the functional index of cardiac performance was established in a variety of clinical settings. Although this measure is not a pure index of contractility and is influenced by preload and afterload, it has excellent accuracy and reproducibility.[21] It can be performed in virtually all patients and is not limited by acoustic window artifacts that can affect ultrasound studies. The technique is fully automated[22] and well standardized and provides the level of reproducible quantitative data necessary for reliable serial application.

In 1979, Alexander and colleagues[4] initially described 55 patients monitored with serial first-pass quantitative radionuclide angiocardiography at rest. They observed a significant relationship between the cumulative dose of doxorubicin and the development of ventricular dysfunction. Five patients in this series had heart failure; all five had an ejection fraction of less than 30% when symptoms occurred (Fig. 31-1). Based on this initial experience, guidelines were suggested.

Schwartz and colleagues, nearly a decade later, reported a larger experience with the monitoring of 1487 patients over a 7-year period.[19] Based on this experience, the initial guidelines were slightly amended. These guidelines remain in place today (Table 31-2). In patients with a normal baseline ejection fraction (>50%), moderate toxicity was defined to include an end point of a decline of more than 10% in absolute ejection fraction, with a final ejection fraction of less than 50%.

Somewhat modified guidelines have been applied to patients with abnormal baseline ventricular function.[23] Initially it was believed that administration of doxorubicin to such patients was contraindicated. In this setting, more frequent monitoring is useful (see Table 31-2). In our initial experience, no identifiable etiology was noted

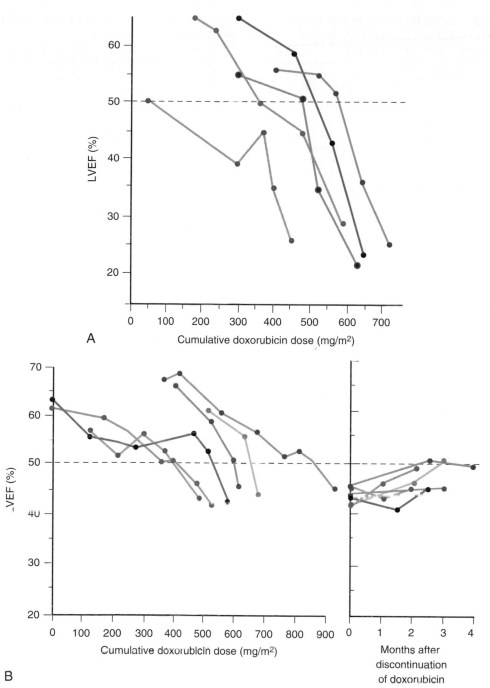

Figure 31-1 A, Sequential measurement of left ventricular ejection fraction (LVEF) in five patients in whom severe cardiotoxicity (congestive heart failure) developed. LVEF is plotted on the vertical axis, and cumulative doxorubicin dose is plotted on the horizontal axis. The *dashed line* represents the lower limit of normal for LVEF (50%). In each patient, congestive heart failure was associated with LVEF of less than 30%. Each patient with congestive heart failure initially had a period of moderate cardiotoxicity, defined by an absolute decrease in LVEF of 15% or more to a level of 45% or less. **B,** Sequential measures of LVEF in six patients in whom doxorubicin was discontinued after the finding of moderate cardiotoxicity. The relationship between LVEF and the cumulative doxorubicin dose up to the time of moderate cardiotoxicity is shown *(left)* as well as that between LVEF at the time of moderate toxicity and LVEF measured sequentially during a follow-up period of 1 to 4 months in the same patients *(right)*. The *dashed line* represents the lower limit of normal for LVEF (50%). LVEF increased modestly in all six patients after discontinuation of doxorubicin. In contrast to the five patients shown in **A**, in whom congestive heart failure developed with continuing dosage, no patient in this group had either congestive heart failure or a progressive decrease in left ventricular function. *(From Alexander J, Dainiak N, Berger HJ, et al: Serial assessment of doxorubicin cardiotoxicity with quantitative radionuclide angiocardiography, N Engl J Med 300:278–283, 1979.)*

in approximately a third of patients with abnormal baseline function.[19] This observation underscores the importance of obtaining baseline measurements in patients before instituting therapy.

In the experience of Schwartz and colleagues,[19] clinical congestive heart failure developed in 46 of 282 (16%) high-risk patients. The total cumulative dosage of doxorubicin that precipitated heart failure varied widely and

Table 31-2   Guidelines for Monitoring Doxorubicin Cardiotoxicity by Serial Radionuclide Angiography

Baseline evaluation: Baseline radionuclide angiocardiography at rest is done to estimate left ventricular ejection fraction (LVEF) before the start of doxorubicin therapy or before 100 mg/m² of doxorubicin has been given.

Subsequent evaluations: Subsequent studies are done 3 weeks after the indicated last dose of doxorubicin and before consideration of the next dose, at the following intervals:

I. Patients with normal baseline LVEF (≥50%)
  A. Obtain a second study after 250–300 mg/m².
  B. Obtain a repeat study after 400 mg/m² in patients with known heart disease, hypertension, radiation exposure, abnormal electrocardiographic findings, or cyclophosphamide therapy; or after 450 mg/m² in the absence of these risk factors.
  C. Obtain sequential studies thereafter before each dose.

Discontinue doxorubicin therapy once functional criteria for cardiotoxicity develop (i.e., absolute decrease in LVEF ≥ 10% to a level < 50% [LVEF units]).

II. Patients with abnormal baseline LVEF (<50%)
  A. With baseline LVEF < 30%, do not start doxorubicin therapy.
  B. With baseline LVEF > 30% and < 50%, perform a study before each dose.

Discontinue doxorubicin in patients with an absolute decrease in LVEF ≥ 10% (EF units) or final LVEF ≤ 30%.

Adapted from Schwartz RG, Zaret B: Diagnosis and treatment of drug-induced myocardial disease. In Muggia FC, Speyer JL (eds): Cardiotoxicity of Anticancer Therapy, Baltimore: Johns Hopkins University Press, 1992, pp 173–197.

ranged from 75 to 1095 mg/m². Clinical congestive heart failure was mild in 46% of patients, moderate in 41%, and severe in 11%. In only one patient could death be attributed to congestive heart failure. There was no worsening of heart failure during 1 year of follow-up. In that study, high-risk patients whose management was in accordance with the guidelines specified in Table 31-2 had a very low of incidence of mild clinical congestive heart failure (2 of 70 patients). In contrast, 20% of patients who were not managed according to guidelines based on serial monitoring had clinical signs of congestive heart failure (Fig. 31-2).

Schwartz and colleagues[19] also compared the experience in community versus university hospitals and found no difference in any of the outcomes. Initial results showed that measures of resting global ventricular function obtained serially clearly provided a means of monitoring patients receiving chemotherapy. Earlier it was suggested that sensitivity could be improved by adding exercise stress to the resting study. Although earlier findings were conflicting with respect to the value of exercise ventricular function and outcome,[24] for several reasons, we believe that data support serial studies in the resting state alone. First, resting studies show excellent sensitivity for detecting problems. Second, patients with malignancy may have excessive discomfort with exercise and may be at risk for pathologic fracture. Third, the reproducibility of exercise over time may be difficult due to systemic factors such as anemia, general debilitation, and changes in blood pressure. Fourth, exercise responses may be nonspecific, particularly in the elderly.

Based on clinical experience obtained in the 1980s and 1990s, the use of serial ventricular function monitoring for assessing patients receiving doxorubicin has

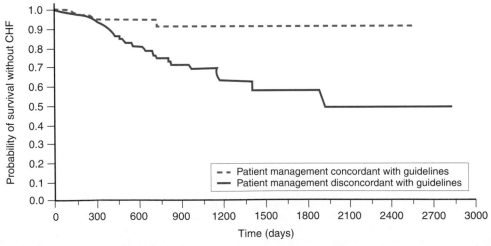

Figure 31-2   The Kaplan-Meier curve describes the probability of survival without clinical congestive heart failure (CHF) in patients whose management was either in accordance or not in accordance with the guidelines proposed in the current study. In patients managed according to the guidelines, the reduction in the incidence of clinical CHF was fourfold, independent of other predictor variables (P < 0.01), as assessed by proportional hazards regression analysis (Cox). Patients managed in accordance with the guidelines had no worse than mild CHF. In contrast, most of the patients who had clinical CHF and were not managed in accordance with the guidelines had worse than mild CHF. *(From Schwartz RG, McKenzie B, Alexander J, et al: Congestive heart failure and left ventricular dysfunction complicating doxorubicin therapy: Seven-year experience using serial radionuclide angiocardiography, Am J Med 82:1109–1118, 1987.)*

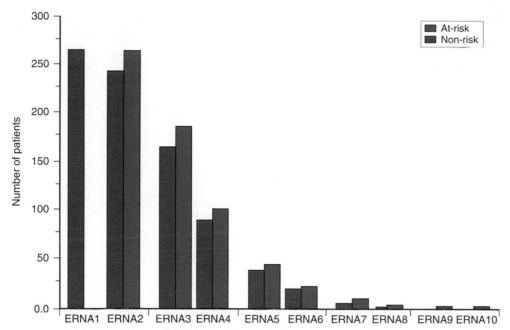

Figure 31-3 The number of patients who underwent each serial equilibrium radionuclide angiocardiogram (ERNA) study. Each patient had 2 to 10 ERNA studies (mean, 3.3 ± 1.3 studies per patient). After the third study, the number of patients decreased remarkably. *(From Mitani I, Jain D, Joska TM, et al: Doxorubicin cardiotoxicity: Prevention of congestive heart failure with serial cardiac function monitoring with equilibrium radionuclide angiocardiography in the current era, J Nucl Cardiol 10:132–139, 2003.)*

become clinically routine. However, it is unclear whether earlier guidelines carry the same importance as they did previously. To evaluate this question, Mitani and colleagues[25] reported a retrospective clinical study at our institution in which 265 patients with malignancy were followed with serial left ventricular ejection fraction measurements. Studies were obtained with serial equilibrium radionuclide angiocardiography on at least two occasions. Each patient underwent an average of 3.3 ± 1.3 studies (Fig. 31-3). Follow-up was complete in 93% of patients. In this retrospective analysis, patients with normal ventricular function at baseline and a 10% or greater absolute decrease in left ventricular ejection fraction, to a final value of 50% or less during doxorubicin therapy, were considered to be "at risk" for heart failure. Over an average follow-up of more than 2 years, seven patients (2.6%) had some form of congestive heart failure (Fig. 31-4). Within the same time frame, 90 patients (34%) died of cancer-related causes. There were no deaths due to heart failure. Comparison of the at-risk group with a low-risk group of patients who did not meet these criteria showed a higher incidence of heart failure, a lower baseline ejection fraction (with the lowest ejection fraction at its lower level), and a high rate of cancer-related deaths in the at-risk group. In 34 patients, doxorubicin was discontinued during the monitoring period. In 20 of these patients (59%), discontinuation was based on ejection fraction criteria for toxicity.

A cost analysis showed that the overall expenditure for serial equilibrium radionuclide angiocardiogram studies was less than the estimated 1-year cost of care for the additional estimated cases of congestive heart failure that theoretically would have developed without

monitoring but were prevented by routine monitoring of left ventricular ejection fraction.[25,26] It was concluded that serial monitoring of left ventricular ejection fraction by radionuclide techniques is both appropriate and cost-effective for predicting and preventing congestive heart failure in this patient cohort. This study showed only a weak inverse relationship between the lowest ejection fraction and the cumulative dose achieved (Fig. 31-5). In addition, congestive heart failure occurred at varying doses, some of which were relatively low, further emphasizing the need for careful monitoring in these patients, even early in the course of chemotherapy.

Other approaches exist for monitoring ventricular function noninvasively. These include echocardiography and magnetic resonance imaging. In neither instance is there either sufficiently large experience or sufficient precision to allow for the effectiveness of monitoring achieved with radionuclide angiocardiography. The invasive technique of serial endomyocardial biopsy, for the reasons described earlier, is neither practical nor feasible for long-term follow-up.

Other nuclear imaging approaches involving the myocardium include indium-111-antimyosin imaging, a marker of myocardial necrosis, and iodine-123-methyliodobenzylguanidine (MIBG), which measures adrenergic neuronal uptake.[27–32] Antimyosin antibody imaging uptake showed high sensitivity but low specificity. Its uptake lacks specificity and is observed in most patients receiving intermediate doses of doxorubicin, even in the absence of left ventricular dysfunction. This technique is no longer available for clinical use in the United States. Data have been obtained primarily in experimental animals.

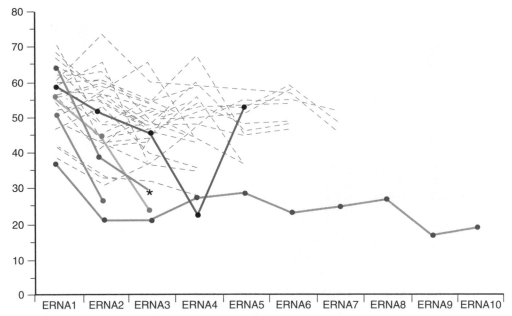

Figure 31-4   Serial changes in left ventricular ejection fraction in 41 patients at risk. *Dashed lines* represent 36 patients who were at risk but did not have congestive heart failure. *Solid lines* represent 5 patients who had overt congestive heart failure. *One patient died of cardiogenic shock in the setting of sepsis. (*From Mitani I, Jain D, Joska TM, et al: Doxorubicin cardiotoxicity: Prevention of congestive heart failure with serial cardiac function monitoring with equilibrium radionuclide angiocardiography in the current era, J Nucl Cardiol 10:132–139, 2003.*)

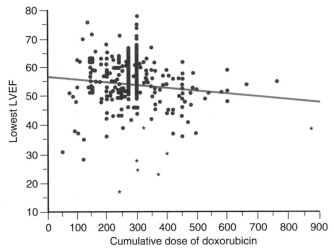

Figure 31-5   Cumulative dose of doxorubicin and lowest left ventricular ejection fraction monitored during follow-up. *Circles* represent patients who did not have CHF, and *asterisks* (*) represent those who had overt CHF. The progression of CHF did not always relate to the cumulative dose, and overt CHF developed in a few patients at a relatively low cumulative dose of doxorubicin. (*From Mitani I, Jain D, Joska TM, et al: Doxorubicin cardiotoxicity: Prevention of congestive heart failure with serial cardiac function monitoring with equilibrium radionuclide angiocardiography in the current era, J Nucl Cardiol 10:132–139, 2003.*)

In conclusion, serial monitoring of radionuclide measures of global left ventricular function continues to provide clinically relevant, time-tested data for monitoring patients for doxorubicin cardiotoxicity. This approach remains a standard clinical procedure in our institution and constitutes the largest current indication for the performance of radionuclide angiocardiography. In patients who achieve long-term success with doxorubicin treatment of malignancy, it will be important to show that late-developing left ventricular dysfunction does not become a clinical problem. Similarly, few data are available on the short- and long-term results in children with malignancy monitored with the same approach.[33] Nevertheless, serial monitoring of left ventricular ejection fraction as a well-standardized measure of global left ventricular function with radionuclide techniques remains a valuable clinical procedure.

TRASTUZUMAB (HERCEPTIN) CARDIOTOXICITY

Trastuzumab was approved by the U.S. Food and Drug Administration (FDA) for clinical use in 1998 and is indicated for the treatment of metastatic breast carcinoma in women with tumors that overexpress the HER2 (human epidermal growth factor receptor 2) protein.[34] Trastuzumab is a humanized monoclonal antibody against HER2. The drug binds to the extracellular juxtamembrane domain of HER2 and inhibits proliferation and survival of HER2-dependent tumors.[35] This overexpression of HER2 occurs in 20% to 25% of breast tumors. For the drug to be chemotherapeutically useful, either HER2 overexpression must be demonstrated by immunohistochemistry, or amplification of the gene must be detected by fluorescence in situ hybridization (FISH). The development of this chemotherapeutic agent represents a prime example of translational research in which molecular mechanisms are first defined and then used as the basis for developing new therapeutic approaches.[35]

Table 31-3 Comparison of Chemotherapy Cardiotoxicity

	Doxorubicin	Trastuzumab
Clinical profile	Myocardial damage permanent Histologic changes No histologic changes	Likely reversible if drug stopped (2–4 months)
Dose relationship	Dose related, cumulative	Not dose related
Likely mechanism	Oxidative stress	Blocked ErbB2 signaling
Rechallenge	Likely progressive cardiac dysfunction	Increasing data showing rechallenge may be safe
Monitoring of ventricular function	Well-established means of following patient's experience	Provides valuable data but less clinical than with doxorubicin

Adapted from Ewer MS, Lippman SM: Type II chemotherapy-related cardiac dysfunction: Time to recognize a new entity, J Clin Oncol 23:2900–2902, 2005.

The *HER2* gene plays an important role in embryonic and postnatal heart function. It is also involved in blunting the effects of stress signaling pathways as well as apoptosis. Several large clinical trials have demonstrated the efficacy of trastuzumab treatment in patients with HER2-positive breast cancer. However, in the course of these studies, the side effects of decreased cardiac function and clinical congestive heart failure have been recognized.[36–42] Although there has not been complete standardization of specific protocols for the monitoring for cardiotoxicity, equilibrium radionuclide angiocardiography (ERNA) has played a major role in evaluating and following such patients. The cardiotoxicity of trastuzumab stands in direct contrast to that of doxorubicin (Table 31-3). Whereas cardiotoxicity with doxorubicin may stabilize and can be detected relatively early in its course, underlying damage appears to be permanent. Trastuzumab cardiotoxicity has a reasonably high likelihood of reversal within 2 to 4 months if medication is discontinued. Doxorubicin effects are generally cumulative and dose related, whereas those of trastuzumab are not. The overall mechanism of doxorubicin toxicity is likely free radical formation and oxidative stress, whereas with trastuzumab the mechanism involves blocked ErbB2 signaling. Permanent changes are detected with electromicrosopy and routine histology in doxorubicin toxicity but are not seen with trastuzumab. Rechallenge with doxorubicin is associated with a high likelihood of recurrent ventricular dysfunction that may result in progressively severe heart failure and death. In contrast, increasing data demonstrate that rechallenge is possible with trastuzumab, without further decline in ventricular function.

Although there is some variation in the literature, the risk for cardiotoxicity is about 4% with trastuzumab when administered as monotherapy, and 25% to 30% when given in association or following treatment with anthracyclines and cyclophosphamide. The findings of asymptomatic falls in left ventricular ejection fraction are far more common than the presence of clinical congestive heart failure. When heart failure occurs, it is often readily treated with standard congestive heart failure regimens. Several risk factors have been related to trastuzumab treatment. These include concomitant or prior treatment with anthracyclines and cyclophosphamide, age older than 60 years, anthracycline doses that exceed 400 mg/n², prior

chest wall irradiation, and preexisting cardiac dysfunction. Left ventricular ejection fraction should be monitored at baseline and then at regular intervals every 2 to 3 months during treatment. If patients develop new signs or symptoms such as persistent sinus tachycardia or symptoms of congestive heart failure, then ejection fraction should be measured immediately. Generally, trastuzumab should be discontinued at least temporarily if left ventricular ejection fraction falls by more than 10% to a level of less than 50%. If function returns to normal and the drug has been effective in treating the malignancy, it likely can be restarted with careful monitoring. It should be noted that severe congestive heart failure has been relatively uncommon, occurring in fewer than 1% of patients. As more clinical experience is obtained with trastuzumab, it is anticipated that more specific guidelines concerning monitoring of ventricular function will become available.

REFERENCES

1. Blum RH, Carter SK: Adriamycin: A new anticancer drug with significant clinical activity, *Ann Intern Med* 80:249–259, 1974.
2. Young RC, Ozols RF, Myers CE: The anthracycline antineoplastic drugs, *N Engl J Med* 305:139–153, 1981.
3. Jain D: Cardiotoxicity of doxorubicin and other anthracycline derivatives, *J Nucl Cardiol* 7:53–62, 2000.
4. Alexander J, Dainiak N, Berger HJ, et al: Serial assessment of doxorubicin cardiotoxicity with quantitative radionuclide angiocardiography, *N Engl J Med* 300:278–283, 1979.
5. Singhal PK, Iliskovic N, Li T, et al: Adriamycin cardiomyopathy: Pathophysiology and prevention, *FASEB J* 11:931–936, 1997.
6. Gianni L, Myers CE: The role of free radical formation in the cardiotoxicity of anthracycline. In Muggia FM, Green MD, Speyer JL, editors: *Cancer Treatment and the Heart,* Baltimore, 1992, Johns Hopkins University Press, pp 9–46.
7. Hershko C, Pinson A, Link G: Prevention of anthracycline cardiotoxicity by iron chelation, *Acta Hematol* 95:87–92, 1996.
8. Halili-Rutman I, Hershko C, Link G, et al: Inhibition of calcium accumulation by the sarcoplasmic reticulum: A putative mechanism for the cardiotoxicity of Adriamycin, *Biochem Pharmacol* 54:211–214, 1997.
9. Harada H, Cusack FJ, Olson RD, et al: Taurine deficiency and doxorubicin: Interaction with the cardiac sarcolemmal calcium pump, *Biochem Pharmacol* 39:745–751, 1990.
10. Ito H, Miller SC, Billingham ME, et al: Doxorubicin selectively inhibits muscle gene expression in cardiac muscle cells in vivo and in vitro, *Proc Natl Acad Sci U S A* 87:4275–4279, 1990.
11. Jeyaseelan R, Poizat C, Wu HY, et al: Molecular mechanisms of doxorubicin-induced cardiomyopathy: Selective suppression of Reiske iron-sulfur protein, ADP/ATP translocase, and phosphofructokinase genes is associated with ATP depletion in rat cardiomyocytes, *J Biol Chem* 272:5828–5832, 1997.
12. Zhang J, Clark JR, Herman EH, et al: Doxorubicin-induced apoptosis in spontaneously hypertensive rats: Differential effects in heart, kidney

and intestine and inhibition by ICRF-187, *J Mol Cell Cardiol* 28: 1931–1943, 1996.

13. Billingham ME, Mason JW, Bristow MR, et al: Anthracycline cardiomy-opathy monitored by morphologic changes, *Cancer Treat Rep* 62: 865–872, 1978.

14. Bristow MR, Mason JW, Billingham ME, et al: Dose-effect and struc-ture-function relationship in doxorubicin cardiomyopathy, *Am Heart J* 102:709–718, 1981.

15. Isner JM, Ferrans VJ, Cohen SR, et al: Clinical and morphologic cardiac findings after anthracycline chemotherapy: Analysis of 64 patients studied at necropsy, *Am J Cardiol* 51:1167–1174, 1983.

16. Young RC, Ozols RF, Myers CE: The anthracycline antineoplastic drugs, *N Engl J Med* 305:139–153, 1981.

17. Lefrak EA, Pitha J, Rosenheim S, et al: A clinicopathologic analysis of Adriamycin cardiotoxicity, *Cancer* 32:302–314, 1973.

18. Saini J, Rich MW, Lyss AP: Reversibility of severe left dysfunction due to doxorubicin cardiotoxicity: Report of three cases, *Ann Intern Med* 106:814–816, 1987.

19. Schwartz RG, McKenzie B, Alexander J, et al: Congestive heart failure and left ventricular dysfunction complicating doxorubicin therapy: Seven-year experience using serial radionuclide angiocardiography, *Am J Med* 82:1109–1118, 1987.

20. Schwartz RG, Zaret BL: Diagnosis and treatment of drug induced myo-cardial disease. In Muggia FC, Speyer JL, editors: *Cardiotoxicity of Anti-cancer Therapy*, Baltimore, 1992, Johns Hopkins University Press, pp 173–197.

21. van Royen N, Jaffe CC, Krumholz HM, et al: Comparison and reproducibility of visual echocardiographic and quantitative radio-nuclide left ventricular ejection fractions, *Am J Cardiol* 77:843–850, 1996.

22. Lee FA, Fetterman R, Zaret BL, et al: Rapid radionuclide derived sys-tolic and diastolic cardiac function using cycle-dependent back-ground correction and Fourier analysis. In *Proceedings of Computers in Cardiology*, Linkoping, Sweden, 1985, IEEE Computer Society, pp 443–446.

23. Choi BW, Berger HJ, Schwartz PE, et al: Serial radionuclide assessment of doxorubicin cardiotoxicity in cancer patients with abnormal base-line resting left ventricular performance, *Am Heart J* 106:638–643, 1983.

24. Palmeri ST, Bonow RO, Myers CE, et al: Prospective evaluation of doxorubicin cardiotoxicity by rest and exercise radionuclide angiogra-phy, *Am J Cardiol* 58:607–613, 1986.

25. Mitani I, Jain D, Joska TM, et al: Doxorubicin cardiotoxicity: Preven-tion of congestive heart failure with serial cardiac function monitoring with equilibrium radionuclide angiocardiography in the current era, *J Nucl Cardiol* 10:132–139, 2003.

26. Schulman KA, Mark DB, Califf RM: Outcomes and costs within a dis-ease management program for advanced congestive heart failure, *Am Heart J* 135:S282–S292, 1998.

27. Estorch M, Carrio I, Berna L, et al: ^{111}In-Antimyosin scintigraphy after doxorubicin therapy in patients with advanced breast cancer, *J Nucl Med* 31:1965–1969, 1990.

28. Carrio I, Lopez-Pousa A, Estorch M, et al: Detection of doxorubicin car-diotoxicity in patients with sarcomas by indium-111-antimyosin monoclonal antibody studies, *J Nucl Med* 34:1503–1507, 1993.

29. Jain D, Zaret BL: Antimyosin cardiac imaging: Will it play a role in the detection of doxorubicin cardiotoxicity? [editorial], *J Nucl Med* 31: 1970–1974, 1990.

30. Carrio I, Estorch M, Berna L, et al: Indium-111-antimyosin and iodine-123-MIBG studies in early assessment of doxorubicin cardiotoxicity, *J Nucl Med* 36:2044–2049, 1995.

31. Lekakis J, Prassopoulos V, Athanassiadis P, et al: Doxorubicin-induced cardiac neurotoxicity: Study with iodine 123-labeled metaiodobenzyl-guanidine scintigraphy, *J Nucl Cardiol* 3:37–41, 1996.

32. Takano H, Ozawa H, Kobayashi I, et al: Myocardial sympathetic dysin-nervation in doxorubicin cardiomyopathy, *J Nucl Cardiol* 27:49–55, 1996.

33. Goorin AM, Chauvenet AR, Perez-Atayda AR, et al: Initial congestive heart failure, six to ten years after doxorubicin chemotherapy for childhood cancer, *J Pediatr* 116:144–147, 1990.

34. Hudis CA: Trastuzumab: Mechanism of action and use in clinical prac-tice, *N Engl J Med* 357:39–51, 2007.

35. Chien KR: Herceptin and the heart: A molecular modifier of cardiac failure, *N Eng J Med* 354:789–790, 2006.

36. Keefe DL: Trastuzumab-associated cardiotoxicity, *Cancer* 95: 1592–1600, 2002.

37. Perez EA, Rodeheffer R: Clinical cardiac tolerability of trastuzumab, *J Clin Oncol* 22:322–329, 2004.

38. Ewer MS, Lippman SM: Type II chemotherapy-related cardiac dysfunc-tion: Time to recognize a new entity? *J Clin Oncol* 2900–2902, 2005.

39. Ewer MS, Vooletich MT, Durand J-B, et al: Reversibility of trastuzumab-related cardiotoxicity: New insights based on clinical course and response to medical treatment, *J Clin Oncol* 23:7820–7826, 2005.

40. Guarnei V, Lenihan DJ, Valero V, et al: Long-term cardiac tolerability of trastuzumab in metastatic breast cancer: The M.D. Anderson Cancer Center Experience, *J Clin Oncol* 24:4107–4115, 2006.

41. Telli ML, Hunt SA, Carlson RW, et al: Trastuzumab-related cardiotoxi-city: Calling into question the concept of reversibility, *J Clin Oncol* 25:3525–3533, 2007.

42. Suter TM, Procter M, van Veldhuisen DJ, et al: Trastuzumab-associated cardiac adverse effects in the Herceptin adjuvant trial, *J Clin Oncol* 25:3859–3865, 2007.

Mechanistic and Methodological Considerations for the Imaging of Mental Stress Ischemia

ROBERT SOUFER, MATTHEW M. BURG
AND ANTONIO B. FERNANDEZ

INTRODUCTION

The role of emotion or stress in the provocation of angina pectoris has been described as far back in ancient history as Celsus, followed by Hunter in the 1700s, and by Osler at the turn of the 20th century.[1] We have an intuitive sense of the importance of these factors, yet gathering empirical data to support or refute this intuition have been slow to unfold. The effort to do so has been hindered by the impact of the philosophical proposition of the duality of the mind and body entrenched in Western culture since Descartes, and by the compartmentalized structure of biomedical research.[2] Modern epistemological/ontological constructs and emerging studies in neuroscience have questioned this duality. The latter enjoined with the expansion of integrative biomedical research will shed further light on the interaction of emotional processing/triggers and biological consequences in the next decade.

In the few short years since the previous edition of this volume, new information regarding the nature of mental stress–provoked ischemia, with refinement of key aspects of the pathophysiologic construct, has emerged. In this edition, we discuss new advances in diagnostic tools available to improve the accuracy of mental stress ischemia (MSI) diagnosis, such as peripheral arterial tonometry (PAT). We review MSI as a vulnerability factor for lethal arrhythmias and arrhythmia-induced implantable cardioverter defibrillator (ICD) shocks. We also describe the phenomenon of myocardial stunning due to sudden emotional stress (variably known as *takotsubo cardiomyopathy* or "broken heart syndrome") as part of the continuum described by stress-provoked cardiac phenomena. In the previous edition, we outlined the importance of parasympathetic withdrawal and endothelial dysfunction in response to stress or emotionally provoked ischemia. We will discuss the possible links between these two consistent observations of MSI (parasympathetic withdrawal and endothelial dysfunction), based upon studies describing a new pathway that may mediate the vascular effects of MSI, termed the *cholinergic antiinflammatory reflex*.[3]

MENTAL STRESS ISCHEMIA

Myocardial ischemia that occurs in response to mental and emotional stress—MSI—is a phenomenon of clinical importance associated with a threefold increased risk of poor outcome in patients with coronary artery disease (CAD).[4–9] The pathophysiology of MSI demonstrates a degree of overlap with that of demand-induced ischemia; however, MSI has distinct physiologic correlates, as suggested by differences in hemodynamic, vascular, and neuroendocrine responses to these distinct forms of stress.[10,11] In addition, certain psychological factors related to the experience and expression of anger and hostility identify patients who are more vulnerable to MSI.[12–15] The history of nuclear cardiology is replete with examples of our creativity in addressing difficult diagnostic challenges in order to demonstrate the manifestation of occult myocardial ischemia. Myocardial ischemia provoked by mental and emotional stress is pervasive and an important presentation within the spectrum of CAD. The overarching goal of this chapter is to provide a working conceptual construct grounded in empirical data on which to base future noninvasive testing for the identification of those at risk for MSI.

Evidence Base for MSI—An Historical Perspective

There are several lines of evidence demonstrating that mental and emotional stress—whether experienced in the context of normal daily routine or occasioned in the laboratory setting under controlled conditions—can provoke myocardial ischemia. This evidence includes the traditional signatures of ischemia as measured by electrocardiographic, functional cardiovascular, and perfusion indices.

ECG Changes During Mental Stress

The ability to detect myocardial ischemia under real-life situations was made possible by the development of the

Holter monitor in the 1960s, which records the ECG in real time on a medium that provides for later examination of a depression in the ST-segment—the marker of ischemia. By the latter part of that decade, cardiologists were using this technology to monitor coronary patients while they drove their car, while they engaged in routine daily activities, and while they performed stressful tasks in the laboratory. Studies using this approach demonstrated that among patients with CAD, ischemia is common during moderate to extreme mental and emotional activity independent of the degree of concurrent physical exertion,[15–18] is most usually without symptoms of angina, and accounts for up to 75% of total ischemic burden (Fig. 32-1).[14,16,19] Most ischemic episodes during mental stress were found to occur at lower heart rate and blood pressure than episodes during physical exertion, supporting the concept of dynamic coronary obstruction (i.e., ischemia caused by changes in arterial tone) as a pathophysiologic mechanism. This does not imply, however, that myocardial demand is not a contributor to MSI as well, since increases in diastolic blood pressure in particular are often seen.[20]

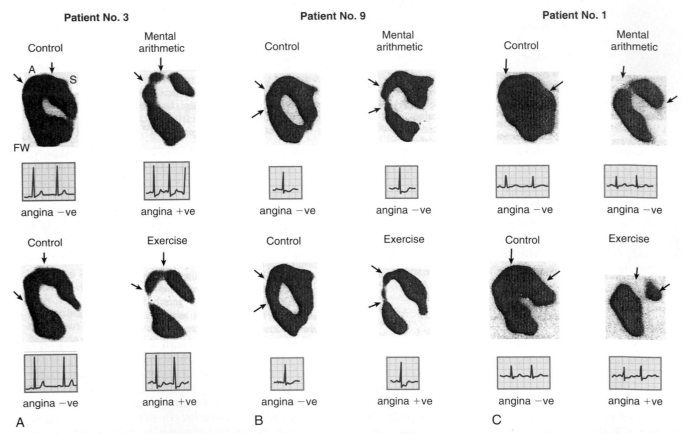

Figure 32-1 Changes in regional myocardial uptake of rubidium-82 and in electrocardiographic findings in relation to chest pain before and after mental arithmetic or exercise stress. Control scans show homogeneous regional cation uptake. **A**, Defects in uptake by the anterior wall are seen with mental arithmetic and exercise stress. These changes are accompanied by ST-segment depression and angina. **B**, Anterior and free wall ischemia and ST-T-segment depression are seen with mental arithmetic and exercise stress, but angina only is seen after exercise. **C**, Transient regional anterior and septal ischemia are seen with mental arithmetic and exercise stress, but ST-segment depression and chest pain are seen after exercise only. In each case, the mental stress–induced perfusion deficit occurs in the same region as the exercise-induced deficit. However, mental stress–induced deficits vary in extent and severity compared with exercise-induced deficits. A, anterior wall; FW, left ventricular free wall; S, interventricular septum. *(Reprinted from Deanfield JE, Shea M, Kensett M, et al: Silent myocardial ischaemia due to mental stress, Lancet 2:1001–1005, 1984, with permission from Elsevier.)*

Left Ventricular Dysfunction During Mental Stress

Assessment of left ventricular ejection fraction (LVEF) provides a sensitive (but potentially less specific) method to evaluate the acute cardiovascular effects of various interventions under controlled conditions. The development of radionuclide- and ultrasound-based methods to assess LVEF provided the opportunity to more directly examine the effects of stress on myocardial function as an index of ischemia, and marked the next step in the emergence of this research. The approaches used for this purpose have included equilibrium radionuclide angiography (ERNA), echocardiography, and volumetric measurement with a nonimaging nuclear probe. ERNA has been used in conjunction with mental stress for determination of LVEF and wall-motion abnormalities (WMAS). This approach is similar to that used for exercise ERNA studies, which are no longer routinely performed. In addition to this more standard approach, left ventricular (LV) function during mental stress has been assessed with a nonimaging nuclear probe after injection of radiolabeled red blood cells. This method has the advantage of providing beat-to-beat global LV volume curves, allowing assessment of rapid changes in LV function over an extended period (Fig. 32-2). The disadvantages are that regional wall motion cannot be assessed, and the technology is not widely available. The criteria used to define MSI by these techniques are similar to those used for other forms of stress: a reduction in LVEF of 5% or more and/or the development of a new regional WMA.

Overall, studies conducted in laboratory settings using such methods clearly established that mental stress induced by having the patient perform any one of several mentally/emotionally demanding tasks—induced transient global and/or regional LV dysfunction in upwards of 50% of patients with CAD. Among patients who demonstrated this dysfunction, it occurred rapidly after the initiation of the stressful task, usually within 1 minute, and recovery was temporally related to the discontinuation of the task and likewise tended to occur rapidly.[21] Consistent with the ambulatory ECG data, these abnormalities developed at a lower heart rate than with exercise, were usually asymptomatic, and occurred predominantly, although not exclusively, in patients with exercise tests that were positive for ischemia.[12]

Studies Using Radionuclide Angiography

Rozanski and colleagues[12] were among the first to describe mental stress–induced LV dysfunction by ERNA in a study of CAD patients and normal controls during mental stress and exercise. Largely asymptomatic WMAs were observed during mental stress in 59% of the CAD patients, and 36% had a decrease in ejection fraction of more than 5%. This occurred at a lower heart rate than ischemia induced during exercise, and ECG changes indicative of ischemia were rarely seen. These researchers using the same criteria subsequently found MSI in up to 75% of CAD patients with exercise-induced ischemia. In other studies using only changes in global

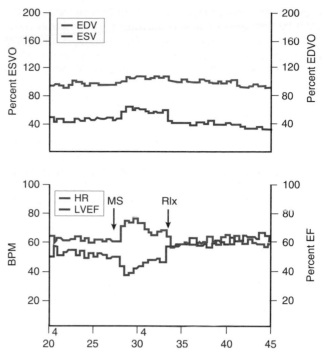

Figure 32-2 Trended data over 25-minute periods for left ventricular ejection fraction (LVEF), heart rate (HR) *(bottom)*, and relative end-diastolic and end-systolic volumes (EDVO and ESVO) *(top)* during mental arithmetic stress (MS) in one patient. With MS, there is a 10% decrease in LVEF, which promptly recovers to baseline with the withdrawal of stimulus and onset of relaxation (Rlx). The decrease in LVEF is accompanied by a small increase in HR (14 beats/min [BPM]), a minimal increase in end-diastolic volume (EDV), and a significant increase in end-systolic volume (ESV). No chest pain or ST-segment depression occurred during the decrease in LVEF. *(From Jain D, Burg M, Soufer R, Zaret BL: Prognostic implications of mental stress–induced silent left ventricular dysfunction in patients with stable angina pectoris, Am J Cardiol 76:31–35, 1995.)*

LV function as evidence of MSI (decrease in LVEF), 50% to 60% of CAD patients demonstrated global LV dysfunction during mental stress.[22,23] These changes were usually *without* ECG changes and—again—asymptomatic.

Studies Using Echocardiography

Data from studies using echocardiography to assess changes in LV function during mental stress have been largely consistent with data from radionuclide-based studies. For example, Modena and colleagues[24] reported mental stress–induced LV dysfunction in 38% of patients with chest pain who were referred for angiography. Gottdiener and colleagues[25] similarly reported over 50% of patients with known CAD had new regional WMA during mental stress echocardiography. Patients with MSI defined in this manner also showed more frequent ischemia by ambulatory ECG monitoring during sedentary activities.

Despite evidence of LV dysfunction induced during mental stress, a number of unresolved issues remained. For example, the specificity of the LV response as an index of ischemia during mental versus physical stress was unclear. Mental stress causes a substantial sympathetic response that leads to an increase in systemic vascular resistance,[11] which may affect LV function independent of ischemia. Indeed the Psychophysiological Investigations of Myocardial Ischemia (PIMI) study[10] found that 41% of older *normal* subjects (43 to 73 years old) exhibited a decrement in LVEF of 5% during mental stress. The reproducibility of LV functional changes during mental stress was and remains a second unresolved issue. The PIMI study data suggest that approximately two-thirds of patients have consistent responses when studied on different days, with the observed reproducibility a function of the type of stressor utilized.[26] Others have corroborated these findings.[27] A third issue concerned the association between LV functional changes and other potentially more specific indicators of ischemia, such as myocardial perfusion defects. These issues have implications for the development of standardized approaches for risk stratification in the clinical setting.

Myocardial Perfusion During Mental Stress

Radionuclide perfusion imaging is another modality used to study the effects of mental stress in patients with CAD. The rapid emergence of this modality and associated technologies has provided greater insight into the pathophysiology of MSI. Since the last edition, perfusion imaging has emerged as the gold standard for the detection of MSI and is preferred over echocardiography with regard to accuracy.

In an early clinical application of positron emission tomography (PET), Deanfield and colleagues[14] found that 75% of patients with positive exercise tests had regional perfusion abnormalities during mental stress. Although the rate-pressure product was lower with mental stress than with exercise, the degree and location of perfusion defect were largely similar between the two forms of stress. A subsequent study by others using planar technetium-99m ^{99m}Tc sestamibi perfusion imaging found that 85% of CAD patients had myocardial perfusion abnormalities in the same vascular territory during both mental and physical stress, though the extent and degree of abnormalities were smaller during mental stress.[28] These studies, using qualitative methods for assessment of myocardial perfusion, demonstrated that regional heterogeneity of blood flow develops in many patients during mental stress.

Quantitative assessment of myocardial blood flow by PET provides particular insights regarding the differential pathophysiology of MSI. This approach allows investigation of effects that may be more subtle than can be observed by more conventional approaches to assessment of LV function or myocardial perfusion. Several groups of investigators have used this approach to assess the effect of mental stress on absolute myocardial blood. For example, studying CAD patients and normal subjects, Schoder and colleagues found that despite similar increases in rate-pressure product in both cohorts, the magnitude of flow increase during mental stress was less in the patients.[29] Subsequently, our group investigated regional differences in blood flow response to mental versus pharmacologic stress in CAD patients

and found that with mental stress, a blunted flow response was observed, primarily in regions without significant epicardial coronary stenosis.[30] These findings suggest that mental stress may more predominantly affect coronary microvascular tone, implicating this as an operative factor in the pathogenesis of myocardial ischemia at relatively low levels of work.

Flow heterogeneity during mental stress may be mild, variable, and perhaps insufficient to generate regional wall motion. Single-photon emission computed tomography (SPECT) myocardial perfusion imaging (MPI), less costly than approaches that rely upon PET, may therefore represent a best and most cost-effective approach to the diagnosis of MSI. Indeed, there is a growing body of research using this modality to study the effects of mental stress. It remains to be determined, however, whether this approach will result in greater sensitivity/specificity in the detection of MSI or incremental prognostic value for patients with CAD. In addition, the relationship of perfusion defects to LV dysfunction during mental stress is unclear. For example, our group has simultaneously assessed perfusion (using SPECT sestamibi) and function (using echocardiography), and has found a significant discordance between perfusion and functional changes during mental stress.[31] Further study is needed to assess the significance of these findings. Nonetheless, MPI defects are a reliable indicator of ischemia (Fig. 32-3).

Comparison Between Mental Stress Imaging and Standard Exercise and Pharmacologic MPI

Although both mental stress and exercise induce hemodynamic changes, differences exist in the magnitude of change between these stressors. For example, the increase in heart rate during mental stress is much less than that during exercise.[11,12] Systolic blood pressure response can be less than or similar to that during exercise, whereas diastolic blood pressure increases more during mental stress.[11,12] Additionally, the rate of increase in the rate-pressure product is accelerated with mental stress and can peak within 1 minute of the onset of stress.[21] These differences in hemodynamic responses likely relate to differential neurohormonal activation and peripheral vascular effects. For example, during mentally stressful tasks, epinephrine levels increase more than norepinephrine levels. The opposite is observed during exercise.[32] Peripheral vascular resistance decreases during exercise but increases or remains constant during mental stress.[11,33] The observation that MSI occurs at relatively low rate-pressure product suggests that other mechanisms such as coronary vasoconstriction and the neurohormonal effects on endothelium-dependent vasomotor tone may be operative. The importance of these findings to any differential pathophysiology between mental stress and exercise-induced ischemia, however, remains to be determined.

Recent studies suggest that vulnerability to either exercise or mental stress–provoked ischemia in the same individual does not reliably predict ischemia to both stimuli. For example, Ramachandruni et al.[34] found that 6

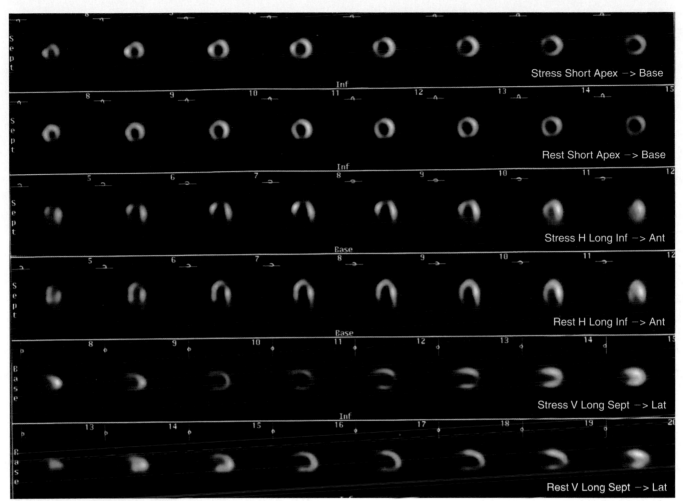

Figure 32-3 Mental stress technetium-99m-tetrofosmin single-photon emission tomography (low-dose rest, high-dose stress) images from a patient who had an apical perfusion defect consistent with mental stress–induced ischemia *(top)* compared with rest images *(bottom)*. Ant, anterior; Inf, inferior; Lat, lateral; Sept, septum.

of 21 CAD patients (29%) who had previously shown no flow defect during exercise or pharmacologic provocation had a reversible flow defect with mental stress. Conversely, as described earlier, only 40% to 60% of CAD patients with exercise-induced or pharmacologically induced ischemia have MSI. More recently, Hassan et al.[35] demonstrated significant intraindividual variability in the *severity and location* of myocardial ischemia provoked by mental versus exercise or pharmacologic stress. This study of 187 patients with CAD found only 71% concordance for the provocation of ischemia between mental versus exercise/pharmacologic stress. In addition, 11% of the cohort demonstrated ischemia to mental but not exercise/pharmacologic stress, while 22% demonstrated ischemia to exercise/pharmacologic but not mental stress. Furthermore, the location of flow defect(s) provoked by mental versus exercise/pharmacologic stress was often different, as was the severity of the flow defect(s) observed. A prior study by Arrighi et al.[30] using regional PET MPI may shed some light on the pathophysiology underlying the Hassan group's results.

In their study, Arrighi and colleagues found that pharmacologic stress caused an expected absolute reduction of myocardial blood flow in regions with significant epicardial disease (compared to regions without significant epicardial disease), and that this decreased flow was associated with a compensatory reduction in distal coronary microvascular resistance. Conversely, during mental stress, absolute myocardial blood flow was lower in regions *without* significant epicardial disease than in regions with significant epicardial disease, and *was associated with an increase in distal coronary microvascular resistance*. The study by Arrighi et al. therefore provides insights into the Hassan et al. findings by suggesting a prominent role for coronary microvascular dysfunction in mental versus exercise/pharmacologic stress–provoked ischemia. Overall, these studies describe contrasts in the coronary vascular response to mental stress and traditional clinical provocations to myocardial ischemia. Differences in CNS activity for these discordant groups are emerging and will be discussed under the heading "Functional PET Brain Imaging."

Prognostic Significance of Myocardial Stress Ischemia

The prognostic significance of MSI has been explored by a number of investigators. In the first published report,[33] there were a significantly greater ($P < 0.025$) number of events (MI, unstable angina) at 2 years in a group of patients who had previously demonstrated LV dysfunction—assessed by radionuclide methods—during mental stress than in the group who did not show this response. In a later study,[36] patients with LV dysfunction—by ERNA—during mental stress were at increased 2-year risk of events (MI, unstable angina, revascularization; risk ratio = 2.40), even after adjusting for age, history of MI, and baseline EF. Similarly, in patients followed over a 4.4-year follow-up period (median = 3.5 years),[37] almost 45% of patients with MSI in the lab—defined by WMA on ECHO or ERNA—experienced an event (death, MI, unstable angina), while less than 25% of patients without MSI experienced an event. Most recently, the PIMI investigators have reported on the prognostic significance of MSI in their multicenter study,[38] with 17 patients dying during an average follow-up of 5.2 years (Fig. 32-4). MSI—defined by WMA on ERNA—had been demonstrated among 40% of those who died but only 17% of those who survived (rate ratio = 3.0; $P < 0.04$). Other indicators of ischemia during MS testing, including LVEF and/or ECG changes, did not predict death.

These studies have consistently shown an increase in major adverse cardiac events among stable CAD patients with mental stress–induced LV dysfunction compared to those who do not show this type of LV dysfunction, although few of the studies were sufficiently powered to include prognostically significant covariates. Furthermore, the existing studies used LV dysfunction as an index of MSI. The prognostic significance of MSI

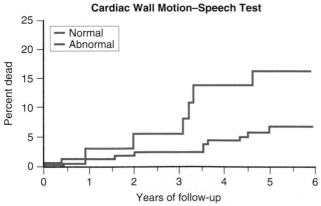

Figure 32-4 Total mortality rate in patients with mental stress–induced ischemia versus those without ischemia. The *red line* represents patients who had wall-motion abnormalities during mental stress; the *blue line* represents patients with normal left ventricular function and no wall-motion abnormalities. *(From Sheps DS, McMahon RP, Becker L, et al: Mental stress–induced ischemia and all-cause mortality in patients with coronary artery disease: Results from the Psychophysiological Investigations of Myocardial Ischemia Study, Circulation 105:1780–1784, 2002.)*

diagnosed by new perfusion abnormalities (a more powerful tool) and the differential prognosis for those patients who show ischemia to both physical and mental stress versus those with ischemia to mental stress alone remains to be determined.

Psychological Factors and Prognosis in Mental Stress Ischemia

The contribution of psychological makeup to prognosis in patients with CAD deserves special mention inasmuch as factors including depression, anxiety, anger, and hostility have broadly been reported. Determination of the specific psychological factors that contribute to risk for MSI may help to determine when mental stress testing is likely to provide important prognostic information. Studies have found, for example, that patients with easily provoked anger and hostility have twice the incidence of CAD and a fivefold increased risk of recurrent MI over an extended follow-up period.[37] High levels of hostility have also been associated with a higher incidence of restenosis after angioplasty[38] and rapid progression of CAD.[39] Similarly, chronic anger is associated with a 2.7 relative risk of cardiovascular death, myocardial infarction, and angina,[40] whereas the experience of moderate to extreme anger increases risk of MI 2.5-fold for up to 2 hours.[41]

Data from our group and others specifically related mental stress–induced LV dysfunction to psychological makeup. In comparing patients with MSI to those without MSI, we found no difference on standard clinical indicators, on measures of cardiovascular performance during mental stress testing and exercise thallium testing, or on measures of CAD severity. Patients with MSI, however, scored higher on measures of emotional arousability, hostility, anger, and aggressive response to perceived provocation, and lower on a measure of anger control. In addition, the duration of ischemia evidenced during a clinical interview used as a measure of emotional arousability was highly correlated with the degree of emotional arousability measured by the interview (0.70, $P < 0.0001$). Hence, a hostile, angry psychological profile was associated with emotional arousability, which increased the risk of MSI.[42]

These data suggest the potential importance of psychological makeup in assessing an individual's risk of MSI. This type of clinical assessment may be used to identify patients for whom mental stress testing can provide useful risk information. Further studies are needed to assess this strategy.

PATHOPHYSIOLOGY OF MENTAL STRESS ISCHEMIA

Mental Stress and Vascular Function

As described, mental stress is associated with significant increases in heart rate and blood pressure, which are indicative of increased myocardial oxygen demand (though the level of increase in these cardiovascular indices is less than that associated with ischemia during physical stress) and of sympathetic nervous system activity, a key pathway by which vascular tone can be modulated. For example, norepinephrine has an important role in local vasomotion during mental stress; it is released at local sympathetic termini in the coronary arteries, and it has a largely vasoconstricting effect on vascular smooth muscle. Therefore, early in the study of MSI, researchers directed their focus predominantly toward supply-side mechanisms.

Coronary angiography studies show direct evidence of epicardial coronary artery segmental vasoconstriction during mental stress[43–45] in concert with a paradoxical vasoconstriction of these segments to intracoronary administration of acetylcholine.[44] This finding suggests that endothelial dysfunction is a substrate upon which mental stress acts. Further evidence from our lab, described earlier, indicates that rather than epicardial vasoconstriction, the greater impact of mental stress is on coronary blood flow in the microvascular bed.[30,45] These findings overall suggest that endothelial dysfunction is a substrate upon which mental stress acts.

Vascular beds are richly innervated by adrenergic fibers[46] through which regulation by sympathetic nervous system activity is accomplished. The performance of vascular beds in the periphery has been found to correlate with the performance of the coronary microvascular bed under given conditions. Therefore, measurement of pulse wave amplitude (PWA) in cutaneous vascular beds by peripheral arterial tonometry (PAT) is being evaluated for its added value as a noninvasive diagnostic tool to identify vulnerability to mental stress.

The EndoPAT-2000 (Itamar Inc.) is a self-contained, computer-operated device that has been validated for use in the assessment of sympathetic activity in the setting of exercise stress testing.[47,48] It has also recently demonstrated moderate correlation between PWA in cutaneous beds and peripheral endothelial function assessed by brachial artery ultrasound.[48] Goor et al. used PAT for the assessment of mental stress effects in patients with stable CAD. During simultaneous assessment of ejection fraction and WMA by ERNA, and PWA assessment by PAT, the PWA began to change as soon as 4 seconds after the transition from rest to stress. A positive PAT tracing—defined as PWA reductions of at least 20% from rest to mental stress—was 88% concordant with ERNA results.[49] Our group has tested the utility of PAT in predicting MSI in patients with CAD. Patients with MSI had significantly lower ratios of PWA during stress to rest than those patients without MSI (0.76 versus 0.91) (Fig. 32-5). This PAT ratio had a sensitivity of 62% and a specificity of 63% in detecting MSI. In patients who were on angiotensin-converting enzyme (ACE) inhibitors, the sensitivity improved to 73% and specificity to 86%.[50] This new diagnostic modality, properly utilized, might serve as a screening tool for primary and secondary prevention of MSI-vulnerable patients.

Several studies have also demonstrated that mental stress can provoke sustained impairment in endothelial function, assessed by forearm hyperemic flow, with one study in particular demonstrating that this effect is mediated by endothelin-A receptors.[51] Using this approach, Cardillo and colleagues[52] found that inhibition of nitric oxide synthesis attenuated a previously observed vasodilator response to mental stress. Each of these findings is consistent with the concept that vasomotor response to mental stress is endothelially mediated. Thus, mental stress–induced transient endothelial dysfunction may be an important factor in the pathogenesis of MSI in patients with known CAD.

Mental Stress and Inflammation

An indicator of chronic inflammation, C-reactive protein (CRP) has been identified as a risk marker for acute coronary syndromes (ACS) and a direct participant in the progression of atherosclerosis.[53,54] Our group[55] has found a positive correlation between serum CRP and MSI ($r = 0.23$; $P = 0.04$) and a dose-response relationship, with 42.7% of patients showing clinically meaningful CRP levels also demonstrating MSI. Each unit (1 mg/L) increase in CRP level was associated with 20% higher risk of MSI (OR 1.2; 95% CI 1.01–1.29; $P = 0.04$) (Fig. 32-6). These findings indicate that inflammatory processes may play a role in the provocation of MSI.

Cholinergic Antiinflammatory Reflex

As described, mental stress provokes an increase in the sympathetic response, often paired with a decrease in parasympathetic tone.[1] The complex interplay between the CNS and the periphery that maintains the balance of homeostasis and mounts responses to both internal and external threats is rich with multiple interacting systems and complex negative-feedback loops. A growing body of evidence points to a role for the autonomic nervous system in the regulation of inflammatory processes germane to CAD. The relationship between autonomic balance and the release of inflammatory factors is complex and dependent upon variables that are presently not fully understood in a human in vivo model. Increased sympathetic activation can play an important proinflammatory role, working through A_2 receptors to increase production of TNF-α and comparable markers. In addition, there is emerging evidence linking decrements in parasympathetic tone to the generation of inflammatory cytokines such as TNF-α.[3] The latter has been described as the *cholinergic antiinflammatory reflex* (Fig. 32-7). The involvement of specific brain regions (including the medial prefrontal cortex) in the vagal component of heart rate regulation during self-generated emotions has been demonstrated,[56] and we have also found these regions activated in concert with parasympathetic withdrawal during mental stress (see later discussion).

TNF-α is a proinflammatory molecule involved in atherosclerotic plaque rupture, coronary artery vasospasm, and ischemic injury.[57] In CAD patients, brief exposure to TNF-α depresses endothelium-dependent relaxation[58–62] and causes coronary vasoconstriction[63] and decreased coronary flow rate.[64] Furthermore, it can provoke release of endothelin-1 (ET-1) from macrophages[65,66] and has been observed in combination with ET-1 to promote constriction in the microvascular bed.[67] The effect is specific for endothelium-dependent vasodilators.[58] In addition to promoting release of ET-1, TNF-α alters endothelial vasomotor responses by blocking the

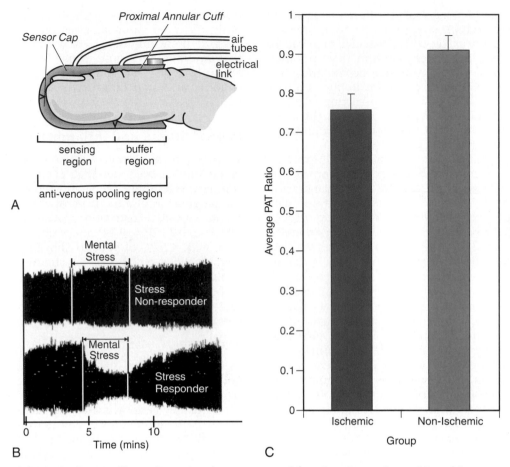

Figure 32-5 **A**, Schematic diagram illustrating sensor's structure and function. Sensor is partitioned into two contiguous sections of equal length, each consisting of an external rigid case bound to an internal latex membrane in an airtight manner. Air tubes connect each segment to a console that controls pressure. Sensor cap is thimble-shaped and longitudinally split so that when pressurized, it imparts a two-point clamping effect to lock sensor firmly to fingertip. This part of the sensor is used to measure pulsatile volume changes in distal phalanx. Volume changes that accompany pulse waves alter pressure in space surrounding fingertip, which is sensed by a pressure transducer within console. An open-ended annular cuff contiguous to sensor tip and pressurized to same level provides a buffering effect against blood volume perturbations. This compartment also extends the effective boundary of sensing compartment. Cuff section is not used for sensing pulsatile volume changes. Both compartments are pressurized to an equal level, which is designed to prevent venous transmural pressure from becoming positive, even if finger is maximally lowered, thereby preventing venous pooling from occurring. **B**, Pulse wave amplitude (PWA) of two patients, *top*, an MS negative and *below*, a patient with MSI. Mental stress time frame shows a narrowing at the PWA in MSI, which is not effected in the PWA immediately above. Ratios of this PWA during MS are derived with the baseline PWA preceding the MS interval. **C**, Average PAT ratio for those with and without mental stress ischemia. Those with ischemia had an average ratio of 0.76 ± 0.04; those with no ischemia had an average ratio of 0.91 ± 0.05 (*P* = 0.03). Those with lower PAT ratios had higher CRP and ET-1 24 hours after stress. (**A**, *From Rozanski A, Qureshi E, Bauman M, et al: Peripheral arterial responses to treadmill exercise among healthy subjects and atherosclerotic patients, Circulation 103:2084–2089, 2001;* **B**, *From Goor DA, Sheffy J, Schnall RP, et al: Peripheral arterial tonometry: A diagnostic method for detection of myocardial ischemia induced during mental stress tests: A pilot study. Clin Cardiol 27:137–141, 2004.)*

activation of endothelial nitric oxide synthase (eNOS), which is essential for flow-dependent relaxation of blood vessels.[68] TNF-α directly degrades eNOS mRNA[69] and contributes to the posttranscriptional inactivation of eNOS.

With these findings in mind, one could describe a model whereby during mental stress, the observed parasympathetic withdrawal would leave macrophages without the cholinergic inhibitory input from the vagus nerve. The resulting increase in local release of cytokines and related vasoactive proteins (e.g., ET-1) would favor vasoconstriction in vascular beds.

Furthermore, the increase of sympathetic output, also evident during metal stress, would lead to an unopposed vasoconstrictive effect of catecholamines. The speed with which this response operates and the wide distribution of macrophages in diseased coronary vessels may implicate this reflex as a mechanism by which the effects of mental stress on coronary microvascular beds are modulated. Preliminary evidence is emerging that CAD patients who demonstrate parasympathetic withdrawal during anger recall in the laboratory are more likely to demonstrate increases in levels of ET-1 during stress.[70]

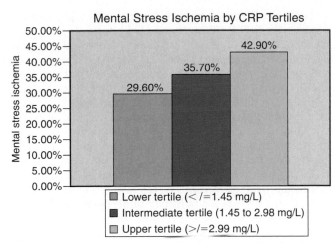

Mental Stress Ischemia by CRP Tertiles

- Lower tertile (</=1.45 mg/L)
- Intermediate tertile (1.45 to 2.98 mg/L)
- Upper tertile (>/=2.99 mg/L)

Figure 32-6 Each unit (1 mg/L) increase in CRP level was associated with 20% higher risk of MSI (OR 1.2; 95% CI 1.01–1.39; $P = 0.04$). (*From Shah R, Burg MM, Vashist A, et al: C-Reactive protein and vulnerability to mental stress–induced myocardial ischemia; Mol Med 12:269–274, 2006.*)

Neurocardiac Central Nervous System Correlates

In addition to the potential role of nuclear imaging to determine the acute cardiac effects of mental stress on perfusion and function, more complex nuclear imaging methods are contributing to the development and elucidation of a neurocardiac model of stress and emotion. These techniques include functional PET brain imaging and imaging of cardiac neuronal integrity.

Functional PET Brain Imaging

We and others have developed techniques to study the effects of mental stress on both brain activity (using ^{15}O-water PET) and cardiac function (using simultaneous echocardiography or SPECT MPI) to investigate the role of the central nervous system (CNS) in MSI. These studies are yielding a number of interesting observations. First, during mental arithmetic stress, cortical frontal-limbic circuits implicated in affect and cognition are activated in patients with CAD but not in healthy subjects.[71] The greater activation in cortical areas may indicate that the task of mental calculation requires more effort in CAD patients than in healthy subjects and may indicate more intense activation of areas associated with emotion and memory as well. Second, comparison of CAD patients with and without MSI showed distinct activation during MSI in the hippocampus and anterior cingulate region, suggesting important influences of the brain regions implicated in mediation of stress, emotion, and memory (Fig. 32-8).[72,73] The cortical regions implicated in these studies may be integral to stress effector systems that transduce cardiovascular reactivity and vasomotor tone. These effector systems are mediated by neurohormonal constituents in vascular

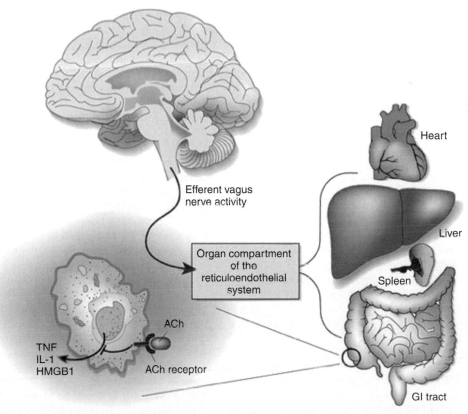

Figure 32-7 The cholinergic antiinflammatory pathway. Efferent activity in the vagus nerve leads to acetylcholine (ACh) release in organs of the reticuloendothelial system, including the liver, heart, spleen and gastrointestinal tract. Acetylcholine interacts with α-bungarotoxin-sensitive nicotinic receptors (ACh receptor) on tissue macrophages, which inhibit the release of TNF, IL-1, HMGB1, and other cytokines. HMGB1, high-mobility group box 1; IL-1, interleukin-1; TNF, tumor necrosis factor. (*From Tracey KJ: The inflammatory reflex, Nature 420:853–859, 2002.*)

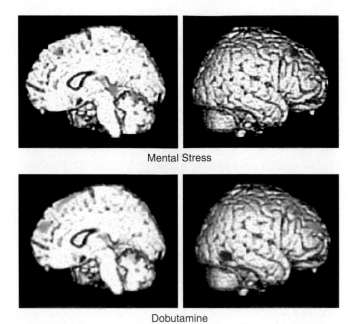

Mental Stress

Dobutamine

Figure 32-8 Panel showing activation *(green)* and deactivation *(red)* in response to mental stress *(top)* and dobutamine *(bottom)*. Activation during mental stress occurs in deep limbic structures, which transduce the visceral effectors to the heart, which determines the myocardial response. Concurrently, there is deactivation in the frontal lobes. Activation during dobutamine does not occur in deep limbic structures but occurs in the somatosensory areas. *(From Vashist A, Burg MM, Arrighi JA, et al: Central nervous system correlates of myocardial ischemia: Neurocardiac distinctions between mental stress and dobutamine provocation, Psychosom Med 67: A8–9, 2005.)*

and tissue compartments. Thus, brain PET imaging is a useful research tool to investigate the effect of the CNS in the pathophysiology of MSI.

Our group evaluated 58 subjects with CAD with simultaneous measurement of cerebral blood flow with ^{15}O PET and cardiac wall-motion analysis with echocardiography during arithmetic mental stress and dobutamine stress.[74] Thirteen patients (22%) were ischemic during mental stress but not during dobutamine stress. When brain PET images were analyzed, cerebral hyperactivation was observed in the frontolimbic circuits and neocortical regions of the brain during mental stress relative to dobutamine stress. These areas are associated with emotion, memory, fear, anxiety, and autonomic regulation. These findings support the notion that mental stress may produce ischemia in some subjects with CAD by different operative mechanisms than those described in exercise or pharmacologic-induced ischemia.[56]

Imaging of Cardiac Neuronal Integrity

Nuclear imaging is well suited to the study of neuronal function and integrity at the level of the myocardium. For example, imaging of labeled catecholamines, such as fluorine-18-fluorodopamine or carbon-11-hydroxyephedrine, can show cardiac sites of sympathetic innervation. Ligands also have been developed to assess muscarinic and β-receptor density. The potential utility

of such imaging and its link to clinically relevant variables is shown most convincingly in patients who have heart failure or undergo cardiac transplantation. These techniques are ideally suited to studying the physiology of MSI and should be a focus of further development in this regard. Given the prominent role of the CNS and peripheral sympathoadrenal effector systems in psychological stress, knowledge of cardiac innervation may be important in understanding the effects of mental stress on hemodynamics, coronary vascular tone, contractile state, propensity for arrhythmias, and proinflammatory effects. Although imaging of neuronal integrity is limited to a few academic centers, the advancement of nuclear cardiology beyond perfusion imaging will likely involve the development of such imaging techniques.

MENTAL STRESS AND DISEASE—EMERGING AREAS

Takotsubo Cardiomyopathy

Reversible myocardial stunning in response to extreme emotional stress—takotsubo cardiomyopathy—is a phenomenon that is attracting growing attention among clinicians and those who study the effects of stress on the heart. This clinical presentation is associated with markedly increased serum catecholamine levels accompanying a transient and profound decrease in LV systolic function, with no angiographic evidence of significant CAD.[75] Takotsubo cardiomyopathy was initially described by Dote in Japan,[76] with subsequent case reports and series around the world demonstrating a similar presentation. Characteristically, there is apical ballooning and compensatory hyperkinesis of the basal segments of the heart.

A number of pathways have been proposed to account for this phenomenon, including multivessel coronary vasospasm, abnormalities in coronary microvascular function, and catecholamine-mediated cardiotoxicity. The definite pathophysiology of this syndrome, however, remains unknown. SPECT MPI with these patients[77–79] consistently shows impairment immediately after hospital admission, with considerable improvement at 3 to 5 days. The presentation seems to be more frequent in Caucasian or Asian females (age > 50). Most of the reports and case series typically describe the absence of significant coronary disease. Nevertheless, evaluations of TIMI frame counts in patients being admitted with transient LV apical ballooning syndrome have shown significant abnormalities in one or more epicardial coronary vessels, compared to matched controls.[78,80] PET studies using nitrogen-13-ammonia and 18-fluorodeoxyglucose have documented a regional transient decrease in myocardial blood flow and coronary flow reserve during the acute phase of takotsubo cardiomyopathy that completely resolves after 3 months (Fig. 32-9).[81–84] The use of iodine-123-metaiodobenzylguanidine (I-123 MIBG) has recently shown regional cardiac denervation in the apex and in the inferior wall of the left ventricle during the acute phase.[85] Takotsubo is

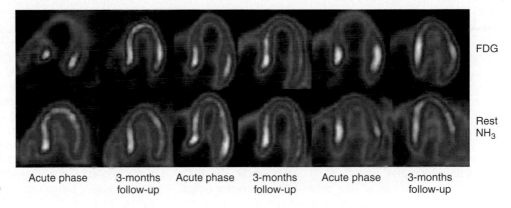

Figure 32-9 FDG/NH$_3$ scans of three patients during the acute phase and 3-month follow-up. During the acute phase, glucose metabolism (FDG)/perfusion (NH$_3$) mismatch is noted. At 3-month follow-up, FDG metabolism normalized. The normalization of FDG/NH$_3$ pattern temporarily coincided with recovery of cardiac function. *(From Feola M, Chauvie S, Rosso GL, et al: Reversible impairment of coronary flow reserve in takotsubo cardiomyopathy: A myocardial PET study, J Nucl Cardiol 15:811–817, 2008.)*

FDG

Rest NH$_3$

Acute phase   3-months follow-up   Acute phase   3-months follow-up   Acute phase   3-months follow-up

a multifaceted and apparently stress-provoked phenomenon that is defined by elements of flow, function, and metabolism. A multimodal imaging approach that captures each of these elements by including echocardiography, coronary angiography with left ventriculography, cardiac magnetic resonance imaging, and PET/SPECT metabolic imaging may allow the precise depiction of the various aspects of the diagnosis. Takotsubo represents a potentially important window into the processes by which mental/psychological stress can profoundly and acutely affect myocardial performance and myocardial perfusion.

Electrophysiologic Abnormalities and Arrhythmic Heart Disease

Case series have described individuals experiencing cardiac arrest or sudden death in the setting of acute grief, fear, or anger,[86,87] while anger and anxiety are described as potent triggers of life-threatening arrhythmias[88] and capable of provoking ICD shock in both the laboratory and natural setting (Fig. 32-10).[89,90] Comparable to findings for the provocation of ischemia, anger appears to be a particularly important emotional component, both as a stressor[89] and as an underlying part of the person's psychological makeup.[90]

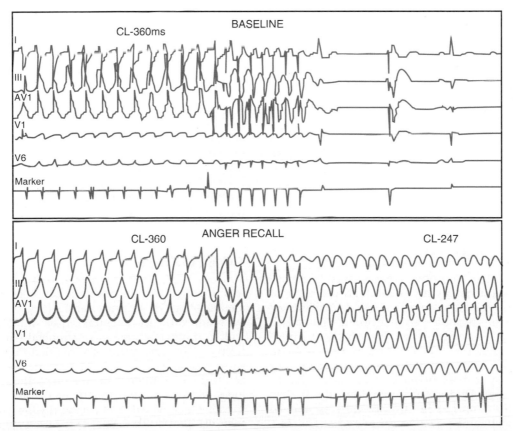

Figure 32-10 The recording of ventricular tachycardia in a subject during baseline conditions *(top)* and during anger recall *(bottom)*. During anger recall, the ventricular tachycardia was more resistant to termination and required cardioversion.

T-wave alternans (TWA) is a marker of repolarization instability[91,92] that is a recognized factor in the development of ventricular fibrillation,[91,93,94] and that immediately precedes development of ventricular fibrillation.[95] TWA increases with heart rate,[91,96,97] and sympathetic activation/catecholamine release play a role.[89] TWA induced by exercise or atrial pacing under controlled conditions predicts subsequent ventricular arrhythmias,[97,98] cardiac arrest,[97,99] and mortality.[100–102] TWA increases during anger in daily life, and experimental studies demonstrate that as the level of TWA increases, the likelihood of developing an arrhythmia increases as well.[103,104] TWA increases in ICD patients during the recall of a previously anger-provoking incident,[89,105] suggesting that mental stress induced in the laboratory predicts increases in TWA with anger in daily life and might predict subsequent arrhythmia.[106]

SUGGESTED PROTOCOL FOR MENTAL STRESS SPECT

The following protocol for mental stress testing is based on the premise that mental stress causes ischemia and that MSI is associated with a worse prognosis. We recommend perfusion measurements over determinations of function because of the potential low specificity of functional changes. Mental arithmetic or anger recall may be used, based on the expertise available. Data suggest that these methods produce ischemia in a similar number of patients.

Imaging

Mental stress SPECT MPI is similar to other stress SPECT imaging (see Chapters 14 and 15). SPECT is performed during two conditions: rest and mental stress. We recommend the use of a ^{99m}Tc-based perfusion agent with low-dose rest and high-dose stress studies. Resting SPECT MPI is performed after intravenous injection of 7 to 10 mCi ^{99m}Tc sestamibi or ^{99m}Tc tetrofosmin. One hour after injection, SPECT MPI is acquired. On completion of resting MPI, the patient is removed from the camera, and mental stress testing may begin. After 90 seconds of mental stress, the patient is injected with 25 to 30 mCi ^{99m}Tc sestamibi or ^{99m}Tc tetrofosmin. SPECT MPI is acquired 30 minutes after radiotracer injection.

Mental Stress Protocol

Various mental stress protocols are described in the literature, but we recommend mental arithmetic and anger recall. For the anger recall technique, the subject is asked to vividly recall a recent incident that caused moderate to extreme anger. The subject is given 1 minute to fully recall the incident and is then told to describe it fully to the experimenter. The subject is asked specifically to "describe it as if you were describing it to a friend." During the description, the subject is prompted for details about actual words exchanged during the event and affective experiences. The task takes approximately 6 minutes to complete. One advantage of this technique is its reproducibility.

Further, in patients with CAD, anger appears to be a particularly potent psychological stressor. In a study by Ironson and colleagues,[107] anger recall reduced LVEF more than exercise and other psychological stressors, and more patients with CAD had a significant reduction in LVEF (7%) during anger (7 of 18) than during exercise (4 of 18). The protocol necessitates that a clinical psychologist or someone with focused training in this technique be present.

The arithmetic task consists of serial subtraction from a specified number. For most subjects, the number 7 is used; however, for patients who cannot perform this task, an easier subtraction task is provided (e.g., subtracting by 4, 3, or 2). Throughout the task, the patient is prompted for faster performance and the base number is changed (e.g., starting with 1013 and changing to 436 after the patient has performed a number of successful serial subtractions). In addition, errors are corrected in a harsh tone, providing an element of harassment and increasing the difficulty of the task. The frequency of prompting the patient and changing the base number is contingent on the patient's performance, with an error rate of approximately 1 error in 10 subtractions as the "goal." These methods correct for individual differences in mathematical ability and maintain a fairly constant stress level across patients. The main advantage of this protocol is its ease of use; however, data suggest that it is somewhat less reproducible than anger recall.

Monitoring during the stress portion of the MPI is identical to that for clinical stress testing. In brief, heart rate, blood pressure, and 12-lead ECG measurements are obtained at 1-minute intervals throughout the stress portion of the study. Indications for early termination of stress are identical to those for clinical stress testing: severe angina, ST-segment depression of more than 3 mm, decrease in systolic blood pressure, and arrhythmia.

Processing and Interpretation

SPECT images are reconstructed in the same way as for exercise or pharmacologic stress perfusion imaging. Myocardial perfusion images are analyzed visually for reversible defects, which indicate ischemia. Quantitative analysis may be performed as well, but reference cohorts have yet to be standardized and validated.

CONCLUSION

It is not often that our specialty can take the lead in the identification of distinct cardiovascular presentations. We outlined the incremental impact of MSI on prognosis and its distinct central and peripheral pathophysiologic features. The emergence of simplified finger probes and stress protocols since the last edition serves as evidence of the growing interest in this phenomenon. Epidemiologic evidence suggests that acute coronary events occur in individuals who do not necessarily have the traditional high-risk profile for CAD.[8] This observation, in concert with the high frequency of myocardial infarction during catastrophic events, suggests that the identification of patients who are vulnerable to MSI is highly relevant. MSI predisposes vulnerable individuals to adverse clinical outcomes, angina, and fatal arrhythmias. In this chapter, we outlined a simplified algorithm for clinicians interested in conducting mental stress examinations. As work in this field progresses, more laboratories will likely incorporate mental stress imaging into the management of patients with CAD. The main economic limitation is a specific Current Procedural Terminology code for testing for ischemia in response to mental stress. Policy guidelines from professional societies are planned, because they are the customary antecedents toward reimbursement. Nonetheless, clinical demand to aid in the identification of such patients has not diminished. The rationale and logistics outlined in this chapter can provide the framework for this testing.

REFERENCES

1. Soufer R: Neurocardiac interaction during stress-induced myocardial ischemia: how does the brain cope? *Circulation* 110:1710–1713, 2004.
2. Damasio AR: Remembering when, *Sci Am* 287:66–73, 2002.
3. Tracey KJ: The inflammatory reflex, *Nature* 420:853–859, 2002.
4. Powell LH, Thoresen CE: Behavioral and physiologic determinants of long term prognosis after myocardial infarction, *J Chron Dis* 38: 253–263, 1985.
5. Jain D, Burg M, Soufer R, et al: Prognostic implications of mental stress-induced silent left ventricular dysfunction in patients with stable angina pectoris, *Am J Cardiol* 76:31–35, 1995.
6. Sheps DS, McMahon RP, Becker L, et al: Mental stress–induced ischemia and all-cause mortality in patients with coronary artery disease: Results from the Psychophysiological Investigations of Myocardial Ischemia study, *Circulation* 105:1780–1784, 2002.
7. Jiang W, Babyak M, Krantz DS, et al: Mental stress–induced myocardial ischemia and cardiac events, *JAMA* 275:1651–1656, 1996.
8. Ruberman W, Weinblatt E, Goldberg JD, et al: Psychosocial influences on mortality after myocardial infarction, *N Engl J Med* 311:552–559, 1984.
9. Rosengren A, Tibblin G, Wilhelmsen L: Self-perceived psychological stress and incidence of coronary artery disease in middle-aged men, *Am J Cardiol* 68:1171–1175, 1991.
10. Becker LC, Pepine CJ, Bonsall R, et al: Left ventricular, peripheral vascular, and neurohumoral responses to mental stress in normal middle-aged men and women. Reference Group for the Psychophysiological Investigations of Myocardial Ischemia (PIMI) Study, *Circulation* 94:2768–2777, 1996.
11. Jain D, Shaker SM, Burg M, et al: Effects of mental stress on left ventricular and peripheral vascular performance in patients with coronary artery disease, *J Am Coll Cardiol* 31:1314–1322, 1998.
12. Rozanski A, Bairey CN, Krantz DS, et al: Mental stress and the induction of silent myocardial ischemia in patients with coronary artery disease, *N Engl J Med* 318:1005–1012, 1988.
13. Specchia G, De Servi S, Falcone C, et al: Mental arithmetic stress testing in patients with coronary artery disease, *Am Heart J* 108:56–63, 1984.
14. Deanfield JE, Shea M, Kensett M, et al: Silent myocardial ischaemia due to mental stress, *Lancet* 2:1001–1005, 1984.
15. Barry J, Selwyn AP, Nabel EG, et al: Frequency of ST-segment depression produced by mental stress in stable angina pectoris from coronary artery disease, *Am J Cardiol* 61:989–993, 1988.
16. Specchia G, Falcone C, Traversi E, et al: Mental stress as a provocative test in patients with various clinical syndromes of coronary heart disease, *Circulation* 83:II-108–II-114, 1991.
17. Schang SJ Jr, Pepine CJ: Transient asymptomatic S-T segment depression during daily activity, *Am J Cardiol* 39:396–402, 1977.
18. Stern S, Tzivoni D: Early detection of silent ischaemic heart disease by 24-hour electrocardiographic monitoring of active subjects, *Br Heart J* 36:481–486, 1974.
19. Bosimini E, Galli M, Guagliumi G, et al: Electrocardiographic markers of ischemia during mental stress testing in postinfarction patients—Role of body surface mapping, *Circulation* 83:II-115–II-127, 1991.
20. Sherwood A, Johnson K, Blumenthal JA, et al: Endothelial function and hemodynamic responses during mental stress, *Psychosom Med* 61:365–370, 1999.
21. LaVeau PJ, Rozanski A, Krantz DS, et al: Transient left ventricular dysfunction during provocative mental stress in patients with coronary artery disease, *Am Heart J* 118:1, 1989.
22. Stone PH, Krantz DS, McMahon RP, et al: Relationship among mental stress-induced ischemia and ischemia during daily life and during
exercise: the Psychophysiologic Investigations of Myocardial Ischemia (PIMI) study, *J Am Coll Cardiol* 33:1476–1484, 1999.
23. Vassiliadis IV, Fountos AI, Papadimitriou AG, et al: Mental stress induced silent myocardial ischemia detected during ambulatory ventricular function monitoring, *Int J Card Imaging* 14:171–177, 1998.
24. Modena MG, Corghi F, Fantini G, et al: Echocardiographic monitoring of mental stress test in ischemic heart disease, *Clin Cardiol* 12:21–24, 1989.
25. Gottdiener JSKD, Howell RH, Hecht GM, et al: Induction of silent myocardial ischemia with mental stress testing: Relation to the triggers of ischemia during daily life activities and to ischemic functional severity, *J Am Coll Cardiol* 24:1645–1651, 1994.
26. Carney RM, McMahon RP, Freedland KE, et al: Reproducibility of mental stress-induced myocardial ischemia in the Psychophysiological Investigations of Myocardial Ischemia (PIMI) study, *Psychosom Med* 60:64–70, 1998.
27. Jain D, Joska T, Lee FA, et al: Day-to-day reproducibility of mental stress-induced abnormal left ventricular function response in patients with coronary artery disease and its relationship to autonomic activation, *J Nucl Cardiol* 8:347–355, 2001.
28. Giubbini R, Galli M, Campini R, et al: Effects of mental stress on myocardial perfusion in patients with ischemic heart disease, *Circulation* 83:II-100–II-107, 1991.
29. Schoder H, Silverman DH, Campisi R, et al: Effect of mental stress on myocardial blood flow and vasomotion in patients with coronary artery disease, *J Nucl Med* 41:11–16, 2000.
30. Arrighi JA, Burg M, Cohen IS, et al: Myocardial blood-flow response during mental stress in patients with coronary artery disease, *Lancet* 356:310–311, 2000.
31. Arrighi JA, Burg M, Cohen IS, et al: Simultaneous assessment of myocardial perfusion and function during mental stress in patients with chronic coronary artery disease, *J Nucl Cardiol* 10:267–274, 2003.
32. Dimsdale JE, Moss J: Plasma catecholamines in stress and exercise, *JAMA* 243:340–342, 1980.
33. Goldberg AD, Becker LC, Bonsall R, et al: Ischemic, hemodynamic, and neurohormonal responses to mental and exercise stress. Experience from the Psychophysiological Investigations of Myocardial Ischemia Study (PIMI), *Circulation* 94:2402–2409, 1996.
34. Ramachandruni S, Fillingim RB, McGorray SP, et al: Mental stress provokes ischemia in coronary artery disease subjects without exercise- or adenosine-induced ischemia, *J Am Coll Cardiol* 47:987–991, 2006.
35. Hassan M, York KM, Li Q, et al: Variability of myocardial ischemic responses to mental versus exercise or adenosine stress in patients with coronary artery disease, *J Nucl Cardiol* 15:518–525, 2008.
36. Krantz DS, Santiago HT, Kop WJ, et al: Prognostic value of mental stress testing in coronary artery disease, *Am J Cardiol* 84:1292–1297, 1999.
37. Rosenman RH, Brand RJ, Jenkins D, et al: Coronary heart disease in Western Collaborative Group Study. Final follow-up experience of 8 1/2 years, *JAMA* 233:872–877, 1975.
38. Goodman M, Quigley J, Moran G, et al: Hostility predicts restenosis after percutaneous transluminal coronary angioplasty, *Mayo Clin Proc* 71:729–734, 1996.
39. Julkunen J, Salonen R, Kaplan GA, et al: Hostility and the progression of carotid atherosclerosis, *Psychosom Med* 56:519–525, 1994.
40. Kawachi I, Sparrow D, Spiro A III, , et al: A prospective study of anger and coronary artery disease, *Circulation* 94:2090–2095, 1996.
41. Mittleman MA, Maclure M, Sherwood JB, et al: Triggering of acute myocardial infarction onset by episodes of anger. Determinants of Myocardial Infarction Onset Study Investigators, *Circulation* 92. 1720–1725, 1995.
42. Burg MM, Jain D, Soufer R, et al: Role of behavioral and psychological factors in mental stress-induced silent left ventricular dysfunction in coronary artery disease, *J Am Coll Cardiol* 22:440–448, 1993.
43. Rebecca G, Wagner R, Zebede T: Pathogenic mechanism causing transient myocardial ischemia with mental arousal in patients with coronary artery disease (abstract), *Clin Res* 34:338A, 1989.
44. Yeung AC, Vekshtein VI, Krantz DS, et al: The effect of atherosclerosis on the vasomotor response of coronary arteries to mental stress, *N Engl J Med* 325:1551–1556, 1991.
45. Kop WJ, Krantz DS, Howell RH, et al: Effects of mental stress on coronary epicardial vasomotion and flow velocity in coronary artery disease: relationship with hemodynamic stress responses, *J Am Coll Cardiol* 37:1359–1366, 2001.
46. Burton A: The range and variability of the blood flow in the human fingers and the vasomotor regulation of body temperature, *Am J Physiol* 127:437–453, 1939.
47. Rozanski A, Qureshi E, Bauman M, et al: Peripheral arterial responses to treadmill exercise among healthy subjects and atherosclerotic patients, *Circulation* 103, 2001.
48. Kuvin JT, Patel AR, Sliney KA, et al: Assessment of peripheral vascular endothelial function with finger arterial pulse wave amplitude, *Am Heart J* 146:168–174, 2003.
49. Goor DA, Sheffy J, Schnall RP, et al: Peripheral arterial tonometry: A diagnostic method for detection of myocardial ischemia induced

during mental stress tests: A pilot study, *Clin Cardiol* 27:137–141, 2004.

50. Burg MM, Graeber B, Vashist A, et al: Noninvasive detection of risk for emotion provoked myocardial ischemia, *Psychosom Med* 71:14–20, 2009.

51. Spieker LE, Hurlimann D, Ruschitzka F, et al: Mental stress induces prolonged endothelial dysfunction via endothelin-A receptors, *Circulation* 105:2817–2820, 2002.

52. Cardillo C, Kilcoyne CM, Quyyumi AA, et al: Role of nitric oxide in the vasodilator response to mental stress in normal subjects, *Am J Cardiol* 80:1070–1074, 1997.

53. Sabatine MS, Morrow DA, Jablonski KA, et al: Prognostic significance of the Centers for Disease Control/American Heart Association high-sensitivity C-reactive protein cut points for cardiovascular and other outcomes in patients with stable coronary artery disease, *Circulation* 115:1528–1536, 2007.

54. Albert MA, Glynn RJ, Ridker PM: Plasma concentration of C-reactive protein and the calculated Framingham Coronary Heart Disease Risk Score, *Circulation* 108:161–165, 2003.

55. Shah R, Burg MM, Vashist A, et al: C-reactive protein and vulnerability to mental stress-induced myocardial ischemia, *Mol Med* 12:269–274, 2006.

56. Soufer R, Burg MM: The heart-brain interaction during emotionally provoked myocardial ischemia: implications of cortical hyperactivation in CAD and gender interactions, *Cleve Clin J Med* 74(Suppl 1): S59–S62, 2007.

57. Mizia-Stec K, Gasior Z, Zahorska-Markiewicz B, et al: Serum tumour necrosis factor-alpha, interleukin-2 and interleukin-10 activation in stable angina and acute coronary syndromes, *Coron Artery Dis* 14:431–438, 2003.

58. Bhagat K, Vallance P: Inflammatory cytokines impair endothelium-dependent dilatation in human veins in vivo, *Circulation* 96: 3042–3047, 1997.

59. Chia S, Qadan M, Newton R, et al: Intra-arterial tumor necrosis factor-alpha impairs endothelium-dependent vasodilatation and stimulates local tissue plasminogen activator release in humans, *Arterioscler Thromb Vasc Biol* 23:695–701, 2003.

60. Nakamura M, Yoshida H, Arakawa N, et al: Effects of tumor necrosis factor-alpha on basal and stimulated endothelium-dependent vasomotion in human resistance vessel, *J Cardiovasc Pharmacol* 36:487–492, 2000.

61. Patel JN, Jager A, Schalkwijk C, et al: Effects of tumour necrosis factor-alpha in the human forearm: blood flow and endothelin-1 release, *Clin Sci (Lond)* 103:409–415, 2002.

62. Rask-Madsen C, Dominguez H, Ihlemann N, et al: Tumor necrosis factor-alpha inhibits insulin's stimulating effect on glucose uptake and endothelium-dependent vasodilation in humans, *Circulation* 108: 1815–1821, 2003.

63. Edmunds NJ, Woodward B: Effects of tumour necrosis factor-alpha on the coronary circulation of the rat isolated perfused heart: a potential role for thromboxane A2 and sphingosine, *Br J Pharmacol* 124: 493–498, 1998.

64. Edmunds NJ, Lal H, Woodward B: Effects of tumour necrosis factor-alpha on left ventricular function in the rat isolated perfused heart: possible mechanisms for a decline in cardiac function, *Br J Pharmacol* 126:189–196, 1999.

65. Woods M, Mitchell JA, Wood EG, et al: Endothelin-1 is induced by cytokines in human vascular smooth muscle cells: evidence for intracellular endothelin-converting enzyme, *Mol Pharmacol* 55:902–909, 1999.

66. Kaheleh MB, Fan PS: Effect of cytokines on the production of endothelin by endothelial cells, *Clin Exp Rheumatol* 15:163–167, 1997.

67. Hohlfeld T, Klemm P, Thiemermann C, et al: The contribution of tumour necrosis factor-alpha and endothelin-1 to the increase of coronary resistance in hearts from rats treated with endotoxin, *Br J Pharmacol* 116:3309–3315, 1995.

68. Dimmeler S, Fleming I, Fisslthaler B, et al: Activation of nitric oxide synthase in endothelial cells by Akt-dependent phosphorylation, *Nature* 399:601–605, 1999.

69. Yoshizumi M, Perrella MA, Burnett JC Jr, et al: Tumor necrosis factor downregulates an endothelial nitric oxide synthase mRNA by shortening its half-life, *Circ Res* 73:205–209, 1993.

70. Soufer A, Ranjbaran H, Graeber B, et al: Parasympathetic withdrawal and sympathetic arousal during anger correlate with elevated endothelin-1 in patients with coronary artery disease, *Psychosom Med* 70, 2008.

71. Soufer R, Bremner JD, Arrighi JA, et al: Cerebral cortical hyperactivation in response to mental stress in patients with coronary artery disease, *Proc Natl Acad Sci U S A* 95:6454–6459, 1998.

72. Bremner JD, Krystal JH, Southwick SM, et al: Functional neuroanatomical correlates of the effects of stress on memory, *J Trauma Stress* 8:527–553, 1995.

73. LeDoux J: *The Emotional Brain*, New York, 1998, Touchstone Books.

74. Vashist A, Burg MM, Arrighi JA, et al: Central nervous system correlates of myocardial ischemia: Neurocardiac distinctions between mental stress and dobutamine provocation, *Psychosom Med* 67:A8–A9, 2005.

75. Gianni M, Dentali F, Grandi AM, et al: Apical ballooning syndrome or takotsubo cardiomyopathy: A systematic review, *Eur Heart J* 27: 1523–1529, 2006.

76. Dote K, Sato H, Tateishi H, et al: Myocardial stunning due to simultaneous multivessel coronary spasms: a review of 5 cases, *J Cardiol* 21:203–214, 1991.

77. Akashi YJ, Nakazawa K, Sakakibara M, et al: 123I-MIBG myocardial scintigraphy in patients with "takotsubo" cardiomyopathy, *J Nucl Med* 45:1121–1127, 2004.

78. Kurisu S, Inoue I, Kawagoe T, et al: Time course of electrocardiographic changes in patients with tako-tsubo syndrome: comparison with acute myocardial infarction with minimal enzymatic release, *Circ J* 68: 77–81, 2004.

79. Ito K, Sugihara H, Katoh S, et al: Assessment of takotsubo (ampulla) cardiomyopathy using ^{99m}Tc-tetrofosmin myocardial SPECT—comparison with acute coronary syndrome, *Ann Nucl Med* 17: 115–122, 2003.

80. Bybee KA, Prasad A, Barsness GW, et al: Clinical characteristics and thrombolysis in myocardial infarction frame counts in women with transient left ventricular apical ballooning syndrome, *Am J Cardiol* 94:343–346, 2004.

81. Feola M, Rosso GL, Casasso F, et al: Reversible inverse mismatch in transient left ventricular apical ballooning: perfusion/metabolism positron emission tomography imaging, *J Nucl Cardiol* 13:587–590, 2006.

82. Feola M, Chauvie S, Rosso GL, et al: Reversible impairment of coronary flow reserve in takotsubo cardiomyopathy: a myocardial PET study, *J Nucl Cardiol* 15:811–817, 2008.

83. Malafronte C, Farina A, Tempesta A, et al: Tako-tsubo: a transitory impairment of microcirculation? A case report, *Ital Heart J* 6:933–938, 2005.

84. Alexanderson E, Cruz P, Talayero JA, et al: Transient perfusion and motion abnormalities in takotsubo cardiomyopathy, *J Nucl Cardiol* 14:129–133, 2007.

85. Scholte AJ, Bax JJ, Stokkel MP, et al: Multimodality imaging to diagnose takotsubo cardiomyopathy, *J Nucl Cardiol* 13:123–126, 2006.

86. Reich P, DeSilva RA, Lown B, et al: Acute psychological disturbances preceding life-threatening ventricular arrhythmias, *JAMA* 246: 233–235, 1981.

87. Engel GL: Sudden and rapid death during psychological stress. Folklore or folk wisdom, *Ann Intern Med* 74:771–782, 1971.

88. Albert CM, Lampert R, Conti JB, et al: Episodes of anger trigger ventricular arrhythmias in patients with implantable cardioverter defibrillators, *Circulation* 114:II-831, 2006.

89. Lampert R, Shusterman V, Burg MM, et al: Effects of psychologic stress on repolarization and relationship to autonomic and hemodynamic factors, *J Cardiovasc Electrophysiol* 16:372–377, 2005.

90. Burg MM, Lampert R, Joska T, et al: Psychological traits and emotion-triggering of ICD shock-terminated arrhythmias, *Psychosom Med* 66: 898–902, 2004.

91. Pastore JM, Girouard SD, Laurita KR, et al: Mechanism linking T-wave alternans to the genesis of cardiac fibrillation, *Circulation* 99: 1385–1394, 1999.

92. Shimizu W, Antzelevitch C: Cellular and ionic basis for t-wave alternans under long-QT conditions, *Circulation* 99:1499–1507, 1999.

93. Han J, Moe GK: Nonuniform recovery of excitability in ventricular muscle, *Circ Res* 14:44–60, 1964.

94. Nearing BD, Verrier RL: Modified moving average analysis of T-wave alternans to predict ventricular fibrillation with high accuracy, *J Appl Physiol* 92:541–549, 2002.

95. Shusterman V, Goldberg A, London B: Upsurge in T-wave alternans and non-alternating repolarization instability precedes spontaneous initiation of ventricular tachyarrhythmias in humans, *Circulation* 113:2880–2887, 2006.

96. Hohnloser SH, Klingenheben T, Zabel M, et al: T wave alternans during exercise and atrial pacing in humans, *J Cardiovasc Electrophysiol* 8: 987–993, 1997.

97. Rosenbaum DS, Jackson LE, Smith JM, et al: Electrical alternans and vulnerability to ventricular arrhythmias, *N Engl J Med* 330:235–241, 1994.

98. Cantillon DJ, Stein KM, Markowitz SM, et al: Predictive value of microvolt t-wave alternans in patients with left ventricular dysfunction, *J Am Coll Cardiol* 50:166–173, 2007.

99. Gold MR, Bloomfield DM, Anderson KP, et al: A comparison of T-wave alternans, signal averaged electrocardiography and programmed ventricular stimulation for arrhythmia risk stratification, *J Am Coll Cardiol* 36:2247–2253, 2000.

100. Bloomfield DM, Steinman RC, Namerow PB, et al: Microvolt T-wave alternans distinguishes between patients likely and patients not likely to benefit from implanted cardiac defibrillator therapy: a solution to the Multicenter Automatic Defibrillator Implantation Trial (MADIT) II conundrum, *Circulation*, 2004.

101. Klingenheben T, Zabel M, D'Agostino RB, et al: Predictive value of T-wave alternans for arrhythmic events in patients with congestive heart failure (letter), *Lancet* 356:651–652, 2000.

102. Nieminen T, Lehtimaki T, Viik J, et al: T-wave alternans predicts mortality in a population undergoing a clinically indicated exercise test, *Eur Heart J* 28:2332–2337.
103. Nearing BD, Huang AH, Verrier RL: Dynamic tracking of cardiac vulnerability by complex demodulation of the T wave, *Science* 252:437–440, 1991.
104. Nearing B, Oesterle S, Verrier R: Quantification of ischaemia induced vulnerability by precordial T wave alternans analysis in dogs and humans, *Cardiovasc Res* 28:1440–1449, 1994.
105. Kop WJ, Krantz DS, Nearing BD, et al: Effects of acute mental stress and exercise on T-wave alternans in patients with implantable cardioverter defibrillators and controls, *Circulation* 109:1864–1869, 2004.
106. Lampert R, Shusterman V, Burg M, et al: Arrhythmias in patients with Implantable cardioverter defibrillators, *J Am Coll Cardiol* 53:774–778, 2009.
107. Ironson G, Taylor CB, Boltwood M, et al: Effects of anger on left ventricular ejection fraction in coronary artery disease, *Am J Cardiol* 70:281–285, 1992.

Chapter 33

Myocardial Blood Flow Measurement: Evaluating Coronary Pathophysiology and Monitoring Therapy

THOMAS HELLMUT SCHINDLER, INES VALENTA
AND HEINRICH R. SCHELBERT

INTRODUCTION

Positron emission tomography (PET) combined with tracer kinetic modeling allows the assessment of regional myocardial blood flow (MBF) of the left ventricle in mL/g/min and adds a new dimension to the noninvasive evaluation and understanding of coronary pathophysiology. Measuring coronary flow responses to sympathetic stimulation with cold pressor testing and/or hyperemic flow increases due to pharmacologic vasodilation enable the noninvasive identification and characterization of coronary circulatory function. These flow responses can identify both functional and structural abnormalities of the coronary circulation, reflecting early stages of developing coronary artery disease (CAD) long before the development of macroscopic morphologic alterations of the arterial wall and the clinical manifestation of CAD. PET measurements of MBF combined with various forms of vasomotor stress, therefore, extend the scope of conventional scintigraphic imaging in the noninvasive delineation of coronary circulatory dysfunction in early subclinical stages of CAD. The identification of the CAD process does not depend on demonstrating regional perfusion defects at rest or during stress on conventional myocardial perfusion imaging. Rather, the extent of coronary flow responses to vasomotor stress or the coronary flow reserve may help identify coronary functional abnormalities that may precede or accompany CAD-related structural alterations of the arterial wall.[1]

This chapter aims to briefly denote technical aspects of PET-measured MBF, reviews the determinants of MBF and flow reserve, comments on the definitions of coronary circulatory function, evaluates the responses of MBF to physiologic and pharmacologic stimuli and their relationship to coronary circulatory function, and assesses the value of measurements of MBF for delineation of coronary risk and monitoring the responses to therapeutic intervention.

METHODOLOGY OF BLOOD FLOW MEASUREMENT

PET approaches for the measurement of regional MBF in mL/g/min entail intravenous administration of positron-emitting tracers of MBF such as nitrogen-13-labeled (^{13}N) ammonia, oxygen-15-labeled (^{15}O) water, or rubidium-82 (^{82}Rb) (Table 33-1) and imaging of the radiotracer's transit time through the central circulatory system and its extraction and retention in the myocardium. ^{13}N-ammonia and ^{15}O-water, the most commonly used flow tracers with PET, are short-lived (physical half-life 9.8 and 2.4 minutes, respectively) and therefore necessitate on-site cyclotron production. Rubidium-82, with an ultrashort physical half-life of 78 seconds, is available through a strontium-82/rubidium-82 generator system with a 4- to 5-week shelf life and thus does not require an on-site cyclotron.

Beginning with the intravenous injection of the radiotracer of blood flow, serial images are acquired to capture the initial transit of the flow tracer through the central circulation and its extraction into the myocardium (see Table 33-1). The serially acquired image data sets are then reformatted into short-axis and long-axis myocardial slices and assembled into polar maps.[2,3] Regions of interest (ROIs) are assigned by the analysis software program to the territories of the three major coronary

Table 33-1   Tracers of Myocardial
Blood Flow

Tracer	Half-Life	Method
O-15 water	2.4 min	Cyclotron
N-13-ammonia	9.8 min	Cyclotron
Rubidium-82	78 sec	Generator

Cyclotron, in-house cyclotron needed; Generator, available through generator; Half-Life, physical half-life.

arteries; a 25 mm^2 ROI is positioned in the left ventricular blood pool on a short-axis slice. The ROIs are then copied to all serially acquired image data sets, and time-activity curves are generated that reflect the arterial radiotracer input function and the myocardial response to it. The time-activity curves are then fitted with operational equations derived from tracer kinetic models, which describe the exchange of radiotracer between tissue compartments and the volume of tracer distribution in each compartment. The operational equations then yield regional MBF in mL/g/min. Tracer kinetic models also correct for physical decay of the radioisotope, partial volume–related underestimations of the true myocardial tissue concentrations (by assuming a uniform myocardial wall thickness of 1 cm),[4] and spillover of radioactivity between the left ventricular blood pool and myocardium.[5]

PET TRACERS OF MYOCARDIAL BLOOD FLOW (See Chapter 19)

Estimates of MBF obtained with ^{13}N-ammonia and ^{15}O-water have been widely validated against independent microsphere blood flow measurements in animals and yielded highly reproducible values of MBF (correlation coefficient for ^{13}N-ammonia: $r = 0.99$ and standard error of the estimate (SEE): 0.17; correlation coefficient for ^{15}O-water: $r = 0.95$).[6,7] Similarly, measurements of MBF with ^{13}N-ammonia and ^{15}O-water in humans yield comparable estimates of MBF,[8,9] but these tracers differ in several aspects in their use to measure MBF.

[13]N-Ammonia

Used as a myocardial flow tracer, ^{13}N-ammonia is selectively retained by the myocardial cells and has a longer physical half-life (9.8 minutes). This allows acquisition of statistically high-count ^{13}N-ammonia images of the myocardium, and thus the relative distribution of the myocardial flow can be denoted with high diagnostic quality in the visual and semiquantitative assessment of myocardial perfusion defects during stress underlying hemodynamically obstructive CAD.[10–15] Although ^{13}N-ammonia becomes metabolically trapped in myocardium, mainly in the form of glutamate and mostly glutamine, alterations in cardiac work or myocardial metabolism do not significantly affect the association between tracer tissue concentrations and MBF.[10] Acute ischemia may moderately reduce the retention fraction of ^{13}N-ammonia in the myocardium, but it does not

significantly affect its use as a flow tracer. The longer physical half-life of ^{13}N-ammonia, however, necessitates longer time intervals ($\approx$45 minutes) between repeat assessments of MBF, restraining the numbers of interventions that can be undertaken during a single PET flow study.

Rubidium-82

As a myocardial flow tracer, [82]Rb is increasingly used for the assessment of myocardial perfusion or its relative radiotracer uptake of the left ventricle during stress and rest in the evaluation of flow-limiting epicardial stenosis.[12,16–22] Recent investigations also suggest the utility of [82]Rb for quantifying MBF in mL/g/min.[23–27] The ultrashort physical half-life of [82]Rb (only 76 seconds) allows serial investigations of myocardial perfusion at short time intervals (e.g., 10 minutes). Yet the ultrashort physical half-life necessitates the delivery of high [82]Rb activity doses (i.e., 60 mCi) for adequate visualization of the myocardial tracer uptake after 1 to 2 physical half-lives for tracer clearance from the blood pool. Clinical investigations report the feasibility and utility of MBF quantification with [82]Rb PET combined with one- or two-compartment tracer kinetic models.[24–27] Initial animal validation studies[24,28] using a two-compartment tracer kinetic model yielded precise MBF values at rest, while the hyperemic flow was generally underestimated and highly variable. Applying [82]Rb with a one-compartment tracer kinetic model, however, appears to be more promising in the quantifications of MBF.[26,27] In 14 healthy volunteers, for example, estimates of MBF both at rest and during dipyridamole-stimulated hyperemia correlated well with flow values obtained with ^{13}N-ammonia ($r = 0.85$). Mean hyperemic MBF values were comparable between both flow tracers (^{13}N-ammonia: 2.71 mL/g/min versus [82]Rb: 2.83 mL/g/min); however, the corresponding standard deviations (SD), as an index for the individual measurement variability between both flow studies, was higher for rubidium-82 with 0.81 mL/g/min when compared to ^{13}N-ammonia with an SD of 0.50 mL/g/min.[27] In another investigation,[25] PET measurements of myocardial blood flow with [82]Rb using a wavelet-based noise-reduction protocol[29] and a two-compartment model were compared to myocardial flows as determined with ^{15}O-water in eleven healthy individuals. For these two approaches to quantify myocardial flow, the authors found a close association of resting and hyperemic MBF ($r = 0.94$; $P < 0.001$) ranging between 0.45 mL/g/min to 2.75 mL/g/min, emphasizing the potential role of [82]Rb in the quantification of myocardial blood flows by PET. Further studies on the interstudy and interobserver variability of [82]Rb-estimated MBF are needed to determine the exact range of measurement-related errors of this approach in the individual person and, thereby, its utility in the assessment of subclinical and clinically manifest CAD.

[15]O-Water

As a myocardial flow tracer, ^{15}O-water distributes into the water spaces of both the myocardium and the blood pool. Thus, ^{15}O-water does not selectively accumulate in the myocardial cells, and corrections for the blood-pool activity are needed. These corrections are commonly performed by blood-pool imaging with ^{15}O water or ^{11}C-labeled red blood cells and subtraction of the blood pool from the ^{15}O water images. Applying a one-compartment tracer kinetic model, estimates of MBF are then determined from the rate of clearance of ^{15}O-water from the left ventricular myocardium.[7,30] The subtraction of the blood pool from the ^{15}O water images, in concert with the rapid clearance of ^{15}O-water and its short half-life, may produce statistically low-count images of the myocardium. Thus, the visual evaluation and semiquantitative analysis of the relative distribution of the myocardial ^{15}O-water uptake ("static" image) may be of limited value in the diagnostic evaluation of flow-limiting epicardial lesions. On the other hand, using ^{15}O-water, with its short physical half-life (2.4 minutes), affords repeat MBF measurements at short intervals of 10 to 15 minutes. This allows a convenient assessment of MBF at rest as well as the response to vasomotor stress before and after intervention during the same study session.

DETERMINANTS OF MYOCARDIAL BLOOD FLOW AND FLOW RESERVE

Coronary Circulatory Function: Definitions

The investigation of coronary vasomotor (circulatory) function is usually confined to patients with chest pain syndromes undergoing coronary angiography. Although the identification of coronary vasomotor dysfunction during coronary angiography entails important diagnostic and prognostic information,[31–36] the invasive nature and time-consuming process to determine this abnormality in vasomotor function pose major limitations. Invasive approaches to assess abnormalities in coronary vasomotor function, therefore, cannot be applied for widespread clinical use.[37–43] A variety of invasive methods for evaluating coronary vasomotor function exist.[37,44,45] Such methods commonly necessitate computer-based measurements of coronary vessel diameter (QCA; quantitative coronary angiography) and intracoronary flow-velocity probes for determining coronary flow alterations in response to infused acetylcholine, bradykinin, or substance P–stimulated release of endothelium-derived nitric oxide (NO), or flow-mediated (and thus endothelium-dependent) alterations of the lumen of the epicardial artery.[37,38,42,44,45] As regards the latter approach, increases in coronary flow can be stimulated either by intracoronary infusion of papaverine or adenosine or by a more physiologic stress test such as sympathetic stimulation with cold pressor testing (CPT).[36–38,40,46]

In more detail, endothelium-dependent vasodilators such as acetylcholine specifically stimulate the muscarinic receptor–mediated release of endothelium-derived NO that induces the epicardial artery to dilate through relaxation of the vascular smooth muscle cells. It is worth noting that such vasodilation in response to acetylcholine can only be partially prevented by inhibitors of endothelial NO synthase (eNOS).[37] Thus there appears to also be a concomitant release of other endothelium-derived vasodilators, such as prostacyclin and/or endothelium-derived hyperpolarizing factors (EDHF) that contribute to the acetylcholine-stimulated normal coronary vasodilation.[37,45] The specific intracoronary infusion of acetylcholine, for example, through an infusion catheter defines normal endothelial function when there is a vasodilation of the epicardial artery. In the presence of dysfunctional epicardial artery endothelium, however, the concurrent smooth muscle cell constrictor effects of acetylcholine overcome the endothelium-mediated vasodilation,[37] and a lack of vasodilation or, more commonly, a paradoxical vasoconstriction ensues.[37,47] For the determination of coronary blood flow to evaluate the responses of the coronary microcirculatory system, an intracoronary Doppler catheter and the placement of a flow wire are necessary.[37,45] Endothelium-dependent vasodilators such as acetylcholine also increase coronary blood flow, paralleling their concurrent vasodilator effects on the coronary arteriolar resistance vessels. Increases in coronary flows to acetylcholine stimulation as measured with the Doppler flow wire, therefore, identify normal endothelium-dependent coronary arteriolar vasomotor function, whereas an impairment or absence of coronary flow is appreciated as endothelial dysfunction of the arteriolar vessels.[37,48] Notably, a similar phenomenon has been described for sympathetically induced coronary flow increases during CPT with immersion of the left hand into ice water.[40,46,48,49] Normally, CPT-induced and metabolically induced vasodilation of the coronary arteriolar vessels induces an increase in flow in the coronary circulatory system. This increase in coronary flow results in an elevation of shear forces on the vascular wall, with a concomitant release of endothelial-derived NO[50,51] and thereby induces a flow-mediated vasodilation of the upstream coronary vessels.[37,38,46] If the endothelium is dysfunctional, however, the sympathetically mediated vasoconstrictor response of the vascular smooth muscle cells during CPT prevails and causes an impairment, absence, or even decrease in coronary flow.[46,52–54] Of note, the CPT-induced coronary vasomotor response closely correlates with the specific determination of coronary vasomotion due to acetylcholine stimulation at the site of the epicardial conduit artery and the coronary microcirculation.[40,48,52,55]

Substances such as nitroglycerin or sodium nitroprusside provide NO directly to the vascular smooth muscle cell layer, causing epicardial vasodilation. Thus, the latter vasomotor response to nitroglycerin or sodium nitroprusside is independent of the functional state of the vascular endothelium and thereby provides specific information on vascular smooth muscle cell function of the epicardial artery.[37] Similarly, adenosine or papaverine relax vascular smooth muscle cells of the coronary vessels and are commonly applied intracoronarily to gain information on the predominantly endothelium-independent hyperemic coronary flows or so-called total coronary vasodilatory capacity. At the same time, determination of flow-mediated epicardial vasodilation by QCA during hyperemic flow increases with adenosine or papaverine may serve as another important and more physiologic index of endothelium-dependent epicardial vasomotion.[37,40,56] Applying such a protocol, a flow-related and NO-mediated epicardial vasodilation during a hyperemic coronary flow increase defines normal endothelial function, whereas an impairment or absence of flow-related epicardial vasodilation is indicative of a dysfunctional state of the coronary endothelium.

NONINVASIVE ASSESSMENT OF CORONARY CIRCULATORY FUNCTION

Myocardial Blood Flow at Rest

PET-measured MBF at rest in healthy volunteers has been reported to range between 0.4 and 1.2 mL/g/min.[23,57–61] Apart from some interstudy variations of PET-measured MBF related to methodologic differences, including radiotracers, tracer kinetic models, and image analysis, the variability in these individual resting blood flows is likely attributable to differences in left ventricular myocardial workload at the time of assessment.[57,62] As observed in several clinical investigations,[57,58,63] there is a close linear correlation between resting MBF and the rate-pressure product (RPP; defined as the product of systolic blood pressure and heart rate) as an index of cardiac work and therefore metabolic oxygen demand. These observations indicate that increases in myocardial work are closely accompanied by commensurate flow increases to adequately meet increases in oxygen demand. Accordingly, MBF is closely coupled to myocardial oxygen demand and myocardial work, both at rest and during physical stress (e.g., bicycle exercise, treadmill exercise, dobutamine stimulation).[14,63] Age-related increase in resting MBF has also been related to increases in cardiac work due to higher systolic blood pressures.[58,61] More controversial are possible differences in MBF at rest between males and females. Some but not all investigations observed higher values of resting MBF,[57,61,64] that are thought to be related to gender-dependent differences in plasma lipid profiles.

Assessment of Coronary Reactivity

Approaches to assessing coronary circulatory function include measurements of MBF with PET at rest and its responses to physiologically or pharmacologically stimulated coronary flow increases, including bicycle exercise, dobutamine stress, sympathetic stimulation with CPT, as well as vascular smooth muscle relaxation with vasodilator agents.[14,46,63,65–71] An additional indicator of coronary function is a heterogeneous perfusion response to pharmacologic or sympathetic stimulation, with a progressive decrease in perfusion from the base to the apex of the left ventricle. This abnormal perfusion response might prove useful as a noninvasive indicator of epicardial coronary dysfunction.[72,73]

Total Integrated Vasodilator Capacity and Coronary Flow Reserve

The most widely and clinically used approach for the assessment of coronary circulatory function is the pharmacologically induced hyperemic MBF.[62,65,70,74,75] Vascular smooth muscle–relaxing substances such as dipyridamole, adenosine, adenosine triphosphate (ATP), or adenosine receptor agonists[76] lower the resistance to flow at the site of the coronary arterioles and produce maximum or submaximum hyperemic MBF. Hyperemic flow is considered a measure of a predominantly endothelium-independent flow response. However, inhibition of eNOS by intravenous infusion of N^G-nitro-L-arginine methyl ester (L-NAME) significantly reduces adenosine-induced MBF increases by 21% to 25%, as measured with PET (Fig. 33-1).[77,78] This attenuation in hyperemic flow responses most likely reflects an impairment of flow-mediated vasodilation during higher coronary flows. Thus, shear-sensitive components of the coronary endothelium contribute, in part, through flow-mediated coronary vasodilation to the overall hyperemic flow during pharmacologic vasodilation.[37,77,78] Since pharmacologically induced hyperemic MBF increases reflect smooth muscle cell and, in part, endothelium-related vasodilatory effects, it is also defined as the "total integrated coronary circulatory function."[44,65,70]

The coronary vasodilatory capacity reflects the ability of the coronary circulatory system to increase flows from baseline in order to meet increases in myocardial metabolic demand. This capacity to increase coronary flow to a maximum from rest is known as *coronary flow reserve* and first described by Coffman and Gregg.[79] A more physiologic framework for the coronary flow reserve was provided by Mosher et al.[80] by adding the concept of *coronary autoregulation*. Within the latter concept, resting coronary blood flow is determined by several factors,

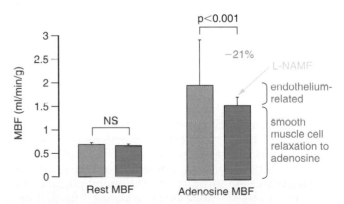

Figure 33-1 Hyperemic MBF increase to adenosine stimulation and its alteration to the intravenous infusion of the nitric oxide (NO) synthase inhibitor, N^G-nitro-L-arginine methyl ester (L-NAME), 4 mg/L/body weight. In the presence of L-NAME, the hyperemic MBF response was attenuated by 21%; that is likely to reflect the impairment of the flow-mediated and thus endothelium-derived and NO-mediated vasodilation by L-NAME. *(Adapted from Buus NH, Bottcher M, Hermansen F, et al: Influence of nitric oxide synthase and adrenergic inhibition on adenosine-induced myocardial hyperemia. Circulation 104:2305-2310, 2001.)*

while myocardial oxygen demand—as a function of heart rate, blood pressure, myocardial contractility, and ventricular preload—is appreciated as the predominant factor in the regulation of resting coronary flows. Given that the metabolic myocardial oxygen demand is widely constant, coronary flow within the range of its autoregulation is widely independent of the coronary perfusion pressure. Consequently, within the range of coronary autoregulation, so-called plateau coronary flow changes little, despite alterations in perfusion pressures. Conversely, a pharmacologically induced dilation of the coronary arteriolar resistance vessels leads to a hyperemic coronary inflow that no longer is governed by autoregulatory mechanisms and that changes linearly with changes in intracoronary perfusion pressure. In this consideration, the ratio of hyperemic to resting coronary flow is defined as the coronary flow reserve. Values for the flow reserve should be interpreted with caution, however. Under certain conditions, the coronary flow reserve does not necessarily indicate the true coronary vasodilator capacity. The coronary flow reserve can decline due to increase in resting flow or decrease in maximum hyperemic flow. Factors that increase the demand for myocardial oxygen, such as arterial hypertension, increased myocardial contractility, increased left ventricular wall stress, and tachycardia, cause an increase in resting flow. On the other hand, maximum hyperemic coronary flow may decline in the presence of a focal flow-limiting epicardial lesion, in the presence of microvascular disease in patients with hypertension or diabetes, or as a consequence of increases in extravascular resistive forces paralleled by increases in left ventricular pressures in patients with congestive heart failure or hypertension. Thus, there are several limitations when interpreting the coronary flow reserve. Nevertheless, the concept of the coronary flow reserve remains an important and useful index for assessing the functional significance or downstream effects of focal epicardial arterial lesions, functional improvement after coronary revascularization, and coronary circulatory function in individuals with subclinical or clinically manifest CAD.[65,81,82]

Sympathetic Stimulation with Cold Pressor Testing

PET measurements of alterations in MBF from rest to sympathetic stimulation by CPT entail specific information on coronary endothelial function.[39,46,48,53,83,84] CPT is performed with immersion of a hand into ice water, which in turn induces a sympathetically mediated increase in heart rate and blood pressure and thus an increase in myocardial workload. The RPP can be used as an index of myocardial workload and oxygen demand. Increases in myocardial workload during CPT are associated with vasodilation of the coronary arteriolar resistance vessels through the release of (presumably) adenosine as a metabolic vasodilator.[85] As a consequence, there is a decrease in coronary vascular resistance that causes an increase in coronary inflow. This increase in coronary inflow causes in turn a flow-mediated, endothelium-dependent dilation of the

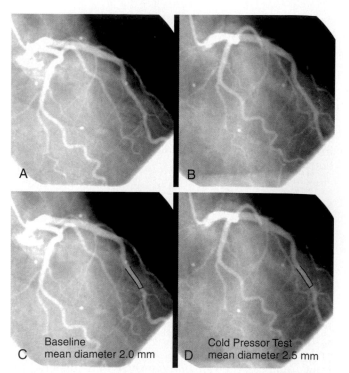

Figure 33-2 **A,** Normal coronary angiogram of the left coronary tree in the RAO view of a healthy individual without coronary risk factors. **B,** Corresponding angiogram during sympathetic stimulation with CPT. **C** and **D,** Quantitative angiographic assessment of the proximal-mid LAD segment (**C**) at rest (mean diameter 2.0 mm) and (**D**) during CPT (mean diameter 2.5 mm). *(From Schindler TH, Nitzsche EU, Olschewski M, et al: PET-measured responses of MBF to cold pressor testing correlate with indices of coronary vasomotion on quantitative coronary angiography, J Nucl Med 45:419–428, 2004. Reprinted with permission.)*

upstream coronary vessel segments. As demonstrated in Figure 33-2, an increase in cardiac work is normally accompanied by commensurate flow-mediated coronary vasodilation, and an increase in MBF is determined with PET.[46,53,54,61] In the presence of coronary endothelial dysfunction, however, the sympathetically induced increase in coronary inflow does not mediate a flow-related vasodilation. Under such conditions, the sympathetically mediated vasoconstrictor effects of the vascular smooth muscle cells predominate and are not overcome by normal flow-related coronary vasodilation (Fig. 33-3).[37,46,86] Myocardial blood flows during CPT are then attenuated, absent, or even paradoxically decreased, which denotes a dysfunction of the coronary endothelium.[46,53,54,84]

Several clinical investigations in the assessment of coronary vasomotor function emphasize the validity and value of PET-measured changes in MBF during CPT from rest as a noninvasive index of coronary endothelial function. For example, coronary flow increases during CPT, as assessed invasively with Doppler wire during coronary angiography, closely correlate with the flow response to acetylcholine stimulation, which is considered a specific probe of endothelial function (Fig. 33-4).[37,48] Coronary flows during sympathetic stimulation with CPT, therefore, may probe endothelium-related vasomotor function

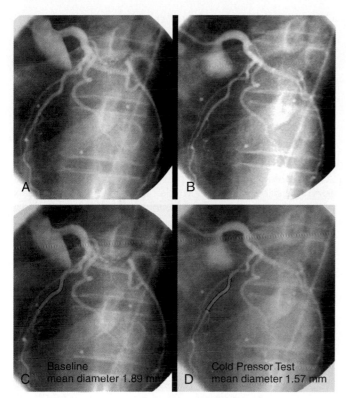

Figure 33-3 **A**, Normal coronary angiogram of the left coronary artery tree in the LAO view in a chronic smoker at rest. **B**, Corresponding coronary angiogram during CPT. **C** and **D**, Quantitative angiographic assessment of the proximal-mid LAD segment (**C**) at rest (mean diameter: 1.89 mm) and (**D**) during CPT (mean diameter: 1.57 mm). *(From Schindler TH, Nitzsche EU, Olschewski M, et al: PET-measured responses of MBF to cold pressor testing correlate with indices of coronary vasomotion on quantitative coronary angiography, J Nucl Med 45:419–428, 2004. Reprinted with permission.)*

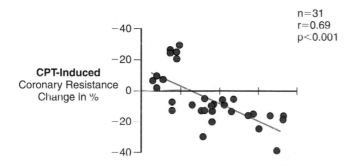

Acetylcholine-Induced Blood Flow Response
(proportion of max papaverine response in %)

Figure 33-4 Association between the coronary flow response to CPT and acetylcholine stimulation during coronary angiography in 12 normal control patients and in 19 patients with diffuse CAD. The CPT-induced changes in coronary vascular resistance inversely and significantly correlated with the extent of endothelial dysfunction of the coronary arteriolar vessels, as determined with acetylcholine stimulation. *(From Zeiher AM, Drexler H, Wollschlager H, et al: Endothelial dysfunction of the coronary microvasculature is associated with coronary blood flow regulation in patients with early atherosclerosis, Circulation 84:1984–1992, 1991. Reprinted with permission.)*

and thereby delineate the functional integrity of the vascular wall.[37,46] In particular, it was observed that the epicardial vasomotor response to CPT was closely paralleled by the acetylcholine-stimulated response, suggesting the epicardial vasomotor response to CPT may be intimately related to the integrity of endothelial function.[37,52] Further, CPT-induced changes in epicardial luminal diameter, as determined by QCA, and PET-measured responses of MBF to CPT, are closely correlated.[46,53,54] More direct evidence for the involvement of the endothelium in CPT-mediated MBF responses has been provided by Campisi et al.[84] In chronic smokers exhibiting an impairment of MBF responses to CPT, intravenous infusion of L-arginine as a substrate of nitric oxide synthase restored the MBF increase to CPT, most likely due to increases in the bioavailability of endothelium-derived NO.

Perfusion Heterogeneity and Base-to-Apex Myocardial Perfusion Gradient

In the last 2 decades, the interrelation of structural and functional determinants of clinically manifest CAD has been extensively studied.[87–92] As shown by previous fundamental work of Gould et al.,[87] focal coronary artery lesions between 60% and 85% diameter stenosis commonly do not affect the resting MBF, as the result of a compensatory vasodilation of the downstream arteriolar resistance vessels.[87] This adaptive vasodilation under resting conditions may fail to compensate for greater increases in epicardial resistance, that is, for cases of severe coronary artery stenoses (greater than 85%), so stress-induced myocardial ischemia may manifest.[69,93] In light of several investigations, it has been widely accepted that hyperemic coronary flows during pharmacologic vasodilation commonly begin to decline when focal epicardial artery narrowing reaches 50% diameter stenosis.[87,88,90,92]

Whether structural changes of the arterial wall in early stages of CAD may also affect the coronary flow is an area of ongoing debate and interest. PET flow studies[1,82,94–96] add evidence that hyperemic flow increases may be mildly diminished in the presence of diffuse CAD with coronary lesions less than 50% and/or coronary circulatory dysfunction. Such observations have raised a new concept that even subclinical CAD-related structural alterations of the arterial wall may exert downstream fluid dynamic effects that, as reported recently, may manifest as mild myocardial perfusion heterogeneity at rest,[97,98] and during vasomotor stress[98] or as longitudinal base-to-apex perfusion gradient during hemodynamic stress.[72,73,94,99] Gould et al.[94] were the first to describe heterogeneity in longitudinal myocardial perfusion during pharmacologically induced hyperemia in patients with diffuse CAD. Other investigators found that PET-determined quantitative estimates of MBF during pharmacologically induced hyperemia also denoted a relative decrease in longitudinal myocardial flow from the mid to the mid-distal part of the left ventricular myocardium in individuals with coronary risk factors but without clinically manifest CAD.[72,73]

It has been argued that fluid dynamic consequences of CAD- related vessel stiffness and/or functional abnormalities of the epicardial conduit vessels may account for the longitudinal heterogeneity in myocardial perfusion. Based on the Hagen-Poiseuille equation, intracoronary resistance relates to the velocity of the blood flow and inversely to the fourth power of the vessel diameter.[91,100,101] Normal function of the vascular endothelium ascertains that increases in flow velocity during exercise or pharmacologic vasodilation are associated with a flow-dependent and nitric-oxide-mediated dilation of the coronary artery, which balances the velocity-induced increase in coronary resistance, so that the resistance is kept low or does not increase.[38,42] Structural and/or functional disturbances of coronary arterial walls in the early development of CAD, however, commonly impair a flow-mediated and thus endothelial-derived NO–mediated dilation of the epicardial artery. In this concept, the absence of a flow-mediated epicardial vasodilation causes an increase in intracoronary resistance during higher coronary flows that leads to a progressive proximal-to-distal decline in intracoronary pressure along the epicardial artery.[100] Such a decrease in intracoronary pressure has been put forth as cause for a gradual base-to-apex, relative decline or heterogeneity in myocardial perfusion or MBF.[72,73,94,100]

There is some direct evidence of a cause-and-effect relationship of structural and/or functional changes of the epicardial artery and downstream hemodynamic effects. As previous investigations have demonstrated, there is a close association between heterogeneity in myocardial perfusion during dipyridamole stimulation and the presence of diffuse CAD.[94] A more recently performed comparative study of patients with coronary risk factors and angina pectoris symptoms provided further insight.[102] Comparisons were made between the invasive assessment of epicardial endothelial function in response to acetylcholine stimulation, and ^{99m}Tc tetrofosmin SPECT-measured myocardial perfusion during both bicycle exercise and dipyridamole stimulation. In these patients without flow-limiting epicardial coronary lesions, a moderate but significant association ($r = 0.49$; $P < 0.002$) between acetylcholine-induced alterations in epicardial artery diameter and the degree of exercise-induced myocardial perfusion defects was observed, suggesting that functional abnormalities of the epicardial artery may indeed account, at least in part, for stress-induced regional myocardial perfusion defects.[102,103] A perfusion heterogeneity in longitudinal (base-to-apex) MBF during sympathetic stimulation with CPT, as measured with PET, was observed to be related to a functional decrease in epicardial luminal diameter as determined with quantitative coronary angiography ($r = 0.77$; $P < 0.0001$).[99] Apart from structural alterations of the coronary arterial wall, an impairment of flow-mediated, endothelium-dependent epicardial coronary vasomotor function may contribute to the manifestation of a longitudinal heterogeneity in MBF during vasomotor stress.[44,103] The assessment of heterogeneity in longitudinal myocardial perfusion or quantitative blood flow with PET could be a promising noninvasive index of early structural and/or functional alterations of the CAD process, predominantly at the site of the epicardial artery. As another noninvasive index of the early stages of the development of CAD, it may carry important predictive information on future cardiovascular events[95,104] but awaits further confirmation through clinical end-point investigations.

Reproducibility of Measurements of Myocardial Blood Flow and Responses to Stressors

As outlined before, an impairment of coronary circulatory function in individuals with subclinical stages of the CAD process has been widely appreciated to carry important diagnostic and prognostic information.[31,32,105–107] If this holds true, then a restoration of abnormalities in coronary circulatory function by lifestyle modifications or therapeutic interventions should lead to an improved clinical outcome, as some preliminary data of the peripheral circulation may indeed suggest.[108–110] PET measurements of MBF responses to cold exposure and pharmacologic vasodilation are increasingly applied to determine and monitor the effects of lifestyle modifications or therapeutic interventions on coronary circulatory function.[53,67,111–117] Such serial PET flow studies raise the need for establishing the reproducibility of repeat PET measurements of MBF.[118] This allows determination of the methodologic measurement error of PET-determined flows in repeat assessments[62,74,118] and also the biological and hemodynamic variability of these flow measurements.[46,58,118–120] By using the mean difference of repeat MBF measurements, the sample size of the study populations needed for adequately powering clinical investigations with serial PET blood-flow measurements can be determined.

A reasonable reproducibility of hyperemic MBF during pharmacologic vasodilation with ^{13}N-ammonia or ^{15}O-labeled water and PET has been demonstrated previously.[66,74,121] As recently shown, CPT-related MBF measurements were also reproducible when determined with ^{15}O-labeled water on a 1-day protocol.[122] Further, in a more detailed and extended investigation,[118] the hemodynamic and endothelium-related MBF responses to CPT or its change from rest (ΔMBF), as measured with ^{13}N-ammonia and PET, were demonstrated to be not only highly reproducible in short-term (1-day protocol) but also in long-term (2 to 3 weeks protocol) measurements (Table 33-2). There are important considerations in interpreting the reproducibility data of PET-measured MBF. For example, the Pearson's correlation coefficient (r) of the least-square regression analysis can be used to denote the strength of agreement between repeat MBF measurements. Notably, the standard error of the estimate (SEE) indicates the tightness of the linear fit of the data and is considered to represent the actual range of method-related measurement error (or its variability). For example, the range of measurement errors, as denoted by the SEE for the endothelium-related change of MBF from rest to CPT, was found to be 0.09 mL/g/min for short-term and 0.17 mL/g/min for long-term repeat measurements (Fig. 33-5). According to the latter values of the SEE, alterations in the change in MBF in serial

Table 33-2 Myocardial Blood Flow and Hemodynamics at Same-Day and 2-Week Measurements*

	m = 1	CV	m = 2	CV	m = 3	CV	Absolute Mean Difference m = 12	Absolute Mean Difference m = 13
MBF in mL/g/min								
At rest	0.67 ± 0.19	0.29	0.66 ± 0.15	0.22	0.63 ± 0.18	0.28	0.09 ± 0.10	0.10 ± 0.10
During CPT	0.88 ± 0.21	0.24	0.85 ± 0.20	0.23	0.82 ± 0.21	0.13	0.11 ± 0.09	0.14 ± 0.10
Δ to CPT	0.21 ± 0.17	0.79	0.19 ± 0.16	0.83	0.19 ± 0.14	0.41	0.08 ± 0.05	0.19 ± 0.10
Hemodynamics at Rest								
Heart rate (beats/min)	61 ± 7	0.12	62 ± 9	0.13	61 ± 9	0.16	2.5 ± 2.2	7.1 ± 5.0
SBP (mm Hg)	116 ± 12	0.11	120 ± 15	0.12	115 ± 13	0.11	5.5 ± 7.6	6.6 ± 5.6
DBP (mm Hg)	71 ± 7	0.10	73 ± 6	0.08	69 ± 8	0.11	3.0 ± 2.6[†]	5.5 ± 5.3
RPP (mm Hg/min)	7113 ± 1161	0.16	7349 ± 1157	0.16	6936 ± 986	0.14	430 ± 445	789 ± 691
Hemodynamics During CPT								
Heart rate (beats/min)	68 ± 8	0.12	67 ± 7	0.11	67 ± 9	0.14	3.5 ± 2.4	5.8 ± 5.1
SBP (mm Hg)	148 ± 22	0.15	152 ± 22	0.15	149 ± 23	0.16	5.8 ± 10	8.3 ± 11
DBP (mm Hg)	86 ± 11	0.13	87 ± 12	0.14	85 ± 13	0.15	2.7 ± 2.1	8.5 ± 6.9
RPP (mm Hg/min)	9982 ± 1798	0.18	10160 ± 1456	0.14	9935 ± 1259	0.18	724 ± 543	1470 ± 1011
Δ RPP (mm Hg/min)	2869 ± 1666	0.58	2811 ± 1300	0.46	2999 ± 1740	0.58	762 ± 517	1046 ± 857

*Measurement 1 (m = 1) and measurement 2 (m = 2) on the same day and measurement 3 (m = 3) after 2 weeks for all study participants (n = 20).
[†]$p \leq 0.05$ for difference by paired t-test; P = NS for intragroup comparisons between coefficients of variation (CV) 1–3 by ANOVA (Levene Test).
Δ, change; beats/min, beats per minute; CPT, cold pressor testing; DBP, diastolic blood pressure; MBF, myocardial blood flow; RPP, rate-pressure product; SBP, systolic blood pressure.

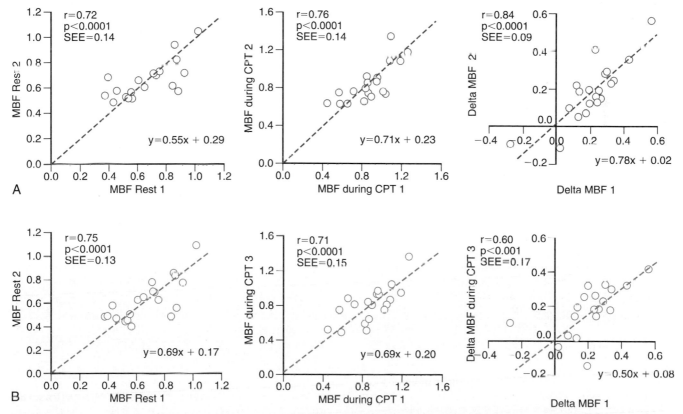

Figure 33-5 Scattergram of short-term (**A**) and long-term (**B**) repeat myocardial blood flow (MBF) measurements. Line of equality is shown, along which points should lie for perfect agreement. As can be seen, individual MBF at rest and its response to CPT did vary between individuals but also, as demonstrated, were found to correlate well between measurements. *(From Schindler TH, Zhang XL, Prior JO, et al: Assessment of intra- and interobserver reproducibility of rest and cold pressor test-stimulated myocardial blood flow with (13)N-ammonia and PET, Eur J Nucl Med Mol Imaging 34:1178–1188, 2007. Reprinted with permission.)*

pharmaceutical studies that are above this range of SEE are likely to be related to beneficial effects of pharmaceutical interventions on coronary endothelial function.[118] In addition, the mean difference and the corresponding standard deviation (SD) of repeat MBF measurements are used to calculate the sample size of a study population needed to sufficiently power a serial flow study. For example, using the longitudinal mean difference and the corresponding SD of the endothelium-related change in MBF from rest to CPT of 0.08 ± 0.05 mL/g/min in the short-term and of 0.19 ± 0.10 mL/g/min in the long-term (see Table 33-2), at a 5% significance level with a power of 87%, a sample size of 14 and 22 individuals would be needed for serial PET flow studies to identify possible intervention-related, statistically significant alterations in MBF responses to CPT.[118] Another important statistical parameter used in the interpretation of reproducibility data is the repeatability coefficient (RPC) as proposed by Bland and Altman.[123] The RPC serves as a useful index to denote the agreement between repeat measurements. Given a normal Gaussian distribution of MBF measurements,[123] the RPC denotes the expected range of measurement error between repeat assessments of myocardial blood flows. It is critical, however, to keep in mind that most PET flow studies have investigated relatively small sample sizes, between 11 and 25 study participants.[66,74,118,124] Given the relatively small sample sizes of these PET flow studies, they may not have fully met the assumption of a normal Gaussian distribution of flow values. Further, the RPC can also be applied as an index of precision of MBF measurements between different studies (Table 33-3). For example, in the aforementioned investigation,[118] the RPC for the endothelium-related change in MBF from rest to CPT was 0.18 mL/g/min for the short-term and 0.27 mL/g/min for the long-term reproducibility measurements with ^{13}N-ammonia and PET. Both RPCs indicate less measurement error in the assessment of endothelium-related MBF responses to CPT with ^{13}N-ammonia PET than was observed with the short-term RPC of CPT-related flows and ^{15}O-water measurements (1-day study protocol)[122] and also for hyperemic flow increases reported in previous studies,[66,74,124] which have

been reported between 0.49 and 1.34 mL/g/min (see Table 33-3).

ALTERED CORONARY CIRCULATORY FUNCTION AND CARDIOVASCULAR EVENTS

Normal endothelium-dependent vasomotor function has been widely appreciated to play an active and central role in the modulation of the integrity and metabolism of the vascular wall, vasomotor tone, and hemostasis.[125,126] The coronary vasomotor tone underlies the endothelium-dependent production and release of vasoactive mediators such as prostacyclin, endothelin-1, endothelium-derived hyperpolarizing factor (EDHF), and in particular, NO. Given normal function of the coronary endothelium, increases in coronary flow with physical exercise lead to a flow-mediated and thus endothelium-dependent release of NO, prompting a NO-mediated relaxation of the vascular smooth muscle cells and vasodilation. This NO-mediated mechanism offsets possible vasoconstrictor effects of elevated endothelin-1 and angiotensin-II levels, and/or sympathetic activation.[37,44,127] Coronary risk factors, however, not only cause a reduction in the bioavailability of endothelial-derived NO and/or prostacyclin but are usually associated with increased activity of vasoconstrictors such as endothelin-1, angiotensin II, and reactive oxygen species (ROS), most likely accounting for the diminished endothelium-dependent coronary vasodilator capacity. Coronary vasomotor function, therefore, constitutes a tenuous balance between vasodilator and vasoconstrictor mechanisms, where the endothelium-mediated vasodilation normally prevails.

Importantly, the flow-mediated release of endothelial-derived NO not only leads to coronary vasodilation during higher flow velocities but also exerts anti-atherosclerotic and antithrombotic effects.[37,126,127] For example, one atheroprotective mechanism of endothelial-derived NO is to act in concert with prostacyclin to prevent platelet aggregation, while another is to reduce expression of cellular adhesion molecules, thereby

Table 33-3 Myocardial Blood Flow Repeatability Coefficient in Different Studies

Radiotracer	SCHINDLER ET AL.[179] ^{13}N-ammonia		SIEGRIST ET AL.[183] ^{15}O-water	KAUFMANN ET AL.[100] ^{15}O-water	WYSS ET AL.[86] ^{15}O-water	JAGATHESAN ET AL.[185] ^{15}O-water	
Period	ST (1 d)	LT (2 wk)	ST (1 d)	ST (1 d)	ST (1 d)	LT (24 wk)	
MBF at baseline	0.26	0.26	—	0.17	0.26	0.30*	0.26**
MBF during CPT	0.28	0.31	0.41	—	—	—	—
Δ MBF to CPT	0.18	0.27	—	—	—	—	—
MBF during ado	—	—	—	0.94	1.34	—	—
MBF to bicycle exercise	—	—	—	—	0.82	—	—
MBF during dob	—	—	—	—	—	0.49	0.58

*Ischemic and **remote myocardium.
Δ, change; ado, adenosine; CPT, cold pressor testing; dob, dobutamine; LT, long term; MBF, myocardial blood flow; ST, short term.

preventing the attachment of neutrophils to the endothelium and their migration into the subintimal space.[37,126,127] NO further inhibits vascular smooth muscle cell proliferation and exerts antiinflammatory and antioxidative effects within the arterial wall. Reductions in the bioavailability of atheroprotective and endothelial-derived NO contribute to the initiation or acceleration of the atherosclerotic process. Risk factors for CAD as diverse as smoking, hypercholesterolemia, hypertension, hyperglycemia, obesity, and a family history of premature atherosclerotic disease have all been shown to be associated with an attenuation or loss of endothelium-dependent vasodilation.[37,105,126] The causes of coronary circulatory dysfunction in patients with coronary risk factors are certainly multifactorial. Increased vascular production of ROS derived from superoxide-producing endothelial enzymes, such as NAD(P)H oxidase, xanthine oxidase, or uncoupled NO synthase, reduces the bioavailability of endothelium-derived NO, which has been implicated as a leading cause and common final pathway of abnormal coronary vasodilatory capacity.[128]

An impairment of endothelium-dependent coronary circulatory function is commonly associated with other active processes such as inflammation, proliferation or apoptosis, and the expression of vascular cellular adhesion molecules (ICAM). This so-called endothelial activation reflects an initial injury of the vascular wall that may initiate and contribute to the development and progression of the atherosclerotic process. In particular, this "endothelial activation" plays an important role in the pathogenesis of acute coronary syndromes characterized by coronary plaque vulnerability and paradoxical vasoconstriction, paralleled by endothelial dysfunction, which is likely to contribute to plaque rupture,[129,130] and increased thrombogenicity due to loss of a potent antithrombotic endothelial surface.[131] An impairment of coronary circulatory function, therefore, is likely to reflect the vulnerability of plaques, which may explain the independent predictive value of coronary circulatory dysfunction for future cardiovascular events.[31,32,105,106] Alterations of coronary circulatory function appear to reflect active processes that modify the functional and structural state of the arterial wall and may serve as an explanation for the independent predictive value of coronary circulatory dysfunction for future cardiovascular events.[32,126,127]

Individuals with traditional and novel coronary risk factors and those with clinically manifest CAD commonly present an impairment of endothelium-dependent vasomotion.[35] The degree of the dysfunctional endothelium probably reflects the cumulative effect of several risk factors on the arterial wall. Nevertheless, there is considerable variability in the extent of endothelial dysfunction in individuals with similar coronary risk factor profiles.[36] It is worth noting that the assessment of peripheral and coronary vasomotor dysfunction has been considered an important marker of the inherent atherosclerotic risk in an individual, reflecting the cumulative risk of various coronary risk factors as well as of yet-unknown variables and genetic

predispositions.[132,133] Of particular interest is that PET-measured flow responses to sympathetic stimulation with CPT, indicative of coronary endothelial dysfunction in patients with angiographically normal coronary vessels but with coronary risk factors, appear to be associated with an increased risk for future cardiovascular events (Fig. 33-6).[106] This appears to be similar to observations by Britten et al.[34] They found, in patients with normal or mildly diseased epicardial coronary arteries, an inverse relationship between the attenuation of the flow response to intracoronary papaverine and a higher risk of future cardiovascular events (Fig. 33-7).

These observations on coronary circulatory dysfunction or of an impairment of the total coronary vasodilator capacity as a predictor of cardiovascular events in patients with normal coronary angiograms or with only mild or subclinical CAD are, at first sight, in contrast to the more favorable outcome of a normal SPECT or PET stress/rest perfusion imaging study.[134–138] Cardiovascular events predicted by the presence of stress-induced perfusion defects on SPECT or PET normally occur within 2 to 3 years, whereas cardiovascular events predicted by PET-determined coronary vasomotor abnormality or by invasively determined measures of endothelial function in patients without epicardial flow-limiting lesions appeared in some studies to have occurred after longer time periods. Thus, it is possible that assessment of coronary circulatory dysfunction by PET may identify individuals without clinically manifest CAD but who may be at risk of developing CAD and its

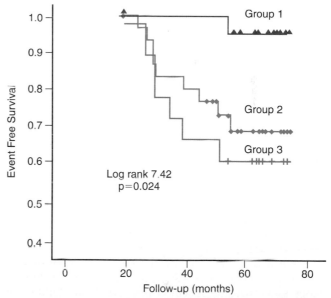

Figure 33-6 Prognostic value of PET-measured, endothelium-related myocardial blood flow responses to sympathetic stimulation with cold pressor testing (CPT). The Kaplan-Meier analysis demonstrates an association between the incidence of cardiovascular events and the degree of diminished myocardial blood flow (MBF) response to CPT (group 1: ΔMBF ≥ 40%; group 2: ΔMBF < 40%; and group 3: ΔMBF ≤ 0%). *(From Schindler TH, Nitzsche EU, Schelbert HR, et al: Positron emission tomography-measured abnormal responses of myocardial blood flow to sympathetic stimulation are associated with the risk of developing cardiovascular events. J Am Coll Cardiol 45(9):1505–1512, 2005.)*

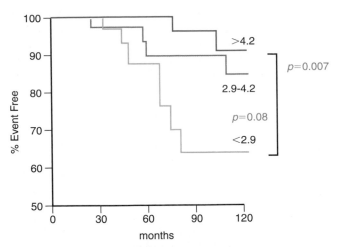

Figure 33-7 Coronary flow reserve as assessed by intracoronary Doppler and quantitative coronary angiography, and long-term prediction of cardiovascular events in 120 patients with angiographically normal or minimally diseased coronary vessels. Kaplan-Meier analysis demonstrating the proportion of patients without cardiovascular events during long-term follow-up according to tertiles of coronary flow reserve. *(From Britten MB, Zeiher AM, Schachinger V: Microvascular dysfunction in angiographically normal or mildly diseased coronary arteries predicts adverse cardiovascular long-term outcome, Coron Artery Dis 15:259–264, 2004. Reprinted with permission.)*

atherothrombotic sequelae. Such functional alterations of the coronary circulation also appear to be superior to CAD-related structural alterations of the epicardial wall in the prediction of future cardiovascular clinical outcome.[139-143]

Of further interest is that impairment in coronary circulatory function may be predictive of future cardiovascular outcome not only in individuals with early stages of the CAD process but also in patients with hypertrophic or idiopathic cardiomyopathy.[107,144] For example, Cecchi et al.[107] stratified the extent of diminished vasodilatory capacity during dipyridamole-stimulated and PET-determined flow increases in patients with hypertrophic cardiomyopathy, which reflected the severity of microvascular dysfunction to functional and/or structural abnormalities of the coronary arteriolar vessels. In 51 patients with hypertrophic cardiomyopathy, a clinical follow-up of 8.1 ± 2.1 years was performed.[107] The authors observed that the extent of reduced hyperemic coronary flow in these patients was independently predictive of death from cardiovascular causes, progression toward severe congestive heart failure, or sustained ventricular arrhythmias requiring the implantation of a cardioverter-defibrillator. Similarly, Neglia et al.[144] observed that in 67 patients with idiopathic cardiomyopathy, severe reductions in hyperemic myocardial blood flows during dipyridamole stimulation of ≤ 1.36 mL/g/min were independently associated with a 3.5 and 3.3 relative risk of death or development or progression of heart failure during a mean follow-up of 45 ± 37 months. These observations clearly suggest that in patients with hypertrophic or idiopathic cardiomyopathy, dysfunction of the coronary arteriolar

vessels may precede clinical deterioration,[70,107] although its diagnostic value and its impact on medical treatment remain uncertain.

Insights Into Mechanisms of Coronary Circulatory Dysfunction by PET

PET measurements of MBF at rest and during various forms of vasomotor stress have added important in vivo insights into mechanisms affecting coronary circulatory function, such as inflammation, vascular oxidation-reduction state in various conditions of coronary risk, insulin resistance, and obesity.

Vascular Inflammatory States

The CAD process is commonly characterized by low-grade inflammation affecting coronary vasomotor function and is associated with increases in C-reactive protein (CRP) serum levels, levels of soluble endothelial cell adhesion molecules, and procoagulant activity.[126,130] The exact mechanism underlying abnormal coronary vasomotion is certainly multifactorial, but it has been attributed in part to an imbalance of the redox equilibrium between endothelial-derived NO and ROS toward oxidative stress. Increases in oxidative stress in turn, apart from reducing the bioavailability of endothelial-derived NO associated with an impairment of endothelium-dependent coronary vasodilatory function, may lead to activation of a whole array of inflammatory genes such as nuclear factor κB (NF-κB), activator protein 1 (AP-1), or peroxisome proliferator, activated receptors (PPARs) involved in the pathogenesis of the CAD process. The inflammatory activation at the site of the arterial system is associated with the production of interleukin 6 (IL-6), which increases systemic markers of inflammation such as CRP.[130,145] Whether elevated CRP levels reflect an alternate mediator to CAD or an epiphenomenon of no pathologic consequence is a matter of ongoing experimental and clinical research. Several studies have demonstrated that increases in CRP serum levels correlated with the degree of endothelial dysfunction in both the peripheral and the coronary circulation.[31,54,146] Such findings suggest that inflammatory mechanisms might indicate, at least in part, the presence of endothelial dysfunction, providing an important link between inflammation and the development of atherosclerosis. Notably, PET flow measurements not only unmask the pathophysiologic consequences of elevated CRP serum levels on the epicardial conduit vessels[31] but also extend into the coronary microcirculation and, in particular, appear to contribute to the effects of coronary risk factors in the initiation and development of CAD.[54] The latter conclusion may also be supported by the independent value of elevated CRP serum levels in the predicting of future cardiovascular events.[147,148]

Smoking, Vascular Oxidation-Reduction State, and Hypertension

Noninvasive PET measurements of MBF have contributed to elucidating the complex relationship between the oxidation-reduction state of the arterial wall and coronary circulatory function.[44,65] For example, Kaufmann et al.[114] demonstrated that acute intravenous antioxidant intervention with vitamin C, given to reduce the oxidative stress burden in smokers, significantly increased hyperemic coronary flows during pharmacologic vasodilation, implicating ROS as a dominant cause of the attenuated total coronary vasodilator function in chronic smokers. In regard to the effects of hypercholesterolemia on coronary circulatory function, hyperemic flows during pharmacologic vasodilation were found to be reduced in individuals with familial hypercholesterolemia or with secondary hypercholesterolemia in comparison to age-matched controls.[149-151] Importantly, the hyperemic flow increases were inversely related to the severity of abnormal plasma lipid levels. The detrimental effects of elevated total plasma cholesterol levels on the coronary circulation are well known, but it appears that LDL cholesterol is also a major determinant of reduced coronary vasodilatory capacity, as observed with PET.[149] Another interesting observation is that a restoration of tetrahydrobiopterin (BH4) deficiency in hypercholesterolemic individuals restored the total hyperemic vasodilatory capacity of the coronary circulation.[112] BH4 deficiency may thus contribute to coronary circulatory dysfunction, most likely through an uncoupling of eNOS,[152] with further increases of ROS in hypercholesterolemia.

Of further interest is that the assessment of coronary vasomotor function by PET[53] unmasked distinct differences in responses of coronary endothelial dysfunction to short-term and long-term antioxidant intervention with vitamin C in patients with different coronary risk factors such as smoking, arterial hypertension, and hypercholesterolemia (Fig. 33-8). These in vivo findings

by PET[53] differed from those in other investigations, that proposed increases in ROS as a primary common pathway underlying endothelial dysfunction,[128,153] and suggested complex mechanisms accounting for abnormalities in coronary circulatory function in humans.[37] In chronic smokers, short-term and long-term antioxidant vitamin C challenges improved abnormalities in endothelium-related MBF responses to CPT, while no such beneficial effect was observed in individuals with hypercholesterolemia. Such observation may indicate that abnormalities in endothelium-related coronary vasomotion in smokers are predominantly mediated by the release of ROS, while other mechanisms appeared to prevail in hypercholesterolemia-related coronary endothelial dysfunction. For example, selective targeting of G protein–dependent signal transduction by oxidized LDL results in a diminished receptor-mediated stimulation of endothelial NO production[154] not affected by antioxidant intervention. Interestingly, although short-term vitamin C challenges did not lead to an improvement in coronary endothelial dysfunction in hypertensive patients, a normalization of the endothelium-related vasodilation was observed after long-term application of vitamin C for 3 months, which was sustained after a 2-year follow-up. The reason for the delayed onset of the beneficial effect of vitamin C challenges on coronary endothelial dysfunction remains uncertain; it may be related to an improvement of the endothelial redox equilibrium, resulting in an increased expression of eNOS or prevention of eNOS uncoupling through enhanced bioavailability of BH4.[152,155,156] Another PET flow study investigated the effects of deferoxamine, an iron chelator that inhibits the generation of hydroxyl radicals, on endothelium-related flow responses to CPT in type 1 diabetes mellitus.[116] Acute intravenous challenges of deferoxamine normalized the abnormality in endothelium-related flow responses to CPT, suggesting that ROS within the endothelium or in the subendothelial space plays a central role in mediating coronary flow abnormalities in type 1 diabetes mellitus.

More recently, PET flow studies also contributed to unmasking heterogeneous effects of drug interventions on endothelium-related coronary vasomotion. Naya et al.[157] studied 26 patients with untreated essential hypertension at baseline and after medical control of blood pressures with the angiotensin II receptor blocker (ARB) olmesartan or with the calcium antagonist amlodipine. The investigators demonstrated that only ARB inhibition improved endothelium-related MBF responses to sympathetic stimulation, while no such effect was observed for the calcium antagonist amlodipine (Fig. 33-9). The study further demonstrated that the elevation of superoxide dismutase (SOD) by ARB inhibition significantly correlated with the improvement of endothelium-dependent vasomotion in essential hypertension ($r = 0.61$; $P < 0.05$). These observations suggest that specific antioxidative effects of ARB inhibition, possibly mediated by inhibition of endothelial NADPH oxidase activation associated with a decrease in ROS or increases in antioxidative superoxide dismutase concentrations,[128] account for the improvement in coronary endothelial function in these hypertensive patients.

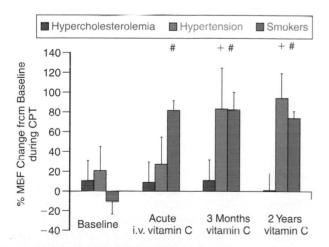

+ p ≤ 0.03 compared to baseline

Figure 33-8 Effects of short-term and long-term antioxidant intervention on endothelium-related myocardial blood flow (MRF) responses to CPT. The graphic demonstrates contrasting MBF responses to challenges in vitamin C in hypercholesterolemic patients, smokers, and hypertensive patients. *(From Schindler TH, Nitzsche EU, Munzel T, et al: Coronary vasoregulation in patients with various risk factors in response to cold pressor testing: Contrasting myocardial blood flow responses to short- and long-term vitamin C administration, J Am Coll Cardiol 42:814–822, 2003. Reprinted with permission.)*

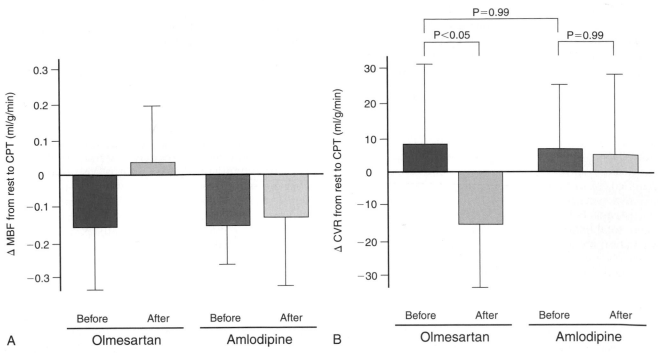

Figure 33-9 Effects of blood pressure–lowering medication in hypertensive patients on endothelium-related change in MBF from rest to CPT (ΔMBF) before and after treatment with olmesartan (n = 13) and amlodipine (n = 13) (**A**) and the corresponding ΔCVR (**B**). *(From Naya M, Tsukamoto T, Morita K, et al: Olmesartan, but not amlodipine, improves endothelium-dependent coronary dilation in hypertensive patients, J Am Coll Cardiol 50:1144–1149, 2007. Reprinted with permission.)*

Obesity, Insulin-Resistance, and Adipocytokines

Obesity, frequently associated with the insulin-resistance syndrome and systemic microinflammation, has been recognized as a risk factor of cardiovascular morbidity and mortality.[158] The exact mechanism by which obesity initiates and accelerates coronary vascular disease is still poorly understood. Coronary flow studies with PET demonstrated that insulin-resistant patients may present abnormalities in coronary circulatory function in the absence of traditional coronary risk factors.[113] In these individuals, the endothelium-related MBF response to CPT was diminished, while hyperemic flows during dipyridamole stimulation were preserved. Thus, abnormalities of coronary circulatory function in insulin-resistant individuals appear to be confined to the coronary vascular endothelium. It should be noted that initial stages of the vascular injury may only involve the endothelium,[54,84,111,159] whereas more advanced stages of coronary risk-factor states, such as increases in oxidative stress burden, may also lead to an impairment in smooth muscle cell vasodilator function.[152] For example, functional alterations of the coronary circulation in individuals with increasing body weight progress from an impairment in endothelium-dependent coronary flow response to CPT, to an impairment of the predominantly endothelium-independent hyperemic flows during dipyridamole stimulation in obesity (Fig. 33-10).[2] Similarly, Prior et al.[3] observed a progressive worsening of functional abnormalities of endothelium-dependent vasomotion with increasing severity of insulin resistance and

carbohydrate intolerance, while an attenuation of the total vasodilator capacity only became apparent in clinical type 2 diabetes. The observations are in agreement with earlier findings in type 1 and type 2 diabetes mellitus patients, with comparable reductions in hyperemic coronary flows.[160–165] These reductions in hyperemic coronary flows were also related to euglycemic control and were correlated inversely with plasma glucose concentrations averaged over several months.

PET flow studies combined with various plasma or metabolic markers of coronary risk factors and evaluated by univariate and multivariate analysis appear to be promising in teasing out adverse or beneficial effects of various factors on coronary circulatory function in complex in vivo conditions in humans.[2,44,166] Assessing coronary circulatory function in overweight individuals with PET demonstrated that an increase in body weight paralleled by an increase in plasma markers of insulin-resistance syndrome, and chronic inflammation was independently associated with abnormal endothelium-related coronary circulatory function.[2] These findings provided first evidence that obesity is indeed an alternate mediator of coronary vascular disease rather than an epiphenomenon related to other traditional coronary risks.[2,167] Of further interest is the role of various adipocytokines such as leptin, adiponectin, or ghrelin affecting the coronary circulation in humans.[168,169] For example, in in vitro studies, leptin released from adipose tissue may stimulate pro-atherosclerotic effects such as increases in ROS in cultured human endothelial cells, acceleration of vascular cell calcification, and smooth muscle cell proliferation and migration.[170] This is in

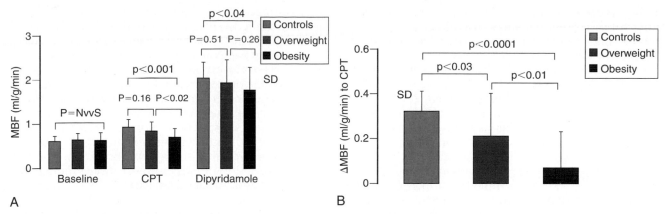

Figure 33-10 **A,** Myocardial blood flow (MBF) at rest, during cold pressor testing (CPT), and during pharmacologic vasodilation with dipyridamole for the three study groups. The dipyridamole-stimulated MBF was lower in overweight subjects than in controls but not significantly. In obesity, the hyperemic MBF during dipyridamole stimulation was lowest. **B,** Change of endothelium-related MBF during CPT (ΔMBF) for the three study groups. As can be appreciated, there is a progressive decrease of the endothelium-related MBF response to CPT from control to overweight and obesity. *(From Schindler TH, Cardenas J, Prior JO, et al: Relationship between increasing body weight, insulin resistance, inflammation, adipocytokine leptin, and coronary circulatory function, J Am Coll Cardiol 47:1188–1195, 2006. Reprinted with permission.)*

contrast to more recent findings of a leptin-induced improvement in both endothelium-dependent and independent vasodilation.[171–173] Notably, intracoronary infusion of leptin in humans with angiographically normal coronary arteries also may directly cause a coronary vasodilation of the conduit and arteriolar vessels.[173] In view of these contradictory observations, PET coronary flow investigations in obese individuals unraveled a significant and positive association between leptin plasma levels and endothelium-related flow responses to CPT ($r = 0.37$; $P < 0.036$). Thus, increases in leptin plasma levels in obesity were associated with relatively higher endothelium-related flow increases to CPT. These observations in humans appear to be in agreement with the reported beneficial effect of leptin substitution on endothelium-dependent and thus nitric-oxide-mediated vasoreactivity in obese leptin knockout mice.[174] The observed positive association between leptin plasma levels in obesity and relatively higher endothelium-related MBF responses to CPT in humans may indeed indicate a beneficial effect of leptin—and/or leptin-related but still undetermined factors—on the coronary endothelium to counteract the adverse effects of increases in body weight on coronary circulatory function.[2] Thus, in vivo imaging with PET may contribute to delineating important associations between coronary risk factors and coronary vascular states that may add to or even contrast with experimental findings to date. In this way, PET flow studies of human coronary circulatory function may also provide information that could aid in defining investigations of more specific direct cause/effect relationships.

DELINEATION OF CORONARY RISK AND MONITORING OF THERAPEUTIC STRATEGIES

According to the Framingham Heart Study,[175] individual persons with a high coronary risk profile (with diabetes or multiple coronary risk factors) are at risk for future cardiovascular events and can substantially benefit from medical intervention in primary and secondary prevention of coronary artery disease.[176–178] The National Health and Nutrition Examination (NHANES) put forth, however, that there is a wide range of individuals (about 40% to 50%) who are estimated to be at intermediate risk for cardiovascular events and yet are not necessarily considered for preventive medical intervention and/or lifestyle modifications.[179] These intermediate-risk individuals could benefit from further risk stratification with surrogates for subclinical CAD such as increases in carotid intima media thickness (IMT) by vascular ultrasound,[180] MDCT-determined coronary artery calcification (CAC),[69,93,181–183] and assessment of peripheral or coronary vasomotor function.[44,65,70,184] Functional measures of vasomotor abnormalities have the advantage that they precede early CAD-related structural alterations of the arterial wall[1] and appear to be more accurate in predicting future cardiovascular outcomes than structural alterations of the arterial wall.[139,140,184] Use of noninvasive methods for identifying and characterizing subclinical stages of the CAD process[44,69,93,185] could in fact lead to more effective primary and secondary prevention. Identification and characterization of functional and/or structural abnormalities of the arterial wall in subclinical stages of the atherosclerotic process in asymptomatic individuals at low or moderate risk could identify those individuals who are in fact at higher cardiac risk.[45,69,93,126,127,179] Whether these individuals would benefit from initiation of or intensified medical preventive therapy remains to be studied.[44,126,186]

Based on the central role of functional abnormalities of the coronary circulation in the development and progression of atherosclerosis, improvement of endothelium-dependent coronary vasomotion by a variety of interventions, such as angiotensin-converting enzyme-inhibitors,[187] β-hydroxymethylglutaryl-coenzyme A reductase inhibitors,[115,188] hormone replacement therapy in postmenopausal women,[111] euglycemic control in diabetes, and physical exercise,[189,190] has become a primary therapeutic strategy for prevention of the atherosclerotic process. Notably, Fichtlscherer et al.[109] reported that normalization of endothelial function of the forearm circulation in patients after an acute coronary syndrome was paralleled by an event-free survival. Similar findings were reported by Modena et al.[108] in hypertensive postmenopausal women. An improvement in brachial artery flow–mediated, endothelium-dependent vasodilation after institution of aggressive antihypertensive therapy resulted in an improved clinical outcome. Although low in numbers, these preliminary results support the evolving concept that improvement in vasomotor function in peripheral and coronary circulation in patients with CAD or at risk of developing CAD may indeed lead to an improved clinical outcome. If this holds true in future clinical studies, then the assessment of coronary circulatory function by PET imaging could be a promising and unique tool to successfully guide preventive therapeutic strategies.

Hormone Replacement Therapy in Postmenopausal Women

Postmenopausal women are commonly at increased risk of developing cardiovascular disease.[191,192] The exact mechanisms underlying the increased risk in developing cardiovascular disease in postmenopausal women have been related to changes in cardiovascular risk profile, such as the metabolic syndrome, insulin resistance, dyslipidemia, arterial hypertension, and deprivation of endogenous estroge, that commonly accompany menopause. Conceptually, insofar as abnormalities in coronary vasomotor function reflect an increased risk for future cardiovascular events, hormone replacement therapy (HRT) in postmenopausal women aiming to maintain or normalize coronary vasomotion should lead to an improved clinical outcome. PET measurements of MBF combined with CPT and pharmacologic stress, therefore, investigated the effects of HRT on coronary vasomotion in postmenopausal women. Long-term estrogen replacement in postmenopausal women without traditional coronary risk factors improved endothelium-related MBF responses to CPT. This beneficial effect, however, was not observed for short-term estrogen administration[111,193,194] or in postmenopausal women with traditional coronary risk factors.[111] Thus it appears that the presence of other coronary risk factors apart from the postmenopausal state may offset potential beneficial effects of HRT on endothelium-dependent coronary vasomotor function. On the other hand, it is intriguing to hypothesize that HRT may exert a beneficial effect on the coronary endothelium when coronary risk factors in postmenopausal women are controlled by medical intervention. Indeed, preliminary results in young postmenopausal women[195] suggest that HRT, in addition to standard management of traditional risk factors, may contribute to maintaining the functional integrity of vascular endothelium.

Regarding the effects of HRT on attenuated hyperemic flows during pharmacologic vasodilation, there is some evidence of a beneficial effect of short-term oral estrogen medication on hyperemic flows in asymptomatic healthy postmenopausal women as well as in symptomatic postmenopausal women, of whom the majority had coronary risk factors.[194] More recently, the effects of 17β-estradiol combined with the progestin, drospirenone on hyperemic flows in symptomatic postmenopausal women, and in part with other cardiovascular pharmaceuticals, were studied.[196] HRT with 17β-estradiol and drospirenone administered for 6 weeks was associated with an improvement of hyperemic MBF when compared to the placebo group. The latter observation[194,196] differs, however, from findings with other PET flow studies and HRT.[111,193,194] The reason for the contradictory observations of a beneficial effect of HRT on hyperemic myocardial blood flows in postmenopausal women remains uncertain but is likely to be multifactorial. For example, differences in the clinical characteristics of postmenopausal women studied, elapsed time after menopause, the state of altered vasomotor function, and/or differences in the use of progestins combined with estrogens could account for differences in the observed effects of HRT on hyperemic flow increases in postmenopausal women.

Responses to Lipid-Lowering Treatments

Multicenter trials have provided convincing evidence of primary and secondary prevention of cardiac events by long-term treatment with reductase inhibitors.[147,197,198] Notably, the beneficial effect in secondary prevention trials was observed despite minimal effects on the anatomic severity of coronary stenosis. Improvement in coronary endothelial dysfunction and stabilization in coronary plaques most likely account for the reported improvement in clinical outcome in hypercholesterolemic patients after long-term treatment with HMG-CoA reductase inhibitors. Several PET flow studies also investigated effects of HMG-CoA reductase inhibitors on diminished vasodilatory coronary capacity as a surrogate marker for early functional stages of developing CAD in hypercholesterolemic patients.

In one study, for example, repeat measurements of MBF were obtained in 51 asymptomatic young men with moderately elevated plasma cholesterol levels who were randomized with placebo or treatment. No significant effect on adenosine hyperemic blood flow was seen after 6 months of treatment with pravastatin (4 mg/day) (Table 33-4).[199] However, average values of hyperemic blood flow and flow reserve were normal at baseline. Post hoc analysis of 15 study participants with diminished hyperemic MBF at baseline (<4 mL/min/g), showed a significant 27% increase in hyperemic MBF and a similar increase in myocardial flow reserve. Similar improvements were reported in asymptomatic patients with familial hypercholesterolemia after 9 to 15 months of treatment with simvastatin (5 to 10 mg/day),[200] as well as in patients with normal or minimally diseased (<30% diameter narrowing or irregular luminal surface) coronary arteries after 6 months of simvastatin (20 mg/day) treatment.[188]

Table 33-4 Effect of Cholesterol-Lowering Treatment on Myocardial Blood Flow

		MBF AT BASELINE (ML/MIN^{-1}/G^{-1})		MBF AT FOLLOW-UP (ML/MIN^{-1}/G^{-1})			
	N	Rest	Stress	Rest	Stress	Change	P
Cardiovascular Conditioning							
Czernin et al., 1995[17]	13*	0.78 ± 0.18	2.06 ± 0.35	0.69 ± 0.14	2.25 ± 0.40	+9.2%	<0.05
HMG-CoA Reductase Inhibitors							
Huggins et al., 1998[213]	12†	0.95 ± 0.35	2.63 ± 0.41	0.83 ± 0.16	2.35 ± 0.64	−10.6%	NS
		0.73 ± 0.19	1.29 ± 0.33	0.74 ± 0.18	1.89 ± 0.79	+46.5%	<0.01
Guethlin et al., 1999[19]	15‡	0.70 ± 0.20	1.70 ± 0.50	0.70 ± 0.20	2.30 ± 0.90	+35.3%	<0.01
Yokoyama et al., 2001[208]	16§	0.77 ± 0.12	1.89 ± 0.75	0.75 ± 0.96	2.26 ± 0.85	+19.6%	<0.05
Baller et al., 1999[198]	23¶	0.87 ± 0.20	1.82 ± 0.36	0.92 + 0.19	2.38 ± 0.58	+30.8%	<0.001
Janatuinen et al., 2001[207]	23#	0.85 ± 0.27	3.61 ± 1.04	0.86 ± 0.23	3.79 ± 1.31	+5%	NS
	15**	0.82 ± 0.20	3.06 ± 0.47	0.81 ± 0.17	3.88 ± 1.34	+26.8%	<0.05

*Normal subjects and patients with coronary artery disease; 6-week course of exercise, cholesterol-lowering diet, and counseling.
**Only in 15 participants with hyperemic blood flow at baseline of less than 4.0 mL·g^{-1}·min^{-1} was there a significant improvement at follow-up.
†No significant effect in patients with coronary artery disease following 4 months of treatment with simvastatin on blood flow in remote myocardium, but a significant effect on blood flow in myocardium supplied by stenosed coronary arteries.
‡Improvements in myocardium supplied by normal and diseased coronary arteries.
§Patients treated with different statins.
¶Patients with hypercholesterolemia but without angiographically significant coronary artery disease.
#Asymptomatic young men with borderline elevated cholesterol levels.
Change, change in hyperemic blood flow; HMG-CoA, hepatic hydroxymethylglutaryl coenzyme A; MBF, myocardial blood flow; NS, not significant.

In these studies, the total cholesterol and LDL plasma cholesterol concentrations in asymptomatic individuals declined by 20% to 30% and 30% to 40%, respectively. Whether the improvement in coronary vasodilator capacity relates directly and quantitatively to reductions in total cholesterol or LDL plasma cholesterol concentrations is uncertain. The improvement in dipyridamole hyperemic MBF within 18 to 20 hours after plasma LDL apheresis suggests such a direct effect.[201] Plasma LDL concentrations in this study were high at baseline (194 ± 38 mg/dL^{-1}) and had decreased by 58%. Hyperemic MBF had increased by 31%. This observation of a significant improvement in coronary vasodilator capacity differs from findings of a delayed improvement in coronary vasoreactivity in patients with hypercholesterolemia who underwent 6 months of fluvastatin treatment (see Table 33-4).[202] After 2 months of treatment, total and LDL plasma cholesterol concentrations had decreased by 28% and 37%, respectively, but hyperemic MBF remained unchanged. When these patients were reevaluated after 6 months, no further changes in plasma lipid levels were noted, but hyperemic MBF had improved by 35%. Unlike the study with LDL plasma apheresis, the delayed increase in coronary vasodilator capacity in the fluvastatin study argues against a direct effect of plasma cholesterol lowering and suggests that the beneficial vasomotor effects of HMG-CoA reductase inhibitors may be independent of plasma cholesterol concentrations. Further, these findings suggest that the effects of reductions in plasma cholesterol levels are mediated by other structural and functional mechanisms. Because of the striking reductions in plasma LDL cholesterol concentrations in the LDL apheresis study, rheologic factors, rather than a direct effect on coronary

vasomotor function, may account for the higher postapheresis hyperemic MBF.[201] Consistent with this possibility is a statistically significant 6.3% decrease in plasma viscosity that would reduce resistance to flow and thus result in higher hyperemic blood flow. It is also possible that the delay in improvement seen in the fluvastatin study was associated with structural improvements of the coronary vessels that required time, e.g., decrease in intima media thickness, and improvement in the bioactivity of or (as postulated by others) down-regulation of angiotensin-II receptors on endothelial cells.[203-205]

Measurements of MBF in other studies also show improvements in hyperemic flow and flow reserve in patients with clinically and angiographically documented CAD.[202,206,207] These studies showed a beneficial effect on blood flow in myocardium subtended by angiographically normal and angiographically diseased coronary arteries. In only one study was the beneficial effect of HMG-CoA reductase inhibitors on hyperemic coronary flow increases confined to myocardial areas supplied by angiographically stenosed coronary arteries.[206] Because the improvement in hyperemic flow was restricted to myocardium subtended by obstructive CAD, an effect on microvascular capacity appears unlikely. Rather, an increase in flow-mediated coronary vasodilation at the site of coronary stenosis may be a possible explanation. Reasons for the lack of improvement in remote myocardial areas include the shorter duration of treatment with HMG-CoA reductase inhibitors (only 4 months compared with 6 months or longer in the other studies), and hyperemic MBF and flow reserves that were essentially normal in the remote myocardium at baseline.

Insulin Resistance, Impaired Glucose Tolerance, and Diabetes Mellitus

More recently, the effects of preventive therapeutic intervention with insulin-sensitizing thiazolidinedione on coronary circulatory function in insulin-resistant patients were studied.[113] The observed abnormalities in coronary endothelial dysfunction normalized with insulin-sensitizing thiazolidinedione treatment in 25 individuals with insulin resistance but without other coronary risk factors. These findings strongly suggest that insulin resistance possibly still has undetermined factors that affect coronary endothelial function. In view of these recent data, insulin-sensitizing pioglitazone application, added to conventional lipid-lowering therapy, did not only lead to an improvement in myocardial glucose utilization but resulted in an increase in resting MBF in nondiabetic patients with combined hyperlipidemia.[166] The pioglitazone-mediated improvements in myocardial glucose utilization and resting MBF in these study participants were associated with a significant decrease in plasma insulin levels; glucose levels, however, were not altered.[166] This might suggest that the insulin-sensitizing effects of pioglitazone accounted for the observed beneficial effects on myocardial metabolism and vascular parameter that go beyond those effects appreciated with conventional lipid-lowering therapy. As observed in the latter study[166] and also in type 2 diabetic patients, pioglitazone medication did not beneficially alter adenosine-induced hyperemic coronary flows.[208] A reasonable explanation for these inconsistent findings is still lacking[113,166,208] but may be related to differences in patient characteristics, differences in the duration of insulin resistance, co-medication, and/or differences in angiopathy and vascular smooth muscle involvement. Another explanation is that in insulin-resistant study participants, alterations of coronary vasomotor function were largely limited to the endothelium and had not yet altered vascular

smooth muscle cell function, as was reported for forearm blood flow measurements in individuals with CAD, new onset type 2 diabetes mellitus, and for the coronary circulation in individuals with increasing body weight or insulin resistance.[2,3,209] In more advanced stages of diabetes, a higher burden of ROS and/or greater abnormalities in LDL subfractions and LDL oxidation within the vascular wall may also directly impair vascular smooth muscle cell function and thereby cause an impairment of the predominantly endothelium-independent hyperemic flow increase.[208,210] The latter possibility may be supported by a recently observed association between PET-measured reductions in hyperemic coronary flows and structural alterations of the retinal arteries in more advanced stages of diabetes mellitus, while the hyperemic flow increase was still preserved in diabetic patients without background retinopathy.[211] The restoration of coronary and peripheral vasomotor function by insulin-sensitizing thiazolidinedione therapy in insulin-resistant and diabetic individuals,[113,166,209] however, may indeed reflect an important mechanistic link between increases in insulin sensitivity and an improvement in cardiovascular outcome in clinically manifest insulin resistance.[178,212]

Effects of glucose lowering therapy on coronary circulatory function in type 2 diabetic patients were investigated as well.[189] Three months of glucose-lowering treatment with glyburide and metformin significantly improved the coronary endothelium-mediated vasomotor function (Fig. 33-11A). The decrease in plasma glucose levels significantly correlated with the improvement in endothelium-related myocardial flow responses to CPT and thus an improvement in coronary vasomotor (dys)function ($r = 0.67$; $P < 0.01$) (see Fig. 33-11B). This association suggests a direct adverse effect of elevated plasma glucose, apart from the adverse effects of the insulin resistance syndrome, on diabetes-related coronary vascular disease in a preclinical state of CAD.

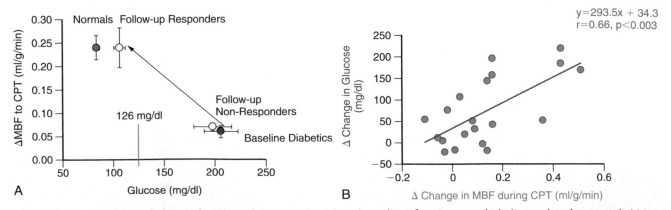

Figure 33-11 **A**, Effects of glucose-lowering therapy with glyburide and metformin on endothelium-related myocardial blood flow to CPT (its change from rest to CPT; ΔMBF) in type 2 diabetes mellitus patients. In type 2 diabetic patients with euglycemic control after 3 months of glucose-lowering treatment, with glucose plasma levels ≤ 126 mg/dL (group of responders), the endothelium-mediated MBF response to CPT significantly increased compared to controls. In patients with glucose plasma levels > 126 mg/dL (group of nonresponders), virtually no change in MBF to CPT was observed. **B**, Association of the endothelium-related ΔMBF to CPT and the change in fasting plasma glucose concentration as defined as difference in ΔMBF and ΔGlucose decrease between 3 months of follow-up and baseline measurements. *(From Schindler TH, Facta AD, Prior JO, et al: Improvement in coronary vascular dysfunction produced with euglycaemic control in patients with type 2 diabetes, Heart 93:345–349, 2007. Reprinted with permission.)*

SUMMARY AND FUTURE DIRECTIONS

Combining cardiac PET perfusion imaging with tracer kinetic models affords the noninvasive assessment of regional myocardial blood flow in mL/g/min which offers important in vivo insight into the complex nature of the mechanisms underlying functional alteration of the coronary circulation. Consequently, cardiac PET imaging may contribute to unraveling the pathophysiology of the early development of the atherosclerotic process. Such in vivo imaging with PET may identify important associations between coronary risk factors and the coronary circulatory function that may complement or even contrast experimental studies that investigate direct cause/effect relationships. By assessing myocardial blood flows at rest and during vasomotor stress and its myocardial flow reserve, the functional consequences of structural and/or functional alterations in the coronary circulation may be identified before hemodynamically significant obstructive CAD may manifest. As the identification of such early structural and/or functional abnormalities of the coronary circulation carries important diagnostic and prognostic information, it remains to be investigated whether preventive medical interventions aiming to restore or to diminish early structural and/or functional abnormalities of the coronary arterial wall will indeed result in an improved clinical outcome.

ACKNOWLEDGMENTS

Some sections of the manuscript are similar to sections of an extensive review of cardiac PET by Schelbert[213] and Schindler et al.[44]

REFERENCES

1. Reddy KG, Nair RN, Sheehan HM, et al: Evidence that selective endothelial dysfunction may occur in the absence of angiographic or ultrasound atherosclerosis in patients with risk factors for atherosclerosis, *J Am Coll Cardiol* 23(4):833–843, 1994.
2. Schindler TH, Cardenas J, Prior JO, et al: Relationship between increasing body weight, insulin resistance, inflammation, adipocytokine leptin, and coronary circulatory function, *J Am Coll Cardiol* 47(6): 1188–1195, 2006.
3. Prior JO, Quinones MJ, Hernandez-Pampaloni M, et al: Coronary circulatory dysfunction in insulin resistance, impaired glucose tolerance, and type 2 diabetes mellitus, *Circulation* 111(18):2291–2298, 2005.
4. Gambhir SS, Schwaiger M, Huang SC, et al: Simple noninvasive quantification method for measuring myocardial glucose utilization in humans employing positron emission tomography and fluorine-18 deoxyglucose, *J Nucl Med* 30(3):359–366, 1989.
5. Weinberg IN, Huang SC, Hoffman EJ, et al: Validation of PET-acquired input functions for cardiac studies, *J Nucl Med* 29(2):241–247, 1988.
6. Kuhle WG, Porenta G, Huang SC, et al: Quantification of regional myocardial blood flow using 13N-ammonia and reoriented dynamic positron emission tomographic imaging, *Circulation* 86(3):1004–1017, 1992.
7. Bergmann SR, Fox KA, Rand AL, et al: Quantification of regional myocardial blood flow in vivo with H215O, *Circulation* 70(4):724–733, 1984.
8. Nitzsche EU, Choi Y, Czernin J, et al: Noninvasive quantification of myocardial blood flow in humans. A direct comparison of the [13N] ammonia and the [15O]water techniques, *Circulation* 93(11): 2000–2006, 1996.
9. Bol A, Melin JA, Vanoverschelde JL, et al: Direct comparison of [13N] ammonia and [15O]water estimates of perfusion with quantification of regional myocardial blood flow by microspheres, *Circulation* 87(2):512–525, 1993.
10. Schelbert HR, Phelps ME, Huang SC, et al: N-13 ammonia as an indicator of myocardial blood flow, *Circulation* 63(6):1259–1272, 1981.
11. Schelbert HR, Wisenberg G, Phelps ME, et al: Noninvasive assessment of coronary stenoses by myocardial imaging during pharmacologic coronary vasodilation. VI. Detection of coronary artery disease in human beings with intravenous N-13 ammonia and positron computed tomography, *Am J Cardiol* 49(5):1197–1207, 1982.
12. Gould KL, Goldstein RA, Mullani NA, et al: Noninvasive assessment of coronary stenoses by myocardial perfusion imaging during pharmacologic coronary vasodilation. VIII. Clinical feasibility of positron cardiac imaging without a cyclotron using generator-produced rubidium-82, *J Am Coll Cardiol* 7(4):775–789, 1986.
13. Gould KL, Schelbert HR, Phelps ME, et al: Noninvasive assessment of coronary stenoses with myocardial perfusion imaging during pharmacologic coronary vasodilatation. V. Detection of 47 percent diameter coronary stenosis with intravenous nitrogen-13 ammonia and emission-computed tomography in intact dogs, *Am J Cardiol* 43(2): 200–208, 1979.
14. Krivokapich J, Czernin J, Schelbert HR: Dobutamine positron emission tomography: absolute quantitation of rest and dobutamine myocardial blood flow and correlation with cardiac work and percent diameter stenosis in patients with and without coronary artery disease, *J Am Coll Cardiol* 28(3):565–572, 1996.
15. Chow BJ, Beanlands RS, Lee A, et al: Treadmill exercise produces larger perfusion defects than dipyridamole stress N-13 ammonia positron emission tomography, *J Am Coll Cardiol* 47(2):411–416, 2006.
16. Go RT, Marwick TH, MacIntyre WJ, et al: A prospective comparison of rubidium-82 PET and thallium-201 SPECT myocardial perfusion imaging utilizing a single dipyridamole stress in the diagnosis of coronary artery disease, *J Nucl Med* 31(12):1899–1905, 1990.
17. Marwick TH, Shan K, Patel S, et al: Incremental value of rubidium-82 positron emission tomography for prognostic assessment of known or suspected coronary artery disease, *Am J Cardiol* 80(7):865–870, 1997.
18. Sampson UK, Dorbala S, Limaye A, et al: Diagnostic accuracy of rubidium-82 myocardial perfusion imaging with hybrid positron emission tomography/computed tomography in the detection of coronary artery disease, *J Am Coll Cardiol* 49(10):1052–1058, 2007.
19. Yoshinaga K, Chow BJ, Williams K, et al: What is the prognostic value of myocardial perfusion imaging using rubidium-82 positron emission tomography? *J Am Coll Cardiol* 48(5):1029–1039, 2006.
20. Chow BJ, Ananthasubramaniam K, dekemp RA, et al: Comparison of treadmill exercise versus dipyridamole stress with myocardial perfusion imaging using rubidium-82 positron emission tomography, *J Am Coll Cardiol* 45(8):1227–1234, 2005.
21. Bateman TM, Heller GV, McGhie AI, et al: Diagnostic accuracy of rest/stress ECG-gated Rb-82 myocardial perfusion PET: comparison with ECG-gated Tc-99m sestamibi SPECT, *J Nucl Cardiol* 13(1):24–33, 2006.
22. Groves AM, Speechly-Dick ME, Dickson JC, et al: Cardiac (82)rubidium PET/CT: initial European experience, *Eur J Nucl Med Mol Imaging* 34(12):1965–1972, 2007.
23. Bergmann SR, Herrero P, Markham J, et al: Noninvasive quantitation of myocardial blood flow in human subjects with oxygen-15-labeled water and positron emission tomography, *J Am Coll Cardiol* 14(3): 639–652, 1989.
24. Herrero P, Markham J, Shelton ME, et al: Noninvasive quantification of regional myocardial perfusion with rubidium-82 and positron emission tomography. Exploration of a mathematical model, *Circulation* 82(4):1377–1386, 1990.
25. Lin JW, Sciacca RR, Chou RL, et al: Quantification of myocardial perfusion in human subjects using 82Rb and wavelet-based noise reduction, *J Nucl Med* 42(2):201–208, 2001.
26. El Fakhri G, Sitek A, Guerin B, et al: Quantitative dynamic cardiac 82Rb PET using generalized factor and compartment analyses, *J Nucl Med* 46(8):1264–1271, 2005.
27. Lortie M, Beanlands RS, Yoshinaga K, et al: Quantification of myocardial blood flow with 82Rb dynamic PET imaging, *Eur J Nucl Med Mol Imaging* 34(11):1765–1774, 2007.
28. Huang SC, Williams BA, Krivokapich J, et al: Rabbit myocardial 82Rb kinetics and a compartmental model for blood flow estimation, *Am J Physiol* 256(4 Pt 2):H1156–H1164, 1989.
29. Lin JW, Laine AF, Akinboboye O, et al: Use of wavelet transforms in analysis of time-activity data from cardiac PET, *J Nucl Med* 42(2): 194–200, 2001.
30. Iida H, Kanno I, Takahashi A, et al: Measurement of absolute myocardial blood flow with H215O and dynamic positron-emission tomography. Strategy for quantification in relation to the partial-volume effect, *Circulation* 78(1):104–115, 1988.
31. Schindler TH, Hornig B, Buser PT, Olschewski M, Magosaki N, Pfisterer EU, Nitzsche EU, Solzbach U, Just H: Prognostic value of abnormal vasoreactivity of epicardial coronary arteries to sympathetic stimulation in patients with normal coronary angiograms, *Arterioscler Thromb Vasc Biol* 23(3):495–501, 2003.
32. Lerman A, Zeiher AM: Endothelial function: cardiac events, *Circulation* 111(3):363–368, 2005.

33. Suwaidi JA, Hamasaki S, Higano ST, et al: Long-term follow-up of patients with mild coronary artery disease and endothelial dysfunction, *Circulation* 101(9):948–954, 2000.

34. Britten MB, Zeiher AM, Schachinger V: Microvascular dysfunction in angiographically normal or mildly diseased coronary arteries predicts adverse cardiovascular long-term outcome, *Coron Artery Dis* 15(5):259–264, 2004.

35. Schachinger V, Britten MB, Zeiher AM: Prognostic impact of coronary vasodilator dysfunction on adverse long-term outcome of coronary heart disease, *Circulation* 101(16):1899–1906, 2000.

36. Halcox JP, Schenke WH, Zalos G, et al: Prognostic value of coronary vascular endothelial dysfunction, *Circulation* 106(6):653–658, 2002.

37. Drexler H: Endothelial dysfunction: clinical implications, *Prog Cardiovasc Dis* 39(4):287–324, 1997.

38. Drexler H, Zeiher AM, Wollschlager H, et al: Flow-dependent coronary artery dilatation in humans, *Circulation* 80(3):466–474, 1989.

39. Zeiher AM, Drexler H, Saurbier B, et al: Endothelium-mediated coronary blood flow modulation in humans. Effects of age, atherosclerosis, hypercholesterolemia, and hypertension, *J Clin Invest* 92(2):652–662, 1993.

40. Zeiher A.M., Drexler H., Wollschlager H., et al: Modulation of coronary vasomotor tone in humans. Progressive endothelial dysfunction with different early stages of coronary atherosclerosis, *Circulation* 83(2):391–401.

41. Zeiher AM, Krause T, Schachinger V, et al: Impaired endothelium-dependent vasodilation of coronary resistance vessels is associated with exercise-induced myocardial ischemia, *Circulation* 91(9):2345–2352, 1995.

42. Cox DA, Vita JA, Treasure CB, et al: Atherosclerosis impairs flow-mediated dilation of coronary arteries in humans, *Circulation* 80(3):458–465, 1989.

43. Gordon JB, Ganz P, Nabel EG, et al: Atherosclerosis influences the vasomotor response of epicardial coronary arteries to exercise, *J Clin Invest* 83(6):1946–1952, 1989.

44. Schindler TH, Zhang XL, Vincenti G, et al: Role of PET in the evaluation and understanding of coronary physiology, *J Nucl Cardiol* 14(4):589–603, 2007.

45. Cohn JN, Quyyumi AA, Hollenberg NK, et al: Surrogate markers for cardiovascular disease: functional markers, *Circulation* 109(25 Suppl 1):IV31–IV46, 2004.

46. Schindler TH, Nitzsche EU, Olschewski M, et al: PET-Measured Responses of MBF to Cold Pressor Testing Correlate with Indices of coronary vasomotion on quantitative coronary angiography, *J Nucl Med* 45(3):419–428, 2004.

47. Ludmer PL, Selwyn AP, Shook TL, et al: Paradoxical vasoconstriction induced by acetylcholine in atherosclerotic coronary arteries, *N Engl J Med* 315(17):1046–1051, 1986.

48. Zeiher AM, Drexler H, Wollschlager H: Endothelial dysfunction of the coronary microvasculature is associated with coronary blood flow regulation in patients with early atherosclerosis, *Circulation* 84(5):1984–1992, 1991.

49. Nitenberg A, Ledoux S, Valensi P, et al: Impairment of coronary microvascular dilation in response to cold pressor–induced sympathetic stimulation in type 2 diabetic patients with abnormal stress thallium imaging, *Diabetes* 50(5):1180–1185, 2001.

50. Dimmeler S, Fleming I, Fisslthaler B, et al: Activation of nitric oxide synthase in endothelial cells by Akt-dependent phosphorylation, *Nature* 399(6736):601–605, 1999.

51. Dimmeler S, Zeiher AM: Exercise and cardiovascular health: get active to "AKTivate" your endothelial nitric oxide synthase, *Circulation* 107(25):3118–3120, 2003.

52. Zeiher AM, Drexler H, Wollschlaeger H, et al: Coronary vasomotion in response to sympathetic stimulation in humans: importance of the functional integrity of the endothelium, *J Am Coll Cardiol* 14(5):1181–1190, 1989.

53. Schindler TH, Nitzsche EU, Munzel T, et al: Coronary vasoregulation in patients with various risk factors in response to cold pressor testing: contrasting myocardial blood flow responses to short- and long-term vitamin C administration, *J Am Coll Cardiol* 42(5):814–822, 2003.

54. Schindler TH, Nitzsche EU, Olschewski M, et al: Chronic inflammation and impaired coronary vasoreactivity in patients with coronary risk factors, *Circulation* 110(9):1069–1075, 2004.

55. Zeiher AM, Drexler H: Coronary hemodynamic determinants of epicardial artery vasomotor responses during sympathetic stimulation in humans, *Basic Res Cardiol* 86(Suppl 2):203–213, 1991.

56. Rossen JD, Quillen JE, Lopez AG, et al: Comparison of coronary vasodilation with intravenous dipyridamole and adenosine, *J Am Coll Cardiol* 18(2):485–491, 1991.

57. Chareonthaitawee P, Kaufmann PA, Rimoldi O, et al: Heterogeneity of resting and hyperemic myocardial blood flow in healthy humans, *Cardiovasc Res* 50(1):151–161, 2001.

58. Czernin J, Muller P, Chan S, et al: Influence of age and hemodynamics on myocardial blood flow and flow reserve, *Circulation* 88(1):62–69, 1993.

59. Tamaki N, Yonekura Y, Senda M, et al: Myocardial positron computed tomography with 13N-ammonia at rest and during exercise, *Eur J Nucl Med* 11(6–7):246–251, 1985.

60. Senneff MJ, Geltman EM, Bergmann SR: Noninvasive delineation of the effects of moderate aging on myocardial perfusion, *J Nucl Med* 32(11):2037–2042, 1991.

61. Prior JO, Schindler TH, Facta AD, et al: Determinants of myocardial blood flow response to cold pressor testing and pharmacologic vasodilation in healthy humans, *Eur J Nucl Med Mol Imaging* 34(1):20–27, 2007.

62. Sawada S, Muzik O, Beanlands RS, et al: Interobserver and interstudy variability of myocardial blood flow and flow-reserve measurements with nitrogen 13 ammonia-labeled positron emission tomography, *J Nucl Cardiol* 2(5):413–422, 1995.

63. Krivokapich J, Smith GT, Huang SC, et al: 13N ammonia myocardial imaging at rest and with exercise in normal volunteers. Quantification of absolute myocardial perfusion with dynamic positron emission tomography, *Circulation* 80(5):1328–1337, 1989.

64. Duvernoy CS, Meyer C, Seifert-Klauss V, et al: Gender differences in myocardial blood flow dynamics: lipid profile and hemodynamic effects, *J Am Coll Cardiol* 33(2):463–470, 1999.

65. Kaufmann PA, Camici PG: Myocardial blood flow measurement by PET: technical aspects and clinical applications, *J Nucl Med* 46(1):75–88, 2005.

66. Wyss CA, Koepfli P, Mikolajczyk K, et al: Bicycle exercise stress in PET for assessment of coronary flow reserve: repeatability and comparison with adenosine stress, *J Nucl Med* 44(2):146–154, 2003.

67. Namdar M, Koepfli P, Grathwohl R, et al: Caffeine decreases exercise-induced myocardial flow reserve, *J Am Coll Cardiol* 47(2):405–410, 2006.

68. Jagathesan R, Barnes E, Rosen SD, et al: Comparison of myocardial blood flow and coronary flow reserve during dobutamine and adenosine stress: Implications for pharmacologic stress testing in coronary artery disease, *J Nucl Cardiol* 13(3):324–332, 2006.

69. Di Carli MF, Hachamovitch R: New technology for noninvasive evaluation of coronary artery disease, *Circulation* 115(11):1464–1480, 2007.

70. Camici PG, Crea F: Coronary microvascular dysfunction, *N Engl J Med* 356(8):830–840, 2007.

71. Alexanderson E, Cruz P, Vargas A, et al: Endothelial dysfunction in patients with antiphospholipid syndrome assessed with positron emission tomography, *J Nucl Cardiol* 14(4):566–572, 2007.

72. Hernandez-Pampaloni M, Keng FY, Kudo T, et al: Abnormal longitudinal, base-to-apex myocardial perfusion gradient by quantitative blood flow measurements in patients with coronary risk factors, *Circulation* 104(5):527–532, 2001.

73. Schindler TH, Facta AD, Prior JO, et al: PET-measured heterogeneity in longitudinal myocardial blood flow in response to sympathetic and pharmacologic stress as a non-invasive probe of epicardial vasomotor dysfunction, *Eur J Nucl Med Mol Imaging* 33(10):1140–1149, 2006.

74. Kaufmann PA, Gnecchi-Ruscone T, Yap JT, et al: Assessment of the reproducibility of baseline and hyperemic myocardial blood flow measurements with 15O-labeled water and PET, *J Nucl Med* 40(11):1848–1856, 1999.

75. Go V, Bhatt MR, Hendel RC: The diagnostic and prognostic value of ECG-gated SPECT myocardial perfusion imaging, *J Nucl Med* 45(5):912–921, 2004.

76. Kubo S, Tadamura E, Toyoda H, et al: Effect of caffeine intake on myocardial hyperemic flow induced by adenosine triphosphate and dipyridamole, *J Nucl Med* 45(5):730–738, 2004.

77. Buus NH, Bottcher M, Hermansen F, et al: Influence of nitric oxide synthase and adrenergic inhibition on adenosine-induced myocardial hyperemia, *Circulation* 104(19):2305–2310, 2001.

78. Tawakol A, Forgione MA, Stuehlinger M, et al: Homocysteine impairs coronary microvascular dilator function in humans, *J Am Coll Cardiol* 40(6):1051–1058, 2002.

79. Coffman JD, Gregg DE: Reactive hyperemia characteristics of the myocardium, *Am J Physiol* 199:1143–1149, 1960.

80. Mosher P, Ross J Jr, McFate PA, et al: Control of coronary blood flow by an autoregulatory mechanism, *Circ Res* 14:250–259, 1964.

81. Morita K, Tsukamoto T, Naya M, et al: Smoking cessation normalizes coronary endothelial vasomotor response assessed with 15O-water and PET in healthy young smokers, *J Nucl Med* 47(12):1914–1920, 2006.

82. Tsukamoto T, Morita K, Naya M, et al: Myocardial flow reserve is influenced by both coronary artery stenosis severity and coronary risk factors in patients with suspected coronary artery disease, *Eur J Nucl Med Mol Imaging* 33(10):1150–1156, 2006.

83. Nabel EG, Ganz P, Gordon JB, et al: Dilation of normal and constriction of atherosclerotic coronary arteries caused by the cold pressor test, *Circulation* 77(1):43–52, 1988.

84. Campisi R, Czernin J, Schoder H, et al: L-Arginine normalizes coronary vasomotion in long-term smokers, *Circulation* 99(4):491–497, 1999.

85. Sato A, Terata K, Miura H, et al: Mechanism of vasodilation to adenosine in coronary arterioles from patients with heart disease, *Am J Physiol Heart Circ Physiol* 288(4):H1633–H1640, 2005.

86. Schindler TH, Schelbert HR: Measurements of myocardial blood flow and monitoring therapy. In Zaret BL, Beller GA, editors: *Nuclear Cardiology: State of the Art and Future Directions*, ed 3, Philadelphia, 2005, Mosby, pp 399–412.

87. Gould KL, Lipscomb K, Calvert C: Compensatory changes of the distal coronary vascular bed during progressive coronary constriction, *Circulation* 51(6):1085–1094, 1975.

88. Di Carli M, Czernin J, Hoh CK, et al: Relation among stenosis severity, myocardial blood flow, and flow reserve in patients with coronary artery disease, *Circulation* 91(7):1944–1951, 1995.

89. Beanlands RS, Muzik O, Melon P, et al: Noninvasive quantification of regional myocardial flow reserve in patients with coronary atherosclerosis using nitrogen-13 ammonia positron emission tomography. Determination of extent of altered vascular reactivity, *J Am Coll Cardiol* 26(6):1465–1475, 1995.

90. Uren NG, Melin JA, De Bruyne B, et al: Relation between myocardial blood flow and the severity of coronary-artery stenosis, *N Engl J Med* 330(25):1782–1788, 1994.

91. Kern MJ: Coronary physiology revisited: practical insights from the cardiac catheterization laboratory, *Circulation* 101(11):1344–1351, 2000.

92. Gould KL, Lipscomb K: Effects of coronary stenoses on coronary flow reserve and resistance, *Am J Cardiol* 34(1):48–55, 1974.

93. Di Carli MF, Dorbala S, Hachamovitch R: Integrated cardiac PET-CT for the diagnosis and management of CAD, *J Nucl Cardiol* 13(2):139–144, 2006.

94. Gould KL, Nakagawa Y, Nakagawa K, et al: Frequency and clinical implications of fluid dynamically significant diffuse coronary artery disease manifest as graded, longitudinal, base-to-apex myocardial perfusion abnormalities by noninvasive positron emission tomography, *Circulation* 101(16):1931–1939, 2000.

95. Gould KL: Assessing progression or regression of CAD: the role of perfusion imaging, *J Nucl Cardiol* 12(6):625–638, 2005.

96. Graf S, Khorsand A, Gwechenberger M, et al: Typical chest pain and normal coronary angiogram: cardiac risk factor analysis versus PET for detection of microvascular disease, *J Nucl Med* 48(2):175–181, 2007.

97. Johnson NP, Gould KL: Clinical evaluation of a new concept: resting myocardial perfusion heterogeneity quantified by Markovian analysis of PET identifies coronary microvascular dysfunction and early atherosclerosis in 1,034 subjects, *J Nucl Med* 46(9):1427–1437, 2005.

98. Schindler TH, Facta AD, Prior JO, et al: Structural alterations of the coronary arterial wall are associated with myocardial flow heterogeneity in type 2 diabetes mellitus, *Eur J Nucl Med Mol Imaging* 36(2):219–229, 2009 (Epub 2008).

99. Schindler TH, Zhang XL, Vincenti G, et al: Diagnostic value of PET-measured heterogeneity in myocardial blood flows during cold pressor testing for the identification of coronary vasomotor dysfunction, *J Nucl Cardiol* 14(5):688–697, 2007.

100. De Bruyne B, Hersbach F, Pijls NH, et al: Abnormal epicardial coronary resistance in patients with diffuse atherosclerosis but "normal" coronary angiography, *Circulation* 104(20):2401–2406, 2001.

101. Lim MJ, Kern MJ: Coronary pathophysiology in the cardiac catheterization laboratory, *Curr Probl Cardiol* 31(8):493–550, 2006.

102. Verna E, Ceriani L, Provasoli S, et al: Larger perfusion defects with exercise compared with dipyridamole SPECT (exercise-dipyridamole mismatch) may reflect differences in epicardial and microvascular coronary dysfunction: when the stressor matters, *J Nucl Cardiol* 14(6):818–826, 2007.

103. Schindler TH, Schelbert HR: "Mismatch" in regional myocardial perfusion defects during exercise and pharmacologic vasodilation: a noninvasive marker of epicardial vasomotor dysfunction, *J Nucl Cardiol* 14(6):769–774, 2007.

104. Sdringola S, Loghin C, Boccalandro F, et al: Mechanisms of progression and regression of coronary artery disease by PET related to treatment intensity and clinical events at long-term follow up, *J Nucl Med* 47(1):59–67, 2006.

105. Bonetti PO, Lerman LO, et al: Endothelial dysfunction: a marker of atherosclerotic risk, *Arterioscler Thromb Vasc Biol* 23:168–175, 2003.

106. Schindler TH, Nitzsche EU, Schelbert HR, et al: Positron emission tomography-measured abnormal responses of myocardial blood flow to sympathetic stimulation are associated with the risk of developing cardiovascular events, *J Am Coll Cardiol* 45(9):1505–1512, 2005.

107. Cecchi F, Olivotto I, Gistri R, et al: Coronary microvascular dysfunction and prognosis in hypertrophic cardiomyopathy, *N Engl J Med* 349(11):1027–1035, 2003.

108. Modena MG, Bonetti L, Coppi F, et al: Prognostic role of reversible endothelial dysfunction in hypertensive postmenopausal women, *J Am Coll Cardiol* 40(3):505–510, 2002.

109. Fichtlscherer S, Breuer S, Zeiher AM: Prognostic value of systemic endothelial dysfunction in patients with acute coronary syndromes: further evidence for the existence of the "vulnerable" patient, *Circulation* 110(14):1926–1932, 2004.

110. Papaioannou GI, Kasapis C, Seip RL, et al: Value of peripheral vascular endothelial function in the detection of relative myocardial

111. Campisi R, Nathan L, Pampaloni MH, et al: Noninvasive assessment of coronary microcirculatory function in postmenopausal women and effects of short-term and long-term estrogen administration, *Circulation* 105(4):425–430, 2002.

112. Wyss CA, Koepfli P, Namdar M, et al: Tetrahydrobiopterin restores impaired coronary microvascular dysfunction in hypercholesterolaemia, *Eur J Nucl Med Mol Imaging* 32(1):84–91, 2005.

113. Quinones MJ, Hernandez-Pampaloni M, Schelbert H, et al: Coronary vasomotor abnormalities in insulin-resistant individuals, *Ann Intern Med* 140(9):700–708, 2004.

114. Kaufmann PA, Gnecchi-Ruscone T, di Terlizzi M, et al: Coronary heart disease in smokers: vitamin C restores coronary microcirculatory function, *Circulation* 102(11):1233–1238, 2002.

115. Wielepp P, Baller D, Gleichmann U, et al: Beneficial effects of atorvastatin on myocardial regions with initially low vasodilatory capacity at various stages of coronary artery disease, *Eur J Nucl Med Mol Imaging* 32(12):1371–1377, 2005.

116. Hattori N, Schnell O, Bengel FM, et al: Deferoxamine improves coronary vascular responses to sympathetic stimulation in patients with type 1 diabetes mellitus, *Eur J Nucl Med Mol Imaging* 29(7):891–898, 2002.

117. Bengel FM, Abletshauser C, Neverve J, et al: Effects of nateglinide on myocardial microvascular reactivity in Type 2 diabetes mellitus–a randomized study using positron emission tomography, *Diabet Med* 22(2):158–163, 2005.

118. Schindler TH, Zhang XL, Prior JO, et al: Assessment of intra- and interobserver reproducibility of rest and cold pressor test-stimulated myocardial blood flow with (13) N-ammonia and PET, *Eur J Nucl Med Mol Imaging* 34:1178–1188, 2007.

119. Panza JA, Quyyumi AA, Diodati JG, et al: Long-term variation in myocardial ischemia during daily life in patients with stable coronary artery disease: its relation to changes in the ischemic threshold, *J Am Coll Cardiol* 19(3):500–506, 1992.

120. el-Tamimi H, Mansour M, Pepine CJ, et al: Circadian variation in coronary tone in patients with stable angina. Protective role of the endothelium, *Circulation* 92(11):3201–3205, 1995.

121. Nagamachi S, Czernin J, Kim AS, et al: Reproducibility of measurements of regional resting and hyperemic myocardial blood flow assessed with PET, *J Nucl Med* 37(10):1626–1631, 1996.

122. Siegrist PT, Gaemperli O, Koepfli P, et al: Repeatability of cold pressor test-induced flow increase assessed with H(2)(15)O and PET, *J Nucl Med* 47(9):1420–1426, 2006.

123. Bland JM, Altman DG: Statistical methods for assessing agreement between two methods of clinical measurement, *Lancet* 1(8476):307–310, 1986.

124. Jagathesan R, Kaufmann PA, Rosen SD, et al: Assessment of the long-term reproducibility of baseline and dobutamine-induced myocardial blood flow in patients with stable coronary artery disease, *J Nucl Med* 46(2):212–219, 2005.

125. Celermajer DS: Endothelial dysfunction: does it matter? Is it reversible, *J Am Coll Cardiol* 30(2):325–333, 1997.

126. Ganz P, Vita JA: Testing endothelial vasomotor function: nitric oxide, a multipotent molecule, *Circulation* 108(17):2049–2053, 2003.

127. Widlansky ME, Gokce N, Keaney JF, et al: The clinical implications of endothelial dysfunction, *J Am Coll Cardiol* 42(7):1149–1160, 2003.

128. Cai H, Harrison DG: Endothelial dysfunction in cardiovascular diseases: the role of oxidant stress, *Circ Res* 87(10):840–844, 2000.

129. Tomai F, Crea F, Gaspardone A, et al: Unstable angina and elevated C-reactive protein levels predict enhanced vasoreactivity of the culprit lesion, *Circulation* 104(13):1471–1476, 2001.

130. Faxon DP, Fuster V, Libby P, et al: Atherosclerotic vascular disease conference: Writing group III: pathophysiology, *Circulation* 109(21):2617–2625, 2004.

131. Topol EJ, Yadav JS: Recognition of the importance of embolization in atherosclerotic vascular disease, *Circulation* 101(5):570–580, 2000.

132. Berliner JA, Navab M, Fogelman AM, Frank JS, Demer LL, Edwards AD, Watson AD, Lusis AJ: Atherosclerosis: basic mechanisms. Oxidation, inflammation, and genetics, *Circulation* 91(9):2488–2496, 1995.

133. Brull DJ, Serrano N, Zito F, et al: Human CRP gene polymorphism influences CRP levels: implications for the prediction and pathogenesis of coronary heart disease, *Arterioscler Thromb Vasc Biol* 23(11):2063–2069, 2003.

134. Hachamovitch R, Hayes SW, Friedman JD, et al: Stress myocardial perfusion single-photon emission computed tomography is clinically effective and cost effective in risk stratification of patients with a high likelihood of coronary artery disease (CAD) but no known CAD, *J Am Coll Cardiol* 43(2):200–208, 2004.

135. Hachamovitch R, Hayes SW, Friedman JD, et al: A prognostic score for prediction of cardiac mortality risk after adenosine stress myocardial perfusion scintigraphy, *J Am Coll Cardiol* 45(5):722–729, 2005.

136. Beller GA: Cardiac imaging: value, cost, and appropriateness, *J Nucl Cardiol* 14(6):763–764, 2007.

137. Beller GA: Nuclear cardiology: where are we and where are we going? *J Nucl Cardiol.* 13(5):601–602, 2006.
138. Berman DS, Wong ND, Gransar H, et al: Relationship between stress-induced myocardial ischemia and atherosclerosis measured by coronary calcium tomography, *J Am Coll Cardiol* 44(4):923–930, 2004.
139. Rozanski A, Gransar H, Wong ND, et al: Clinical outcomes after both coronary calcium scanning and exercise myocardial perfusion scintigraphy, *J Am Coll Cardiol* 49(12):1352–1361, 2007.
140. Nishimura RA, Lerman A, Chesebro JH, et al: Epicardial vasomotor responses to acetylcholine are not predicted by coronary atherosclerosis as assessed by intracoronary ultrasound, *J Am Coll Cardiol* 26(1):41–49, 1995.
141. Schuijf J.D., Wijns W., Jukema J.W., et al: A comparative regional analysis of coronary atherosclerosis and calcium score on multislice CT versus myocardial perfusion on SPECT, *J Nucl Med* 47(11):1749–1755.
142. Madjid M, Toutouzas K, Stefanadis C, et al: Coronary thermography for detection of vulnerable plaques, *J Nucl Cardiol* 14(2):244–249, 2007.
143. Cury RC, Nieman K, Shapiro MD, et al: Comprehensive cardiac CT study: evaluation of coronary arteries, left ventricular function, and myocardial perfusion–is it possible?*J Nucl Cardiol* 14(2):229–243, 2007.
144. Neglia D, Michelassi C, Trivieri MG, et al: Prognostic role of myocardial blood flow impairment in idiopathic left ventricular dysfunction, *Circulation* 105(2):186–193, 2002.
145. Szmitko PE, Wang CH, Weisel RD, et al: New markers of inflammation and endothelial cell activation: Part I, *Circulation* 108(16):1917–1923, 2003.
146. Fichtlscherer S, Rosenberger G, Walter DH, et al: Elevated C-reactive protein levels and impaired endothelial vasoreactivity in patients with coronary artery disease, *Circulation* 102(9):1000–1006, 2000.
147. Blake GJ, Ridker PM: C-reactive protein, subclinical atherosclerosis, and risk of cardiovascular events, *Arterioscler Thromb Vasc Biol* 22(10):1512–1513, 2002.
148. Tracy RP, Lemaitre RN, Psaty BM, et al: Relationship of C-reactive protein to risk of cardiovascular disease in the elderly. Results from the cardiovascular health study and the rural health promotion project, *Arterioscler Thromb Vasc Biol* 17(6):1121–1127, 1997.
149. Kaufmann PA, Gnecchi-Ruscone T, Schafers KP, et al: Low density lipoprotein cholesterol and coronary microvascular dysfunction in hypercholesterolemia, *J Am Coll Cardiol* 36(1):103–109, 2000.
150. Yokoyama I, Ohtake T, Momomura S, et al: Reduced coronary flow reserve in hypercholesterolemic patients without overt coronary stenosis, *Circulation* 94(12):3232–3238, 1996.
151. Pitkanen OP, Nuutila P, Raitakari OT, et al: Coronary flow reserve in young men with familial combined hyperlipidemia, *Circulation* 99(13):1678–1684, 1999.
152. Munzel T, Daiber A, Ullrich V, et al: Vascular consequences of endothelial nitric oxide synthase uncoupling for the activity and expression of the soluble guanylyl cyclase and the cGMP-dependent protein kinase, *Arterioscler Thromb Vasc Biol* 25(8):1551–1557, 2005.
153. Munzel T, Keaney JF Jr, : Are ACE inhibitors a "magic bullet" against oxidative stress? *Circulation* 104(13):1571–1574, 2001.
154. Ohgushi M, Kugiyama K, Fukunaga K, et al: Protein kinase C inhibitors prevent impairment of endothelium-dependent relaxation by oxidatively modified LDL, *Arterioscler Thromb Vasc Biol* 13(10):1525–1532, 1993.
155. May JM: How does ascorbic acid prevent endothelial dysfunction? *Free Radic Biol Med* 28(9):1421–1429, 2000.
156. Heller R, Unbehaun A, Schellenberg B, et al: L-ascorbic acid potentiates endothelial nitric oxide synthesis via a chemical stabilization of tetrahydrobiopterin, *J Biol Chem* 276(1):40–47, 2001.
157. Naya M, Tsukamoto T, Morita K, et al: Olmesartan, but not amlodipine, improves endothelium-dependent coronary dilation in hypertensive patients, *J Am Coll Cardiol* 50(12):1144–1149, 2007.
158. Eckel RH, Daniels SR, Jacobs AK, et al: America's children: a critical time for prevention, *Circulation* 111(15):1866–1868, 2005.
159. Campisi R, Czernin J, Schoder H, et al: Effects of long-term smoking on myocardial blood flow, coronary vasomotion, and vasodilator capacity, *Circulation* 98(2):119–125, 1998.
160. Yokoyama I, Momomura S, Ohtake T, et al: Reduced myocardial flow reserve in non-insulin-dependent diabetes mellitus, *J Am Coll Cardiol* 30(6):1472–1477, 1997.
161. Pitkanen OP, Nuutila P, Raitakari OT, et al: Coronary flow reserve is reduced in young men with IDDM, *Diabetes* 47(2):248–254, 1998.
162. Di Carli MF, Bianco-Batlles D, Landa ME, et al: Effects of autonomic neuropathy on coronary blood flow in patients with diabetes mellitus, *Circulation* 100(8):813–819, 1999.
163. Di Carli MF, Janisse J, Grunberger G, et al: Role of chronic hyperglycemia in the pathogenesis of coronary microvascular dysfunction in diabetes, *J Am Coll Cardiol* 41(8):1387–1393, 2003.
164. Srinivasan M, Herrero P, McGill JB, et al: The effects of plasma insulin and glucose on myocardial blood flow in patients with type 1 diabetes mellitus, *J Am Coll Cardiol* 46(1):42–48, 2005.
165. Herrero P, Peterson LR, McGill JB, et al: Increased myocardial fatty acid metabolism in patients with type 1 diabetes mellitus, *J Am Coll Cardiol* 47(3):598–604, 2006.
166. Naoumova RP, Kindler H, Leccisotti L, et al: Pioglitazone improves myocardial blood flow and glucose utilization in nondiabetic patients with combined hyperlipidemia: a randomized, double-blind, placebo-controlled study, *J Am Coll Cardiol* 50(21):2051–2058, 2007.
167. Al Suwaidi J, Higano ST, Holmes DR Jr, et al: Obesity is independently associated with coronary endothelial dysfunction in patients with normal or mildly diseased coronary arteries, *J Am Coll Cardiol* 37(6):1523–1528, 2001.
168. Matsuzawa Y: Therapy Insight: adipocytokines in metabolic syndrome and related cardiovascular disease, *Nat Clin Pract Cardiovasc Med* 3(1):35–42, 2006.
169. Avogaro A, de Kreutzenberg SV: Mechanisms of endothelial dysfunction in obesity, *Clin Chim Acta* 360(1–2):9–26, 2005.
170. Bouloumie A, Marumo T, Lafontan M, et al: Leptin induces oxidative stress in human endothelial cells, *Faseb J* 13(10):1231–1238, 1999.
171. Vecchione C, Maffei A, Colella S, et al: Leptin effect on endothelial nitric oxide is mediated through Akt-endothelial nitric oxide synthase phosphorylation pathway, *Diabetes* 51(1):168–173, 2002.
172. Lembo G, Vecchione C, Fratta L, et al: Leptin induces direct vasodilation through distinct endothelial mechanisms, *Diabetes* 49(2):293–297, 2000.
173. Matsuda K, Teragawa H, Fukuda Y, et al: Leptin causes nitric-oxide independent coronary artery vasodilation in humans, *Hypertens Res* 26(2):147–152, 2003.
174. Winters B, Mo Z, Brooks-Asplund E, et al: Reduction of obesity, as induced by leptin, reverses endothelial dysfunction in obese (Lep (ob)) mice, *J Appl Physiol* 89(6):2382–2390, 2000.
175. Wilson PW, D'Agostino RB, Levy D, et al: Prediction of coronary heart disease using risk factor categories, *Circulation* 97(18):1837–1847, 1998.
176. Yusuf S, Sleight P, Pogue J, et al: Effects of an angiotensin-converting-enzyme inhibitor, ramipril, on cardiovascular events in high-risk patients. The Heart Outcomes Prevention Evaluation Study Investigators, *N Engl J Med* 342(3):145–153, 2000.
177. Randomised trial of cholesterol lowering in 4444 patients with coronary heart disease: the Scandinavian Simvastatin Survival Study (4S), *Lancet* 344(8934):1383–1389, 1994.
178. Dormandy JA, Charbonnel B, Eckland DJ, et al: Secondary prevention of macrovascular events in patients with type 2 diabetes in the PROactive Study (PROspective pioglitAzone Clinical Trial In macroVascular Events): a randomised controlled trial, *Lancet* 366(9493):1279–1289, 2005.
179. Verma S, Buchanan MR, Anderson TJ: Endothelial function testing as a biomarker of vascular disease, *Circulation* 108(17):2054–2059, 2003.
180. Graner M, Varpula M, Kahri J, et al: Association of carotid intima-media thickness with angiographic severity and extent of coronary artery disease, *Am J Cardiol* 97(5):624–629, 2006.
181. Hoffmann U, Ferencik M, Cury RC, et al: Coronary CT angiography, *J Nucl Med* 47(5):797–806, 2006.
182. Hoffmann U, Nagurney JT, Moselewski F, et al: Coronary multidetector computed tomography in the assessment of patients with acute chest pain, *Circulation* 114(21):2251–2260, 2006.
183. Schepis T., Gaemperli O., Koepfli P., et al: Added value of coronary artery calcium score as an adjunct to gated SPECT for the evaluation of coronary artery disease in an intermediate-risk population, *J Nucl Med* 48(9):1424–1430..
184. Chan SY, Mancini GB, Kuramoto L, et al: The prognostic importance of endothelial dysfunction and carotid atheroma burden in patients with coronary artery disease, *J Am Coll Cardiol* 42(6):1037–1043, 2003.
185. Husmann L, Valenta I, Gaemperli O, et al: Feasibility of low-dose coronary CT angiography: first experience with prospective ECG-gating, *Eur Heart J* 29(2):191–197, 2008.
186. Quyyumi AA: Prognostic value of endothelial function, *Am J Cardiol* 91(12A):19H–24H, 2003.
187. Mancini GB, Henry GC, Macaya C, et al: Angiotensin-converting enzyme inhibition with quinapril improves endothelial vasomotor dysfunction in patients with coronary artery disease. The TREND (Trial on Reversing Endothelial Dysfunction) Study, *Circulation* 94(3):258–265, 1996.
188. Baller D, Notohamiprodjo G, Gleichmann U, et al: Improvement in coronary flow reserve determined by positron emission tomography after 6 months of cholesterol-lowering therapy in patients with early stages of coronary atherosclerosis, *Circulation* 99(22):2871–2875, 1999.
189. Schindler TH, Facta AD, Prior JO, et al: Improvement in coronary vascular dysfunction produced with euglycaemic control in patients with type 2 diabetes, *Heart* 93(3):345–349, 2007.
190. Czernin J, Barnard RJ, Sun KT, et al: Effect of short-term cardiovascular conditioning and low-fat diet on myocardial blood flow and flow reserve, *Circulation* 92(2):197–204, 1995.

191. Gordon T, Kannel WB, Hjortland MC, et al: Menopause and coronary heart disease. The Framingham Study, *Ann Intern Med* 89(2):157–161, 1978.
192. Rossi R, Nuzzo A, Origliani G, et al: Prognostic role of flow-mediated dilation and cardiac risk factors in post-menopausal women, *J Am Coll Cardiol* 51(10):997–1002, 2008.
193. Peterson LR, Eyster D, Davila-Roman VG, et al: Short-term oral estrogen replacement therapy does not augment endothelium-independent myocardial perfusion in postmenopausal women, *Am Heart J* 142(4):641–647, 2001.
194. Duvernoy CS, Rattenhuber J, Seifert-Klauss V, et al: Myocardial blood flow and flow reserve in response to short-term cyclical hormone replacement therapy in postmenopausal women, *J Gend Specif Med* 4(3):21–27, 47, 2001.
195. Schindler TH, Campisi R, Dorsey D, et al: Effect of hormone replacement therapy on vasomotor function of the coronary microcirculation in postmenopausal women with medically treated cardiovascular risk factors, *Eur Heart J* 30(8):978–986, 2009.
196. Knuuti J, Kalliokoski R, Janatuinen T, et al: Effect of estradiol-drospirenone hormone treatment on myocardial perfusion reserve in postmenopausal women with angina pectoris, *Am J Cardiol* 99(12):1648–1652, 2007.
197. Collins R, Armitage J, Parish S, et al: MRC/BHF Heart Protection Study of cholesterol-lowering with simvastatin in 5963 people with diabetes: a randomised placebo-controlled trial, *Lancet* 361(9374):2005–2016, 2003.
198. Collins R, Armitage J, Parish S, et al: Effects of cholesterol-lowering with simvastatin on stroke and other major vascular events in 20536 people with cerebrovascular disease or other high-risk conditions, *Lancet* 363(9411):757–767, 2004.
199. Janatuinen T, Laaksonen R, Vesalainen R, et al: Effect of lipid-lowering therapy with pravastatin on myocardial blood flow in young mildly hypercholesterolemic adults, *J Cardiovasc Pharmacol* 38(4):561–568, 2001.
200. Yokoyama I, Yonekura K, Inoue Y, et al: Long-term effect of simvastatin on the improvement of impaired myocardial flow reserve in patients with familial hypercholesterolemia without gender variance, *J Nucl Cardiol* 8(4):445–451, 2001.
201. Mellwig KP, Baller D, Gleichmann U, et al: Improvement of coronary vasodilatation capacity through single LDL apheresis, *Atherosclerosis* 139(1):173–178, 1998.
202. Guethlin M, Kasel AM, Coppenrath K, et al: Delayed response of myocardial flow reserve to lipid-lowering therapy with fluvastatin, *Circulation* 99(4):475–481, 1999.
203. Kaesemeyer WH, Caldwell RB, Huang J, et al: Pravastatin sodium activates endothelial nitric oxide synthase independent of its cholesterol-lowering actions, *J Am Coll Cardiol* 33(1):234–241, 1999.
204. Laufs U, La Fata V, Plutzky J, et al: Upregulation of endothelial nitric oxide synthase by HMG CoA reductase inhibitors, *Circulation* 97(12):1129–1135, 1998.
205. Nickenig G, Baumer AT, Temur Y, et al: Statin-sensitive dysregulated AT1 receptor function and density in hypercholesterolemic men, *Circulation* 100(21):2131–2134, 1999.
206. Huggins GS, Pasternak RC, Alpert NM, et al: Effects of short-term treatment of hyperlipidemia on coronary vasodilator function and myocardial perfusion in regions having substantial impairment of baseline dilator reverse, *Circulation* 98(13):1291–1296, 1998.
207. Yokoyama I, Momomura S, Ohtake T, et al: Improvement of impaired myocardial vasodilatation due to diffuse coronary atherosclerosis in hypercholesterolemics after lipid-lowering therapy, *Circulation* 100(2):117–122, 1999.
208. McMahon GT, Plutzky J, Daher E, et al: Effect of a peroxisome proliferator-activated receptor-gamma agonist on myocardial blood flow in type 2 diabetes, *Diabetes Care* 28(5):1145–1150, 2005.
209. Sourij H, Zweiker R, Wascher TC: Effects of pioglitazone on endothelial function, insulin sensitivity, and glucose control in subjects with coronary artery disease and new-onset type 2 diabetes, *Diabetes Care* 29(5):1039–1045, 2006.
210. Tan KC, Ai VH, Chow WS, et al: Influence of low density lipoprotein (LDL) subfraction profile and LDL oxidation on endothelium-dependent and independent vasodilation in patients with type 2 diabetes, *J Clin Endocrinol Metab* 84(9):3212–3216, 1999.
211. Sundell J, Janatuinen T, Ronnemaa T, et al: Diabetic background retinopathy is associated with impaired coronary vasoreactivity in people with Type 1 diabetes, *Diabetologia* 47(4):725–731, 2004.
212. Erdmann E, Dormandy JA, Charbonnel B, et al: The effect of pioglitazone on recurrent myocardial infarction in 2,445 patients with type 2 diabetes and previous myocardial infarction: results from the PROactive (PROactive 05) Study, *J Am Coll Cardiol* 49(17):1772–1780, 2007.
213. Schelbert HR: Positron emission tomography of the heart: Methodology, findings in the normal and the diseased heart, and clinical applications. In Phelps M, editor. *PET: Molecular imaging and its biological applications*, New York, 2005, Springer-Verlag, pp 389–508.

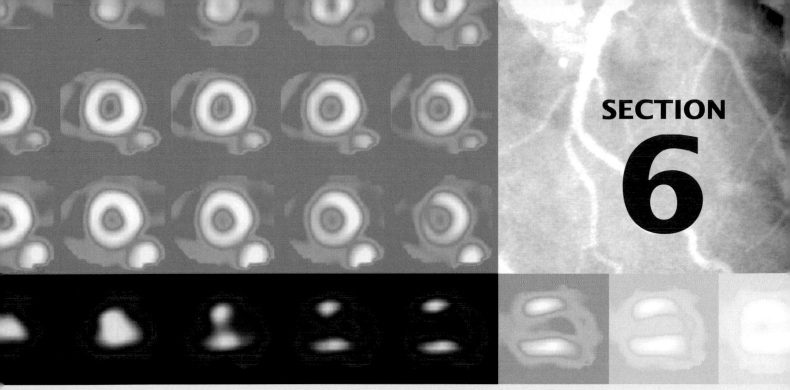

Acute Coronary Syndromes

Chapter 34

Imaging Patients with Chest Pain in the Emergency Department

MICHAEL C. KONTOS

INTRODUCTION

Patients with acute chest pain or symptoms consistent with myocardial ischemia involve a broad clinical spectrum of risk and are a common emergency department (ED) problem. This group accounts for approximately 8% to 10% of all ED visits and represents approximately 10 to 15 million ED visits yearly. At one end of the spectrum are those who have ischemic ECG changes indicating acute myocardial infarction (MI) or ischemia and require rapid pharmacologic and invasive diagnostic procedures and, when appropriate, coronary intervention. Effective implementation of treatments that can reduce the risk of subsequent cardiovascular complications in these patients requires timely and accurate identification.

At the other end of the spectrum are patients with atypical and noncardiac chest discomfort who can be safely sent home. However, these patients represent only a small minority of patients with potential acute coronary syndrome (ACS). The majority of patients presenting with chest pain have an initial evaluation that is insufficient to either diagnose or exclude myocardial ischemia, and thus further evaluation is required. This group accounts for nearly two-thirds of ED chest pain patients.[1,2]

Standard tools and techniques currently used for the evaluation of all chest pain patients include the ECG, the history, and myocardial markers. The ECG is the first test performed for the evaluation of patients with potential myocardial ischemia. Although the presence of ischemic ECG findings can identify patients who will benefit from more aggressive pharmacologic and interventional treatment, diagnostic ECG changes are present in only a minority of patients with ACS.[3] The history can be useful for risk stratifying patients into higher- and lower-risk groups, but in most cases, the substantial overlap prevents it use for determining who can be safely discharged from the ED.[3]

Another key component in the evaluation of chest pain patients are myocardial markers, particularly the troponins, which are considered the gold standard for diagnosing MI. Current recommendations are that all patients presenting with chest pain in the ED should undergo cardiac biomarker sampling, with repeat or serial sampling 6 to 8 hours later in those with initially negative markers (class I), with troponin being the preferred marker.[3] However, as with the ECG, there are important limitations. First, all markers have a time-dependent rise and fall from their release to detection in the bloodstream, which takes at least 2 to 4 hours after MI onset. Second, by definition, markers of necrosis require myocardial damage to be released; therefore, they will be negative in patients who have ischemia only.

Because of these limitations, the standard evaluation process for patients who have a nonischemic ECG and a low-risk presentation typically involves admission to a chest pain observation area where serial biomarkers are performed to exclude MI. If negative, the patient subsequently undergoes provocative testing (typically treadmill testing without imaging) and is discharged if negative. If any part of the evaluation is positive, the patient is admitted for further evaluation. This approach has limitations because a significant minority of patients have an intermediate likelihood of coronary artery disease, or an abnormal rest ECG, or are unable to exercise adequately,[4] limiting the number of chest pain patients eligible for an observational admission.

In an attempt to overcome these limitations, a variety of newer diagnostic techniques and tools have been evaluated to identify the few high-risk patients among the large number of low-risk patients in a rapid, accurate, cost-effective, and time-sensitive process. Advantages include early initiation of appropriate therapy in those with ACS, reduction in the inadvertent discharge of patients with ongoing ischemia, and shortened length of stay and reduced admissions for patients with noncardiac chest pain. The ability to do so has become increasingly important in the current setting of ED and hospital overcrowding, now commonplace in large urban centers.

Prior to implementing any new diagnostic tool or test, a number of features need to be demonstrated. These include the accuracy (sensitivity and specificity) of the test, the incremental diagnostic information it adds to that already available, and, increasingly important, its overall cost-effectiveness.

ACUTE MYOCARDIAL PERFUSION IMAGING

When patients develop ischemia, abnormal blood flow is the first event to occur, with the subsequent development of diastolic and systolic dysfunction, ECG changes, and lastly, symptoms. Because it provides a direct assessment of blood flow, myocardial perfusion imaging (MPI) is an optimal tool for identifying ischemia or infarction in patients who initially appear at low risk based on clinical and ECG criteria.

The first studies to evaluate the ability of rest MPI to identify ACS in chest pain patients were performed in the 1970s. Wackers et al.[5] found a high diagnostic accuracy when planar thallium-201 (^{201}Tl) imaging was performed in 203 patients admitted for possible MI. Images were abnormal in all 34 patients who had MI, as well as in 27 of the 47 (58%) patients who had unstable angina. (Fig. 34-1). In contrast, none of the 98 patients diagnosed with stable angina or atypical chest pain had abnormal studies. Others, also using ^{201}Tl in chest pain patients, subsequently confirmed these results.[6]

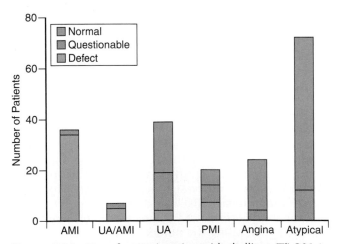

Figure 34-1 Use of acute imaging with thallium (Tl)-201 in patients admitted to cardiac care unit. Categorization of patients based on whether images were interpreted as having a defect, questionable, or normal. AMI, acute MI; UA, unstable angina; UA/AMI, unstable angina progressing to acute MI; PMI, previous MI. *(Modified with permission from Wackers FJ, Lie KI, Liem KL, et al: Potential value of thallium-201 scintigraphy as a means of selecting patients for the coronary care unit, Br Heart J 41:111–117, 1979).*

Although imaging of chest pain patients using ^{201}Tl appeared to be a promising tool, a number of limitations precluded its widespread adoption. Planar imaging has a lower sensitivity for detecting small areas of ischemia and ischemia in the posterior distribution, an area not often associated with diagnostic ECG changes. Because of its energy characteristics, relatively rapid redistribution, and imaging limitations in large patients, ^{201}Tl is not an optimal agent for acute imaging. Although some attempted to overcome the logistical problems by using portable gamma cameras placed in the ED,[7,8] these efforts were unsuccessful.

The development of single-photon emission computed tomography (SPECT) imaging, in combination with the availability of the technetium-labeled myocardial perfusion agents and their superior image quality, subsequently led to observational studies, followed by clinical trials demonstrating the utility of acute ED MPI. Technetium-99m (^{99m}Tc)-labelled sestamibi and tetrofosmin are taken up by the myocardium in proportion to blood flow, similar to thallium, but they lack significant redistribution.[9] Therefore, patients can be injected while experiencing symptoms and imaged up to several hours later, making it possible to perform high-quality SPECT imaging outside of the ED setting in the absence of dedicated equipment.

The favorable energy and dosimetry of ^{99m}Tc allows for gated reconstructions, an advantage not available at that time with ^{201}Tl imaging. The ability to quantitate ejection fraction[10] adds an additional prognostic component, identifying patients who may have unsuspected systolic dysfunction. More important, correlating wall motion and thickening with perfusion defects can be used to determine whether a defect reflects true ischemia or infarction or is the result of artifact or tissue attenuation.[11] In the setting of acute infarction or ischemia, wall motion is typically abnormal; in contrast, an apparent perfusion defect in the presence of normal wall motion and thickening on gated SPECT usually indicates an artifact such as tissue attenuation (Fig. 34-2). The ability to perform simultaneous wall motion and perfusion significantly improves specificity[12] and is particularly valuable in the acute setting where serial images are not available. Theoretically a patient could be injected during symptoms, and if imaged after symptom resolution, the wall-motion abnormality could resolve, and the defect could be misinterpreted as resulting from attenuation rather than ischemia. However, this appears to be infrequent in practice. Kontos et al. reported that for 2286 consecutive patients who were admitted for exclusion of ischemia following acute rest MPI, the proportion of patients who had troponin I (TnI) elevations (4.0 vs 3.5%), creatine kinase (CK)-MB MI (1.7 vs 1.5%), or who underwent revascularization (5.5 vs 5.2%), was not different between those who had normal perfusion and function and those who had perfusion defects but had normal wall motion in that area. In contrast, those who had perfusion defects associated with abnormal wall motion were significantly more likely to have TnI elevations (15%), CK-MB MI (10%), and undergo revascularization (17%) (Fig. 34-3).[12] A potential explanation is that the severity of ischemia

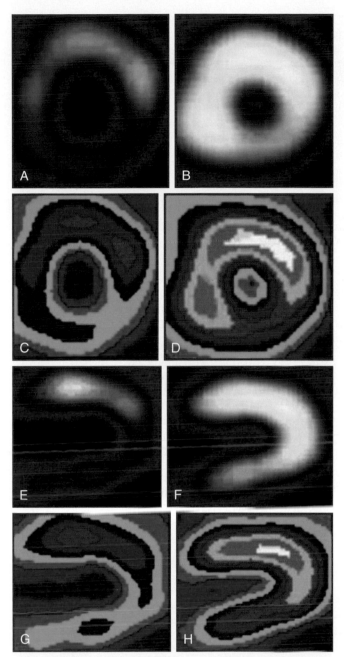

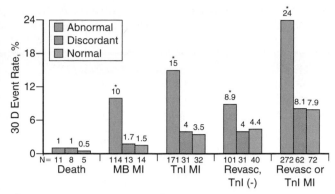

Figure 34-3 Comparison of 30-day outcomes based on initial myocardial perfusion imaging results in (**A**) all patients and (**B**) after excluding patients with prior myocardial infarction. There were no significant differences in patients with images interpreted as normal and discordant. For all end points other than mortality, both were significantly different ($P < 0.001$) when compared to images interpreted as abnormal. *Light bars*: abnormal; *gray bars*: discordant; *dark bars*: normal. * = $P < 0.001$ compared to discordant and normal. MI, myocardial infarction; Revasc, revascularization; TnI, troponin I.

DIAGNOSTIC VALUE

Sensitivity in Acute Myocardial Infarction

The first studies to demonstrate the high diagnostic accuracy using SPECT imaging with sestamibi for evaluating chest pain patients were performed in select populations of admitted patients. In a proof-of-concept study, Christian et al. performed early MPI in 14 patients without ST-segment elevation (most of whom had ST-segment depression) who were diagnosed with MI and who later underwent coronary angiography.[16] Abnormal studies were found in 13 of the 14 patients. The amount of myocardium at risk averaged 20% ± 15% (range 2% to 53%) of the left ventricle, and half had either the left circumflex or a ramus branch as the culprit artery.

In one of the first studies to evaluate ED patients, Hilton et al. imaged 102 patients who presented to the ED with typical angina and a nonischemic ECG.[17] Only 1 of the 70 patients with a normal MPI had an event, compared to 2 of the 15 with an equivocal MPI (13%), and 12 of the 17 (71%) with abnormal MPI. In a multivariate analysis, the only independent predictor of cardiac events was abnormal MPI.

Numerous subsequent studies that included single-center and multicenter observational studies, as well as a randomized trial, were performed in large numbers of heterogenous patients undergoing an ED chest pain evaluation. They consistently found a high sensitivity (90% to 100%) for detecting acute MI (Table 34-1). Because sensitivity is not perfect, the results of acute MPI cannot be interpreted in isolation but must be placed in context with the clinical evaluation. However, infarcts that are present despite normal acute MPI are typically small, non-Q-wave infarcts and associated with an uncomplicated clinical course.

In contrast to most diagnostic tools that have not been evaluated in a randomized trial, the ability to safely

Figure 34-2 Example of a patient with abnormal perfusion but normal wall motion and thickening in the inferior/posterior wall. In both the short-axis and long-axis slices, the perfusion defect is seen to thicken normally, especially on the step 10 color coding (each color change indicates a 10% change in thickening). Subsequent evaluation was negative for coronary disease. *Images*: short-axis: warm: (**A**) diastole and (**B**) systole; short-axis step 10: (**C**) diastole and (**D**) systole. Long-axis warm: (**E**) diastole and (**F**) systole; long-axis step 10: (**G**) diastole and (**H**) systole.

that occurs with an ACS event is associated with underlying myocardial stunning[13,14] and persistence of wall motion abnormalities.

The combination of perfusion and wall motion has prognostic value. In a recent multicenter study reported by Kaul et al., perfusion plus regional function provided significantly greater diagnostic and prognostic value when compared to perfusion alone for predicting outcomes in 163 patients with possible ACS.[15]

Table 34-1   Diagnostic Accuracy of Rest Myocardial Perfusion Imaging in Patients with Acute Chest Pain Syndrome and Normal or Nonischemic Rest Electrocardiograms

	Year	N =	Tracer	Sens	Spec	NPV	Endpoint
Wackers et al.[53]	1979	203	Tl-201	100%	72%	100%	AMI
Varetto et al.[51]	1993	64	Tc-mibi	100%	92%	100%	CAD
Hilton et al.[16]	1994	102	Tc-mibi	94%	83%	99%	CAD/AMI
Tatum et al.[47]	1997	438	Tc-mibi	100%	78%	100%	AMI
Kontos et al.[29]	1997	532	Tc-mibi	93%	71%	99%	AMI
Heller et al.[13]	1998	357	Tc-tetro	90%	60%	99%	AMI
Kontos et al.[28]	1999	620	Tc-mibi	92%	67%	99%	AMI
Udelson et al.[49]	2002	1215	Tc-mibi	96%	NR	99%	AMI
Schaeffer et al.[46]	2007	479	Tc-mibi	77%	92%	99%	ACS

AMI, acute myocardial infarction; CAD, coronary artery disease (angiographic); Sens, sensitivity; Spec, specificity; NPV, negative predictive value; NR, not reported; Tc-mibi, ^{99m}Tc-sestamibi; Tc-tetro, ^{99m}Tc-tetrofosmin; Tl-201, thallium-201.

discharge a patient after negative acute MPI was confirmed in the Emergency Room Assessment of Sestamibi for Evaluating Chest Pain (ERASE) study.[18] A total of 2475 patients were randomized to routine care or ED MPI, in which patients were injected with sestamibi in the ED and then underwent acute imaging, with the results called back to the ED physician.[18] All patients, whether admitted or discharged, underwent subsequent marker analysis and further diagnostic evaluation with either stress testing or coronary angiography. There was no difference between the two groups, in the percentage of ACS patients with MI (97% versus 96%) or unstable angina (83% versus 81%) who were admitted with one MI patient from each group discharged from the ED. However, there was a significantly lower admission rate and a higher rate of direct discharge from the ED in the ED MPI arm of the study compared to the standardized care arm. Importantly, this was a consistent effect seen at six of the seven institutions involved in the trial.

These results were confirmed in a subsequent smaller randomized trial. Candell-Riera et al. randomized 222 low-risk chest pain patients to either acute rest MPI or conventional management in the ED. Fewer patients undergoing rest MPI were admitted (18% versus 33%; $P < 0.03$), and overall ED time was shorter (13 ± 6 versus 16 ± 9 hours; $P < 0.01$).[19]

A limitation of the mentioned studies is that acute MPI was performed predominantly in low-risk patients, so relatively small numbers of patients who had MI were included in any one study, resulting in an imprecise estimate of sensitivity. To address this, Kontos et al. analyzed results from 141 consecutive patients who underwent ED MPI and were subsequently diagnosed with CK-MB MI.[20] Overall sensitivity was 89% (95% CI: 83% to 94%), consistent with prior studies but with smaller confidence intervals. Similar to prior studies, patients with negative MPI had small MIs, with an average peak CK of 313 ± 227 U/L, compared to 590 ± 620 U/L ($P < 0.001$) in those with positive MPI. In addition, nonsignificant disease was found in the majority of patients with negative MPI who sunderwent coronary angiography.

Acute Coronary Syndrome Without Myocardial Infarction

Although specificity of acute MPI appears low when MI is the only end point considered, this in part relates to one of its important advantages, the ability to identify patients who have ischemia alone. Bilodeau et al.[21] imaged 45 patients without a history of MI who were admitted for unstable angina. The presence of a perfusion defect had a high accuracy (sensitivity 96%, specificity 79%) for predicting angiographic coronary disease in patients injected during an episode of pain, compared to a sensitivity of only 65% for the ECG. In another study Kontos et al. found that in 532 patients admitted after acute rest MPI in the ED, acute MI, as assessed by CK-MB elevations, was present in only 15% of patients with positive MPI (Fig. 34-4).[22] However, the majority of patients with positive MPI had an end point consistent

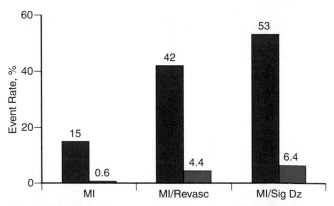

Figure 34-4   Outcomes associated with results of acute rest myocardial perfusion imaging (MPI). Patients with positive rest MPI *(dark bars)* had significantly ($P < 0.0001$) more myocardial infarction (MI), MI or revascularization (MI/Revasc), and MI, revascularization, or significant coronary artery disease (MI/Sig Dz) (>70% stenosis) than patients with negative rest MPI *(white bars)*. *(Modified with permission from Kontos MC, Jesse RL, Schmidt KL, et al: Value of acute rest sestamibi perfusion imaging for evaluation of patients admitted to the emergency department with chest pain, J Am Coll Cardiol 30:976–982, 1997.)*

with ACS, including acute MI, subsequent revascularization, or significant coronary disease (>70% stenosis) on coronary angiography. Considering these as positive end points improved positive predictive value to 53%.

NEGATIVE PREDICTIVE VALUE AND PROGNOSIS

The negative predictive value in clinical studies has been consistently high and has typically exceeded 99% (see Table 34-1).[18,23-26] The high negative predictive value for excluding significant ischemia allows effective identification of those who can be evaluated in lower-intensity settings other than the coronary care unit (CCU) or who can be discharged home. Patients with negative MPI have a low risk for both short- and long-term cardiac complications as well. Hilton et al.[17] found that patients with normal MPI had an excellent prognosis, with no late events at 90-day follow-up. Similarly, Tatum et al. reported that patients with negative acute MPI had a cardiac event rate of only 3% during the subsequent year.[26]

INCREMENTAL DIAGNOSTIC VALUE

In the current cost-conscious environment, even though a new test may offer high diagnostic value, an additional requirement before adoption is that it also provides significant incremental value over the current standard of care. Kontos et al. found that in a multivariate analysis, abnormal MPI was the most important independent predictor of MI or revascularization in 532 patients who underwent acute ED MPI.[22] Similarly, Heller et al. found that that abnormal SPECT was the most important multivariate predictor of MI in 357 patients who underwent acute MPI. In addition, acute MPI added significant incremental diagnostic value after consideration of demographic, clinical, and ECG variables (Fig. 34-5).[23]

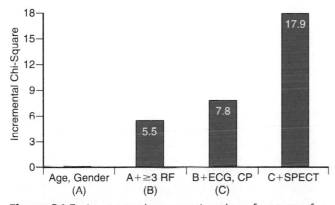

Figure 34-5 Incremental prognostic value of rest tetrofosmin SPECT imaging over clinical variables. Model **A**: clinical variables; model **B**: A + three or more risk factors (RF); model **C**: B + admission ECG and chest pain (CP) at the time of tetrofosmin injection. *(Modified from Heller GV, Stowers SA, Hendel RC, et al: Clinical value of acute rest technetium-99m tetrofosmin tomographic myocardial perfusion imaging in patients with acute chest pain and nondiagnostic electrocardiograms, J Am Coll Cardiol 31:1011-1017, 1998.)*

In an interesting intent-to-treat survey study, Knott et al. performed acute MPI in 120 ED patients.[27] The requesting physician completed a questionnaire before imaging, asking what the proposed management would be had the test not been available. They found there would have been a 34% reduction in overall hospital admissions and a 59% reduction in planned CCU admissions. Interestingly, overall CCU admissions were not reduced, because 17 patients initially considered low risk were admitted to the CCU after MPI was found to be abnormal, indicating a more appropriate utilization of resources.

COST-EFFECTIVENESS

Despite the application of relatively complex and expensive technology, ED MPI can be cost effective if the number of patients admitted is decreased.[23,28,29,30] Several observational studies have confirmed that cost reductions occur when rest MPI is used as an integral part of patient management. In addition, a preliminary analysis from the ERASE study confirms that using ED MPI as a key part of the initial diagnostic strategy was indeed cost-effective, since costs were reduced a mean $70 per patient.[31]

Costs are reduced by a number of mechanisms. One obvious mechanism is discharging more low-risk patients directly from the ED rather than the patient being admitted or undergoing a more prolonged observation. Second, by identifying patients with atypical symptoms and a nonischemic ECG who have MI, inappropriate discharges can be averted. A third mechanism is more appropriate selection of diagnostic procedures, reducing the rate of coronary angiography in low-risk patients.[27,28]

Comparison with Troponin

Because most of the studies evaluating the use of acute MPI were performed in the 1990s, CK or CK-MB were typically used to diagnose MI. However, because of its high sensitivity and specificity for detecting myocardial necrosis, current guidelines recommend that cardiac troponin should be the diagnostic standard for MI.[32] Since approximately 3% to 4% of the left ventricle must be ischemic to allow detection by MPI,[33] it would be expected that use of a more sensitive cardiac marker such as troponin would identify more patients who have necrosis than would acute MPI. This has been supported by a number of small studies that reported that although the sensitivity of MPI was high, it was significantly lower than that of TnI or TnT.[25,34] In a larger study, Kontos et al. analyzed outcomes in 319 patients who were initially considered low risk for ACS and underwent acute rest MPI as part of standard chest pain evaluation protocol. They subsequently were found to have elevated TnI values,[35] thus meeting the American College of Cardiology/European Society of Cardiology (ACC/ESC) definition for MI. A total of 77 patients had negative MPI, giving a sensitivity of only 76%. However, more than half (n = 47 [61%]) had a peak CK-MB of < 8 ng/mL and therefore did not meet the previous

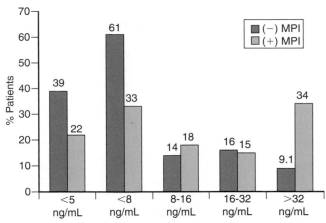

Figure 34-6 Proportion of patients with positive *(black bars)* and negative *(white bars)* rest myocardial perfusion imaging and levels of creatine kinase (CK)-MB elevations. Of 104 patients with CK-MB level less than 8 ng/mL, 61% had normal images, whereas of 192 patients with CK-MB greater than 8 ng/mL, only 27% had normal images (sensitivity 83%). *(Modified with permission from Kontos MC, Fratkin MJ, Jesse RL, et al: Sensitivity of acute rest myocardial perfusion imaging for identifying patients with myocardial infarction based on a troponin definition, J Nucl Cardiol 11:12–19, 2004.)*

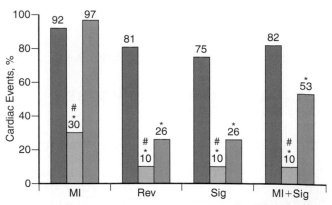

Figure 34-7 Sensitivity of myocardial perfusion imaging *(dark bars),* the initial troponin I *(open bars),* and peak troponin I *(light bars)* for identifying endpoints. * = P < 0.001 compared to perfusion imaging; # = P < 0.001 compared to serial troponin. MI, myocardial infarction; Rev, revascularization; Sig, significant disease (>70% stenosis). *(Adapted from Kontos MC, Jesse RL, Anderson FP, et al: Comparison of myocardial perfusion imaging and cardiac troponin I in patients admitted to the emergency department with chest pain, Circulation 99:2073–2078, 1999.)*

CK-MB MI definition (Fig. 34-6). Patients with negative MPI had significantly lower peak CK-MB values (15 ± 25 ng/mL versus 45 ± 78 ng/mL; P < 0.001), had higher ejection fractions (56 ± 15% versus 47 ± 13%; P < 0.01) and were more likely to have nonsignificant disease (45% versus 30%; P < 0.001) than those with positive MPI.

Rather than being considered as competing diagnostic tools, markers and MPI offer complementary information. Despite the higher sensitivity of troponin, rest MPI has some important advantages over using markers alone. By definition, myocardial markers are abnormal only in patients with necrosis and therefore are negative in patients who have ischemia alone. However, in both settings, perfusion will be abnormal. Second, after the onset of infarction, it typically takes a few hours before markers of necrosis can be detected in the bloodstream. Given the additional time for laboratory processing and reporting (blood-to-brain time),[36] this may be as long as 4 to 6 hours after MI onset. In contrast, despite the time required for imaging and processing, acute MPI results can be available within 1 to 2 hours after injection. Thus, the sensitivity of MPI is significantly higher than that of the initial troponin. These two advantages were demonstrated in a study of 620 consecutive patients who underwent serial marker sampling with TnI and CK-MB after having acute ED MPI performed. The sensitivity of TnI and MPI were similar for identifying patients who had CK-MB MI. However, sensitivity of MPI was higher when compared to the initial TnI, and was superior for identifying patients who underwent revascularization or who had significant disease on coronary angiography (Fig. 34-7).[25]

Another advantage of acute MPI is the ability to quantify risk area, which may be a better way to assess overall ischemic risk than markers alone. For example, two patients with similar low peak TnI values, one

secondary to occlusion of a small branch vessel, the other resulting from a brief occlusion of the proximal portion of a major vessel, have markedly different areas at risk and the potential for significantly different outcomes, which can be readily determined using MPI (discussed next).

RISK AREA

An important prognostic parameter provided by acute MPI is that it provides quantitative information on the ischemic risk area in ACS patients. The most important determinant of infarct size is the ischemic risk zone, or the amount of myocardium in jeopardy.[37] The ischemic risk area is a validated measure of prognosis; patients with larger defects have a worse long-term prognosis.[38,39] The ischemic risk area in patients with non-ST-elevation ACS is often large, even in the absence of ischemic ECG changes. Kontos et al.[40] reported that in a group of 87 patients diagnosed with MI after undergoing ED acute MPI, the ischemic risk area ranged from 0% to 62% of the left ventricle, with a mean risk area of 18% ± 11%. These results were similar to those reported by Christian et al.[16] in the initial group of 14 patients studied. Patients with normal ECGs at the time of presentation had risk areas similar to those of patients with abnormal but nonischemic ECGs (16% ± 12% versus 19% ± 12%; P = 0.25).[41]

In a follow-up study, 69 patients who had acute MPI in the ED were diagnosed with MI and subsequently underwent repeat MPI.[42] The initial risk area was 19% ± 9.7% of the left ventricle. Only two patients had a risk area = 6%. When performed, revascularization occurred more than 9 hours after presentation (mean time 3.0 ± 3.5 days [median 2 days]). Repeat MPI was performed a median of 5 days after acute MPI. The amount of salvage averaged 45% ± 34%, although variations in area at risk,

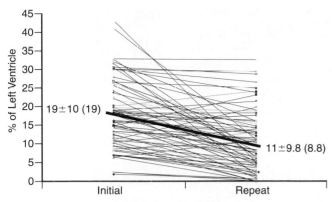

Figure 34-8 Initial and repeat perfusion defect sizes in patients who had acute rest myocardial perfusion imaging with subsequent follow up imaging (median 2 days later). No patient had revascularization <9 hours after presentation. The amount of salvage averaged 45 ± 34%, with, 67% having >25% decrease in defect size, and 46% with >50% defect size reduction. *(Adapted from Kontos MC, Kurdziel KA, Ornato JP, Jesse RL, Tatum JL. Myocardial salvage in patients with non-ST-elevation myocardial infarction: results using technetium-99m sestamibi myocardial perfusion imaging. Am J Cardiol. 2005; 95:398–401.)*

final infarct size, and degree of salvage were high (see Fig. 34-8). Forty-six patients (67%) had significant salvage, defined as a greater than 25% decrease in defect size, 32 (46%) of whom had over 50% salvage (see Fig. 34-7). In those who had significant salvage, the initial defect size was 19% ± 10% (median 16%), which decreased to 6.5% ± 5.1% (5.6%) on repeat imaging. An example of a patient with significant salvage is shown in Figure 34-9. Fifty patients (73%) had EF measured on the initial and repeat images. Initial mean EF was 49% ± 12% (median 50%), which showed a trend toward improvement on repeat imaging by increasing to 53% ± 10% (P = 0.06; median 54%). Fifty percent of patients had an abnormal EF at the time of initial imaging, whereas only 34% had an abnormal EF

on repeat MPI. EF increased significantly in patients who had significant salvage, from 50% ± 14% (51%) to 55% ± 7.7% (55%) (15% increase; P < 0.01) but was unchanged in patients who did not have significant salvage, from 50% ± 14% (51%) to 49% ± 13% (52%) (2% decrease; P = NS). Consistent with prior studies, the area at risk was substantial, was similar to that of patients with inferior ST-elevation MI,[42,43] and occurred despite late revascularization, outside the time frame typically considered necessary for myocardial salvage. A case with significant salvage is shown in Figure 34-9.

One explanation for this is that MI in these patients is often due to occlusion of the left circumflex coronary artery. Because it usually supplies the lateral and posterior walls of the left ventricle, thus areas not well represented by the surface ECG,[44] infarcts from this artery are much less likely to have ischemic ECG changes. In a study of consecutive patients with MI, left circumflex occlusion was associated with ST-segment elevation less than 50% of the time, and diagnostic ECG changes occurred significantly less frequently than infarctions resulting from occlusion of the left anterior descending or right coronary artery.[44] O'Keefe found that risk area was not significantly different in patients who had left circumflex occlusion associated with ST-segment elevation, left circumflex occlusion without ST elevation, and right coronary artery occlusion.[43]

OTHER ISSUES

Radiopharmaceuticals

The limitations of thallium as an imaging agent for acute chest pain evaluation have been discussed. However, one alternative in some institutions is that in the chest pain–free patient, rest thallium rather than technetium is used.[45] If negative, the patient can then undergo immediate stress MPI, an option not available if a high-dose-technetium injection had been used instead.

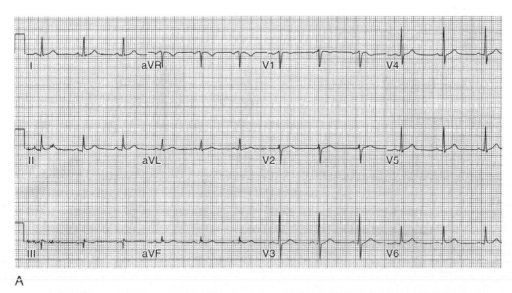

A

Figure 34-9 Example of patient who presented with acute chest pain: a 40-year-old male with atypical chest pain and a non-ischemic ECG (**A**).

Continued

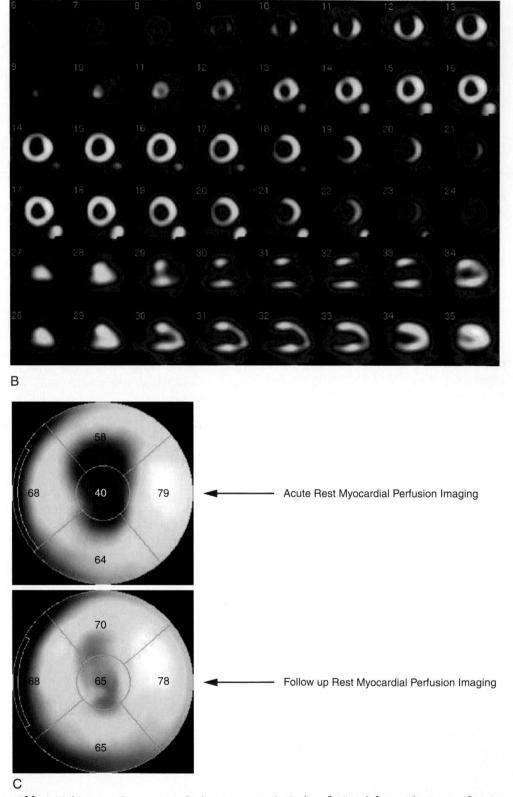

B

C

Acute Rest Myocardial Perfusion Imaging

Follow up Rest Myocardial Perfusion Imaging

Figure 34-9—cont'd   Initial images demonstrated a large anterior/apical perfusion defect with ejection fraction of 37%, and he was subsequently admitted. Peak creatine kinase was 424 U/L. The next day, coronary angiography demonstrated significant left anterior coronary disease, and revascularization was performed. Repeat imaging was performed 2 days later prior to revascularization. Images demonstrated significant resolution of the defect (**B** and **C**), with improvement of ejection fraction to 52%.

Although most studies were performed with sestamibi, comparable results have been obtained with tetrofosmin. In a multicenter study, Heller et al. found a sensitivity of 90% in 357 patients who underwent acute MPI.[23] Negative predictive value (NPV) was equally high (99%), with only two patients who had small non-Q-wave MIs having negative acute MPI. In the study in which 319 patients had TnI elevations, sensitivity of acute MPI with sestamibi (75%) and tetrofosmin (80%) was similar, as was the proportion who had CK-MB MI (84% versus 87%).[35]

Timing of Tracer Injection

For optimal diagnostic accuracy, it is important to inject a radiotracer as soon as possible after presentation and prior to symptom resolution. Although it would be expected that as time progresses after resolution of symptoms that the diagnostic yield of rest MPI in patients with ischemia alone would decrease, this has not been a consistent finding. Studies in which patients were injected within 6 hours of symptom resolution have not found a significant decrease in diagnostic accuracy.[21,22,46,47] Kontos et al. found that when patients were injected within 6 hours of symptoms, sensitivity was similar for identifying patients who had MI, revascularization, or significant coronary disease between those with and without symptoms who were injected.[22]

However, the longer the symptom-free interval, the more likely rest MPI will be negative. Wackers et al.[47] performed ^{201}Tl scintigraphy in 98 patients admitted with chest pain who had MI excluded. Sensitivity was 57% when patients were imaged within 6 hours of the last anginal symptoms; however, it decreased to only 8% when patients were imaged after 12 hours. Bilodeau et al.[21] found that the sensitivity of MPI for detection of coronary artery disease was 96% in 45 patients injected with tracer during chest pain. When the same patients were reinjected later while pain free, the sensitivity had decreased to 65%. In both cases, the sensitivity was significantly higher than that of the initial ECG.

One explanation relates to the difference in the underlying mechanisms causing perfusion defects in ACS patients as compared to those undergoing stress testing. Rather than causing true ischemia, stress perfusion defects result from flow heterogeneity between areas supplied by coronary arteries with and without significant stenoses. The perfusion tracer is injected at the time of maximal flow imbalance, with a rapid return of coronary flow to baseline once the patient stops exercising. In contrast, in ACS patients, perfusion defects result from the combination of intermittent thrombotic occlusion and vasoconstriction in the setting of complex coronary morphology,[48] resulting in marked decreased coronary blood flow[49] and persistently decreased regional myocardial perfusion.[48] Because regional hypoperfusion is one of the first steps in the ischemic cascade, symptoms of chest discomfort are often a late clinical manifestation, so regional hypoperfusion will frequently be present even in the absence of symptoms.

Perfusion defects may also result from distal embolization of a proximal thrombus, leading to downstream microvascular obstruction.[50] In a study of 75 patients who underwent sestamibi injection during rotational atherectomy, a procedure in which distal embolization of microparticles is frequent, perfusion defects were present in 65% of patients.[50]

Another potential mechanism was reported in an interesting study of 40 patients who had a percutaneous intervention. Fram et al. found that perfusion abnormalities persisted in patients injected with ^{99m}Tc-sestamibi at varying time intervals after balloon inflation, although the size of the perfusion defect decreased as the time interval after the procedure increased.[51] They hypothesized that the pharmacodynamics of sestamibi are dependent on both membrane and mitochondrial functional integrity, which may be depressed as a result of lingering metabolic alterations, especially in high-energy metabolites, which occur after transient ischemia. In summary, the sensitivity of acute MPI will be dependent on a number of factors, including the time interval after symptom cessation, the severity of ischemia, the severity of the underlying degree of stenosis, and presence or absence of necrosis.

One new imaging agent, β-methyl-p-[^{123}I]-iodophenyl pentadecanoic acid (BMIPP), which relies on the change from free fatty acid to glucose metabolism in the heart, may offer advantages for identifying ACS in chest pain–free patients. Free fatty acids are the preferred substrate for high-energy ATP production in the normal myocardium.[52] In the setting of myocardial ischemia, suppression of fatty acid metabolism and a switch to glucose utilization occur. This switch in metabolism, known as *metabolic stunning*, offers advantages for imaging the chest-pain patient in whom symptoms have resolved, a group of patients who represent a significant proportion of ED chest-pain patients. BMIPP is a methyl branched-chained fatty acid that is not easily metabolized and thus is retained in myocardial cells.[53] When labeled with ^{123}I, iodofiltic acid provides excellent images of the myocardium.

The feasibility of BMIPP imaging was recently evaluated in a pilot study in which 105 patients presenting with possible ACS were injected with BMIPP within 30 hours of symptom cessation.[54] Quantitative BMIPP imaging plus initial diagnosis increased sensitivity for identifying ischemia by 30% (from 54% to 84%; $P = 0.003$) and for ACS by 17% (from 83% to 100%; $P = NS$), without significantly changing specificity. Further studies are in progress that will more fully evaluate the potential of this technique.

Special Populations

In selected subgroups of patients with known coronary artery disease, although they are not normally considered candidates for acute MPI because of their higher pretest likelihood of ischemia, rest MPI can provide useful additional diagnostic information. This includes patients with a nonischemic ECG who have atypical symptoms, particularly if they are different from their typical angina, those who have had a recent negative cardiac evaluation, or those in whom the risk of coronary angiography is increased, such the presence of significant renal disease. In patients who have multivessel disease or prior bypass surgery, the ability to determine the ischemic risk area can be used to identify the culprit lesion.

Patients with prior MI, especially those with Q waves, are likely to have perfusion defects, and subsequent repeat rest imaging after a pain-free period is required to differentiate new ischemia from old infarction. Alternatively, if prior images are available, they can be used for comparison to determine the significance of perfusion defects.

Another group of patients in whom ED rest MPI can be useful are those presenting with cocaine-associated chest pain. In the absence of ischemic ECG changes or known coronary disease, the risk of ACS is low.[55] In a study of 216 consecutive patients with chest pain after recent cocaine use who underwent ED MPI, only 5 patients (2.3%) had abnormal studies, including 2 with acute MI.[56] None of the 38 patients with normal MPI had subsequently acute MI by biomarkers after admission to the CCU, and only 7% of the 67 patients undergoing subsequent stress MPI had reversible myocardial perfusion defects. At 30-day follow-up, there were no cardiac events in patients with normal rest MPI. This indicates that rest MPI can be used as an alternative to either hospital or observation admission.

LIMITATIONS OF ACUTE MYOCARDIAL PERFUSION IMAGING

Acute MPI has some limitations when used to assess chest pain patients. Acute MI, acute ischemia, and prior MI all cause perfusion defects, and differentiation is not possible based on the images alone. However, patients with prior MI are at higher risk for acute events and are usually not candidates for primary triage to an outpatient evaluation. Sensitivity for identifying necrosis is imperfect for MPI, since at least 3% to 5% of the left ventricle must be ischemic for a defect to be visible. However, many patients who have negative rest MPI despite marker elevations have nonsignificant disease on coronary angiography[35] and are therefore at low risk for short-term adverse outcomes, although aggressive risk-factor modification would still be indicated. Therefore, rather than being seen as competitive diagnostic tools for evaluating ED chest-pain patients, markers and MPI should be considered complementary.

Some of these perceived limitations have led to consideration of other techniques for evaluating ED chest-patients and include coronary computed tomographic angiography (CTA). Improvements in technology have dramatically increased overall sensitivity and specificity, and have reduced the number of coronary segments that cannot be accurately assessed. Using current 64-slice technology, CTA has a reported sensitivity and specificity that exceeds 90% and a negative predictive value of 99%.[57,58] This high negative predictive value of CTA, because of its ability to rapidly exclude clinically significant coronary artery disease, has the potential to

more efficiently diagnose and triage ED chest pain patients.

A randomized trial of low-risk patients with acute chest pain evaluated by either early CTA or a standard diagnostic protocol has been reported.[59] Patients randomized to immediate CTA were eligible for discharge with normal or minimally abnormal results (<25%), patients with severe stenosis (>70%) were referred for immediate invasive angiography, and patients with intermediate-grade stenosis underwent additional stress testing. Among patients randomized to CTA, 75% could be triaged by CTA alone. Importantly, of the 67% of CTA patients who were discharged immediately, no major adverse cardiac events occurred over the next 6 months. Overall, the diagnostic accuracy of CTA was 94%, and the negative predictive value was 100%. However, a number of limitations were demonstrated in this study: 46% of potential subjects were excluded for a reason that would have precluded imaging, and 24% of those who did undergo CTA had to have further diagnostic testing with stress MPI because of equivocal CTA results.

There are other potential limitations that will need to be addressed prior to widespread use of this technology. These include the potential for higher doses of radiation, the relatively high lung and breast radiation exposure, the need for further diagnostic testing in patients with unevaluable coronary segments, a high proportion of patients who are unacceptable candidates for imaging due to underlying renal insufficiency or inability to take β-blockers (often required on older scanners to decrease heart rate sufficiently), and the potential for identifying other noncardiac abnormalities (e.g., lung nodules, "incidentalomas") that will require multiple repeat imaging.

Although in many patients, CTA provides anatomic data regarding the coronary lumen and the presence of stenoses, such data alone do not necessarily provide insight regarding the physiologic impact of a given lesion on coronary blood flow; therefore, the significance of intermediate-severity lesions (25% to 75%) requires physiologic testing.

INCORPORATION INTO EMERGENCY DEPARTMENT CHEST-PAIN EVALUATION

The consistently favorable results of observational and clinical trials on the efficacy of acute rest MPI in the ED have formed the basis of current recommendations and guidelines (Table 34-2).[60] The recommended patient selection criteria are similar to those used for admission to a chest-pain observation unit. Patients should be low risk (no ischemic ECG changes or history of coronary disease) and hemodynamically stable. The optimal use of MPI as a triage tool is in patients who will be discharged home and have stress testing on an outpatient basis if imaging is negative.[61]

In low-risk patients injected during symptoms, the presence of normal rest images makes an ACS unlikely, and in the younger patient, subsequent stress testing

Table 34-2 Guidelines for the Use of Acute Rest Myocardial Perfusion Imaging in the Emergency Department

Indication	Test	Class	Level of Evidence
Assessment of myocardial risk in possible ACS patients with nondiagnostic ECG and initial serum markers, if available	Rest MPI	I	A
Diagnosis of CAD in possible ACS patients with chest pain with nondiagnostic ECG and negative serum markers or normal resting scan	Same-day rest/stress perfusion imaging	I	B
Routine imaging of patients with myocardial ischemia/necrosis already documented clinically, by ECG and serum markers	Rest MPI	III	C

ACS, acute coronary syndrome; CAD, coronary artery disease; ECG, electrocardiogram; MPI, myocardial perfusion imaging.

may not be necessary. If the likelihood of having coronary artery disease based on clinical variables is relatively low and the rest ECG normal, rest MPI can be followed by standard ECG exercise testing. However, a significant proportion of patients have an intermediate likelihood of coronary artery disease and an abnormal rest ECG, or are unable to adequately exercise.[4] In these patients, stress testing with imaging, either echocardiography or (more commonly) SPECT imaging, using exercise or pharmacologic stress would be appropriate.

One limitation of using rest MPI is for the patient whose symptoms resolved prior to or shortly after arrival at the ED. In patients injected while pain free, although risk in the subsequent 2 to 3 days is low, ACS has not necessarily been excluded. Some centers have elected to perform acute MPI only in patients with ongoing symptoms, resulting in a higher prevalence of abnormal images. Symptom-free patients, rather than undergoing imaging, are admitted for observation; serial biomarkers of myocardial injury are obtained and patients undergo stress testing.

The ability to have imaging available during all hours is a potential logistic issue. In a study from Schaeffer et al. addressing this issue, patients presenting from 12 AM to 6 AM were injected with sestamibi, and imaging was delayed until that morning.[62] There was no difference in diagnostic accuracy in patients who waited to be imaged compared to those who presented during other time periods.

One of the first programs to incorporate rest MPI as a diagnostic strategy for ED chest-pain patients was at Virginia Commonwealth University Medical Center (formerly Medical College of Virginia). In contrast to most chest-pain programs, the systematic chest-pain protocol developed and implemented is designed for all chest pain patients, with MPI used for the evaluation of lower-risk patients (Table 34-3).[26] All patients presenting to the ED with chest pain or other symptoms consistent with myocardial ischemia undergo rapid evaluation with assignment to a triage risk level, which is based on the probability of having MI or ischemia as derived from clinical and ECG variables. After the initial evaluation, patients thought to be at high risk (ST-segment elevation [level 1], ST-segment depression, or ischemic T-wave inversion [level 2]) or those with known coronary disease experiencing typical symptoms (level 2)

are admitted directly to the CCU. Patients considered low to moderate risk for ACS (e.g., absence of ischemic ECG changes or history of coronary disease) undergo further risk stratification using acute rest MPI.[26] Level 3 patients are admitted as observation patients and undergo a rapid rule-in protocol. Level 4 patients are evaluated in the ED. If images are either negative or unchanged from previous studies, patients are discharged home and scheduled for outpatient stress testing. If MPI is positive, they are admitted and advanced to the level 2 treatment protocol.

The role of acute rest MPI is different between level 3 and level 4 patients. In level 3 patients, the presence of a significant perfusion defect identifies a high-risk patient in whom early initiation of aggressive treatment is indicated, with the potential for early intervention. The combination of negative MPI and negative markers, on the other hand, identifies patients who can safely undergo early stress testing and discharge. Although the identification of higher-risk patients is usually considered the primary focus, the ability to better risk stratify intermediate-risk patients into a low-risk group who can be stressed safely is an important advantage. In contrast, the role of MPI in the level 4 patients is to diagnose unsuspected ACS and prevent the inadvertent discharge of these patients from the ED. Follow-up stress testing is used to exclude significant coronary disease.

This simple risk-stratification scheme accurately separates patients into high-, intermediate-, and low-risk groups. The ability of MPI to further risk stratify lower-risk patients was confirmed; outcomes in patients with positive MPI were similar to those in the high-risk level 2 patients (Fig. 34-10).[26] Close collaboration of the ED, CCU, and nuclear medicine staff can lead to patients without prior MI who have large perfusion defects at the time of imaging being successfully triaged directly to coronary angiography and revascularization.

Fesmire and colleagues have used a similar protocol with a slight modification.[45] Patients presenting with chest pain are evaluated similar to the MCV protocol. Patients who present without chest pain undergo rest SPECT thallium imaging. If images are negative, subsequent stress SPECT ^{99m}Tc-sestamibi imaging is immediately performed. If rest images are abnormal, the patient is reevaluated for possible ACS prior to stress testing.

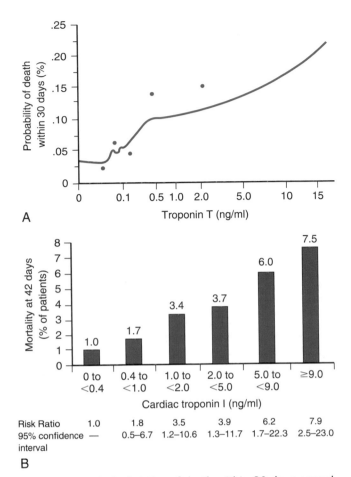

A

B

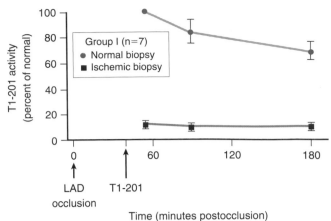

Figure 35-5 Myocardial thallium (Tl)-201 time activity curves in dogs after 3 hours of sustained coronary artery occlusion. Note the constancy of low counts in the area of the infarct zone (ischemic biopsy) versus the decrease in counts from the normal myocardium over time. *(From Granato JE, Watson DD, Flanagan TL, et al: Myocardial thallium-201 kinetics during coronary occlusion and reperfusion: Influence of method of reflow and timing of thallium-201 administration, Circulation 73:150, 1986.)*

Figure 35-4 **A,** Probability of death within 30 days according to the troponin T level at hospital admission. Smoothed nonparametric estimates are shown. The troponin T levels are plotted on a cube-root scale. The density of the data is indicated at the *top,* with each mark representing one patient, The *dots* represent simple estimates of mortality derived from ranges of the troponin T level that included at least 70 patients. **B,** Mortality rates at 42 days, according to the level of cardiac troponin I measured at enrollment. Mortality rates at 42 days (without adjustment for baseline characteristics) are shown for ranges of cardiac troponin I levels measured at baseline. The numbers at the *bottom* of each bar are the percentages. *P* < 0.001 for the increase in the mortality rate (and the risk ratio for mortality) with increasing levels of cardiac troponin I at enrollment. *(A, From Ohman EM, Armstrong PW, Christenson RH, et al. for the GUSTO-IIa Investigators: Cardiac troponin T levels for risk stratification in acute myocardial ischemia, N Engl J Med 335:1333, 1996. B, From Antman EM, Tanasijevic MJ, Thompson B, et al: Cardiac-specific troponin I levels to predict the risk of mortality in patients with acute coronary syndromes, N Engl J Med 335:1342, 1996.)*

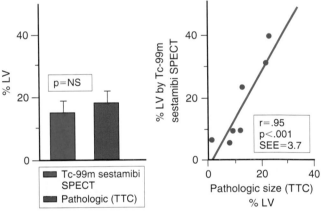

Figure 35-6 Comparison of tomographic (SPECT) and pathologic infarct sizes in 13 dogs with permanent coronary occlusion. LV, left ventricle; Tc, technetium; TTC, triphenyltetrazolium chloride. *(From Verani MS, Jeroudi MO, Mahmarian JJ, et al: Quantification of myocardial infarction during coronary occlusion and myocardial salvage after reperfusion using cardiac imaging with technetium-99m hexakis 2-methoxyisobutyl isonitrile, J Am Coll Cardiol 12:1573, 1988.)*

radionuclide angiography was performed within the first 2 weeks of AMI, and patients with an LVEF less than 40% were randomized to receive either placebo or captopril therapy.[39] One-third of all patients had thrombolytic therapy during AMI. The mean LVEF in patients randomized to placebo was 31%, and the associated 1-year mortality approximately 12%—similar to the 15% mortality reported by the MPRG in patients with an LVEF less than 40%.[10] Likewise, in the Western Washington Streptokinase Trials, LVEF measured 8.7 ± 6 weeks after enrollment was the best univariate and

multivariate predictor of survival.[6] In the 20% of patients with an LVEF less than 35%, the 1-year mortality was 15%, which increased to 22% by 3 years—virtually identical to the 22% placebo mortality reported in SAVE (Fig. 35-10).

Similar results are reported by Simoons and coworkers in 422 patients randomized to intracoronary streptokinase versus placebo, where the LVEF was measured 10 to 40 days after AMI.[11] In patients with LVEF greater than 40%, the 3-year mortality rate remained low (4.3%). Conversely, in patients with an LVEF less than 40%, the 1- and 3-year mortality rates increased with worsening LVEF, but irrespective of initial therapy

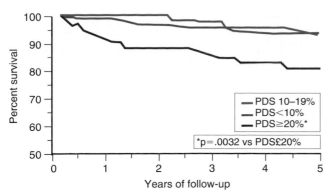

Figure 35-7 Kaplan-Meier survival curves based on cutoffs of total resting left ventricular perfusion defect size as assessed by thallium-201 tomography. Patients with a greater than 20% perfusion defect size had a significantly higher mortality rate than those with smaller infarct sizes. *(From Cerqueira MD, Maynard C, Ritchie JL, et al: Long-term survival in 618 patients from the Western Washington Streptokinase in Myocardial Infarction trials, J Am Coll Cardiol 20:1452, 1992.)*

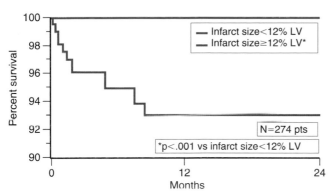

Figure 35-8 Kaplan-Meier survival curves based on infarct size as assessed by Tc-99m sestamibi tomography. LV, left ventricle. *(From Miller TD, Christian TF, Hopfenspirger MR, et al: Infarct size after acute myocardial infarction measured by quantitative tomography Tc-99m sestamibi imaging predicts subsequent mortality, Circulation 92:334, 1995.)*

(Fig. 35-11). Mortality was strongly influenced by LVEF and the extent of angiographic coronary artery disease (CAD) (Fig. 35-12), the latter presumably an indicator of the extent of jeopardized myocardium. In the series by Dakik and colleagues, the LVEF was the only significant predictor of infarct-free survival. The relative risk of death or nonfatal MI doubled for every 10% decrease in LVEF (RR = 2.06, 95% CI, 1.17–3.64; $P = 0.01$) (Fig. 35-13).[35]

The TIMI-II[36] and Grupo Italiano per lo Studio della Streptochinase Nell'Infarcto Miocardico (GISSI-2)[37] trials indicate that survival at any given LVEF is better in patients who receive thrombolytic therapy compared to historical controls in the prethrombolytic era (see Fig. 35-9).[10] This may be due to differing patient characteristics, refinements in risk stratification, therapeutic improvements, or the use of thrombolytics, which may prevent long-term remodeling by maintaining arterial patency. In addition, patients who achieve early coronary reperfusion during AMI frequently exhibit regional

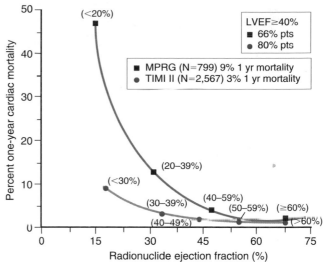

Figure 35-9 Impact of left ventricular ejection fraction (LVEF) on mortality after myocardial infarction. Comparison of Multicenter Postinfarction Research Group (MPRG) with Thrombolysis in Myocardial Infarction (TIMI) trial. *(Adapted from The Multicenter Postinfarction Research Group: Risk stratification and survival after myocardial infarction, N Engl J Med 309:331, 1983; and Zaret BL, Wackers FJT, Terrin ML, et al., for the TIMI Study Group: Value of radionuclide rest and exercise left ventricular ejection fraction in assessing survival of patients after thrombolytic therapy for acute myocardial infarction: Results of Thrombolysis in Myocardial Infarction (TIMI) Phase II Study, J Am Coll Cardiol 26:73, 1995.)*

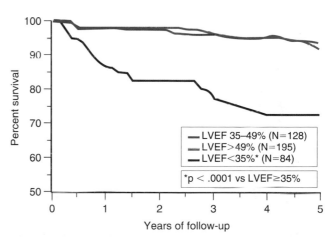

Figure 35-10 Kaplan-Meier survival curves based on cutoffs of left ventricular ejection fraction (LVEF) assessed by gated radionuclide angiography. Patients with an LVEF less than 35% had a significantly higher mortality rate than those with better preserved LV function. *(From Cerqueira MD, Maynard C, Ritchie JL, et al: Long-term survival in 618 patients from the Western Washington Streptokinase in Myocardial Infarction trials, J Am Coll Cardiol 20:1452, 1992.)*

myocardial stunning that can persist for weeks.[27,30] Patients with minimal LV dysfunction (i.e., LVEF > 40%) are expected to have a low subsequent mortality rate. The TIMI-II[36] and GISSI-2[37] data confirm a similar and comparably low mortality rate in patients with normal LV function (LVEF > 50%; 1.2%), as reported earlier by the MPRG (see Fig. 35-9).[10] However, if the LVEF is

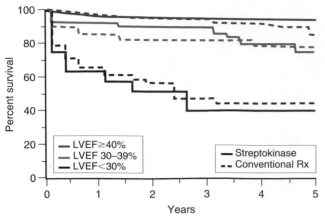

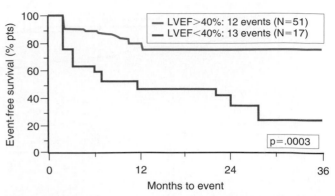

Figure 35-11 Survival of patients based on various LVEF cut-offs and initial therapy during acute infarction. No difference in survival was observed between patients treated with streptokinase *(solid lines)* or conventional therapy *(dashed lines)* within a given range of LVEF. *(From Simoons ML, Vos J, Tijssen JG, et al: Long-term benefit of early thrombolytic therapy in patients with acute myocardial infarction: 5 year follow-up of a trial conducted by the Interuniversity Cardiology Institute of the Netherlands, J Am Coll Cardiol 14:1609, 1989.)*

Figure 35-13 Kaplan-Meier curves showing event-free survival as a function of left ventricular ejection fraction (LVEF). Events were defined as cardiac death, myocardial re-infarction, unstable angina, or congestive heart failure. *(Adapted from Dakik HA, Mahmarian JJ, Kimball KT, et al: Prognostic value of exercise thallium-201 tomography in patients treated with thrombolytic therapy during acute myocardial infarction, Circulation 94:2735, 1996.)*

of stunning and offer a more reliable estimate of risk. Despite these caveats, the final LVEF remains an important predictor of long-term survival irrespective of initial therapy during STEMI.

Left Ventricular Volumes

Left ventricular enlargement increases mortality in patients with AMI and particularly when coexisting myocardial dysfunction is present. White and colleagues showed that survival decreased with progressive LV dilation and a decrease in LVEF.[13] However, LV dilation influenced survival only in patients with LVEF less than 50% (Fig. 35-14). Likewise, the SAVE investigators demonstrated in 512 patients with LVEF less than 40% that 1-year survivors had a significantly smaller increase in LV dimensions, compared to patients who died.[14] LV enlargement is also known to increase mortality in patients with chronic CAD who have a depressed LVEF less than 45%.[40]

Left ventricular dilation develops early in patients after AMI, presumably as a compensatory mechanism for maintaining stroke volume.[41] This is particularly true in patients with anterior infarction, who generally have the greatest degree of initial LV dysfunction and are therefore most likely to develop early infarct zone expansion.[41,42] Over the ensuing months, structural and geometric changes occur that entail scar formation and thinning of the infarct zone as well as hypertrophy and dilation of noninfarcted regions.[43-45] The initial loss of myocardium, if large enough, leads to progressive LV dilation, increasing wall stress, further LV dysfunction, and ultimately end-stage heart failure. One study in survivors of AMI reported a progressive increase in both LV end-diastolic and end-systolic volumetric indices over a 6-month period, but this occurred almost exclusively in those with an initial LVEF less than 40% (Fig. 35-15).[46] Various therapies that limit LV dilation can improve survival in patients with LV dysfunction.[14,46] LV volumes can be accurately measured with

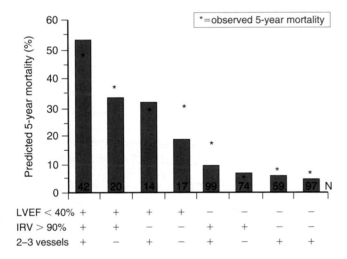

Figure 35-12 Prediction of the 5-year mortality rate (%) by Cox regression analysis based on left ventricular ejection fraction (LVEF), the status of the infarct-related vessel (IRV) (>90% stenosis), and the extent of coronary artery disease as assessed at hospital discharge in 422 patients with angiography between days 10 and 40. 2–3 vessels, patients with double- or triple-vessel coronary artery disease. *(From Simoons ML, Vos J, Tijssen JG, et al: Long-term benefit of early thrombolytic therapy in patients with acute myocardial infarction: 5 year follow-up of a trial conducted by the Interuniversity Cardiology Institute of the Netherlands, J Am Coll Cardiol 14:1609–1615, 1989.)*

reduced due to extensive myocardial stunning that later resolves, cardiac risk could be spuriously overestimated. This may partially explain the lower 1-year mortality rate in patients with LV dysfunction in the TIMI-II and GISSI-2 studies compared to the MPRG. Measuring LVEF 1 to 2 months after infarction rather than within the first 2 weeks would reduce the confounding influence

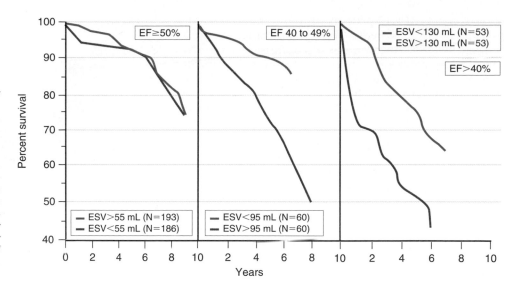

Figure 35-14 Interaction of end-systolic volume (ESV) and left ventricular ejection fraction (LVEF) on survival in patients with acute myocardial infarction. In patients with an abnormal LVEF (<50%), LV dilation resulted in a significantly higher mortality rate. *(From White HD, Norris RM, Brown MA, et al: Left ventricular end-systolic volume as the major determinant of survival after recovery from myocardial infarction, Circulation 76:44, 1987.)*

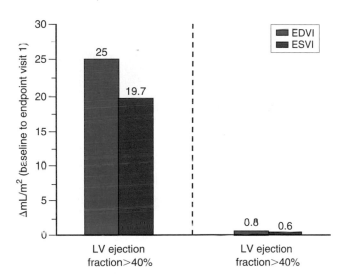

Figure 35-15 Changes in placebo left ventricular (LV) end-diastolic volume index (EDVI) and end-systolic volume index (ESVI) from baseline to end point Visit 1 (6-month analysis) based on initial left ventricular ejection fraction (LVEF). *(Adapted from Mahmarian JJ, Moye LA, Chinoy DA, et al: Transdermal nitroglycerin patch therapy improves left ventricular function and prevents remodeling after acute myocardial infarction: Results of a multicenter prospective randomized double-blind placebo controlled trial, Circulation 97:2017, 1998.)*

both gated radionuclide angiography[47] and gated SPECT[48] techniques.

Myocardial Ischemia

The presence and extent of myocardial ischemia are strong predictors of both fatal and nonfatal cardiac events and improve risk stratification beyond the information gleaned from clinical variables[15-18] or the extent of CAD.[17,35,49,50] The detection of myocardial ischemia using exercise electrocardiography[51-59] has been largely supplanted by more sensitive techniques, including stress echocardiography,[60,61] exercise radionuclide

angiography,[62,63] and most important, stress myocardial perfusion scintigraphy.[15-18]

RISK STRATIFICATION FOLLOWING ACUTE MYOCARDIAL INFARCTION

Exercise Stress Testing

Exercise stress testing has been extensively studied for identifying high- and low-risk survivors of AMI.[51-59] Predictors of high risk include a poor exercise effort (<4 METs) and exercise-induced angina, ischemic (>1 mm) ST-segment depression, hypotension, and ventricular arrhythmias. Inability to perform a predischarge exercise test is, in itself, a poor prognostic finding.[37,64] In the TIMI-II trial, the mortality rate at 1 year was 7.7% in those who did not perform an exercise test, compared to 1.8% in those who did ($P < 0.001$).[64] In GISSI-2, the mortality rate at 6 months increased from 1.3% to 9.8% based on whether patients could perform an exercise test.[37]

Electrocardiographic (ECG) ischemia during submaximal exercise predicts subsequent cardiac death.[51] In an early study from the Montreal Heart Institute, the 1-year mortality rate among all patients was 9.5%, but death occurred almost exclusively in the 30% of patients with ECG ischemia. Patients without ischemia had only a 2.1% mortality, compared to a 27% mortality in those with ST-segment depression.[51]

Low-level exercise ECG testing predicts mortality in seemingly low-risk groups after AMI, but it is of limited value in predicting other morbid events. The stress ECG is insensitive for detecting significant CAD,[52,65] particularly in patients who perform only submaximal exercise.[66] The exercise ECG is much less accurate in risk stratification than myocardial perfusion scintigraphy.[16,18,49] Furthermore, an ischemic ECG response during treadmill exercise currently occurs less frequently than previously reported. In the prethrombolytic era, approximately 31% of patients with uncomplicated AMI exhibited ECG ischemia on predischarge exercise testing.[15,16,67,68] However, this has decreased to approximately 15% among patients evaluated in the thrombolytic era.[35,50,64,69–71] All of these factors limit the ability of the treadmill test to accurately predict which stable patients after AMI are at increased risk for subsequent events (Fig. 35-16).

Gated Radionuclide Angiography

Gated radionuclide angiography allows assessment of LVEF at rest and during dynamic bicycle exercise (see Chapter 11). The resting LVEF identifies patients at high risk for death,[6,10–12,35–37] and the presence of exercise-induced ischemia may further improve risk stratification, depending on the population studied and the types of subsequent events considered (Table 35-1).[62,63,72–77] Morris and coworkers studied 106 patients, of whom 24 died and an additional 38 had either recurrent AMI, readmission for unstable angina, or refractory angina necessitating coronary revascularization.[77] The resting and exercise LVEF both predicted mortality but no other cardiac event. The lack of change in LVEF from resting to exercise identified patients at high risk for developing refractory angina who then underwent coronary revascularization. Abraham and colleagues reported a 58% event rate at 2 years in patients with an exercise LVEF less than 50%, compared to a 17% event rate among those with normal LV function.[72] A more than 5% increase in the LVEF during exercise identified a very low-risk group for subsequent cardiac events, particularly if the resting function was greater than 40%.

In a study by Hung and colleagues, 115 patients had resting/exercise radionuclide angiography 3 weeks after AMI.[74] Twenty-two patients subsequently died (n = 3) or had recurrent infarction (n = 5), readmission for unstable angina (n = 4), congestive heart failure (n = 1), or need for bypass surgery (n = 9), primarily due to refractory angina. The change in LVEF during exercise was a significant predictor of both hard (i.e., death,

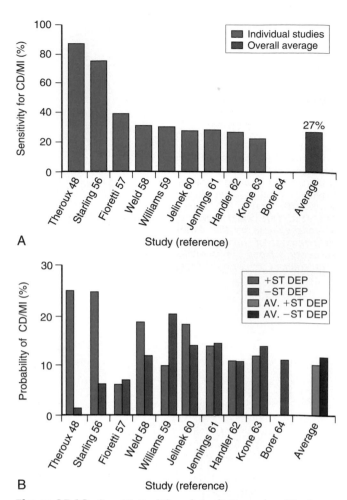

A

B

Figure 35-16 Sensitivity (**A**) and predictive value (**B**) of predischarge exercise electrocardiography after acute myocardial infarction (MI) for detection of patients who had subsequent cardiac death (CD) or recurrent MI. The overall sensitivity (27%) and predictive value of the exercise electrocardiogram were low for identifying patients at risk for events. DEP, depression; ST, ST segment. *(From Brown KA: Prognostic value of myocardial perfusion imaging: State of the art and new developments, J Nucl Cardiol 3:516, 1996.)*

Table 35-1 Gated Exercise Radionuclide Angiography for Risk Assessment after Acute Myocardial Infarction

	N	Follow-Up (mo)	Events	Predictor	Positive Predictive Accuracy (%)	Negative Predictive Accuracy (%)	Overall Accuracy (%)
Candell-Riera et al.[62]	115	12	D/RMI/A/ CHF/REV	EX LVEF <40%	—	—	82
Corbett et al.[63]	61	9.6	D/RMI/A/ UA/CHF	Δ LVEF <5%	97	92	95
Corbett et al.[73]	117	8.3	D/RMI/A/ UA/CHF	Δ LVEF <5%	95	91	93
Nicod et al.[75]	42	8	D/RMI/UA	Δ LVEF <5%	46	86	52
Roig et al.[76]	93	16	D/RMI/UA	Δ LVEF <5%	26	94	62
Hung et al.[74]	115	11.6	D/RMI/UA/ CHF/REV	Δ LVEF <5%	63	84	83

A, exertional angina; CHF, congestive heart failure; D, death; EX, exercise; LVEF, left ventricular ejection fraction; REV, revascularization; RMI, recurrent myocardial infarction; UA, unstable angina.

recurrent infarction) and all cardiac events. Corbett and coworkers showed that 97% of patients who failed to increase their LVEF during exercise returned with a cardiac event by 6 months; however, most of these events were ischemic (i.e., angina or recurrent infarction).[63] Conversely, in the series by Nicod and coworkers, where the majority of events were death or recurrent infarction (65%), the exercise LVEF was less discriminating (positive predictive accuracy = 46%).[75] Knowing the extent of resting and inducible LV dysfunction appears to identify patients who might best be further evaluated with coronary angiography.

Patients who receive thrombolytic therapy frequently have exercise-induced ischemic LV dysfunction. In the TIMI-II trial, 59% of 2143 patients who had resting and exercise radionuclide angiography prior to hospital discharge had an ischemic response, defined as either a less than 5% increase (48%) or a greater than 5% decrease (11%) in exercise LVEF.[36] The 1-year mortality rate in the total TIMI cohort of 3197 patients was 3%, which decreased to 2.2% in the 2567 who underwent gated radionuclide angiography and 1.7% in those who had both resting and exercise radionuclide angiography. Although the resting (see Fig. 35-9), peak exercise (Fig. 35-17), and change in LVEF with exercise all predicted survival, the exercise variables did not improve predictive accuracy over the resting LVEF alone. This result may partially be explained by the exclusion of 1045 patients who could not exercise and had a high mortality rate of 5.8% (see Fig. 35-17). The exercise LVEF variables may also better predict nonfatal ischemic cardiac events, which were not evaluated in this trial. Although important from an historical perspective, exercise gated radionuclide angiography has been largely supplanted by gated SPECT perfusion imaging for risk stratification.

Exercise Myocardial Perfusion Scintigraphy

Exercise myocardial perfusion scintigraphy can accurately define risk in stable survivors of AMI

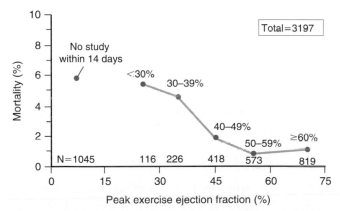

Figure 35-17 Relation of all-cause mortality to peak exercise ejection fraction. *(From Zaret BL, Wackers FJT, Terrin ML, et al, for the TIMI Study Group: Value of radionuclide rest and exercise left ventricular ejection fraction in assessing survival of patients after thrombolytic therapy for acute myocardial infarction: Results of Thrombolysis in Myocardial Infarction (TIMI) Phase II Study, J Am Coll Cardiol 26:73, 1995.)*

(Table 35-2).[15,16,50,68,78] Patients without scintigraphic ischemia have a very low cardiac event rate (<5%), whereas 40% to 50% of patients with ischemia will develop subsequent cardiac events. Early reports demonstrated increased lung uptake of ^{201}Tl and ischemia in multiple vascular territories as additional high-risk predictors.[16] With the advent of quantitative SPECT analysis, the size of the stress-induced perfusion defect, in relation to the presence and quantified extent of scintigraphic ischemia, has added a new dimension to risk stratification.[17] Furthermore, with gated SPECT, the important prognostic variables of LVEF and LV volumes can be calculated directly from the perfusion images (see Chapter 12).

In a landmark study from Gibson and colleagues, 140 seemingly low-risk patients were evaluated with submaximal exercise ^{201}Tl scintigraphy and coronary angiography.[16] Over 15 ± 12 months of follow-up, 36% of patients either died (n = 7), had recurrent AMI (n = 9), or had readmission for unstable angina (n = 34). The presence of scintigraphic ischemia, particularly when involving multiple vascular territories, was the most powerful prognosticator. The scintigraphic variables were superior to the treadmill exercise variables in defining high- and low-risk individuals. Fifty-nine percent of patients with evidence of ^{201}Tl redistribution and 86% of those with redistribution in multiple vascular beds (an indicator of multivessel CAD) had a subsequent cardiac event (Fig. 35-18), compared to only 49% of those with ECG ischemia. Moreover, only 6% of patients without scintigraphic ischemia had a cardiac event versus 26% of those with a low-risk exercise test (see Fig. 35-18).

More recently, Travin and colleagues demonstrated the value of exercise ^{99m}Tc sestamibi SPECT in stratifying risk after AMI.[50] Submaximal exercise SPECT was performed in 134 stable patients within 14 days (mean, 7.5 ± 2 days) of AMI. Ischemic ECG changes were observed in only 23% of patients, whereas 70% had scintigraphic ischemia. Thirty-three patients who had early coronary revascularization were excluded from analysis, and most (79%) of these patients had ischemia by SPECT. Cardiac events occurred in 13 patients over 15 ± 10 months of follow-up. Patients without scintigraphic ischemia had a very low 7% event rate. In patients with ischemia, both the presence and extent of this variable predicted outcome. Overall, 19% of patients with ischemia had a subsequent cardiac event, but this increased from 12% in those with one or two ischemic defects to 38% in patients with more than three ischemic defects. By Cox regression analysis of clinical, exercise treadmill, and scintigraphic variables, only the number of ischemic defects on SPECT predicted outcome.

Pharmacologic Stress Perfusion Scintigraphy

Dipyridamole and adenosine stress are effective and preferable to exercise SPECT as methods for assessing risk in stable patients after AMI.[17,67,79-81] Pharmacologic vasodilators maximize heterogeneity in coronary blood

Table 35-2 Comparison of Exercise Versus Pharmacologic Coronary Vasodilators for Risk Assessment after Acute Myocardial Infarction

	N	Follow-Up (mo)	Events	Predictor	Positive Predictive Accuracy (%)	Negative Predictive Accuracy (%)
Exercise						
Wilson et al.[68]	97	39	Death/MI/unstable angina	IZRD	42	77
Brown et al.[78]	59	37	Death/MI/unstable angina	IZRD	28	100
Gibson et al.[15]	140	15	Death/MI/unstable angina	RD	59 (86)*	94
Gibson et al.[16]	241	27	Death/MI	IZRD	31	97
Travin et al.[50]	87	15	Death/MI/unstable angina	RD	20	96
Overall	624				37	93
Dipyridamole						
Gimple et al.[67]	36	6	Death/MI/unstable angina	NIZRD	26 (42)*	88
Younis et al.[79]	68	12	Death/MI	RD	22	94
Leppo et al.[80]	51	19	Death/MI	RD	33	94
Brown et al.[81]	50	12	Death/MI/unstable angina	RD	45	100
Overall	205				30	94
Adenosine						
Mahmarian et al.[17]	92	15	Death/MI/unstable angina/ CHF	RD (5% LV)	50	97

*Numbers in parentheses describe positive predictive accuracy for ischemia in multiple vascular territories.
IZ, infarct zone; LV, left ventricle; MI, myocardial infarction; NIZ, noninfarct zone; RD, redistribution.
Adapted from Mahmarian JJ: Prediction of myocardium at risk: Clinical significance during acute infarction and in evaluating subsequent prognosis, Cardiol Clin 13:355–378, 1995.

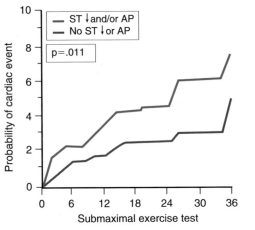

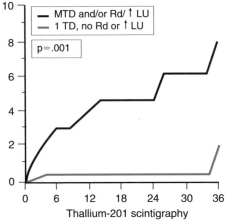

Figure 35-18 Kaplan-Meier event-free survival curves in 140 stable patients with acute myocardial infarction, based on the presence of ischemia as assessed by the submaximal exercise test and thallium-201 scintigraphy. The thallium-201 scintigraphic results best predicted risk for subsequent cardiac events. RD, redistribution. *(Adapted from Gibson RS, Watson DD, Craddock GB, et al: Prediction of cardiac events after uncomplicated myocardial infarction: A prospective study comparing predischarge exercise thallium-201 scintigraphy and coronary angiography, Circulation 68:321, 1983.)*

flow and can thereby accurately identify the extent of LV hypoperfusion and residual ischemia.[82,83] Adenosine induces a similar perfusion defect size as observed with maximal exercise stress.[84] Since these tests can be safely performed even within 1 to 2 days after AMI, patients can be rapidly triaged to early coronary angiography or hospital discharge.[85–88] The scintigraphic risk variables identified with exercise stress have been confirmed in studies using dipyridamole and adenosine (see Table 35-2).

Dipyridamole SPECT

In the initial series by Leppo and colleagues, dipyridamole ^{201}Tl scintigraphy was performed in 51 patients 1 to 2 weeks after uncomplicated AMI.[80] The presence of ^{201}Tl redistribution was the only significant predictor of cardiac death or recurrent AMI. Brown and coworkers safely performed dipyridamole imaging in 50 stable patients very early (mean, 62 ± 121 hours) after hospitalization.[81] The only significant predictor of in-hospital and late cardiac events among clinical, scintigraphic, and angiographic variables was the presence of infarct zone ^{201}Tl redistribution. Conversely, none of the patients without redistribution had a subsequent cardiac event over the ensuing year. Other investigators have confirmed the prognostic importance of ^{201}Tl redistribution on dipyridamole imaging after AMI.[89,90]

Brown and associates reported the results of a large multicenter trial evaluating dipyridamole SPECT for predicting early and late cardiac events.[18] Stable patients postinfarction underwent 3:1 randomization to either early (2 to 4 days) dipyridamole ^{99m}Tc sestamibi SPECT followed by exercise SPECT (at 6 to 12 days) (n = 284) or submaximal exercise SPECT alone (n = 309). Twenty-nine patients who had in-hospital cardiac events and 24 who had early coronary revascularization were excluded from long-term follow-up. Following hospital discharge, death or recurrent AMI occurred in 37 patients assigned to dipyridamole testing and in 31 who had submaximal exercise SPECT. A semiquantitative summed stress score (SSS) and summed difference score (SDS) were generated to assess the size of the stress-induced perfusion defect and the extent of scintigraphic ischemia, respectively. Multivariate predictors of in-hospital events among clinical, dipyridamole stress ECG, and scintigraphic variables were only the SSS, SDS, and peak creatine kinase. Multivariate predictors of death or MI following hospital discharge were the dipyridamole SPECT-derived SSS and SDS, as well as anterior infarction location. The extent of scintigraphic ischemia (i.e., SDS) further improved risk stratification—particularly in patients with intermediate-size perfusion defects (Fig. 35-19). Risk stratification was significantly better with dipyridamole than with submaximal exercise SPECT (Fig. 35-20). This study emphasizes that pharmacologic stress testing after infarction is safe and effective at identifying low- and high-risk groups

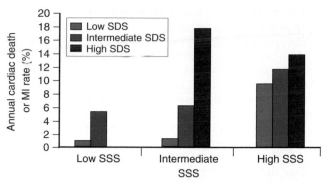

Figure 35-19 Annual cardiac death or myocardial infarction (MI) rate as a function of summed difference score (SDS) for a given summed stress score (SSS). For each SSS subgroup, cardiac event risk increased as SDS increased. The effect of SDS was greatest in the intermediate SSS group. *(Adapted from Brown KA, Heller GV, Landin RS, et al: Early dipyridamole 99mTc-sestamibi single photon emission computed tomographic imaging 2 to 4 days after acute myocardial infarction predicts in-hospital and postdischarge cardiac events: Comparison with submaximal exercise imaging, Circulation 100:2060, 1999.)*

based on the extent of stress-induced hypoperfusion and scintigraphic ischemia. This is the first study to demonstrate improved risk stratification with dipyridamole stress, compared to submaximal treadmill exercise in the same patients.

Adenosine SPECT

Adenosine is a potent direct coronary artery vasodilator that predictably induces maximal hyperemia[82,83] and thereby produces a similar perfusion defect extent as observed with maximal exercise stress in patients who have CAD.[84] Based on these considerations, its high safety profile,[87,88] and exceedingly short half-life,[82] this

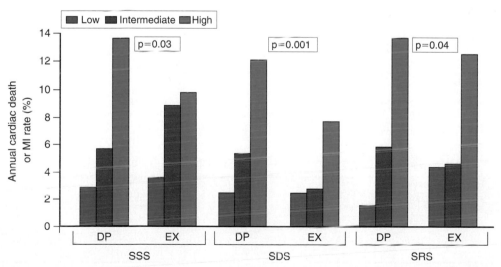

Figure 35-20 Annual cardiac death or recurrent myocardial infarction (MI) rate as a function of summed stress score (SSS), summed difference score (SDS), and summed rest score (SRS) for dipyridamole (DP) and submaximal exercise (EX) Tc-99m sestamibi tomographic imaging. Event rate increased as scores increased. The ability to predict cardiac events was better for dipyridamole studies than for exercise studies for each summed score (*P* value depicted). All event rates are derived from risk-adjusted Cox survival scores. *(Adapted from Brown KA, Heller GV, Landin RS, et al: Early dipyridamole 99mTc-sestamibi single photon emission computed tomographic imaging 2 to 4 days after acute myocardial infarction predicts in-hospital and postdischarge cardiac events: Comparison with submaximal exercise imaging, Circulation 100:2060, 1999.)*

agent is well suited for evaluating patients after AMI for residual myocardial ischemia.

The role of adenosine ^{201}Tl SPECT for detecting residual ischemia and predicting in-hospital cardiac events was first reported in 120 stable survivors of AMI who were imaged early (5 ± 3 days) after infarction.[86] The overall sensitivity for detecting significant (>50%) CAD was 87%. Sixty-three percent of patients with double-vessel and 91% of patients with triple-vessel CAD were accurately predicted to have multivessel involvement. Scintigraphic ischemia was common within the infarct zone (59%) but also in noninfarct-zone (63%) territories in patients with multivessel CAD. Neither angiographic patency of the infarct and noninfarct-related arteries (Table 35-3) nor the presence of collaterals (Table 35-4) predicted the presence of scintigraphic ischemia.

The adenosine-induced LV perfusion defect size was significantly larger in the 41 patients with in-hospital complications (45 ± 15%) compared to those without such complications (22 ± 15%) (Table 35-5). No patient with a small (<10%) LV perfusion defect size had an in-hospital cardiac event, compared to 51% of those with larger defects. A positive predictive value of 43% and a negative predictive value of 91% were observed when the ischemic perfusion defect size was dichotomized at 12%. This study emphasized that (1) adenosine SPECT can readily identify patients with multivessel CAD, (2) the scintigraphic total and ischemic perfusion defect size can identify patients at high and low risk for in-hospital events, and (3) the angiographic information alone is a poor predictor of myocardial viability and may be misleading when trying to decide the appropriateness of coronary revascularization.

A subsequent trial[17] from the same group studied 92 stable patients with adenosine ^{201}Tl SPECT 5 ± 3 days after AMI. Cardiac events occurred in 30 (33%) patients over 15.7 ± 4.9 months of follow-up (8 deaths, 12

Table 35-3 Redistribution Patterns in Infarct and Noninfarct Zones: Relation to Vessel Patency

	PATENT ARTERY (N = 86)			OCCLUDED ARTERY (N = 54)		
	Complete R	Partial R	No R	Complete R	Partial R	No R
Infarct zone	8 (13%)	27 (45%)	25 (42%)	5 (13%)	19 (47%)	16 (40%)
Noninfarct zone	13 (50%)*	12 (46%)	1 (4%)†	6 (43%)†	6 (43%)	2 (14%)
Infarct/noninfarct zones	21 (24%)	39 (45%)	26 (31%)	11 (21%)	25 (46%)	18 (33%)

*$P = 0.0005$ versus infarct zone.
†$P = 0.02$ versus infarct zone.
R, redistribution.
From Mahmarian JJ, Pratt CM, Nishimura S, et al: Quantitative adenosine Tl-201 single-photon emission computed tomography for the early assessment of patients surviving acute myocardial infarction, Circulation 87:1197–1210, 1993.

Table 35-4 Prevalence of Redistribution Associated with Occluded Infarct and Noninfarct Arteries: Relation to Coronary Collaterals

COLLATERALS (N = 43)			NO COLLATERALS (N = 11)		
IRA	NIRA	Total	IRA	NIRA	Total
22/31 (71%)*	11/12 (92%)	33/43 (77%)†	2/9 (22%)	1/2 (50%)	3/11 (27%)

*$P = 0.009$ versus no collaterals.
†$P = 0.002$ versus no collaterals.
IRA, infarct-related artery; NIRA, noninfarct-related artery.
From Mahmarian JJ, Pratt CM, Nishimura S, et al: Quantitative adenosine Tl-201 single-photon emission computed tomography for the early assessment of patients surviving acute myocardial infarction, Circulation 87:1197–1210, 1993.

Table 35-5 Adenosine SPECT Perfusion Defect Size: Cardiac Events

	No Complications (N = 52)	Chest Pain (N = 14)	CHF/Death/VT (N = 25/1/2)	Total Complications (N = 41)
PDS (total)	22 ± 15%	33 ± 19%*	51 ± 14%‡	45 ± 18%‡
PDS (ischemia)	10 ± 10%	21 ± 16%†	18 ± 14%§	19 ± 14¶
PDS (scar)	12 ± 10%	12 ± 8%	33 ± 10‡	26 ± 16%‡

*$P = 0.047$ versus no complications.
†$P = 0.0001$ versus no complications.
‡$P = 0.01$ versus no complications.
§$P = 0.001$ versus no complications.
¶$P = 0.004$ versus no complications.
CHF, congestive heart failure; PDS, perfusion defect size; VT, ventricular tachycardia.
From Mahmarian JJ, Pratt CM, Nishimura S, et al: Quantitative adenosine Tl-201 single-photon emission computed tomography for the early assessment of patients surviving acute myocardial infarction, Circulation 87:1197–1210, 1993.

recurrent infarctions, 7 admissions for unstable angina, and 3 for congestive heart failure). Clinical predictors of risk were patient age, gender, prior history of AMI, and prior coronary revascularization. Scintigraphic risk predictors were the LVEF ($P < 0.0001$), the quantified LV perfusion defect size ($P < 0.0001$), and absolute extent of scintigraphic ischemia ($P < 0.000001$) (Fig. 35-21).

Multivariate analysis incorporating clinical, angiographic, and scintigraphic variables identified several models for predicting risk. The most powerful model was based on the absolute extent of scintigraphic ischemia and LVEF, where 10% increments in these variables increased risk by 82% or decreased risk by 24%, respectively. Only female gender added to the model, at a P value of 0.03. At any given LVEF, risk increased dramatically according to the extent of LV ischemia (Fig. 35-22).

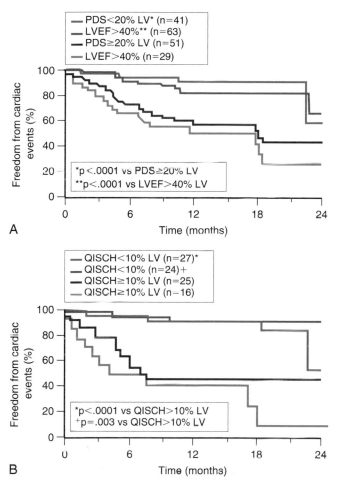

A

B

Figure 35-21 Kaplan-Meier curves depicting freedom from cardiac events on the basis of (**A**) left ventricular (LV) perfusion defect size (PDS) and ejection fraction (EF) and (**B**) quantified extent of left ventricular ischemia (QISCH). The total PDS and global LVEF were inversely related and provided similar prognostic information. QISCH was the best univariate predictor of risk and did so irrespective of initial therapy during acute infarction. *Blue and green lines* in **B** represent early reperfusion therapy; *red and purple lines* represent no early reperfusion therapy. (*From Mahmarian JJ, Mahmarian AC, Marks GF, et al: Role of adenosine thallium 201 tomography for defining long-term risk in patients after acute myocardial infarction, J Am Coll Cardiol 25:1333, 1994.*)

A second risk model was based solely on the scintigraphic perfusion variables of total LV perfusion defect size and infarct-zone ischemia (see Fig. 35-22). Chi-square analysis using a baseline model of clinical variables demonstrated improved risk stratification when LVEF as well as total and ischemic perfusion defect size were added in an incremental fashion. The addition of coronary angiographic findings did not improve the clinical model (Fig. 35-23).

To further validate these retrospective results, 133 stable patients after AMI were prospectively risk stratified according to their initial perfusion defect size and the extent of scintigraphic ischemia (Fig. 35-24).[91] Patients with a small (<20%) adenosine-induced LV perfusion defect size were classified as low risk, those with a large (>20%) but predominantly nonischemic (<10%) perfusion defect size as intermediate risk, and patients with a large (>20%) and predominantly ischemic (>10%) LV perfusion defect size as high risk. High-risk patients who were considered good revascularization candidates following coronary angiography underwent randomization to receive either intensive antiischemic medical therapy or coronary revascularization, whereas the remainder received medical therapy as tolerated.

Patients classified as low risk had a relatively low overall cardiac event rate (17%) with no deaths and few reinfarctions (7%) over 11 ± 5 months; patients classified as intermediate risk had an overall higher event rate (29%). The patients with large ischemic defects who were not randomized to intensive antiischemic therapy had a significantly higher event rate than those with scintigraphic scar (78% versus 29%, $P < 0.001$, respectively), despite a comparable LVEF of 36%. This was also true when events were limited to death and nonfatal reinfarction (see Fig. 35-24). These data imply that stable patients after AMI who have a small or nonischemic perfusion defect size can generally be managed conservatively, with aggressive antiischemic therapy reserved for those with large reversible defects who are at high risk for subsequent cardiac events. This paradigm is further supported by a study that focused primarily on patients with a remote (>6 months) history of AMI. In this study of 1413 patients, the defect size and extent of ischemia again predicted outcome, with the lowest annual event rate in patients who had a small MI and no inducible ischemia (0.6%), and the greatest prognostic impact of ischemia observed among those with an intermediate-size perfusion defect (Fig. 35-25).[92]

RISK STRATIFICATION IN THE THROMBOLYTIC ERA

Nuclear cardiac imaging is an accurate method for risk stratifying patients following acute reperfusion therapy. Much of the initial controversy surrounding the prognostic accuracy of scintigraphy in this population grew from the low mortality rate reported in patients who received acute reperfusion therapy and the unproven sensitivity of scintigraphy for detecting residual ischemia in such patients.

or thrombolytic therapy) during AMI.[69] The positive predictive value of exercise-induced scintigraphic ischemia for predicting subsequent events was similar in both groups (36% versus 33%, respectively). The presence of scintigraphic ischemia identified 80% (4 out of 5) of intervened patients who died or had recurrent infarction. Travin and colleagues followed 87 patients after submaximal exercise SPECT, of whom 34 received thrombolytic therapy.[50] The number of ischemic segments predicted subsequent cardiac events equally well, irrespective of initial therapy.

Dakik and coworkers studied 71 patients who received thrombolytic therapy during AMI and had exercise ^{201}Tl SPECT and coronary angiography prior to hospital discharge.[35] Twenty-five (37%) patients either died (n = 2), had recurrent MI (n = 5), or were rehospitalized due to unstable angina (n = 11) or heart failure (n = 7). The LVEF ($P < 0.005$) (see Fig. 35-13) as well as the exercise-induced total ($P = 0.002$) and ischemic ($P < 0.0005$) SPECT perfusion defect size (Fig. 35-26) were all strong univariate predictors of subsequent cardiac events over 26 ± 18 months of follow-up. This is despite the fact that 45% of patients had coronary revascularization prior to SPECT imaging. None of the treadmill exercise variables predicted subsequent outcome. By multivariate analysis, the best predictors of risk were the LVEF (RR 1.85 for a 10% decrease) and quantified ischemic perfusion defect size (RR 1.38 for a 5% increase). The LVEF and scintigraphic variables significantly contributed to predicting risk beyond the clinical variables alone, with no additional information gained from the angiographic results (Fig. 35-27).

These results with submaximal exercise testing have been confirmed in patients studied with pharmacologic vasodilators. Brown and colleagues[18] reported better separation of high and low risk with dipyridamole sestamibi SPECT in patients who received thrombolytic therapy ($P = 0.02$). Mahmarian and colleagues likewise showed that adenosine ^{201}Tl SPECT imaging could predict events comparably well in patients who did or did not receive thrombolytic therapy during AMI, based on the quantified ischemic perfusion defect size (see Fig. 35-21B).[17]

The prognostic value of SPECT is evident even in seemingly very low-risk patients.[49] In one study, 203 clinically stable enrolled patients (of whom 62% received thrombolytic therapy) had a normal submaximal exercise treadmill test prior to dipyridamole SPECT. Most patients, by coronary angiography, had either no significant CAD (23%) or only single-vessel involvement (52%). Over a mean follow-up of 15 ± 3 months, cardiac events occurred in 69 patients (34%), with 1 cardiac death, 7 recurrent infarctions, 26 admissions for unstable angina, and 35 subsequent revascularization procedures. Multivariate predictors of all events were the angiographic extent of CAD and presence of scintigraphic ischemia (Fig. 35-28). The scintigraphic data provided greater prognostic value than the angiographic results (Fig. 35-29). These data all indicate that the resultant extent of residual scintigraphic ischemia, rather than the initial thrombolytic strategy per se, best predicts future cardiac risk. Since patients postthrombolysis who lack ischemia by noninvasive testing have an excellent prognosis, it seems unlikely that coronary revascularization in this population would further improve outcome.[98]

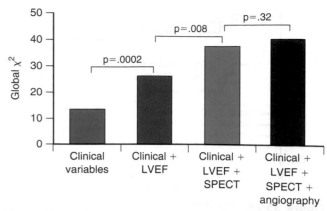

Figure 35-27 Incremental prognostic value of left ventricular ejection fraction (LVEF) and thallium-201 single-photon emission computed tomography (SPECT) variables. *(From Dakik HA, Mahmarian JJ, Kimball KT, et al: Prognostic value of exercise thallium-201 tomography in patients treated with thrombolytic therapy during acute myocardial infarction, Circulation 94:2735, 1996.)*

RISK STRATIFICATION WITH NUCLEAR CARDIAC IMAGING IN THE ERA OF INTERVENTIONAL CARDIOLOGY

The cornerstone of risk stratification in stable survivors of STEMI is to identify (1) high-risk individuals who might benefit from coronary revascularization and (2) low-risk individuals in whom medical therapy and early hospital discharge is warranted. It is generally accepted

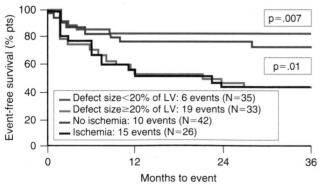

Figure 35-26 Kaplan-Meier curves showing event-free survival as a function of left ventricular (LV) perfusion defect size and presence of myocardial ischemia. Events were defined as cardiac death, myocardial re-infarction, unstable angina, or congestive heart failure. *(Adapted from Dakik HA, Mahmarian JJ, Kimball KT, et al: Prognostic value of exercise thallium-201 tomography in patients treated with thrombolytic therapy during acute myocardial infarction, Circulation 94:2735, 1996.)*

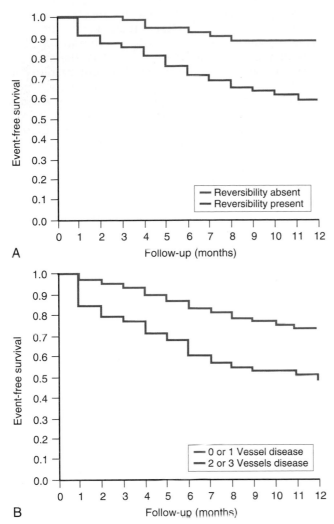

Figure 35-28 Event-free survival based on presence or absence of scintigraphic reversibility (**A**) and number of coronary arteries with greater than 70% stenosis (**B**). *(From Chiamvimonvat V, Goodman SG, Langer A, et al: Prognostic value of dipyridamole SPECT imaging in low-risk patients after myocardial infarction, J Nucl Cardiol 8:136, 2001.)*

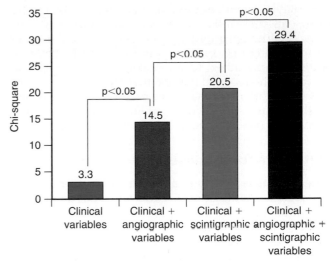

Figure 35-29 Incremental prognostic power (depicted by global chi-square on *y*-axis) of angiographic and scintigraphic variables over clinical model in predicting all cardiac events after myocardial infarction. *(From Chiamvimonvat V, Goodman SG, Langer A, et al: Prognostic value of dipyridamole SPECT imaging in low-risk patients after myocardial infarction, J Nucl Cardiol 8:136, 2001.)*

that patients admitted with AMI who have signs of clinical instability are a high-risk group who should undergo coronary angiography with the intent to revascularize. These patients generally have ongoing or recurrent ischemic chest pain despite medical therapy, congestive heart failure, or hemodynamic instability and thereby incorporate many of the variables contained within the TIMI risk score.[3] Patients with a high TIMI risk score (>5) have a reported in-hospital mortality of approximately 21% but fortunately represent only a relatively small (<20%) percentage of patients with STEMI. Importantly, these patients have been typically, and appropriately, excluded from trials assessing the role of nuclear cardiac imaging in risk stratification.

A further level of complexity exists in patients who receive acute PCI as the initial treatment of STEMI, where the coronary anatomy is, by default, revealed. Primary PCI is increasingly recognized as the treatment of choice for restoring coronary blood flow, preventing reinfarction, and improving survival.[99-101] The Danish

Multicenter Randomized Study on Fibrinolytic Therapy versus Acute Coronary Angioplasty in Acute Myocardial Infarction (DANAMI-2) study showed a significant reduction in the 30-day composite end point of death, recurrent MI, and disabling stroke among the 1572 patients who were randomized to PCI (8.0%) versus alteplase (13.7%).[99] However, despite growing support for performing PCI over thrombolytic therapy in STEMI, for various reasons, only 18% of patients currently undergo primary PCI in the United States, with most either receiving thrombolytic agents (52%) or no reperfusion therapy (30%).[102] Patients not treated with primary PCI would be good candidates for noninvasive risk stratification using nuclear cardiac imaging techniques. In those who do have primary PCI, nuclear cardiac imaging could still be selectively used to identify viable myocardium within the infarct zone, to assess for ischemia outside the infarct zone in patients with multivessel CAD, and to predict recovery in LV function in patients with myocardial stunning.

Rationale for an Invasive Approach

Beyond the benefits of coronary reperfusion during the early stages of STEMI, the rationale behind a routine invasive approach is to identify patients with a high-risk coronary anatomy where appropriate revascularization can be readily performed. Implicit to this approach is that coronary revascularization following AMI will improve survival and reduce morbidity from CAD, and do so more effectively than intensive medical therapy. If so, this should result in a more cost-effective strategy by limiting initial hospital stay and preventing subsequent admissions due to recurrence of clinical instability. Currently, only one trial has directly compared the relative efficacy of medical therapy versus coronary revascularization in patients surviving AMI who had stress-induced ischemia by noninvasive testing.[103] Although mortality rates were similar over 2.4 years, infarct-free survival was significantly better in patients randomized to revascularization (90.5%) than in those who received medical therapy (85.1%).[103] However, this difference may have occurred because of suboptimal use of medical therapy rather than a significant beneficial effect from revascularization per se.

Rationale for a Conservative Approach

The rationale behind a noninvasive conservative approach is that (1) most patients with AMI do not have subsequent cardiac events, (2) the subset of high-risk patients who are likely to benefit from revascularization can be accurately identified by noninvasive testing, and (3) intensive medical therapy can prevent anginal symptoms, and do so as well as routine revascularization. For a conservative approach to be effective, patients must undergo early risk stratification and with an accurate technique such as stress MPI. Exercise treadmill testing alone is insensitive for detecting high-risk patients with residual myocardial ischemia, but when combined with perfusion scintigraphy, it readily identifies ischemic patients and those with multivessel CAD.[86] This is a critical issue, since patients who have preserved LV function and no residual ischemia are at very low risk, which is not further reduced with coronary revascularization.[98] Likewise, coronary angioplasty and stenting of an occluded infarct-related artery does not improve outcome over medical therapy in patients who have depressed LV function and minimal or no residual ischemia.[104] Based on the total and ischemic PDS and LVEF by gated SPECT, individual patient risk can be determined, followed by appropriate selection of patients for either invasive procedures or medical therapy and early hospital discharge.[88,105] With the introduction of pharmacologic vasodilators, in lieu of exercise stress, perfusion imaging can be performed safely within 1 to 2 days of admission, thereby providing rapid risk stratification to guide patient-management decisions.[17,18,85,87,88] Imaging early after admission is of paramount importance, since cardiac instability in susceptible patients tends to recur within days of the initial event.[106,107] The TIMI investigators reported a significant reduction in overall survival among the approximately 4% of patients who received thrombolytic therapy for acute ST-segment elevation and had subsequent in-hospital reinfarction.[106] This has also been shown in patients admitted with an ACS where prolonged antithrombotic therapy prior to a diagnostic procedure to assess risk leads to a higher event rate.[107]

Clinical Trial Support for Either Strategy

The widespread acceptance of an invasive strategy as the community standard of care for patients following AMI has largely been fueled by favorable results reported from trials in acute coronary syndromes (Table 35-8).[108–115] Trials demonstrating an outcome advantage with a routine invasive approach have generally compared "state-

of-the-art" interventional strategies to one of submaximal treadmill testing.[110,112] Other trials have not even included routine noninvasive risk stratification in their study design (see Table 35-8).[111,113,114] Furthermore, in many of these trials, such as the Fast Revascularization during Instability in Coronary artery disease (FRISC) and Treat Angina with Aggrastat and Determine Cost of Therapy with an Invasive or Conservative Strategy (TACTICS)-TIMI 18 trials, it is unclear the degree to which medical therapy was administered in patients with residual ischemia.[110,112] This is particularly relevant, since patients in the conservative strategy only crossed over to coronary angiography when ischemia was considered severe by treadmill testing. Since exercise treadmill testing was the stressor used in both of these trials, many patients randomized to the conservative strategy suffered a recurrent cardiac event during the "watchful waiting" period—before the index stress test could be safely performed.

A more recent study disputes the finding from TACTICS[112] and FRISC-II[110] in ACS patients who all had enzymatic evidence of non-ST-elevation AMI. The Invasive versus Conservative Treatment in Unstable Coronary Syndromes (ICTUS) trial randomized 1200 patients to either a routine invasive strategy or a conservative strategy where coronary angiography was selectively performed based on clinical criteria and predischarge exercise stress test results.[115] Similar to other trials, the primary end point was a composite of death, reinfarction, or rehospitalization for angina at 1 year. Coronary revascularization was performed by 1 year in 79% of patients assigned to the early invasive strategy and in 54% randomized to the selectively invasive group. Most PCI procedures were performed with stents (88%) and abciximab. The study was powered at 80% to detect a 25% risk reduction between the two groups at an alpha level of 0.05. The 1-year cumulative event rate was similar in the two groups, balanced by the higher reinfarction rate in the invasive (15%) versus the conservative (10%) group (RR 1.50, 95% CI 1.10–2.04, $P = 0.005$), but the higher rehospitalization rate in the conservative versus invasive limb (10.9% versus 7.4%, $P = 0.04$) (Fig. 35-30). Subgroup analysis based on age, gender, diabetes status, ST-segment deviation, and baseline troponin T showed no advantage of the early invasive over the conservative strategy. The results did not change when the more strict definitions of reinfarction used in FRISC-II and TACTICS were applied to the ICTUS population.

Beyond these trials in acute coronary syndromes, several studies in patients with STEMI showed no significant prognostic advantage with an invasive versus a conservative strategy. In the TIMI-IIB study, 3339 patients with acute STEMI received thrombolytic therapy and were then randomized to either early coronary angiography or a conservative strategy where coronary angiography was performed only in patients who had spontaneous ischemia or inducible ischemia on treadmill testing.[116] Although twice as many patients had either angioplasty or coronary artery bypass surgery by 1 year in the invasive (72%) versus the conservative limb (35%), 1-year[71] and 3-year[94] infarct-free survival were virtually identical in both groups.

Similar results were reported in the Should We Intervene Following Thrombolysis (SWIFT) study, where

Table 35-8 Trials in Non-ST-Elevation Acute Coronary Syndromes

Trial	Yr	# Pts	% with AMI	Stress Testing	CORONARY REVASC		FU Mos	DEATH/AMI		Risk Ratio	P Value
					INV	CONS		INV	CONS		
TIMI-IIIb[21]	1995	1473	33%	Yes	64%*	58%	12	80/740 (10.8%)	89/733 (12.2%)	.89 (.67-1.18)	.42
VANQWISH[23]	1998	920	100%	Yes	44%†	33%	23	138/462 (29.8%)	123/458 (26.9%)	1.15 (.91-1.4)	.35
FRISC-II[22]	1999	2457	58%	Yes	77%‡	37%	12	127/1222 (10.4%)	174/1235 (14.1%)	.74 (.6-.92)	.005
TRUCS[147]	2000	148	0%	No	78%§	38%	12	6/76 (7.6%)	12/72 (16.7%)	.47 (.19-1.2)	.27
TACTICS[24]	2001	2220	54%	Yes	60%‡	44%	6	81/1114 (7.3%)	105/1106 (9.5%)	.74 (.54-1.0)	<.05
RITA-3[149]	2002	1810	75%	No	57%*	28%	12	68/895 (7.6%)	76/915 (8.3%)	.91 (.67-1.25)	.58
VINO[148]	2002	131	100%	No	73%†	39%	6	4/64 (6.3%)	15/67 (22.4%)	.30 (.10-.83)	.001
ICTUS[150]	2005	1200	100%	Yes	79%*	54%	12	92/604 (15.3%)	61/596 (10.3%)	1.49 (1.1-2.0)	.002

*1 year
†23 months
‡6 months
§In hospital
AMI, acute myocardial infarction; CONS, conservative strategy; FU, follow-up; INV, invasive strategy; Mos, months; Pts, patients; Revasc, revascularization; Yr, year.

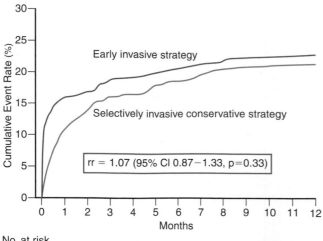

Figure 35-30 ICTUS results: Kaplan-Meier estimates of the cumulative rate of the composite primary end point of death, nonfatal myocardial infarction, or rehospitalization for anginal symptoms within 1 year. *(From de Winter RJ, Windhausen F, Cornel JH, et al., for the Invasive versus Conservative Treatment in Unstable Coronary Syndromes (ICTUS) Investigators: Early invasive versus selectively invasive management for acute coronary syndromes, N Engl J Med 353:1095–1104, 2005.)*

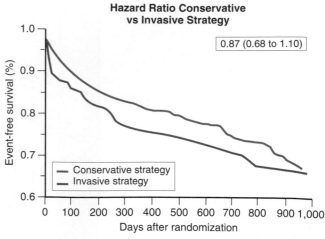

Figure 35-31 Kaplan-Meier infarct-free survival curves in patients randomized to the invasive and conservative strategies of VANQWISH. *(From Boden WE, O'Rourke RA, Crawford MH, et al: Outcomes in patients with acute non-Q-wave myocardial infarction randomly assigned to an invasive as compared with a conservative management strategy. Veterans Affairs Non-Q-Wave Infarction Strategies in Hospital [VANQWISH] Trial Investigators, N Engl J Med 338:1785, 1998.)*

800 patients with STEMI received anistreplase and were then randomized to either a conservative or invasive strategy.[117] Coronary revascularization was performed in 57% of patients randomized to the invasive strategy, which increased to 61% by 1 year. In the conservative strategy group, 5% of patients had coronary revascularization at hospital discharge and only 15% by 1 year. As in TIMI-IIB, the conservative therapy group did as well as those assigned to an invasive strategy, with a 1-year infarct-free survival of 83.4% versus 80.9% (*P* = NS), respectively.

In the Medicine versus Angiography in Thrombolytic Exclusion (MATE) trial, 201 patients with STEMI who were ineligible for thrombolysis were randomized.[118] In the invasive strategy, 58% of patients were revascularized, compared to 37% in the conservative medical therapy limb (*P* = 0.004). Of note, 27 of 54 patients who underwent coronary angiography in the conservative limb did so as a result of physician preference and not because of clinical instability. After 21 months of follow-up, no significant differences in death (11% versus 10%) or infarct-free survival (14% versus 12%) were observed between the two groups.

The Veterans Affairs Non-Q-Wave Infarction Strategies in Hospital (VANQWISH) trial is the only one that selected myocardial perfusion scintigraphy as the noninvasive testing modality in 920 patients randomized to either an invasive or conservative strategy following non-Q-wave AMI.[109] In this study, 30% of randomized patients had STE on the initial ECG.[119] During the trial, significantly higher rates of coronary angiography (94% versus 48%) and revascularization (44% versus 33%) were observed in the invasive versus conservative limbs, despite a comparable 1-year infarct-free survival (76% versus 81%; Fig. 35-31). A recent analysis from the VANQWISH investigators demonstrated that the conservative strategy was more cost-effective than the routine invasive approach.[120]

These large randomized trials are further supported by subgroup analyses from the SAVE[121] and GUSTO-I trials,[122] which showed comparable infarct-free survival among patients treated in the United States and Canada, despite a two- to threefold higher rate of coronary revascularization in the former country. In SAVE, only effort-related angina was less frequent in the United States than Canada (27% versus 33%).[122] Data from the Organization to Assess Strategies for Ischemic Syndromes (OASIS) registry also show no difference in 6-month outcome among patients admitted to hospitals in countries where coronary angiography and revascularization are more frequently performed.[123] In addition, a recent substudy from the OASIS-5 trial in 184 women with non-STE AMI showed no added benefit to an early invasive versus a selective-invasive approach.[124] In fact in this study, as in ICTUS, there was a strong trend for a higher event rate (death, AMI, stroke) in women randomized to the invasive versus the conservative limb (HR 1.46, 95% CI 0.73–2.94). Consistent with current clinical practice, most patients in the conservative limb were administered aspirin (98.9%), an angiotensin receptor blocker (80.4%), a β-blocker (93.5%), and lipid-lowering therapy (85.9%). The sum of these trials indicate that a routine invasive approach may be most appropriate in the clinically highest-risk patients and particularly when timely noninvasive risk stratification is not available and/or appropriate intensive medical therapy is not administered.

THE INSPIRE TRIAL—IMPLICATIONS FOR RISK STRATIFICATION

The Adenosine Sestamibi SPECT Post-Infarction Evaluation (INSPIRE) trial was a large prospective multicenter randomized study that enrolled 728 stabilized patients with ST-elevation (60%) or non-ST-elevation (40%) AMI.[88,105,125] Adenosine ^{99m}Tc sestamibi SPECT was used as an initial noninvasive method to assess risk and guide subsequent therapeutic decision making early after AMI. INSPIRE is the only prospective trial other than VANQWISH[109] to use myocardial perfusion scintigraphy for risk stratification. Unlike previous studies, all patients in INSPIRE were assigned to a conservative strategy of stress SPECT, with subsequent triage to invasive procedures based on the imaging results. Imaging was performed early after AMI, with online study interpretation by a central core laboratory within 24 hours. This was a critical study design feature, recognizing that cardiac events tend to recur early after both ST-elevation[106] and non-ST-elevation AMI.[107] In TACTICS[112] and FRISC,[110] exercise stress testing in the conservative limb led to an unavoidable delay in identifying ischemia. In INSPIRE, over half the patients at U.S. sites were safely imaged with adenosine within 2 days of hospital admission so as to facilitate subsequent patient care and avoid the pitfalls of these earlier trials. No cardiac events occurred in INSPIRE patients prior to noninvasive testing, due in part to the expedited imaging protocol.

Based on previous preliminary studies,[17,91,126] patient risk and management decisions were prospectively defined by the scintigraphic findings (Fig. 35-32).[125] Patients with a small quantified PDS (<20%) were considered low risk with an anticipated greater than 95%

infarct-free survival at 1 year. These patients were medically managed and targeted for early hospital discharge. Patients with large (>20%) primarily nonischemic (<10%) defects were recognized to be at higher (intermediate) risk but thought unlikely to benefit from coronary revascularization. Patients with large (>20%) and ischemic (>10%) perfusion defects who had an LVEF less than 35% were defined as high risk and encouraged to have coronary angiography with the intent to revascularize, whereas those with an LVEF greater than 35% were randomized to receive either intensive medical therapy or coronary revascularization.[125] Following optimization of therapy, SPECT was repeated at 6 to 8 weeks to assess the relative effect of therapy on total and ischemic PDS and subsequent patient outcome. Follow-up was complete at 1 year in 98% of patients.

As anticipated, overall cardiac and death/reinfarction event rates significantly increased across INSPIRE risk groups (Fig. 35-33).[88] However, a very low 1.8% death and re-infarction rate was observed at 1 year in the prospectively defined low-risk group, even though 38% were at intermediate or high clinical risk based on their TIMI score, and their mean troponin T was elevated at 1.1 ± 1 µg/mL. Adenosine SPECT identified this low-risk population irrespective of age, gender, site of infarction, or clinical risk. The total and ischemic defect sizes were the best multivariate risk predictors and allowed estimation of risk in individual patients (Fig. 35-34). This was true both in patients with STEMI and in those with non-ST-elevation MI.

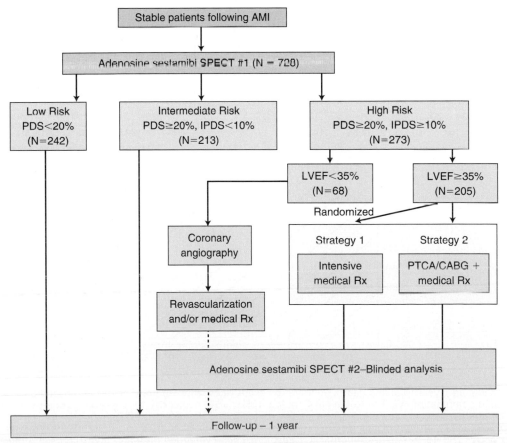

Figure 35-32 The adenosine Sestamibi Post-Infarction Evaluation (INSPIRE) trial study design. AMI, acute myocardial infarction; CABG, coronary artery bypass surgery; IPDS, ischemic perfusion defect size; PDS, perfusion defect size; PTCA, percutaneous transluminal coronary angioplasty; SPECT, single-photon emission computed tomography.

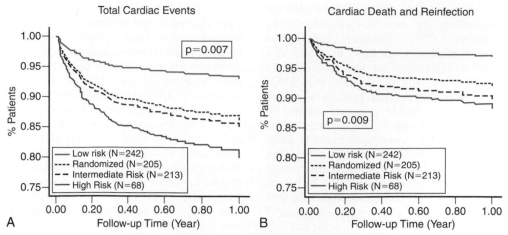

Figure 35-33 Total (**A**) and cardiac death/re-infarction (**B**) rates based on Adenosine Sestamibi Post-Infarction Evaluation (INSPIRE) risk categories. *(From Mahmarian JJ, Shaw LJ, Filipchuk NG, et al., for the Adenosine Sestamibi SPECT Post-Infarction Evaluation (INSPIRE) Investigators: A multinational study to establish the value of early adenosine technetium-99m sestamibi myocardial perfusion imaging in identifying a low-risk group for early hospital discharge following acute myocardial infarction, J Am Coll Cardiol 48:2448–2457, 2006.)*

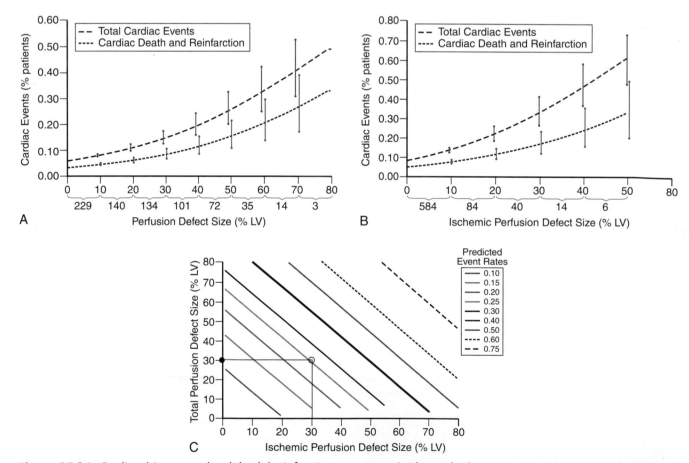

Figure 35-34 Predicted 1-year total and death/re-infarction event rates (with standard error bars) based on total (**A**) and ischemic (**B**) PDS and their combination (**C**). The isobars in **C** (range: 10% to 75%) depict risk for any event. For a patient with a 30% non-ischemic PDS, the predicted event rate is 11% *(filled circle)*, versus 25% if the defect is all ischemic *(empty circle)*. IPDS, ischemic perfusion defect size; LVEF, left ventricular ejection fraction; SPECT, single-photon tomography. *(From Mahmarian JJ, Shaw LJ, Filipchuk NG, et al, for the Adenosine Sestamibi SPECT Post-Infarction Evaluation (INSPIRE) Investigators: A multinational study to establish the value of early adenosine technetium-99m sestamibi myocardial perfusion imaging in identifying a low-risk group for early hospital discharge following acute myocardial infarction, J Am Coll Cardiol 48:2448–2457, 2006.)*

The results from INSPIRE,[88] ICTUS,[115] and the Occluded Artery Trial (OAT)[104] question the recommendations from TACTICS[112,127] that all patients with an elevated troponin should undergo routine coronary angiography, since it is unlikely that coronary revascularization will further benefit scintigraphically low-risk patients or those with minimal or no residual ischemia. The prospectively defined low-risk group in INSPIRE, which represented one-third of all enrolled patients, had the lowest rate of coronary revascularization, the shortest hospital stay, the lowest hospital-related costs, and yet the lowest overall event rate (Table 35-9). Coronary revascularization did not improve outcome in this group (Table 35-10). Based on the cost-analysis approach used in TACTICS,[128] the cost savings in this group would have been approximately 65% compared to a routine invasive approach.

It must be emphasized that the purpose of risk stratification is not only to identify high-risk patients but also to determine in whom risk can be reduced. The INSPIRE intermediate-risk group represented an additional 29% of patients who were at higher clinical risk for events but unlikely to benefit from coronary revascularization, since they had minimal residual ischemia.[104,129,130] The recently published OAT trial demonstrated no prognostic advantage to dilating and stenting occluded infarct-related arteries over medical therapy alone in patients with minimal or no residual ischemia (Fig. 35-35).[104] In fact, a disturbing trend toward a higher reinfarction rate was observed in those randomized to PCI. The intermediate-risk group in INSPIRE also showed similar event rates among those who were or were not revascularized (see Table 35-10). The high-risk INSPIRE group who had extensive residual ischemia and significantly depressed LV function were generally selected for coronary revascularization but represented only 9% of all enrolled patients. As supported by retrospective analyses,[129-130] those who were revascularized had a significantly lower overall 1-year event rate than the remainder who received medical therapy alone (10% versus 32%, $P = 0.049$) (see Table 35-10). The Surgical Treatment for Ischemic Heart Failure (STICH) trial is a prospective randomized trial comparing medical therapy to cardiac surgery in similar patients but who have chronic ischemic cardiomyopathy and an LVEF less than 35%.[131]

Among the randomized patients with preserved LV function, intensive medical therapy was as effective as coronary revascularization in reducing total and ischemic PDS, as determined by serial SPECT imaging pre- and post-therapy (Table 35-11) (Fig. 35-36).[105] Patients with ischemia in the conservative limbs of other trials have generally been referred for coronary angiography with the intent to revascularize. Similar to ICTUS,[115] FRISC-II,[110] and TACTICS,[112] most patients randomized to the interventional arm had coronary revascularization (81%) with over 80% of significantly (>70%) stenosed arteries revascularized. Stents were placed in 94% of arteries undergoing PCI. However, unlike most trials, patients randomized to medical therapy had

Table 35-9 Event Rates, Length of Hospital Stay, and Cost Analysis in the INSPIRE Risk Groups

INSPIRE Risk Category	Total Event Rate at 1 Year	CCU Stay (Days)	Hospital Stay (Days)	Hospital Costs (USA Dollars)
Low risk	5.4%	2.1 ± 1.5	5.5 ± 1.8	5,609 ± 3,632
Intermediate risk	14.0%	3.5 ± 3.1	8.0 ± 5.4	9,967 ± 7,344
High risk	18.6%	3.6 ± 2.0	13.9 ± 13.3	13,269 ± 6,432
P Value	0.0007	0.0001	0.0001	0.0001

CCU, coronary care unit; INSPIRE, Adenosine Sestamibi SPECT Post-Infarction Evaluation trial.
Adapted from Mahmarian JJ, Shaw LJ, Filipchuk NG, et al, for the Adenosine Sestamibi SPECT Post-Infarction Evaluation (INSPIRE) Investigators: A multinational study to establish the value of early adenosine technetium-99m sestamibi myocardial perfusion imaging in identifying a low-risk group for early hospital discharge following acute myocardial infarction, J Am Coll Cardiol 48:2448–2457, 2006.

Table 35-10 Coronary Angiography, Revascularization, and Event Rates in the INSPIRE Risk Groups

INSPIRE Risk Group	CORONARY ANGIOGRAPHY (% PATIENTS)			CORONARY REVASCULARIZATION (% PATIENTS)			EVENT RATES (%)		
	1 month	3 months	1 year	1 month	3 months	1 year	REV	No REV	P Value
Low risk	15	18	21	11	13	16	6.9	7.0	0.97
Intermediate risk	31	34	35	17	20	21	13.9	14.7	0.84
High risk	75	82	82	50	62	64	10.0	32.0	0.049

REV, coronary revascularization.
From Mahmarian JJ, Shaw LJ, Filipchuk NG, et al., for the Adenosine Sestamibi SPECT Post-Infarction Evaluation (INSPIRE) Investigators: A multinational study to establish the value of early adenosine technetium-99m sestamibi myocardial perfusion imaging in identifying a low-risk group for early hospital discharge following acute myocardial infarction, J Am Coll Cardiol 48:2448–2457, 2006.

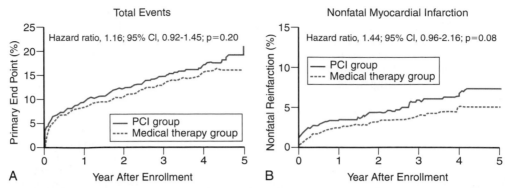

Figure 35-35 Kaplan-Meier curves depicting the total (**A**) and nonfatal myocardial infarction (**B**) event rates in patients randomized to percutaneous coronary intervention versus medical therapy in the Occluded Artery Trial (OAT). *(From Hochman JS, Lamas GA, Buller CE, et al., for the Occluded Artery Trial Investigators: Coronary intervention for persistent occlusion after myocardial infarction, N Engl J Med 355:2395–407, 2006.)*

Table 35-11 Changes in Gated SPECT Results in the Medical Versus Revascularization Strategies in INSPIRE

	Strategy 1 (Medical Therapy) (N = 83)	Strategy 2 (Revascularization Therapy) (N = 86)	*P* Value	Difference in Treatment Effect Strategy 1 vs Strategy 2
Total LV PDS (absolute % change)	−16.2 ± 10 (−35.8 to 3.4)	−17.8 ± 12 (−41.3 to 5.7)	0.36	1.6 ± 11 (−20.0 to 23.3)
Ischemic LV PDS (absolute % change)	−15.0 ± 9 (−32.6 to 2.6)	−16.2 ± 9 (−33.8 to 1.4)	0.44	1.2 ± 9 (−16.4 to 18.8)
Scar LV PDS (absolute % change)	−1.2 ± 8 (−16.9 to 14.5)	−1.6 ± 7 (−15.3 to 12.1)	0.73	0.4 ± 7 (−14.3 to 15.1)
% Patients ≥ 9% decrease				
Total LV PDS	75%	79%	0.50	
Ischemic LV PDS	80%	81%	0.76	
LVEF (absolute % change)	4.7 ± 7	4.6 ± 8	0.93	

95% confidence intervals in parentheses.
LV, left ventricular; LVEF, left ventricular ejection fraction; PDS, perfusion defect size; SPECT, single-photon emission computed tomography.
From Mahmarian JJ, Dakik HA, Filipchuk NG, et al., for the INSPIRE Investigators: An initial strategy of intensive medical therapy is comparable to that of coronary revascularization for suppression of scintigraphic ischemia in high-risk but stable survivors of acute myocardial infarction, J Am Coll Cardiol 48:2458–2467, 2006.

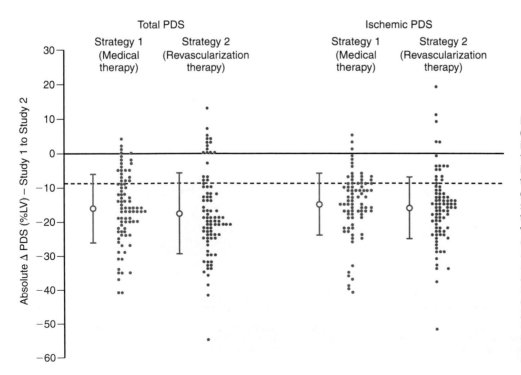

Figure 35-36 Absolute mean (±SD) and individual changes in total and ischemic LV PDS from SPECT-1 to SPECT-2 study in patients randomized to the two INSPIRE treatment strategies. The *dashed line* represents a 9% reduction in PDS, that is, a 95% confidence interval for a real patient change. *(From Mahmarian JJ, Dakik HA, Filipchuk NG, et al, for the INSPIRE Investigators: An initial strategy of intensive medical therapy is comparable to that of coronary revascularization for suppression of scintigraphic ischemia in high-risk but stable survivors of acute myocardial infarction, J Am Coll Cardiol 48:2458–2467, 2006.)*

prospectively defined intensive treatment with antiplatelet (100%), β-blocker (93%), ACE inhibitor (77%), and statin (84%) medications so as to ensure a fair comparison to coronary revascularization. The suppression of scintigraphic ischemia with medical therapy is consistent with earlier small reports in patients with chronic CAD[132] and similar to the findings from the pilot study to INSPIRE.[126] The comparable event rates in the two groups support the scintigraphic findings and indicate that currently available intensive medical therapy may be a reasonable alternative in stable AMI patients who are not optimal revascularization candidates (Fig. 35-37). The pilot study to INSPIRE also indicated improved event-free survival in patients who had a significant (>9%) reduction in PDS following either medical therapy or PCI (Fig. 35-38).[126] These data suggest that MPI may be used not only to assess initial risk but also to track subsequent risk by evaluating the efficacy of various therapies on myocardial ischemia. A larger adequately powered prospective randomized event trial in ischemic patients after AMI is warranted.

The INSPIRE results are consistent with over 2 decades of clinical studies evaluating a broad spectrum of patients with ACS in whom stress myocardial perfusion scintigraphy provided accurate risk stratification.[15–18,35,49–50,80–81,91] The implications from INSPIRE are that "state-of-the-art" adenosine SPECT imaging performed very early after AMI can safely and reliably identify a large patient cohort unlikely to benefit from

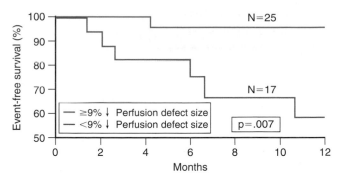

Figure 35-38 Kaplan-Meier curves depicting event-free survival based on changes in perfusion defect size after antiischemic therapy. *(From Dakik HA, Kleiman NS, Farmer JA, et al: Intensive medical therapy versus coronary angioplasty for suppression of myocardial ischemia in survivors of acute myocardial infarction. A prospective, randomized pilot study, Circulation 98:2017, 1998, with permission.)*

an invasive evaluation, either because of their low-risk scintigraphic profile or lack of inducible ischemia. Conversely, adenosine SPECT can also identify the subset of high-risk patients with extensive ischemia where intensive medical and/or interventional therapies are appropriate. The INSPIRE results complement the findings from earlier randomized clinical trials comparing invasive approaches to conservative approaches, which have incorporated either routine noninvasive risk stratification as a method for triaging patients and/or used current medical therapy approaches.

Figure 35-37 The beneficial effect of intensive medical therapy for treating ischemia. The pre-therapy adenosine SPECT study (**A**) shows a large defect *(arrows)* in the inferior and lateral walls *(upper panels)* that improves with rest imaging *(lower panels)*. The total perfusion defect size (PDS) is 43%, with predominance of ischemia *(green area on polar map)*. This patient was randomized to revascularization but was not an optimal candidate. Following intensive medical therapy (**B**), there is a significant improvement in myocardial perfusion, with only an 8% residual defect. LV, left ventricle; SPECT, single-photon emission computed tomography.

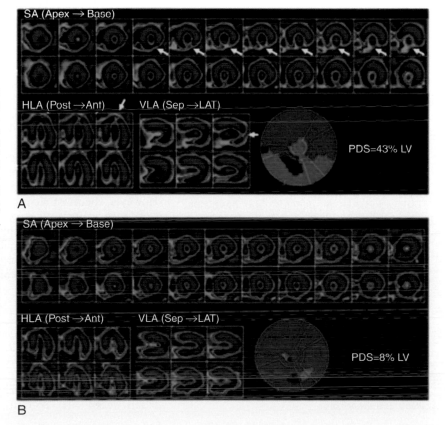

CURRENT GUIDELINES FOR STRATIFYING RISK IN ST-ELEVATION AMI

Exercise MPI is recommended in stable patients with ST-elevation AMI who have not yet undergone in-hospital coronary angiography and who have an uninterpretable ECG for assessing ischemia.[5] This would include patients who receive thrombolytics or patients who have not had reperfusion therapy (Table 35-12). Treadmill testing alone is still recommended in patients with an interpretable ECG. This may change in subsequent guidelines, since treadmill testing is inferior to exercise SPECT for detecting residual ischemia[18] and predicting subsequent outcome,[16,18,35,49,50] and cannot localize ischemia to the culprit coronary artery.

Table 35-12 Current Practice Guidelines: Risk Stratification Following ST-Elevation AMI[5]

Class I

1. In patients not selected for cardiac catheterization and who are without high risk features, exercise testing prior to or early after hospital discharge to assess for myocardial ischemia. (Level of Evidence: B)

2. In patients with baseline abnormalities that compromise ECG interpretation, myocardial perfusion imaging should be added to standard exercise testing. (Level of Evidence: B)

3. In patients unable to exercise who are not undergoing cardiac catheterization, dipyridamole or adenosine myocardial perfusion imaging prior to or early after discharge to look for inducible ischemia. (Level of Evidence: B)

Class IIa

Myocardial perfusion imaging in hemodynamically and electrocardiographically stable patients 4–10 days after ST-elevation AMI to assess myocardial viability when required to define the potential benefit of revascularization. (Level of Evidence: C)

Class IIb

Stress myocardial perfusion imaging to evaluate the functional significance of a coronary lesion primarily identified at angiography. (Level of Evidence: C)

Class III

1. Exercise testing should not be performed within 2–3 days of ST-elevation AMI in patients who have not undergone successful reperfusion. (Level of Evidence: C)

2. Exercise testing should not be performed to evaluate patients who have unstable postinfarction angina, decompensated CHF, life-threatening cardiac dysrhythmias, noncardiac conditions that limit exercise capability, or other absolute contraindications to exercise. (Level of Evidence: C)

3. Exercise testing should not be used to risk stratify patients scheduled for cardiac catheterization. (Level of Evidence: C)

AMI, acute myocardial infarction; CHF, congestive heart failure; ECG, electrocardiogram.
From Antman EM: 2004 Update: A report of the American College of Cardiology/American Heart Association Task Force on Practice Guidelines (Committee on Management of Acute Myocardial Infarction). Available at www.acc.org.

Pharmacologic vasodilators are currently recommended with SPECT only in patients who cannot exercise, even though submaximal exercise SPECT is less sensitive for detecting ischemia[18] and cannot be performed earlier than 3 to 4 days after admission. This latter issue significantly limits the value of a noninvasive approach, since events recur early after AMI.[106–107] INSPIRE corroborates earlier trial data attesting to the safety of adenosine in assessing risk even when administered within 24 hours of admission.[88] Future guidelines may liberalize the use of pharmacologic vasodilators to patients regardless of their exercise capability so as to expedite risk stratification.

Clinically unstable patients with postinfarction angina, decompensated CHF, life-threatening cardiac dysrhythmias, or hemodynamic instability are recommended for coronary angiography.[5] Such patients are appropriately excluded from a noninvasive assessment but represent a small minority (15% to 20%) of those with AMI. However, the guidelines also categorize patients with an LVEF less than 40% as a uniformly high-risk group who will benefit from routine catheterization. This recommendation may also change based on the recent OAT results, where PCI did not improve outcome in patients who had significant LV dysfunction[104] but minimal or no ischemia. Gated adenosine SPECT can readily identify which patients have depressed LV function and whether there is ischemic or nonviable myocardium present so as to guide management.[88]

CURRENT GUIDELINES FOR STRATIFYING RISK IN NON-ST-ELEVATION AMI

The most recent practice guidelines addressing management of patients with unstable angina and non-ST-elevation AMI have been strongly influenced by the FRISC-II[110] and TACTICS-TIMI 18[112] results. Prior to these trials, a routine conservative approach was considered an acceptable alternative to an invasive strategy except in the clinically highest-risk unstable patients. Since then, coronary angiography has been recommended as a frontline approach in all but the most stable lowest-risk patients and in all who are troponin positive. However, the most recent ACC/AHA 2007 guideline revision once again lends stronger support for a noninvasive conservative strategy (Table 35-13).[133] The INSPIRE,[88] ICTUS,[115] and OAT[104] trial results should further promote this philosophy and emphasize the role of perfusion imaging in patient evaluation.

CONCLUSION

Although the complexion of STEMI and non-ST-elevation MI continues to change, present studies and the results from INSPIRE should further solidify the important role of nuclear cardiac imaging, particularly when used in combination with pharmacologic

Table 35-13 Current Practice Guidelines: Risk Stratification Following Non-ST-Elevation AMI and Unstable Angina

Class I

1. An early invasive strategy (i.e., diagnostic angiography with intent to perform revascularization) is indicated in UA/NSTEMI patients who have refractory angina or hemodynamic or electrical instability (without serious comorbidities or contraindications to such procedures). (Level of Evidence: B)

2. An early invasive strategy (i.e., diagnostic angiography with intent to perform revascularization) is indicated in initially stabilized UA/NSTEMI patients (without serious comorbidities or contraindications to such procedures) who have an elevated risk for clinical events. (Level of Evidence: A)

Class IIb

1. In initially stabilized patients, an initially conservative (i.e., a selectively invasive) strategy may be considered as a treatment strategy for UA/NSTEMI patients (without serious comorbidities or contraindications to such procedures) who have an elevated risk for clinical events, including those who are troponin positive. (Level of Evidence:B)

    The decision to implement an initial conservative (versus initial invasive) strategy in these patients may be made by considering physician and patient preference. (Level of Evidence: C)

2. An invasive strategy may be reasonable in patients with chronic renal insufficiency. (Level of Evidence: C)

AMI, acute myocardial infarction; NSTEMI, non-ST-elevation infarction; UA, unstable angina.
From Anderson JL, Adams CD, Antman EM, et al: ACC/AHA 2007 Guidelines for the management of patients with unstable angina/non-ST-elevation myocardial infarction: A report of the American College of Cardiology/American Heart Association Task Force on Practice Guidelines (Writing Committee to Revise the 2002 Guidelines for the Management of Patients with Unstable Angina/Non-ST-Elevation Myocardial Infarction), developed in collaboration with the American College of Emergency Physicians, the Society for Cardiovascular Angiography and Interventions, and the Society of Thoracic Surgeons, endorsed by the American Association of Cardiovascular and Pulmonary Rehabilitation and the Society for Academic Emergency Medicine, J Am Coll Cardiol 50:e1–e157, 2007.

vasodilator stressors, in initial risk stratification of patients with MI and their appropriate triage to medical or interventional strategies.

REFERENCES

1. Detailed diagnoses and procedures. National Hospital Discharge Survey, 1996. National Center for Health Statistics, *Vital Health Stat* 13:138, 1998.
2. Lee KL, Woodlief LH, Topol EJ: for the GUSTO-I Investigators: Predictors of 30-day mortality in the era of reperfusion for acute myocardial infarction. Results from an international trial of 41,021 patients, *Circulation* 91:1659–1668, 1995.
3. Morrow DA, Antman EM, Charlesworth A, et al: TIMI risk score for ST-elevation myocardial infarction: A convenient, bedside, clinical score for risk assessment at presentation. An Intravenous nPA for Treatment of Infarcting Myocardium Early II trial substudy, *Circulation* 102:2031–2037, 2000.
4. Morrow DA, Antman EM, Parsons L, et al: Application of the TIMI risk score for ST-elevation MI in the National Registry of Myocardial Infarction 3, *JAMA* 286:1356–1359, 2001.
5. Antman EM: 2004 update: a report of the American College of Cardiology/American Heart Association Task Force on Practice Guidelines (Committee on Management of Acute Myocardial Infarction), Available at www.acc.org.
6. Cerqueira MD, Maynard C, Ritchie JL, et al: Long-term survival in 618 patients from the Western Washington Streptokinase in Myocardial Infarction trials, *J Am Coll Cardiol* 20:1452–1459, 1992.
7. Miller TD, Christian TF, Hopfenspirger MR, et al: Infarct size after acute myocardial infarction measured by quantitative tomography Tc-99m sestamibi imaging predicts subsequent mortality, *Circulation* 92:334–341, 1995.
8. Ohman EM, Armstrong PW, Christenson RH, et al: for the GUSTO-IIa Investigators: Cardiac troponin T levels for risk stratification in acute myocardial ischemia, *N Engl J Med* 335:1333–1341, 1996.
9. Antman EM, Tanasijevic MJ, Thompson B, et al: Cardiac-specific troponin I levels to predict the risk of mortality in patients with acute coronary syndromes, *N Engl J Med* 335:1342–1349, 1996.
10. The Multicenter Postinfarction Research Group: Risk stratification and survival after myocardial infarction, *N Engl J Med* 309:331–336, 1983.
11. Simoons ML, Vos J, Tijssen JG, et al: Long-term benefit of early thrombolytic therapy in patients with acute myocardial infarction: 5-year follow-up of a trial conducted by the Interuniversity Cardiology Institute of the Netherlands, *J Am Coll Cardiol* 14:1609–1615, 1989.
12. Sanz G, Castaner A, Betriu A, et al: Determinants of prognosis in survivors of myocardial infarction. A prospective clinical angiographic study, *N Engl J Med* 306:1065–1070, 1987.
13. White HD, Norris RM, Brown MA, et al: Left ventricular end-systolic volume as the major determinant of survival after recovery from myocardial infarction, *Circulation* 76:44–51, 1987.
14. St John Sutton M, Pfeffer MA, Plappert T, et al, for the SAVE investigators: Quantitative two-dimensional echocardiographic measurements are major predictors of adverse cardiovascular events after acute myocardial infarction. The protective effects of captopril, *Circulation* 89:68–75, 1994.
15. Gibson RS, Beller GA, Gheorghiade M, et al: The prevalence and clinical significance of residual myocardial ischemia 2 weeks after uncomplicated non-Q wave infarction: A prospective natural history study, *Circulation* 73:1186–1198, 1986.
16. Gibson RS, Watson DD, Craddock GB, et al: Prediction of cardiac events after uncomplicated myocardial infarction: A prospective study comparing predischarge exercise thallium-201 scintigraphy and coronary angiography, *Circulation* 68:321–336, 1983.
17. Mahmarian JJ, Mahmarian AC, Marks GF, Pratt CM, Verani MS: Role of adenosine thallium-201 tomography for defining long-term risk in patients after acute myocardial infarction, *J Am Coll Cardiol* 25:1333–1340, 1995.
18. Brown KA, Heller GV, Landin RS, et al: Early dipyridamole 99mTc-sestamibi single photon emission computed tomographic imaging 2 to 4 days after acute myocardial infarction predicts in-hospital and postdischarge cardiac events: Comparison with submaximal exercise imaging, *Circulation* 100:2060–2066, 1999.
19. Leppo JA, Meerdink DA: Comparison of the myocardial uptake of a technetium-labeled isonitrile analogue and thallium, *Circ Res* 65:632–639, 1989.
20. Nishiyama H, Adolph RJ, Gabel M, et al: Effect of coronary blood flow on thallium-201 uptake and washout, *Circulation* 65:534–542, 1982.
21. Okada RD, Glover D, Gaffney T, et al: Myocardial kinetics of technetium-99m-hexakis-2-methoxy-2-methylpropyl-isonitrile, *Circulation* 77: 491–498, 1988.
22. Granato JE, Watson DD, Flanagan TL, et al: Myocardial thallium-201 kinetics during coronary occlusion and reperfusion: Influence of method of reflow and timing of thallium-201 administration, *Circulation* 73:150–160, 1986.
23. DeCoster PM, Wijns W, Cauwe F, et al: Area-at-risk determination by technetium-99m-hexakis-2-methoxyisobutyl isonitrile in experimental reperfused myocardial infarction, *Circulation* 82:2152–2162, 1990.
24. Liu P, Houle S, Mills L, et al: Kinetics of Tc-99m MIBI in clearance in ischemia-reperfusion: Comparison with Tl-201 (abstr), *Circulation* 76(Suppl IV):216, 1987.
25. Sinusas AJ, Trautman KA, Bergin JD, et al: Quantification of area at risk during coronary occlusion and degree of myocardial salvage after reperfusion with technetium-99m methoxyisobutyl isonitrile, *Circulation* 82:1424–1437, 1990.
26. Verani MS, Jeroudi MO, Mahmarian JJ, et al: Quantification of myocardial infarction during coronary occlusion and myocardial salvage after reperfusion using cardiac imaging with technetium-99m hexakis 2-methoxyisobutyl isonitrile, *J Am Coll Cardiol* 12:1573–1581, 1988.
27. Christian TF, Behrenbeck T, Pellikka PA, et al: Mismatch of left ventricular function and infarct size demonstrated by technetium-99m isonitrile imaging after reperfusion therapy for acute myocardial infarction: Identification of myocardial stunning and hyperkinesia, *J Am Coll Cardiol* 16:1632–1638, 1990.
28. Gibbons RJ, Verani MS, Behrenbeck T, et al: Feasibility of tomographic 99mTc-hexakis-2-methoxy-2-methylpropyl-isonitrile imaging for the

assessment of myocardial area at risk and the effect of treatment in acute myocardial infarction, *Circulation* 80:1277–1286, 1989.

29. Gibbons RJ, Holmes DR, Reeder GS, et al: Immediate angioplasty compared with the administration of a thrombolytic agent followed by conservative treatment for myocardial infarction, *N Engl J Med* 328:685–691, 1993.

30. Santoro GM, Bisi G, Sciagra R, et al: Single photon emission computed tomography with technetium-99m hexakis 2-methoxyisobutyl isonitrile in acute myocardial infarction before and after thrombolytic treatment: Assessment of salvaged myocardium and prediction of late functional recovery, *J Am Coll Cardiol* 15:301–314, 1990.

31. Dixon SR, Whitbourn RJ, Dae MW, et al: Induction of mild systemic hypothermia with endovascular cooling during primary percutaneous coronary intervention for acute myocardial infarction, *J Am Coll Cardiol* 40:1928–1934, 2002.

32. Kopecky SL, Aviles RJ, et al, for the AmP579 Delivery for Myocardial Infarction REduction Study: A randomized, double-blinded, placebo-controlled, dose-ranging study measuring the effect of an adenosine agonist on infarct size reduction in patients undergoing primary percutaneous transluminal coronary angioplasty: The ADMIRE (AmP579 Delivery for Myocardial Infarction REduction) study, *Am Heart J* 146:146–152, 2003.

33. Angeja BG, Gunda M, Murphy SA, et al, TIMI myocardial perfusion grade and ST segment resolution: Association with infarct size as assessed by single photon emission computed tomography imaging, *Circulation* 105:282–285, 2002.

34. Faxon DP, Gibbons RJ, Chronos NA, et al, for the HALT-MI Investigators: The effect of blockade of the CD11/CD18 integrin receptor on infarct size in patients with acute myocardial infarction treated with direct angioplasty: The results of the HALT-MI study, *J Am Coll Cardiol* 40:1199–1204, 2002.

35. Dakik HA, Mahmarian JJ, Kimball KT, et al: Prognostic value of exercise thallium-201 tomography in patients treated with thrombolytic therapy during acute myocardial infarction, *Circulation* 94: 2735–2742, 1996.

36. Zaret BL, Wackers FJT, Terrin ML, et al, for the TIMI Study Group: Value of radionuclide rest and exercise left ventricular ejection fraction in assessing survival of patients after thrombolytic therapy for acute myocardial infarction: Results of Thrombolysis in Myocardial Infarction (TIMI) Phase II Study, *J Am Coll Cardiol* 26:73–79, 1995.

37. Volpi A, DeVita C, Franzosi MG, et al, the Ad hoc Working Group of the Gruppo Italiano per lo Studio della Sopravivienza nell'Infarto Miocardico (GISSI)-2 Data Base: Determinants of 6-month mortality in survivors of myocardial infarction after thrombolysis: Results of the GISSI-2 Data Base, *Circulation* 88:416–429, 1993.

38. The GUSTO: Angiographic Investigators: The effects of tissue plasminogen activator, streptokinase, or both on coronary-artery patency, ventricular function, and survival after acute myocardial infarction, *N Engl J Med* 329:1615–1622, 1993.

39. Pfeffer MA, Braunwald E, Moye LA, et al: Effect of captopril on mortality and morbidity in patients with left ventricular dysfunction after myocardial infarction. Results of the Survival and Ventricular Enlargement Trial, *N Engl J Med* 327:669–677, 1992.

40. Sharir T, Germano G, Kavanagh PB, et al: Incremental prognostic value of post-stress left ventricular ejection fraction and volume by gated myocardial perfusion single photon emission computed tomography, *Circulation* 100:1035–1042, 1999.

41. Seals AA, Pratt CM, Mahmarian JJ, et al: Relation of left ventricular dilation during acute myocardial infarction to systolic performance, diastolic dysfunction, infarct size and location, *Am J Cardiol* 61: 224–229, 1988.

42. Pfeffer MA, Lamas GA, Vaughan DE, et al: Effect of captopril on progressive left ventricular dilation after anterior myocardial infarction, *N Engl J Med* 319:80–86, 1988.

43. Pfeffer MA, Braunwald E: Ventricular remodeling after myocardial infarction. Experimental observations and clinical implications, *Circulation* 81:1161–1172, 1990.

44. Erlebacher JA, Weiss JL, Weisfeldt ML, et al: Early dilation of the infarcted segment in acute transmural myocardial infarction: Role of infarct expansion in acute left ventricular enlargement, *J Am Coll Cardiol* 4:201–208, 1984.

45. Erlebacher JA, Weiss JL, Eaton LW, et al: Late effects of acute infarct dilation on heart size: A two-dimensional echocardiographic study, *Am J Cardiol* 49:1120–1126, 1982.

46. Mahmarian JJ, Moye LA, Chinoy DA, et al: Transdermal nitroglycerin patch therapy improves left ventricular function and prevents remodeling after acute myocardial infarction: Results of a multicenter prospective randomized double-blind placebo controlled trial, *Circulation* 97:2017–2024, 1998.

47. Mahmarian JJ, Moye L, Verani MS, et al: Criteria for the accurate interpretation of changes in left ventricular ejection fraction and cardiac volumes as assessed by rest and exercise gated radionuclide angiography, *J Am Coll Cardiol* 18:112–119, 1991.

48. Hyun IY, Kwan J, Park KS, et al: Reproducibility of Tl-201 and Tc-99m sestamibi gated myocardial perfusion SPECT measurement of myocardial function, *J Nucl Cardiol* 8:182–187, 2001.

49. Chiamvimonvat V, Goodman SG, Langer A, et al: Prognostic value of dipyridamole SPECT imaging in low-risk patients after myocardial infarction, *J Nucl Cardiol* 8:136–143, 2001.

50. Travin MI, Dessouki A, Cameron T, et al: Use of exercise technetium-99m sestamibi SPECT imaging to detect residual ischemia and for risk stratification after acute myocardial infarction, *Am J Cardiol* 75: 665–669, 1995.

51. Theroux P, Waters DD, Halphen C, et al: Prognostic value of exercise testing soon after myocardial infarction, *N Engl J Med* 301:341–345, 1979.

52. Starling MR, Crawford MH, Kennedy GT, et al: Exercise testing early after myocardial infarction: Predictive value of subsequent unstable angina and death, *Am J Cardiol* 46:909–914, 1980.

53. Fioretti P, Brower RW, Simoons ML, et al: Prediction of mortality during the first year after acute myocardial infarction from clinical variables and stress test at hospital discharge, *Am J Cardiol* 55: 1313–1318, 1984.

54. Weld FM, Chu K-L, Bigger JT, et al: Risk stratification with low-level exercise testing 2 weeks after acute myocardial infarction, *Circulation* 64:306–314, 1981.

55. Williams WL, Nair RC, Higginson LA, et al: Comparison of clinical and treadmill variables for the prediction of outcome after myocardial infarction, *J Am Coll Cardiol* 4:477–486, 1984.

56. Jelinek VM, McDonald IG, Ryan WF, et al: Assessment of cardiac risk 10 days after uncomplicated myocardial infarction, *BMJ* 284: 227–230, 1982.

57. Jennings K, Reid DS, Hawkins T, et al: Role of exercise testing early after myocardial infarction in identifying candidates for coronary surgery, *BMJ* 288:185–187, 1984.

58. Handler CE: Submaximal predischarge exercise testing after myocardial infarction: Prognostic value and limitations, *Eur Heart J* 6:510–517, 1985.

59. Krone RJ, Gillespie JA, Weld FM, et al: Low-level exercise testing after myocardial infarction: Usefulness in enhancing clinical risk stratification, *Circulation* 71:80–89, 1985.

60. Applegate RJ, Dell'Italia LJ, Crawford MH: Usefulness of two-dimensional echocardiography during low-level exercise testing early after uncomplicated acute myocardial infarction, *Am J Cardiol* 60:10–14, 1987.

61. Picano E, Landi P, Bolognese L, et al: Prognostic value of dipyridamole echocardiography early after uncomplicated myocardial infarction: A large-scale, multicenter trial, *Am J Med* 95:608–618, 1993.

62. Candell-Riera J, Permanyer-Miralda G, Castell J, et al: Uncomplicated first myocardial infarction: Strategy for comprehensive prognostic studies, *J Am Coll Cardiol* 18:1207–1219, 1991.

63. Corbett JR, Nicod P, Lewis SE, et al: Prognostic value of submaximal exercise radionuclide ventriculography after myocardial infarction, *Am J Cardiol* 52:82A–91A, 1983.

64. Chaitman BR, McMahon RP, Terrin M, et al: Impact of treatment strategy on predischarge exercise test in the Thrombolysis in Myocardial Infarction (TIMI) II Trial, *Am J Cardiol* 71:131–138, 1993.

65. Gianrossie R, Detrano R, Mulvihill D, et al: Exercise induced ST depression in the diagnosis of coronary artery disease: A meta-analysis, *Circulation* 80:87–98, 1989.

66. Heller GV, Ahmed I, Tilkemeier PL, et al: Influence of exercise intensity on the presence, distribution, and size of thallium-201 defects, *Am Heart J* 123:909–916, 1992.

67. Gimple LW, Hutter Am, Guiney TE, et al: Prognostic utility of predischarge dipyridamole-thallium imaging after uncomplicated acute myocardial infarction, *Am J Cardiol* 64:1243–1248, 1989.

68. Wilson WW, Gibson RS, Nygaard TW, et al: Acute myocardial infarction associated with single vessel coronary artery disease. An analysis of clinical outcome and the prognostic importance of vessel patency and residual ischemic myocardium, *J Am Coll Cardiol* 11:223–234, 1988.

69. Tilkemeier PL, Guiney TE, LaRaia PJ, et al: Prognostic value of predischarge low-level exercise thallium testing after thrombolytic treatment of acute myocardial infarction, *Am J Cardiol* 66:1203–1207, 1990.

70. Haber HL, Beller GA, Watson DD, et al: Exercise thallium-201 scintigraphy after thrombolytic therapy with or without angioplasty for acute myocardial infarction, *Am J Cardiol* 71:1257–1261, 1993.

71. Williams DO, Braunwald E, Knatterud G, et al: One-year results of the Thrombolysis in Myocardial Infarction Investigation (TIMI) Phase II trial, *Circulation* 85:533–542, 1992.

72. Abraham RD, Harris PJ, Roubin GS, et al: Usefulness of ejection fraction response to exercise one month after acute myocardial infarction in predicting coronary anatomy and prognosis, *Am J Cardiol* 60:225–230, 1987.

73. Corbett JR, Dehmer GJ, Lewis SE, et al: The prognostic value of submaximal exercise testing with radionuclide ventriculography before

hospital discharge in patients with recent myocardial infarction, *Circulation* 64:535–544, 1981.

74. Hung J, Goris ML, Nash E, et al: Comparative value of maximal treadmill testing, exercise thallium myocardial perfusion scintigraphy and exercise radionuclide ventriculography for distinguishing high- and low-risk patients soon after acute myocardial infarction, *Am J Cardiol* 53:1221–1227, 1984.

75. Nicod P, Corbett JR, Firth BG, et al: Prognostic value of resting and submaximal exercise radionuclide ventriculography after acute myocardial infarction in high-risk patients with single and multivessel disease, *Am J Cardiol* 52:30–36, 1983.

76. Roig E, Magrina J, Armengol X, et al: Prognostic value of exercise radionuclide angiography in low-risk acute myocardial infarction survivors, *Eur Heart J* 14:213–218, 1993.

77. Morris KG, Palmeri ST, Califf RM, et al: Value of radionuclide angiography for predicting specific cardiac events after acute myocardial infarction, *Am J Cardiol* 55:318–324, 1985.

78. Brown KA, Weiss RM, Clements JP, et al: Usefulness of residual ischemic myocardium within prior infarct zone for identifying patients at high risk late after acute myocardial infarction, *Am J Cardiol* 60:15–19, 1987.

79. Younis LT, Byers S, Shaw L, et al: Prognostic value of intravenous dipyridamole-thallium scintigraphy after acute myocardial ischemic events, *Am J Cardiol* 64:161–166, 1989.

80. Leppo JA, O'Brien J, Rothendler JA, et al: Dipyridamole-thallium-201 scintigraphy in the prediction of future cardiac events after acute myocardial infarction, *N Engl J Med* 310:1014–1018, 1984.

81. Brown KA, O'Meara J, Chambers CE, et al: Ability of dipyridamole-thallium-201 imaging 1 to 4 days after acute myocardial infarction to predict in-hospital and late recurrent myocardial ischemic events, *Am J Cardiol* 65:160–167, 1990.

82. Wilson RF, Wyche K, Christensen BV, Zimmer S, Laxson DD: Effects of adenosine on human coronary arterial circulation, *Circulation* 82:1595–1606, 1990.

83. Rossen JD, Quillen JE, Lopez AG, Stenberg RG, Talman CL, Winniford MD: Comparison of coronary vasodilation with intravenous dipyridamole and adenosine, *J Am Coll Cardiol* 18:485–491, 1991.

84. Nishimura S, Mahmarian JJ, Verani MS: Effect of exercise level on equivalence between adenosine and exercise thallium-201 myocardial tomography in coronary artery disease (abstr), *J Nucl Med* 34:95P, 1993.

85. Heller GV, Brown KA, Landin RJ, et al: and the Early Post MI IV Dipyridamole Study (EPIDS): Safety of early intravenous dipyridamole technetium 99m sestamibi SPECT myocardial perfusion imaging after uncomplicated first myocardial infarction, *Am Heart J* 134:105–111, 1997.

86. Mahmarian JJ, Pratt CM, Nishimura S, et al: Quantitative adenosine Tl-201 single-photon emission computed tomography for the early assessment of patients surviving acute myocardial infarction, *Circulation* 87:1197–1210, 1993.

87. Abreu A, Mahmarian JJ, Nishimura S, et al: Tolerance and safety of pharmacologic coronary vasodilation with adenosine in association with thallium-201 scintigraphy in patients with suspected coronary artery disease, *J Am Coll Cardiol* 18:730–735, 1991.

88. Mahmarian JJ, Shaw LJ, Filipchuk NG, et al: for the Adenosine Sestamibi SPECT Post-Infarction Evaluation (INSPIRE) Investigators: A multinational study to establish the value of early adenosine technetium-99m sestamibi myocardial perfusion imaging in identifying a low-risk group for early hospital discharge following acute myocardial infarction, *J Am Coll Cardiol* 48:2448–2457, 2006.

89. Bosch X, Magrina J, March R, et al: Prediction of in-hospital cardiac events using dipyridamole-thallium scintigraphy performed very early after acute myocardial infarction, *Clin Cardiol* 19:189–196, 1996.

90. Pirelli S, Inglese E, Suppa M, et al: Dipyridamole-thallium-201 in the early post-infarction period: Safety and accuracy in predicting the extent of coronary disease and future recurrence of angina in patients suffering from their first myocardial infarction, *Eur Heart J* 9:1324–1331, 1988.

91. Dakik HA, Wendt JA, Kimball K, Pratt CM, Mahmarian JJ: Prognostic value of adenosine Tl-201 myocardial perfusion imaging after acute myocardial infarction: results of a prospective clinical trial, *J Nucl Cardiol* 12:276–283, 2005.

92. Zellweger MJ, Dubois EA, Lai S, et al: Risk stratification in patients with remote prior myocardial infarction using rest-stress myocardial perfusion SPECT: Prognostic value and impact on referral to early catheterization, *J Nucl Cardiol* 9:23–32, 2002.

93. Grines CL, Browne KF, Marco J, et al: A comparison of immediate angioplasty with thrombolytic therapy for acute myocardial infarction, *N Engl J Med* 328:673–679, 1993.

94. Terrin ML, Williams DO, Kleiman NS, et al: Two- and three-year results of the Thrombolysis in Myocardial Infarction (TIMI) Phase II clinical trial, *J Am Coll Cardiol* 22:1763–1772, 1993.

95. Califf RM, White HD, VandeWerf F, et al: for the GUSTO-I Investigators: One-year results from the Global Utilization of Streptokinase and TPA for Occluded Coronary Arteries (GUSTO-I) Trial, *Circulation* 94:1233–1238, 1996.

96. Krone RJ, Gregory JJ, Freedland KE, et al: Limited usefulness of exercise testing and thallium scintigraphy in evaluation of ambulatory patients several months after recovery from an acute coronary event: Implications for management of stable coronary heart disease. Multicenter Myocardial Ischemia Research Group, *J Am Coll Cardiol* 24:1274–1281, 1994.

97. Miller TD, Gersh BJ, Christian TF, et al: Limited prognostic value of thallium-201 exercise treadmill testing early after myocardial infarction in patients treated with thrombolysis, *Am Heart J* 130:259–266, 1995.

98. Ellis SG, Mooney MR, George BS, et al: Randomized trial of late elective angioplasty versus conservative management for patients with residual stenoses after thrombolytic treatment of myocardial infarction. Treatment of Post Thrombolytic Stenoses (TOPS) Study Group, *Circulation* 86:1400–1406, 1992.

99. Andersen HR, Nielsen TT, Rasmussen K, et al: for the DANAMI-2 Investigators: A comparison of coronary angioplasty with fibrinolytic therapy in acute myocardial infarction, *N Engl J Med* 349:733–742, 2003.

100. Zijlstra F, de Boer MJ, Hoorntje JC, et al: A comparison of immediate coronary angioplasty with intravenous streptokinase in acute myocardial infarction, *N Engl J Med* 328:680–684, 1993.

101. Keeley EC, Boura JA, Grines CL: Primary angioplasty versus intravenous thrombolytic therapy for acute myocardial infarction: A quantitative review of 23 randomised trials, *Lancet* 361(9351):3–20, 2003.

102. Rogers WJ, Canto JG, Lambrew CT, et al: Temporal trends in the treatment of over 1.5 million patients with myocardial infarction in the US from 1990 through 1999: The National Registry of Myocardial Infarction 1, 2 and 3, *J Am Coll Cardiol* 36:2056–2063, 2000.

103. Madsen JK, Grande P, Saunamaki K, et al: Danish multicenter randomized study of invasive versus conservative treatment in patients with inducible ischemia after thrombolysis in acute myocardial infarction (DANAMI). DANish trial in Acute Myocardial Infarction, *Circulation* 96:748–755, 1997.

104. Hochman JS, Lamas GA, Buller CE, Dzavik V, Reynolds HR, Abramsky SJ, Forman S, Ruzyllo W, Maggioni AP, White H, Sadowski Z, Carvalho AC, Rankin JM, Renkin JP, Steg PG, Mascette AM, Sopko G, Pfisterer ME, Leor J, Fridrich V, Mark DB, Knatterud GL: Occluded Artery Trial Investigators. Coronary intervention for persistent occlusion after myocardial infarction, *N Engl J Med* 355:2395–2407, 2006.

105. Mahmarian JJ, Dakik HA, Filipchuk NG, Shaw LJ, Iskander SS, Ruddy TD, Keng F, Henzlova MJ, Allam A, Moye LA, Pratt CM, INSPIRE: Investigators. An initial strategy of intensive medical therapy is comparable to that of coronary revascularization for suppression of scintigraphic ischemia in high-risk but stable survivors of acute myocardial infarction, *J Am Coll Cardiol* 48:2458–2467, 2006.

106. Gibson CM, Karha J, Murphy SA, James D, Morrow DA, Cannon CP, Giugliano RP, Antman EM, Braunwald E: TIMI Study Group. Early and long-term clinical outcomes associated with reinfarction following fibrinolytic administration in the Thrombolysis in Myocardial Infarction trials, *J Am Coll Cardiol* 42:7–16, 2003.

107. Neumann FJ, Kastrati A, Pogatsa-Murray G, Mehilli J, Bollwein H, Bestehorn HP, Schmitt C, Seyfarth M, Dirschinger J, Schomig A: Evaluation of prolonged antithrombotic pretreatment ("cooling-off" strategy) before intervention in patients with unstable coronary syndromes: a randomized controlled trial, *JAMA* 290:1593–1599, 2003.

108. The TIMI IIIB Investigators: Effects of tissue plasminogen activator and a comparison of early invasive and conservative strategies in unstable angina and non-Q-wave myocardial infarction. Results of the TIMI IIIB Trial, *Circulation* 89:1545–1556, 1994.

109. Boden WE, O'Rourke RA, Crawford MH, et al: Outcomes in patients with acute non-Q-wave myocardial infarction randomly assigned to an invasive as compared with a conservative management strategy. Veterans Affairs Non-Q-Wave Infarction Strategies in Hospital (VANQWISH) Trial Investigators, *N Engl J Med* 338:1785–1792, 1998.

110. FRagmin and Fast Revascularisation during InStability in Coronary artery disease (FRISC II) Investigators: Invasive compared with noninvasive treatment in unstable coronary-artery disease: FRISC II prospective randomised multicentre study, *Lancet* 354:708–715, 1999.

111. Michalis LK, Stroumbis CS, Pappas K, Sourla E, Niokou D, Goudevenos JA, Siogas C, Sideris DA: Treatment of refractory unstable angina in geographically isolated areas without cardiac surgery. Invasive versus conservative strategy (TRUCS study), *Eur Heart J* 21:1954–1959, 2000.

112. Cannon CP, Weintraub WS, Demopoulos LA, et al, for the TACTICS-Thrombolysis in Myocardial Infarction 18 Investigators: Comparison of early invasive and conservative strategies in patients with unstable coronary syndromes treated with the glycoprotein IIb/IIIa inhibitor tirofiban, *N Engl J Med* 344:1879–1887, 2001.

Pathophysiologic Basis of Hibernating Myocardium

JOHN M. CANTY, JR. AND JAMES A. FALLAVOLLITA

INTRODUCTION

Nuclear cardiology is increasingly used to identify viable chronically dysfunctional myocardium, and imaging is frequently the most significant factor in the decision to pursue coronary revascularization in patients with left ventricular dysfunction and ischemic cardiomyopathy. As summarized in Table 36-1, multiple pathophysiologies can account for viable dysfunctional myocardium in chronic coronary artery disease, and not all of these are the result of chronic repetitive ischemia distal to a coronary stenosis. Reversible dyssynergy has become lumped into a general category termed *hibernating myocardium*, but there appear to be important aspects of cellular remodeling, adaptation, and maladaptation that differ among entities responsible for viable dysfunctional myocardium. These can influence functional recovery, heart failure symptoms, and cardiovascular mortality, including sudden cardiac death. This chapter reviews our current understanding of the functional and metabolic consequences of ischemia. It also summarizes intrinsic mechanisms responsible for viable dysfunctional myocardium with an emphasis on how the physiologic changes impact the interpretation of viability imaging using single-photon emission computed tomography (SPECT), positron emission tomography (PET), and other imaging modalities.

IRREVERSIBLE ISCHEMIA AND THE EVOLUTION OF MYOCARDIAL INFARCTION

The high rate of myocardial metabolism and the near-maximal extraction of oxygen in the coronary circulation dictate that a sudden loss of blood flow due to an acute coronary occlusion quickly leads to the cessation of aerobic metabolism, depletion of creatine phosphate, and anaerobic glycolysis. This is followed by a progressive reduction in tissue adenosine triphosphate (ATP) levels,

with the accumulation of lactate and other catabolites. These metabolic derangements cause a progressive decline in regional contraction within several heartbeats, reaching dyskinesis within 1 minute. Regional dysfunction leads to a reduction in global left ventricular (LV) contractility, a progressive rise in LV end-diastolic pressure, and a fall in systolic pressure. The magnitude of these changes is dependent upon the severity and extent of ischemic myocardium. Electrocardiographic ST-segment changes follow within minutes as the efflux of potassium into the extracellular space reaches a critical level. Anginal symptoms are variable and are usually the last event to occur in the evolution of ischemia. Eventually, ATP levels fall below those required to maintain critical membrane function, resulting in myocyte death.

Evolution of Acute Myocardial Injury

The temporal evolution and extent of irreversible myocardial injury after coronary occlusion is quite variable and strongly dependent on the magnitude of residual coronary flow, the hemodynamic determinants of oxygen consumption, and any endogenous protection afforded by preconditioning.[1,2] Reimer and Jennings demonstrated that in the absence of significant collaterals, irreversible injury begins approximately 20 minutes after coronary occlusion[3] and progresses in a wavefront from the subendocardium to the subepicardium (Fig. 36-1).[4] This susceptibility of the subendocardium to injury reflects its higher oxygen consumption and the redistribution of collateral flow to the outer layers of the heart by the compressive determinants of flow at reduced coronary pressure.[5] In experimental infarction, the entire subendocardium is irreversibly injured within 1 hour of occlusion, and the transmural progression of infarction is largely complete within 4 to 6 hours. Factors that increase myocardial oxygen consumption (e.g., tachycardia, hypertension) or reduce oxygen delivery (e.g., anemia, hypotension) accelerate the progression to irreversible injury. In contrast,

Table 36-1   Viable Dysfunctional Myocardium: Patterns of Contractile Reserve, Resting Perfusion, and Temporal Recovery of Function after Revascularization

	Contractile Reserve	Resting Flow	Extent of Functional Recovery	Time Course of Recovery
Transient Reversible Ischemia				
Postischemic stunning	Present	Normal	Normalizes	<24 Hours
Short-term hibernation	Present	Normal	Normalizes	<7 Days
Chronic Repetitive Ischemia				
Chronic stunning	Present	Normal	Improves	Days to weeks
Chronic hibernating myocardium	Variable	Reduced	Improves	Up to 12 Months
Structural Remodeling				
Remodeled/tethered myocardium	Present	Normal	Improves	Months
Subendocardial infarction	Variable	Reduced	Variable	Weeks

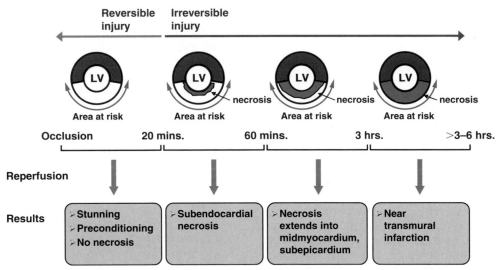

Figure 36-1   Wavefront of necrosis in infarction. Total coronary occlusions of less than 20 minutes do not cause irreversible injury but can cause myocardial stunning, as well as precondition the heart and protect against recurrent ischemic injury. Irreversible myocyte injury begins after 20 minutes and progresses as a wavefront from subendocardium to subepicardium. After 60 minutes, the inner third of the LV wall is irreversibly injured. After 3 hours, there is a subepicardial rim of tissue remaining, with the transmural extent of infarction completed between 3 to 6 hours after occlusion. The most important factor delaying the progression of irreversible injury is the magnitude of collateral flow, which is primarily directed to the outer layers of the heart. *(Modified from Kloner RA, Jennings RB: Consequences of brief ischemia: Stunning, preconditioning, and their clinical implications: Part 1, Circulation 104:2981–2989, 2001, Reprinted with permission.)*

repetitive reversible ischemia prior to occlusion can limit irreversible injury through a preconditioning effect.[1]

Residual Coronary Flow Limits Infarction

The magnitude of residual coronary flow, either due to subtotal coronary occlusion or the presence of intercoronary collaterals, is the most important determinant of the actual time course of irreversible injury. Ultimate infarct size as a percent of the area at risk of ischemia during a total occlusion is inversely related to collateral flow.[6] Subendocardial flow of as little as 30% of resting values can prevent infarction during ischemic periods exceeding an hour. More moderate subendocardial

ischemia (e.g., flow reduced by 50%) can persist for hours without resulting in significant irreversible injury.[7] This phenomenon explains how the signs and symptoms of ischemia can be present for prolonged periods without producing significant myocardial necrosis. It also accounts for the observation that late coronary reperfusion can salvage myocardium beyond the 6-hour limit predicted from experimental models.

Mechanisms of Myocyte Death

During prolonged ischemia with myocardial infarction, cell death arises from two distinct mechanisms. Oxidative stress associated with reperfusion immediately causes myocyte necrosis, characterized by sarcolemmal disruption with the leakage of cell contents into the extracellular space. The associated damage is further amplified by leukocyte-mediated injury arising from reperfusion that can variably produce intravascular occlusion and the "no-reflow phenomenon." After initial survival from ischemia and reperfusion, there is a second wave of myocyte loss due to programmed cell death or apoptosis. This is an energy-dependent and coordinated involution of critically damaged cells that circumvents the inflammation associated with necrotic cell death. The relative importance of each mechanism of cell death in myocardial infarction continues to be controversial.

FUNCTIONAL CONSEQUENCES OF ACUTE REVERSIBLE ISCHEMIA

Fortunately, reversible ischemia is considerably more common than irreversible injury. The functional consequences of acute ischemia are summarized in Figure 36-2. Transient coronary occlusion as a result of coronary vasospasm or temporary thrombosis produces supply-mediated ischemia similar to that present at the onset of infarction (vide supra). Upon reperfusion, regional function can remain depressed as a result of myocardial stunning (vide infra). Demand-induced ischemia develops when regional perfusion is unable to sufficiently increase in response to increases in

myocardial oxygen demand; this predominantly affects the subendocardium. Interestingly, these two mechanisms of acute ischemia have fundamentally different effects on myocardial diastolic relaxation, with supply-mediated ischemia increasing LV compliance and demand-induced ischemia reducing it. Because of the temporal delay in the development of angina, many episodes of acute myocardial ischemia associated with ST-segment depression are symptomatically silent. Very brief episodes of ischemia (as reflected by more sensitive indices such as regional dysfunction or elevations in end-diastolic pressure) can even be electrocardiographically silent.

Stunned Myocardium

There is a temporal delay in the recovery of function after single episodes of ischemia lasting more than 2 minutes. This regional dysfunction occurs despite the restoration of perfusion, with the time course of recovery determined by the duration and severity of the antecedent ischemia. Heyndrickx et al. were the first to demonstrate that regional dysfunction could persist for hours following a 15-minute occlusion, despite complete reperfusion (Fig. 36-3),[8] a phenomenon that Kloner and Braunwald subsequently called *stunned myocardium.*[9] The physiologic hallmark of stunned myocardium is a dissociation of the usual close relation between subendocardial flow and function, where

Consequences of Acute Ischemia

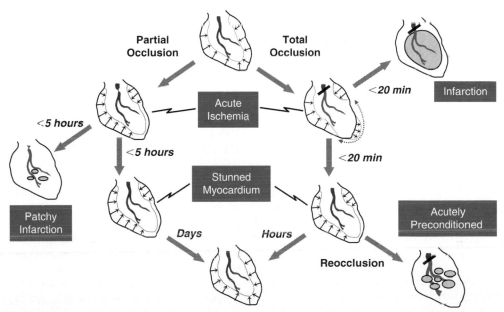

Figure 36-2 Effects of single episodes of acute ischemia on left ventricular function and injury. The ventriculograms illustrate contractile dysfunction *(dotted lines and arrows)*. A brief total occlusion *(right)* or a prolonged partial occlusion (due to an acute high-grade stenosis; *left*) leads to acute contractile dysfunction that is proportional to the reduction in blood flow. Irreversible injury commences 20 minutes after a total coronary occlusion. This progression can be delayed for up to 5 hours in the setting of partial coronary occlusion (or with significant collaterals) due to perfusion-contraction matching or "short-term hibernation." When reperfusion is established before the onset of irreversible injury, stunned myocardium develops, and the time required for recovery of function increases with the duration and severity of ischemia. Brief episodes of ischemia also precondition the heart against infarction by up-regulating a variety of intrinsic protective pathways. *(Modified from Canty JM Jr: Coronary blood flow and myocardial ischemia. In Libby P, Bonow RO, Mann DL, et al (eds): Braunwald's Heart Disease, 8th ed. Philadelphia: Elsevier, 2007, pp 1167–1194.)*

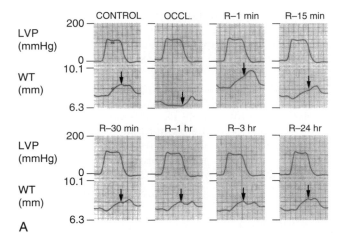

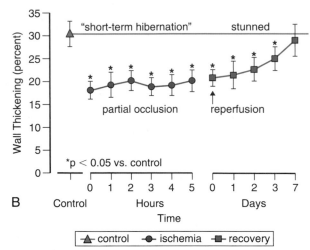

Figure 36-3 Experimental findings in stunned myocardium. **A,** Myocardial stunning following a brief total occlusion. During a 15-minute total occlusion (OCCL), wall thickening measured by ultrasonic crystals (WT) is dyskinetic, with systolic thinning. After reperfusion (R), function is initially depressed but normalizes after 24 hours. **B,** Myocardial stunning following a prolonged partial occlusion. During acute ischemia *(red circles)*, there was perfusion-contraction matching or "short-term hibernation." With reperfusion *(blue squares)*, wall thickening remains depressed and only returns to normal after several days. (**A,** *Modified from Heyndrickx et al.[84] and republished with permission from the American Physiological Society.* **B,** *From Matsuzaki M, Gallagher KP, Kemper WS, et al: Sustained regional dysfunction produced by prolonged coronary stenosis: Gradual recovery after reperfusion, Circulation 68:170–182, 1983. Reprinted with permission.*)

regional dysfunction is present despite normal levels of resting perfusion. Stunned myocardium can also occur after demand-induced ischemia. For example, in the presence of a coronary stenosis, exercise can result in depressed regional function that persists for hours after perfusion is restored, and repetitive ischemia can lead to cumulative stunning.[10] From a clinical perspective, the identification of stunned myocardium is important, since unlike other dysfunctional states, regional function will spontaneously normalize in the absence of recurrent ischemia. Furthermore, contractile reserve is invariably present with inotropic stimulation (e.g.,

dobutamine infusion), usually normalizing regional function (see Table 36-1). In contrast to animal models, acutely stunned myocardium in patients is not always a "pure entity" and frequently coexists with irreversibly injured and viable, chronically dysfunctional myocardium (i.e., chronically stunned and hibernating myocardium, vide infra).

Short-Term Hibernation During Prolonged Moderate Ischemia

When coronary pressure distal to a stenosis falls below the lower limit of autoregulation, flow reserve is exhausted, resulting in subendocardial ischemia during which reductions in subendocardial flow are closely coupled to reductions in regional contractile function.[11] When moderate ischemia persists, the close matching between perfusion and contraction results in a new steady-state with reduced regional oxygen consumption and energy utilization, a phenomenon termed *short-term hibernation*.[7,11] Despite persistent hypoperfusion, the balance between oxygen supply and demand is reestablished, as reflected by regeneration of creatine phosphate and ATP as well as the resolution of lactate production (Fig. 36-4).[12] Importantly, this ability to restore an energetic balance allows myocyte viability to be maintained for a much longer period of time than when flow is absent. Reperfusion of short-term hibernation also leads to stunning, which may take up to a week to resolve (see Fig. 36-3).[13]

While short-term hibernation was originally hypothesized to be the mechanism of chronic hibernating myocardium, it is now clear that short-term hibernation is an extremely tenuous condition, with small increases in myocardial oxygen demand precipitating recurrent ischemia and a rapid deterioration in function and metabolism.[6] Thus, the reversible nature of short-term hibernation is limited by the severity and duration of ischemia, with irreversible injury frequently occurring after more than 12 to 24 hours.[14]

PATHOPHYSIOLOGY OF CHRONIC REPETITIVE ISCHEMIA

Over 60% of patients with ischemic cardiomyopathy have regional dysfunction as a result of repetitive episodes of myocardial ischemia. This dysfunction is part of a pathophysiologic continuum from chronically stunned myocardium with normal resting perfusion to chronic hibernating myocardium with reduced resting perfusion, which appears to be related to the functional significance of the underlying coronary disease and therefore its propensity to cause ischemia (Fig. 36-5).[15,16] The distinguishing physiologic features differentiating chronically stunned from hibernating myocardium are described in the following sections.

Chronically Stunned Myocardium

Basic studies have clearly shown that repetitive episodes of myocardial ischemia with[17-19] and without a residual stenosis[20,21] can result in chronic regional

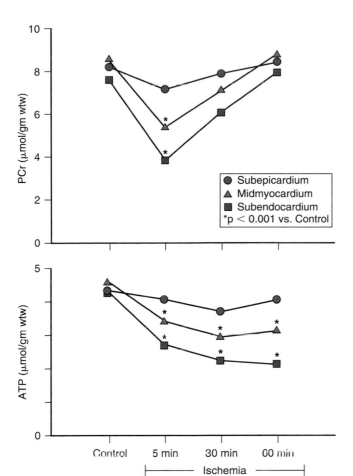

Figure 36-4 Metabolic matching during short-term hibernation. During moderate ischemia, contractile function falls to a new steady state and is accompanied by adaptations in myocardial energy metabolism. These are characterized by an initial fall in creatine phosphate (PCr) and adenosine triphosphate (ATP). The transmural metabolite changes are greatest in the subendocardium *(red squares)*, reflecting the transmural variations in flow. With persistent ischemia, metabolism stabilizes with a regeneration of PCr that prevents further ATP depletion. Although not shown, tissue lactate is transiently increased but normalizes with persistent ischemia. *(Adapted from Pantely GA, Malone SA, Rhen WS, et al: Regeneration of myocardial phosphocreatine in pigs despite continued moderate ischemia, Circ Res 67:1481–1493, 1990.)*

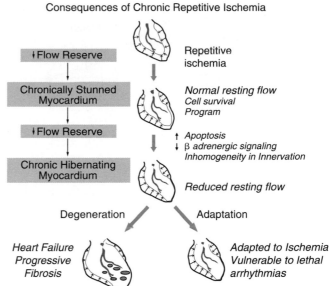

Figure 36-5 Functional consequences of repetitive ischemia. With the progression in severity of a stenosis, coronary flow reserve decreases, and ischemia becomes more frequent. Repetitive ischemia initially leads to chronic preconditioning against infarction and stunning (see Fig. 36-2), which maintains resting function and prevents the development of infarction. As stenosis severity and the frequency of spontaneous ischemia increase further, there is a gradual progression from contractile dysfunction with normal resting flow (chronically stunned myocardium) to contractile dysfunction with depressed resting flow (hibernating myocardium). This transition is related to the physiologic significance of a coronary stenosis and can occur in a time frame as short as 1 week. Alternatively, it can develop chronically and progress in the absence of symptomatic ischemia. The cellular responses during the progression to chronic hibernating myocardium are quite variable. While some patients exhibit little cell death and fibrosis (Adaptation), others develop a picture characterized by degenerative changes that include progressive fibrosis and myocyte death that is difficult to distinguish from subendocardial infarction (Degeneration). The factors that determine the variable progression have not been resolved. *(Modified from Canty JM Jr: Coronary blood flow and myocardial ischemia. In Libby P, Bonow RO, Mann DL, et al (eds): Braunwald's Heart Disease, 8th ed. Philadelphia: Elsevier, 2007, pp 1167–1194.)*

dysfunction with normal resting perfusion. In experimental animal models with a progressive stenosis, chronically stunned myocardium precedes the development of hibernating myocardium.[18,22] Although resting flow is normal in chronically stunned myocardium, the regional uptake of the glucose analog, fluorine-18 2-fluorodeoxyglucose (FDG), is variably increased and appears to be related to the physiologic severity of a coronary stenosis. For example, pigs chronically instrumented with a fixed-diameter left anterior descending (LAD) coronary artery stenosis have regional dysfunction with normal resting perfusion at both 1 and 2 months after initial instrumentation (Fig. 36-6).[18] Regional FDG uptake is initially normal, but it becomes increased as the reduction in flow reserve progresses, and this persists with the transition to hibernating myocardium.

From a clinical perspective, it is important to recognize that viable, chronically dysfunctional myocardium with normal resting perfusion is much more common than hibernating myocardium,[23,24] and it can develop independently of ischemia. For example, in patients with ischemic cardiomyopathy, regional dysfunction with normal resting perfusion may occur distant from a large dysfunctional region (viable or infarcted) as a result of pathologic remodeling. Dysfunction in this remodeled myocardium will not improve with regional revascularization, since it is not a direct result of ischemia. Thus, normal resting perfusion does not necessarily translate into reversible dyssynergy, and it is not surprising that noninfarcted but remodeled segments sometimes have persistent dysfunction after coronary revascularization.[25]

Chronic Hibernating Myocardium

Hibernating myocardium is characterized by contractile dysfunction with reduced resting flow, in the absence

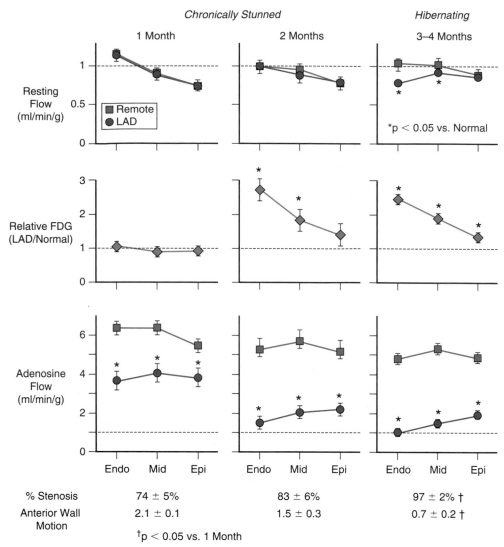

Figure 36-6 Physiologic progression from chronically stunned to hibernating myocardium. Transmural microsphere flow measurements from pigs instrumented with a progressive LAD stenosis at rest and during adenosine vasodilation are shown, along with transmural variations in FDG uptake (fasting conditions) obtained by ex vivo counting. Angiographic stenosis severity and anterior wall motion score (3 normal, 2 mild hypokinesis, 1 severe hypokinesis) at each time point are summarized below the graphs. As stenosis severity increases over time, there is a reduction in vasodilated flow (adenosine) to the LAD region, reflecting a functionally significant coronary lesion. Initially (1 and 2 months after instrumentation), anterior hypokinesis develops, with normal resting flow consistent with chronically stunned myocardium. After 3 months, the stenosis frequently progresses to total occlusion with collateral-dependent myocardium and a critical impairment in coronary flow reserve. At this time, resting flow to the inner two-thirds of the LAD myocardium becomes reduced, compared to normally perfused remote myocardium. The latter findings are consistent with hibernating myocardium and develop without evidence of infarction in this animal model. The temporal progression of abnormalities demonstrates that chronic stunning precedes the development of hibernating myocardium. In contrast to short-term hibernation resulting from acute ischemia, the reduction in resting flow is a consequence rather than cause of the contractile dysfunction. FDG, fluorine-18 2-fluorodeoxyglucose; LAD, left anterior descending coronary artery. *(Modified from Fallavollita JA, Canty JM Jr: Differential 18F-2-deoxyglucose uptake in viable dysfunctional myocardium with normal resting perfusion: Evidence for chronic stunning in pigs, Circulation 99:2798–2805, 1999.)*

of acute ischemia or significant necrosis. It is common in patients with ischemic cardiomyopathy,[26] where it frequently coexists with nontransmural infarction and can also occur in the absence of heart failure or global LV dysfunction. The best clinical example of isolated hibernating myocardium is in patients with chronic coronary occlusions and collateral-dependent myocardium (Fig. 36-7).[27,28] A similar constellation of findings has been reproduced in pigs in the absence of infarction or heart failure, which has facilitated the investigation of the underlying adaptations to ischemia that result in

hibernating myocardium.[22] Studies examining these key physiologic adaptations are summarized later.

The unpredictable progression of clinical coronary disease precludes defining the temporal evolution of hibernating myocardium in patients, and it was originally thought that hibernating myocardium arose from a primary reduction in flow in a fashion similar to experimental models of prolonged moderate ischemia and short-term hibernation.[7] While this is a plausible mechanism for the development of hibernating myocardium in association with an acute coronary syndrome, more

Hibernating Myocardium

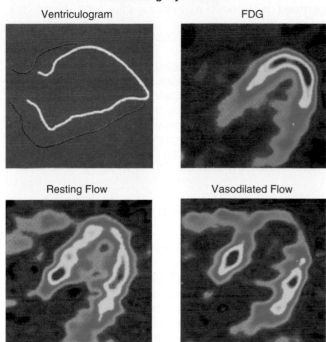

Figure 36-7 Clinical imaging of chronic LAD occlusion and collateral-dependent hibernating myocardium. The RAO tracings of the left ventriculogram show anterior akinesis *(upper left)*. Transaxial PET scans illustrate $^{13}NH_3$ flow measurements at rest *(lower left)* and following pharmacologic vasodilation with dipyridamole *(lower right)*. Resting flow is reduced compared to normal regions in the same heart. The perfusion deficit during vasodilation is even more severe, and quantitative analysis demonstrates that LAD flow reserve is critically impaired. Viability is identified by increased FDG uptake (following an oral glucose load) in the anterior wall *(upper right)*. FDG, fluorine 18 2-fluorodeoxyglucose; LAD, left anterior descending coronary artery. *(Modified from Vanoverschelde J-LJ, Wijns W, Depre C, et al: Mechanisms of chronic regional postischemic dysfunction in humans: New insights from the study of noninfarcted collateral-dependent myocardium, Circulation 87:1513–1523, 1993.)*

recent studies have highlighted the role of the physiologic severity of a coronary stenosis and repetitive ischemia as the major determinants of the progression from stunned to hibernating myocardium. This paradigm developed from animal studies with a slowly progressive stenosis that clearly demonstrated that regional dysfunction with normal resting flow (chronically stunned myocardium) preceded the development of hibernating myocardium, with the down-regulation in resting flow associated with a critical impairment in subendocardial flow reserve (see Fig. 36-6).[15,18,22,29] This progression is not merely a function of time, since the transition from chronically stunned to hibernating myocardium can be experimentally produced in as little as 1 week after placement of a critical stenosis which exhausts coronary flow reserve.[19] A common conclusion of all serial studies is that reduced resting flow in hibernating myocardium is a result rather than a cause of the contractile dysfunction. As will be discussed, the down-regulation of resting flow in hibernating myocardium appears to be a physiologic marker reflecting numerous intrinsic metabolic

adaptations of the heart to repetitive episodes of ischemia.

Metabolic and Energetic Adaptations to Chronic Ischemia

Myocardial Glucose Uptake

Acute myocardial ischemia is obviously associated with acute reductions in oxidative metabolism and an increased dependence on anaerobic glycolysis. This is facilitated by the mobilization of glycogen stores, as well as an increase in myocardial glucose uptake secondary to the translocation of the glucose transporter GLUT4 from intracellular vesicles. This underlies the basis of "hot spot" imaging with the glucose analog FDG for exercise-induced ischemia and acute coronary syndromes[30] and is likely responsible for the enhanced FDG uptake in viable dysfunctional myocardium following dobutamine infusion.[31] Chronically dysfunctional myocardium also demonstrates enhanced basal glucose utilization,[32] and this adaptation can occur in chronically stunned myocardium.[21] Although the mechanism by which glucose utilization is increased in viable dysfunctional myocardium is still under investigation, studies in chronically instrumented pigs have shown an increase in membrane-bound GLUT4, likely due to an up-regulation in p38 mitogen-activated protein kinase.[33] Preliminary studies had suggested a role for up-regulation of glucose transporters in chronic ischemia[34]; however, maximal FDG uptake during insulin stimulation was not altered in pigs with hibernating myocardium (Fig. 36-8).[35] A small decrease in maximal insulin-stimulated FDG uptake has been reported in humans.[36]

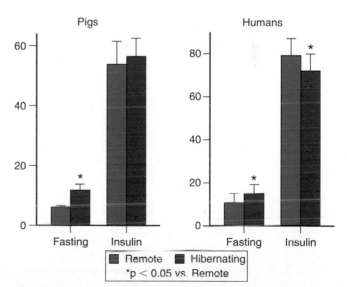

Figure 36-8 Differential FDG uptake in hibernating myocardium in the fasting and insulin-stimulated state. Data summarize fasting and maximal insulin-stimulated glucose uptake estimated in pigs and humans with a chronic coronary occlusion and collateral-dependent myocardium. Whereas regional FDG uptake was increased in the fasting state, quantitative values were well below those attained after insulin infusion. Despite regional increases in the fasting state, maximum insulin-stimulated FDG uptake is not increased in hibernating myocardium. FDG, fluorine-18 2-fluorodeoxyglucose.

Oxygen Consumption

Since myocardial oxygen extraction is near maximal at rest, resting oxygen consumption must also be reduced in hibernating myocardium, and this has been clearly documented using invasive techniques in animals (Fig. 36-9).[37] Other investigators have noninvasively documented regionally reduced oxygen consumption in viable, chronically dysfunctional myocardium using PET and carbon-11 acetate.[27] Most but not all[32,38] studies have shown an energetic balance despite hypoperfusion and some ability to increase metabolism during submaximal stress. For example, in pigs with hibernating myocardium, there was net lactate uptake and normal venous pH during submaximal increases in heart rate, despite the fact that flow and function were lower than in normal myocardium.[37] In humans, coronary venous lactate levels[39] and myocardial tissue lactate concentrations in biopsy specimens were normal.[40] Both basic and clinical studies have also demonstrated preserved creatine phosphate/ATP ratios[41,42] and ATP/adenosine diphosphate (ADP) ratios in hibernating myocardium.[40,42] Absolute ATP levels are mildly reduced in hibernating myocardium,[41] but these alterations are also present in the remote, normally perfused myocardium,[42,43] similar to those occurring in normally perfused periinfarct regions of pigs with myocardial infarction.

Fatty Acid Metabolism

Coincident with the increase in glucose utilization during acute ischemia is a down-regulation in fatty acid utilization, which can be imaged with PET using carbon-11 palmitic acid[44] and other tracers.[45] This down-regulation persists in acute and chronically stunned myocardium,[21] but the limited data currently available suggest that fatty acid metabolism can normalize in chronically dysfunctional myocardium.[46]

Pathologic Remodeling in Hibernating Myocardium

Myocardial biopsy specimens obtained from patients at the time of coronary bypass surgery have demonstrated a broad array of cellular changes that could contribute to the phenotype of hibernating myocardium. The heterogeneity of these findings has led to controversy over whether the myocyte pathologic alterations represent an adaptive or maladaptive response to chronic

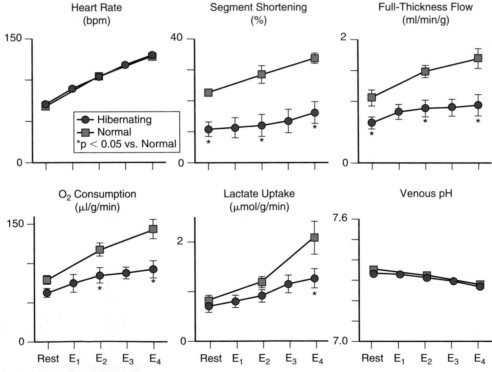

Figure 36-9 Attenuated functional and metabolic responses to submaximal increases in myocardial metabolism in swine with hibernating myocardium. Graphs depict steady-state physiologic parameters after β-adrenergic stimulation with submaximal epinephrine infusion (E_1-E_4) to increase heart rate up to approximately 150 beats/min. In hibernating myocardium, LAD subendocardial-segment shortening, flow, and oxygen consumption were depressed at rest compared to normal control animals. At each level of β-adrenergic stimulation, regional function, flow, and oxygen consumption were reduced compared to normal myocardium. Nevertheless, there was no functional or metabolic evidence of ischemia. LAD segment shortening did not deteriorate, and there was no lactate release or reduction in anterior interventricular vein pH. These findings indicate that the adaptations in hibernating myocardium allow it to operate at a lower point on the relation between myocardial oxygen consumption and external workload. This intrinsic adaptation protects the heart against the development of an acute supply/demand imbalance during submaximal increases in workload, at the expense of reduced resting function and oxygen consumption. LAD, left anterior descending coronary artery. *(Reprinted from Fallavollita JA, Malm BJ, Canty JM Jr: Hibernating myocardium retains metabolic and contractile reserve despite regional reductions in flow, function, and oxygen consumption at rest, Circ Res 92:48–55, 2003.)*

repetitive ischemia. Many studies have supported adaptation, with a reversion to a fetal cellular phenotype and a protein expression pattern that would serve to protect hibernating cardiac myocytes from ischemic stress.[47,48] In contrast, other investigators have found a degenerative phenotype characterized by progressive cell death and marked fibrosis.[49,50] The range of findings reported in human biopsies is illustrated in Figure 36-10. The factors that determine a path of progressive structural degeneration, as opposed to successful adaptation to chronic repetitive ischemia, are currently unknown. Nevertheless, degenerative changes appear to be more common when global LV dysfunction and heart failure are present, and adaptation is more common in stable patients with only regional cardiac dysfunction. This suggests that adaptive changes may be importantly modified by neurohormonal activation. The subsequent discussion of potential mechanisms will primarily focus on observations from animals and humans where hibernating myocardium occurs regionally in the absence of heart failure.

Myofibrillar Loss and Glycogen Accumulation

Biopsies from patients with hibernating myocardium reveal several prototypical features that include myofibrillar loss or myolysis, increased glycogen content, and small mitochondria.[51] While highly affected areas can be identified, less than 40% of the myocytes in a hibernating region exhibit these morphologic changes, so normal myocytes still predominate. In addition, when the myofibrillar volume fraction was quantified, there was less than 10% loss of myofibrils (Fig. 36-11).[19] Many of the cellular changes reported are consistent with a reversion to a fetal myocyte phenotype.[47] The extent that this reflects dedifferentiated adult myocytes versus regenerating myocytes from resident cardiac stem cells is unknown. Nevertheless, these cellular changes can develop rapidly and be recapitulated in animal models in a period of as little as 2 weeks.[19,52,53] They are also seen in disease states such as atrial fibrillation, dilated cardiomyopathy, and in the border zone between

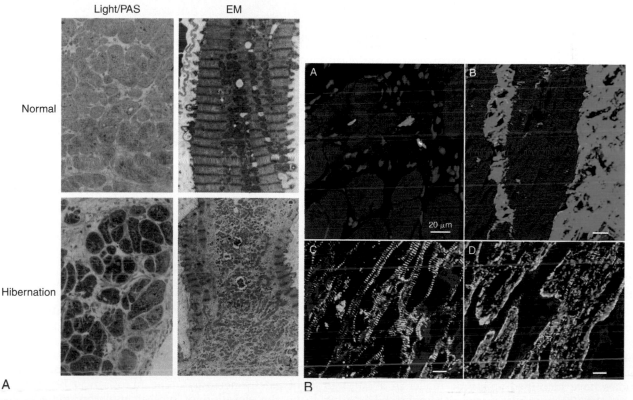

Figure 36-10 Diversity of pathologic findings from transmural biopsies of humans with hibernating myocardium. **A,** Adapted myocyte phenotype. In patients selected so as to avoid the confounding effects of superimposed infarction, Borgers et al. have reported ultrastructural characteristics that suggest reversion to a fetal phenotype.[48] The major electron microscopic features (EM; *right* photomicrographs) are myofibrillar loss and mini-mitochondria. At the light microscopy level, there is increased glycogen content and minimal interstitial fibrosis (Light/PAS; *left* photomicrographs). Necrosis, apoptosis, and autophagy are absent. **B,** Degenerative myocyte phenotype. In consecutive unselected patients with viable dysfunctional myocardium and heart failure, the amount of fibrosis associated with reversible dyssynergy is substantially greater. Myocardial biopsies reveal apoptotic *(panel A)* and autophagic myocyte cell death, as well as interstitial remodeling with increased collagen *(panel B)* and fibronectin *(panels C and D)* that averages as much as 30% of the biopsy. The physiologic and clinical variables determining the progression to each of the two phenotypes is currently unclear. *(A, Adapted from Vanoverschelde J-L, Wijns W, Borgers M, et al: Chronic myocardial hibernation in humans. From bedside to bench, Circulation 95:1961–1971, 1997. B, Panel A adapted from Elsasser A, Vogt AM, Nef H, et al: Human hibernating myocardium is jeopardized by apoptotic and autophagic cell death, J Am Coll Cardiol 43:2191–2199, 2004. Panels B-D adapted from Elsasser A, Schlepper M, Klovekorn WP, et al: Hibernating myocardium: An incomplete adaptation to ischemia, Circulation 96:2920–2931, 1997.)*

Reticular Collagen	Myocyte Hypertrophy	Myolysis	Glycogen

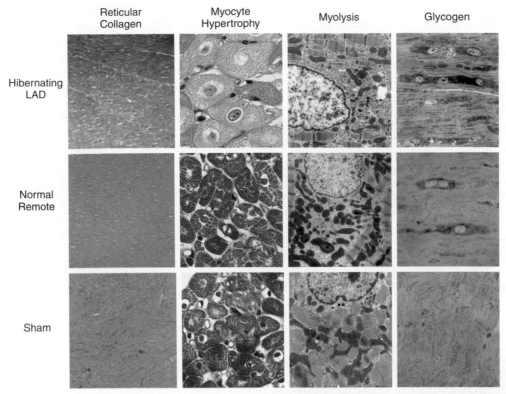

Figure 36-11 Myocyte cellular changes in swine with hibernating myocardium in the absence of heart failure. Swine with hibernating myocardium from a chronic LAD occlusion and collateral-dependent myocardium without infarction or heart failure develop an adapted phenotype. Like the results described by Borgers et al., there is increased reticular connective tissue that is only about 2% greater than values in the remote normally perfused region *(left column)*. Hearts appear grossly normal, but there is cellular hypertrophy in the hibernating region that reflects the consequences of apoptosis-induced myocyte loss *(second column)*. The electron microscopic characteristics of hibernating myocardium are similar to humans with an adapted phenotype and demonstrate myofibrillar loss (Myolysis), numerous small mitochondria, and increased glycogen content *(right column)*. Interestingly, while these are markedly different from normal hearts, biopsies of remote nonischemic segments show similar morphologic changes. Global ultrastructural changes are also seen for other structural proteins.[52] These data indicate that the "cellular hibernating phenotype" is not directly related to ischemia, nor is it the cause of regional contractile dysfunction. This accounts for its presence in disease states not associated with myocardial ischemia. LAD, left anterior descending coronary artery. *(Adapted from Canty JM Jr, Fallavollita JA: Chronic hibernation and chronic stunning: A continuum, J Nucl Cardiol 7:509–527, 2000.)*

normal and infarcted segments of the heart, reviewed elsewhere.[16]

Myocardial Fibrosis, Cell Death, and Myocyte Hypertrophy

In patients with single-vessel disease and hibernating myocardium, there is no necrosis, and interstitial fibrosis averages less than 15% of the tissue volume.[51] The limited number of myocytes in a clinical biopsy precludes accurate quantification of cell death, but porcine studies have identified apoptotic nuclei in about 1 to 2 per 10,000 myocyte nuclei. Although hibernating myocardium appears grossly normal, the chronic nature of apoptosis results in an approximately 30% regional loss of myocytes, with compensatory cellular hypertrophy occurring to maintain normal wall thickness.[54] In contrast to some clinical studies that have suggested that cell death and fibrosis inexorably progress over time,[55,56] pigs with hibernating myocardium demonstrate stable function and connective-tissue staining for at least 2 months.[57,58] Some clinical studies have also demonstrated stability rather than deterioration in function and viability.[59] The intrinsic molecular

adaptations discussed later eventually serve to abrogate myocyte apoptosis (Fig. 36-12). Nevertheless, myocyte loss and/or remodeling, even in the absence of fibrosis, may ultimately limit functional recovery after revascularization.[60,61]

When biopsies are obtained from patients with ischemic cardiomyopathy and heart failure, reversible dyssynergy can be demonstrated, with fibrosis comprising as much as 30% of the sample.[49] In this setting, myocyte death is more evident, with autophagy and even areas of patchy necrosis.[50] The fibrosis may be exacerbated by the elevation of pro-inflammatory cytokines associated with active interstitial remodeling.[62–64] Owing to the heterogeneous nature of the histologic changes in ischemic cardiomyopathy and the frequent association with patchy infarction, it is difficult to determine whether there is myocyte adaptation superimposed on nontransmural infarction or an incomplete adaptation to chronic ischemia in hibernating myocardium. In addition, interstitial fibrosis following repetitive ischemia and stunning may actually be reversible after reperfusion in some experimental models,[65] similar to the reduction in scar volume after myocardial infarction.[66]

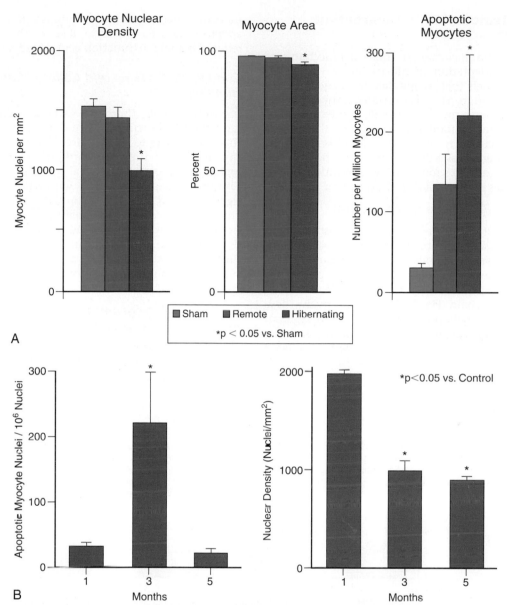

Figure 36-12 Apoptosis and regional myocyte loss in hibernating myocardium. Data from hibernating LAD regions are compared to remote regions as well as LAD regions from normal animals. **A,** The progression from chronically stunned to hibernating myocardium is accompanied by regional apoptosis-induced myocyte loss. Apoptosis is increased approximately sevenfold, yet only affects about 1 in 5000 myocyte nuclei. Nevertheless, since this is a chronic phenomenon, there is an approximately 30% reduction in LAD myocyte nuclear number. This occurs without significant fibrosis, as reflected by the fact that the myocyte area remains nearly normal. **B,** Temporal progression of myocyte apoptosis in swine with viable chronically dysfunctional myocardium. As resting dysfunction develops in response to repetitive ischemia, myocyte apoptosis increases and peaks at 3 months with the transition to hibernating myocardium. While the physiologic features of hibernating myocardium remain unchanged up to 5 months, the intrinsic adaptations to ischemia limit further apoptosis. LAD, left anterior descending coronary artery. *(Adapted from Lim et al.,[54] Fallavollita et al.,[05] and Suzuki et al.[58])*

Global Versus Regional Changes

The cellular alterations described earlier were originally felt to be pathognomonic of hibernating myocardium, but it is now clear that identical changes occur in a variety of disease states associated with elevated preload, such as nonischemic cardiomyopathy and atrial fibrillation.[16] Indeed, when remote normally perfused regions from patients as well as pigs with hibernating myocardium were evaluated, there were identical pathologic findings in both regions (see Fig. 36-11).[19,52,40] Thus, it appears that the majority of histologic changes reflect myocyte stretch rather than the consequences of ischemia. It is also clear that there is a continuum of changes as the heart progresses from chronically stunned to hibernating myocardium, and although cellular dedifferentiation had been emphasized as a mechanism of adaptation, the ultrastructural changes are probably not causally related to the regional responses to ischemia in hibernating myocardium.[16,14]

Molecular Remodeling in Hibernating Myocardium

Recent studies have elucidated the molecular mechanisms responsible for adaptation in hibernating myocardium using animal models that recapitulate the major physiologic features found in patients. In general, these adaptations serve to preserve myocyte viability at the expense of a depressed contractile function. Collectively, the cellular changes that occur in response to regional ischemia in the setting of single-vessel disease are very similar to the global molecular changes found in hypertrophied, nonischemic myocytes in patients with heart failure.

Mitochondrial Proteins and Metabolism

A key target of the intrinsic adaptations of the myocyte to repetitive ischemia appears to be mitochondrial function. Proteomic analysis demonstrates numerous down-regulated proteins, including the entry points to oxidative metabolism and members of the mitochondrial electron-transport chain (Fig. 36-13).[67] Collectively, these changes reduce mitochondrial respiration and regional oxygen consumption at any external workload[37] and protect myocytes from oxidative injury following simulated ischemia in vitro. One potential mechanism is through the up-regulation of uncoupling protein 2.[68] The

mitochondrial adaptations eventually prevent progressive apoptosis-induced myocyte loss at the expense of a reduced contractile function and metabolism.

Contractile Proteins and Cellular Calcium Handling

In swine models, there are variable reductions in the sarcoplasmic reticulum (SR) calcium uptake proteins that are similar to global alterations in cardiomyopathy. In hibernating myocardium, these changes are regional and occur in the absence of heart failure.[69] Like other adaptations, they vary with the physiologic significance of the stenosis and are initially absent in chronically stunned myocardium.[70] Isolated myocytes from swine with viable dysfunctional myocardium demonstrate that changes in SR calcium proteins are functionally significant,[71] and human studies also support an important role of the SR in the depressed contractile response.[72]

Cell Survival Program and Antiapoptotic Program in Response to Repetitive Ischemia

Cell survival pathways are also induced by repetitive ischemia and appear to be particularly prominent during the transition from stunned to hibernating

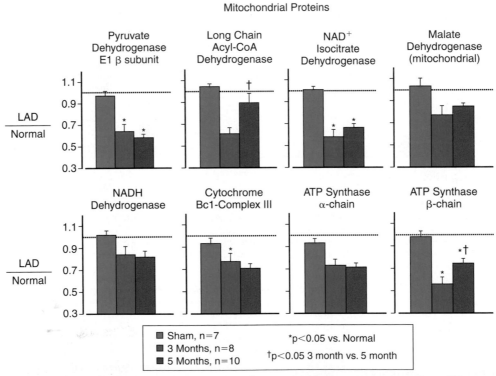

Figure 36-13 Mitochondrial protein remodeling in animals with persistent hibernating myocardium. There were no differences in proteomic profiles between the LAD region of normal sham animals compared to remote myocardium. In contrast, animals with hibernating myocardium developed a down-regulation in mitochondrial proteins, including some of the entry points to oxidative metabolism and selected components of the electron-transport chain. These changes did not reflect mitochondrial loss or increased connective tissue. Like the physiologic changes, most of the mitochondrial proteomic changes persisted in animals with hibernating myocardium that were studied 5 months after instrumentation. Exceptions included long-chain acyl-CoA dehydrogenase and the ATP-synthase β-chain, which tended to normalize. While not shown, increases in stress proteins remained persistently elevated, but increases in cytoskeletal proteins normalized in animals with longer-term hibernation (5 months). LAD, left anterior descending coronary artery. *(Adapted from Page B, Young R, Iyer V, et al: Persistent regional downregulation in mitochondrial enzymes and upregulation of stress proteins in swine with chronic hibernating myocardium, Circ Res 102:103–112, 2008.)*

myocardium. Although the specific pathways vary depending upon model and physiologic state, they include up-regulation of heat shock proteins[69] and down-regulation of glycogen synthase kinase-3β.[21] There is variability in antiapoptotic protein expression in degenerating tissue, with proapoptotic proteins such as Bax increased when a profile of progressive cell death and fibrosis are present in human biopsies.[50] It is likely that the variability of findings among studies reflect differences in the frequency and severity of ischemia, as well as the complex temporal expression of myocardial responses to chronic repetitive ischemia.

Inhomogeneity in Sympathetic Innervation and β-Adrenergic Signaling

Although contractile reserve to β-adrenergic stimulation is present in hibernating myocardium, compared to normal, the response is attenuated,[37] which likely accounts for the underestimation of viability with inotropic stimulation as compared to nuclear imaging.[73] Despite a critical limitation in subendocardial flow reserve, increases in regional function can occur in the absence of acute metabolic ischemia during steady-state submaximal stimulation.[37] At a cellular and molecular level, there are profound regional alterations in myocardial sympathetic innervation, with attenuation of both pre- and post synaptic adrenergic function. Previous studies in isolated vesicular preparations have demonstrated a reduction in cyclic adenosine monophosphate (cAMP) production, as well as a shift from a high- to low affinity β-receptor subtype.[74] In addition, there is partial sympathetic denervation[75] associated with profound reductions in presynaptic sympathetic norepinephrine uptake, as assessed using iodine-131 metaiodobenzylguanidine (MIBG)[76] or carbon-11 metahydroxyephedrine (HED) with PET imaging (Fig. 36-14).[77] The magnitude of these changes is similar to those reported in infarcted myocardium and lead to profound inhomogeneity in myocardial sympathetic innervation. They are functionally significant and attenuate in vivo responses to sympathetic nerve stimulation as well as exogenous β-adrenergic stimulation.[75] The temporal development of these changes and their potential reversibility are currently under study. As will be discussed, inhomogeneity in sympathetic nerve function in hibernating myocardium may identify a myocardial substrate at risk of lethal ventricular arrhythmias, even in the absence of infarction.[78]

TRANSLATION OF MECHANISTIC STUDIES TO THE CLINICAL ASSESSMENT OF VIABILITY

Clinical and basic studies directed at understanding the mechanisms responsible for hibernating myocardium have provided insight into how the heart adapts to ischemia. We will review how some of these mechanisms may impact the ability of imaging to predict myocardial viability, functional recovery, and clinical prognosis.

Blunted Contractile Reserve in Viable Myocardium

It is clear that contractile reserve during β-adrenergic stimulation has a high positive predictive value for functional recovery. However, the molecular alterations in hibernating myocardium that are responsible for the adaptation to chronic ischemia attenuate inotropic responsiveness. For example, the blunted contractile response in pigs with hibernating myocardium[37,79,80] reflects a reduction in cAMP production due to a shift in the β-adrenergic receptor to a low-affinity subtype.[74] In addition, reductions in the SR calcium-handling proteins reduce calcium uptake and release for any level of inotropic stimulation.[19,69] These intrinsic responses in hibernating myocardium may underlie the clinical observation that contractile reserve generally underestimates the frequency of viable dysfunctional myocardium.[73]

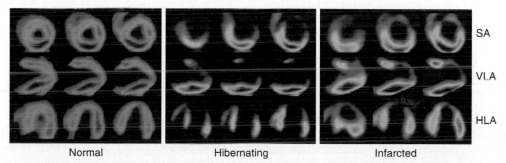

Normal	SA
Hibernating	VLA
Infarcted	HLA

Figure 36-14 PET tomograms of carbon-11 metahydroxyephedrine (HED) uptake in pigs with hibernating myocardium. In normal pigs *(left panel)*, HED uptake was homogeneous. The *middle panel* shows HED uptake in hibernating myocardium. Even though there was no infarction or pathologic fibrosis, there was a prominent reduction in HED uptake in the anterior wall. The *right panel* summarizes findings in a pig with a chronic myocardial infarction, demonstrating the well-known reduction in sympathetic nerves typical of irreversible injury. These findings indicate that there are profound abnormalities in myocardial sympathetic innervation in hibernating myocardium that can contribute to inhomogeneity in myocardial electrophysiologic responses during stress. *(From Luisi AJ Jr, Suzuki G, deKemp R, et al: Regional ^{11}C-hydroxyephedrine retention in hibernating myocardium: Chronic inhomogeneity of sympathetic innervation in the absence of infarction, J Nucl Med 46:1368-1374, 2005. Reprinted with permission of the Society of Nuclear Medicine.)*

Roles of Myocyte Loss and Cellular Remodeling in Limiting Functional Recovery

When resting perfusion is normal, the myocardium is always viable. Nevertheless, contractile dysfunction does not always improve after revascularization of these segments. There are several potential explanations. First, some of these segments may actually exhibit myocyte loss and molecular remodeling typical of hibernating myocardium, but routine clinical imaging may be too insensitive to detect the modest (~20%) relative reductions in flow identified in experimental studies. In addition, the assessment of resting perfusion may not detect infarction confined to the subendocardium, where small amounts of fibrosis can disproportionately reduce regional contraction.

Even when myocardial scarring is carefully excluded with gadolinium magnetic resonance imaging (MRI),[25] up to 25% of noninfarcted segments fail to improve after revascularization. The reasons for persistent dysfunction in the absence of recurrent ischemia or scar are not entirely clear but likely reflect the importance of irreversible myocyte remodeling. In support of this, pigs with hibernating myocardium and apoptosis-induced myocyte loss exhibit persistent dysfunction following revascularization, in the absence of any infarction. Similar myocardial changes can result in irreversible LV dysfunction after surgical intervention for advanced valvular regurgitation. This cellular remodeling is likely a major contributor to the LV dysfunction in advanced ischemic cardiomyopathy, where roughly 80% of the left ventricle is viable and less than 20% irreversibly scarred. Thus, developing approaches to identify myocyte remodeling in the absence of fibrosis may be useful in identifying the likelihood of reversible dyssynergy.

The Impact of Hibernating Myocardium on Prognosis (See Chapters 37 and 38)

While nonrandomized clinical studies have demonstrated the profound negative effect of hibernating myocardium on survival and the amelioration of this risk with revascularization,[26] cause-specific mortality remains undefined. Studies have primarily focused on the potential reversibility of myocardial dysfunction and heart failure; however, some data suggest that the major impact of hibernating myocardium may relate to an increased risk of sudden death.[81] Basic studies support this contention[78] and have demonstrated inhomogeneity in cellular myocyte remodeling and regional inhomogeneity in presynaptic and postsynaptic sympathetic nerve function, which can lead to a substrate that is electrically unstable. Indeed, sudden death from ventricular tachycardia/ventricular fibrillation (VT/VF) develops in pigs with chronic collateral-dependent myocardium in the absence of heart failure (Fig. 36-15). This has given rise to the notion that although adapted to ischemia, the myocyte cellular alterations associated with hibernating myocardium lead to vulnerability to lethal arrhythmias. Since asymptomatic myocardial

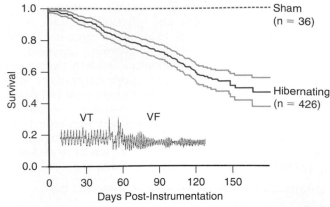

Figure 36-15 Increased risk of arrhythmic death in pigs with hibernating myocardium. Kaplan-Meier survival analysis demonstrated a progressive reduction in survival due to sudden death. There was no mortality in sham-operated control animals. Using implantable Reveal-Plus loop recorders or telemetry, the mechanism of sudden death was almost always ventricular tachycardia (VT) degenerating into ventricular fibrillation (VF) *(inset)*. Postmortem analysis showed that more than 90% of the animals developing sudden death had no pathologic evidence of acute or healed infarction. Total coronary occlusion and physiologic features consistent with hibernating myocardium could be demonstrated several weeks prior to sudden death in a subset of animals. These data indicate that the myocardial adaptive response to ischemia may be a two-edged sword. While protecting myocytes from acute ischemia, they may lead to a substrate characterized by electrical instability and a high risk of lethal ventricular arrhythmias. *(From Canty JM Jr, Suzuki G, Banas MD, et al: Hibernating myocardium: Chronically adapted to ischemia but vulnerable to sudden death, Circ Res 94:1142–1149, 2004.)*

ischemia is so common, it is plausible that similar neural and myocyte remodeling underlie the progression of coronary artery disease and development of sudden death.[82] Thus, while the amount of hibernating myocardium can predict the likelihood of improvement from the standpoint of myocardial dysfunction and heart failure, even small amounts may increase the risk of sudden death. This hypothesis is the basis of an ongoing prospective study to determine whether the presence of hibernating myocardium and/or regional inhomogeneity in sympathetic innervation can predict an increased risk of sudden death in patients who are candidates to receive an implantable cardiac defibrillator (Fig. 36-16).[83]

SUMMARY

In summary, the advent of careful clinical studies in focused patient populations, as well as the development of chronic animal models of hibernating myocardium, have allowed us to make considerable progress in our understanding of the pathophysiologic basis of hibernating myocardium. Previously identified pathologic changes appear to be globally induced and are therefore unrelated to myocardial ischemia and not responsible for the chronic contractile dysfunction. Novel molecular adaptations have been identified that

Viable, Denervated Myocardium

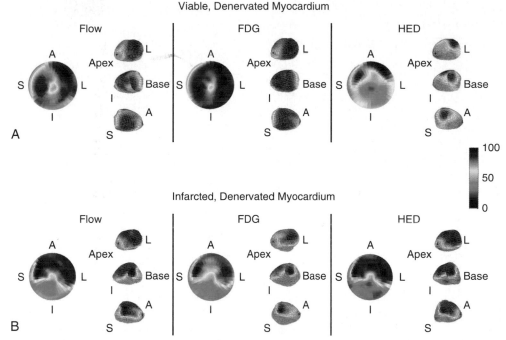

Infarcted, Denervated Myocardium

Figure 36-16 Patterns of viability and sympathetic denervation in patients with ischemic heart failure. Like pigs, humans exhibit variable amounts of viable but denervated myocardium. The upper images are from a patient with a large HED defect that is completely viable, demonstrating a mismatch between viability and denervation. The lower images show a similar HED defect in a patient with a myocardial scar. Here the denervation is matched with a reduction in FDG. The hypothesis that PET imaging can be used to predict the risk of sudden cardiac death in patients who are candidates for primary prevention with an ICD is being tested in the PAREPET study (Prediction of Arrhythmic Events with Positron Emission Tomography). FDG, fluorine-18 2-fluoro-deoxyglucose; HED, carbon-11 hydroxyephedrine; ICD, implantable cardioverter-defibrillator; PET, positron emission tomography. *(From Fallavollita JA, Luisi AJ Jr, Michalek SM, et al: Prediction of arrhythmic events with positron emission tomography: PAREPET study design and methods, Contemp Clin Trials 27:374–388, 2006.)*

collectively indicate that the adapted myocytes take on a regional phenotype similar to that of myocytes in advanced heart failure. This regional response appears to arise as a result of cellular hypertrophy secondary to apoptotic myocyte loss, which can occur in the absence of heart failure. While considerable clinical attention has been directed at identifying hibernating myocardium as a reversible cause of myocardial dysfunction and heart failure, its more significant impact may be in providing a substrate that, while protected against progressive ischemic injury, is vulnerable to the development of lethal ventricular arrhythmias. This could explain the profound impact of revascularization on survival when hibernating myocardium is identified. Ongoing clinical studies should provide more insight into the prevalence of hibernating myocardium in patients with ischemic cardiomyopathy and its impact on prognosis and cause-specific mortality.

REFERENCES

1. Downey JM, Cohen MV: Reducing infarct size in the setting of acute myocardial infarction, *Prog Cardiovasc Dis* 48:363–371, 2006.
2. Cokkinos DV, Pantos C: Myocardial protection in man–from research concept to clinical practice, *Heart Fail Rev* 12:345–362, 2007.
3. Reimer KA, Jennings RB: The "wavefront phenomenon" of myocardial ischemic cell death. II. Transmural progression of necrosis within the framework of ischemic bed size (myocardium at risk) and collateral flow, *Lab Invest* 40:633–644, 1979.
4. Kloner RA, Jennings RB: Consequences of brief ischemia: stunning, preconditioning, and their clinical implications: part 1, *Circulation* 104:2981–2989, 2001.
5. Canty JM Jr: Coronary blood flow and myocardial ischemia. In Libby RO, Bonow RO, Mann DL, et al: *Braunwald's heart disease*, ed 8, Philadelphia, 2007, Elsevier, pp 1167–1194.
6. Schulz R, Rose J, Martin C, et al: Development of short-term myocardial hibernation: Its limitation by the severity of ischemia and inotropic stimulation, *Circulation* 88:684–695, 1993.
7. Heusch G: Hibernating myocardium, *Physiol Rev* 78:1055–1085, 1998.
8. Heyndrickx GR, Millard RW, McRitchie RJ, et al: Regional myocardial functional and electrophysiological alterations after brief coronary artery occlusion in conscious dogs, *J Clin Invest* 56:978–985, 1975.
9. Kloner RA, Jennings RB: Consequences of brief ischemia: stunning, preconditioning, and their clinical implications: part 2, *Circulation* 104:3158–3167, 2001.
10. Homans DC, Laxson DD, Sublett E, et al: Cumulative deterioration of myocardial function after repeated episodes of exercise-induced ischemia, *Am J Physiol* 256:H1462–H1471, 1989.
11. Ross J Jr: Myocardial perfusion-contraction matching: Implications for coronary heart disease and hibernation, *Circulation* 83: 1076–1083, 1991.
12. Pantely GA, Malone SA, Rhen WS, et al: Regeneration of myocardial phosphocreatine in pigs despite continued moderate ischemia, *Circ Res* 67:1481–1493, 1990.
13. Matsuzaki M, Gallagher KP, Kemper WS, et al: Sustained regional dysfunction produced by prolonged coronary stenosis: Gradual recovery after reperfusion, *Circulation* 68:170–182, 1983.
14. Heusch G, Schulz R, Rahimtoola SH: Myocardial hibernation: a delicate balance, *Am J Physiol Heart Circ Physiol* 288:H984–H999, 2005.
15. Canty JM Jr., Fallavollita JA: Chronic hibernation and chronic stunning: a continuum, *J Nucl Cardiol* 7:509–527, 2000.
16. Canty JM, Fallavollita JA: Hibernating myocardium, *J Nucl Cardiol* 12:104–119, 2005.
17. Shen Y-T, Vatner SF: Mechanism of impaired myocardial function during progressive coronary stenosis in conscious pigs: Hibernation versus stunning? *Circ Res* 76:479–488, 1995.
18. Fallavollita JA, Canty JM Jr: Differential ^{18}F-2-deoxyglucose uptake in viable dysfunctional myocardium with normal resting perfusion: Evidence for chronic stunning in pigs, *Circulation* 99:2798–2805, 1999.

19. Thomas SA, Fallavollita JA, Borgers M, et al: Dissociation of regional adaptations to ischemia and global myolysis in an accelerated swine model of chronic hibernating myocardium, *Circ Res* 91:970–977, 2002.
20. Bolli R: Myocardial 'stunning' in man, *Circulation* 86:1671–1691, 1992.
21. Kim SJ, Peppas A, Hong SK, et al: Persistent stunning induces myocardial hibernation and protection: flow/function and metabolic mechanisms, *Cir Res* 92:1233–1239, 2003.
22. Fallavollita JA, Perry BJ, Canty JM Jr: ^{18}F-2-deoxyglucose deposition and regional flow in pigs with chronically dysfunctional myocardium: Evidence for transmural variations in chronic hibernating myocardium, *Circulation* 95:1900–1909, 1997.
23. Melon PG, de Landsheere CM, Degueldre C, et al: Relation between contractile reserve and positron emission tomographic patterns of perfusion and glucose utilization in chronic ischemic left ventricular dysfunction: implications for identification of myocardial viability, *J Am Coll Cardiol* 30:1651–1659, 1997.
24. Sawada S, Elsner G, Segar DS, et al: Evaluation of patterns of perfusion and metabolism in dobutamine-responsive myocardium, *J Am Coll Cardiol* 29:55–61, 1997.
25. Kim RJ, Wu E, Rafael A, et al: The use of contrast-enhanced magnetic resonance imaging to identify reversible myocardial dysfunction, *New Engl J Med* 343:1445–1453, 2000.
26. Allman KC, Shaw LJ, Hachamovitch R, et al: Myocardial viability testing and impact of revascularization on prognosis in patients with coronary artery disease and left ventricular dysfunction: a meta-analysis, *J Am Coll Cardiol* 39:1151–1158, 2002.
27. Vanoverschelde J-LJ, Wijns W, Depre C, et al: Mechanisms of chronic regional postischemic dysfunction in humans: New insights from the study of noninfarcted collateral-dependent myocardium, *Circulation* 87:1513–1523, 1993.
28. Arani DT, Greene DG, Bunnell IL, et al: Reductions in coronary flow under resting conditions in collateral-dependent myocardium of patients with complete occlusion of the left anterior descending coronary artery, *J Am Coll Cardiol* 3:668–674, 1984.
29. Canty JM, Jr., Klocke FJ: Reductions in regional myocardial function at rest in conscious dogs with chronically reduced regional coronary artery pressure, *Circ Res* 61(Suppl II):II–107–II–116, 1987.
30. He ZX, Shi RF, Wu YJ, et al: Direct imaging of exercise-induced myocardial ischemia with fluorine-18-labeled deoxyglucose and Tc-99m-sestamibi in coronary artery disease, *Circulation* 108:1208–1213, 2003.
31. McFalls EO, Murad B, Haspel HC, et al: Myocardial glucose uptake after dobutamine stress in chronic hibernating swine myocardium, *J Nucl Cardiol* 10:385–394, 2003.
32. Vogt AM, Elsasser A, Nef H, et al: Increased glycolysis as protective adaptation of energy depleted, degenerating human hibernating myocardium, *Mol Cell Biochem* 242:101–107, 2003.
33. McFalls EO, Hou M, Bache RJ, et al: Activation of p38 MAPK and increased glucose transport in chronic hibernating swine myocardium, *Am J Physiol Heart Circ Physiol* 287:H1328–H1334, 2004.
34. Brosius FC, Nguyen N, Egert S, et al: Increased sarcolemmal glucose transporter abundance in myocardial ischemia, *Am J Cardiol* 80:77A–84A, 1997.
35. Fallavollita JA: Spatial heterogeneity in fasting and insulin-stimulated 18F-2-deoxyglucose uptake in pigs with hibernating myocardium, *Circulation* 102:908–914, 2000.
36. Maki M, Luotolahti M, Nuutila P, et al: Glucose uptake in the chronically dysfunctional but viable myocardium, *Circulation* 93:1658–1666, 1996.
37. Fallavollita JA, Malm BJ, Canty JM Jr: Hibernating myocardium retains metabolic and contractile reserve despite regional reductions in flow, function, and oxygen consumption at rest, *Circ Res* 92:48–55, 2003.
38. Elsasser A, Muller KD, Skwara W, et al: Severe energy deprivation of human hibernating myocardium as possible common pathomechanism of contractile dysfunction, structural degeneration and cell death, *J Am Coll Cardiol* 39:1189–1198, 2002.
39. Indolfi C, Piscione F, Perrone-Filardi P, et al: Inotropic stimulation by dobutamine increases left ventricular regional function at the expense of metabolism in hibernating myocardium, *Am Heart J* 132:542–549, 1996.
40. Wiggers H, Noreng M, Paulsen PK, et al: Energy stores and metabolites in chronic reversibly and irreversibly dysfunctional myocardium in humans, *J Am Coll Cardiol* 37:100–108, 2001.
41. McFalls EO, Baldwin D, Palmer B, et al: Regional glucose uptake within hypoperfused swine myocardium as measured by positron emission tomography, *Am J Physiol* 272:H343–H349, 1997.
42. Hu Q, Suzuki G, Young RF, et al: Reductions in mitochondrial O_2 consumption and preservation of high energy phosphate levels after simulated ischemia in chronic hibernating myocardium, *Am J Physiol Heart Circ Physiol* 297:H223–H232, 2009.
43. McFalls EO, Kelly RF, Hu Q, et al: The energetic state within hibernating myocardium is normal during dobutamine despite inhibition of ATP-dependent potassium channel opening with glibenclamide, *Am J Physiol Heart Circ Physiol* 293:H2945–H2951, 2007.
44. Schwaiger M, Schelbert HR, Keen R, et al: Retention and clearance of C-11 palmitic acid in ischemic and reperfused canine myocardium, *J Am Coll Cardiol* 6:311–320, 1985.
45. Shoup TM, Elmaleh DR, Bonab AA, et al: Evaluation of trans-9-^{18}F-fluoro-3,4-methyleneheptadecanoic acid as a PET tracer for myocardial fatty acid imaging, *J Nucl Med* 46:297–304, 2005.
46. Maki MT, Haaparanta MT, Luotolahti MS, et al: Fatty acid uptake is preserved in chronically dysfunctional but viable myocardium, *Am J Physiol* 273:H2473–H2480, 1997.
47. Ausma J, Schaart G, Thon F, et al: Chronic ischemic viable myocardium in man: Aspects of dedifferentiation, *Cardiovasc Pathol* 4:29–37, 1995.
48. Vanoverschelde J-L, Wijns W, Borgers M, et al: Chronic myocardial hibernation in humans. From bedside to bench, *Circulation* 95:1961–1971, 1997.
49. Elsasser A, Schlepper M, Klovekorn WP, et al: Hibernating myocardium: an incomplete adaptation to ischemia, *Circulation* 96:2920–2931, 1997.
50. Elsasser A, Vogt AM, Nef H, et al: Human hibernating myocardium is jeopardized by apoptotic and autophagic cell death, *J Am Coll Cardiol* 43:2191–2199, 2004.
51. Maes A, Flameng W, Nuyts J, et al: Histological alterations in chronically hypoperfused myocardium: Correlation with PET findings, *Circulation* 90:735–745, 1994.
52. Thijssen VL, Borgers M, Lenders M-H, et al: Temporal and spatial variations in structural protein expression during the progression from stunned to hibernating myocardium, *Circulation* 110:3313–3321, 2004.
53. Chen C, Liu J, Hua D, et al: Impact of delayed reperfusion of myocardial hibernation on myocardial ultrastructure and function and their recoveries after reperfusion in a pig model of myocardial hibernation, *Cardiovasc Pathol* 9:67–84, 2000.
54. Lim H, Fallavollita JA, Hard R, et al: Profound apoptosis-mediated regional myocyte loss and compensatory hypertrophy in pigs with hibernating myocardium, *Circulation* 100:2380–2386, 1999.
55. Schwarz ER, Schaper J, vom DJ, et al: Myocyte degeneration and cell death in hibernating human myocardium, *J Am Coll Cardiol* 27:1577–1585, 1996.
56. Elsasser A, Decker E, Kostin S, et al: A self-perpetuating vicious cycle of tissue damage in human hibernating myocardium, *Mol Cell Biochem* 213:17–28, 2000.
57. Fallavollita JA, Logue M, Canty JM Jr: Stability of hibernating myocardium in pigs with a chronic left anterior descending coronary artery stenosis: Absence of progressive fibrosis in the setting of stable reductions in flow, function and coronary flow reserve, *J Am Coll Cardiol* 37:1989–1995, 2001.
58. Suzuki G, Lee TC, Fallavollita JA, et al: Adenoviral gene transfer of FGF-5 to hibernating myocardium improves function and stimulates myocytes to hypertrophy and reenter the cell cycle, *Circ Res* 96:767–775, 2005.
59. Wiggers H, Nielsen SS, Holdgaard P, et al: Adaptation of nonrevascularized human hibernating and chronically stunned myocardium to long-term chronic myocardial ischemia, *Am J Cardiol* 98:1574–1580, 2006.
60. Angelini A, Maiolino G, La Canna G, et al: Relevance of apoptosis in influencing recovery of hibernating myocardium, *Eur J Heart Fail* 9:377–383, 2007.
61. Banas MD, Page B, Young RF, et al: Residual dysfunction after revascularization of hibernating myocardium is independent of fibrosis and secondary to myocyte loss and persistent regional reduction in mitochondrial oxidative enzymes, *Circulation* 114(Suppl II):II–66, 2006.
62. Frangogiannis NG, Shimoni S, Chang SM, et al: Active interstitial remodeling: an important process in the hibernating human myocardium, *J Am Coll Cardiol* 39:1468–1474, 2002.
63. Frangogiannis NG, Shimoni S, Chang SM, et al: Evidence for an active inflammatory process in the hibernating human myocardium, *Am J Pathol* 160:1425–1433, 2002.
64. Frangogiannis NG: The pathological basis of myocardial hibernation, *Histol Histopathol* 18:647–655, 2003.
65. Dewald O, Frangogiannis NG, Zoerlein M, et al: Development of murine ischemic cardiomyopathy is associated with a transient inflammatory reaction and depends on reactive oxygen species, *Pro Natl Acad Sci U S A* 100:2700–2705, 2003.
66. Fieno DS, Hillenbrand HB, Rehwald WG, et al: Infarct resorption, compensatory hypertrophy, and differing patterns of ventricular remodeling following myocardial infarctions of varying size, *J Am Coll Cardiol* 43:2124–2131, 2004.
67. Page B, Young R, Iyer V, et al: Persistent regional downregulation in mitochondrial enzymes and upregulation of stress proteins in swine with chronic hibernating myocardium, *Circ Res* 102:103–112, 2008.
68. McFalls EO, Sluiter W, Schoonderwoerd K, et al: Mitochondrial adaptations within chronically ischemic swine myocardium, *J Mol Cell Cardiol* 41:980–988, 2006.

69. Fallavollita JA, Jacob SC, Young RF, et al: Regional alterations in SR Ca^{2+}-ATPase, phospholamban, and HSP-70 expression in chronic hibernating myocardium, *Am J Physiol* 277:H1418–H1428, 1999.

70. Fallavollita JA, Lim H, Canty JM Jr: Myocyte apoptosis and reduced SR gene expression precede the transition from chronically stunned to hibernating myocardium, *J Mol Cell Cardiol* 33:1937–1944, 2001.

71. Bito V, van der Velden J, Claus P, et al: Reduced force generating capacity in myocytes from chronically ischemic, hibernating myocardium, *Circ Res* 100:229–237, 2007.

72. Nef HM, Mollmann H, Skwara W, et al: Reduced sarcoplasmic reticulum Ca^{2+}-ATPase activity and dephosphorylated phospholamban contribute to contractile dysfunction in human hibernating myocardium, *Mol Cell Biochem* 282:53–63, 2006.

73. Underwood SR, Bax JJ, vom Dahl J, et al: Imaging techniques for the assessment of myocardial hibernation. Report of a Study Group of the European Society of Cardiology, *Eur Heart J* 25:815–836, 2004.

74. Iyer V, Canty JM Jr: Regional desensitization of β-adrenergic receptor signaling in swine with chronic hibernating myocardium, *Circ Res* 97:789–795, 2005.

75. Ovchinnikov V, Canty JM Jr, Fallavollita JA: Hibernating myocardium leads to an upregulation in nerve growth factor and partial subendocardial sympathetic denervation, *J Am Coll Cardiol* 49(Suppl A):34A, 2007.

76. Luisi AJ Jr, Fallavollita JA, Suzuki G, et al: Spatial inhomogeneity of sympathetic nerve function in hibernating myocardium, *Circulation* 106:779–781, 2002.

77. Luisi AJ Jr., Suzuki G, deKemp R, et al: Regional ^{11}C-hydroxyephedrine retention in hibernating myocardium: Chronic inhomogeneity of sympathetic innervation in the absence of infarction, *J Nucl Med* 46:1368–1374, 2005.

78. Canty JM Jr, Suzuki G, Banas MD, et al: Hibernating myocardium: Chronically adapted to ischemia but vulnerable to sudden death, *Circ Res* 94:1142–1149, 2004.

79. Malm BJ, Suzuki G, Canty JM Jr, et al: Variability of contractile reserve in hibernating myocardium: Dependence on the method of stimulation, *Cardiovasc Res* 56:422–433, 2002.

80. Ovchinnikov V, Suzuki G, Canty JM Jr, et al: Blunted functional responses to pre- and postjunctional sympathetic stimulation in hibernating myocardium, *Am J Physiol Heart Circ Physiol* 289:H1719–H1728, 2005.

81. Di Carli MF, Maddahi J, Rokhsar S, et al: Long-term survival of patients with coronary artery disease and left ventricular dysfunction: implications for the role of myocardial viability assessment in management decisions, *J Thorac Cardiovasc Surg* 116:997–1004, 1998.

82. Burke AP, Kolodgie FD, Farb A, et al: Healed plaque ruptures and sudden coronary death: evidence that subclinical rupture has a role in plaque progression, *Circulation* 103:934–940, 2001.

83. Fallavollita JA, Luisi AJ, Michalek SM, et al: Prediction of Arrhythmic Events with Positron Emission Tomography: PAREPET study design and methods, *Contemp Clin Trials* 27:374–388, 2006.

84. Heyndrickx GR, Baig H, Nellens P, et al: Depression of regional blood flow and wall thickening after brief coronary occlusions, *Am J Physiol* 234:H653–H659, 1978.

85. Fallavollita JA, Lim H, Canty JM Jr: Apoptosis and reduced SR gene expression precede the transition from chronically stunned to hibernating myocardium, *J Mol and Cell Cardiol* 33:1937–1944, 2001.

Chapter 37

Assessment of Myocardial Viability with Thallium-201 and Technetium-Based Agents

THOMAS A. HOLLY AND ROBERT O. BONOW

INTRODUCTION (See Chapter 36)

In the current era of revascularization surgery and interventional cardiology, the assessment of myocardial viability has become an integral component of the diagnostic evaluation of patients with coronary artery disease (CAD) and depressed left ventricular (LV) function. It is now well established that LV dysfunction is not always an irreversible process related to previous infarction, as once was widely believed. Regional and global ventricular function may improve substantially and even normalize after reperfusion therapy for acute myocardial infarction[1-5] and after myocardial revascularization procedures in patients with chronic CAD.[6-9] This potentially reversible form of LV dysfunction is known as *myocardial hibernation*, indicating a condition in which myocardial contractility has been reduced in the setting of a sustained reduction in myocardial blood supply.[9-12] The conceptual framework of hibernation has been challenged in recent years, and an alternative concept has been proposed of persistent LV dysfunction caused by repeated episodes of myocardial ischemia leading to repetitive stunning.[13,14] This latter mechanism for reversible LV dysfunction in chronic CAD has gathered support from excellent experimental models of repetitive ischemia in the setting of a chronic coronary artery stenosis.[15-18] Independent of the mechanism, which is difficult to determine clinically in individual patients, the important clinical issue is that viable but dysfunctional myocardium in patients with chronic CAD will improve in function only if identified and revascularized. Imaging to evaluate the presence and extent of viable but dysfunctional myocardium has become an important component of the clinical

assessment of patients with CAD and impaired LV function,[19,20] particularly among patients who are possible candidates for myocardial revascularization. These procedures are often accompanied by high operative morbidity and mortality rates in this subset of patients. On the other hand, the large subgroup of patients with moderate to severe LV dysfunction is at considerable risk for death during the course of medical therapy, and these patients potentially have the most to gain from successful revascularization in terms of survival (Fig. 37-1).[21]

Although the percentage of patients showing an important reversal of LV dysfunction after revascularization varies among reported series (probably as a result of patient selection factors and revascularization techniques), it is not inconsequential. It is estimated that 25% to 40% of patients with chronic CAD and LV dysfunction have the potential for significant improvement in LV function after revascularization (Fig. 37-2).[6-8,22,23] These findings have several implications. First, given the important relationship between LV function and survival (see Fig. 37-1), the improvement in LV function after revascularization may translate into an improvement in survival. Although definitive data tying improved function to improved survival are lacking, many recent retrospective studies have begun to establish this point, as discussed later. Second, the decision to proceed with revascularization in patients with moderate to severe LV dysfunction is often difficult. These patients undergo coronary artery bypass surgery or percutaneous coronary intervention with considerable risk of procedure-related morbidity and mortality. The perioperative mortality rate associated with surgical revascularization of patients with severe LV dysfunction is as high as 10%. Hence, accurate methods to detect viable myocardium distal to a coronary stenosis,

594

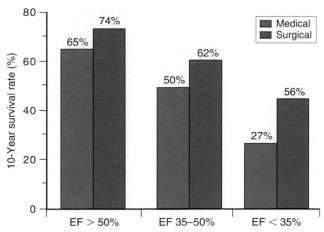

Figure 37-1 Influence of left ventricular ejection fraction (EF) on survival in patients with coronary artery disease. Data from the Duke database are shown for patients with normal left ventricular function *(left)*, mild to moderate left ventricular dysfunction *(center)*, and severe left ventricular dysfunction *(right)*. For each subgroup, survival rates in patients undergoing coronary artery bypass surgery are compared with those in patients treated medically. Although survival rates are higher with surgery compared with medical therapy across the spectrum of left ventricular function, the incremental benefit of surgery is greatest in patients with the most severe left ventricular dysfunction. *(From Muhlbaier LH, Pryor DB, Rankin JS, et al: Observational comparison of event-free survival with medical and surgical therapy in patients with coronary artery disease. 20 years of follow-up, Circulation 86[5 suppl]:II198II–204, 1992.)*

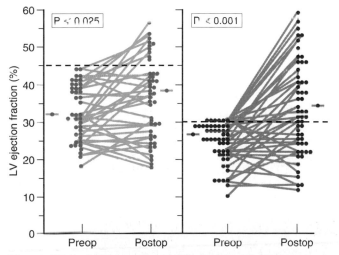

Figure 37-2 Left ventricular (LV) ejection fraction at rest shown by radionuclide ventriculography before (Preop) and after (Postop) coronary artery bypass surgery in patients with preoperative LV dysfunction in two surgical series.[8,20] Although surgery resulted in only a small increase in mean ejection fraction, substantial increases were observed in a substantial subset of patients, with normalization of ejection fraction occurring in many patients. *(From Elefteriades JA, Tolis G Jr, Levi E, et al: Coronary artery bypass grafting in severe left ventricular dysfunction: Excellent survival with improved ejection fraction and functional state, J Am Coll Cardiol 22:1411–1417, 1993; and Bonow RO, Dilsizian V: Thallium-201 for assessment of myocardial viability, Semin Nucl Med 21:230–241, 1991.)*

with the potential for reversal of LV dysfunction, are essential to select prospective patients in whom these risks are justified.

Several clinically reliable physiologic markers can be used to assess myocardial viability. Indexes of regional coronary blood flow, regional wall motion, and regional systolic wall thickening are accurate markers of viability if they are normal or near normal. However, these indexes have major limitations in identifying viable myocardium when they are reduced or absent. By definition, regional perfusion and systolic function (regional wall motion and wall thickening) are severely reduced or absent in patients with hibernating myocardium,[7,9–11,24] despite maintenance of tissue viability. Other patients have preserved blood flow at rest but recurrent ischemic episodes during stress that lead to persistent contractile dysfunction from repetitive stunning.[1,25–29] In these latter patients, indexes of wall motion and wall thickening are also imprecise markers of viability. More recently, cardiac magnetic resonance imaging (MRI) has become a valuable tool for the assessment of myocardial viability. In addition to functional information, areas of hyperenhancement on delayed imaging after gadolinium injection correlate well with areas of scarring.[30–32]

Techniques to assess intact cellular metabolic processes or cell membrane integrity have intrinsic advantages over indices of resting function and blood flow. During the last 2 decades, many studies have shown that nuclear cardiology techniques involving single-photon methods, as well as positron emission tomography (PET), can be used to investigate perfusion, cell membrane integrity, and metabolic activity. Thus, they provide critically important viability information in patients with LV dysfunction. This chapter focuses on the assessment of myocardial viability with thallium- and technetium-based agents.

THALLIUM-201 IMAGING TO ASSESS MYOCARDIAL VIABILITY

Cellular viability requires intact sarcolemmal function to maintain electrochemical gradients across the cell membrane and preserved metabolic activity to generate high-energy phosphates. These processes require adequate myocardial blood flow to deliver substrates and washout metabolites. The retention of ^{201}Tl is an active process that is a function of cell viability and cell membrane activity as well as blood flow. Therefore, in theory, ^{201}Tl should be taken up and retained by viable myocardium regardless of whether systolic function is preserved. Thus, regional thallium activity, even in asynergic regions, should be an accurate marker of viability and should predict improvement of regional contraction after revascularization.[19,27,33–37]

Stress-Redistribution Imaging

Several recent studies of patients with chronic CAD showed that blood flow under basal conditions may be normal or near normal in myocardial regions, despite severe segmental dysfunction, and that this regional dysfunction improves after myocardial revascularization.[1,25,26,28,29] In these patients with perfusion-contraction mismatch, the segmental dysfunction is believed to arise from repeated episodes of myocardial ischemia that lead to repetitive stunning, rather than true myocardial hibernation, which, by definition, requires reduced blood flow under basal conditions. Although the relative prevalence of stunning versus hibernation as a causative mechanism for reversible contractile dysfunction in patients with chronic CAD is uncertain, it appears that both processes occur, but most patients have a form of repetitive stunning. In these patients, the finding of reversible ischemia may be the key to determining the viability of dysfunctional segments, which is readily accomplished with stress thallium imaging. Thus, thallium redistribution in an asynergic region with a defect shown on stress imaging predicts improvement of regional contraction after revascularization (Fig. 37-3).[37,38] However, many regions of severely ischemic or hibernating myocardium appear to have irreversible thallium defects on standard exercise-redistribution imaging; hence, the negative predictive value of an irreversible ^{201}Tl defect is relatively poor. Up to 50% of regions with "irreversible" thallium defects improve in function after revascularization.[38–43] Thus, standard stress-redistribution thallium imaging has an excellent positive predictive value, but a suboptimal negative predictive value. It is generally accepted that stress 4-hour redistribution imaging does not provide satisfactory precision in differentiating between LV dysfunction arising from infarcted versus hibernating myocardium. This technique often underestimates the presence of viable myocardium and hence the potential for recovery after revascularization.

This concept is supported by studies directly comparing the results of PET imaging and exercise-redistribution thallium scintigraphy. In four studies, between 38% and 47% of apparently irreversible thallium defects (that would have been identified as scar by stress-redistribution thallium imaging) were identified as viable on the basis of regional uptake of fluorine-18 (^{18}F)-fluorodeoxyglucose (FDG).[44–47] Although these data suggest that metabolic imaging with PET is superior to thallium imaging in the detection of viable myocardium, two limitations of these studies must be emphasized. First, the severity of the

reduction in thallium activity within the irreversible thallium defects was not assessed. The importance of quantitative analysis of regional thallium activity is discussed later. Second, the previous comparative studies of thallium scintigraphy and PET all used postexercise thallium imaging followed by a single redistribution study 3 to 4 hours later. As noted earlier, the limitations of 4-hour redistribution imaging are well established.

Modifications in imaging protocols with ^{201}Tl considerably enhance the ability of ^{201}Tl imaging to detect viable myocardium.[12,20,35] These include late redistribution imaging and ^{201}Tl reinjection techniques.

Late Thallium-Redistribution Imaging

In many patients, late imaging at 24 to 72 hours elicits ^{201}Tl redistribution in many defects that appear to be irreversible at 3 to 4 hours. This late ^{201}Tl redistribution is evidence of viable myocardium.[39,40,48,49] As many as 54% of defects that appear irreversible at 3 to 4 hours show reversibility at 24 hours, although this number is as low as 22% in some studies. [201]Tl redistribution is a continual process,[50] and a truly irreversible defect shown on early redistribution images will not reverse later. However, in many viable regions, defect reversal at 3 to 4 hours may be minimal and poorly detected. Hence, the defect may not reverse appreciably on qualitative interpretation, and the increase in relative tracer activity also may not exceed the reproducibility limit on quantitative analysis. In these regions, late redistribution imaging may confirm that defect reversibility has occurred.

Several studies show that late imaging at 8 to 72 hours shows substantial thallium redistribution in many defects that appear to be irreversible at 3 to 4 hours,[39,40,48,49] and that this late thallium redistribution is consistent with viable myocardium.[40,49] Kiat et al.[40] reported in 21 patients undergoing myocardial revascularization procedures that 61% of apparently irreversible defects seen at 4 hours reversed at the time of late (18- to 72-hour) redistribution imaging. The revascularization results in this latter study, as assessed by postintervention repeat thallium imaging, provided additional important insights. Of all regions that appeared irreversible at 4 hours, 72% showed improvement after revascularization, confirming earlier studies that found that standard 3- to 4-hour thallium

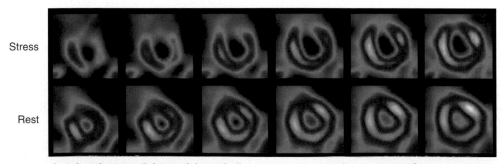

Stress

Rest

Figure 37-3 Stress and redistribution (3-hour delay) thallium-201 tomographic images after maximal treadmill exercise, showing a reversible perfusion abnormality in the septal, anterior, and apical regions in a patient with high-grade stenosis of the left anterior descending coronary artery. The finding of reversibly ischemic myocardium is an accurate indicator of viable myocardium.

redistribution imaging overestimates the prevalence and severity of irreversible myocardial damage. However, when these 4-hour irreversible defects were further analyzed with the results of late imaging, 95% of regions with late redistribution improved after revascularization, compared with only 37% of regions that remained irreversible on late imaging.[40] These findings indicate that myocardial segments that show late thallium redistribution represent viable myocardium and that late imaging may considerably improve the identification of viable myocardium in thallium defects that appear irreversible at 3 to 4 hours. The implications of late thallium redistribution for myocardial viability are similar to those of 3- to 4-hour redistribution. Many persistent defects seen at 3 to 4 hours show late redistribution. The positive predictive value of late redistribution is excellent, but the negative predictive value remains poor. The positive predictive value of late redistribution is more than 90%[40] in predicting improvement after revascularization; thus, defect reversibility with late imaging is an excellent marker of viable myocardium. The negative predictive value of an irreversible defect at 24 hours appears to be only marginally better than that of an irreversible defect at 3 to 4 hours. For example, 37% of irreversible defects seen at 24 hours improve after revascularization,[40] and 39% of irreversible defects seen at 24 hours show improvement by quantitative analysis when ^{201}Tl is reinjected at rest.[51] Moreover, nearly 50% of these defects are metabolically active on PET imaging.[52] This finding suggests that some ischemic regions may never redistribute, even on late imaging, no matter how long the redistribution period, unless serum thallium levels are augmented.

Thallium-Reinjection Techniques

The reinjection of thallium at rest immediately after the standard 4-hour redistribution image may overcome several of these limitations and may be used to assess myocardial viability in apparently irreversible thallium defects on standard early or late-redistribution images (Fig. 37-4).[53–55] Up to 49% of apparently irreversible defects on 3- to 4-hour redistribution images[53] and 39% of these defects on 24-hour redistribution

images[51,56,57] show improved or normal uptake after thallium reinjection.[53] Additional redistribution imaging obtained hours after the reinjected thallium dose appears to provide no information beyond that obtained by imaging immediately after reinjection.[58] Fewer than 5% of myocardial regions with persistent defects on 3- to 4-hour redistribution plus reinjection images show evidence of late redistribution. However, late redistribution imaging is important when reinjection is performed at 4 hours without an intervening redistribution study. A simple exercise-reinjection protocol without redistribution imaging may miss unique and important viability information provided by redistribution. Hence, if reinjection protocols are used, it is essential to perform routine 3- to 4-hour redistribution imaging before the reinjection or to perform late-redistribution imaging in patients with persistent defects on stress-reinjection images.[59]

The observation that thallium uptake after reinjection represents viable myocardium is substantiated in three subgroups of patients. First, in nine studies[43,53,60–66] reporting on 295 patients with LV dysfunction who were evaluated again 3 to 6 months after revascularization, improved wall motion occurred in 69% of segments identified as viable by thallium reinjection before revascularization. Such improvement occurred in only 11% of segments considered nonviable by redistribution or reinjection images (Fig. 37-5). Second, in comparative studies with thallium reinjection and PET imaging with FDG, most myocardial segments that were identified as viable by reinjection had metabolic evidence of myocardial viability.[67–69] The concordance between data on thallium reinjection and FDG uptake was excellent, with 51% of regions with severe irreversible thallium defects on 4-hour redistribution studies identified as viable by both thallium reinjection and PET.[67] Third, in patients who underwent gated MRI to assess regional systolic function, excellent correlation was observed between regional thallium activity and FDG activity in myocardial regions with severely reduced or absent wall thickening.[68]

These PET data are in keeping with previous studies indicating that up to 50% of regions with apparently

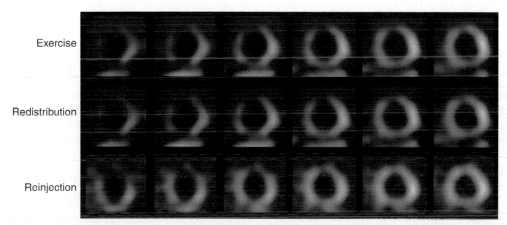

Figure 37-4 Thallium reinjection imaging. Short-axis thallium single-photon emission tomography images obtained after exercise show extensive abnormalities in anterior and septal perfusion that persist on 4-hour redistribution images but improve substantially after reinjection.

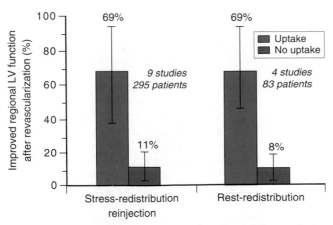

Figure 37-5 Likelihood of improved regional left ventricular (LV) function after revascularization based on thallium-201 single-photon emission tomography imaging. Data are summarized from nine studies done with stress-redistribution-reinjection imaging[43,53,60–66] and four studies done with rest-redistribution imaging.[71,73–75] The range of values reported in the individual studies is shown by the *horizontal bars connected by vertical lines*. The *blue bars* represent the positive predictive value, and the *red bars* represent the inverse of the negative predictive value.

irreversible thallium defects have metabolic activity by PET and thus evidence of viability.[44–47] These data also indicate that thallium reinjection is a convenient, clinically accurate, and relatively inexpensive method with which to identify viable myocardium in patients with chronic CAD and LV dysfunction. Thus, thallium reinjection at rest after 3- to 4-hour redistribution imaging provides most of the clinically relevant information on myocardial viability in regions with apparently irreversible thallium defects. Thallium reinjection may be used instead of 24-hour imaging in most patients with a persistent thallium defect on conventional redistribution images.

Rest-Redistribution Thallium Imaging

The finding of exercise-induced ischemia in a patient with LV dysfunction has important prognostic implications that usually identify the patient as a candidate for revascularization therapy. Thus, exercise-redistribution-reinjection thallium protocols are attractive because they provide important information about both jeopardized myocardium and viable myocardium. However, in many patients, the sole clinical issue is the viability of one or more regions of dysfunctional LV myocardium, not whether there is also inducible ischemia. In others, the coronary anatomy is known to be at high risk, and stress testing is contraindicated, although the determination of viability may establish the potential benefit of revascularization. In these patients, rest-redistribution thallium imaging is a practical approach that can yield accurate viability data. It is essential to obtain both initial images (indicating regional perfusion) and subsequent redistribution images. Although early thallium studies yielded mixed results on the predictive accuracy of rest-redistribution imaging,[33,36]

subsequent studies show that a quantitative analysis of regional thallium activity in rest-redistribution studies predicts recovery of regional LV function with accuracy that is virtually identical to that achieved with thallium exercise-redistribution-reinjection imaging (see Fig. 37-5).[56,70–75] These results are also comparable to those with PET imaging with FDG. PET achieves a higher positive predictive value, and thallium single-photon emission tomography (SPECT) imaging achieves a higher negative predictive value.

The available data comparing rest-redistribution imaging and stress-redistribution-reinjection imaging indicate comparable positive and negative predictive values for recovery of regional function after revascularization. Both techniques have high sensitivity, yielding a negative predictive value of approximately 90% (see Fig. 37-5). However, specificity is much lower, yielding a positive predictive value of less than 70%. A limitation of this analysis is that thallium data are considered binomially, rather than as a continuum.

In laboratories using dual-isotope imaging for stress/rest imaging, with a technetium-99m (^{99m}Tc) tracer for stress imaging and ^{201}Tl for rest imaging, the rest-redistribution thallium technique for viability assessment can be easily incorporated into the evaluation of patients with LV dysfunction, as discussed subsequently in this chapter. This can be done by performing rest-redistribution thallium imaging before the ^{99m}Tc stress test (Fig. 37-6). Alternatively, if irreversible defects are detected after routine stress/rest imaging, late imaging of thallium redistribution at a time when the technetium has decayed provides additional information regarding viability of myocardium with reduced flow under resting conditions.

Quantitative Analysis of Thallium Data

In 12 of the 13 SPECT studies summarized in Figure 37-5, regional thallium activity was analyzed quantitatively rather than with a visual scoring system. It is unclear whether a subjective interpretation of images can replicate these results. However, in most cases, the criteria for viability in these quantitative studies were based on a threshold level of thallium activity such that a thallium level greater than 50% or 60% of the activity in normal myocardial segments was considered viable. This black-and-white approach to the thallium data, classifying myocardial areas simply as viable or nonviable, achieves reasonable results. However, it does not take advantage of one of the greatest strengths of perfusion imaging: the ability to view regional tracer activity as a continuum rather than a simple binary function. Several studies show the nearly linear relationship (Fig. 37-7) between regional thallium activity and the likelihood of recovery of regional function after revascularization.[73–75] This continuous relationship between thallium activity and myocardial viability is confirmed by histologic studies of myocardial biopsy specimens obtained at surgery[76] that show a significant inverse relationship between thallium uptake and the degree of myocardial interstitial fibrosis (Fig. 37-8). For example, all myocardial segments with thallium activity greater

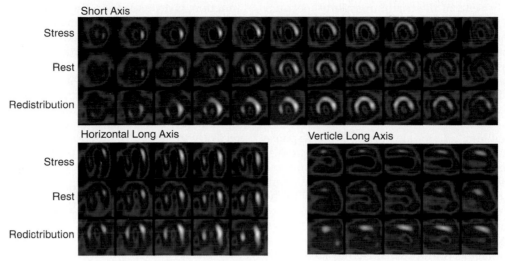

Figure 37-6 Rest-redistribution thallium imaging performed as part of a dual-isotope technetium-thallium stress imaging protocol in a 55-year-old patient with severe heart failure and left ventricular dysfunction (ejection fraction 30%). The initial thallium images at rest demonstrate several areas of reduced resting blood flow involving the septum, anteroapical wall, and inferior wall. Thallium redistribution imaging 4 hours later demonstrates substantial redistribution of thallium in the septal, anteroapical, and inferior regions of the left ventricle, indicating myocardial viability, with only the basal portion of the inferolateral wall representing irreversibly damaged myocardium. Following the thallium-redistribution image acquisition, stress imaging with technetium-99m sestamibi demonstrates inducible ischemia in the septum and anterior wall. However, without the redistribution images, routine stress/rest imaging would have given misleading information about viability because of the irreversible defects in the inferior and anteroapical walls.

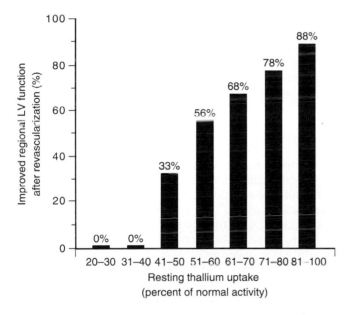

Figure 37-7 The nearly linear relationship between the percentage of peak thallium activity on rest-redistribution imaging and the likelihood of segmental improvement after revascularization. Although various cutoff values have been proposed as "thresholds" for viability, this figure shows the continuous nature of this relationship. LV, left ventricular. *(From Perrone-Filardi P, Pace L, Prastaro M, et al: Assessment of myocardial viability in patients with chronic coronary artery disease: Rest-4 hour-24-hour ^{201}thallium tomography versus dobutamine echocardiography, Circulation 94: 2712–2719, 1996.)*

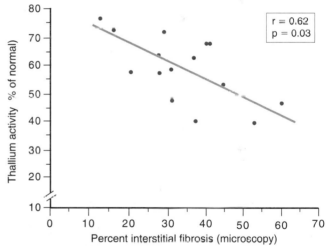

Figure 37-8 Regional thallium activity assessed on single-photon emission tomography imaging in dysfunctional myocardial regions plotted as a function of the percentage of interstitial fibrosis on myocardial biopsy specimens obtained from the same regions. *(From Zimmermann R, Mall G, Rauch B, et al: Residual ^{201}Tl activity in irreversible defects as a marker of myocardial viability: Clinicopathological study, Circulation 91:1016–1021, 1995.)*

than 50% of normal were considered viable in the study of Perrone-Filardi et al.[73] However, 56% of segments with thallium activity of 50% to 60% improved after revascularization, whereas 88% of segments with

thallium activity greater than 80% showed functional improvement after revascularization (see Fig. 37-7). This important factor may explain the wide range of positive predictive values of thallium imaging reported in the individual studies summarized in Figure 37-5; there may have been considerable differences in relative thallium activity in regions considered viable in these studies. A corollary to this argument is that relative regional thallium activity provides a high degree of certainty at either end of the thallium-activity spectrum (see Fig. 37-7), but important uncertainty exists for intermediate thallium levels. Recent data suggest that late redistribution imaging (using a rest-redistribution protocol) may provide greater confidence about the potential for recovery of function in a myocardial region with intermediate thallium activity at 3 to 4 hours; 21% of such regions show increased relative thallium activity at 24 hours.[74]

Regional thallium activity also predicts the response of dysfunctional myocardium to dobutamine stimulation. Dobutamine echocardiography to assess inotropic reserve in viable myocardium shows considerable promise in assessing myocardial viability, in keeping with the presence of residual inotropic reserve in stunned or hibernating myocardium that may be elicited through catecholamine stimulation.[60,71,73,74,77–84] Data suggest that thallium imaging is more sensitive but less specific in identifying which myocardial regions and which patients will show improved function after revascularization.[20] Relative regional thallium activity can be used to determine the likelihood that an asynergic myocardial segment will show contractile reserve with dobutamine (Fig. 37-9).[74,85]

Several studies show another advantage of quantitative analysis. The level of regional thallium activity on delayed redistribution images appears to be a more important determinant of functional recovery after revascularization and a stronger determinant of dobutamine responsiveness than is the change in regional activity between the initial resting images and the redistribution study.[56,74] Thus, the severity of a thallium defect on redistribution images is more predictive of functional outcome than is reversibility of the defect.

Finally, the likelihood of a meaningful increase in LV ejection fraction after revascularization, rather than merely an improvement in regional ventricular

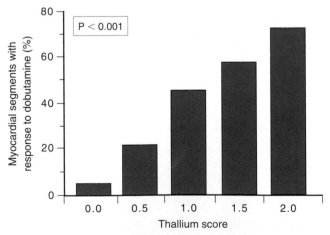

Figure 37-9 Relationship between regional thallium activity (graded on a 5-point visual scale) and the likelihood of inotropic reserve during dobutamine echocardiography. Inotropic reserve is significantly related to regional thallium activity. *(From Panza JA, Dilsizian V, Laurienzo JM, et al: Relation between thallium uptake and contractile response to dobutamine: Implications regarding myocardial viability in patients with chronic coronary artery disease and left ventricular dysfunction, Circulation 91:990–998, 1995.)*

function, is dependent on the mass of myocardium with potentially reversible asynergy. In the study of Ragosta and colleagues,[56] revascularization of seven or more viable but dysfunctional myocardial segments was required for a postoperative increase in LV ejection fraction. This observation is consistent with previous data derived with preoperative PET imaging with FDG.[86,87] Thus, the extent of viable myocardium in a patient with LV dysfunction can be used to predict the magnitude of recovery in global LV function after revascularization.

TECHNETIUM-99ᴍ PERFUSION IMAGING TO ASSESS VIABILITY

^{99m}Tc sestamibi, like ^{201}Tl, requires intact sarcolemmal and mitochondrial processes for retention. This agent is an excellent marker of cellular viability (see Chapters 2 and 3).[88–90] In both experimental and clinical settings in which ^{99m}Tc sestamibi delivery is adequate to dysfunctional myocardium, such as after reperfusion of previously ischemic or damaged myocardium, the uptake and retention of ^{99m}Tc sestamibi tracks with markers of myocardial viability rather than with pure markers of perfusion.[89,91] However, ^{99m}Tc sestamibi does not redistribute as rapidly or as completely as ^{201}Tl after its initial uptake, either during exercise or at rest. Thus, compared with ^{201}Tl, ^{99m}Tc sestamibi appears to have inherent weaknesses for viability assessment when blood flow is severely impaired and tracer delivery is reduced.[92] This observation was supported by initial studies comparing rest/exercise ^{99m}Tc sestamibi imaging with exercise-redistribution-reinjection ^{201}Tl imaging that reported that Tc-99m sestamibi underestimates viable myocardium in patients with chronic CAD and LV dysfunction.[81,93–95]

However, many subsequent studies provided consistent, convincing evidence of the potential use of ^{99m}Tc sestamibi for viability assessment in patients with LV dysfunction. First, ^{99m}Tc sestamibi is well established as an excellent perfusion tracer for detecting inducible myocardial ischemia, determining whether LV function is normal, and assessing the viability of ischemic myocardium. As with ^{201}Tl imaging, myocardial regions with systolic dysfunction and reversible (ischemic) defects on ^{99m}Tc sestamibi imaging have a very high likelihood of recovery of function after revascularization. Moreover, many studies show that a quantitative analysis of ^{99m}Tc sestamibi activity in regions with perfusion defects at rest provides important insights into the potential for improved function with revascularization.[75,96–100] Udelson et al.[75] showed a high concordance (87%) between quantitative resting ^{201}Tl and ^{99m}Tc sestamibi activity in viable segments of myocardium in patients with regional LV dysfunction. Of greater importance, however, was the finding that ^{99m}Tc sestamibi activity at 60% of peak activity had high positive and negative predictive values for the recovery of ventricular function after coronary revascularization (80% and 96%, respectively). These values were similar to those obtained in the same study with ^{201}Tl

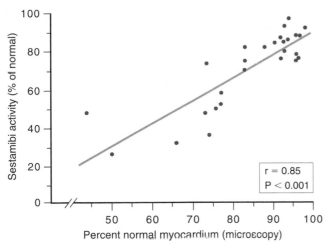

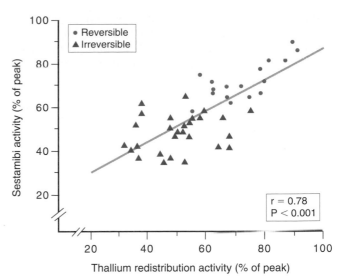

Figure 37-10 Regional sestamibi activity assessed by single-photon emission tomography imaging in dysfunctional myocardial regions plotted as a function of the percentage of viable myocardium on myocardial biopsy specimens obtained from the same regions. *(From Dakik HA, Howell JF, Lawria GM, et al: Assessment of myocardial viability with ^{99m}Tc-sestamibi tomography before coronary bypass graft surgery: Correlation with histopathology and postoperative improvement in cardiac function, Circulation 96:2892–2898, 1997.)*

Figure 37-11 Comparison of regional sestamibi activity at rest and redistribution thallium activity on rest-redistribution imaging in dysfunctional myocardium in patients before coronary bypass surgery. Both tracers show a continuous relationship relative to the likelihood of functional improvement after revascularization. *(From Udelson JE, Coleman PS, Metherall J, et al: Predicting recovery of severe regional ventricular dysfunction: Comparison of resting scintigraphy with ^{201}Tl and ^{99}Tc-sestamibi, Circulation 89:2552–2561, 1994.)*

imaging.[75] As with ^{201}Tl imaging, there is a continuous inverse relationship between regional ^{99m}Tc sestamibi activity and the extent of interstitial fibrosis measured in myocardial biopsy specimens (Fig. 37-10).[98,99] This observation indicates a continuous relationship, similar to that seen with ^{201}Tl imaging, between regional ^{99m}Tc sestamibi activity and the likelihood of improvement in regional function after revascularization (Fig. 37-11).[75] Regional ^{99m}Tc sestamibi activity at rest correlates more strongly with ^{201}Tl redistribution activity than with initial uptake of ^{201}Tl, when resting ^{99m}Tc sestamibi imaging is compared directly with rest-redistribution ^{201}Tl imaging in the same patients.[75,101,102]

Another approach with which to optimize viability assessment with ^{99m}Tc sestamibi is nitroglycerin administration (Fig. 37-12). Several studies show that nitrates improve the detection of viable myocardium by

reducing the size and intensity of the perfusion defect in most viable regions.[100,103–107] Sciagra and colleagues[107] showed that a significant decrease in global defect score after nitroglycerin infusion was noted only in patients who had functional recovery after revascularization. There was a strong correlation between changes in ejection fraction after revascularization and change in defect size after nitroglycerin administration. The mechanism of this phenomenon is unclear, but it may be related to improvement in blood flow and contractility, reducing the partial volume effect of thin, poorly contracting myocardium.[108,109]

Adding ECG gating and dobutamine allows simultaneous assessment of myocardial cellular integrity with perfusion imaging and contractile reserve to potentially reduce the need for echocardiographic assessment.[110,111]

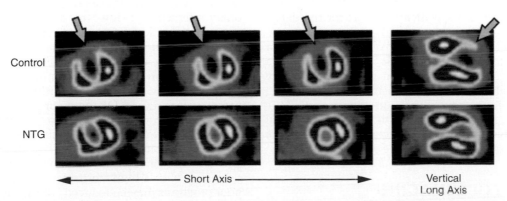

Figure 37-12 Nitrate-enhanced sestamibi imaging showing enhanced tracer uptake in the anterior wall and apex in areas of diminished sestamibi uptake at rest *(arrows)* after nitrate (NTG) administration. *(Images courtesy of Drs. S. Maurea and A. Cuocolo.)*

Leoncini et al.,[112] using nitrate rest and dobutamine SPECT perfusion stress imaging, found that the sensitivity of 99mTc sestamibi for assessing viability, as measured by improved wall motion after revascularization, was 85%, with a specificity of 55%. The use of contractile reserve data alone reduced sensitivity to 64%, but specificity rose to 85%. This study showed that in the subgroup with hypokinetic segments, the sensitivity of the contractile reserve assessment alone compared with perfusion was not affected as much as in the dyskinetic segments, but specificity remained unchanged. Consequently, dobutamine-gated SPECT enhanced the reliability of nitrate-enhanced 99mTc sestamibi in hypokinetic segments, whereas perfusion quantification remained superior in the akinetic segments.

Thus, 99mTc sestamibi may be used for viability assessment with one or a combination of these approaches: assessing the reversibility of stress-induced defects, determining the severity of resting defects with or without nitroglycerin, and assessing contractile reserve with dobutamine administration. The combination of these approaches would optimize the use of 99mTc sestamibi for detecting viable but dysfunctional myocardium.

Other Technetium-99m-Based Tracers

Studies with 99mTc tetrofosmin to assess myocardial viability are somewhat limited. Both agents require active processes for mitochondrial uptake; therefore, 99mTc tetrofosmin should perform in a similar manner to 99mTc sestamibi. Despite some of the limitations of 99mTc tetrofosmin as a perfusion tracer,[113] it can be used in a similar manner to 99mTc sestamibi[114–117] to show viability. A study by He and coworkers[118] showed that Tc-99m tetrofosmin imaging after nitroglycerin administration correlated well with the results of PET imaging with FDG. Similarly, Giorgetti et al. demonstrated that perfusion defects seen when tetrofosmin was administered during an infusion of nitroglycerin correlated well with the areas of hyperenhancement (infarction) seen on contrast-enhanced MRI.[119] Apparently 99mTc tetrofosmin can be used similarly to 99mTc sestamibi for the assessment of myocardial viability.

99mTc NOET is a neutral lipophilic imaging agent that appears to undergo redistribution similar to that of 201Tl.[120] In a small clinical study, 99mTc NOET showed similar sensitivity and specificity to 201Tl for the detection of CAD.[121] However, animal studies show conflicting data on the potential utility of 99mTc NOET for assessing viability.[122,123] Although isolated heart data suggest that 99mTc NOET retention may be affected by myocardial viability,[122] a study using a canine model of reperfused myocardial infarction found that 99mTc NOET uptake reflected reperfusion myocardial blood flow rather than viability.[123] Larger clinical trials are necessary before conclusions can be drawn.

DUAL-ISOTOPE IMAGING

Dual-isotope imaging with separate acquisition of 201Tl images at rest and 99mTc sestamibi or tetrofosmin for

stress imaging is used in many laboratories for the routine evaluation of CAD.[124,125] Viability assessments with these protocols use resting thallium images. Viability determination can be performed in two ways. The choice of protocol usually depends on the pretest likelihood of the need for such a determination. When myocardial viability is a concern before the stress test because of known LV dysfunction, the test can be performed so that thallium rest-redistribution imaging is performed before the stress test (see Fig. 37-6). However, more often, the viability of one or more myocardial regions becomes an issue after the stress test is performed and severe, fixed defects are seen. In this case, 24-hour thallium redistribution imaging can be performed after the stress test, because enough of the technetium has decayed or cleared from the myocardium so that it does not contaminate the thallium images (crosstalk). Some laboratories prefer to give an additional dose of thallium before the 24-hour redistribution images, but simply increasing the acquisition time (25 to 40 seconds per stop in our laboratory) increases the counts and improves image quality. Although comparative data[126] or data on predictive value[127] are limited, results should be similar to those obtained with standard thallium rest-redistribution (4-hour or 24-hour) imaging.

CLINICAL IMPLICATIONS

Viability Assessment and Patient Outcome

The recovery of LV function after revascularization in patients with evidence of myocardial viability also appears to indicate an improved prognosis. PET imaging shows that myocardial revascularization in patients with FDG–blood flow mismatch significantly improves survival, compared with patients who have medical therapy. In two separate studies[128,129] involving a total of 87 patients with LV dysfunction (mean ejection fraction, 31%) the 1-year mortality rate in patients treated medically was 33% in one study and 41% in the other. In contrast, the mortality rate was reduced to 4% in the first study and 12% in the second in patients treated with coronary artery bypass surgery or percutaneous coronary intervention. However, these studies have limitations that should be addressed. They are retrospective, nonrandomized studies with relatively small numbers of patients. The factors used to select some patients for revascularization and others for medical therapy are unspecified, and it is unclear if other predictors of outcome, such as severity of angina or inducible myocardial ischemia, were used to guide the selection for revascularization. However, the overall concordance of the results supports the concept that patients with LV dysfunction and evidence of myocardial viability represent a high-risk group with a high cardiac event rate, and that this poor prognosis may be reduced considerably by revascularization of the viable but underperfused myocardium.

Conversely, thallium imaging may identify patients with LV dysfunction who should not undergo myocardial revascularization. Patients with impaired LV function who have no evidence of residual myocardial viability in dysfunctional regions, or who have only a small number of viable regions, appear to have significantly greater short-term and long-term postoperative mortality risk than patients who undergo revascularization with evidence of extensive viable myocardium in the dysfunctional segments.[130,131] These data show that assessment of myocardial viability with ^{201}Tl imaging may provide critically important data for risk stratification and revascularization decision making in patients with CAD and LV dysfunction.

The clinical utility of viability determination was shown in a meta-analysis by Allman and colleagues.[132] The authors analyzed 24 studies that used thallium imaging, PET imaging, or dobutamine echocardiography to determine myocardial viability in patients with chronic CAD and LV dysfunction. They showed a strong association between viability as determined by these tests and survival after revascularization (Fig. 37-13). In patients with viable myocardium, the annual mortality rate after revascularization was 3.2% compared with 16.0% per year for patients treated medically. However, there was no significant difference in mortality rate between patients undergoing revascularization and those treated medically who did not have viable myocardium (7.7% versus 6.2%, respectively). When the type of treatment was compared, revascularized patients had greater survival rates if they had viable myocardium (annual mortality rate, 3.2% versus 7.7%, respectively), whereas medically treated patients had worse outcomes if they had viable myocardium (16.0% versus 6.2%, respectively). Although the study has several limitations,

it does indicate that using these techniques to determine myocardial viability may help to identify patients who will benefit from revascularization.

A recent review by Camici et al.[133] addressed the phenomena of stunning and hibernation and the assessment of myocardial viability. By pooling data from 11 nonrandomized studies published between 1998 and 2006 that examined long-term survival of patients with LV dysfunction, the authors examined the outcome of four patient groups based on the type of therapy (medical or revascularization) and by the presence or absence of myocardial viability by various techniques (Fig. 37-14). Similar to the results from the meta-analysis of Allman et al., the analysis of Camici et al. demonstrated a survival benefit in patients with viable myocardium who underwent revascularization (weighted average annual mortality 3.71% [95% CI 2.31–5.12] in the viable group versus 10.64% [8.17–13.12] in the nonviable group). However, in those patients without evidence of viable myocardium, there was no significant difference between the treatment groups (weighted average annual mortality 11.69% [8.87–14.51] for medical therapy versus 8.45% [5.80–11.10] for revascularization). In this review of the literature, there was no significant difference in survival between patients with or without evidence of viable myocardium who were treated medically.

The results from the CHRISTMAS (Carvedilol Hibernating Reversible Ischemia Trial: Marker of Success) study showed the ability of SPECT myocardial perfusion imaging to predict improvement in ejection fraction in patients with ischemic LV dysfunction treated with carvedilol.[134] Patients received ^{99m}Tc sestamibi after the administration of sublingual nitroglycerin spray. SPECT imaging was performed at rest. On a separate day, stress imaging was performed, and the myocardial regions were assessed for areas of ischemia and hibernating myocardium (dysfunctional but with preserved tracer uptake). The patients were randomized to receive carvedilol or placebo for 6 months. Overall, the mean

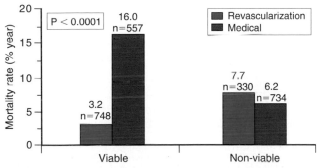

Figure 37-13 Death rates for patients with and without myocardial viability treated by revascularization or medical therapy. This meta-analysis combines data from 24 studies involving 3088 patients who underwent viability testing with thallium-201, dobutamine echocardiography, or positron emission tomography. The annual mortality rate after revascularization in patients with viable myocardium was significantly lower than that for patients treated medically. There was no significant difference in mortality rates between patients undergoing revascularization and those treated medically who did not have viable myocardium. Revascularized patients had significantly greater survival rates if they had viable myocardium. Medically treated patients had worse outcomes if they had viable myocardium. (*From Allman KC, Shaw LJ, Hachamovitch R, et al: Myocardial viability testing and impact of revascularization on prognosis in patients with coronary artery disease and left ventricular dysfunction: A meta-analysis, J Am Coll Cardiol 39:1151–1158, 2002.*)

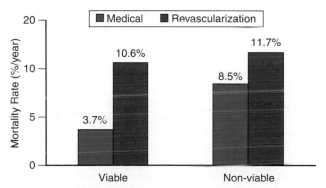

Figure 37-14 Mortality rates for patients with and without myocardial viability treated by revascularization or medical therapy. This analysis involves data from 11 studies involving 2217 patients who underwent viability testing with thallium-201, technetium-99m perfusion tracers, echocardiography, or positron emission tomography. (*Data taken from Table 2 in Camici, Prasad SJ, Rimoldi OE: Stunning, hibernation, and the assessment of myocardial viability, Circulation 117:103–114, 2008.*)

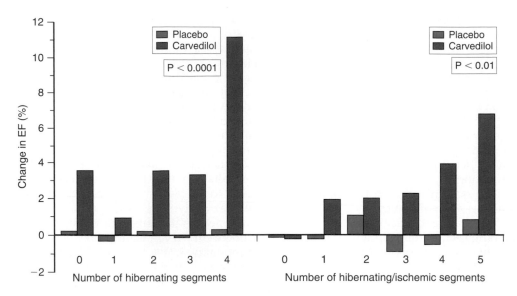

Figure 37-15 Change in left ventricular ejection fraction (EF) according to the number of segments at baseline with hibernating *(left)* or hibernating or ischemic *(right)* myocardium. A significant linear trend was noted between the number of segments affected by either hibernation or ischemia and the response to carvedilol. *(From Cleland JG, Pennell DJ, Ray SG, et al: Carvedilol hibernating reversible ischaemia trial: Marker of success investigators. Myocardial viability as a determinant of the ejection fraction response to carvedilol in patients with heart failure [CHRISTMAS trial]: Randomised controlled trial, Lancet 362:14–21, 2003.)*

improvement in ejection fraction was 2.8% in the carvedilol group (compared with −0.4% in the placebo group), and the degree of improvement in ejection fraction was related to the amount of myocardium that was hibernating, ischemic, or both (Fig. 37-15).

The assessment of myocardial viability is an area of intense interest for several reasons. Among these is the unique potential of nuclear cardiology techniques to identify viable regions on the basis of perfusion, cell membrane integrity, and metabolic activity, thereby providing greater precision than can be achieved by assessment of regional anatomy or function. However, there are unresolved issues regarding the clinical applications of such techniques. Recovery of regional LV function after revascularization, long the gold standard against which noninvasive imaging techniques have been compared, may not be the only, or even the most important, benefit of revascularization of viable but dysfunctional myocardium. Even in the absence of improved LV systolic function, revascularization of viable myocardium downstream from a critical coronary artery stenosis may provide clinical benefit by attenuating LV dilation and remodeling, reducing ventricular arrhythmias, and decreasing the risk of subsequent fatal ischemic events.

Whether a clinically relevant change in ventricular performance occurs after myocardial revascularization, and whether this change translates into improved lifestyle and prognosis, depends on a number of factors, many of which are poorly defined. The amount of dysfunctional but viable myocardium is certainly one such factor, but at the current time, the identification of viable myocardium is not in and of itself an indication for revascularization. Large randomized, controlled clinical trials are needed to address the role of revascularization and viability assessment in the management of patients with ischemic cardiomyopathy. The STICH trial (Surgical Treatment for Ischemic Heart Failure) is a National Heart, Lung and Blood Institute–sponsored study to examine such questions.[135] Results regarding viability determination are anticipated to be available in 2010. Based on the currently available data, assessing for viability/ischemia is listed as an appropriate indication (with a score of 8.5) in the American College of Cardiology SPECT Appropriateness Criteria.[136] In addition, the assessment of viability for consideration of revascularization in patients with CAD and LV systolic dysfunction who do not have angina is a class I indication for the use of radionuclide imaging with SPECT or PET.[137]

As in any other patient with CAD, the decision to revascularize should be based on clinical presentation, coronary anatomy, LV function, and evidence of inducible ischemia. The knowledge that a large region of LV myocardium is viable rather than irreversibly damaged will aid in this decision-making process, but it should not be the primary indication for revascularization.

REFERENCES

1. Bolli R: Myocardial "stunning" in man, *Circulation* 86:1671–1691, 1992.
2. Braunwald E, Kloner RA: The stunned myocardium: Prolonged, postischemic ventricular dysfunction, *Circulation* 66:1146–1149, 1982.
3. Sheehan FH, Doerr R, Schmidt WG, et al: Early recovery of left ventricular function after thrombolytic therapy for acute myocardial infarction: An important determinant of survival, *J Am Coll Cardiol* 12: 289–300, 1988.
4. Stack RS, Phillips HR 3rd, Grierson DS, et al: Functional improvement of jeopardized myocardium following intracoronary streptokinase infusion in acute myocardial infarction, *J Clin Invest* 72:84–95, 1983.
5. Topol EJ, Weiss JL, Brinker JA, et al: Regional wall motion improvement after coronary thrombolysis with recombinant tissue plasminogen activator: Importance of coronary angioplasty, *J Am Coll Cardiol* 6:426–433, 1985.
6. Bonow RO: The hibernating myocardium: Implications for management of congestive heart failure, *Am J Cardiol* 75:17A–25A, 1995.
7. Dilsizian V, Bonow RO, Cannon RO 3rd, , et al: The effect of coronary artery bypass grafting on left ventricular systolic function at rest: Evidence for preoperative subclinical myocardial ischemia, *Am J Cardiol* 61:1248–1254, 1988.
8. Elefteriades JA, Tolis G Jr, Levi E, et al: Coronary artery bypass grafting in severe left ventricular dysfunction: Excellent survival with improved ejection fraction and functional state, *J Am Coll Cardiol* 22:1411–1417, 1993.

9. Ross J Jr: Myocardial perfusion-contraction matching: Implications for coronary artery disease and hibernation, *Circulation* 83:1076–1083, 1991.
10. Braunwald E, Rutherford JD: Reversible ischemic left ventricular dysfunction: Evidence for "hibernating" myocardium, *J Am Coll Cardiol* 8:1467–1470, 1986.
11. Rahimtoola SH: The hibernating myocardium, *Am Heart J* 117:211–213, 1989.
12. Dilsizian V, Bonow RO: Current diagnostic techniques of assessing myocardial viability in hibernating and stunned myocardium, *Circulation* 87:1–20, 1993.
13. Camici PG, Wijns W, Borgers M, et al: Pathophysiology of chronic reversible left ventricular dysfunction due to coronary artery disease (hibernating myocardium), *Circulation* 96:3205–3214, 1997.
14. Wijns W, Vatner SF, Camici PG: Mechanisms of disease: Hibernating myocardium, *N Engl J Med* 339:173–181, 1998.
15. Fallovollita JA, Malm BJ, Canty JM Jr: Hibernating myocardium retains metabolic and contractile reserve despite regional reductions in flow, function, and oxygen consumption at rest, *Circ Res* 92:48–55, 2003.
16. Thijssen VLJL, Borgers M PhD, Lenders MH, et al: Temporal and spatial variations in structural protein expression during the progression from stunned to hibernating myocardium, *Circulation* 110:3313–3321, 2004.
17. Canty JM Jr, Suzuki G, Banas MD, Verheyen F, Borgers M, Fallavollita JA: Hibernating myocardium: chronically adapted to ischemia but vulnerable to sudden death, *Circ Res* 94:1142–1149, 2004.
18. Iyer VS, Canty JM Jr: Regional desensitization of β-adrenergic receptor signaling in swine with chronic hibernating myocardium, *Circ Res* 97:789–795, 2005.
19. Beller GA: Comparison of thallium-201 scintigraphy and low-dose dobutamine echocardiography for the noninvasive assessment of myocardial viability, *Circulation* 94:2681–2684, 1996.
20. Bonow RO: Identification of viable myocardium, *Circulation* 94:2674–2680, 1996.
21. Muhlbaier LH, Pryor DB, Rankin JS, et al: Observational comparison of event-free survival with medical and surgical therapy in patients with coronary artery disease. 20 years of follow-up, *Circulation* 86(Suppl 5):II-198–II-204, 1992.
22. Brundage BH, Massie BM, Botvinick EH: Improved regional ventricular function after successful surgical revascularization, *J Am Coll Cardiol* 3:902–908, 1984.
23. Rozanski A, Berman D, Gray R, et al: Preoperative prediction of reversible myocardial asynergy by postexercise radionuclide ventriculography, *N Engl J Med* 307:212–213, 1982.
24. Rahimtoola SH: A perspective on the three large multicenter randomized clinical trials of coronary bypass surgery for chronic stable angina, *Circulation* 72(6 Pt 2):V123–V135, 1985.
25. Buxton DB: Dysfunction in collateral-dependent myocardium: Hibernation or repetitive stunning? *Circulation* 87:1756–1758, 1993.
26. Gerber BL, Vanoverschelde JL, Bol A, et al: Myocardial blood flow, glucose uptake, and recruitment of inotropic reserve in chronic left ventricular ischemic dysfunction: Implications for the pathophysiology of chronic myocardial hibernation, *Circulation* 94:651–659, 1996.
27. Hendel RC, Chaudhry FA, Bonow RO: Myocardial viability, *Curr Probl Cardiol* 21:145–224, 1996.
28. Sawada S, Elsner G, Segar DS, et al: Evaluation of patterns of perfusion and metabolism in dobutamine-responsive myocardium, *J Am Coll Cardiol* 29:55–61, 1997.
29. Vanoverschelde JL, Wijns W, Depre C, et al: Mechanisms of chronic regional postischemic dysfunction in humans: New insights from the study of noninfarcted collateral-dependent myocardium, *Circulation* 87:1513–1523, 1993.
30. Kim RJ, Wu E, Rafael A, et al: The use of contrast-enhanced magnetic resonance imaging to identify reversible myocardial dysfunction, *N Engl J Med* 343:1445–1453, 2000.
31. Bucciarelli-Ducci C, Wu E, Lee DC, Holly TA, Klocke FJ, Bonow RO: Contrast-enhanced cardiac magnetic resonance in the evaluation of myocardial infarction and myocardial viability in patients with ischemic heart disease, *Curr Probl Cardiol* 31:125–168, 2006.
32. Wu E, Ortiz J, Tejedor P, et al: Infarct size by contrast enhanced cardiac magnetic resonance is a stronger predictor of outcomes than left ventricular ejection fraction or end-systolic volume index: prospective cohort study, *Heart* 94:730–736, 2008.
33. Berger BC, Watson DD, Burwell LR, et al: Redistribution of thallium at rest in patients with stable and unstable angina and the effect of coronary artery bypass surgery, *Circulation* 60:1114–1125, 1979.
34. Bonow RO, Dilsizian V: Thallium-201 for assessing myocardial viability, *Semin Nucl Med* 21:230–241, 1991.
35. Hendel RC: Single-photon perfusion imaging for the assessment of myocardial viability, *J Nucl Med* 35(Suppl):23S–31S, 1994.
36. Iskandrian AS, Hakki AH, Kane SA, et al: Rest and redistribution thallium-201 myocardial scintigraphy to predict improvement in left

ventricular function after coronary artery bypass grafting, *Am J Cardiol* 51:1312–1316, 1983.
37. Rozanski A, Berman DS, Gray R, et al: Use of thallium-201 redistribution scintigraphy in the preoperative differentiation of reversible and nonreversible myocardial asynergy, *Circulation* 64:936–944, 1981.
38. Gibson RS, Watson DD, Taylor GJ, et al: Prospective assessment of regional myocardial perfusion before and after coronary revascularization surgery by quantitative thallium-201 scintigraphy, *J Am Coll Cardiol* 1:804–815, 1983.
39. Gutman J, Berman DS, Freeman M, et al: Time to completed redistribution of thallium-201 in exercise myocardial scintigraphy: Relationship to the degree of coronary artery stenosis, *Am Heart J* 106:989–995, 1983.
40. Kiat H, Berman DS, Maddahi J, et al: Late reversibility of tomographic myocardial thallium-201 defects: An accurate marker of myocardial viability, *J Am Coll Cardiol* 12:1456–1463, 1988.
41. Liu P, Kiess MC, Okada RD, et al: The persistent defect on exercise thallium imaging and its fate after myocardial revascularization: Does it represent scar or ischemia? *Am Heart J* 110:996–1001, 1985.
42. Manyari DE, Knudtson M, Kloiber R, et al: Sequential thallium-201 myocardial perfusion studies after successful percutaneous transluminal coronary artery angioplasty: Delayed resolution of exercise induced scintigraphic abnormalities, *Circulation* 77:86–95, 1988.
43. Ohtani H, Tamaki N, Yonekura Y, et al: Value of thallium-201 reinjection after delayed SPECT imaging for predicting reversible ischemia after coronary artery bypass grafting, *Am J Cardiol* 66:394–399, 1990.
44. Brunken R, Schwaiger M, Grover-McKay M, et al: Positron emission tomography detects tissue metabolic activity in myocardial segments with persistent thallium perfusion defects, *J Am Coll Cardiol* 10:557–567, 1987.
45. Brunken RC, Kottou S, Nienaber CA, et al: PET detection of viable tissue in myocardial segments with persistent defects at Tl-201 SPECT, *Radiology* 65:65–73, 1989.
46. Tamaki N, Yonekura Y, Yamashita K, et al: Relation of left ventricular perfusion and wall motion with metabolic activity in persistent defects on thallium-201 tomography in healed myocardial infarction, *Am J Cardiol* 62:202–208, 1988.
47. Tamaki N, Yonekura Y, Yamashita K, et al: SPECT thallium-201 tomography and positron tomography using N-13 ammonia and F-18 fluorodeoxyglucose in coronary artery disease, *Am J Cardiac Imaging* 3:3–9, 1987.
48. Cloninger KG, DePuey EG, Garcia EV, et al: Incomplete redistribution in delayed thallium-201 single photon emission computed tomographic (SPECT) images: An overestimation of myocardial scarring, *J Am Coll Cardiol* 12:955–963, 1988.
49. Yang LD, Berman DS, Kiat H, et al: The frequency of late reversibility in SPECT thallium-201 stress-redistribution studies, *J Am Coll Cardiol* 15:334–340, 1990.
50. Watson DD: Methods for detection of myocardial viability and ischemia. In Zaret BL, Beller GA, editors: *Nuclear cardiology*, St. Louis, 1992, CV Mosby, pp 65–76.
51. Kayden DS, Sigal S, Soufer R, et al: Thallium-201 for assessment of myocardial viability: Quantitative comparison of 24-hour redistribution imaging with imaging after reinjection at rest, *J Am Coll Cardiol* 18.1480–1486, 1991.
52. Brunken RC, Mody FV, Hawkins RA, et al: Positron emission tomography detects metabolic activity in myocardium with persistent 24-hour single photon emission computed tomography ^{201}Tl defects, *Circulation* 86:1357–1369, 1992.
53. Dilsizian V, Rocco TP, Freedman NM, et al: Enhanced detection of ischemic but viable myocardium by the reinjection of thallium after stress-redistribution imaging, *N Engl J Med* 323:141–146, 1990.
54. Rocco TP, Dilsizian V, McKusick KA, et al: Comparison of thallium redistribution with rest "reinjection" imaging for detection of viable myocardium, *Am J Cardiol* 66:158–163, 1990.
55. Tamaki N, Ohtani II, Yonekura Y, et al: Significance of fill-in after thallium-201 reinjection following delayed imaging: Comparison with regional wall motion and angiographic findings, *J Nucl Med* 31:1617–1623, 1990.
56. Ragosta M, Beller GA, Watson DD, et al: Quantitative planar rest-redistribution ^{201}Tl imaging in detection of myocardial viability and prediction of improvement in left ventricular function after coronary bypass surgery in patients with severely depressed left ventricular function, *Circulation* 87:1630–1641, 1993.
57. Mori T, Minamiji K, Kurogane H, et al: Rest-injected thallium-201 imaging for assessing viability of severe asynergic regions, *J Nucl Med* 32:1718–1724, 1991.
58. Dilsizian V, Smeltzer WR, Freedman NM, et al: Thallium reinjection after stress-redistribution imaging: Does 24-hour delayed imaging following reinjection enhance detection of viable myocardium? *Circulation* 83:1247–1255, 1991.
59. Dilsizian V, Bonow RO: Differential uptake and apparent thallium-201 "washout" after thallium reinjection: Options regarding early redistribution imaging before reinjection or late redistribution imaging after reinjection, *Circulation* 85:1032–1038, 1992.

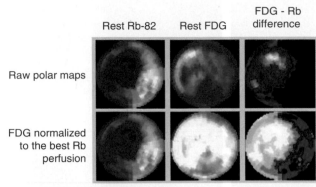

Figure 38-6 Quantification of relative myocardial perfusion and FDG uptake using circumferential profile analysis. FDG, fluorine-18-deoxyglucose; Rb-82, rubidium-82. *(Courtesy of Dr. Cesar Santana, Emory University.)*

Gated FDG Study

Parameters of global and regional left ventricular (LV) function derived from gated FDG PET images correlate closely with those obtained by MRI.[24] As mentioned earlier, gated images are particularly useful when FDG PET patterns are interpreted in relation to non-attenuation-corrected SPECT perfusion images.[25] In addition, measures of global LV function and remodeling (i.e., LVEF and volumes) are also useful for predicting improvement in LV function after revascularization.[26] Myocardial infarction (MI), especially one that is large and transmural, can produce alterations in both the infarcted and noninfarcted regions that result in changes in LV architecture known as *remodeling*.[27] Increased LV volumes and cavity size are important predictors of poor outcome in patients after infarction[28] and may offset the potential benefits from revascularization on ventricular function and survival even if there is evidence of viable (ischemic) myocardium.[29–32]

Hybrid FDG Positron Emission Tomography and Computed Tomography

Since modern PET scanners now include a multislice CT scanner, an attractive approach could be performing FDG PET imaging with CT (Fig. 38-7). CT could be used for attenuation correction, calcium score measurement, and visualization of coronary arteries and accompanying stenoses. Recently, multislice CT has been found to have sufficient accuracy to image coronary arteries and assess the coronary stenoses.[30] An example of such a viability study using FDG and PET/CT hybrid imaging is displayed in Figure 38-7. The application of contrast-enhanced CT angiography in heart failure patients who need viability investigation may be problematic, owing to advanced coronary atherosclerosis and concomitant problems such as kidney disease. The clinical value of hybrid imaging is at this time still open, and feasibility needs to be explored.

Carbon-11-Acetate

Physiologic Basis

The consumption of oxygen by the myocardium is required for the continued generation of high-energy phosphates to maintain contractile function and other

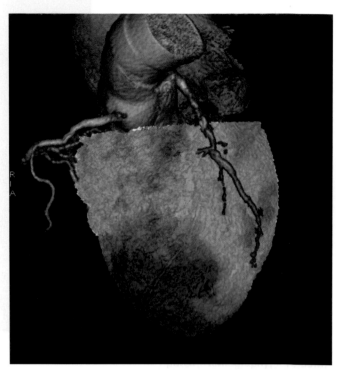

Figure 38-7 Example of viability study using FDG and PET/CT hybrid imaging. FDG PET images are overlaid with CT angiography. Scarred region is visualized as *blue* color. CT, computed tomography; FDG, fluorine-18-deoxyglucose; PET, positron emission tomography.

cellular processes. As mentioned, the heart uses a variety of substrates to support overall oxidative metabolism and thus fulfill its energy requirements.[7] PET imaging with ^{11}C-acetate offers a direct approach to evaluating myocardial oxygen consumption (MVO$_2$) and oxidative metabolism.[31,32] Indeed, the clearance of ^{11}C-acetate from myocardium on PET imaging reflects overall regional myocardial oxidative metabolism. Acetate is a short-chained fatty acid that is readily extracted by myocardial tissue. The extracted acetate is then converted into acetyl-CoA within the mitochondria and undergoes near-complete oxidation by the tricarboxylic acid (TCA) cycle and oxidative phosphorylation.

Quantification of Myocardial Carbon-11-Acetate Kinetics (See Chapter 40)

Dynamic imaging following the intravenous administration of [^{11}C]acetate demonstrates the passage of the radioactive bolus through the cardiac chambers, followed by the extraction and accumulation of the radiotracer in the myocardium and its clearance from the blood pool, and finally the clearance of the radiotracer from the myocardial tissue, reflecting the rate of oxidative metabolism (Fig. 38-8). The rapid tissue clearance rate (K$_{mono}$) is determined by monoexponential least-squares fitting of the initial portion of the time-activity curve. K$_{mono}$ values are then compared to reference normal values and used to determine the amount of residual viability within a dysfunctional myocardial segment.[33]

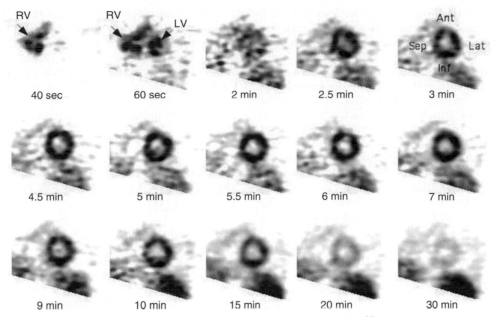

Figure 38-8 Serial mid-short-axis images following the administration of carbon-11 (^{11}C)-acetate. Images were acquired for 30 minutes, starting at the time of ^{11}C-acetate injection. The first image demonstrates the first pass of the radioactive bolus through the right (RV) and left (LV) ventricular chambers. The subsequent images show the clearance of ^{11}C-acetate from the blood pool, followed by the uptake of the radiotracer in the myocardium, and finally the washout of ^{11}C-acetate over time.

ACCURACY AND IMPACT OF VIABILITY ASSESSMENT BY PET

The term *viable* commonly refers to the myocardial region that has compromised function but is alive and has potential to recover function after revascularization. In patients with chronic LV dysfunction, the frequency of segmental recovery of function after revascularization, as well as the proportion of patients showing functional recovery, has been estimated to be 50% to 60%, even in patients with baseline ejection fraction below 40%.[34,35] However, the true prevalence of recoverable dysfunction is likely even higher, because the revascularization is seldom complete, and it may take up to a year to recover function.[36-38]

The goal of viability assessment in the setting of severe LV dysfunction after MI is to identify patients in whom revascularization can potentially improve LV function, symptoms, and survival. Then viability assessment would be of critical clinical importance in patients with the highest clinical risk after MI (i.e., LVEF < 30%), those who would derive the highest potential benefit from revascularization. Even in patients being considered for cardiac transplantation, viability assessment can alter the initial choice of treatment in majority of the patients.[39] However, the vast majority of the published data documenting the accuracy of noninvasive methods for diagnosing viability and predicting functional recovery have been obtained in patients with normal, mild, or moderate LV dysfunction (i.e., LVEF > 30%).[34] This is important because the accuracy of noninvasive methods for predicting functional recovery after revascularization appears to decrease significantly with worsening LV function (Fig. 38-9). Consequently,

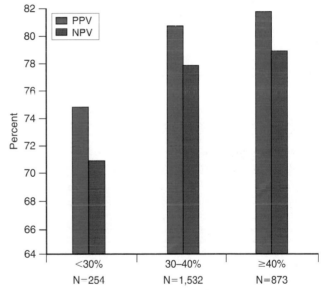

Figure 38-9 Accuracy of methods of viability assessment for predicting a change in left ventricular (LV) function after revascularization by the level of LV ejection fraction before revascularization. NPV, negative predictive value; PPV, positive predictive value. *(Reproduced from Di Carli M: The quest for myocardial viability: Is there a role for nitrate-enhanced imaging? J Nucl Cardiol 10:599–606, 2003.)*

the direct extrapolation of the excellent results obtained in patients with regional or mild to moderate LV dysfunction to patients with very low EF is problematic, and it often results in suboptimal clinical results.

Furthermore, it is not always clear whether the dominant symptom is angina or heart failure. Viability testing is of course more relevant in patients with heart failure but without limiting angina, because the main indication for revascularization would be to improve LV function rather than to abolish symptoms or ischemia.

It is important to also realize that various imaging techniques measure different characteristics of viability, such as nuclear function, metabolic function, contractile function, membrane function, and so forth. It is also important to note that although individual myocytes may only be viable or nonviable, the macroscopic myocardium has a continuum from fully viable, through areas of partial infarction, to areas of scar with no remaining myocytes. It should also be kept in mind that although a large majority of studies have assessed the accuracy of the imaging technique against the recovery of regional function, clinically more important parameters are global LV function, exercise capacity, quality of life, and long-term survival, and these are less often assessed (Table 38-1).[40]

The focus on viability information alone seems to ignore the multifactorial influences on improvement in LV function after revascularization.[41] From a clinical standpoint, it is likely that relying even on the most accurate of these multiple indexes of tissue viability or its absence in isolation will lead to suboptimal prediction of outcomes.[42] It is now evident that multiple other factors—including the presence and magnitude of stress-induced ischemia, the stage of cellular degeneration within viable myocytes, mitral insufficiency, the degree of LV remodeling, the timing and success of

revascularization procedures, the adequacy of the target coronary vessels, and the timing of LV functional assessment after revascularization—can affect functional outcome after revascularization. Indeed, recent evidence suggests that integrating many of these factors influencing functional recovery after revascularization in multivariable models results in improved clinical predictions, as compared to approaches that are based only on a single index of tissue viability.[43]

PREDICTING IMPROVEMENT IN REGIONAL LEFT VENTRICULAR FUNCTION

Myocardial Perfusion

The experience using PET tracers of blood flow, including ^{15}O-water, ^{11}C-acetate, and ^{13}N-ammonia, for predicting recovery of function has been documented in 6 studies including 182 patients with LV dysfunction (Table 38-2).[44] Contractile dysfunction was predicted to be reversible after revascularization when regional blood flow was only mild or moderately reduced (>50% of normal) and irreversible when regional blood flow was severely reduced (<50% of normal). Using these criteria, the average positive predictive accuracy of blood flow estimates for predicting functional recovery after revascularization is 63% (range, 45% to 78%), whereas the average negative predictive accuracy is 63% (range, 45% to 100%). While normal or near-normal blood flow in a dysfunctional region served by a stenosed coronary artery indicates tissue viability and that function can be improved with revascularization, a severe blood flow deficit generally (although not always) reflects mostly nonviable myocardium that is unlikely to show improved function with revascularization. However, blood flow deficits of intermediate severity are more difficult to interpret. They may represent the coexistence of extensive subendocardial necrosis with normal myocardium, a condition unlikely to show improved function with revascularization. Alternatively, they may reflect the coexistence of extensive areas of ischemic but viable with normal and/or scar tissue, a condition likely to show improved function with revascularization. Patients with low ejection fraction and relatively normal

Table 38-1 End points Used in Various Studies in Assessing the Accuracy of Viability Imaging

- Improvement of regional LV function
- Improvement of global LV function (i.e., LVEF)
- Improvement in symptoms
- Improvement of exercise capacity
- Reduction in hospital readmissions for CHF
- Reverse LV remodeling
- Long-term prognosis

CHF, congestive heart failure; LV, left ventricular; LVEF, left ventricular ejection fraction.

Table 38-2 Predictive Values for Segmental Functional Recovery After Revascularization Using Estimates of Regional Myocardial Perfusion With PET

Author	N	LVEF %	Criteria for Viability	PPV % (Segs)	NPV % (Segs)	Diagnostic Accuracy
Gropler[74]	34	NR	ACE ± 2 SD	45 (34/75)	68 (28/41)	53 (62/116)
Maes[75]	20	48 ± 9	NH3 > 50%	53 (10/19)	100 (1/1)	55 (11/20)
Grandin[76]	25	49 ± 11	NH3 > 50%	78 (14/18)	57 (4/7)	72 (18/25)
Tamaki[77]	43	41	NH3 > 50%	48 (47/98)	87 (28/32)	58 (75/130)
Wolpers[33]*	30	42 ± 11	MBF > 50%	78	85	—
Marinho[78]	30	35 ± 11	MBF ± 2 SD	55 (53/96)	45 (5/11)	54 (58/107)
Mean ± SD	**182**			**63 ± 14**	**63 ± 28**	**58 ± 8**

*Segmental data not reported.
ACE, [^{11}C]acetate; LVEF, left ventricular ejection fraction; MBF, myocardial blood flow (mL/min/g); N, number of patients; NH3, [^{13}N]ammonia; NPV, negative predictive value; NR, not reported; PPV, positive predictive value; SD, standard deviation; Segs, segments.

Table 38-3 Predictive Values for Segmental Functional Recovery after Revascularization Using Combined Estimates of Myocardial Perfusion and FDG Metabolism with PET

Author	N	LVEF %	Criteria for Viability	PPV % (Segs)	NPV % (Segs)	Diagnostic Accuracy
Tillisch[1]	17	32 ± 14	Mismatch	85 (35/41)	92 (24/26)	88 (59/67)
Tamaki[79]	22	NR	Mismatch	78 (18/23)	78 (18/23)	78 (36/46)
Tamaki[80]	11	NR	Mismatch	80 (40/50)	100 (0/6)	82 (46/56)
Carrel[81]	23	34	Mismatch	84 (16/19)	75 (3/4)	83 (19/23)
Lucignani[82]	14	38 ± 5	Mismatch	95 (37/39)	80 (12/51)	91 (49/54)
Gropler[46]	16	NR	Mismatch	79 (19/24)	83 (24/29)	81 (43/53)
Marwick[83]	16	NR	FDG > 2 SD	67 (25/37)	79 (38/48)	74 (63/85)
Gropler[74]	34	NR	FDG > 2 SD	52 (38/73)	81 (35/43)	63 (73/116)
Vanoverschelde[84]	12	55 ± 7	Mismatch	100 (12/12)	—	100 (12/12)
vom Dahl[85]	37	34 ± 10	Mismatch	53 (29/55)	86 (90/105)	74 (119/160)
Knuuti[86]	48	53 ± 11	FDG > 85%	70 (23/33)	93 (53/57)	84 (76/90)
Maes[75]	20	48 ± 9	Mismatch	75 (9/12)	75 (6/8)	75 (15/20)
Grandin[76]	25	49 ± 11	Mismatch	79 (15/19)	67 (4/6)	76 (19/25)
Tamaki[72]	43	41	FDG UI	76 (45/59)	91 (65/71)	85 (110/130)
Baer[87]	42	40 ± 13	FDG > 50%	72 (167/232)	91 (126/139)	79 (293/371)
vom Dahl[36]	52	47 + 10	Mismatch	68 (19/28)	96 (25/26)	81 (44/54)
Wolpers[33]*	30	42 ± 11	FDG > 50%	78	85	—
Schmidt[88]	40	42 ± 10	FDG > 50%	86 (25/29)	100 (11/11)	90 (36/40)
Kuhl[89]	29	32 ± 10	Mismatch	78 (83/107)	84 (67/80)	80 (150/187)
Mean ± SD	**531**			**77 ± 12**	**85 ± 9**	**81 ± 8**

*Segmental data not reported.
FDG, fluorine-18-deoxyglucose; LVEF, left ventricular ejection fraction; N, number of patients; NPV, negative predictive value; NR, not reported; PET, positron emission tomography; PPV, positive predictive value; SD, standard deviation; UI, uptake index.

perfusion at rest should undergo stress imaging to determine whether reversible ischemia (followed by stunning) is the likely cause of LV dysfunction.

FDG With and Without Myocardial Perfusion

Experience with the combined blood flow–FDG approach using PET or the PET-SPECT hybrid technique (SPECT perfusion with PET FDG imaging) has been extensively documented in 19 studies including 531 patients (Table 38-3). Contractile dysfunction was predicted to be reversible after revascularization in regions with increased FDG uptake or a perfusion-metabolism mismatch, and irreversible in those with reduced FDG uptake or a perfusion-metabolism match pattern. Using these criteria, the average positive predictive accuracy for predicting improved segmental function after

revascularization is 77% (range, 52% to 100%), whereas the average negative predictive accuracy is 85% (range, 67% to 100%). In a recent meta-analysis by Schinkel et al.,[45] very similar values were reported (weighted positive predictive value was 74% and negative predictive value 87%).

Measures of Myocardial Oxidative Metabolism

The experience with ^{11}C-acetate and PET for identifying viability and predicting functional recovery after revascularization has been documented in 5 studies, of which only 3 studies including 83 patients provided sufficient data to estimate predictive accuracies for regional functional recovery (Table 38-4). Of note, most of these studies come from the same institution,[46,47,48] indicating that assessment of myocardial viability using ^{11}C-acetate

Table 38-4 Predictive Values for Segmental Functional Recovery After Revascularization Using Estimates of Regional Myocardial MVO$_2$ with ^{11}C-Acetate and PET

Author	N	LVEF %	Criteria for Viability	PPV % (Segs)	NPV % (Segs)	Diagnostic Accuracy
Gropler[74]	34	NR	Mean MVO$_2$ ± 2 SD	67 (40/60)	89 (50/56)	78 (90/116)
Rubin[48]	19	NR	Mean MVO$_2$ ± 2 SD	88 (28/32)	73 (16/22)	81 (44/54)
Wolpers[33]*	30	42 ± 11	MVO$_2$ (k$_2$) > 0.09/min	62	65	—
Mean ± SD	**83**			**72 ± 14**	**76 ± 12**	

*Segmental data not reported.
[11]C, Carbon-11, LVEF, left ventricular ejection fraction; MVO$_2$, myocardial oxygen consumption; N, number of patients; NPV, negative predictive value; NR, not reported; PET, positron emission tomography; PPV, positive predictive value; SD, standard deviation.

has had less widespread validation compared to the FDG PET approach. Relatively preserved quantitative measures of oxidative metabolism in dysfunctional myocardial regions were predictive of improved function after revascularization; severely decreased oxidative metabolism was predictive of irreversible damage. Using these criteria, the average positive predictive accuracy for predicting improved segmental function after revascularization is 72% (range, 62% to 88%), whereas the average negative predictive accuracy is 76% (range, 65% to 89%) (see Table 38-4). Similar to regional perfusion measures, estimates of MVO$_2$ (which are closely coupled with myocardial perfusion) accurately predict functional outcome when they are either normal or severely decreased. In individual patients, intermediate reductions in estimates of MVO$_2$ are more difficult to interpret because they could represent nontransmural scar or hibernating myocardium. To overcome this limitation, it has been suggested that the magnitude of improvement (from baseline) in estimates for MVO$_2$ during low-dose dobutamine stimulation (a measure of myocardial "oxidative reserve") may be a more accurate predictor of functional recovery than PET measurements of MVO$_2$ performed at rest.[49] In 28 patients with chronic MI and mild to moderate LV dysfunction, Hata et al. demonstrated excellent discrimination (with virtually no overlap) between viable and nonviable myocardium using estimates of MVO$_2$ in response to low-dose dobutamine stimulation, assessed by ^{11}C-acetate and PET.[49]

PREDICTING IMPROVEMENT IN GLOBAL LEFT VENTRICULAR FUNCTION

An important question in patients with severely depressed LV function is whether revascularization will provide a clinically meaningful improvement in global cardiac function that can translate into improved exercise capacity, symptoms, and survival. Several studies using different PET approaches have shown that the gain in global LV systolic function after revascularization is related to the magnitude of viable myocardium assessed preoperatively (Table 38-5).[44] These data demonstrate that clinically meaningful changes in global LV function can be expected after revascularization only in patients with relatively large areas of hibernating and/or stunned myocardium ($\geq$17% of the LV mass). Similar results have been reported using estimates of myocardial scar with PET.[43] These results are in agreement with those obtained with SPECT,[50] dobutamine echocardiography,[51] and contrast-enhanced MRI.[52] In a recent meta-analysis,[45] the positive predictive value of FDG PET for improvement of global LV function was 68%, with negative predictive value of 80%.

Predicting Improvement in Symptoms and Exercise Capacity

An important challenge in the management of patients with poor cardiac function under consideration for

Table 38-5 Relation Between the Extent of Viability and the Change in LVEF after Revascularization*

Author	N	Criteria for Viability	Pre LVEF (%)	Post LVEF (%)
Tillisch[1]	17	Mismatch $\geq$ 25% LV	30 ± 11	45 ± 14
Carrel[81]	23	Mismatch $\geq$ 17% LV	34 ± 14	52 ± 11
Vanoverschelde[90]	12	Anterior wall mismatch	55 ± 7	65 ± 8
Maes[75]	20	Anterior wall mismatch	51 ± 11	60 ± 10
Grandin[76]	25	Mismatch $\geq$ 20% LV	51 ± 12	63 ± 18
Schwarz[91]	24	Anterior wall mismatch	44 ± 12	54 ± 9
Wolpers[33]	30	Anterior wall mismatch	39 ± 10	49 ± 17
vom Dahl[87]	82	Mismatch $\geq$ 1 CAT	46 ± 9	54 ± 11

*Using combined estimates of myocardial perfusion and FDG metabolism with positron emission tomography.
CAT, coronary artery territory; LV, left ventricle; LVEF, left ventricular ejection fraction; N, number of patients.

bypass surgery is to identify those in whom revascularization can provide a significant alleviation of anginal and, especially, heart failure symptoms, which is often their primary functional limitation.[53] Several studies have documented the association of viability with improvement of symptoms (NYHA class).[54-56] The magnitude of post revascularization improvement in heart failure symptoms correlates with the preoperative extent of viable myocardium.[57]

A few studies have also documented that improvement in exercise capacity after revascularization is linked with viability in FDG PET study.[57,58,59] In one study of 23 patients with LV dysfunction (LVEF: 35% ± 14%) and impaired functional capacity (70% in NYHA classes II-III), investigators have shown that the amount of viable myocardium before revascularization was predictive of a significant improvement in exercise parameters after revascularization.[58] In this study, peak rate-pressure product, maximal heart rate, and exercise capacity increased significantly after revascularization only in patients with multiple viable regions on preoperative PET imaging.

Di Carli et al. demonstrated a significant linear correlation between the global extent of a preoperative perfusion-metabolism PET mismatch and the percent improvement in functional capacity after CABG in 36 patients with ischemic cardiomyopathy (LVEF: 28% ± 6%) (Fig. 38-10).[57] In this study, a perfusion-metabolic PET mismatch involving $\geq$ 18% of the LV on quantitative analysis was associated with a sensitivity of 76% and a specificity of 78% for predicting a significant improvement in heart failure class following bypass surgery. In these patients, exercise capacity improved by

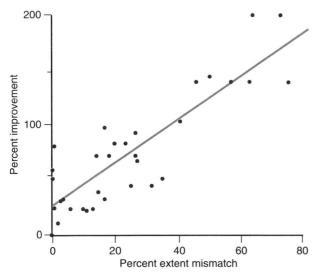

Figure 38-10 Relation between the anatomic extent of the perfusion-FDG PET mismatch (% of the LV) and the change in functional capacity after CABG in patients with severe LV dysfunction ($r = 0.87$, $P < 0.001$). CABG, coronary artery bypass graft; FDG, fluorine-18-deoxyglucose; LV, left ventricular; PET, positron emission tomography *(Reprinted from Di Carli MF, Asgarzadie F, Schelbert HR, et al: Quantitative relation between myocardial viability and improvement in heart failure symptoms after revascularization in patients with ischemic cardiomyopathy, Circulation 92:3436–3444, 1995.)*

107% after CABG, compared to only 34% improvement in patients without significant viability (<5% of the left ventricle).

Predicting a Reduction In Hospital Readmissions for Congestive Heart Failure

Frequent hospital readmissions for decompensated CHF are a major source of morbidity and increased health care costs in patients with CHF. Thus, the notion that preoperative viability imaging may be able to identify patients with a high likelihood of improvement in LV function and CHF symptoms is of great clinical importance because it would also prevent costly hospitalizations for CHF. A study by Rohatgi et al. examined the interaction between the extent of preoperative viability, the mode of treatment (i.e., medical therapy versus CABG), and the frequency of hospital readmissions during a mean follow-up of 25 months after the PET scan in 99 patients with severe LV dysfunction (LVEF: 22% ± 6%).[60] They found that among patients with relatively large areas of viable myocardium preoperatively, high-risk revascularization provided a significant reduction in hospital readmissions for CHF compared to medical therapy alone (3% versus 31%, respectively). In contrast, hospital admissions for CHF were similarly high regardless of the mode of treatment in patients without significant amounts of viability by PET (50% versus 48% for revascularization and medical therapy, respectively).

Predicting Improvement in Survival

A major goal of viability imaging is to identify patients with low EF who are at the highest clinical risk, in whom revascularization may offer the greatest survival benefit.[44] Table 38-6 summarizes the results of five published reports[61-65] evaluating the risk of cardiovascular events in patients with viable myocardium treated medically compared to those without viability. In 288 patients with CAD and moderate or severe LV dysfunction, patients with viable myocardium had a consistently higher event rate than those without viability. The odds ratios were consistently greater than 1 in all reports, suggesting an increased risk of a cardiac event for those subjects with viable myocardium treated medically. In a recent meta-analysis,[45] annualized mortality rates in patients with viable and nonviable myocardium assessed by PET and FDG of 10 studies and 1046 patients were reported. In patients with viability and who were revascularized, annual mortality rate was 4% but it was 17% in patients who were not revascularized (Fig. 38-11). The corresponding values in patients without viability were 6% and 8%. These data suggest that the presence of ischemic but viable myocardium as assessed by FDG PET is able to identify patients with LV dysfunction who are at high risk for cardiac events when treated with medical therapy alone.

These findings with FDG PET have been confirmed by virtually all subsequent studies using noninvasive imaging with either nuclear testing or echocardiography. Indeed, Allman and colleagues recently reported

Table 38-6 Risk of Cardiac Events for Patients with Moderate to Severe LV Dysfunction and Hibernating Myocardium*

Author	Year	Viability Assessment	Patients	LVEF (%)	FU (mos)	OR	Lower 95% CI	Upper 95% CI
Eitzman[88]	1992	PET	42	34 ± 13	12	7.00	1.53	32.08
Di Carli[89]	1994	PET	50	24 ± 7	13	7.00	1.51	32.33
Lee[90]	1994	PET	61	38 ± 16	17	7.66	2.31	25.44
vom Dahl[87]	1997	MIBI/FDG	77	≤50	29	1.21	0.22	6.51
Rohatgi[91]	2001	PET	58	22 ± 6	25	1.27	0.44	3.66

*Compared with those without hibernating myocardium.
CI, confidence interval; FDG, fluorine-18-deoxyglucose; FU, follow-up (reflects reported average); LVEF, left ventricular ejection fraction; MIBI, technetium-99m-sestamibi single-photon emission computed tomography; mos, months; OR, odds ratio; PET, positron emission tomography.

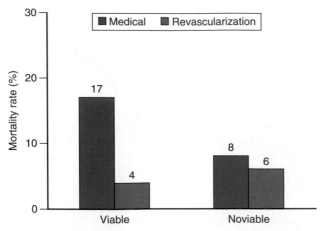

Figure 38-11 Annualized mortality rates in patients with viable and nonviable myocardium assessed by FDG PET in relation to treatment (revascularization or medical therapy). FDG, fluorine-18-deoxyglucose; PET, positron emission tomography. *(From Schinkel AF, Bax JJ, Poldermans D, et al: Hibernating myocardium: Diagnosis and patient outcomes, Curr Probl Cardiol 32:375–410, 2007. Reprinted with permission.)*

a meta-analysis of 24 studies that documented long-term patient outcomes after viability imaging by SPECT, PET, or dobutamine echocardiography in 3088 patients (2228 men, 860 women) with a mean ejection fraction of 32% ± 8% and follow-up for 25 ± 10 months.[66] The results demonstrated that in patients with evidence of viable myocardium, a strong association was present between revascularization and improved outcomes, particularly in patients with severe LV dysfunction. There was no apparent benefit for revascularization over medical therapy in the absence of demonstrated viability, and there was a trend toward higher death and nonfatal event rates with revascularization, which could reflect the higher procedural risk for patients with severe LV impairment associated with the revascularization itself in the absence of a balancing clinical benefit. Multivariate modeling (meta-regression) of the pooled study data in patients with viable myocardium demonstrated an inverse relationship between ejection fraction and the prognostic benefit associated with revascularization. That is, as the severity of LV dysfunction increased, the potential benefit (reduction in risk of death as well as nonfatal events) associated with revascularization of patients with viable myocardium increased as well. This finding implies that despite an increasing risk of revascularization with worsening LV dysfunction, noninvasive imaging evidence of preserved viability may provide information on clinical benefit to balance against that risk, informing clinical decision making.

In a recent study,[67] it was found that the extent of perfusion-metabolism mismatch of greater than 20% was predictive for cardiac death, but when the extent was smaller, no difference was detected in prognosis, indicating that large areas of viable myocardium on PET indicate a high risk for cardiac death. Zhang et al.[68] studied the prognostic value of myocardial viability in the LV aneurysms in 70 patients. It was detected that viable aneurysm predicted cardiac events if treated medically, as compared with patients with a viable aneurysm treated surgically.

In a recent randomized trial, the effectiveness of FDG PET–assisted management in patients with severe ventricular dysfunction was studied in 430 patients.[69] The study could not demonstrate a significant reduction in cardiac events in patients with LV dysfunction and suspected coronary disease for FDG PET–assisted management versus standard care in a general population. However, in those who adhered to PET recommendations, significant benefits were observed (hazard ratio 0.62; 95% CI 0.42 to 0.93; $P = 0.019$).

RELATIVE VALUE OF FDG PET VERSUS SPECT IN MANAGEMENT DECISIONS

In a relatively small prospective randomized clinical trial, Siebelink et al. compared management decisions and clinical outcomes based on either PET or SPECT image-guided management in patients with chronic CAD and LV dysfunction.[70] Although all patients underwent both PET and SPECT imaging, each patient was randomized to have information from only one of the modalities revealed to the clinical decision-making physicians. Management decisions were made on the basis of the data provided, and the patients were followed for an average of 28 months. The end point in this study was cardiac event-free survival. Events recorded were cardiac death, MI, and unintended revascularization. The results demonstrated no significant differences in the proportions of patients sent to revascularization (PCI or CABG) or medical therapy, or in event-free survival between the groups managed based on results from the two techniques. One of the important limitations of the study by Siebelink and colleagues is that only one-third of the patients had severe LV dysfunction (i.e., LVEF ≤ 30%), which in practice comprises the majority of patients in whom the viability question is of most clinical relevance. Although they reported no difference in outcomes in the subgroup of patients with very low LVEF using the two different imaging modalities, the numbers in each group were too small to provide a definite answer as to relative value of each technique. This is important because FDG imaging appears to improve the detection of viability in patients with very low EF (<25%) when compared to thallium SPECT scintigraphy.[71]

In a more recent study,[72] dual-isotope simultaneous acquisition (DISA) SPECT was compared against PET. PET and DISA SPECT had comparable predictive values for improvement in regional and global LV function and for the prediction of LV reverse remodeling after revascularization.

CONCLUSIONS AND FUTURE DIRECTIONS

The experimental and clinical evidence presented in this chapter indicate that PET is an accurate and reproducible technique for the evaluation of myocardial viability. Although several methods have been proposed, the FDG approach has undergone extensive validation worldwide and is commonly used in clinical practice. For successful application, appropriate patient preparation is mandatory to optimize diagnostic accuracy, especially in patients with diabetes. The available evidence suggests that this approach can provide accurate predictions of functional, symptomatic, and prognostic improvement after revascularization and thus improve management decisions in patients with poor cardiac function.

Despite the robust and extensive body of evidence supporting the use of viability information for selecting patients for high-risk revascularization, several issues remain unresolved. There appears to be a rather significant reduction in the accuracy of viability testing, including PET, for predicting functional recovery in patients with severely depressed LV function (LVEF < 30%). As discussed, this is likely related to the fact that clinical predictions of functional recovery based on viability information alone are inadequate because they ignore the multifactorial influences affecting changes in LV function after revascularization.[41] Clinically important factors such as the degree of LV remodeling and the severity of morphologic alterations within viable but dysfunctional myocytes (and likely others) may influence clinical outcomes, even in the presence of relatively large areas of viable myocardium.[26,29,54,73] Future studies should focus on understanding the complex links between viability and ischemia, as well as the molecular changes leading to altered myocyte function, progressive tissue damage, and LV remodeling. This type of information will be of great pathophysiologic interest and will likely have important diagnostic implications.

REFERENCES

1. Tillisch J, Brunken R, Marshall R, et al: Reversibility of cardiac wall-motion abnormalities predicted by positron tomography, *N Engl J Med* 314:884–888, 1986.
2. Kitsiou AN, Bacharach SL, Bartlett ML, et al: [^{13}N]ammonia myocardial blood flow and uptake: relation to functional outcome of asynergic regions after revascularization, *J Am Coll Cardiol* 33(3):678–686, 1999.
3. Gould KL: Identifying and measuring severity of coronary artery stenosis. Quantitative coronary arteriography and positron emission tomography, *Circulation* 78(2):237–245, 72, 1988.
4. Grover-McKay M, Ratib O, Schwaiger M, et al: Detection of coronary artery disease with positron emission tomography and rubidium 82, *Am Heart J* 123(3):646–652, 1992.
5. De Silva R, Yamamoto Y, Rhodes CG, et al: Preoperative prediction of the outcome of coronary revascularization using positron emission tomography, *Circulation* 86(6):1738–1742, 1992.
6. Yamamoto Y, De Silva R, Rhodes CG, et al: A new strategy for the assessment of viable myocardium and regional myocardial blood flow using ^{15}O-water and dynamic positron emission tomography, *Circulation* 86(1):167–178, 1992.
7. Opie LH: *The heart. Physiology and metabolism*, ed 2, New York, 1991, Raven Press.
8. Young LH, Coven DL, Russell RR 3rd: Cellular and molecular regulation of cardiac glucose transport, *J Nucl Cardiol* 7:267–276, 2000.
9. Opie LH: Effects of regional ischemia on metabolism of glucose and fatty acids, *Circ Res* 38:152–174, 1976.
10. Liedtke AJ: Alterations of carbohydrate and lipid metabolism in the acutely ischemic heart, *Prog Cardiovasc Dis* 23:321–336, 1981.
11. Camici P, Araujo LI, Spinks T, et al: Increased uptake of ^{18}F-fluorodeoxyglucose in postischemic myocardium of patients with exercise-induced angina, *Circulation* 74:81–88, 1986.
12. Phelps ME, Hoffman EJ, Selin C, et al: Investigation of [^{18}F]2-fluoro-2-deoxyglucose for the measure of myocardial glucose metabolism, *J Nucl Med* 19:1311–1319, 1978.
13. Knuuti MJ, Nuutila P, Ruotsalainen U, Teräs M, Saraste M, Härkönen R, Ahonen A, Wegelius U, Haapanen A, Bergman J, Haaparanta M, Voipio-Pulkki L-M: The Value of Quantitative Analysis of Glucose Utilization in Detection of Myocardial Viability by PET, *J Nucl Med* 34:2068–2075, 1993.
14. Gerber BL, Ordoubadi FF, Wijns W, et al: Positron emission tomography using(18)F-fluoro-deoxyglucose and euglycaemic hyperinsulinaemic glucose clamp: optimal criteria for the prediction of recovery of post-ischaemic left ventricular dysfunction. Results from the European Community Concerted Action Multicenter study on use of (18) F-fluoro-deoxyglucose Positron Emission Tomography for the Detection of Myocardial Viability, *Eur Heart J* 22(18):1691–1701, 2001.
15. Bacharach SL, Bax JJ, Case J, et al: PET myocardial glucose metabolism and perfusion imaging with ^{18}FDG, ^{13}NH$_3$ and ^{82}Rb. Part 1—Guidelines for data acquisition and patient preparation, *J Nucl Cardiol* 10(5):543–556, 2003.
16. Hesse B, Tagil K, Cuocolo A, Anagnostopoulos C, Bardies M, Bax J, Bengel F, Busemann Sokole E, Davies G, Dondi M, Edenbrandt L, Franken P, Kjaer A, Knuuti J, Lassmann M, Ljungberg M, Marcassa C, Marie PY, McKiddie F, O'Connor M, Prvulovich E, Underwood R, van Eck-Smit B: EANM/ESC procedural guidelines for myocardial perfusion imaging in nuclear cardiology, *Eur J Nucl Med Mol Imaging* 32 (7):855–897, 2005.
17. Schoder H, Campisi R, Ohtake T, et al: Blood flow-metabolism imaging with positron emission tomography in patients with diabetes mellitus for the assessment of reversible left ventricular contractile dysfunction, *J Am Coll Cardiol* 33:1328–1337, 1999.
18. Knuuti MJ, Nuutila P, Ruotsalainen U, Saraste M, Härkönen R, Ahonen A, Teräs M, Haaparanta M, Wegelius U, Haapanen A, Hartiala J, Voipio-Pulkki L-M: Euglycemic Hyperinsulinemic Clamp and Oral Glucose Load in Stimulating Myocardial Glucose Utilization During Positron Emission Tomography, *J Nucl Med* 33:1255–1256, 1992.
19. Bax JJ, Veening MA, Visser FC, et al: Optimal metabolic conditions during fluorine-18 fluorodeoxyglucose imaging; a comparative study using different protocols, *Eur J Nucl Med* 24:35–41, 1997.
20. Knuuti MJ, Yki-Järvinen H, Voipio-Pulkki L-M, Mäki M, MD, Ruotsalainen U, Härkönen R, Teräs M, Haaparanta M, Bergman J, Hartiala U, Wegelius U, Nuutila P: Enhancement of Myocardial 18-FDG Uptake by Nicotinic Acid Derivative, *J Nucl Med* 35:989–998, 1994.
21. Stone CK, Holden JE, Stanley W, Perlman SB: Effect of nicotinic acid on exogenous myocardial glucose utilization, *J Nucl Med* 36(6):996–1002, 1995.
22. Di Carli MF, Prcevski P, Singh TP, et al: Myocardial blood flow, function, and metabolism in repetitive stunning, *J Nucl Med* 41: 1227–1234, 2000.
23. Nowak B, Sinha AM, Schaefer WM, et al: Cardiac resynchronization therapy homogenizes myocardial glucose metabolism and perfusion in dilated cardiomyopathy and left bundle branch block, *J Am Coll Cardiol* 41:1523–1528, 2003.
24. Schaefer WM, Lipke CS, Nowak B, et al: Validation of an evaluation routine for left ventricular volumes, ejection fraction and wall motion from gated cardiac FDG PET: a comparison with cardiac magnetic resonance imaging, *Eur J Nucl Med Mol Imaging* 30:545–553, 2003.
25. Slart RH, Bax JJ, van Veldhuisen DJ, et al: Prediction of functional recovery after revascularization in patients with coronary artery disease and left ventricular dysfunction by gated FDG-PET, *J Nucl Cardiol* 13(2):210–219, 2006.
26. Yamaguchi A, Ino T, Adachi H, Mizuhara A, Murata S, Kamio H: Left ventricular end-systolic volume index in patients with ischemic cardiomyopathy predicts postoperative ventricular function, *Ann Thorac Surg* 60:1059–1062, 1995.
27. Pfeffer MA, Braunwald E: Ventricular remodeling after myocardial infarction. Experimental observations and clinical implications, *Circulation* 81:1161–1172, 1990.
28. White HD, Norris RM, Brown MA, Brandt PW, Whitlock RM, Wild CJ: Left ventricular end-systolic volume as the major determinant of survival after recovery from myocardial infarction, *Circulation* 76:44–51, 1987.
29. Yamaguchi A, Ino T, Adachi H, et al: Left ventricular volume predicts postoperative course in patients with ischemic cardiomyopathy, *Ann Thorac Surg* 65:434–438, 1998.
30. Schroeder S, Achenbach S, Bengel F, et al: Cardiac computed tomography: indications, applications, limitations, and training requirements: Report of a Writing Group deployed by the Working Group Nuclear Cardiology and Cardiac CT of the European Society of Cardiology and the European Council of Nuclear Cardiology, *Eur Heart J* 29(4):531–556, 2008.
31. Armbrecht JJ, Buxton DB, Schelbert HR: Validation of [1–11C]acetate as a tracer for noninvasive assessment of oxidative metabolism with positron emission tomography in normal, ischemic, postischemic, and hyperemic canine myocardium, *Circulation* 81: 1594–1605, 1990.

32. Sun KT, Chen K, Huang SC, et al: Compartment model for measuring myocardial oxygen consumption using [1–11C]acetate, *J Nucl Med* 38:459–466, 1997.

33. Wolpers HG, Burchert W, van den Hoff J, Weinhardt R, Meyer GJ, Lichtlen PR: Assessment of myocardial viability by use of 11C-acetate and positron emission tomography. Threshold criteria of reversible dysfunction, *Circulation* 95:1417–1424, 1997.

34. Bax JJ, Poldermans D, Elhendy A, Boersma E, Rahimtoola SH: Sensitivity, specificity, and predictive accuracies of various noninvasive techniques for detecting hibernating myocardium, *Curr Probl Cardiol* 26:141–186, 2001.

35. Schinkel AF, Bax JJ, Sozzi FB, Boersma E, Valkema R, Elhendy A, Roelandt JR, Poldermans D: Prevalence of myocardial viability assessed by single photon emission computed tomography in patients with chronic ischaemic left ventricular dysfunction, *Heart* 88(2):125–130, 2002.

36. vom Dahl J, Altehoefer C, Sheehan FH, et al: Recovery of regional left ventricular dysfunction after coronary revascularization. Impact of myocardial viability assessed by nuclear imaging and vessel patency at follow-up angiography, *J Am Coll Cardiol* 28:948–958, 1996.

37. Vanoverschelde JL, Depre C, Gerber BL, et al: Time course of functional recovery after coronary artery bypass graft surgery in patients with chronic left ventricular ischemic dysfunction, *Am J Cardiol* 85:1432–1439, 2000.

38. Auerbach MA, Sch€oder H, Hoh C, et al: Prevalence of myocardial viability as detected by positron emission tomography in patients with ischemic cardiomyopathy, *Circulation* 99:2921–2926, 1999.

39. Beanlands RS, deKemp RA, Smith S, et al: F-18 fluorodeoxyglucose PET imaging alters clinical decision making in patients with impaired ventricular function, *Am J Cardiol* 79:1092–1095, 1997.

40. Underwood SR, Bax JJ, vom Dahl J, et al: Study Group of the European Society of Cardiology. Imaging techniques for the assessment of myocardial hibernation. Report of a Study Group of the European Society of Cardiology, *Eur Heart J* 25(10):815–836, 2004.

41. Di Carli MF, Hachamovitch R, Berman D: The Art and Science of Predicting Post-revascularization Improvement in LV Function in Patients With Severely Depressed LV Function (Editorial), *J Am Coll Cardiol* 40:1744–1747, 2002.

42. Di Carli MF, Hachamovitch R, Berman DS: The art and science of predicting postrevascularization improvement in left ventricular (LV) function in patients with severely depressed LV function, *J Am Coll Cardiol* 40:1744–1747, 2002.

43. Beanlands RS, Ruddy TD, deKemp RA, et al: Positron emission tomography and recovery following revascularization (PARR-1): the importance of scar and the development of a prediction rule for the degree of recovery of left ventricular function, *J Am Coll Cardiol* 40:1735–1743, 2002.

44. Di Carli MF: Predicting improved function after myocardial revascularization, *Curr Opin Cardiol* 13:415–424, 1998.

45. Schinkel AF, Bax JJ, Poldermans D, Elhendy A, Ferrari R, Rahimtoola SH: Hibernating myocardium: diagnosis and patient outcomes, *Curr Probl Cardiol* 32(7):375–410, 2007.

46. Gropler RJ, Geltman EM, Sampathkumaran K, et al: Functional recovery after coronary revascularization for chronic coronary artery disease is dependent on maintenance of oxidative metabolism, *J Am Coll Cardiol* 20:569–577, 1992.

47. Gropler RJ, Bergmann SR: Flow and metabolic determinants of myocardial viability assessed by positron-emission tomography, *Coron Artery Dis* 4:495–504, 1993.

48. Rubin PJ, Lee DS, Davila-Roman VG, et al: Superiority of C-11 acetate compared with F-18 fluorodeoxyglucose in predicting myocardial functional recovery by positron emission tomography in patients with acute myocardial infarction, *Am J Cardiol* 78:1230–1235, 1996.

49. Hata T, Nohara R, Fujita M, et al: Noninvasive assessment of myocardial viability by positron emission tomography with 11C acetate in patients with old myocardial infarction, *Circulation* 94:1834–1841, 1996.

50. Ragosta M, Beller GA, Watson DD, Kaul S, Gimple LW: Quantitative planar rest-redistribution 201Tl imaging in detection of myocardial viability and prediction of improvement in left ventricular function after coronary bypass surgery in patients with severely depressed left ventricular function, *Circulation* 87:1630–1641, 1993.

51. Perrone-Filardi P, Pace L, Prastaro M, et al: Dobutamine echocardiography predicts improvement of hypoperfused dysfunctional myocardium after revascularization in patients with coronary artery disease, *Circulation* 91:2556–2565, 1995.

52. Kim RJ, Wu E, Rafael A, et al: The use of contrast-enhanced magnetic resonance imaging to identify reversible myocardial dysfunction, *N Engl J Med* 343:1445–1453, 2000.

53. Dreyfus GD, Duboc D, Blasco A, et al: Myocardial viability assessment in ischemic cardiomyopathy: benefits of coronary revascularization, *Ann Thorac Surg* 57:1402–1408, 1994.

54. Beanlands RS, Hendry PJ, Masters RG, deKemp RA, Woodend K, Ruddy TD: Delay in revascularization is associated with increased mortality rate in patients with severe left ventricular dysfunction and viable myocardium on fluorine 18-fluorodeoxyglucose positron emission tomography imaging, *Circulation* 98:II51–II56, 1998.

55. Haas F, Haehnel CJ, Picker W, et al: Preoperative positron emission tomographic viability assessment and perioperative and postoperative risk in patients with advanced ischemic heart disease, *J Am Coll Cardiol* 30:1693–1700, 1997.

56. Schwarz ER, Schoendube FA, Kostin S, et al: Prolonged myocardial hibernation exacerbates cardiomyocyte degeneration and impairs recovery of function after revascularization, *J Am Coll Cardiol* 31:1018–1026, 1998.

57. Di Carli MF, Asgarzadie F, Schelbert HR, et al: Quantitative relation between myocardial viability and improvement in heart failure symptoms after revascularization in patients with ischemic cardiomyopathy, *Circulation* 92:3436–3444, 1995.

58. Marwick TH, Nemec JJ, Lafont A, Salcedo EE, MacIntyre WJ: Prediction by postexercise fluoro-18 deoxyglucose positron emission tomography of improvement in exercise capacity after revascularization, *Am J Cardiol* 69:854–859, 1992.

59. Marwick TH, Zuchowski C, Lauer MS, et al: Functional status and quality of life in patients with heart failure undergoing coronary bypass surgery after assessment of myocardial viability, *J Am Coll Cardiol* 33:750–758, 1999.

60. Rohatgi R, Epstein S, Henriquez J, et al: Utility of positron emission tomography in predicting cardiac events and survival in patients with coronary artery disease and severe left ventricular dysfunction, *Am J Cardiol* 87:1096–1099, 2001 A6.

61. vom Dahl J, Altehoefer C, Sheehan FH, et al: Effect of myocardial viability assessed by technetium-99m-sestamibi SPECT and fluorine-18-FDG PET on clinical outcome in coronary artery disease, *J Nucl Med* 38:742–748, 1997.

62. Eitzman D, al-Aouar Z, Kanter HL, et al: Clinical outcome of patients with advanced coronary artery disease after viability studies with positron emission tomography [commentary], *J Am Coll Cardiol* 20:559–565, 1992.

63. Di Carli MF, Davidson M, Little R, et al: Value of metabolic imaging with positron emission tomography for evaluating prognosis in patients with coronary artery disease and left ventricular dysfunction, *Am J Cardiol* 73:527–533, 1994.

64. Lee KS, Marwick TH, Cook SA, et al: Prognosis of patients with left ventricular dysfunction, with and without viable myocardium after myocardial infarction. Relative efficacy of medical therapy and revascularization, *Circulation* 90:2687–2694, 1994.

65. Rohatgi R, Epstein S, Henriquez J, et al: Utility of positron emission tomography in predicting cardiac events and survival in patients with coronary artery disease and severe left ventricular dysfunction, *Am J Cardiol* 87:1096–1099, A6, 2001.

66. Allman K, Shaw LJ, Hachamovitch R, Udelson JE: Myocardial viability testing and impact of revascularization on prognosis in patients with coronary artery disease and left ventricular dysfunction: a meta-analysis, *J Am Coll Cardiol* 39(7):1151–1158, 2002.

67. Desideri A, Cortigiani L, Christen AI, et al: The extent of perfusion-F18-fluorodeoxyglucose positron emission tomography mismatch determines mortality in medically treated patients with chronic ischemic left ventricular dysfunction, *J Am Coll Cardiol* 46(7):1264–1269, 2005.

68. Zhang X, Liu XJ, Hu S, et al: Long-term survival of patients with viable and nonviable aneurysms assessed by 99mTc-MIBI SPECT and 18F-FDG PET: a comparative study of medical and surgical treatment, *J Nucl Med* 49(8):1288–1298, 2008, Epub 2008 Jul 16.

69. Beanlands RS, Nichol G, Huszti E, et al: F-18-fluorodeoxyglucose positron emission tomography imaging-assisted management of patients with severe left ventricular dysfunction and suspected coronary disease: a randomized, controlled trial (PARR-2), *J Am Coll Cardiol* 50(20):2002–2012, 2007, Epub 2007 Oct 1.

70. Siebelink HM, Blanksma PK, Crijns HJ, et al: No difference in cardiac event-free survival between positron emission tomography-guided and single-photon emission computed tomography-guided patient management: a prospective, randomized comparison of patients with suspicion of jeopardized myocardium, *J Am Coll Cardiol* 37:81–88, 2001.

71. Srinivasan G, Kitsiou AN, Bacharach SL, Bartlett ML, Miller-Davis C, Dilsizian V: 18F-Deoxyglucose SPECT: can it replace PET and thallium SPECT for the assessment of myocardial viability? *Circulation* 97:843–850, 1998.

72. Slart RH, Bax JJ, van Veldhuisen DJ, et al: Prediction of functional recovery after revascularization in patients with chronic ischaemic left ventricular dysfunction: head-to-head comparison between 99mTc-sestamibi/18F-FDG DISA SPECT and 13N-ammonia/ 18F-FDG PET, *Eur J Nucl Med Mol Imaging* 33(6):716–723, 2006, Epub 2006 Mar 8.

73. Elsasser A, Schlepper M, Klovekorn WP, et al: Hibernating myocardium: an incomplete adaptation to ischemia, *Circulation* 96:2920–2931, 1997.

74. Gropler RJ, Geltman EM, Sampathkumaran K, et al: Comparison of carbon-11-acetate with fluorine-18-fluorodeoxyglucose for delineating

viable myocardium by positron emission tomography, *J Am Coll Cardiol* 22:1587–1597, 1993.

75. Maes A, Borgers M, Flameng W, Nuyts JL, van de Werf F, Ausma JJ, Sergeant P, Mortelmans LA: Assessment of myocardial viability in chronic coronary artery disease using technetium-99m sestamibi SPECT, *J Am Coll Cardiol* 29:62–68, 1997.
76. Grandin C, Wijns W, Melin JA, et al: Delineation of myocardial viability with PET, *J Nucl Med* 36:1543–1552, 1995.
77. Tamaki N, Kawamoto M, Tadamura E, et al: Prediction of reversible ischemia after revascularization. Perfusion and metabolic studies with positron emission tomography, *Circulation* 91:1697–1705, 1995.
78. Marinho NV, Keogh BE, Costa DC, Lammerstma AA, Ell PJ, Camici PG: Pathophysiology of chronic left ventricular dysfunction. New insights from the measurement of absolute myocardial blood flow and glucose utilization, *Circulation* 93:737–744, 1996.
79. Tamaki N, Yonekura Y, Yamashita K, et al: Positron emission tomography using fluorine-18 deoxyglucose in evaluation of coronary artery bypass grafting, *Am J Cardiol* 64:860–865, 1989.
80. Tamaki N, Ohtani H, Yamashita K, et al: Metabolic activity in the areas of new fill-in after thallium-201 reinjection: comparison with positron emission tomography using fluorine-18-deoxyglucose, *J Nucl Med* 32:673–678, 1991.
81. Carrel T, Jenni R, Haubold-Reuter S, Von Schulthess G, Pasic M, Turina M: Improvement in severely reduced left ventricular function after surgical revascularization in patients with preoperative myocardial infarction, *Eur J Cardiothorac Surg* 6:479–484, 1992.
82. Lucignani G, Schwaiger M, Melin J, Fazio F: Assessing hibernating myocardium: an emerging cost-effectiveness issue [editorial], *Eur J Nucl Med* 24:1337–1341, 1997.
83. Marwick TH, MacIntyre WJ, Lafont A, Nemec JJ, Salcedo EE: Metabolic responses of hibernating and infarcted myocardium to revascularization. A follow-up study of regional perfusion, function, and metabolism, *Circulation* 85:1347–1353, 1992.
84. Vanoverschelde JL, Wijns W, Depre C, et al: Mechanisms of chronic regional postischemic dysfunction in humans. New insights from the study of noninfarcted collateral-dependent myocardium [commentary], *Circulation* 87:1513–1523, 1993.
85. vom Dahl J, Eitzman DT, al-Aouar ZR, et al: Relation of regional function, perfusion, and metabolism in patients with advanced coronary artery disease undergoing surgical revascularization, *Circulation* 90:2356–2366, 1994.
86. Knuuti MJ, Saraste M, Nuutila P, et al: Myocardial viability: fluorine-18-deoxyglucose positron emission tomography in prediction of wall motion recovery after revascularization, *Am Heart J* 127:785–796, 1994.
87. Baer FM, Voth E, Deutsch HJ, et al: Predictive value of low dose dobutamine transesophageal echocardiography and fluorine-18 fluorodeoxyglucose positron emission tomography for recovery of regional left ventricular function after successful revascularization, *J Am Coll Cardiol* 28:60–69, 1996.
88. Schmidt M, Voth E, Schneider CA, et al: F-18-FDG uptake is a reliable predictor of functional recovery of akinetic but viable infarct regions as defined by magnetic resonance imaging before and after revascularization, *Magn Reson Imaging* 22:229–236, 2004.
89. Kuhl HP, Lipke CS, Krombach GA, et al: Assessment of reversible myocardial dysfunction in chronic ischaemic heart disease: comparison of contrast-enhanced cardiovascular magnetic resonance and a combined positron emission tomography single photon emission computed tomography imaging protocol, *Eur Heart J* 27:846–853, 2006.
90. Vanoverschelde JL, Wijns W, Depre C, et al: Mechanisms of chronic regional postischemic dysfunction in humans. New insights from the study of noninfarcted collateral-dependent myocardium, *Circulation* 87:1513–1523, 1993.
91. Schwarz ER, Schaper J, vom Dahl J, et al: Myocyte degeneration and cell death in hibernating human myocardium, *J Am Coll Cardiol* 27:1577–1585, 1996.

Myocardial Viability: Comparison with Other Techniques

AREND F.L. SCHINKEL, DON POLDERMANS, ERNST E. VAN DER WALL AND JEROEN J. BAX

INTRODUCTION

Coronary artery disease (CAD) is the most common cause of chronic heart failure.[1] Over the last decades, significant progress in the treatment of patients with chronic ischemic heart failure has been made. Advances in pharmacologic therapy, the introduction of device therapy, and developments in cardiac surgery have led to improved prognosis in these patients (Table 39-1). Pharmacologic therapy in ischemic left ventricular (LV) dysfunction typically consists of angiotensin-converting enzyme (ACE) inhibitors, β-blockers, and spironolactone and may improve symptoms and clinical outcome. However, pharmacologic therapy is a partial success. In general, patients with chronic ischemic heart failure have a history of myocardial infarction, multivessel CAD, and a variable degree of LV dysfunction. The primary question in these patients is whether they will benefit from surgical revascularization. In patients with a substantial amount of viable myocardium, coronary revascularization may improve heart failure symptoms, left ventricular ejection fraction (LVEF), and long-term prognosis. On the other hand, patients without viable myocardium are unlikely to benefit from surgical revascularization and are at increased risk for perioperative complications.[2,3]

Various noninvasive imaging techniques have been used to evaluate myocardial viability in patients with ischemic LV dysfunction considered for coronary revascularization, including nuclear imaging, stress echocardiography, and magnetic resonance imaging (MRI). The most frequently used modality is nuclear imaging with positron emission tomography (PET) or single-photon emission computed tomography (SPECT); the value of nuclear imaging is discussed extensively elsewhere in this book. In the current chapter, the role of other imaging modalities for assessment of myocardial viability is discussed, focusing on echocardiography and MRI.

DEFINITION OF MYOCARDIAL VIABILITY (See Chapter 36)

Patients with ischemic cardiomyopathy often have a variable degree of coexisting hibernating and stunned myocardium and nonviable scar tissue.[4] The term *myocardial hibernation* was first described by Rahimtoola[5] to explain the condition of chronic LV dysfunction attributable to chronically reduced blood flow in patients with CAD in whom coronary revascularization may result in recovery of LV contractility. *Myocardial stunning* refers to reversible myocardial contractile dysfunction in the presence of normal myocardial blood flow at rest.[6] Repetitive stunning is a condition that may be caused by repeated ischemic periods inducing chronic dysfunction in the presence of normal or mildly reduced myocardial blood flow at rest; coronary flow reserve, however, is reduced. It has been suggested that a temporal progression exists from stunning, characterized by normal blood flow at rest, to repetitive stunning with normal or mildly reduced blood flow at rest (but reduced flow reserve), to hibernation with reduced blood flow at rest.

Biopsy samples obtained in patients with ischemic LV dysfunction undergoing coronary revascularization revealed that myocardial stunning and hibernation are not just pathophysiologic concepts. Hibernating myocardium shows signs of energy depletion and downregulation of energy turnover, which may cause and maintain contractile dysfunction, tissue degeneration, and loss of cardiomyocytes.[7] Structural dedifferentiation of cardiomyocytes has been observed in hibernating

Table 39-1 Therapeutic Options in Ischemic Cardiomyopathy

Medical Therapy
ACE inhibitors
Amiodarone
AT-II receptor blockers
β-blockers
Diuretics
Digoxin
Spironolactone
Despite new drugs, survival on medical therapy is poor
Device Therapy
Biventricular pacing
Internal cardiac defibrillator (ICD)
Left ventricular assist device (as bridge to transplantation)
Heart Transplantation
Limited number of donor hearts does not meet large demand
Excessive comorbidity in potential recipients
Good long-term survival
Surgery
Revascularization if viable myocardium present, but associated risk is high
Additional Surgery
Mitral valve repair
Left ventricular aneurysmectomy
Left ventricular restoration

Table 39-2 Characteristics of Dysfunctional but Viable Myocardium in Relation to Imaging Modalities

Imaging Modality	Characteristics of Viability
Echocardiography at rest	Wall thickness
Echocardiography with dobutamine	Contractile reserve
Echocardiography using contrast	Perfusion
Magnetic resonance imaging at rest	Wall thickness
Magnetic resonance imaging with dobutamine	Contractile reserve
Magnetic resonance with intravenous contrast	Scar tissue
PET or SPECT with FDG	Glucose utilization
SPECT with thallium-201	Perfusion and cell membrane integrity
SPECT with technetium-99m	Perfusion and cell membrane/mitochondrial integrity

FDG, fluorine-18 2-fluorodeoxyglucose; PET, positron emission tomography; SPECT, single-photon emission computed tomography.

Accordingly, it may be more appropriate to state "jeopardized but viable myocardium" when revascularization is considered.

NONINVASIVE IMAGING TECHNIQUES (See Chapters 37 and 38)

Assessment of viability has become an integrated part of the clinical evaluation of patients with chronic ischemic LV dysfunction. Based on the presence/absence of viability, it is possible to predict improvement of regional and global LV function, heart failure symptoms, and exercise capacity after revascularization. In addition, viability assessment carries important prognostic information. A large variety of imaging techniques has been developed to evaluate myocardial viability in patients with ischemic LV dysfunction. These techniques probe different characteristics of dysfunctional but viable myocardium. Nuclear imaging techniques are frequently used to assess myocardial viability, and PET is often considered as the reference technique for assessing myocardial viability. Both echocardiography and MRI have been extensively evaluated and are alternative tests for viability assessment. The methodology and the clinical value of these different modalities for the detection of myocardial viability are discussed in the next paragraphs. Also, their relative merits compared to nuclear imaging methods are addressed. Currently, dobutamine stress echocardiography and contrast-enhanced MRI are the most frequently used alternative techniques for nuclear imaging.

Echocardiography

Echocardiography at Rest

A crude differentiation between viable and nonviable myocardium can be made using measurement of

myocardium, characterized by a loss of contractile filaments, small mitochondria, nuclei with uniformly distributed chromatin, and a nearly absent sarcoplasmic reticulum.[8] It appears that cardiomyocytes adapt their activity level to prevailing circumstances. This may explain why in hibernating myocardium some characteristics (e.g., contractile reserve) can be lost, whereas more basal characteristics such as cell membrane integrity and glucose metabolism are still intact. Several noninvasive imaging techniques have been developed to probe the different characteristics of dysfunctional but viable myocardium. Some techniques address rather basic characteristics such as cell membrane integrity and glucose metabolism, and other techniques rely on assessment of contractile reserve; this (in part) explains the differences in diagnostic accuracy of the various techniques (Table 39-2). The general term *viability* includes both hibernation and repetitive stunning but also includes segments with subendocardial scar tissue. These segments are indeed viable, but they contain a mixture of subendocardial necrosis and normal, viable myocardium in the epicardial layers. Whereas both hibernation and repetitive stunning benefit from revascularization (with functional recovery, and potentially improve long-term outcome), dysfunctional segments with subendocardial scar tissue and normal, viable myocardium do not benefit from revascularization.

end-diastolic wall thickness with echocardiography at rest. Schinkel et al.[9] evaluated 150 consecutive patients with ischemic LV dysfunction and demonstrated that the end-diastolic wall thickness was reduced (<6 mm) in 2% of the dysfunctional region and preserved (≥6 mm) in 309 dysfunctional regions. Regions with a reduced end-diastolic wall thickness virtually never exhibited contractile reserve during dobutamine stress echocardiography. In regions with a wall thickness equal to 6 mm, the response to dobutamine varied; approximately 60% of these segments were viable on dobutamine stress echocardiography, and the remaining 40% were nonviable. Conceivably, the regions with an end-diastolic wall thickness less than 6 mm consist of scarred and fibrotic tissue and do not improve in function following revascularization. Assessment of LV end-diastolic wall thickness can be used as an initial evaluation for myocardial viability: Dysfunctional segments with an end-diastolic thickness less than 6 mm are nonviable and may not need further evaluation; segments with a preserved end-diastolic wall thickness (≥6 mm) can be further classified as viable and nonviable myocardium based on the presence/absence of contractile reserve during dobutamine challenge.

Dobutamine Stress Echocardiography

Methodology. Extensive clinical experience has been obtained with dobutamine stress echocardiography to assess myocardial viability.[2,3] Dobutamine is a β_1-specific agonist that increases myocardial oxygen demand by increasing heart rate, contractility, and arterial blood pressure. The safety of dobutamine stress echocardiography was evaluated by Secknus et al.,[10] reporting an incidence of 7.6% side effects in 3011 patients undergoing dobutamine stress echocardiography. β-blockers can be used as antidotes. Infusion of low-dose dobutamine (5 to 10 mcg/kg/min) has been demonstrated to increase contractility (without a substantial increase in heart rate) in dysfunctional but viable myocardium, which has been referred to as *contractile reserve*. Segments without viable myocardium do not show contractile reserve. The protocol can be extended with high-dose dobutamine infusion (with infusions up to 40 mcg/kg/min with addition of atropine if needed), which allows assessment of myocardial ischemia.[12] With the low-high dobutamine dose stress protocol, four response patterns can be observed:

1. No change (no change in wall motion during the entire study)
2. Worsening (direct deterioration of wall motion without initial improvement)
3. Sustained improvement (improvement of wall motion without subsequent deterioration)
4. Biphasic response (initial improvement followed by worsening of wall motion)

Pattern 1 represents transmural scar, whereas pattern 2 represents severe ischemia in a region subtended by a critically stenosed artery. Pattern 3, on the other hand, is probably related to subendocardial scar tissue, whereas pattern 4 represents viability with superimposed ischemia. An example of a patient with myocardial ischemia during dobutamine stress echocardiography is shown in Figure 39-1.

Accuracy. Stress echocardiography has been evaluated extensively for the detection of viable myocardium in patients with chronic ischemic LV dysfunction. Forty-one studies with dobutamine stress echocardiography have reported on the sensitivity and specificity for detection of myocardial viability and prediction of recovery of regional function following revascularization.[11–51] A total of 1849 patients were included in these 41 studies. The weighted mean sensitivity and specificity respectively were 80% and 78%, with a positive and negative predictive value of 75% and 83% (Fig. 39-2; Table 39-3).

For the prediction of recovery of global LV function, 6 studies including 287 patients are available, using dobutamine stress echocardiography.[45–47,50,52,53] Pooled analysis of these six studies revealed a weighted mean

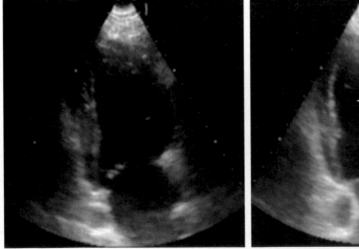

Figure 39-1 Echocardiography (apical two-chamber view, end-systolic frame) at rest *(left panel)* and during dobutamine stress *(right)*. The inferior wall *(arrow)* was contracting normally at rest and became dyskinetic (outward motion) during high-dose dobutamine stress.

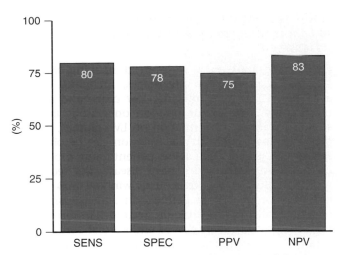

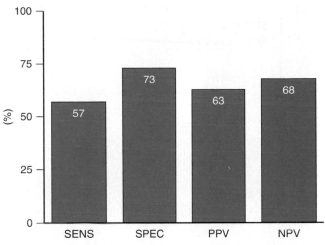

Figure 39-2 Accuracy of 41 studies using dobutamine stress echocardiography to detect viability and predict improvement of regional function after revascularization. NPV, negative predictive value; PPV, positive predictive value; SENS, sensitivity; SPEC, specificity. (*Data based on Bax JJ, Poldermans D, Elhendy A, et al: Sensitivity, specificity, and predictive accuracies of various noninvasive techniques for detecting hibernating myocardium, Curr Probl Cardiol 26:142–186, 2001; and Schinkel AF, Bax JJ, Poldermans D, et al: Hibernating myocardium: Diagnosis and patient outcomes, Curr Probl Cardiol 32:375–410, 2007.)*

Figure 39-3 Accuracy of six studies using dobutamine stress echocardiography to detect viability and predict improvement of global function after-revascularization. NPV, negative predictive value; PPV, positive predictive value; SENS, sensitivity; SPEC, specificity. (*Data based on Schinkel AF, Bax JJ, Poldermans D, et al: Hibernating myocardium: Diagnosis and patient outcomes, Curr Probl Cardiol 32:375–410, 2007.)*

Table 39-3 Pooled Data from Viability Studies Using Different Techniques to Predict Improvement of Regional Contractility After Revascularization*

Technique	N	Sens (%)	Spec (%)	PPV (%)	NPV (%)
DSE	41	80	78	75	83
MRI (wall thickness)	3	95	41	56	92
MRI (dobutamine stress)	9	74	82	78	78
Contrast MRI	5	84	63	72	78
FDG PET	24	92	63	74	87
Thallium-201	40	87	54	67	79
Technetium-99m	25	83	65	74	76

DSE, dobutamine stress echocardiography; FDG PET, fluorine-18 2-fluorodeoxyglucose and positron emission tomography; MRI, magnetic resonance imaging; N, number of studies; NPV, negative predictive value; PPV, positive predictive value; Sens, sensitivity; Spec, specificity.
*Data based on Bax JJ, Poldermans D, Elhendy A, et al: Sensitivity, specificity, and predictive accuracies of various noninvasive techniques for detecting hibernating myocardium, Curr Probl Cardiol 26:142–186, 2001; and Schinkel AF, Bax JJ, Poldermans D, et al: Hibernating myocardium: Diagnosis and patient outcomes, Curr Probl Cardiol 32:375–410, 2007.

Table 39-4 Pooled Data from Viability Studies Using Different Techniques Predicting Improvement of Global Left Ventricular Function After Revascularization*

Technique	N	Sens (%)	Spec (%)	PPV (%)	NPV (%)
DSE	6	57	73	63	68
FDG PET	3	83	64	68	80
Thallium-201	3	84	53	76	64
Technetium-99m	2	84	68	74	80

DSE, dobutamine stress echocardiography; FDG PET, fluorine-18 2-fluorodeoxyglucose and positron emission tomography; N, number of studies; NPV, negative predictive value; PPV, positive predictive value; Sens, sensitivity; Spec, specificity.
*Data based on Schinkel AF, Bax JJ, Poldermans D, et al: Hibernating myocardium: Diagnosis and patient outcomes, Curr Probl Cardiol 32:375–410, 2007.

sensitivity and specificity of 57% and 73%, respectively with a positive and negative predictive value of 63% and 68% (Fig. 39-3; Table 39-4).

The prognostic value of viability assessment using dobutamine stress echocardiography was addressed in 11 studies that included 1753 patients (5 studies used

high-dose dobutamine, 5 low-dose dobutamine, 1 low-high dose dobutamine).[54-63] The event rates in relation to viability and therapy are presented in four groups:

1. Patients with viability who underwent revascularization
2. Patients with viability who received medical treatment
3. Patients without viability who underwent revascularization
4. Patients without viability who received medical treatment

Patients with viable myocardium undergoing revascularization had the best survival, while the highest annualized mortality rates were noted in patients receiving medical therapy, either with or without viable myocardium. An intermediate mortality rate was observed in patients without viable myocardium who underwent revascularization (Fig. 39-4).

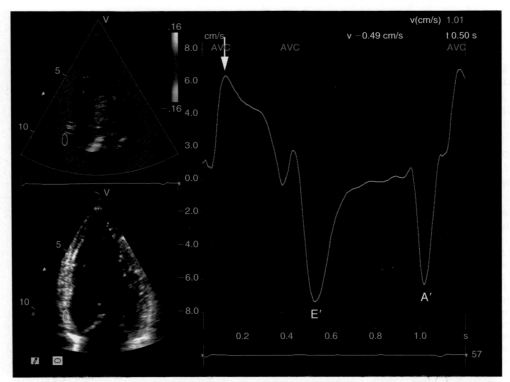

Figure 39-8 Tissue Doppler imaging allows quantification of systolic and diastolic myocardial velocities. In this tracing of the interventricular septum, the peak systolic velocity *(arrow)* was 6.3 cm/sec, and the diastolic velocities (E' and A') were 7.3 cm/sec and 6.2 cm/sec, respectively.

tissue as assessed with contrast-enhanced MRI. Radial strain allowed differentiation between nontransmural and transmural infarction with a sensitivity of 70.0% and a specificity of 71.2%, when a cutoff value for radial strain of 16.5% was used. In a subsequent study, 53 patients underwent two-dimensional (2D) radial strain imaging to assess viability; these patients underwent revascularization with assessment of functional recovery at 9 ± 2 months of follow-up.[72] Segments with recovery of function had more preserved radial strain (22.6% ± 6.3% versus 15.2% ± 7.5%, $P < 0.001$); using a cutoff of 17.2% for peak systolic radial strain, functional recovery could be predicted with a sensitivity of 70.2% and a specificity of 85.1%). The quantification of strain during low-dose dobutamine stress to assess viability has also been explored. In 55 patients undergoing revascularization, the quantification of strain during low-dose dobutamine stress echocardiography yielded a sensitivity ranging from 74% to 80%, with a specificity around 77%, to predict improvement of function after revascularization.[73] Finally, postsystolic thickening can be derived from tissue Doppler imaging and has been proposed as a marker for viability.[74] Some groups argued that postsystolic thickening is an accurate marker of viability and demonstrated good agreement with viability on metabolic imaging with FDG,[75] whereas others suggested that postsystolic shortening represents scar tissue. Lim et al.[76] evaluated 25 patients with chronic LV dysfunction (mean ejection fraction 32% ± 10%) with tissue Doppler imaging (to assess postsystolic thickening) and contrast-enhanced MRI. The authors demonstrated

that postsystolic thickening was most often observed in segments with transmural scar formation on MRI.

Echocardiography with Intravenous Contrast

Methodology. The improved technical properties of the myocardial contrast agents now allow for assessment of myocardial perfusion (Fig. 39-10). In early studies, intracoronary injection of contrast was still needed, but with the newer generation of contrast agents, intravenous administration is possible. The recent contrast agents are composed of high-molecular-weight inert gases. The microbubbles stay in the vascular space and do not enter the extravascular space. Within the vascular space, microbubbles behave like red cells in terms of rheology and can be used in combination with echocardiography to directly visualize the myocardial perfusion. Since myocardial perfusion is a prerequisite for myocardial viability, myocardial contrast echocardiography has been used to assess myocardial viability. It has been shown that echo contrast parameters of myocardial perfusion correlate positively with the microvascular density and the capillary area and inversely with the extent of fibrosis.[77] In the clinical setting, myocardial perfusion by myocardial contrast echocardiography is evaluated qualitatively, and segments are visually classified as being viable with normal or patchy perfusion, and nonviable when perfusion is absent (see Fig. 39-10).

Accuracy. The number of studies using contrast echocardiography for the prediction of functional recovery is limited. A small direct comparison between

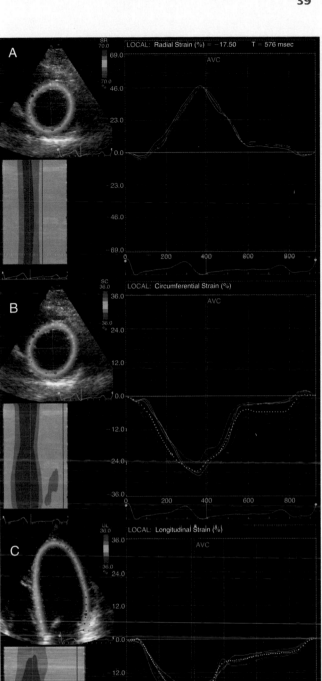

Figure 39-9 Multidirectional assessment of myocardial deformation by two-dimensional speckle tracking imaging. **(A)** Radial strain and **(B)** circumferential strain from the left ventricular short-axis view and **(C)** longitudinal strain from the 4-chamber apical view of the left ventricle.

dobutamine stress echocardiography, thallium-201 imaging, and contrast echocardiography was performed in 18 patients undergoing revascularization.[41] Both thallium-201 imaging and contrast echocardiography had a high sensitivity with a relatively low specificity, whereas dobutamine stress echocardiography had a

lower sensitivity with a relatively high specificity for the prediction of improvement of regional function after revascularization. In that particular study, contrast echocardiography had a sensitivity of 89% with a specificity of 51%. Two other studies using contrast echocardiography confirmed this observation and showed a high sensitivity with a lower specificity.[78,79] The lower specificity is related to the inability to identify subendocardial scar, resulting in "over-prediction of functional recovery": Segments that contain subendocardial scar are indeed partially viable, but will not improve in function after revascularization. These segments consist of a mixture of scar and viable but normal myocardium, and since jeopardized but viable myocardium is not present, recovery of function will not occur. One study demonstrated that patients with three or more viable segments on contrast echocardiography had a high likelihood of improvement in global LV function post revascularization.[41] At present, no studies with contrast echocardiography are available on the improvement in symptoms or long-term outcome.

Many more studies using echo contrast for viability assessment have been performed in patients with acute myocardial infarction. It has been shown that the extent and severity of perfusion defects after acute infarction correlated (inversely) with the likelihood of functional recovery at follow-up. Pooled analyses of 23 studies (including > 1,100 patients) revealed high sensitivity (approximately 85%) but lower specificity (approximately 74%) to predict recovery of regional and/or global function after acute infarction.[80] The lack of viability after acute infarction on contrast echocardiography was also related to development of LV remodeling at longer follow-up. Galiuto and colleagues[81] demonstrated in the Acute Myocardial Infarction Contrast Imaging (AMICI) study that 27% of 110 patients developed LV dilation at 6 months follow-up, and this was related mainly to no-reflow and absence of viability on contrast echocardiography. Finally, the prognostic value of contrast echocardiography after acute infarction has been demonstrated. Dwivedi et al.[82] evaluated 95 patients with contrast echocardiography after acute infarction and demonstrated that among the clinical, biochemical, electrocardiographic, echocardiographic, and coronary angiographic markers of prognosis, the absence of viability on contrast echocardiography was independently predictive of cardiac death or acute infarction.

Magnetic Resonance Imaging

Methodology. Substantial progress has been made in the development of MRI protocols for the assessment of myocardial viability. Currently, three techniques are frequently used in clinical practice:

1. Resting MRI can be used to assess end-diastolic wall thickness and contractile function at rest. The excellent spatial resolution of the technique allows precise determination of both global function (LVEF) and regional function (wall thickness and thickening). An example of the modified center-line method to precisely determine regional

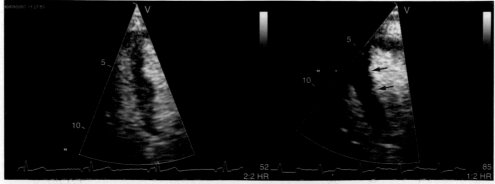

Figure 39-10 *Left,* Contrast echocardiography showing fill-in of the entire left ventricular myocardium, indicating normal perfusion. *Right,* Contrast echocardiography showing a perfusion defect indicated by the *arrows.*

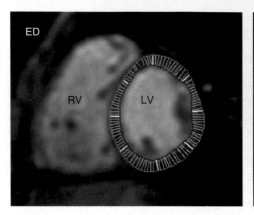

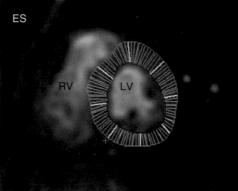

Figure 39-11 Modified center-line method used to assess, from a left ventricular (LV) short-axis magnetic resonance imaging (MRI) slice, the precise wall thickness and thickening. Based on epicardial and endocardial contours drawn on the end-diastolic (ED, *left*) and end-systolic (ES, *right*) frames and placement of chords, it is possible to calculate the precise thickening per chord. When results are added for all short-axis slices, LV volumes and LV ejection fraction can be precisely calculated. RV, right ventricle.

wall thickness and thickening is demonstrated in Figure 39-11. Segments with an end-diastolic wall thickness less than 6 mm most likely represent transmural scar formation (Fig. 39-12), and contractile function will not improve after myocardial revascularization.

2. Dobutamine stress MRI can be used to evaluate contractile reserve in a similar manner to dobutamine echocardiography. Detection of increased systolic thickening during low-dose dobutamine infusion can be detected easily with MRI, and the advantage of MRI is the relative simplicity in quantification of systolic wall thickening.

3. Contrast-enhanced MRI, using gadolinium-based contrast agents, permits precise detection of the extent and transmurality of scar tissue. This technique is referred to as *delayed contrast-enhanced imaging;* the contrast is accumulated in the infarcted area, and these areas appear hyperenhanced (bright) on the MR images. With the new imaging sequences, the intensities in the hyperenhanced areas are 400% to 500% higher than in the remote, viable myocardium.[83] This approach was validated in animal studies, demonstrating excellent agreement between the extent and transmurality of infarct tissue on MRI and on triphenyltetrazolium chloride–stained specimens.[84] In Figures 39-13 and 39-14, various examples of patients with different extent and transmurality of infarction are demonstrated. The majority of

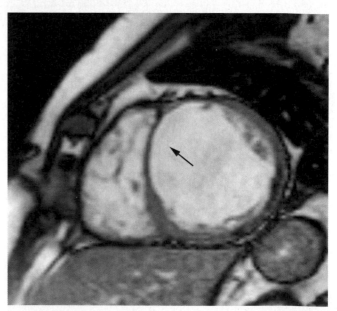

Figure 39-12 MRI short-axis slice of a patient with a previous anteroseptal infarction. The thinned wall in the infarcted region *(arrow)* indicates scar tissue without viable myocardium. MRI, magnetic resonance imaging.

the studies have used visual analysis of the extent and transmurality of the infarcted tissue, but precise quantification is also possible. An automated algorithm has been developed for this purpose (Fig. 39-15).[85] The entire set of short-axis slices is

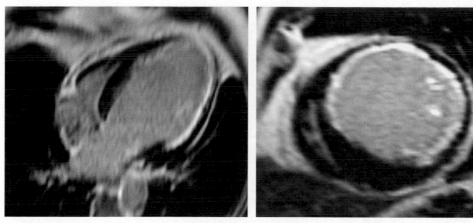

Figure 39-13 Contrast-enhanced MRI, 4-chamber view *(left)*. The region with high signal intensity *(white)* represents a subendocardial infarction extending from the apex to the lateral wall. The short-axis view *(right)* demonstrates a large subendocardial anterior infarction also extending to the septum and the lateral wall. MRI, magnetic resonance imaging.

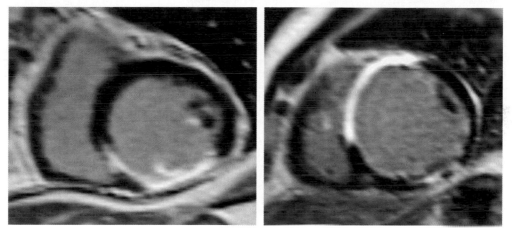

Figure 39-14 Contrast-enhanced MRI, short-axis view. A large transmural infarction *(white area)* is visible in the inferior wall *(left panel)*. The short-axis view *(right panel)* demonstrates a large anteroseptal infarction. MRI, magnetic resonance imaging.

selected, and epicardial and endocardial contours are drawn. In one representative slice, two regions of interest are manually drawn: one in a region showing the highest signal intensity (center of infarction) and another equally sized region of interest in normal myocardium (with normal wall motion). A threshold value is calculated by dividing the sum of the signal intensities in both regions by 2. Myocardial tissue showing signal intensity equal or higher than the threshold value is considered scar tissue. The extent of transmurality is then subsequently determined by the use of the modified center-line method. The obtained information can be presented in a polar map format, and the extent of infarction throughout the LV can readily be appreciated. Of note, the use of multislice computed tomography for detection of scar tissue has also been reported, with preliminary data suggesting comparable accuracy to contrast-enhanced MRI for detection of scar tissue.[86] However, the use of multislice computed tomography is associated with substantial radiation and may not be preferred at this stage for detection of scar tissue.

Accuracy. The described MRI techniques have been evaluated for assessment of myocardial viability in patients with chronic ischemic LV dysfunction (Fig. 39-16). For the prediction of recovery of regional contractile function following revascularization, 3 studies including 100 patients used end-diastolic wall thickness assessment by MRI.[87–89] Pooled analysis resulted in a weighted mean sensitivity and specificity of 95% and 41%, respectively, whereas the positive predictive value and negative predictive value were 56% and 92%, respectively. Nine studies[87,88,90–96] including 272 patients, employed dobutamine stress MRI. In these studies, the mean sensitivity and specificity to predict recovery of function post revascularization were 74% and 82%, respectively; positive predictive value and negative predictive value were both 78%. Contrast-enhanced MRI was used in 5 studies,[95–99] including 178 patients, resulting in a weighted mean sensitivity and specificity of 84% and 63%, respectively, with positive and negative predictive values of 72% and 78%, respectively. No studies are currently available using MRI for the prediction of recovery of global LV function or for evaluation of prognosis following revascularization.

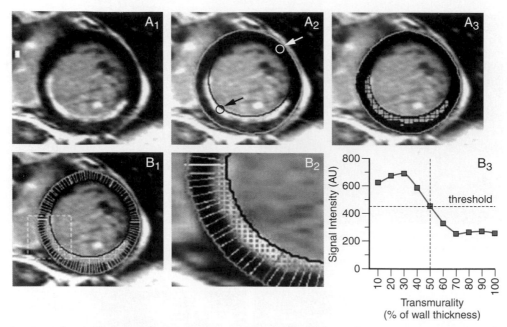

Figure 39-15 Automated quantitative analysis of transmurality of infarction. **A₁,** Representative contrast-enhanced, short-axis slice. **A₂,** Two manually drawn regions of interest: one in the center of infarction *(black arrow)* and another in normal myocardium *(white arrow).* **A₃,** Contrast-enhanced slice after application of the threshold value. **B₁,** Application of the modified center-line method, resulting in 100 equidistant chords along the left ventricular (LV) wall. **B₂,** Enlargement of the dashed box in B₁. **B₃,** A signal-intensity curve of one of these center-line chords, showing the signal intensity in 10 points along this particular center-line chord, revealing an infarction of 50% of LV wall thickness. *(From Schuijf JD, Kaandorp TA, Lamb HJ, et al: Quantification of myocardial infarct size and transmurality by contrast-enhanced magnetic resonance imaging in men, Am J Cardiol 94:284–288, 2004. Reprinted with permission.)*

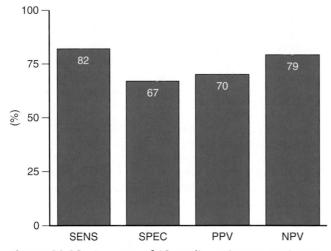

Figure 39-16 Accuracy of 13 studies using magnetic resonance imaging to detect viability and predict improvement of regional function post revascularization. NPV, negative predictive value; PPV, positive predictive value; SENS, sensitivity; SPEC, specificity. *(Data based on Schinkel AF, Bax JJ, Poldermans D, et al: Hibernating myocardium: Diagnosis and patient outcomes. Curr Probl Cardiol 32:375–410, 2007.)*

Additional Information Provided by Echocardiography and MRI

In patients with severe heart failure, the left ventricle dilates and becomes less elliptical and more spherical, a process referred to as *LV remodeling.* LV volumes will increase and LVEF will decline. LV volumes are important to determining the likelihood of functional improvement after revascularization. It has been shown previously that patients with severely dilated left ventricles have a low likelihood of improved function, despite the presence of viable tissue. For example, among 61 patients with substantial viability (= 4 viable segments), the likelihood of improvement in LVEF was minimal when the LV end-systolic volume exceeded 153 mL.[100] Accordingly, precise information on LV volumes and size, and LVEF is needed. This can be obtained by both echocardiography (using 3D approaches with or without intravenous contrast to improve endocardial border opacification) and MRI (see Figs. 39-7, 39-11, and Fig. 39-17). Surgical resection of dysfunctional myocardium and/or scar tissue is increasingly used in patients with ischemic cardiomyopathy. It has been demonstrated that these procedures can reduce LV size and restore the normal geometry of the left ventricle. In the RESTORE study, surgical ventricular restoration was applied in 1198 patients with a previous infarction.[101] A clear reduction in LV volumes with an improvement in LV shape was obtained. The LV end-systolic volume index decreased from 80.4 ± 51.4 mL/m^2 before surgery to 56.6 ± 34.3 mL/m^2 after surgery ($P < 0.001$); in these patients, the 5-year survival was $68.6\% \pm 2.8\%$. Prior to these surgical procedures, precise information on the presence, location, and extension of LV aneurysms is needed. This can be obtained by transthoracic echocardiography, preferably in combination with intravenous. In addition, MRI is extremely suited to depict LV aneurysms. The excellent spatial resolution of MRI

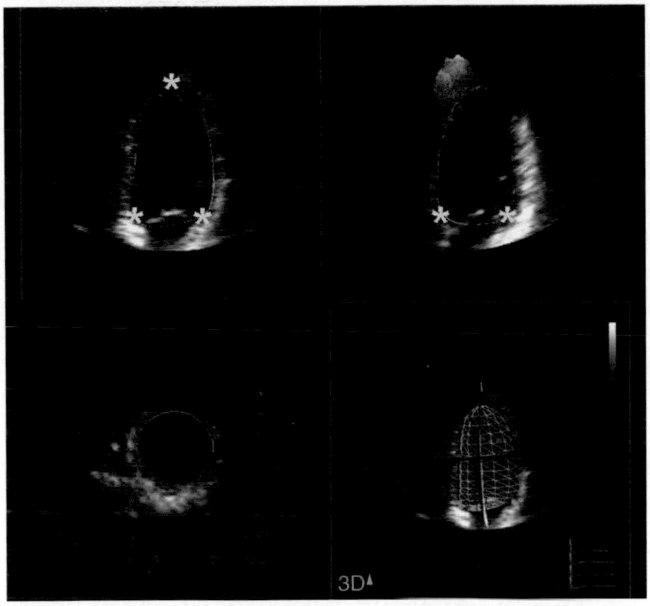

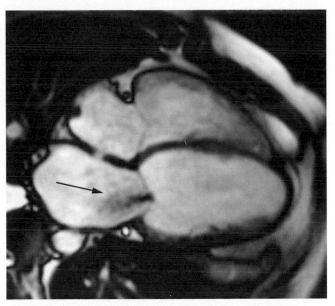

Figure 39-17 Three-dimensional left ventricular (LV) volumes obtained from the post processing of real-time three-dimensional echocardiographic data (*top*: long-axis views, *bottom-left*: short-axis, *bottom-right*: reconstructed 3D LV permitting precise quantification of LV volumes and LV ejection fraction).

Figure 39-18 Magnetic resonance imaging can also provide information on mitral regurgitation. In this 4-chamber view, the regurgitant jet *(arrow)* is clearly visible, which is the result of left ventricular dilation, mitral annular dilation, and systolic retraction of the leaflets.

permits measurement of precise wall thickness at the aneurismal regions; the use of contrast-enhanced MRI permits detection of scar tissue in these regions.

Another area of importance concerns the presence of ischemic mitral regurgitation, which is frequently observed in patients with ischemic heart failure, as a consequence of mitral annular dilation and systolic retraction of the mitral leaflets. Chronic ischemic mitral regurgitation causes volume overload, resulting in further LV dilation and progressive mitral regurgitation, which is associated with poor long-term outcome. It has also been shown that surgical correction of severe mitral regurgitation (mitral valve repair) at the time of revascularization resulted in reverse LV remodeling, a reduction in left atrial size, and good outcome.[102] Accordingly, information on the presence, severity, and etiology of mitral regurgitation in patients with ischemic cardiomyopathy is needed. Transthoracic echocardiography is the technique of choice and permits quantification of regurgitant volume. Transesophageal echocardiography may be preferred for determination of etiology of regurgitation and to determine the feasibility of surgical mitral valve repair. Eventually, MRI may provide superior information on valve anatomy (to determine precise etiology of mitral regurgitation) and regurgitant volume (Fig. 39-18), but, at present, availability and post processing of data hamper routine use of MRI to evaluate ischemic mitral regurgitation.

Finally, information on the presence, location, shape, and size of LV thrombi is important. This information can be provided either with echocardiography (using intravenous contrast, Fig. 39-19) or (contrast-enhanced) MRI.

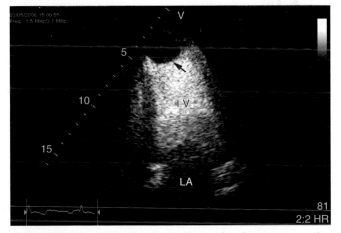

Figure 39-19 Contrast echocardiography demonstrates the presence of an apical thrombus as a contrast defect *(arrow)*. LA, left atrium; LV, left ventricle.

COMPARISON OF THE DIFFERENT TECHNIQUES

It is important to realize that the different viability techniques detect different aspects of myocardial viability (see Table 39-2). Nuclear imaging with technetium-99m-labeled agents or thallium-201 detects cell membrane integrity, intact mitochondria, or preserved perfusion, whereas imaging with FDG detects preserved glucose metabolism. Dobutamine stress echocardiography can detect contractile reserve. Previous comparative studies have shown that severely damaged myocardium may still have preserved perfusion or glucose utilization, or intact cell membranes/mitochondria, but may no longer have contractile reserve, secondary to the severely damaged contractile apparatus. Indeed, head-to-head comparisons between nuclear imaging with thallium-201 or FDG and dobutamine stress echocardiography demonstrated that about 50% of the dysfunctional segments considered viable on nuclear imaging did not have contractile reserve. For example, 114 patients with ischemic cardiomyopathy underwent perfusion imaging with technetium-99m-tetrofosmin and dobutamine stress echocardiography.[103] Of the 1336 dysfunctional segments, perfusion was preserved in 51% of segments and contractile reserve in 31% ($P <$ 0.05); 47% of the segments with perfusion did not exhibit contractile reserve.

Contrast-enhanced MRI detects scar tissue; with great precision, the extent and location of scar tissue is delineated. The remaining myocardium, however, is alive but it cannot be derived whether this is normal myocardium or ischemically jeopardized myocardium (chronic stunning, hibernation). Indeed, in direct comparisons between nuclear imaging and contrast-enhanced MRI, it was observed that great agreement existed between the two techniques for assessment of scar tissue.[104–106] Ibrahim and coworkers[105] compared contrast-enhanced MRI with technetium-99m-sestamibi SPECT in 78 patients imaged within 7 days after acute infarction. The authors demonstrated that contrast-enhanced MRI was superior to SPECT to detect small regions of scar tissue; particularly in non-Q-wave infarctions, contrast-enhanced MRI was more sensitive to detect scar formation.

Klein and colleagues[106] evaluated 31 patients with chronic ischemic LV dysfunction using both FDG PET and contrast-enhanced MRI. The authors demonstrated that the sensitivity to detect FDG-perfusion matches (indicating scar tissue) was excellent (96% on a patient level and 100% on a segment level). However, Roes et al.[104] recently demonstrated in another head-to-head comparison between FDG SPECT and contrast-enhanced MRI that in the non-scarred myocardium on contrast-enhanced MRI, FDG imaging showed a mixture of normal, chronically stunned, and hibernating myocardium. To enhance the detection of viability with MRI (and better identify jeopardized but viable myocardium and discriminate this from normal, viable myocardium), the combined assessment of contrast-enhanced MRI and low-dose dobutamine MRI has been proposed. While contrast-enhanced MRI provides the information on the scar tissue, the addition of low-dose dobutamine MRI helps to differentiate in the non scarred myocardium among normal, chronically stunned, and hibernating myocardium.[107]

The diagnostic accuracies of the noninvasive imaging modalities for the prediction of recovery of regional dysfunction after revascularization (Fig. 39-20) are summarized in Table 39-3. In general, FDG PET had the highest sensitivity (92%, $P < 0.05$ versus other techniques) and is therefore often considered the reference technique. The specificities of all imaging techniques are lower compared to the sensitivities. Dobutamine stress echocardiography has the highest specificity for the prediction of recovery of regional dysfunction (78%, $P < 0.05$ versus other techniques).

For the prediction of improvement of global LV function after revascularization (Fig. 39-21), the diagnostic accuracy of the techniques is summarized in Table 39-4. Currently, no studies are available using MRI for the prediction of recovery of global LV function. Pooling of the data showed that all techniques have a relatively good sensitivity, whereas dobutamine stress echocardiography has a somewhat lower sensitivity. On the other hand, this technique appeared to have a higher specificity for the prediction of improvement of global function, although the differences compared to the other techniques were not statistically significant.

Accordingly, noninvasive imaging generally provides a high sensitivity for the prediction of improvement of function post revascularization. The specificity for all

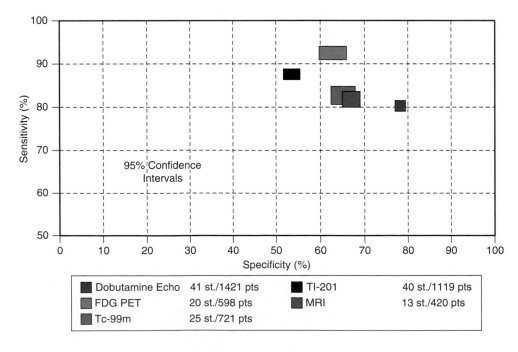

Figure 39-20 Comparison of sensitivities and specificities with 95% confidence intervals of the various techniques for the prediction of recovery of regional function after revascularization. FDG PET, fluorine-18-deoxyglucose and positron emission tomography; MRI, magnetic resonance imaging; Tc-99m, technetium-99m-labeled tracers; Tl-201, thallium-201. *(From Schinkel AF, Bax JJ, Poldermans D, et al: Hibernating myocardium: Diagnosis and patient outcomes, Curr Probl Cardiol 32:375–410, 2007. Reprinted with permission.)*

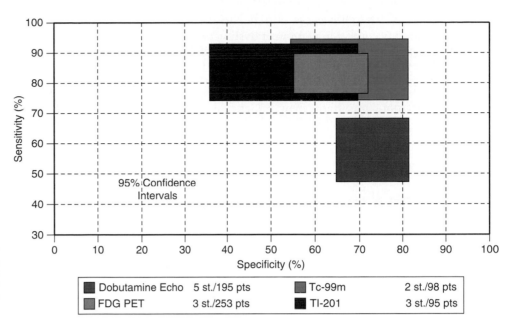

Figure 39-21 Comparison of sensitivities and specificities with 95% confidence intervals of the various techniques for the prediction of recovery of global left ventricular function after revascularization. The number of available studies and patients are indicated per technique. FDG PET, fluorine-18-deoxyglucose and positron emission tomography; MRI, magnetic resonance imaging; Tc-99m, technetium-99m-labeled tracers; TI-201, thallium-201. *(From Schinkel AF, Bax JJ, Poldermans D, et al: Hibernating myocardium: Diagnosis and patient outcomes, Curr Probl Cardiol 32:375–410, 2007. Reprinted with permission.)*

techniques is lower, however, which means that some segments that are classified as viable do not improve in function after revascularization. A variety of reasons can be considered to understand this phenomenon. These are summarized in Table 39-5 and can be divided into factors influencing specificity before, during, and after revascularization.

Factors before revascularization include the imperfect assessment of jeopardized but viable myocardium; a substantial number of dysfunctional segments are classified as viable but contain only a mixture of subendocardial scar and normal (viable) myocardium, with jeopardized

(viable) myocardium. These segments are indeed viable, but they cannot improve in function after revascularization. It has been discussed, however, whether revascularization of these segments may have other beneficial effects (instead of improvement in function)—for example, prevention of ventricular arrhythmias and prevention of LV remodeling. This remains to be determined. In addition, often ischemic events occur after imaging and before revascularization. Accordingly, viable segments may become damaged and progress to scar formation prior to revascularization, thereby preventing recovery of function post revascularization. The duration of hibernation before revascularization is also important. Various studies have demonstrated that hibernation is an unstable substrate, and delay in revascularization may result in progress from hibernation to scar tissue, without recovery of function post revascularization.[108,109] The extent of LV dilation is also important. It has been shown that too-severely dilated ventricles will not improve in function post revascularization, despite the presence of substantial viable tissue. During revascularization, prolonged ischemia and incomplete revascularization may also prevent recovery of function after revascularization. The severity of CAD and coronary anatomy may hamper complete revascularization. Finally, after revascularization, the most important factor is that almost every study has performed assessment of functional recovery within 6 months post revascularization. It has been shown, however, that more severely damaged myocardium needs a longer time to improve in function. Bax et al.[109] demonstrated that hibernating myocardium may need up to 1 year to improve in function after revascularization, whereas chronically stunned myocardium (which is less damaged myocardium) may improve within 3 months post revascularization. In addition, the natural progression of CAD may result in ischemic events during follow-up, preventing dysfunctional but viable myocardium from recovering after revascularization, or

Table 39-5 Influences on the Specificity of Noninvasive Imaging Techniques for Predicting Functional Recovery After Revascularization

Factors Before Revascularization

Imperfect assessment of jeopardized but viable myocardium (partial scar/fibrosis: subendocardial scar)

Ischemic events in the time interval between viability assessment and revascularization

Duration of hibernation before revascularization

Too extensive left ventricular remodeling

Presence of large scar adjacent to area of viable myocardium

Factors During Revascularization

Incomplete revascularization

Perioperative ischemic events

Factors After Revascularization

Too short follow-up for functional recovery assessment after revascularization (≤6 months)

Ischemic events during follow-up

Bypass graft occlusion

inducing new dysfunctional areas. In a similar way, early or late bypass graft occlusion may prevent dysfunctional but viable myocardium from recovering. All these different factors may have an impact on the recovery of regional and global contractile dysfunction and as a result, reduce the specificity of the noninvasive imaging techniques and, more important, may influence patient outcome.

CONCLUSIONS

For the assessment of jeopardized but viable myocardium, a variety of imaging techniques are available. Nuclear imaging is probably the most sensitive approach to assess viable myocardium, but dobutamine stress echocardiography and MRI are good alternative techniques. It is important to realize that contrast-enhanced MRI detects (with high precision) scar tissue but does not provide information on the status of the non-scarred myocardium (i.e., it does not differentiate between normal, viable myocardium and jeopardized, viable myocardium).

All imaging techniques have a fairly low specificity to predict improvement of function post revascularization, but there are reasons to explain this low specificity, as outlined in this chapter. From a practical, clinical point of view, it may therefore be preferred, once jeopardized but viable myocardium is detected, to continue with revascularization.

REFERENCES

1. Gheorghiade M, Bonow RO: Chronic heart failure in the United States. A manifestation of coronary artery disease, *Circulation* 97:282–289, 1998.
2. Bax JJ, Poldermans D, Elhendy A, et al: Sensitivity, specificity, and predictive accuracies of various noninvasive techniques for detecting hibernating myocardium, *Curr Probl Cardiol* 26:142–186, 2001.
3. Schinkel AF, Bax JJ, Poldermans D, et al: Hibernating myocardium: Diagnosis and patient outcomes, *Curr Probl Cardiol* 32:375–410, 2007.
4. Schinkel AF, Bax JJ, van Domburg R, et al: Dobutamine-induced contractile reserve in stunned, hibernating, and scarred myocardium in patients with ischemic cardiomyopathy, *J Nucl Med* 44:127–133, 2003.
5. Rahimtoola SH: The hibernating myocardium, *Am Heart J* 117:211–221, 1989.
6. Braunwald E, Kloner RA: The stunned myocardium: prolonged, post-ischemic ventricular dysfunction, *Circulation* 66:1146–1149, 1982.
7. Elsasser A, Muller KD, Skwara W, Bode C, Kubler W, Vogt AM: Severe energy deprivation of human hibernating myocardium as possible common pathomechanism of contractile dysfunction, structural degeneration and cell death, *J Am Coll Cardiol* 39:1189–1198, 2002.
8. Depre C, Vanoverschelde J, Gerber B, et al: Correlation of functional recovery with myocardial blood flow, glucose uptake, and morphologic features in patients with chronic left ventricular ischemic dysfunction undergoing coronary artery bypass grafting, *J Thorac Cardiovasc Surg* 113:371–378, 1997.
9. Schinkel AF, Bax JJ, Boersma E, et al: Assessment of residual myocardial viability in regions with chronic electrocardiographic Q-wave infarction, *Am Heart J* 144:865–869, 2002.
10. Secknus M, Marwick TH: Evolution of dobutamine echocardiography protocols and indications: Safety and side effects in 3011 studies over 5 years, *J Am Coll Cardiol* 29:1234–1240, 1997.
11. Gerber BL, Vanoverschelde J-LJ, Bol A, Michel C, Labar D, Wijns W, et al: Myocardial blood flow, glucose uptake and recruitment of inotropic reserve in chronic left ventricular ischemic dysfunction. Implications for the pathophysiology of chronic hibernation, *Circulation* 94:651–659, 1996.
12. Charney R, Schwinger ME, Chun J, Cohen MV, Nanna M, Menegus MA, et al: Dobutamine echocardiography and resting-redistribution thallium-201 scintigraphy predicts recovery of

hibernating myocardium after coronary revascularization, *Am Heart J* 128:864–869, 1994.
13. Arnese M, Cornel JH, Salustri A, Maat APWM, Elhendy A, Reijs AEM, et al: Prediction of improvement of regional left ventricular function after surgical revascularization: a comparison of low-dose dobutamine echocardiography with 201-TL SPECT, *Circulation* 91:2748–2752, 1995.
14. Perrone-Filardi P, Pace L, Prastaro M, Squame F, Betocchi S, Soricelli A, et al: Assessment of myocardial viability in patients with chronic coronary artery disease. Rest-4-hour-24-hour ^{201}Tl tomography versus dobutamine echocardiography, *Circulation* 94:2712–2719, 1996.
15. Vanoverschelde J-LJ, D'Hondt A-M, Marwick T, Gerber BL, De Kock R, Dion R, et al: Head-to-head comparison of exercise-redistribution-reinjection thallium single-photon emission computed tomography and low dose dobutamine echocardiography for prediction of reversibility of chronic left ventricular ischemic dysfunction, *J Am Coll Cardiol* 28:432–442, 1996.
16. Marzullo P, Parodi O, Reisenhofer B, Sambuceti G, Picano E, Distante A, et al: Value of rest thallium-201/technetium-99m sestamibi and dobutamine echocardiography for detecting myocardial viability, *Am J Cardiol* 71:166–172, 1993.
17. Bax JJ, Cornel JH, Visser FC, Fioretti PM, van Lingen A, Reijs AEM, et al: Prediction of recovery of myocardial dysfunction following revascularization: comparison of F18-fluorodeoxyglucose/thallium-201 single photon emission computed tomography, thallium-201 stress-reinjection single photon emission computed tomography and dobutamine echocardiography, *J Am Coll Cardiol* 28:558–564, 1996.
18. Senior R, Glenville B, Basu S, Sridhara BS, Anagnostou E, Stanbridge R, et al: Dobutamine echocardiography and thallium-201 imaging predict functional improvement after revascularization in severe ischaemic left ventricular dysfunction, *Br Heart J* 74:358–364, 1995.
19. Perrone-Filardi P, Pace L, Prastaro M, Piscione F, Betocchi S, Squame F, et al: Dobutamine echocardiography predicts improvement of hypoperfused dysfunctional myocardium after revascularization in patients with coronary artery disease, *Circulation* 91:2556–2565, 1995.
20. Alfieri O, La Canna G, Giubinni R, Pardini A, Zogno M, Fucci C: Recovery of myocardial function, *Eur J Cardiothorac Surg* 7:325–330, 1993.
21. La Canna G, Alfieri O, Giubbini R, Gargano M, Ferrari R, Visioli O: Echocardiography during infusion of dobutamine for identification of reversible dysfunction in patients with chronic coronary artery disease, *J Am Coll Cardiol* 23:617–626, 1994.
22. Haque T, Furukawa T, Takahashi M, Kinoshita M: Identification of hibernating myocardium by dobutamine stress echocardiography: comparison with thallium-201 reinjection imaging, *Am Heart J* 130:553–563, 1995.
23. Baer FM, Voth E, Deutsch HJ, Schneider CA, Horst M, de Vivie ER, et al: Predictive value of low dose dobutamine transesophageal echocardiography and fluorine-18 fluorodeoxyglucose positron emission tomography for recovery of regional left ventricular function after successful revascularization, *J Am Coll Cardiol* 28:60–69, 1996.
24. DeFilippi CR, Willett DWL, Irani WN, Eichhorn EJ, Velasco CE, Grayburn PA: Comparison of myocardial contrast echocardiography and low-dose dobutamine stress echocardiography in predicting recovery of left ventricular function after coronary revascularization in chronic ischemic heart disease, *Circulation* 92:2863–2868, 1995.
25. Elhendy A, Cornel JH, Roelandt JRTC, van Domburg RT, Fioretti PM: Akinesis becoming dyskinesis during dobutamine stress echocardiography. A predictor of poor functional recovery after revascularization, *Chest* 110:155–158, 1996.
26. Kostopoulos KG, Kranidis AI, Bouki KP, Antonellis JP, Kappos KG, Rodogianni FE, et al: Detection of myocardial viability in the prediction of improvement in left ventricular function after successful coronary revascularization by using the dobutamine stress echocardiography and quantitative SPECT rest-redistribution-reinjection ^{201}Tl imaging after dipyridamole infusion, *Angiology* 47:1039–1046, 1996.
27. Cornel JH, Bax JJ, Fioretti PM, Visser FC, Maat APWM, Boersma E, et al: Prediction of improvement of left ventricular function after revascularization. ^{18}F-fluorodeoxyglucose SPECT vs low-dose dobutamine echocardiography, *Eur Heart J* 18:941–948, 1997.
28. Scognamiglio R, Fasoli G, Casarotto D, Miorelli M, Nistri S, Palisi M, et al: Postextrasystolic potentiation and dobutamine echocardiography in predicting recovery of myocardial function after coronary bypass revascularization, *Circulation* 96:816–820, 1997.
29. Pagano D, Bonser RS, Townend JN, Ordoubadi F, Lorenzoni R, Camici PG: Predictive value of dobutamine echocardiography and positron emission tomography in identifying hibernating myocardium in patients with postischaemic heart failure, *Heart* 79:281–288, 1998.
30. Baer FM, Theissen P, Schneider CA, Voth E, Sechtem U, Schicha H, et al: Dobutamine magnetic resonance imaging predicts contractile recovery of chronically dysfunctional myocardium after successful revascularization, *J Am Coll Cardiol* 31:1040–1048, 1998.

31. Voci P, Bilotta F, Caretta Q, Mercanti C, Marino B: Low-dose dobutamine echocardiography predicts the early response of dysfunctioning myocardial segments to coronary artery bypass grafting, *Am Heart J* 129:521–526, 1995.

32. Picano E, Ostojic M, Varga A, Sicari R, Djordjevic-Dikic A, Nedeljkovic I, et al: Combined low dose dipyridamole-dobutamine stress echocardiography to identify myocardial viability, *J Am Coll Cardiol* 27:1422–1428, 1996.

33. Elhendy A, Cornel JH, Roelandt JRTC, Nierop PR, Van Domburg RT, Geleijnse ML, et al: Impact of severity of coronary artery stenosis and the collateral circulation on the functional outcome of dyssynergic myocardium after revascularization in patients with healed myocardial infarction and chronic left ventricular dysfunction, *Am J Cardiol* 79:883–888, 1997.

34. Cornel JH, Bax JJ, Elhendy A, Poldermans D, Vanoverschelde JLJ, Fioretti PM: Predictive accuracy of echocardiographic response of mildly dyssynergic myocardial segments to low-dose dobutamine, *Am J Cardiol* 80:1481–1484, 1997.

35. Pace L, Perrone-Filardi P, Mainenti P, Prastaro M, Vezzuto P, Varrone A, et al: Combined evaluation of rest-redistribution thallium-201 tomography and low-dose dobutamine echocardiography enhances the identification of viable myocardium in patients with chronic coronary artery disease, *Eur J Nucl Med* 25:744–750, 1998.

36. Sayad DE, Willett DL, Hundley G, Grayburn PA, Peshock RM: Dobutamine magnetic resonance imaging with myocardial tagging quantitatively predicts improvement in regional function after revascularization, *Am J Cardiol* 82:1149–1151, 1998.

37. Sicari R, Varga A, Picano E, Borges AC, Gimelli A, Marzullo P: Comparison of combination of dipyridamole and dobutamine during echocardiography with thallium scintigraphy to improve viability detection, *Am J Cardiol* 83:6–10, 1999.

38. Gunning MG, Anagnostopoulos C, Knight CJ, Pepper J, Burman ED, Davies G, et al: Comparison of ^{201}Tl, 99mTc-tetrofosmin, and dobutamine magnetic resonance imaging for identifying hibernating myocardium, *Circulation* 98:1869–1874, 1998.

39. Afridi I, Kleiman NS, Raizner AE, Zoghbi WA: Dobutamine echocardiography in myocardial hibernation. Optimal dose and accuracy in predicting recovery of ventricular function after coronary angioplasty, *Circulation* 91:663–670, 1995.

40. Qureshi U, Nagueh SF, Afridi I, Vaduganathan P, Blaustein A, Verani MS, et al: Dobutamine echocardiography and quantitative rest-redistribution ^{201}Tl tomography in myocardial hibernation. Relation of contractile reserve to ^{201}Tl uptake and comparative prediction of recovery of function, *Circulation* 95:626–635, 1997.

41. Nagueh SF, Vaduganathan P, Ali N, Blaustein A, Verani MS, Winters WL, et al: Identification of hibernating myocardium: comparative accuracy of myocardial contrast echocardiography, rest-redistribution thallium-201 tomography and dobutamine echocardiography, *J Am Coll Cardiol* 29:985–993, 1997.

42. Cornel JH, Bax JJ, Elhendy A, Maat APWM, Kimman GJP, Geleijnse ML, et al: Biphasic response to dobutamine predicts improvement of global left ventricular function after surgical revascularization in patients with stable coronary artery disease. Implications of time course of recovery on diagnostic accuracy, *J Am Coll Cardiol* 31:1002–1010, 1998.

43. Dellegrottaglie S, Perrone-Filardi P, Pace L, et al: Prediction of long-term effects of revascularization on regional and global left ventricular function by dobutamine echocardiography and rest Tl-201 imaging alone and in combination in patients with chronic coronary artery disease, *J Nucl Cardiol* 9:174–182, 2002.

44. Leoncini M, Sciagra R, Bellandi F, et al: Low-dose dobutamine nitrate-enhanced technetium 99m sestamibi gated SPECT versus low-dose dobutamine echocardiography for detecting reversible dysfunction in ischemic cardiomyopathy, *J Nucl Cardiol* 9:402–406, 2002.

45. Piscione F, De Luca G, Perrone-Filardi P, et al: Relationship between contractile reserve, Tl-201 uptake, and collateral angiographic circulation in collateral-dependent myocardium: implications regarding the evaluation of myocardial viability, *J Nucl Cardiol* 10:17–27, 2003.

46. Piscione F, Perrone-Filardi P, De Luca G, et al: Low dose dobutamine echocardiography for predicting functional recovery after coronary revascularisation, *Heart* 86:679–686, 2001.

47. Pace L, Filardi PP, Cuocolo A, et al: Diagnostic accuracy of low-dose dobutamine echocardiography in predicting post-revascularisation recovery of function in patients with chronic coronary artery disease: relationship to thallium-201 uptake, *Eur J Nucl Med* 28:1616–1623, 2001.

48. Cwajg JM, Cwajg E, Nagueh SF, et al: End-diastolic wall thickness as a predictor of recovery of function in myocardial hibernation: relation to rest-redistribution Tl-201 tomography and dobutamine stress echocardiography, *J Am Coll Cardiol* 35:1152–1161, 2000.

49. Ling LH, Christian TF, Mulvagh SL, et al: Determining myocardial viability in chronic ischemic left ventricular dysfunction: a prospective comparison of rest-redistribution thallium 201 single-photon emission computed tomography, nitroglycerin-dobutamine

50. Hanekom L, Jenkins C, Jeffries L, et al: Incremental value of strain rate analysis as an adjunct to wall-motion scoring for assessment of myocardial viability by dobutamine echocardiography: a follow-up study after revascularization, *Circulation* 112:3892–3900, 2005.

51. Zaglavara T, Karvounis HI, Haaverstad R, et al: Dobutamine stress echocardiography is highly accurate for the prediction of contractile reserve in the early postoperative period, but may underestimate late recovery in contractile reserve after revascularization of the hibernating myocardium, *J Am Soc Echocardiogr* 19:300–306, 2006.

52. Wiggers H, Egeblad H, Nielsen TT, Botker HE: Prediction of reversible myocardial dysfunction by positron emission tomography, low-dose dobutamine echocardiography, resting ECG, and exercise testing, *Cardiology* 96:32–37, 2001.

53. Carluccio E, Biagioli P, Alunni G, et al: Patients with hibernating myocardium show altered left ventricular volumes and shape, which revert after revascularization: evidence that dyssynergy might directly induce cardiac remodeling, *J Am Coll Cardiol* 47:969–977, 2006.

54. Bax JJ, Poldermans D, Elhendy A, et al: Improvement of left ventricular ejection fraction, heart failure symptoms and prognosis after revascularization in patients with chronic coronary artery disease and viable myocardium detected by dobutamine stress echocardiography, *J Am Coll Cardiol* 34:163–169, 1999.

55. Meluzin J, Cerny J, Frelich M, et al: Prognostic value of the amount of dysfunctional but viable myocardium in revascularized patients with coronary artery disease and left ventricular dysfunction. Investigators of this Multicenter Study, *J Am Coll Cardiol* 32:912–920, 1998.

56. Afridi I, Grayburn PA, Panza JA, et al: Myocardial viability during dobutamine echocardiography predicts survival in patients with coronary artery disease and severe left ventricular systolic dysfunction, *J Am Coll Cardiol* 32:921–926, 1998.

57. Anselmi M, Golia G, Cicoira M, et al: Prognostic value of detection of myocardial viability using low-dose dobutamine echocardiography in infarcted patients, *Am J Cardiol* 81:21G–38G, 1998.

58. Senior R, Kaul S, Lahiri A: Myocardial viability on echocardiography predicts long-term survival after revascularization in patients with ischemic congestive heart failure, *J Am Coll Cardiol* 33:1848–1854, 1999.

59. Chaudhry FA, Tauke JT, Alessandrini RS, et al: Prognostic implications of myocardial contractile reserve in patients with coronary artery disease and left ventricular dysfunction, *J Am Coll Cardiol* 34:730–738, 1999.

60. Meluzin J, Cerny J, Spinarova L, et al: Prognosis of patients with chronic coronary artery disease and severe left ventricular dysfunction. The importance of myocardial viability, *Eur J Heart Fail* 5:85–93, 2003.

61. Sicari R, Picano E, Cortigiani L, et al, VIDA (Viability Identification with Dobutamine Administration) Study Group: Prognostic value of myocardial viability recognized by low-dose dobutamine echocardiography in chronic ischemic left ventricular dysfunction, *Am J Cardiol* 92:1263–1266, 2003.

62. Rambaldi R, Bax JJ, Rizzello V, et al: Post-systolic shortening during dobutamine stress echocardiography predicts cardiac survival in patients with severe left ventricular dysfunction, *Coron Artery Dis* 16:141–145, 2005.

63. Rizzello V, Poldermans D, Schinkel AFL, et al: Long term prognostic value of myocardial viability and ischaemia during dobutamine stress echocardiography in patients with ischaemic cardiomyopathy undergoing coronary revascularisation, *Heart* 92:239–244, 2006.

64. Sozzi FB, Poldermans D, Bax JJ, et al: Second harmonic imaging improves sensitivity of dobutamine stress echocardiography for the diagnosis of coronary artery disease, *Am Heart J* 142:153–159, 2001.

65. Grayburn PA, Mulvagh S, Crouse L: Left ventricular opacification at rest and during stress, *Am J Cardiol* 90:21J–27J, 2002.

66. Reilly JP, Tunick PA, Timmermans RJ, et al: Contrast echocardiography clarifies uninterpretable wall motion in intensive care unit patients, *J Am Coll Cardiol* 35:485–490, 2000.

67. Aggeli C, Giannopoulos G, Roussakis G, et al: Safety of myocardial flash-contrast echocardiography in combination with dobutamine stress testing for the detection of ischaemia in 5250 studies, *Heart* 94:1571–1577, 2008.

68. Nucifora G, Marsan NA, Siebelink HM, et al: Safety of contrast-enhanced echocardiography within 24 h after acute myocardial infarction, *Eur J Echocardiogr* 9:816–818, 2008.

69. Marwick TH: Quantitative techniques for stress echocardiography: dream or reality? *Eur J Echocardiogr* 3:171–176, 2002.

70. Rambaldi R, Poldermans D, Bax JJ, et al: Doppler tissue velocity sampling improves diagnostic accuracy during dobutamine stress echocardiography for the assessment of viable myocardium in patients with severe left ventricular dysfunction, *Eur Heart J* 21:1091–1098, 2001.

71. Becker M, Hoffmann R, Kuhl HP, et al: Analysis of myocardial deformation based on ultrasonic pixel tracking to determine transmurality in chronic myocardial infarction, *Eur Heart J* 27:2560–2566, 2006.

72. Becker M, Lenzen A, Ocklenburg C, et al: Myocardial deformation imaging based on ultrasonic pixel tracking to identify reversible myocardial dysfunction, *J Am Coll Cardiol* 51(15):1473–1481, 2008.

73. Hanekom L, Jenkins C, Jeffries L, et al: Incremental value of strain rate analysis as an adjunct to wall-motion scoring for assessment of myocardial viability by dobutamine echocardiography: a follow-up study after revascularization, *Circulation* 112:3892–3900, 2005.

74. Brown MA, Norris RM, Takayama M, White HD: Post-systolic shortening: a marker of potential for early recovery of acutely ischaemic myocardium in the dog, *Cardiovasc Res* 21:703–716, 1987.

75. Rambaldi R, Bax JJ, Rizzello V, et al: Post-systolic shortening during dobutamine stress echocardiography predicts cardiac survival in patients with severe left ventricular dysfunction, *Coron Artery Dis* 16:141–145, 2005.

76. Lim P, Pasquet A, Gerber B, et al: Is postsystolic shortening a marker of viability in chronic left ventricular ischemic dysfunction? Comparison with late enhancement contrast magnetic resonance imaging, *J Am Soc Echocardiogr* 21:452–457, 2008.

77. Shimoni S, Frangogiannis NG, Aggeli CJ, et al: Microvascular structural correlates of myocardial contrast echocardiography in patients with coronary artery disease and left ventricular dysfunction: Implications for the assessment of myocardial hibernation, *Circulation* 106:950–956, 2002.

78. DeFilippi CR, Willett DL, Irani WN, Eichhorn EJ, Velasco CE, Grayburn PA: Comparison of myocardial contrast echocardiography and low-dose dobutamine stress echocardiography in predicting recovery of left ventricular function after coronary revascularization in chronic ischemic heart disease, *Circulation* 92:2863–2868, 1995.

79. Shimoni S, Frangogiannis NG, Aggeli CJ, et al: Identification of hibernating myocardium with quantitative intravenous myocardial contrast echocardiography: comparison with dobutamine echocardiography and thallium-201 scintigraphy, *Circulation* 107: 538–544, 2003.

80. Hayat SA, Senior R: Myocardial contrast echocardiography in ST elevation myocardial infarction: ready for prime time? *Eur Heart J* 29:299–314, 2008.

81. Galiuto L, Garramone B, Scara A, et al: The extent of microvascular damage during myocardial contrast echocardiography is superior to other known indexes of post-infarct reperfusion in predicting left ventricular remodeling: results of the multicenter AMICI study, *J Am Coll Cardiol* 51:552–559, 2008.

82. Dwivedi G, Janardhanan R, Hayat SA, et al: Prognostic value of myocardial viability detected by myocardial contrast echocardiography early after acute myocardial infarction, *J Am Coll Cardiol* 50: 327–334, 2007.

83. Fieno DS, Kim RJ, Chen EL, Lomasney JW, Klocke FJ, Judd RM: Contrast-enhanced magnetic resonance imaging of myocardium at risk: distinction between reversible and irreversible injury throughout infarct healing, *J Am Coll Cardiol* 36:1985–1991, 2000.

84. Wu E, Judd RM, Vargas JD, Klocke FJ, Bonow RO, Kim RJ: Visualisation of presence, location, and transmural extent of healed Q-wave and non-Q-wave myocardial infarction, *Lancet* 357:21–28, 2001.

85. Schuijf JD, Kaandorp TA, Lamb HJ, et al: Quantification of myocardial infarct size and transmurality by contrast-enhanced magnetic resonance imaging in men, *Am J Cardiol* 94:284–288, 2004.

86. Gerber BL, Belge B, Legros GJ, et al: Characterization of acute and chronic myocardial infarcts by multidetector computed tomography: comparison with contrast-enhanced magnetic resonance, *Circulation* 113:823–833, 2006.

87. Schmidt M, Voth E, Schneider CA, et al: F-18-FDG uptake is a reliable predictor of functional recovery of akinetic but viable infarct regions as defined by magnetic resonance imaging before and after revascularization, *Magn Reson Imaging* 22:229–236, 2004.

88. Baer FM, Theissen P, Schneider CA, et al: Dobutamine magnetic resonance imaging predicts contractile recovery of chronically dysfunctional myocardium after successful revascularization, *J Am Coll Cardiol* 31:1040–1048, 1998.

89. Klow NE, Smith HJ, Gullestad L, Seem E, Endresen K: Outcome of bypass surgery in patients with chronic ischemic left ventricular dysfunction. Predictive value of MR imaging, *Acta Radiol* 38:76–82, 1997.

90. Baer FM, Theissen P, Crnac J, et al: Head to head comparison of dobutamine-transoesophageal echocardiography and dobutamine-magnetic resonance imaging for the prediction of left ventricular functional recovery in patients with chronic coronary artery disease, *Eur Heart J* 21:981–991, 2000.

91. Gunning MG, Anagnostopoulos C, Knight CJ, et al: Comparison of 201Tl, 99mTc-tetrofosmin, and dobutamine magnetic resonance imaging for identifying hibernating myocardium, *Circulation* 98:1869–1874, 1998.

92. Sayad DE, Willett DL, Hundley WG, Grayburn PA, Peshock RM: Dobutamine magnetic resonance imaging with myocardial tagging quantitatively predicts improvement in regional function after revascularization, *Am J Cardiol* 82:1149–1151, 1998.

93. Sandstede JJ, Bertsch G, Beer M, et al: Detection of myocardial viability by low-dose dobutamine Cine MR imaging, *Magn Reson Imaging* 17:1437–1443, 1999.

94. Trent RJ, Waiter GD, Hillis GS, McKiddie FI, Redpath TW, Walton S: Dobutamine magnetic resonance imaging as a predictor of myocardial functional recovery after revascularisation, *Heart* 83:40–46, 2000.

95. Wellnhofer E, Olariu A, Klein C, et al: Magnetic resonance low-dose dobutamine test is superior to SCAR quantification for the prediction of functional recovery, *Circulation* 109:2172–2174, 2004.

96. Van Hoe L, Vanderheyden M: Ischemic cardiomyopathy: value of different MRI techniques for prediction of functional recovery after revascularization, *AJR Am J Roentgenol* 182:95–100, 2004.

97. Kim RJ, Wu E, Rafael A, et al: The use of contrast-enhanced magnetic resonance imaging to identify reversible myocardial dysfunction, *N Engl J Med* 343:1445–1453, 2000.

98. Selvanayagam JB, Kardos A, Francis JM, et al: Value of delayed-enhancement cardiovascular magnetic resonance imaging in predicting myocardial viability after surgical revascularization, *Circulation* 110:1535–1541, 2004.

99. Kuhl HP, Lipke CS, Krombach GA, et al: Assessment of reversible myocardial dysfunction in chronic ischaemic heart disease: comparison of contrast-enhanced cardiovascular magnetic resonance and a combined positron emission tomography-single photon emission computed tomography imaging protocol, *Eur Heart J* 27:846–853, 2006.

100. Schinkel AF, Poldermans D, Rizzello V, Vanoverschelde JL, Elhendy A, Boersma E, et al: Why do patients with ischemic cardiomyopathy and a substantial amount of viable myocardium not always recover in function after revascularization? *J Thorac Cardiovasc Surg* 127: 385–390, 2004.

101. Athanasuleas CL, Buckberg GD, Stanley AW, et al, RESTORE group: Surgical ventricular restoration in the treatment of congestive heart failure due to post-infarction ventricular dilation, *J Am Coll Cardiol* 44:1439–1445, 2004.

102. Bax JJ, Braun J, Somer S, et al: Restrictive annuloplasty and coronary revascularization in ischemic mitral regurgitation results in reverse left ventricular remodeling, *Circulation* 110(11 Suppl 1):II-103–II-108, 2004.

103. Bax JJ, Poldermans D, Schinkel AF, et al: Perfusion and contractile reserve in chronic dysfunctional myocardium: relation to functional outcome after surgical revascularization, *Circulation* 106(12 Suppl 1): I14–I18, 2002.

104. Roes SD, Kaandorp TA, Ajmone Marsan N, et al: Agreement and disagreement between contrast-enhanced magnetic resonance imaging and nuclear imaging for assessment of myocardial viability, *Eur J Nucl Med Mol Imaging* 36:594–601, 2009.

105. Ibrahim T, Bülow HP, Hackl T, et al: Diagnostic value of contrast-enhanced magnetic resonance imaging and single-photon emission computed tomography for detection of myocardial necrosis early after acute myocardial infarction, *J Am Coll Cardiol* 49:208–216, 2007.

106. Klein C, Nekolla SG, Bengel FM, et al: Assessment of myocardial viability with contrast-enhanced magnetic resonance imaging: Comparison with positron emission tomography, *Circulation* 105:162–167, 2002.

107. Kaandorp TA, Bax JJ, Schuijf JD, et al: Head-to-head comparison between contrast-enhanced magnetic resonance imaging and dobutamine magnetic resonance imaging in men with ischemic cardiomyopathy, *Am J Cardiol* 93:1461–1464, 2004.

108. Beanlands RS, Hendry PJ, Masters RG, deKemp RA, Woodend K, Ruddy TD: Delay in revascularization is associated with increased mortality rate in patients with severe left ventricular dysfunction and viable myocardium on fluorine 18-fluorodeoxyglucose positron emission tomography imaging, *Circulation* 98(Suppl 19):II51–II56, 1998.

109. Bax JJ, Schinkel AF, Boersma E, et al: Early versus delayed revascularization in patients with ischemic cardiomyopathy and substantial viability: impact on outcome, *Circulation* 108(Suppl 1):II39–II42, 2003.

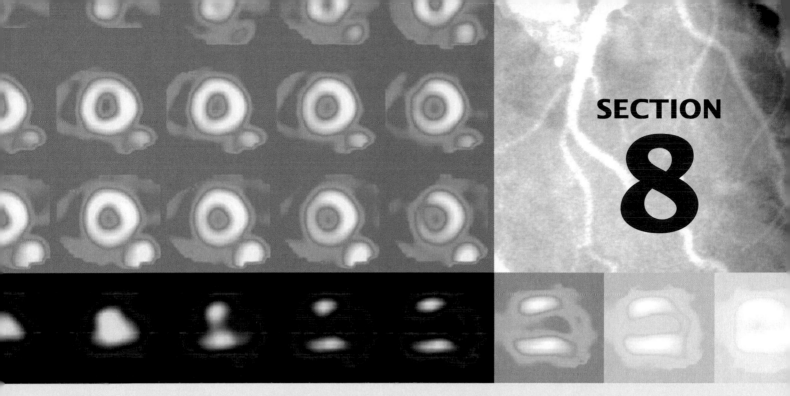

Tracer Specific Imaging Techniques

Chapter 40

Imaging of Myocardial Metabolism

ROBERT J. GROPLER AND LINDA R. PETERSON

INTRODUCTION

Flexibility in myocardial substrate metabolism for energy production is fundamental to cardiac health. The loss in flexibility leads to an overdependence on the metabolism of an individual category of substrates. Prime examples include the predominance in fatty acid metabolism characteristic of diabetic heart disease and the accelerated glucose use associated with dilated cardiomyopathy. Because of the pleiotropic actions of myocardial substrate metabolism, an overdependence on the metabolism of a category of substrates can potentially have detrimental effects on myocardial health that extend beyond impairment in energy production. Important unresolved questions include the extent to which these metabolic perturbations are adaptive and have the propensity to become maladaptive; what are the key determinants of these metabolic alterations, how do they impact prognosis, and do they make robust targets for novel therapeutics? Although numerous transgenic models targeting key aspects of myocardial substrate use continue to be developed, their relevance to the corresponding human condition is frequently unclear. In addition, applied genomics have identified numerous gene variants intimately involved in the regulation of myocardial substrate use. Yet, identifying the clinically significant genetic variants remains elusive. As a consequence, there is a strong demand for accurate noninvasive imaging approaches of myocardial substrate metabolism that provide linkage between the bench and the bedside leading to improved patient management paradigms. Currently, the most successful example is the detection of ischemic but viable myocardium with positron emission tomography (PET) and fluorine-18 (^{18}F)-fluorodeoxyglucose (FDG) for the management of patients with ischemic cardiomyopathy. In this chapter, potential future applications of noninvasive metabolic imaging for the assessment of cardiovascular disease are discussed.

METHODS TO IMAGE MYOCARDIAL METABOLISM

There are currently three methods to image myocardial metabolism noninvasively: magnetic resonance spectroscopy (MRS), single-photon emission computed tomography (SPECT), and PET. A summary of each technique follows.

Magnetic Resonance Spectroscopy

Magnetic resonance spectroscopy offers the advantages of the ability to measure multiple metabolic pathways simultaneously, the relative ease in performing serial measurements, and the lack of ionizing radiation. Moreover, when combined with MRI, near-simultaneous measurements of myocardial perfusion and mechanical function are possible. A number of biologically important nuclei can be measured, including phosphorous (^{31}P), hydrogen (^{1}H), carbon (^{13}C), sodium (^{23}Na), nitrogen (^{15}N), and fluorine (^{19}F). The fundamental principle of MRS is that the chemical environment of nuclei induces local magnetic fields that shift their resonance frequency. The different frequency shift for different metabolites results in a signal consisting of one or more discrete resonance frequencies. The Fourier transform of the acquired signal produces a spectrum with peaks at distinct frequencies. The MRS spectrum displays the signal intensity as a function of frequency measured in parts per million, relative to the frequency of a reference compound. The signal intensity at a given frequency is proportional to the amount of the respective metabolite and can be used to determine the absolute concentration of the metabolite using appropriate calibrating reference signal.[1,2]

MRS is limited by low signal-to-noise, concomitant limited spatial resolution, intravoxel signal contamination, and long acquisition times. Compared with nuclear imaging methods, MRS has a much lower sensitivity (detecting millimolar as opposed to nanomolar concentrations). As a consequence, the initial success of imaging of cardiac metabolism using Carbon-13 labeled agents in intact animals has not been translated to the study of humans.[3] Of note, cardiac applications for MRS become more limited as one moves from rodent to man as opposed to nuclear methods where the reverse occurs. This appears to be a function of both the higher field strength in the small-bore systems and the use of radiofrequency coils that are in closer proximity to the entire heart used in small-animal imaging. In contrast to rodent hearts, where measurements of the entire left ventricular (LV) myocardium are obtained, measurements in human myocardium are typically limited to the anterior myocardium. Currently, only ^{31}P and ^{1}H have been widely used for in vivo clinical cardiac examinations focusing on myocardial energetics (^{31}P) and lipid accumulation (^{1}H).[1,3,4]

Single-Photon Emission Computed Tomography (SPECT) (See Chapter 2)

There are numerous advantages to SPECT, including the inherent high sensitivity of the radionuclide method to measure metabolic processes; wide availability of the technology; with ECG-gating, the ability to measure myocardial function simultaneously; and the long physical half-life of SPECT radiopharmaceuticals, allowing delivery to multiple sites, which facilitates the performance of multicenter studies that incorporate measurements of myocardial substrate metabolism. Small-animal SPECT and SPECT/CT systems are rapidly advancing, allowing the performance of myocardial metabolic studies in rodent models of cardiac disease. The major disadvantage of SPECT is the inability to quantify cellular metabolic processes, primarily because of the technical limitations of SPECT (relatively poor temporal resolution and inaccurate correction for photon attenuation).

Metabolic processes that can be measured by SPECT include:

1. Glucose metabolism: No specific SPECT radiotracers are currently available to measure myocardial glucose metabolism. However, when combined with the appropriate detection scheme or collimator design, myocardial glucose metabolism can be measured with SPECT and FDG.[5]
2. Fatty acid metabolism: One of the earliest and most promising SPECT radiotracers of fatty acid metabolism was 15-(p-iodophenyl)-pentadecanoic acid (IPPA).[6-8] This radiotracer demonstrated rapid accumulation in the heart and exhibited clearance kinetics that followed a biexponential function characteristic for ^{11}C-palmitate. Moreover, the clearance rates correlated directly with β-oxidation. Initial studies in humans with coronary atherosclerosis demonstrated reduced uptake and washout in regions subtended by occluded arteries, consistent with ischemia.[9] Unfortunately, the poor temporal resolution of SPECT systems did not take advantage of the rapid turnover of IPPA. As a consequence, quantification of myocardial fatty acid metabolism

was not possible, and image quality was reduced. This led to the development of branched-chain analogs of IPPA, such as [^{123}I]β-methyl-P-iodophenyl pentadecanoic acid (BMIPP) (Fig. 40-1).[8-11] Alkyl branching inhibits β-oxidation, shunting radiolabel to the triglyceride pool, thereby increasing radiotracer retention and improving image quality.

Positron Emission Tomography (PET) (See Chapter 3)

The major advantages of PET are its intrinsic quantitative capability and the use of radiopharmaceuticals labeled with the positron-emitting radionuclides. The PET detection scheme permits accurate quantification of activity in the field of view. The positron-emitting radionuclides of the biologically ubiquitous elements oxygen (^{15}O), carbon (^{11}C), and nitrogen (^{13}N), as well as fluorine (^{18}F) substituting for hydrogen, can be incorporated into a wide variety of substrates or substrate analogs that participate in diverse biochemical pathways without altering the biochemical properties of the substrate of interest (see Fig. 40-1). By combining the knowledge of the metabolic pathways of interest with kinetic models that faithfully describe the fate of the tracer in tissue, an accurate interpretation of the tracer kinetics as they relate to the metabolic process of interest can be achieved. The major disadvantages of PET are its complexity in both radiotracer design and image quantification schemes and expense. Metabolic processes that are typically measured with PET are myocardial oxygen consumption (MVO_2), carbohydrate metabolism, and fatty acid metabolism.

Myocardial Oxygen Consumption (MVO_2) (See Chapter 38)

Because oxygen is the final electron acceptor in all pathways of aerobic myocardial metabolism, PET with ^{15}O-oxygen has also been used to measure MVO_2. The approach provides a measure of myocardial oxygen extraction and measures MVO_2 directly. Due to its short physical half-life, ^{15}O-oxygen is readily applicable in studies requiring repetitive assessments, such as those with an acute pharmacologic intervention. Its major disadvantages are the need for a multiple-tracer study (to account for myocardial blood flow and blood volume) and fairly complex compartmental modeling to obtain the measurements.[12-14]

PET using ^{11}C-acetate is the preferred method of measuring MVO_2 noninvasively. After initial extraction, acetate, a two-carbon-chain free fatty acid, is rapidly converted to acetyl-CoA. The primary metabolic fate of acetyl-CoA is metabolism through the tricarboxylic acid (TCA) cycle. Because of the tight coupling of the TCA cycle and oxidative phosphorylation, the myocardial turnover of ^{11}C-acetate reflects overall flux in the TCA cycle and thus overall oxidative metabolism, or MVO_2. Either exponential curve fitting or compartmental modeling is used to calculate MVO_2. The latter is typically preferable in situations of low cardiac output where marked splaying of the input function and spillover of activity from the lungs to the myocardium can decrease the accuracy of the curve-fitting method.[15-19]

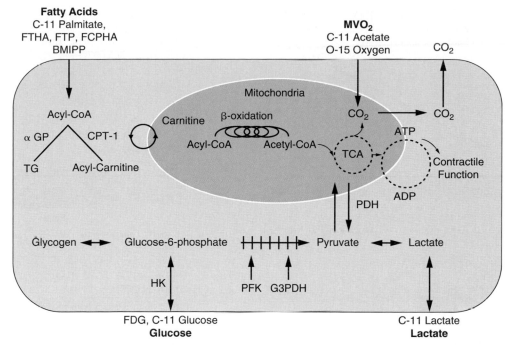

Figure 40-1 Summary of the various PET and SPECT radiopharmaceuticals to assess myocardial substrate metabolism. ADP, adenosine diphosphate; αGP, alpha-glycerol phosphate; BMIPP, [^{123}I]β-methyl-P-iodophenyl pentadecanoic acid; FCPHA, *trans*-9 (RS)-^{18}F-fluoro-3,4(RS,RS) methylene heptadecanoic acid; FTHA, fluorine-18 fluoro-6-thiaheptadecanoic acid; G3PDH, glyceraldehyde 3-phosphate dehydrogenase; HK, hexokinase; PDH, pyruvate dehydrogenase; PFK, phosphofructokinase; TCA, tricarboxylic acid cycle; TG, triglyceride. *(From Herrero P, Gropler R: Imaging of myocardial metabolism, J Nucl Cardiol 12:345–358, 2005. Reproduced with permission.)*

Carbohydrate Metabolism (See Chapter 38)

Most studies of myocardial glucose metabolism with PET have used FDG. This radiotracer competes with glucose for facilitated transport into the sarcolemma, then for hexokinase-mediated phosphorylation. The resultant FDG-6-phosphate is trapped in the cytosol, and the myocardial uptake of FDG is thought to reflect overall anaerobic and aerobic myocardial glycolytic flux.[20–23] The myocardial kinetics of FDG have been well characterized, the acquisition scheme is relatively straightforward, and its production has become routine, owing in part to the rapid growth of its clinical use in oncology. As such, it remains the most widely used tracer for determination of myocardial glucose metabolism. Regional myocardial glucose utilization can be assessed in either relative or absolute terms (i.e., in nmol/g^{-1}/min^{-1}). For quantification, a mathematical correction for the kinetic differences between FDG and glucose called the *lumped constant* must be used to calculate rates of glucose metabolism. Of note, this value may vary depending upon the prevailing plasma substrate and hormonal conditions, decreasing the accuracy of the measurement.[22,24–26] Other disadvantages of FDG include the limited metabolic fate of FDG in tissue, precluding determination of the metabolic fate (i.e., glycogen formation versus glycolysis) of the extracted tracer and glucose, and limitations on the performance of serial measurements of myocardial glucose utilization because of the relatively long physical half-life of ^{10}F.

More recently, quantification of myocardial glucose utilization has been performed with PET using glucose radiolabeled in the 1-carbon position with carbon-11 glucose (^{11}C-glucose). Because ^{11}C-glucose is chemically identical to unlabeled glucose, it has the same metabolic fate as glucose, thus obviating the need for the lumped constant correction. It has been demonstrated that measurements of myocardial glucose utilization based on compartmental modeling of tracer kinetics are more accurate with ^{11}C-glucose than with FDG, and can provide estimates of glycogen synthesis, glycolysis, and glucose oxidation (Figs. 40-2 and 40-3).[27–29] Disadvantages of this method include compartmental modeling that is more demanding with ^{11}C-glucose than it is with FDG, the need to correct the arterial input function for the production of ^{11}CO$_2$ and ^{11}C-lactate, a fairly complex synthesis of the tracer, and the short physical half-life of ^{11}C, requiring an on-site cyclotron.

Lactate metabolism in the heart is a key source of energy production, particularly during periods of increased cardiac work. However, to date, the ability to measure myocardial lactate has been limited by the lack of availability of an appropriate radiotracer and analysis scheme. Recently, a multicompartment model was developed for the assessment of myocardial lactate metabolism using PET and *L-3-^{11}C-lactate*. PET-derived extraction of lactate correlated well with lactate oxidation measured by arterial and coronary sinus sampling over a wide range of conditions (Fig. 40-4).[30] This approach may help delineate the clinical role of lactate metabolism in a variety of pathologic conditions such as diabetes mellitus and myocardial ischemia. Moreover, when combined with either FDG or ^{11}C-glucose, it

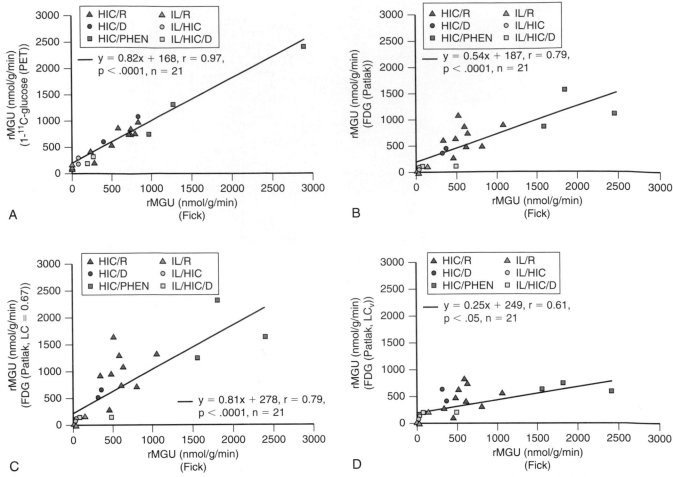

Figure 40-2 Correlation in dog hearts between Fick-derived (*x*-axis) measurements of the rate of myocardial glucose utilization (rMGU) and PET-derived (*y*-axis) rMGU using (**A**)1-^{11}C-glucose, (**B**) FDG before correcting PET values for the lumped constant (LC), (**C**) FDG after correcting PET values by the LC, and (**D**) FDG after correcting PET values by a variable LC (LC$_v$) that accounts for varying substrate, hormonal, and work environments. Correlation with Fick-derived values was significantly closer when 1-^{11}C-glucose *(panel A)*, as opposed to ^{18}F-FDG, was used, regardless of whether an LC was used or the type of LC used *(panels B-D)*. FDG, fluorine-18-deoxyglucose; PET, positron emission tomography. *(From Herrero P, Sharp TL, Dence C, Haraden BM, Gropler RJ: Comparison of 1-(11)C-glucose and (18)F-FDG for quantifying myocardial glucose use with PET, J Nucl Med 43:1530–1541, 2002. Reproduced with permission.)*

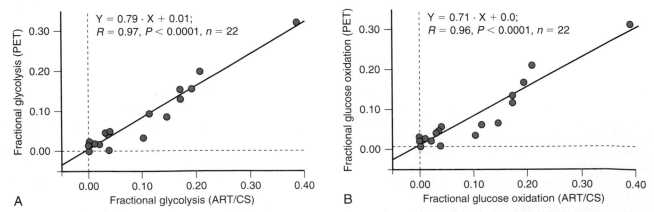

Figure 40-3 Correlation between positron emission tomography and arterial and coronary sinus (ART/CS) measurement of fractional glycolysis (**A**) and glucose oxidation (**B**). *(From Herrero P, Kisrieva-Ware Z, Dence CS, et al: PET measurements of myocardial glucose metabolism with 1-^{11}C-glucose and kinetic modeling, J Nucl Med 48:955–964, 2007. Reproduced with permission.)*

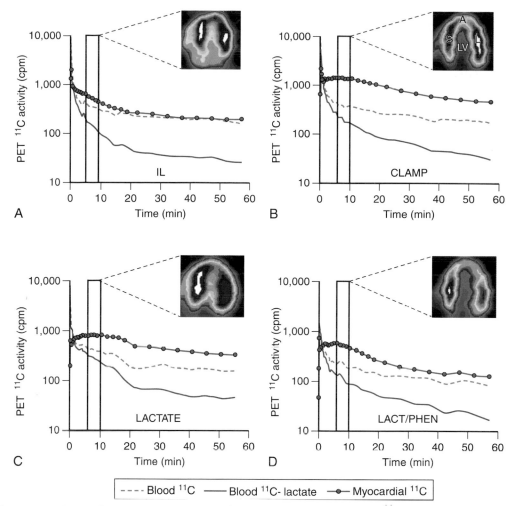

Figure 40-4 Representative positron emission tomography time-activity curves of L-3-^{11}C-lactate obtained from Intralipid (IL), insulin clamp (CLAMP), lactate infusion (LACTATE), or lactate and phenylephrine (LAC/PHEN) studies and corresponding myocardial images obtained 5 to 10 minutes after tracer injection, primarily depicting early tracer uptake. Images are displayed on horizontal long axis. Blood [11]C = [11]C time-activity curves obtained from region of interest (ROI) placed on left atrium; Blood ^{11}C-lactate = blood ^{11}C time-activity curves after removing [11]CO2, ^{11}C-neutral, and ^{11}C-basic metabolites; Myocardial [11]C = [11]C time-activity curves obtained from ROI placed on lateral wall. A, apical wall; L, lateral wall; LV, left ventricle; S, septal wall. *(From Herrero P, Dence CS, Coggan AR, et al: L-3-^{11}C-lactate as a PET tracer of myocardial lactate metabolism: A feasibility study, J Nucl Med 48:2046–2055, 2007. Reproduced with permission.)*

permits a more comprehensive measurement of myocardial carbohydrate metabolism.

Fatty Acid Metabolism

The major advantage of ^{11}C-palmitate is that its myocardial kinetics are identical to labeled palmitate. With appropriate mathematical modeling techniques, its use permits the assessment of various aspects of myocardial fatty acid metabolism such as uptake, oxidation, and storage.[31–34] This level of metabolic detail is important because exactly which component of myocardial fatty acid metabolism is the main contributor to a pathologic process is frequently unclear. However, this method does suffer from several disadvantages, including reduced image quality and specificity, a more complex analysis, and the need for an on-site cyclotron and radiopharmaceutical production capability.

Most of the PET tracers in the category of fatty acid tracers that are trapped have been designed to reflect

myocardial β-oxidation. One of the first radiotracers developed using this approach was 14-(R,S)-^{18}F-fluoro-6-thiaheptadecanoic acid (FTHA). Initial results were promising, with uptake and retention in the myocardium according with changes in substrate delivery, blood flow, and workload in animal models.[35,36] Moreover, PET with FTHA was used to evaluate the effects of various diseases such as coronary artery disease and cardiomyopathy on myocardial fatty acid metabolism.[37,38] However, uptake and retention of FTHA has been shown to be insensitive to the inhibition of β-oxidation by hypoxia, reducing enthusiasm for this radiotracer to measure myocardial fatty acid metabolism.[39] To circumvent this problem, 16-^{18}F-fluoro-4-thiapalmitate (FTP) has been developed. This modification retains the metabolic trapping function of the radiotracer, which is proportional to fatty acid oxidation under normal oxygenation and hypoxic conditions.[39,40] Similar to FDG, quantification of myocardial fatty acid metabolism with FTP

114. Herrero P, McGill JB, Lesniak D, et al: Pet dection of the impact of dobutamine on myocardial glucose metabolism in women with type 1 diabetes mellitus, *J Nucl Cardiol* 15(6):598–604, 2008.

115. Peterson LR, Herrero P, McGill J, et al: Fatty acids and insulin modulate myocardial substrate metabolism in humans with type 1 diabetes, *Diabetes* 57(1):32–40, 2008.

116. Zhou YT, Grayburn P, Karim A, et al: Lipotoxic heart disease in obese rats: implications for human obesity, *Proc Natl Acad Sci U S A* 97(4):1784–1789, 2000.

117. Hallsten K, Virtanen KA, Lonnqvist F, et al: Enhancement of insulin-stimulated myocardial glucose uptake in patients with Type 2 diabetes treated with rosiglitazone, *Diabet Med* 21(12):1280–1287, 2004.

118. Commerford SR, Pagliassotti MJ, Melby CL, Wei Y, Gayles EC, Hill JO: Fat oxidation, lipolysis, and free fatty acid cycling in obesity-prone and obesity-resistant rats, *Am J Physiol Endocrinol Metab* 279(4):E875–E885, 2000.

119. Ogawa M, Ishino S, Mukai T, et al: (18)F-FDG accumulation in atherosclerotic plaques: immunohistochemical and PET imaging study, *J Nucl Med* 45(7):1245–1250, 2004.

120. Rudd JH, Warburton EA, Fryer TD, et al: Imaging atherosclerotic plaque inflammation with [18F]-fluorodeoxyglucose positron emission tomography, *Circulation* 105(23):2708–2711, 2002.

121. Tahara N, Kai H, Ishibashi M, et al: Simvastatin attenuates plaque inflammation: evaluation by fluorodeoxyglucose positron emission tomography, *J Am Coll Cardiol* 48(9):1825–1831, 2006.

122. Tawakol A, Migrino RQ, Bashian GG, et al: In vivo 18F-fluorodeoxyglucose positron emission tomography imaging provides a noninvasive measure of carotid plaque inflammation in patients, *J Am Coll Cardiol* 48(9):1818–1824, 2006.

Cardiac Neurotransmission Imaging: Single-Photon Emission Computed Tomography

ALBERT FLOTATS AND IGNASI CARRIÓ

INTRODUCTION

The heart, like most internal organs, is innervated by the autonomic nervous system (ANS) in a highly integrated circuitry at multiple levels. The ANS provides innervation through fibers originating from autonomic ganglia located outside the central nervous system (CNS), in response to the preganglionic cholinergic stimulation coming from the CNS. The ANS has great influence on cardiovascular physiology by controlling the cardiac performance (contractility, conduction, and heart rate) to respond quickly and effectively to changing demands.

The ANS is divided into two efferent components, the sympathetic system (noradrenergic or cervicothoracic, SNS) and the parasympathetic system (cholinergic or craniosacral, PNS). The main differences between the SNS and PNS relate to: (1) the principal neurotransmitter released by postganglionic fibers (norepinephrine [NE] for the SNS; acetylcholine [ACh] for the PNS), (2) the location of the ganglia (near the spinal cord, either paravertebral [22 pairs] or prevertebral [unpaired] for the SNS; near or within the end-innervated organs for the PNS), (3) the degree of divergence and convergence of preganglionic input to postganglionic neurons (considerable for the SNS; very little for the PNS), and (4) the opposite functional roles (stimulatory for the SNS; inhibitory for the PNS).

Afferent tracts arising from myocardial nerve terminals and reflex receptors (e.g., baroreceptors) are integrated centrally within hypothalamic and medullary cardiostimulatory and cardioinhibitory brain centers, and on central modulation of sympathetic and parasympathetic outflow at the level of the spinal cord and within cervical and thoracic ganglia. There are additional levels of intricate processing within the

extraspinal cervical and thoracic ganglia and within the cardiac ganglionic plexus, where interneurons provide noncentral integration.[1]

The SNS is dominant in the heart, principally in the ventricles. Sympathetic nerve fibers travel along the vascular structures, penetrating into the myocardium from the epicardium toward the endocardium. There is a gradient distribution of nerve terminals from the base to the apex of the left ventricle (LV).[2]

NE is synthesized, stored, and metabolized within the sympathetic nerve terminal. Upon neurostimulation, NE is released by exocytosis within the synaptic cleft. A small portion of the released NE interacts with α- and β-adrenergic receptors in the myocardial cell; β_1-receptors are the predominant receptors in the heart.

Most of the released NE undergoes reuptake in the presynaptic neurons by the NE transporter (NET), a saturable and sodium-, energy-, and temperature-dependent transport protein, cocaine and desipramine sensitive, with high affinity to catecholamines and catecholamine analogs, in a process known as *uptake-1*.[3] In addition, there is NE uptake by a second, corticosterone- and clonidine-sensitive, low-affinity, high-capacity, extraneuronal transport system known as *uptake-2*.[4] Uptake-1 predominates at low concentrations of catecholamines, whereas uptake-2 predominates at higher concentrations,[5] but its contribution in humans is low.[6]

Once NE is again inside the nerve terminal, it is either metabolized by monoamine oxidase (MAO) or stored in vesicles by the vesicular monoamine transporter (VMAT), a proton-dependent transport protein localized in the vesicle membrane. Neuronal uptake-1 regulates the concentration of adrenergic neurotransmitters in the synaptic cleft, playing important physiologic and pathophysiologic roles in modifying signal transduction and extraneuronal catecholamine concentration. It is of paramount importance in protecting the heart from the deleterious effects of elevated levels of circulating catecholamines.[7,8]

The PNS fibers are found most predominantly in the atria. The nerve fibers travel along endocardial layers within the right and left ventricles. There is a high density of muscarinic receptors (predominantly M2), which interact with ACh released by the parasympathetic nerve terminals.

Neurotransmitters released from postganglionic autonomic neurons interact with their respective adrenergic/muscarinic receptors in the myocardial membrane cell. This interaction leads to stimulation (for the SNS) or inhibition (for the PNS) of adenylcyclase or phospholipase C through intermediary GTP–associated regulatory proteins (G proteins: stimulatory for the SNS, inhibitory for the PNS), which results in increase or decrease of cyclic AMP and calcium and activation or inactivation of different protein kinases, respectively. The resultant degree of protein phosphorylation modifies the activity of enzymes and the function of other proteins that control ionic channels, pumps, and exchangers, leading to the cellular response.

Cardiac presynaptic reuptake and storage of sympathetic neurotransmitters in different disorders of the heart can be imaged in vivo using radiolabeled metaiodobenzylguanidine (MIBG). In patients with ischemic heart disease, heart transplantation, dysautonomias, and drug-induced cardiotoxicity, the assessment of neuronal function can be helpful in the characterization of the disease and may improve prognostic stratification. In patients at risk of sudden cardiac death (SCD), such as those with idiopathic ventricular fibrillation (IVF), cardiac neurotransmission imaging demonstrates altered neuronal function when no other structural abnormality is seen. In patients with heart failure (HF), the assessment of sympathetic activity has important prognostic implications, which may result in better therapy and outcome.

METAIODOBENZYLGUANIDINE
(See Chapter 30)

MIBG is an iodinated aromatic analog of the hypotensive false neurotransmitter, guanethidine, which in its turn, is an analog of NE. MIBG and NE have similar molecular structures, and both utilize the same uptake, storage, and release mechanisms in the sympathetic nerve endings. However, MIBG is neither metabolized at nor interacts with postsynaptic receptors. Owing to these characteristics, the labeling of MIBG with iodine-123 (^{123}I) enables in vivo scintigraphic visualization of the sympathetic postganglionic presynaptic fibers,[9-14] thus allowing the assessment of both anatomic integrity[12,13] and function of the nerve terminals.[13] The ability of sympathetic nerves to take up radiolabeled catecholamines was shown to be a more sensitive indicator of intact neuronal function than cardiac NE content.[15]

MIBG, like catecholamines, is primarily removed from the circulation by the uptake-1 system. Blocking

experiments have shown that uptake-2 is responsible for up to 61% of cardiac MIBG uptake.[11-13] For clinical studies, the production of ^{123}I-MIBG involves isotopic exchange, which results in a low specific activity (lower ratio of radiolabeled to nonradiolabeled MIBG), with considerable amount of carrier in the final product. Since uptake-2 predominates at higher concentrations of MIBG,[5] scintigraphic images do not improve by increasing the dose of ^{123}I-MIBG, which might even lead to saturation of the uptake-1. Reduction of the total amount of MIBG in combination with a higher specific activity (no-carrier-added MIBG) improves myocardial uptake of MIBG through uptake-1, leading to better contrast between specific and nonspecific MIBG uptake as compared with carrier-added MIBG.[16]

Planar and SPECT Cardiac Imaging with ^{123}I-MIBG

Before the administration of the radiotracer, it is necessary to withdraw medications known to interfere with the accumulation of MIBG (Table 41-1), taking into account their respective blood half-lives.[17]

Usually, ^{123}I-MIBG (185 to 370 MBq) is administered intravenously 30 minutes after thyroid blockade by oral administration of 500 mg potassium perchlorate, though this could be avoided, considering that ^{123}I is a gamma emitter with a short half-life (13 hours). Planar and SPECT images of the thorax are acquired 15 minutes (early image) and 4 hours (late image) after injection, using a low-energy, high-resolution, parallel-hole collimator. A 20% window is usually used, centered over the 159-keV ^{123}I photopeak. Planar images are acquired for 10 minutes in the anterior and 45-degree left anterior oblique views and stored in 128×128 or 256×256 matrix. SPECT images are acquired by a single pass of 60 steps at 30 seconds per step (64×64 matrix), starting at 45-degree right anterior oblique projection and proceeding anticlockwise to the 45-degree left posterior oblique projection. The data are reconstructed in short-axis, horizontal long-axis, and vertical long-axis tomograms, and scatter or attenuation correction may be applied.

Table 41-1 Drugs Known or Expected to Reduce MIBG Neuronal Accumulation

Drugs	Mechanism of Interference
Tricyclic antidepressants, cocaine, labetalol	Inhibition of uptake-1
Reserpine, tetrabenazine	Inhibition of vesicular uptake
Norepinephrine, serotonin, guanethidine	Competition for vesicular uptake
Reserpine, guanethidine, labetalol, sympathicomimetic amines (e.g., phenylpropanolamines, anorectics)	Depletion of content from storage vesicles
Calcium antagonists	Calcium mediated

^{123}I-MIBG uptake is semiquantified by calculating a heart-to-mediastinum ratio (HMR)[18-20] after drawing regions of interest (ROIs) over the heart (including or not including the cavity) and the upper mediastinum (avoiding the thyroid gland) in the planar anterior view. Average counts per pixel in the myocardium are divided by average counts per pixel in the mediastinum.[21] The myocardial washout rate (WR) from initial to late images is also calculated; WR is expressed in percentage as the rate of decrease in myocardial counts over time between early and late imaging (normalized to mediastinal activity) (Fig. 41-1). The late HMR reflects the relative distribution of sympathetic nerve terminals, offering the global information about neuronal function resulting from uptake, storage, and release.[22] The WR reflects the neuronal integrity or sympathetic tone, mainly representing the uptake-1.[22] More studies are needed to establish the differences in early HMR, late HMR, and WR. Intraobserver and interobserver variabilities of these

calculations are less than 5%.[21] Normal values for late HMR and WR are ≥ 2.5 ± 0.3 and ≤ 20% ± 10, respectively,[23] but vary related to age (late HMR inversely, WR directly).[20,24] Moreover, these parameters fluctuate significantly due to lack of validation and standardization of acquisition parameters such as acquisition duration and type of collimation used (in relation to the additional photo peak of ^{123}I at 529 keV, capable of septal penetration when using the common low-energy collimators). Improved standardization of cardiac ^{123}I-MIBG imaging parameters would contribute to increased clinical applicability for this procedure.[25]

SPECT images can be scored using a point scale for visual evaluation of ^{123}I-MIBG concentration in given cardiac segments, comparable to a myocardial perfusion imaging scoring approach. Careful interpretation should be performed, with knowledge of normal variants and potential artifacts. Normal cardiac ^{123}I-MIBG distribution includes a relatively low uptake in the inferior wall,[26] which is more pronounced in the elderly (Figs. 41-2 and 41-3).[20] In addition, there may be substantial ^{123}I-MIBG uptake in the liver, which overlaps the inferior LV wall. Moreover, scattering from the lung field to the lateral LV wall may also occur. Polar maps (see Fig. 41-3)[27] can be generated from SPECT data and compared with those of normal individuals. Scores of the extension and severity of ^{123}I-MIBG eventual defects and calculation of the mean global and regional WR of the LV are feasible. However, it has to be taken into account that in some pathophysiologic conditions, cardiac ^{123}I-MIBG uptake may be severely reduced, hampering the acquisition and processing of the tomographic slices (Fig. 41-4).

^{123}I-MIBG Imaging in Coronary Artery Disease

The sympathetic nervous tissue is more sensitive to the effects of ischemia than the myocardial tissue.[28-30] It has been shown that the uptake of ^{123}I-MIBG is significantly reduced in areas of myocardial infarction (MI)[31-33] and adjacent noninfarcted regions (see Fig. 41-4),[34,35] as well as in areas with acute and chronic ischemia.[36,37] It is likely that ischemia induces damage to sympathetic neurons, which may take a long time to regenerate, and that episodes of ischemia result in decreased ^{123}I-MIBG uptake.[38] Gaudino et al.[39] provided evidence of good correspondence between ^{123}I-MIBG imaging and the presence or absence of sympathetic cardiac nerves by direct immunohistochemical staining in patients with LV aneurysms due to long-lasting anterior MI.

Reinnervation late after MI in periinfarct regions has been demonstrated by reappearance of ^{123}I-MIBG uptake, which may be in part responsible for the improvement of function. However, reinnervation may be incomplete as late as 3 months after acute MI.[40] Hartikainen et al.[41] examined ^{123}I-MIBG uptake at 3 and 12 months after a first MI and found no difference in ^{123}I-MIBG activity over time within the infarcted zone but an increase in activity in the peri-infarcted region, without a change in perfusion.

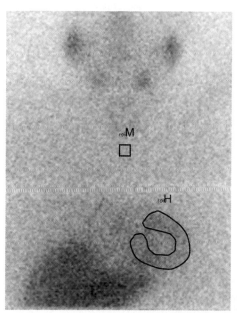

$$\bullet HMR = \frac{\{H\}}{\{M\}}$$

$\{\} = $ mean counts per pixel
$^* = $ [123]I decay correction for 3 hr and 45 min (1 ÷ 0.8213)

$$\bullet WR = \frac{\{H\}_e - (\{H\}_l \times 1.21^*)}{\{H\}_e} \times 100$$

$$\bullet WR_{BKG\ corrected} = \frac{(\{H\}_e - \{M\}_e) - ((\{H\}_l - \{M\}_l) \times 1.21^*)}{(\{H\}_e - \{M\}_e)} \times 100$$

Normal values
HMR$_l$ > 2.5 ± 0.3
WR < 20% ± 10%

Figure 41-1 Semiquantification of ^{123}I-MIBG uptake on the planar anterior view. Heart-to-mediastinum ratio (HMR) and myocardial washout rate (WR) are calculated after drawing a region of interest (ROI) over the heart (H) and the upper mediastinum (M) in the early and late images. ^{123}I-MIBG, iodine-123-labeled metaiodobenzylguanidine.

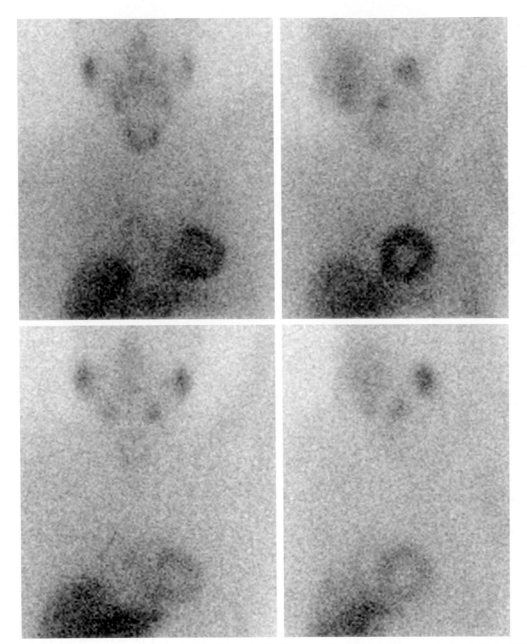

Figure 41-2 Planar images in the anterior *(left side)* and 45-degree left anterior oblique views *(right side)*, acquired at 15 minutes (early images, *top*), and at 4 hours (late images, *bottom*) after ^{123}I-MIBG injection, representing cardiac sympathetic innervation of a 78-year-old woman. Homogeneous distribution of the radiotracer over the left ventricle is observed, except for the relatively low uptake in the inferior wall, which is more often normally observed in the elderly. Heart-to-mediastinum ratios, early 1.86 and late 1.66; washout rate 24%. ^{123}I-MIBG, iodine-123-labeled metaiodobenzylguanidine.

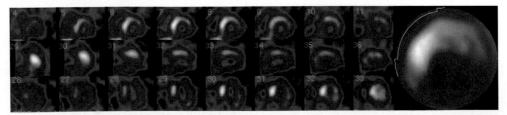

Figure 41-3 Late ^{123}I-MIBG SPECT images of the subject shown in Figure 41-2. Both the SPECT slices and the polar map show reduced tracer uptake in the inferior wall and apex, which is more apparent than on planar images and should be considered a normal variant in the elderly. *Upper row:* short-axis slices (extending from apex to base). *Middle row:* vertical long-axis slices (extending from septum to lateral wall). *Bottom row:* horizontal long-axis slices (extending from inferior wall to anterior wall). ^{123}I-MIBG, iodine-123-labeled metaiodobenzylguanidine; SPECT, single-photon emission computed tomography.

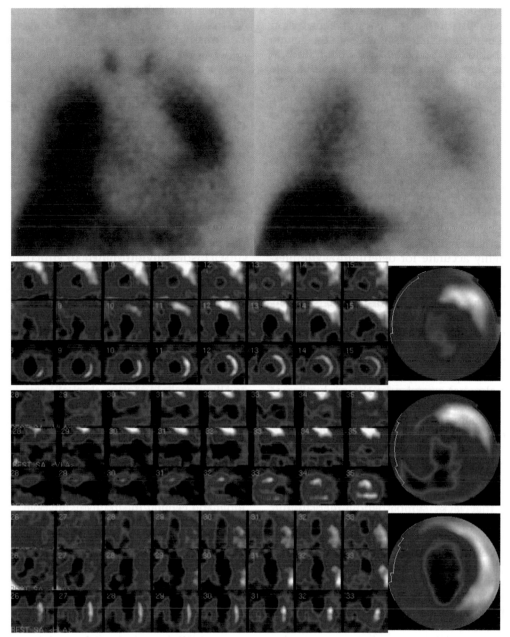

Figure 41-4 Combined ^{123}I-MIBG and ^{99m}Tc-tetrofosmin imaging of a 74-year-old male with three-vessel ischemic dilated heart disease, history of large apical myocardial infarction, and heart failure (NYHA class II, left ventricular ejection fraction 23%). *Upper part of the figure:* planar early *(left)* and late *(right)* anterior ^{123}I-MIBG scans (heart-to-mediastinum ratios, early 1.26 and late 1.18; washout rate 26%). SPECT slices correspond respectively to ^{123}I-MIBG early and late acquisitions and ^{99m}Tc-tetrofosmin study, displayed in the short-axis *(upper row)*, vertical long axis *(middle row)*, and horizontal long axis *(bottom row)*. Polar maps correspond respectively to ^{123}I-MIBG early and late studies and ^{99m}Tc-tetrofosmin study, *from top to bottom of the figure.* Note that ^{123}I-MIBG uptake is severely reduced (hampering the acquisition and processing of the tomographic images) compared with the uptake of ^{99m}Tc-tetrofosmin. ^{123}I-MIBG, iodine 123 labeled metaiodobenzylguanidine; NYHA, New York Heart Association; ^{99m}Tc, technetium-99m.

Dissociation between recovery of myocardial perfusion after an ischemic event and myocardial innervation, as determined with ^{123}I-MIBG SPECT, was reported by Matsunari et al.[42] Despite considerable myocardial salvage following coronary artery reperfusion, ^{123}I-MIBG images obtained a mean of 11 days after MI and reperfusion demonstrated a persistent area of myocardial denervation within the LV. This area was comparable to the area of ischemic myocardium at risk, as determined by myocardial perfusion SPECT during the acute ischemic event.[42] Such modifications of cardiac neuronal function may have an important role in the pathophysiology of HF and arrhythmias, but further studies are warranted to determine the clinical value of innervation imaging in ischemic heart disease.

Concordance between the extent of ^{123}I-MIBG defect at rest and perfusion defect at exercise has been shown in patients with coronary artery disease (CAD).[43] This

any structural or functional cardiac disorder that impairs the ability of the LV to fill with or eject blood. It is a common, costly, disabling, and potentially fatal disorder. The prevalence and incidence of HF are increasing rapidly in the Western world because of the aging of the population and an ever-increasing number of acute coronary syndrome survivals (CAD is the most prevalent underlying etiology, affecting about 70% of cases), despite advances in different pharmacologic and nonpharmacologic therapies.[71]

The development of HF initiates with some injury to, or stress on, the myocardium, which usually produces progressive changes in the geometry and structure of the LV with pathologic hypertrophic growth. This pathologic remodeling involves a shift toward glycolytic metabolism, disorganization of the sarcomere, alterations in calcium handling, changes in contractility, loss of myocytes, fibrotic replacement, LV dilation, systolic or diastolic dysfunction, and electrical remodeling (i.e., alterations in the expression or function of ion-transporting proteins, or both) with propensity to malignant ventricular arrhythmia.[72] Although several factors can accelerate this process, there is evidence of the important role played by the activation of endogenous neurohormonal systems. Patients with HF have elevated circulating or tissue levels of NE, angiotensin II, aldosterone, endothelin, vasopressin, and cytokines, which can adversely affect the structure and function of the heart.[71,72] These neurohormonal factors not only increase the hemodynamic stresses on the LV by causing sodium retention and peripheral vasoconstriction but may also exert direct noxious effects on cardiomyocytes (apoptosis and regression to a fetal phenotype) and changes in the nature of the extracellular matrix (stimulation of myocardial fibrosis), which can further alter the architecture and impair the performance of the failing heart.[73,74]

The hyperadrenergic state present in HF results in down-regulation and uncoupling of cardiac β-adrenergic receptors, which contributes to progressive impairment of LV systolic function by altering postsynaptic signal transduction. Increased sympathetic tone in HF is directly linked to disease progression, prognosis, and risk of SCD.[75] Therefore, noninvasive strategies to determine the state of cardiac autonomic regulation are of significant interest.

The most recent definition of cardiomyopathies makes reference to the presence of HF or electrical disorder. Specifically, they are defined as "a heterogeneous group of diseases of the myocardium associated with mechanical and/or electrical dysfunction that usually (but not invariably) exhibit inappropriate ventricular hypertrophy or dilation and are due to a variety of causes that frequently are genetic. Cardiomyopathies either are confined to the heart or are part of generalized systemic disorders, often leading to cardiovascular death or progressive HF-related disability."[76] Several studies have shown reduced cardiac ^{123}I-MIBG uptake and increased WR in different cardiomyopathies, which could reflect the contribution of the altered cardiac sympathetic nervous function to the development of the myocardial disorder (see Fig. 41-4).

In patients with dilated cardiomyopathy (DCM) and hypertrophic cardiomyopathy (HCM), Zhao et al.[77] found significant correlations of LV function and perfusion with cardiac sympathetic nervous function by means of cardiac ^{123}I-MIBG and ^{99m}Tc-tetrofosmin imaging. WR and early uptake of ^{123}I-MIBG resulted in the most significant factors for predicting LV function and LV perfusion, respectively. These investigators indicated that impairment of neuronal uptake function might not be dominant in HCM, since early ^{123}I-MIBG uptake in the nondilated phase of HCM was preserved and correlated significantly with blood flow. On the other hand, in DCM, early ^{123}I-MIBG uptake was decreased, but it was doubtful whether this phenomenon was caused by the low perfusion other than the impaired neuronal uptake function. In patients with DCM, decreased early ^{123}I-MIBG uptake was closely associated with low perfusion. These findings suggest that the kinetics of ^{123}I-MIBG might be different in these two types of cardiomyopathies. It is still unclear whether the decrease of ^{123}I-MIBG uptake is due to sympathetic denervation or to the impairment of neuronal uptake function. ^{123}I-MIBG WR could reflect cardiac functional impairment, whereas early ^{123}I-MIBG uptake might be determined by myocardial perfusion.

In patients with HCM, Shimizu et al.[78] analyzed early and late HMR and WR of ^{123}I-MIBG in planar images, as well as the dispersion and standard deviation (SD) of uptake and the WR from the polar maps of the LV obtained by the SPECT. The late HMR was significantly lower and the WR of the whole heart was significantly higher in patients with HCM than those in the control group. In patients with HCM, the late HMR, early uptake dispersion, and SD of early uptake showed good correlation with the LV end-diastolic and end-systolic dimensions and the percentage of fractional shortening. In other words, patients with larger regional variations of early ^{123}I-MIBG had larger LV volumes and a lower percentage of fractional shortening. The SD of early uptake was a powerful determinant for the percentage of fractional shortening in patients with HCM. Therefore the heterogeneity of regional cardiac sympathetic nerve activity may be correlated with cardiac dysfunction in patients with HCM. Sipola et al.[79] studied patients with HCM due to the same gene mutation and have described that the degree of LV hypertrophy is related to ^{123}I-MIBG WR, suggesting that cardiac adrenergic activity may modify phenotypic expression in HCM. Global ^{123}I-MIBG WR correlated with the LV mass and LV maximal wall thickness. The mean ^{123}I-MIBG WR was higher in LV segments equal to or greater than 15 mm thick than in LV segments less than 15 mm thick. It has been recently suggested that the primary abnormality in the pathogenesis of HCM is a decreased contractility of cardiac myocytes, producing increased cell stress and expression of stress-responsive trophic factors, including cardiac adrenergic activation, which in turn induces LV hypertrophy.[80] Accordingly, the findings of Sipola et al.[79] suggest that accelerated myocardial adrenergic activity is an important factor contributing to LV hypertrophy in HCM.

Terai et al.[81] evaluated the relationship between cardiac sympathetic nerve activity and the occurrence of VT in patients with HCM. The global WR of ^{123}I-MIBG was significantly higher in patients with VT than in those without VT, and it was the most powerful predictor of VT. In contrast, indices of regional ^{123}I-MIBG uptake were not different between the two groups. Thus, the occurrence of malignant VT in HCM may be associated with global cardiac sympathetic nerve activity rather than with the heterogeneity of such activity.

Resting cardiac ^{123}I-MIBG imaging can noninvasively evaluate LV functional reserve in patients with nonobstructive HCM, as reported by Isobe and colleagues.[82] The percentage of increase from rest to exercise in LV isovolumic contraction (LV dP/dt_{max}) and the percentage shortening of LV pressure half-time ($T_{1/2}$) as an index of isovolumic relaxation were significantly less in patients with decreased late HMR (= 1.8) than in patients with HMR greater than 1.8. The percentage increase of LV dP/dt_{max} and $T_{1/2}$ significantly correlated with both early and late HMR. Similarly, in another study in patients with DCM, a relation between decreased late HMR, impaired LV contractile reserve (determined by LV dP/dt_{max}), and down-regulation of SERCA2 mRNA was reported by Ohshima et al.,[83] establishing possibilities for a new noninvasive assessment of myocardial contractile reserve in patients with DCM.

Stress cardiomyopathy (takotsubo syndrome, or "apical ballooning") is a clinical entity characterized by acute but rapidly reversible LV systolic dysfunction, with midventricular wall-motion abnormalities, apical akinesia or dyskinesia, and preserved or hyperkinetic contractile function of the basal LV segments in the absence of atherosclerotic CAD, triggered by acute emotional or physical stress.[84] Several hypotheses have been advocated as possible pathophysiologic mechanisms, including catecholamine-mediated multivessel epicardial spasm, microvascular coronary spasm, and direct catecholamine-mediated myocyte toxicity. However, it remains unclear whether these abnormalities are the primary cause of the disorder or secondary events. Since the entity is much more common in postmenopausal women, important influences of sex hormones on the sympathetic neurohormonal axis and on coronary vasoreactivity have been suggested. ^{123}I-MIBG SPECT imaging has shown reduced uptake in the akinetic LV apex, with normal or only mildly reduced perfusion within this region.[85]

Assessment of Prognosis

Currently, long-term prognosis of patients with HF remains poor, with a 5-year mortality rate of 59% for men and 45% for women.[86] Furthermore, prognosis in HF can be determined reliably only in populations and not in individuals. To improve survival, adequate risk stratification is needed. The most significant predictors of survival in clinical management include: decreasing left ventricular ejection fraction (LVEF), worsening New York Heart Association (NYHA) functional status, degree of hyponatremia, decreasing peak exercise oxygen uptake (VO₂), decreasing hematocrit, widened QRS on 12-lead ECG, chronic hypotension, resting tachycardia,

renal insufficiency, intolerance to conventional therapy, and refractory volume overload. Routine use of ambulatory ECG monitoring, T-wave alternans analysis, HRV measurement, and signal-averaged electrocardiography do not show incremental value in assessing overall prognosis, although ambulatory ECG monitoring and T-wave alternans can be useful in decision making regarding placement of ICDs.[71,87,88]

Impaired cardiac adrenergic innervation as assessed by ^{123}I-MIBG imaging is strongly related to mortality in patients with HF,[18,89,90] independently of its cause.[22] Merlet et al.[18] studied the prognostic value of ^{123}I-MIBG scintigraphy compared with that of other noninvasive cardiac imaging indices in 90 patients suffering from either ischemic (n = 24) or idiopathic (n = 66) cardiomyopathy. During a follow-up period of 1 to 27 months, 10 patients underwent cardiac transplantation, and 22 died. Among all clinical and imaging variables (cardiac ^{123}I-MIBG uptake, radionuclide LVEF, x-ray cardiothoracic ratio, and echographic end-diastolic diameter), the late HMR was the best predictor of event-free survival. These authors[90] subsequently evaluated 112 patients with HF and DCM (NYHA classes II-IV, LVEF < 40%, LV end-diastolic diameter 70 ± 8 mm, and pulmonary capillary wedge pressure 19 ± 8 mm Hg). Among all variables (cardiac ^{123}I-MIBG uptake, circulating NE concentration, LVEF, peak VO₂, x-ray cardiothoracic ratio, M-mode echographic end-diastolic diameter, and right-sided heart catheterization parameters), only the late HMR and LVEF were independent predictors for mortality (mean follow-up 27 ± 20 months). In addition, ^{123}I-MIBG uptake and circulating NE concentration were the only independent predictors for life duration. In both studies,[18,90] a late HMR of 1.2 was used to identify reduced ^{123}I-MIBG uptake.

In a study of 93 HF patients (LVEF < 45%), Cohen-Solal et al.[91] showed that late HMR was reduced and correlated with other predictors of prognosis such as LVEF, cardiac index, pulmonary wedge pressure, and peak VO₂. Moreover, a late HMR less than or equal to 1.2 and peak VO₂ were predictive of death or cardiac transplantation over 10 ± 8 months follow-up, whereas the early HMR and WR were not. Nakata et al.[92] studied 414 patients (42% with symptomatic HF) with ^{123}I-MIBG scintigraphy. Over a mean follow-up of 22 ± 7 months, 37 cardiac deaths occurred. Late HMR was the most powerful predictor of cardiac mortality among the variables. A late HMR less than or equal to 1.74, age older than 60 years, a history of MI, and NYHA class III or IV strongly indicated poor clinical outcomes.

Wakabayashi et al.[22] reported ^{123}I-MIBG imaging as the most powerful independent long-term prognostic value for both ischemic (n = 76) and idiopathic (n = 56) cardiomyopathy patients, which hints at cardiac autonomic dysfunction as a common end point leading to cardiac death, regardless of the underlying etiology of the cardiac disease. Late HMR was the most powerful independent predictor of cardiac mortality in both groups of patients (superior to early HMR and WR) and had an identical threshold (1.82) for both groups for identifying patients at risk of cardiac death. Nevertheless, when analyzing patients with LVEF less than 40%, the upper cutoff value of late HMR was 1.50 for ischemic patients and 2.02 for idiopathic patients, which may suggest that the underlying etiology of HF relates that the threshold of the late HMR for the differentiation of high-risk patients. This study was designed, however, before optimal up-to-date HF treatment, and derived results may not translate to current cohorts of HF patients.

Kyuma et al.[93] reported that plasma brain natriuretic peptide (BNP) level significantly but roughly correlated with cardiac sympathetic nerve innervation in 158 patients with HF. Univariate analysis identified BNP level, HMR, chronic renal dysfunction, diabetes mellitus, age, and use of nitrates as significant predictors of fatal pump failure, and multivariate Cox analysis showed that BNP level was the most powerful predictor cardiac death. Patients with both plasma BNP level of equal to or greater than 172 pg/mL and late HMR less than or equal to 1.74 had a greater annual rate of fatal pump failure than had those without. The hazard ratio of BNP level (7.2) or cardiac ^{123}I-MIBG activity (10.1) increased to 34.4 when both variables were used, and prevalence of fatal pump failure significantly increased from 22% to 62.5% when diabetes mellitus and chronic renal dysfunction were present with a higher BNP level and low cardiac ^{123}I-MIBG activity.

All these results suggest that the late HRM may be the best prognostic parameter that can be obtained from planar ^{123}I-MIBG imaging.[94] The results of a recent retrospective study with the participation of six centers from five European countries confirm the strong prognostic value of late HMR in patients with HF.[95] Blind review and prospective quantitative reanalysis of the late HMR of 290 patients with ischemic and nonischemic HF (NYHA class II-IV, 262 patients with LVEF < 50%) with follow-up data for 2 years permitted the identification of potential late HMR threshold values for defining groups with high and very low likelihood of major cardiac events. The mean HMR was significantly different between patients with and without events (1.51 versus 1.97). Based on receiver operating characteristic (ROC) curve analysis, a threshold value for MHR of 1.75 yielded a sensitivity of 84% with a specificity of 60% to predict events. Based on this threshold value, the 2-year event-free survival was 62% for late HMR less than 1.75, versus 95% for late HMR of 1.75. Logistic regression showed late HMR and LVEF as the only significant predictors of major cardiac events. When the late HMRs were divided into quartiles, the 2-year event-free survival rates in the lowest quartile (1.45) and the highest quartile (2.17) were 52% and 98%, respectively.[95] Further and larger studies with standardization of data acquisition and data analysis of ^{123}I-MIBG imaging are needed to obtain the optimal threshold value of late HMR for accurate risk stratification of patients with HF.

Besides the late HMR, the prognostic value of other ^{123}I-MIBG parameters has also been reported. Ogita and coworkers[96] evaluated 79 HF patients with LVEF less than 40% with planar ^{123}I-MIBG imaging during a follow-up period between 1 and 52 months. A WR less than 27% was a strong predictor of survival. Kioka et al.[97] studied 97 outpatients with HF (mean LVEF

29%) by means of cardiac ^{123}I-MIBG. Forty-eight patients had abnormal WR (=27%), whereas the remaining 49 patients had normal WR (<27%). During a mean follow-up of 65 ± 29 months, 12 patients with abnormal WR and 2 patients with normal WR died suddenly. SCD was significantly more frequent in patients with abnormal WR than those with normal WR. ^{123}I-MIBG WR and both early and late HMR were significantly associated with SCD.

Yamada et al.[98] prospectively compared the prognostic value of cardiac ^{123}I-MIBG imaging with that of time and frequency domain parameters of HRV in patients with mild to moderate chronic HF (65 outpatients with a radionuclide LVEF < 40%). WR, late HMR, and normalized very low-frequency power (n-VLFP) showed a significant association with the cardiac events after a follow-up of 34 ± 19 months on univariate analysis. Multivariate analysis showed that WR was the only independent predictor of cardiac events, although the predictive accuracy for the combination of abnormal WR and n-VLFP significantly increased, so such a combination would identify a higher-risk subset of patients for cardiac events in chronic HF. In contrast to previous studies that showed a higher predictive value of HMR over WR, these results may be due to differences in the method used to calculate the WR, such as the application of background subtraction. Anastasiou-Nana et al.[99] studied 52 HF patients with LVEF less than 40% and demonstrated that the early HMR was the best predictor for long-term (2-year) outcome. Importantly, the early HMR was obtained at 1 hour after tracer injection, whereas most studies used a 10- to 20-minute interval to obtain the early images.

Recently, Tamaki et al.[100] prospectively compared the predictive value of cardiac ^{123}I-MIBG imaging for SCD with that of the signal-averaged electrocardiogram (SAECG), HRV, and QT dispersion in 106 consecutive outpatients with mild-to moderate stable HF due to ischemic heart disease in 55 patients and idiopathic DCM in 51 patients. During a follow-up period of 65 ± 31 months, 18 of 106 patients died suddenly. A multivariate Cox analysis revealed that only WR and LVEF were significantly and independently associated with SCD. Patients with an abnormal WR (>27%) had a significantly higher risk of SCD (adjusted hazard ratio: 4.79, 95% CI: 1.55 to 14.76). Even when confined to the patients with LVEF >35%, SCD was significantly more frequently observed in the patients with than without an abnormal WR.

A recent systematic review by Verberne et al.[101] on 18 published studies regarding survival in 1755 patients with HF stratified by semiquantitative ^{123}I-MIBG myocardial parameters, showed that patients with HF and decreased cardiac ^{123}I-MIBG uptake or increased WR have a worse prognosis compared with those with normal ^{123}I-MIBG parameters. The pooled hazard ratio estimates for cardiac death and cardiac events associated with WR showed no significant heterogeneity and were 1.72 (95% CI: 1.72–2.52; P = 0.006) and 1.08 (95% CI: 1.03–1.12; P < 0.001), respectively. The pooled hazard ratio estimates for cardiac death and cardiac events associated with early and late HMR showed significant heterogeneity ($I^2 > 75\%$). Limiting the pooling to the qualitative best three studies rendered I^2 insignificant ($I^2 = 0$) and resulted in a pooled hazard ratio of late HMR for cardiac death of 1.82 (95% CI: 0.80−4.12; P = 0.15) and for cardiac events of 1.98 (95% CI: 1.57−2.50; P < 0.001).

In the near future, potential valuable data may be obtained from two currently ongoing identical prospective open-label, multicenter international, phase 3, industry sponsored studies, evaluating the prognostic usefulness of cardiac ^{123}I-MIBG imaging for identifying subjects with HF (NYHA class II and III and LVEF less than or equal to 35%) who will experience a major adverse cardiac event.[102] In these so called ADMIRE-HF trials, subjects are being monitored on a regular basis for 2 years. Time to first occurrence of one of the following NYHA class progression, potentially life-threatening arrhythmic event (including ICD discharge), or cardiac death will be analyzed in comparison to quantitative parameters derived from ^{123}I-MIBG imaging.

Assessment of Treatment

Neurohormonal blockers (β-blockers, angiotensin-converting enzyme inhibitors [ACEIs], angiotensin receptor blockers [ARBs], and aldosterone antagonists) are basic in the management of patients with HF. However, the appropriate time to initiate treatment and the best sequence and combination of medications are uncertain at present. The severity of symptoms typically fluctuates, even in the absence of changes in medications, and changes in medications and diet can have either favorable or adverse effects on functional capacity in the absence of measurable changes in LV function.

Cardiac ^{123}I-MIBG imaging can detect drug-induced changes in cardiac adrenergic activity. Somsen et al.[103] reported that enalapril improves cardiac sympathetic uptake function but did not affect plasma NE levels in a group of patients with HF, supporting the concept that a restoration of cardiac neuronal uptake of NE is one of the beneficial effects of enalapril treatment in these patients.

Characterization of the sympathetic denervation of the heart with ^{123}I-MIBG could also be useful for selecting HF patients for β-blocker therapy. Fukuoka et al. observed that patients with DCM who showed improvement of LVEF equal to 5% after 3 months of treatment with metoprolol had previously shown decrease in regional WR of ^{123}I-MIBG (at 1-month of β-blocker therapy).[104] Watanabe and colleagues[105] studied the cardioprotective features of long-term treatment with carvedilol in a rat model of DCM after autoimmune myocarditis. They measured cardiac uptake of ^{125}I-MIBG in the LV by means of autoradiography and found that late uptake of ^{125}I-MIBG increased after treatment, while the WR decreased. These changes appeared together with a decrease in heart weight, myocardial fibrosis, and LV end diastolic pressure, supporting the beneficial effects of the drug and the protection of cardiac adrenergic neurons in DCM.

Gerson and coworkers[106] studied the effect of chronic carvedilol treatment in patients with HF and cardiac sympathetic nerve dysfunction of varying severity due to idiopathic cardiomyopathy. Most patients showed a favorable response in LV function to the treatment, regardless of the baseline level of cardiac sympathetic nervous system function, as assessed by cardiac ^{123}I-MIBG imaging. Patients with relatively advanced cardiac sympathetic dysfunction (baseline late HMR < 1.40 in ^{123}I-MIBG studies) were the most likely to show evidence of improved cardiac sympathetic nervous system function in response to carvedilol treatment. Conversely, Suwa et al.[107] in a study with patients treated with bisoprolol (β₁-specific blocker) reported that only those patients who showed a late HMR greater than 1.7 had a significant improvement in LV size and clinical status (sensitivity of 91% and specificity of 92% for predicting response to β-blocker therapy). Other studies showing improvement of cardiac ^{123}I-MIBG uptake in response to β-blocker treatment did not show any relationship between the severity of baseline cardiac ^{123}I-MIBG uptake and subsequent improvement in adrenergic function.[108,109] The discordance between these studies may reflect the different properties of various β-blockers. Similar increase in cardiac ^{123}I-MIBG uptake has been observed after treatment with ACEIs[103,110] and ARBs[111] in patients with chronic HF.

Aldosterone prevents the uptake of NE and promotes structural remodeling of the heart. Spironolactone is an aldosterone receptor blocker that improves LV remodeling in patients with DCM. Kasama and coworkers[112] assessed the influence of aldosterone treatment on cardiac sympathetic nerve activity. These investigators compared two groups of patients with DCM treated with an ACEI and a loop diuretic, but differing in the addition of spironolactone only in one group. After 6 months of treatment with spironolactone, the late HMR of ^{123}I-MIBG and LVEF significantly increased, and the late total defect score as well as the WR of ^{123}I-MIBG significantly decreased, with parallel reduction of the LV end-diastolic volume. There were no significant changes in these parameters in the control group. Moreover, significant correlation between changes in the ^{123}I-MIBG kinetics and changes in LV end-diastolic volume with spironolactone treatment was found. The functional class improved in both groups but showed a greater improvement in the spironolactone group than in the control group, indicating the beneficial effect of spironolactone on cardiac sympathetic activity and LV remodeling.

Approximately 40% of patients with severe HF die suddenly, probably of arrhythmia.[113] In patients with HF and frequent episodes of tachyarrhythmias the association of β-blockers and amiodarone is recommended.[71] It is unclear how amiodarone exerts its effects on LV remodeling and cardiac sympathetic nerve function in HF. Amiodarone, unlike most antiarrhythmic agents, has neither cardiodepressant nor proarrhythmic effects[114] and has been shown not to adversely affect survival of patients with HF. However, association of β-blockers and amiodarone may cause bradyarrhythmia. This is important, since it has been recently suggested that SCD in these patients may come from bradyarrhythmia or electrical-mechanical dissociation. Toyama et al.[115] described a prospective 1-year cohort study comparing amiodarone to β-blockers in the treatment of patients with idiopathic DCM. The authors reported similar improvement in cardiac symptoms, function, and sympathetic nerve activity with both drugs, raising the possibility of substituting β-blockers with amiodarone in the treatment of patients with DCM, avoiding the induction of bradyarrhythmias while having comparable beneficial effects. Further and larger clinical studies using the standard doses of amiodarone and with different severity of baseline cardiac ^{123}I-MIBG uptake are needed to confirm these auspicious data. Tachikawa et al.[116] reported that long-term amiodarone treatment on a rat model of DCM (healed cardiac myosin-induced autoimmune myocarditis) prevented LV remodeling, improved cardiac function, and restored cardiac sympathetic tone (late HMR of ^{123}I-MIBG increased, and WR decreased) to hold NE in the heart.

Recently, Kasama and colleagues,[117] taking into account that ^{123}I-MIBG imaging improves by the current medical treatment for HF, analyzed the usefulness of serial ^{123}I-MIBG studies for prognostication in 208 patients with stabilized mild to moderate HF and LVEF less than 45% of both ischemic and nonischemic origin. ^{123}I-MIBG and echocardiographic studies were performed once patients were stabilized and after 6 months of treatment, which included ACEIs, ARBs, β-blockers, loop diuretics, and spironolactone. Treatment did not change during the follow-up. Fifty-six patients experienced fatal cardiac events during the study period (13 died from SCD). Clinical characteristics were similar in both noncardiac death and cardiac death groups. With respect to pharmacotherapy in the two groups, only the use of β-blockers in the noncardiac death group was significantly higher than in the cardiac death group. The variation in the WR between the sequential ^{123}I-MIBG (Δ-WR) was the only independent predictor of cardiac death. The Δ-WR was significantly lower in the noncardiac death group (less than −5%) than that in the cardiac death group (more than or equal to −5%). Moreover, this parameter was also useful for predicting SCD in patients with HF, indicating that serial ^{123}I-MIBG imaging is useful for predicting cardiac death and SCD in stabilized patients with HF.

^{123}I-MIBG Imaging in Heart Transplantation

During orthotopic heart transplantation, the allograft becomes completely denervated since, except for the posterior atrial walls to which the donor atria are anastomosed, the entire recipient heart is excised. Therefore, the transplanted heart provides a model for studying intraindividually the effects of denervation and the process of re-innervation on myocardial biology; it also provides a basis for the application of neuronal imaging in other cardiovascular diseases.

Lack of autonomic nerve supply is associated with major physiologic alterations such as increased baseline heart rate, chronotropic incompetence during exercise (the sinus node is denervated), and reduced diastolic ventricular function. As a result, exercise capacity is reduced compared with that in healthy, normal subjects.[118] In addition, the decreased ability to perceive pain may not allow symptomatic recognition of accelerated allograft vasculopathy, and heart transplant patients often develop acute ischemic events or LV dysfunction or die suddenly. Furthermore, loss of vasomotor tone may adversely affect the physiologic adaptations in blood flow in different circumstances. Scintigraphic uptake of ^{123}I-MIBG supports the concept of spontaneous re-innervation taking place after transplantation.[6,119,120] All studies performed up to 5 years after heart transplantation suggest that re-innervation is likely to be a slow process and partially occurs only after 1 year posttransplantation.[121]

Sympathetic re-innervation, measured by regional distribution and intensity of cardiac ^{123}I-MIBG uptake, increases with time after transplantation, with a positive correlation between HMR and time after transplantation. Serial ^{123}I-MIBG studies over time show that re-innervation begins from the base of the heart and spreads towards the apex. ^{123}I-MIBG uptake is seen primarily in the anterior, anterolateral, and septal regions, and it is usually not apparent in the inferior wall (except for some uptake in basal segments). Complete re-innervation of the transplanted heart is not seen on scintigraphic studies, even up to 12 years posttransplantation. Therefore, sympathetic re-innervation after cardiac transplantation is not simply a function of time. It has been observed by means of PET with the catecholamine analog ^{11}C-hydroxyephedrine (^{11}C-HED) that re-innervation is more likely with young age of the donor and recipient, fast and uncomplicated surgery, and low rejection frequency.[122]

^{123}I-MIBG Imaging in Dysautonomias

Cardiac ^{123}I-MIBG uptake may be impaired in some patients with disorders of the central and peripheral nervous system with autonomic dysfunction.

Diabetes Mellitus

The sympathetic nervous system appears to be activated during the early stages of diabetes, with elevated plasma catecholamine levels. This prolonged exposure to catecholamines leads to down-regulation of adrenergic receptors and to alterations in adrenergic nervous fibers in the myocardium. Hyperglycemia and insulin deficiency may also contribute to the abnormalities in cardiac innervation in diabetes.

Development of diabetic autonomic neuropathy is associated with the advent of orthostatic hypotension, resting tachycardia, exercise intolerance, derangement in myocardial blood flow regulation, LV dysfunction, and silent myocardial ischemia/infarction. Thus, development of autonomic neuropathy is associated with an increased rate of morbidity and mortality in diabetic patients. Kim et al.[123] reported decreased ^{123}I-MIBG uptake associated with autonomic dysfunction in diabetic patients and have correlated decreased cardiac ^{123}I-MIBG uptake with increased mortality. It seems that ^{123}I-MIBG scintigraphy is more sensitive than autonomic nervous function tests for the detection of dysautonomia in diabetes, particularly in early stages of the disease. Atherosclerosis of the large coronary arteries is not a prerequisite cause for these findings, since ^{123}I-MIBG defects are present even in the absence of CAD. However, the role of microvascular disease in adrenergic dysfunction has not been well defined.

Scognamiglio et al.[124] showed that in diabetic patients the impairment of cardiac sympathetic innervation, as shown by ^{123}I-MIBG studies, correlates with abnormal response to exercise and may contribute to LV dysfunction before the appearance of irreversible damage and overt HF. Hattori et al.[125] reported that diabetic patients in whom there is scintigraphic evidence of severe myocardial denervation present with hyperreaction to dobutamine stress, which may in part explain the high incidence of SCD in patients with advanced diabetes mellitus.

Increased incidence of SCD has been related to QT-interval prolongation and QT dispersion, particularly in patients with diabetes. These abnormalities indicate variation in repolarization in different myocardial regions and may reflect inhomogeneities in LV sympathetic innervation. They are more pronounced in patients with diabetic dysautonomia than in healthy control subjects, but there are no consistent differences between diabetic patients with and without dysautonomia. Most studies have failed to show a relationship between ^{123}I-MIBG uptake and the presence or absence of QT abnormalities.[126,127]

Neurodegenerative Disorders

In clinical practice, it is often difficult to identify the cause of a parkinsonian syndrome, particularly when symptoms have begun recently and are confined to the extrapyramidal system. Even with longer duration of symptoms, about 24% of patients with parkinsonian syndrome are misdiagnosed as having Parkinson's disease (PD) and subsequently discovered to have alternative diseases, such as multiple system atrophy (MSA), striatonigral degeneration (SND), and progressive supranuclear palsy (PSP). The differentiation is particularly difficult in patients with PD who show symptoms of autonomic failure.

In PD, autonomic failure is caused by damage and Lewy body (intraneuronal cytoplasmic inclusions that stain with periodic acid–Schiff and ubiquitin) deposition in the postganglionic part of the autonomic nervous system,[128] whereas in MSA, degeneration of preganglionic and central autonomic neurons is revealed histopathologically. The assumption that selective investigation of postganglionic cardiac neurons possibly enables a safe differentiation between both entities is supported by a study of Braune et al.[129] in which patients with PD showed reduced late HMR of ^{123}I-MIBG uptake independent of duration and severity of autonomic and parkinsonian symptoms, whereas it was normal in patients MSA. Similarly, Yoshita et al.[130] described that the mean value of HMR in patients with PD was significantly lower than those with SND, PSP, or no disease, regardless of disease severity or intensity of antiparkinsonian treatment. The mean value of HMR in patients with SND and orthostatic hypotension was lower than that in patients with SND but without orthostatic hypotension.

Although the mean value of HMR in PSP with amitriptyline treatment was significantly lower than that in PSP patients without this treatment, there was no significant difference between the mean value of HMR in PSP patients without amitriptyline treatment and that in control patients. Takatsu and colleagues[131] also described reduced early and late cardiac ^{123}I-MIBG uptake in PD, even at the earlier stages of physical activity or disease duration, and also in patients with normal blood pressure response and normal circadian patterns of variation in blood pressure. Additionally, they observed that cardiac ^{123}I-MIBG uptake in PD patients with normal blood pressure patterns was lower than that in patients with MSA and also normal blood pressure response and variation, which suggests that the decrease in cardiac ^{123}I-MIBG accumulation may be specific for PD among the akinetic-rigid syndromes, independent of clinical stage, disease duration, and systemic sympathetic dysfunction. Furthermore, these investigators determined ^{125}I-MIBG accumulation in an experimental murine model of PD in which the animals were pretreated with the standard dose of 1-methyl-4-phenyl 1,2,3,6-tetrahydropyridine (MPTP) used to destroy dopaminergic neurons. The MPTP significantly reduced cardiac ^{125}I-MIBG accumulation. However, the decrease of ^{125}I-MIBG uptake was still significant with greatly reducing MPTP dose, which may reflect early damage of the postganglionic sympathetic nerves in PD, probably because dopaminergic neurons and sympathetic nerves are substantially similar in their plasma membrane transporters. Therefore, cardiac scintigraphy with ^{123}I-MIBG may be used in the diagnosis and characterization of akinetic-rigid syndromes, especially PD.

In a meta-analysis that included 246 cases of PD and 45 cases of MSA, Braune[132] reported that quantification of cardiac ^{123}I-MIBG uptake is a valuable tool to identify patients with PD and to discriminate PD from MSA early in the course of the disease, with an overall sensitivity of 89.7% and specificity of 94.6%. However, in another study that included 391 outpatients with parkinsonian-like symptoms (PD 122, MSA 14, dementia with Lewy bodies [DLB] 5, PSP 7, senile dementia of Alzheimer type [AD] 15, cerebrovascular disease 129, other disorders 81, and unknown diagnosis 18), the sensitivity and specificity of ^{123}I-MIBG scintigraphy for detecting PD were 87.7% and 37.4%, respectively.[133] Therefore, reduced uptake of ^{123}I-MIBG can be present in autonomic failure disorders other than PD, although the reductions reported are smaller than those in PD.[133,134] Recently, Raffel et al.,[135] using PET and ^{11}C-HED, showed that cardiac sympathetic denervation occurs not only in PD but also in MSA and PSP, thus implying that ^{123}I-MIBG scintigraphy may not be used independently to discriminate PD from other movement disorders such as MSA and PSP. These authors also investigated the relationship between cardiac denervation (with ^{11}C-HED) and nigrostriatal denervation by measuring striatal presynaptic monoaminergic nerve density with PET and ^{11}C-dihydrotetrabenazine (^{11}C-DTBZ), a radioligand for the VMAT, to determine whether the central and peripheral nervous system degenerative processes occur in parallel. Cardiac sympathetic denervation was not correlated with striatal denervation, suggesting that the pathophysiologic processes underlying cardiac denervation and striatal denervation occur independently in patients with parkinsonian syndromes. These findings provide novel information about central and peripheral denervation in patients with neurodegenerative disorders and should be confirmed by additional and larger clinical studies.

Dementia with Lewy bodies is the second most common cause of dementia after AD. Differential diagnosis between these two degenerative senile dementias is clinically challenging. Cardiac ^{123}I-MIBG imaging has been advocated to be useful in this setting because of the similitude between PD and DLB.[136,137] Decreased cardiac ^{123}I-MIBG uptake in DLB has been reported, whereas the uptake is normal or near normal in AD. Moreover, these findings are not related to the presence of autonomic failure or parkinsonism.[137,138] An advantage of cardiac ^{123}I-MIBG imaging over other functional studies is the short acquisition time and comfortable planar imaging, which is appreciated by patients and their caregivers.[139] Randomized controlled multicenter clinical trials should confirm these results.

^{123}I-MIBG Imaging in Drug-Induced Cardiotoxicity

Anthracycline therapy provokes cardiotoxicity, probably owing to stimulation of reactive oxygen metabolism, with free radical–mediated myocyte cell damage. Acute toxicity is generally subclinical, with transitory hypotension, tachycardia, arrhythmias, and pericarditis. Chronic cardiotoxicity is dose related and usually irreversible. It is characterized by development of progressive ventricular dysfunction that may result in fatal HF. The incidence of HF is related not only to the dose of the drug but also to the presence or absence of several risk factors, although there is considerable interindividual variation susceptibility. Predictable biological markers of its appearance and development have not yet been identified. Although serial resting LVEF measurements may remain the method of choice to monitor anthracycline cardiotoxicity, these do not seem to be sensitive enough to detect patients at risk of significant cardiotoxicity at an early stage of chemotherapy administration.

^{123}I-MIBG studies have been used to assess adrenergic innervation impairment due to anthracycline cardiotoxicity. Decreased cardiac ^{123}I-MIBG uptake has been observed after doxorubicin administration, with limited morphologic damage and preceding LVEF deterioration.[140] Valdés Olmos et al.[141] reported decreased cardiac ^{123}I-MIBG uptake in patients with severely decreased LVEF after doxorubicin administration. Correlation with parameters derived from radionuclide angiocardiography suggested a global process of cardiac adrenergic derangement.

A decrease in cardiac ^{123}I-MIBG uptake has also been reported regardless of the patient's functional status. The decrease in cardiac ^{123}I-MIBG accumulation parallels the evolution of LVEF.[142] At intermediate cumulative doses of 240 to 300 mg/m^2, 25% of patients present with some

decrease in ^{123}I-MIBG uptake. At maximal cumulative doses, there is a significant decrease in ^{123}I-MIBG uptake consistent with impaired cardiac adrenergic activity. A moderate to marked decrease in cardiac ^{123}I-MIBG uptake at high cumulative doses was observed in all but one patient with decrease in LVEF more than or equal to 10%.[142] These data suggest that the assessment of drug-induced sympathetic damage could be used to select patients at risk of severe functional impairment and who might benefit from cardioprotective agents or changes in the schedule or administration technique of antineoplastic drugs.

CONCLUSIONS

^{123}I-MIBG cardiac imaging provides significant insights into sympathetic innervation of the heart and its functional role in physiologic and pathophysiologic states, identifying the repercussions of presynaptic sympathetic denervation in CAD and establishing the relationship between heterogeneous autonomic innervation and arrhythmia. ^{123}I-MIBG scintigraphy has also provided evidence of the implication of the sympathetic nervous system in the development and progression of heart failure and the process of reinnervation on heart transplantation. Furthermore, cardiac neurotransmission imaging has established links between disorders of the central and peripheral nervous systems and the presence of autonomic dysfunction. Besides, it has been used to assess adrenergic innervation impairment due to anthracycline cardiotoxicity.

Advance of cardiac neurotransmission SPECT imaging includes the development of tracers for adrenergic receptors, which may allow differentiation of structural denervation (loss of nerve terminals) from dysinnervation (down-regulation of the uptake-1 mechanism). Future challenges include development of tracers for parasympathetic neurotransmission and other receptor systems, as well as targeting second messenger molecules.

Further studies assessing the role of pharmacologic intervention on ^{123}I-MIBG cardiac imaging are warranted. Identification of different responses to pharmacologic challenge may unmask subclinical neuronal dysfunctional states.[143] In addition, large-scale clinical trials are required to ascertain the clinical value of cardiac neurotransmission imaging in various specific indications, such as the assessment of prognosis and prediction of the effectiveness of therapy in patients with HF. Progress in the prevention and treatment of HF is now accelerating rapidly. Expensive therapies for HF (e.g., biventricular pacemakers, ICDs, and ventricular assist devices) are currently being used, and cardiac neurotransmission imaging could be one of the means to identify those patients who would benefit the most.

REFERENCES

1. Verrier RL, Antzelevitch C: Autonomic aspects of arrhythmogenesis: the enduring and the new, *Curr Opin Cardiol* 19:2–11, 2004.
2. Kawano H, Okada R, Yano K: Histological study on the distribution of autonomic nerves in the human heart, *Heart Vessels* 18:32–39, 2003.

3. Pacholczyk T, Blakely RD, Amara SG: Expression cloning of a cocaine- and antidepressant-sensitive human noradrenaline transporter, *Nature* 350:350–354, 1991.

4. Iversen LL: The uptake of catecholamines at high perfusion concentrations in the rat isolated heart: a novel catecholamine uptake process, *Br J Pharmacol* 25:18–33, 1965.

5. DeGrado TR, Zalutsky MR, Vaidyanathan G: Uptake mechanisms of meta-[123I]iodobenzylguanidine in isolated rat heart, *Nucl Med Biol* 22:1–12, 1995.

6. Dae MW, De-Marco T, Botvinick EH, et al: Scintigraphic assessment of MIBG uptake in globally denervated human and canine hearts: implications for clinical studies, *J Nucl Med* 33:1444–1450, 1992.

7. Bristow MR, Minobe W, Rasmussen R, et al: Beta-adrenergic neuroeffector abnormalities in the failing human heart are produced by local rather than systemic mechanisms, *J Clin Invest* 89:803–815, 1992.

8. Bristow MR, Anderson FL, Port JD, et al: Differences in beta-adrenergic neuroeffector mechanisms in ischemic versus idiopathic dilated cardiomyopathy, *Circulation* 84:1024–1039, 1991.

9. Wieland DM, Wu J, Brown LE, et al: Radiolabeled adrenergic neuron-blocking agents: Adrenomedullary imaging with 123I-iodobenzylguanidine, *J Nucl Med* 21:349–353, 1980.

10. Wieland DM, Brown LE, Rogers WL, et al: Myocardial imaging with a radioiodinated norepinephrine storage analog, *J Nucl Med* 22:22–31, 1981.

11. Sisson JC, Shapiro B, Meyers L, et al: Metaiodobenzylguanidine to map scintigraphically the adrenergic nervous system in man, *J Nucl Med* 28:1625–1636, 1987.

12. Dae MW, O'Connell J, Botvinick EH, et al: Scintigraphic assessment of regional cardiac innervation, *Circulation* 79:634–644, 1989.

13. Sisson JC, Wieland DM, Sherman P, et al: Metaiodobenzylguanidine as an index of adrenergic nervous system integrity and function, *J Nucl Med* 28:1620–1624, 1987.

14. Sisson JC, Bolgos G, Johnson J: Measuring acute changes in adrenergic nerve activity of the heart in the living animal, *Am Heart J* 121:1119–1123, 1991.

15. Kaye MP, Tyce GM: Norepinephrine uptake as an indicator of cardiac reinnervation in dogs, *Am J Physiol* 235:H289–H294, 1978.

16. Verberne HJ, de Bruin K, Habraken JBA, et al: No-carrier-added versus carrier-added 123I-metaiodobenzylguanidine for the assessment of cardiac sympathetic nerve activity, *Eur J Nucl Med Mol Imaging* 33: 483–490, 2006.

17. Solanki KK, Bomanji J, Moyes J, et al: A pharmacological guide to medicines which interfere with the biodistribution of radiolabelled meta-iodobenzylguanidine (MIBG), *Nucl Med Commun* 13:513–521, 1992.

18. Merlet P, Valette H, Dubois-Rande JL, et al: Prognostic value of cardiac metaiodobenzylguanidine imaging in patients with heart failure, *J Nucl Med* 33:471–477, 1992.

19. Flotats A, Carrió I: Cardiac neurotransmission SPECT imaging, *J Nucl Cardiol* 11:587–602, 2004.

20. Estorch M, Carrio I, Berna L, et al: Myocardial iodine-labeled metaiodobenzylguanidine uptake relates to age, *J Nucl Cardiol* 2:126–132, 1995.

21. Somsen GA, Verberne HJ, Fleury E, Righetti A: Normal values and within-subject variability of cardiac I-123 MIBG scintigraphy in healthy individuals: implications for clinical studies, *J Nucl Cardiol* 11:126–133, 2004.

22. Wakabayashi T, Nakata T, Hashimoto A, et al: Assessment of underlying etiology and cardiac sympathetic innervation to identify patients at high risk of cardiac death, *J Nucl Med* 42:1757–1767, 2001.

23. Patel AD, Iskandrian AE: MIBG imaging, *J Nucl Cardiol* 9:75–94, 2002.

24. Chen W, Botvinick EH, Alavi A, et al: Age-related decrease in cardiopulmonary adrenergic neuronal function in children as assessed by I-123 metaiodobenzylguanidine imaging, *J Nucl Cardiol* 15:73–79, 2008.

25. Verberne HJ, Habraken JB, van Eck-Smit BL, et al: Variations in (123)I-metaiodobenzylguanidine (MIBG) late heart mediastinal ratios in chronic heart failure: a need for standardisation and validation, *Eur J Nucl Med Mol Imaging* 35:547–553, 2008.

26. Gill JS, Hunter GJ, Gane G, Camm AJ: Heterogeneity of the human myocardial sympathetic innervation: In vivo demonstration by iodine 123-labeled metaiodobenzylguanidine scintigraphy, *Am Heart J* 126:390–398, 1993.

27. Yamazaki J, Muto H, Ishiguro K, et al: Quantitative scintigraphic analysis of 123I-MIBG by polar map in patients with dilated cardiomyopathy, *Nucl Med Commun* 3:219–229, 1997.

28. Dae MW, O'Connell JW, Botvinick E, Chin MC: Acute and chronic effects of transient myocardial ischemia on sympathetic nerve activity, density, and norepinephrine content, *Cardiovasc Res* 30:270–280, 1995.

29. Agostini D, Lecluse E, Belin A, et al: Impact of exercise rehabilitation on cardiac neuronal function in heart failure: an iodine-123 metaiodobenzylguanidine scintigraphy study, *Eur J Nucl Med* 25:235–241, 1998.

30. Estorch M, Flotats A, Serra-Grima R, et al: Influence of exercise rehabilitation on myocardial perfusion and sympathetic heart innervation in ischemic heart disease, *Eur J Nucl Med* 3:333–339, 2000.

31. Fagret D, Wolf JE, Comet M: Myocardial uptake of meta-[123I]-iodobenzylguanidine ([123I]-MIBG) in patients with myocardial infarct, *Eur J Nucl Med* 15:624–628, 1989.

32. McGhie AI, Corbett JR, Akers MS, et al: Regional cardiac adrenergic function using I-123 meta-iodobenzylguanidine tomographic imaging after acute myocardial infarction, *Am J Cardiol* 67:236–242, 1991.

33. Nishimura T, Oka H, Sago M, et al: Serial assessment of denervated but viable myocardium following acute myocardial infarction in dogs using iodine-123 MIBG and thallium-201 chloride myocardial single photon emission tomography, *Eur J Nucl Med* 19:25–29, 1992.

34. Hartikainen J, Mäntysaari M, Kuikka J, et al: Extent of cardiac autonomic denervation in relation to angina on exercise test in patients with recent acute myocardial infarction, *Am J Cardiol* 74:760–763, 1994.

35. Kramer CM, Nicol PD, Rogers WJ, et al: Reduced sympathetic innervation underlies adjacent noninfarcted region dysfunction during left ventricular remodelling, *J Am Coll Cardiol* 30:1079–1085, 1997.

36. Hartikainen J, Mustonen J, Kuikka J, et al: Cardiac sympathetic denervation in patients with coronary artery disease without previous myocardial infarction, *Am J Cardiol* 80:273–277, 1997.

37. Nakata T, Nagao K, Tsuchihashi K, et al: Regional cardiac sympathetic nerve dysfunction and the diagnostic efficacy of metaiodobenzylguanidine tomography in stable coronary artery disease, *Am J Cardiol* 78:292–297, 1996.

38. Minardo JD, Tuli MM, Mock BH, et al: Scintigraphic and electrophysiological evidence of canine myocardial sympathetic denervation and reinnervation produced by myocardial infarction or phenol application, *Circulation* 78:1008–1019, 1988.

39. Gaudino M, Giordano A, Santarelli P, et al: Immunohistochemical-scintigraphic correlation of sympathetic cardiac innervation in post-ischemic left ventricular aneurysms, *J Nucl Cardiol* 9:601–607, 2002.

40. Simula S, Lakka T, Kuikka J, et al: Cardiac adrenergic innervation within the first 3 months after acute myocardial infarction, *Clin Physiol* 20:366–373, 2000.

41. Hartikainen J, Kuikka J, Mäntysaari M, Länsimies E, Pyörälä K: Sympathetic reinnervation after acute myocardial infarction, *Am J Cardiol* 77:5–9, 1996.

42. Matsunari I, Schricke U, Bengel FM, et al: Extent of cardiac sympathetic neuronal damage is determined by the area of ischemia in patients with acute coronary syndromes, *Circulation* 22:2579–2585, 2000.

43. Estorch M, Narula J, Flotats A, et al: Concordance between rest MIBG and exercise tetrofosmin defects: possible use of rest MIBG imaging as a marker of reversible ischaemia, *Eur J Nucl Med* 28: 614–619, 2001.

44. Watanabe K, Takahashi T, Miyajima S, et al: Myocardial sympathetic denervation, fatty acid metabolism, and left ventricular wall motion in vasospastic, *J Nucl Med* 43:1476–1481, 2002.

45. Tsutsui H, Ando S, Fukai T, et al: Detection of angina-provoking coronary stenosis by resting iodine 123 metaiodobenzylguanidine scintigraphy in patients with unstable angina pectoris, *Am Heart J* 129:708–715, 1995.

46. Johnson LL, Thambar S, Donahay T, et al: Effect of endomyocardial laser channels on regional innervation shown with 125I-MIBG and autoradiography, *J Nucl Med* 43:551–555, 2002.

47. Muxi A, Magrina J, Martin F, et al: Technetium 99m-labeled tetrofosmin and iodine 123-labeled metaiodobenzylguanidine scintigraphy in the assessment of transmyocardial laser revascularization, *J Thorac Cardiovasc Surg* 125:1493–1498, 2003.

48. Huikuri HV, Castellanos A, Myerberg RJ: Sudden death due to cardiac arrhythmias, *N Engl J Med* 345:1473–1482, 2001.

49. Myerburg RJ, Mitrani R, Interian A Jr, Castellanos A: Interpretation of outcomes of antiarrhythmic clinical trials: design features and population impact, *Circulation* 97:1514–1521, 1998.

50. Schwartz PJ, La Rovere MT, Vanoli E: Autonomic nervous system and sudden cardiac death. Experimental basis and clinical observations for post-myocardial infarction risk stratification, *Circulation* 85(Suppl 1):I77–I91, 1992.

51. Chen LS, Zhou S, Fishbein MC, Chen PS: New perspectives on the role of autonomic nervous system in the genesis of arrhythmias, *J Cardiovasc Electrophysiol* 18:123–127, 2007.

52. Inoue H, Zipes DP: Results of sympathetic denervation in the canine heart: supersensitivity that may be arrhythmogenic, *Circulation* 75: 877–887, 1987.

53. Kammerling JJ, Green FJ, Watanabe AM, et al: Denervation supersensitivity of refractoriness in noninfarcted areas apical to transmural myocardial infarction, *Circulation* 76:383–393, 1987.

54. Singh SN, Fletcher RD, Fisher SG, et al: Amiodarone in patients with congestive heart failure and asymptomatic ventricular arrhythmia. Survival Trial of Antiarrhythmic Therapy in Congestive Heart Failure, *N Engl J Med* 333:77–82, 1995.

55. Kuck KH, Cappato R, Siebels J, Ruppel R: Randomized comparison of antiarrhythmic drug therapy with implantable defibrillators in patients resuscitated from cardiac arrest : the Cardiac Arrest Study Hamburg (CASH), *Circulation* 102:748–754, 2000.

56. Moss AJ, Zareba W, Hall WJ, et al: Multicenter Automatic Defibrillator Implantation Trial II Investigators. Prophylactic implantation of a defibrillator in patients with myocardial infarction and reduced ejection fraction, *N Engl J Med* 346:877–883, 2002.

57. Bigger JT: Expanding indications for implantable cardiac defibrillators, *N Engl J Med* 346:931–932, 2002.

58. Hallstrom AP, McAnulty JH, Wilkoff BL, et al: Antiarrhythmics Versus Implantable Defibrillator (AVID) Trial Investigators. Patients at lower risk of arrhythmia recurrence: a subgroup in whom implantable defibrillators may not offer benefit. Antiarrhythmics Versus Implantable Defibrillator (AVID) Trial Investigators, *Circulation* 37:1093–1099, 2001.

59. Arora R, Ferrick KJ, Nakata T, et al: ^{123}I-MIBG imaging and heart rate variability analysis to predict the need for an implantable cardioverter defibrillator, *J Nucl Cardiol* 10:121–131, 2003.

60. Schäfers M, Wichter T, Lerch H, et al: Cardiac ^{123}I-MIBG uptake in idiopathic ventricular tachycardia and fibrillation, *J Nucl Med* 40:1–5, 1999.

61. Paul M, Schafers M, Kies P, et al: Impact of sympathetic innervation on recurrent life-threatening arrhythmias in the follow-up of patients with idiopathic ventricular fibrillation, *Eur J Nucl Med Mol Imaging* 33:866–870, 2006.

62. Simões MV, Barthel P, Matsunari I, et al: Presence of sympathetically denervated but viable myocardium and its electrophysiologic correlates after early revascularised, acute myocardial infarction, *Eur Heart J* 25:551–557, 2004.

63. Bax JJ, Kraft O, Buxton AE, et al: ^{123}I-mIBG Scintigraphy to predict inducibility of ventricular arrhythmias on cardiac electrophysiology testing: a prospective multicenter pilot study, *Circ Cardiovasc Imaging* 1:131–140, 2008.

64. Muller KD, Jakob H, Neuzner J, et al: ^{123}I-metaiodobenzylguanidine scintigraphy in the detection of irregular regional sympathetic innervation in long QT syndrome, *Eur Heart J* 14:316–325, 1993.

65. Yamanari H, Nakayama K, Morita H, et al: Effects of cardiac sympathetic innervation on regional wall motion abnormality in patients with long QT syndrome, *Heart* 83:295–300, 2000.

66. Wichter T, Matheja P, Eckardt L, et al: Cardiac autonomic dysfunction in Brugada syndrome, *Circulation* 105:702–706, 2002.

67. Basso C, Thiene G, Corrado D, et al: Arrhythmogenic right ventricular cardiomyopathy. Dysplasia, dystrophy, or myocarditis, *Circulation* 94:983–991, 1996.

68. Lerch H, Bartenstein P, Wichter T, et al: Sympathetic innervation of the left ventricle is impaired in arrhythmogenic right ventricular disease, *Eur J Nucl Med* 20:207–212, 1993.

69. Wichter T, Hindricks G, Lerch H, et al: Regional myocardial sympathetic dysinnervation in arrhythmogenic right ventricular cardiomyopathy. An analysis using ^{123}I-MIBG scintigraphy, *Circulation* 89:667–683, 1994.

70. Wichter T, Schafers M, Rhodes CG, et al: Abnormalities of cardiac sympathetic innervation in arrhythmogenic right ventricular cardiomyopathy: quantitative assessment of presynaptic norepinephrine reuptake and postsynaptic beta-adrenergic receptor density with positron emission tomography, *Circulation* 101:1552–1558, 2000.

71. Hunt SA, Abraham WT, Chin MH, et al: ACC/AHA 2005 guideline update for the diagnosis and management of chronic heart failure in the adult: a report of the American College of Cardiology/American Heart Association Task Force on Practice Guidelines (Writing Committee to Update the 2001 Guidelines for the Evaluation and Management of Heart Failure). American College of Cardiology Web Site, *Circulation* 20(112):e154–e235, 2005. Available at:http://www.acc.org/clinical/guidelines/failure//index.pdf.

72. Hill JA, Olson EN: Cardiac plasticity, *N Engl J Med* 358:1370–1380, 2008.

73. Ungerer M, Bohm M, Elce J, et al: Altered expression of beta-adrenergic receptor kinase and beta-adrenergic receptors in the failing human heart, *Circulation* 87:454–463, 1993.

74. Henderson EB, Kahn JK, Corbet JR, et al: Abnormal I-123-MIBG myocardial wash-out and distribution may reflect myocardial adrenergic derangement in patients with congestive cardiomyopathy, *Circulation* 78:1192–1199, 1988.

75. Cohn JN, Levine TB, Olivari MT, et al: Plasma norepinephrine as a guide to prognosis in patients with chronic congestive heart failure, *N Engl J Med* 311:819–823, 1984.

76. Maron BJ, Towbin JA, Thiene G, et al: Contemporary definitions and classification of the cardiomyopathies: an American Heart Association Scientific Statement from the Council on Clinical Cardiology, Heart Failure and Transplantation Committee; Quality of Care and Outcomes Research and Functional Genomics and Translational Biology Interdisciplinary Working Groups; and Council on Epidemiology and Prevention, *Circulation* 113:1807–1816, 2006.

77. Zhao C, Shuke N, Yamamoto W, et al: Comparison of cardiac sympathetic nervous function with left ventricular function and perfusion in cardiomyopathies by ^{123}I-MIBG SPECT and 99mTc-tetrofosmin electrocardiographically gated SPECT, *J Nucl Med* 42:1017–1024, 2001.

78. Shimizu M, Ino H, Yamaguchi M, et al: Heterogeneity of cardiac sympathetic nerve activity and systolic dysfunction in patients with hypertrophic cardiomyopathy, *J Nucl Med* 43:15–20, 2002.

79. Sipola P, Vanninen E, Aronen HJ, et al: Cardiac adrenergic activity is associated with left ventricular hypertrophy in genetically homogeneous subjects with hypertrophic cardiomyopathy, *J Nucl Med* 44:487–493, 2003.

80. Marian AJ: Pathogenesis of diverse clinical and pathological phenotypes in hypertrophic cardiomyopathy, *Lancet* 355:58–60, 2000.

81. Terai H, Shimizu M, Ino H, et al: Cardiac sympathetic nerve activity in patients with hypertrophic cardiomyopathy with malignant ventricular tachyarrhythmias, *J Nucl Cardiol* 10:304–310, 2003.

82. Isobe S, Izawa H, Iwase M, et al: Cardiac ^{123}I-MIBG reflects left ventricular functional reserve in patients with nonobstructive hypertrophic cardiomyopathy, *J Nucl Med* 46:909–916, 2005.

83. Ohshima S, Isobe S, Izawa H, et al: Cardiac sympathetic dysfunction correlates with abnormal myocardial contractile reserve in dilated cardiomyopathy patients, *J Am Coll Cardiol* 46:2061–2068, 2005.

84. Gianni M, Dentali F, Grandi AM, et al: Apical ballooning syndrome or takotsubo cardiomyopathy: a systematic review, *Eur Heart J* 27:1523–1529, 2006.

85. Burgdorf C, von Hof K, Schunkert H, Kurowski V: Regional alterations in myocardial sympathetic innervation in patients with transient left-ventricular apical ballooning (Tako-Tsubo cardiomyopathy), *J Nucl Cardiol* 15:65–72, 2008.

86. Levy D, Kenchaiah S, Larson MG, et al: Long-term trends in the incidence of and survival with heart failure, *N Engl J Med* 347:1397–1402, 2002.

87. Zipes DP, Camm AJ, Borggrefe M, et al: ACC/AHA/ESC 2006 guidelines for management of patients with ventricular arrhythmias and the prevention of sudden cardiac death-executive summary: a report of the American College of Cardiology/American Heart Association Task Force and the European Society of Cardiology Committee for Practice Guidelines (Writing Committee to Develop Guidelines for Management of Patients with Ventricular Arrhythmias and the Prevention of Sudden Cardiac Death), *Eur Heart J* 27:2099–2140, 2006.

88. Chow T, Kereiakes DJ, Bartone C, et al: Microvolt T-wave alternans identified patients with ischemic cardiomyopathy who benefit from implantable cardioverter-defibrillator therapy, *J Am Coll Cardiol* 49:50–58, 2007.

89. Nakata T, Miyamoto K, Doi A, et al: Cardiac death prediction and impaired cardiac sympathetic innervation assessed by metaiodobenzylguanidine in patients with failing and non-failing hearts, *J Nucl Cardiol* 5:579–590, 1998.

90. Merlet P, Benvenuti C, Moyse D, et al: Prognostic value of MIBG imaging in idiopathic dilated cardiomyopathy, *J Nucl Med* 40:917–923, 1999.

91. Cohen-Solal A, Esanu Y, Logeart D, et al: Cardiac metaiodobenzylguanidine uptake in patients with moderate chronic heart failure: relationship with peak oxygen uptake and prognosis, *J Am Coll Cardiol* 33:759–766, 1999.

92. Nakata T, Miyamoto K, Doi A, et al: Cardiac death prediction and impaired cardiac sympathetic innervation assessed by MIBG in patients with failing and nonfailing hearts, *J Nucl Cardiol* 5:579–590, 1998.

93. Kyuma M, Nakata T, Hashimoto A, et al: Incremental prognostic implications of brain natriuretic peptide, cardiac sympathetic nerve innervation, and noncardiac disorders in patients with heart failure, *J Nucl Med* 45:155–163, 2004.

94. Bax JJ, Boogers M, Henneman MM: Can cardiac iodine-123 metaiodobenzylguanidine imaging contribute to risk stratification in heart failure patients? *Eur J Nucl Med Mol Imaging* 35:352–354, 2008.

95. Agostini D, Verberne HJ, Burchert W, et al: I-123-mIBG myocardial imaging for assessment of risk for a major cardiac event in heart failure patients: insights from a retrospective European multicenter study, *Eur J Nucl Med Mol Imaging* 35:535–546, 2008.

96. Ogita H, Shimonagata T, Fukunami M, et al: Prognostic significance of cardiac (123)I metaiodobenzylguanidine imaging for mortality and morbidity in patients with chronic heart failure: a prospective study, *Heart* 86:656–660, 2001.

97. Kioka H, Yamada T, Mine T, et al: Prediction of sudden death in patients with mild to moderate chronic heart failure by using cardiac iodine-123 metaiodobenzylguanidine imaging, *Heart* 93:1213–1218, 2007.

98. Yamada T, Shimonagata T, Fukunami M, et al: Comparison of the prognostic value of cardiac iodine-123 metaiodobenzylguanidine imaging and heart rate variability in patients with chronic heart failure. A prospective study, *J Am Coll Cardiol* 41:231–238, 2003.

99. Anastasiou-Nana MI, Terrovitis JV, et al: Prognostic value of iodine-123-metaiodobenzylguanidine myocardial uptake and heart rate variability in chronic congestive heart failure secondary to ischemic

or idiopathic dilated cardiomyopathy, *Am J Cardiol* 96:427–431, 2005.

100. Tamaki S, Yamada T, Okuyama Y, et al: Cardiac iodine-123 metaiodobenzylguanidine imaging predicts sudden cardiac death independently of left ventricular ejection fraction in patients with chronic heart failure and left ventricular systolic dysfunction, *J Am Coll Cardiol* 53:426–435, 2009.

101. Verberne HJ, Brewster LM, Somsen GA, et al: Prognostic value of myocardial ^{123}I-metaiodobenzylguanidine (MIBG) parameters in patients with heart failure: a systematic review, *Eur Heart J* 29:1147–1159, 2008.

102. Jacobson AF, Lombard J, Banerjee G, Camici PG: ^{123}I-mIBG scintigraphy to predict risk for adverse cardiac outcomes in heart failure patients: Design of two prospective multicenter international trials, *J Nucl Cardiol* 16:113–121, 2009.

103. Somsen GA, van Vlies B, de Milliano PA, et al: Increased myocardial [123-I]-metaiodobenzylguanidine uptake after enalapril treatment in patients with chronic heart failure, *Heart* 76:218–222, 1996.

104. Fukuoka S, Hayashida K, Hirose Y: Use of iodine-123 metaiodobenzylguanidine myocardial imaging to predict the effectiveness of beta-blocker therapy in patients with dilated cardiomyopathy, *Eur J Nucl Med* 24:523–529, 1997.

105. Watanabe K, Takahashi T, Nakazawa M, et al: Effects of carvedilol on cardiac function and cardiac adrenergic neuronal damage in rats with dilated cardiomyopathy, *J Nucl Med* 43:531–535, 2002.

106. Gerson MC, Craft LL, McGuire N, et al: Carvedilol improves left ventricular function in heart failure patients with idiopathic dilated cardiomyopathy and a wide range of sympathetic nervous system function as measured by iodine123 metaiodobenzylguanidine, *J Nucl Cardiol* 9:608–615, 2002.

107. Suwa M, Otake Y, Moriguchi A, et al: Iodine-123 metaiodobenzylguanidine myocardial scintigraphy for prediction of response to beta-blocker therapy in patients with dilated cardiomyopathy, *Am Heart J* 133:353–358, 1997. Erratum in: Am Heart J 134: 1141, 1997.

108. Agostini D, Belin A, Amar MH, et al: Improvement of cardiac neuronal function after carvedilol treatment in dilated cardiomyopathy: a ^{123}I-MIBG scintigraphic study, *J Nucl Med* 41:845–851, 2000.

109. Lotze U, Kaepplinger S, Kober A, et al: Recovery of the cardiac adrenergic nervous system after long-term beta blocker therapy in idiopathic dilated cardiomyopathy: assessment by increase in myocardial ^{123}I-metaiodobenzylguanidine uptake, *J Nucl Med* 42:49–54, 2001.

110. Gilbert EM, Sandoval A, Larrabee P, et al: Lisinopril lowers cardiac adrenergic drive and increases beta-receptor density in the failing human heart, *Circulation* 88:472–480, 1993.

111. Kasama S, Toyama T, Kumakura H, et al: Effects of candesartan on cardiac sympathetic nerve activity in patients with congestive heart failure and preserved left ventricular ejection fraction, *J Am Coll Cardiol* 45:661–667, 2005.

112. Kasama S, Toyama T, Kumakura H, et al: Effect of spironolactone on cardiac sympathetic nerve activity and left ventricular remodeling in patients with dilated cardiomyopathy, *J Am Coll Cardiol* 41:574–581, 2003.

113. Francis G: Development of arrhythmias in the patient with congestive heart failure: pathophysiology, prevalence and prognosis, *Am J Cardiol* 57:3B–7B, 1986.

114. Packer M: Hemodynamic consequences of antiarrhythmic drug therapy in patients with chronic heart failure, *J Cardiovasc Electrophysiol* 2:S240–S247, 1991.

115. Toyama S, Hoshizaki H, Seki R, et al: Efficacy of amiodarone treatment on cardiac symptom, function and sympathetic nerve activity in patients with dilated cardiomyopathy: comparison with beta-blocker therapy, *J Nucl Cardiol* 11:134–141, 2004.

116. Tachikawa H, Kodama M, Watanabe K, et al: Amiodarone improves cardiac sympathetic nerve function to hold norepinephrine in the heart, prevents left ventricular remodeling, and improves cardiac function in rat dilated cardiomyopathy, *Circulation* 111:894–899, 2005.

117. Kasama S, Toyama T, Sumino H, et al: Prognostic value of serial cardiac ^{123}I-MIBG imaging in patients with stabilized chronic heart failure and reduced left ventricular ejection fraction, *J Nucl Med* 49:907–914, 2008.

118. Mancini D: Surgically denervated cardiac transplant. Rewired or permanently unplugged, *Circulation* 96:6–8, 1997.

119. De Marco T, Dae M, Yuen-Green MS, et al: Iodine-123 MIBG scintigraphic assessment of the transplanted human heart: evidence for late reinnervation, *J Am Coll Cardiol* 25:927–931, 1995.

120. Schwaiger M, Hutchins GB, Kalff V: Evidence for regional catecholamine uptake and storage sites in the transplanted human heart by positron emission tomography, *J Clin Invest* 87:1681–1690, 1991.

121. Estorch M, Camprecios M, Flotats A, et al: Sympathetic reinnervation of cardiac allografts evaluated by ^{123}I-MIBG imaging, *J Nucl Med* 40:911–916, 1999.

122. Bengel FM, Ueberfuhr P, Hesse T, et al: Clinical determinants of ventricular sympathetic reinnervation after orthotopic heart transplantation, *Circulation* 106:831–835, 2002.

123. Kim SJ, Lee JD, Ryu YH, et al: Evaluation of cardiac sympathetic neuronal integrity in diabetic patients using iodine-123 MIBG, *Eur J Nucl Med* 23:401–406, 1996.

124. Scognamiglio R, Avogaro A, Casara D, et al: Myocardial dysfunction and adrenergic cardiac innervation in patients with insulin-dependent diabetes, *J Am Coll Cardiol* 31:404–412, 1998.

125. Hattori N, Tamaki N, Hayashi T, et al: Regional abnormality of iodine-123-MIBG in diabetic hearts, *J Nucl Med* 37:1985–1990, 1996.

126. Bellavere F, Ferri M, Guarini L, et al: Prolonged QT period in diabetic autonomic neuropathy: a possible role in sudden cardiac death? *Br Heart J* 59:379–383, 1989.

127. Wei K, Dorian P, Newman D, Langer A: Association between QT dispersion and autonomic dysfunction in patients with diabetes mellitus, *J Am Coll Cardiol* 26:859–863, 1995.

128. Wakabayashi K, Takahashi H: Neuropathology of autonomic nervous system in Parkinson's disease, *Eur Neurol* 38(Suppl 2):2–7, 1997.

129. Braune S, Reinhardt M, Schnitzer R, Riedel A, Lücking CH: Cardiac uptake of ^{123}I]MIBG separates Parkinson's disease from multiple system atrophy, *Neurology* 53:1020–1025, 1999.

130. Yoshita M: Differentiation of idiopathic Parkinson's disease from striatonigral degeneration and progressive supranuclear palsy using iodine-123 meta-iodobenzylguanidine myocardial scintigraphy, *J Neurol Sci* 155:60–67, 1998.

131. Takatsu H, Nishida H, Matsuo H, et al: Cardiac sympathetic denervation from the early stage of Parkinson's disease: Clinical and experimental studies with radiolabeled MIBG, *J Nucl Med* 41:71–77, 2000.

132. Braune S: The role of cardiac metaiodobenzylguanidine uptake in the differential diagnosis of parkinsonian syndromes, *Clin Auton Res* 11:351–355, 2001.

133. Nagayama H, Hamamoto M, Ueda M, et al: Reliability of MIBG myocardial scintigraphy in the diagnosis of Parkinson's disease, *J Neurol Neurosurg Psychiatry* 76:249–251, 2005.

134. Hirayama M, Hakusui S, Koike Y, et al: A scintigraphical qualitative analysis of peripheral vascular sympathetic function with meta-^{123}I]iodobenzylguanidine in neurological patients with autonomic failure, *J Auton Nerv Syst* 53:230–234, 1995.

135. Raffel DM, Koeppe RA, Little R, et al: PET measurement of cardiac and nigrostriatal denervation in parkinsonian syndromes, *J Nucl Med* 47:1769–1777, 2006.

136. Watanabe H, Ieda T, Katayama T, et al: Cardiac ^{123}I-meta-iodobenzylguanidine (MIBG) uptake in dementia with Lewy bodies: comparison with Alzheimer's disease, *J Neurol Neurosurg Psychiatry* 70:781–783, 2001.

137. Yoshita M, Taki J, Yokoyama K, et al: Value of ^{123}I-MIBG radioactivity in the differential diagnosis of DLB from AD, *Neurology* 66:1850–1854, 2006.

138. Kashihara K, Ohno M, Kawada S, Okumura Y: Reduced cardiac uptake and enhanced washout of ^{123}I-MIBG in pure autonomic failure occurs conjointly with Parkinson's disease and dementia with Lewy bodies, *J Nucl Med* 47:1099–1101, 2006.

139. Estorch M, Camacho V, Paredes P, et al: Cardiac (123)I-metaiodobenzylguanidine imaging allows early identification of dementia with Lewy bodies during life, *Eur J Nucl Med Mol Imaging* 2008. [Epub ahead of print].

140. Wakasugi S, Fischman AJ, Babich JW, et al: Metaiodobenzylguanidine: evaluation of its potential as a tracer for monitoring doxorubicin cardiomyopathy, *J Nucl Med* 34:1283–1286, 1993.

141. Valdés Olmos RA, ten Bokkel Huinink WW, ten Hoeve RF, et al: Assessment of anthracycline related myocardial adrenergic derangement by ^{123}I-MIBG scintigraphy, *Eur J Cancer* 31A.26–31, 1995.

142. Carrio I, Estorch M, Berna L, et al: 111In-antimyosin and ^{123}I-MIBG studies in the early assessment of doxorubicin cardiotoxicity, *J Nucl Med* 36:2044–2049, 1995.

143. Estorch M, Carrió I, Mena E, et al: MIBG imaging and pharmacologic intervention. effect of a single dose of oral amitriptyline on regional cardiac MIBG uptake, *Eur J Nucl Med Mol Imaging* 31:1575–1580, 2004.

Cardiac Neurotransmission Imaging: Positron Emission Tomography

FRANK M. BENGEL, HOSSAM M. SHERIF, ANTTI SARASTE
AND MARKUS SCHWAIGER

INTRODUCTION

The autonomic nervous system plays a central role in regulation of cardiac performance under various physiologic and pathophysiologic conditions. In recent years, the importance of alterations of autonomic innervation in the pathophysiology of heart diseases such as congestive heart failure (CHF), ischemia, and arrhythmia has been increasingly emphasized. Nuclear imaging techniques provide noninvasive information about global and regional myocardial autonomic innervation. They have substantially facilitated and refined the study of the heart's nervous system in health and disease and significantly contributed to a continuous improvement of the understanding of cardiac pathophysiology. Conventional nuclear imaging using the catecholamine analog, iodine-123-labeled metaiodobenzylguanidine (^{123}I-MIBG), is available for mapping of myocardial presynaptic sympathetic innervation on a broad clinical basis. Positron emission tomography (PET) is methodologically more demanding and less widely available but provides advantages for studying the autonomic nervous system of the heart. Owing to high spatial and temporal resolution and routine attenuation correction, tracer kinetics can be defined in detail, and absolute quantification is feasible. Radiolabeled catecholamines and catecholamine analogs are available for PET imaging; they are more physiologic than MIBG and well understood with regard to their tracer physiologic properties. Neurotransmitter PET imaging has been successfully applied to gain unique new insights into mechanisms of myocardial biology and pathology. This chapter summarizes currently available information on the use of cardiac PET imaging of autonomic innervation. First, a brief overview on biology of the sympathetic and parasympathetic nervous system, in the heart is given. Then, available radiolabeled neurotransmitters for PET imaging are discussed with regard to their properties and usefulness. Finally, PET-based observations in experimental and human studies of diseases that involve cardiac sympathetic innervation are described.

THE CARDIAC AUTONOMIC NERVOUS SYSTEM

The autonomic nervous system, referred to as the *visceral nervous system*, consists of two divisions: sympathetic and parasympathetic innervation. The two systems differ in their major neurotransmitters—norepinephrine and acetylcholine—which define the stimulatory and inhibitory effects of each system.[1] Sympathetic and parasympathetic innervation of the heart facilitates its electrophysiologic and hemodynamic adaptation to changing cardiovascular demands. Both sympathetic and parasympathetic tone control the rate of electrophysiologic stimulation and conduction, while contractile performance is primarily modulated by sympathetic neurotransmission. This functional characterization is reflected by the anatomic distribution of nerve fibers and terminals. Sympathetic fibers include multiple nerve endings that are filled with vesicles containing norepinephrine. They travel along epicardial vascular structures and penetrate into underlying myocardium much like coronary vessels. Based on tissue norepinephrine content, the mammalian heart is characterized by dense sympathetic innervation with a gradient from atria to base of the heart and from base to apex of the ventricles.[2]

In contrast to sympathetic nerve fibers, parasympathetic innervation is most prevalent in the atria, the atrioventricular (AV) node, and to a lesser degree within ventricular myocardium. Parasympathetic fibers in the ventricles appear to travel close to the endocardial surface, in contrast to sympathetic innervation. The enzyme choline acetyltransferase has been used as a reliable marker of cholinergic innervation.[3] Choline acetyltransferase concentration is highest in the atria and decreases sharply in the right and left ventricular myocardium.

Figure 42-1 depicts neurotransmitter synthesis and turnover in the sympathetic and parasympathetic nerve terminal. Integrity and growth of both sympathetic and parasympathetic neurons are dependent on neurotrophins such as neuronal growth factor, which are secreted by myocardial target tissue and bind on nerve fibers via tyrosine kinase receptors, thereby inducing expression of growth-associated genes.[4]

Sympathetic Nerve Terminal

Norepinephrine, the dominant sympathetic transmitter, is synthesized from the amino acid tyrosine by several enzymatic steps. Generation of dopa from tyrosine is the rate-limiting step in catecholamine biosynthesis. Following dopa conversion to dopamine by dopa decarboxylase, dopamine is transported into storage vesicles by the energy-requiring vesicular monoamine transporter. Norepinephrine is synthesized by dopamine β-hydroxylase within storage vesicles. Nerve stimulation leads to norepinephrine release, which occurs as the

vesicles fuse with the neuronal membrane and expel their content by exocytosis. Single nerve stimulation leads to exocytosis of only a small fraction of storage vesicles. The average adrenergic neuron has approximately 25,000 vesicles, with each containing approximately 250 pg of norepinephrine.[5] Although most norepinephrine is thought to be released by exocytosis, nonvesicular release also occurs. Apart from neuronal stimulation, release is also regulated by a number of receptor systems. The α_2-adrenergic receptors on the membrane surface provide negative feedback for exocytosis, which can thus be inhibited by presynaptic α_2-agonists such as clonidine, guanabenz, and guanfacine.[6] Muscarinic and adenosine receptors also have antiadrenergic effects. Neuropeptide Y is stored and released together with norepinephrine from the nerve terminal and is thought to inhibit neurotransmitter release.[7] Presynaptic angiotensin II receptors and β-adrenergic receptors, on the other hand, mediate facilitation of norepinephrine release from sympathetic nerve endings so that antihypertensive agents such as angiotensin-converting enzyme (ACE) inhibitors or β-blockers can inhibit excessive norepinephrine release. The complex modulation of sympathetic neurotransmission[6] obviously involves many systems, including dopamine, prostaglandin, and histamine. Only a small amount of norepinephrine release by the nerve terminal is actually available to activate receptors on the myocyte surface.

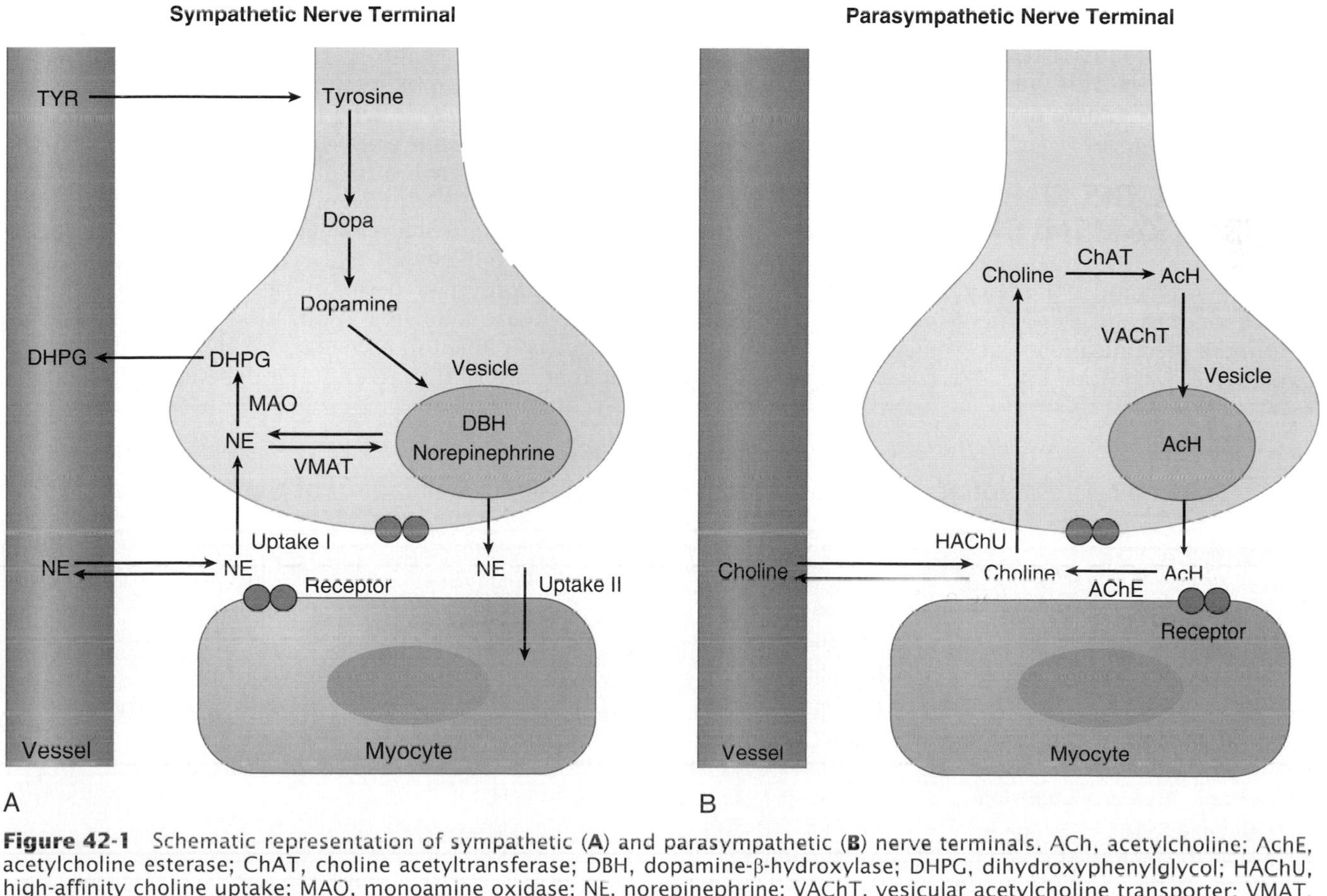

Figure 42-1 Schematic representation of sympathetic (**A**) and parasympathetic (**B**) nerve terminals. ACh, acetylcholine; AchE, acetylcholine esterase; ChAT, choline acetyltransferase; DBH, dopamine-β-hydroxylase; DHPG, dihydroxyphenylglycol; HAChU, high-affinity choline uptake; MAO, monoamine oxidase; NE, norepinephrine; VAChT, vesicular acetylcholine transporter; VMAT, vesicular monoamine transporter.

Most norepinephrine undergoes reuptake into nerve terminals by the presynaptic norepinephrine transporter (uptake-1 mechanism) and recycles into vesicles or is metabolized in cytosol. The uptake-1 mechanism is characterized as saturable and sodium, energy, and temperature dependent.[8] It can be inhibited by cocaine and desipramine.[9] Structurally related amines such as epinephrine, guanethidine, and metaraminol are also transported by this system. In addition to neuronal uptake-1, the uptake-2 system removes norepinephrine into nonneuronal tissue.[10] The uptake-2 mechanism is characterized as nonsaturable and not sodium, energy, or temperature dependent. It can be inhibited by, for example, steroids and clonidine.[11] Free cytosolic norepinephrine is degraded rapidly to dihydroxyphenylglycol (DHPG) by monoamine oxidase (MAO). Only a small fraction of the released norepinephrine diffuses into vascular space, where it can be measured as norepinephrine spillover in coronary sinus vein blood.

Parasympathetic Nerve Terminal

Acetylcholine is synthesized within the parasympathetic nerve terminal. Choline is transported into the cytosol of nerve endings via a high-affinity choline uptake system,[12] is then rapidly acetylated by choline acetyltransferase, and subsequently shuttled into storage vesicles. In contrast to amine uptake in sympathetic terminals, the choline uptake system is restrictive. Even close structural analogs are poor substrates for the high-affinity choline uptake system. Upon nerve stimulation, acetylcholine is released into the synaptic cleft, where it interacts with muscarinic receptors. Free acetylcholine is rapidly metabolized by acetylcholine esterase.

PET TRACERS FOR CARDIAC NEUROTRAMSMITTER IMAGING

Radiolabeled ligands for α- and β-adrenergic receptors, as well as for muscarinic cholinergic receptors, are available and under preclinical/clinical evaluation. Although little experience with imaging of cardiac parasympathetic

neurons is documented, several radiotracers for the sympathetic neuron have been developed. Radiopharmaceutical strategies involve either labeling of true adrenergic neurotransmitters or synthesis of catecholamine analogs ("false neurotransmitters"). Radiolabeled true neurotransmitters follow the entire metabolic catecholamine pathway, but radiolabeled analogs often are resistant to specific steps of catecholamine degradation.

Available tracers of sympathetic innervation differ in their specificity for uptake-1 and vesicular storage. Additionally, their usefulness is defined by the low complexity of radiochemical synthesis and by the resulting specific radioactivity and chemical purity. Low specific activity and/or chemical impurity result in concomitant exposure to nonlabeled catecholamines during tracer injection, which may compete with the radiotracer for specific uptake and storage and increase the likelihood of pharmacologic adrenergic effects. Table 42-1 summarizes currently available PET tracers for imaging of presynaptic adrenergic innervation. Specific tracers, which differ in their kinetic behavior (Fig. 42-2),[13] are described subsequently in an order following the amount of published clinical experience.

Carbon-11-Hydroxyephedrine

Carbon-11 (^{13}C)-labeled metahydroxyephedrine (mHED, or simply HED) is the most frequently used PET tracer for mapping of sympathetic neurons. It is synthesized by N-methylation of metaraminol, which reliably yields HED at high specific activity.[14] HED is resistant to metabolism by MAO or catechol-O-methyltransferase (COMT) and has a high affinity to uptake-1. Nonspecific myocardial uptake is low, as demonstrated in isolated perfused rat hearts following desipramine blockade[15] and in denervated human hearts early after cardiac transplantation.[16] Although vesicular storage seems to occur, binding inside vesicles is reduced, owing to the higher lipophilicity of HED compared to norepinephrine.[17] Addition of desipramine or norepinephrine to the perfusate following application of HED in isolated rat hearts resulted in accelerated HED washout, suggesting that cardiac HED retention is dependent on reuptake

Table 42-1 Radiotracers for Positron Emission Tomography Imaging of the Sympathetic Neuron

Compound	Type	Intraneuronal Metabolism	Uptake-1 Selectivity*
[11]C-metahydroxyephedrine	Analog	No	92%
[18]F-6-fluorodopamine	Catecholamine	Yes	79%
[11]C-epinephrine	Catecholamine	Yes	92%
[11]C-phenylephrine	Analog	Yes	77%
[18]F-6-fluorometaraminol	Analog	No	82%
[18]F-(−)-6-fluoronorepinephrine	Catecholamine	Yes	—
[18]F-para-fluorobenzylguanidine	Analog	No	—
[18]F-fluoroiodobenzylguanidine	Analog	No	43%
[76]Br-metabromobenzylguanidine	Analog	No	64%

*Uptake-1 selectivity in percent reduction of uptake by desipramine blockade in perfused rat hearts.
From Langer O, Halldin C: PET and SPECT tracers for mapping the cardiac nervous system. Eur J Nucl Med Mol Imaging 29:416–434, 2002.

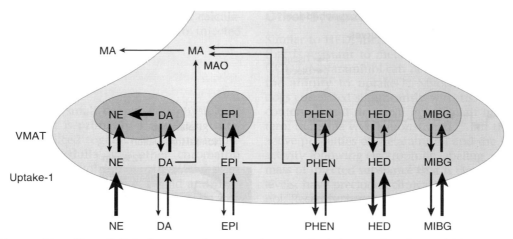

Figure 42-2 Neuronal handling of clinical tracers of presynaptic sympathetic innervation. Arrow thickness represents relative approximate magnitude of rate constants for uptake-1 membrane transporter and vesicular monoamine transporter (VMAT). DA, dopamine; EPI, epinephrine; HED, hydroxyephedrine; MA, monoamine; MAO, monoamine oxidase; MIBG, metaiodobenzylguanidine; NE, norepinephrine; PHEN, phenylephrine. *(From Raffel DM, Wieland DM: Assessment of cardiac sympathetic nerve integrity with positron emission tomography, Nucl Med Biol 28:541–559, 2001.)*

by the norepinephrine transporter. HED is thus believed to undergo continuous release and reuptake by sympathetic neurons.[15]

In contrast to single-photon emission computed tomography (SPECT) imaging using ^{123}I-MIBG, where lower uptake in the inferior myocardium has been observed, distribution of HED throughout the left ventricular (LV) myocardium in healthy, normal individuals is regionally homogeneous, with high uptake in all myocardial segments (Fig. 42-3).[16] For imaging, 400 to 700 MBq of ^{11}C-HED are typically injected intravenously as a bolus, followed by a dynamic acquisition lasting 40 to 60 minutes. For quantification, a "retention index" is commonly calculated by dividing myocardial radioactivity concentration in the final image by the integral of the time-activity curve in arterial blood (which is derived from a region of interest in the LV chamber and needs correction for presence of radiolabeled plasma metabolites). Typical time-activity curves of dynamic HED PET studies are depicted in Figure 42-4. High neuronal affinity of HED makes compartmental modeling of its kinetics difficult, because in addition to norepinephrine transporter density, perfusion and transcapillary transport may significantly influence tracer uptake. An experimental, albeit complex, approach for truly quantitative kinetic modeling of HED has been introduced in the research setting[18] but has not yet been transferred to human studies. In a rat model of varying degrees of cardiac sympathetic nerve denervation, semiquantitative measurement using HED retention was found to have a strong linear correlation with sympathetic nerve density, as reflected by cardiac norepinephrine transport (NET) density.[19] Another experimental animal study aimed to investigate the feasibility of quantitation of ^{11}C-HED PET retention in comparison to ^{123}I-MIBG uptake by in vivo imaging. There was a close correlation between two quantitative parameters—myocardial ^{11}C-HED retention fraction and the normalized ^{11}C-HED activity (% ID/kg/g)—and ^{123}I-MIBG uptake.[20] These results would improve the

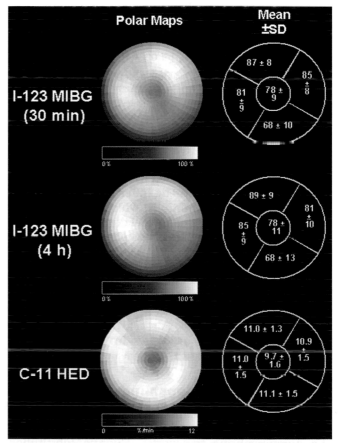

Figure 42-3 Myocardial distribution of the SPECT tracer, iodine-123-labeled metaiodobenzylguanidine (I-123 MIBG), and the PET tracer, carbon-11-hydroxyephedrine (C-11 HED), in healthy normal individuals, depicted in polar maps of the left ventricle. Also shown are segmental mean ± standard deviation in percentage of normalized uptake for MIBG and percent/min retention for HED. There is mildly lower uptake of MIBG in inferior wall of normals, but no such heterogeneity is observed for PET and HED.

73. Schäfers M, Dutka D, Rhodes CG, et al: Myocardial presynaptic and postsynaptic autonomic dysfunction in hypertrophic cardiomyopathy, *Circ Res* 82:57–62, 1998.

74. Li ST, Tack CJ, Fananapazir L, et al: Myocardial perfusion and sympathetic innervation in patients with hypertrophic cardiomyopathy, *J Am Coll Cardiol* 35:1867–1873, 2000.

75. Higuch T, Schwaiger M: Imaging cardiac neuronal function and dysfunction, *Curr Cardiol Rep* 8:131–138, 2006.

76. Calkins H, Allman K, Bolling S, et al: Correlation between scintigraphic evidence of regional sympathetic neuronal dysfunction and ventricular refractoriness in the human heart, *Circulation* 88:172–179, 1993.

77. Calkins H, Lehmann MH, Allman K, et al: Scintigraphic pattern of regional cardiac sympathetic innervation in patients with familial long QT syndrome using positron emission tomography, *Circulation* 87:1616–1621, 1993.

78. Mazzadi AN, Andre-Fouet X, Duisit J, et al: Heterogeneous cardiac retention of ^{11}C-hydroxyephedrine in genotyped long QT patients. A potential amplifier role for severity of the disease, *Am J Physiol Heart Circ Physiol* 285:H1286–H1293, 2003.

79. Schäfers M, Lerch H, Wichter T, et al: Cardiac sympathetic innervation in patients with idiopathic right ventricular outflow tract tachycardia, *J Am Coll Cardiol* 32:181–186, 1998.

80. Wichter T, Schäfers M, Rhodes CG, et al: Abnormalities of cardiac sympathetic innervation in arrhythmogenic right ventricular cardiomyopathy: Quantitative assessment of presynaptic norepinephrine reuptake and postsynaptic beta-adrenergic receptor density with positron emission tomography, *Circulation* 101:1552–1558, 2000.

81. Brugada J, Brugada R, Brugada P: Right bundle-branch block and ST-segment elevation in leads V1 through V3: A marker for sudden death in patients without demonstrable structural heart disease, *Circulation* 97(5):457–460, 1998.

82. Kies P, Wichter T, Schäfers M, et al: Abnormal myocardial presynaptic norepinephrine recycling in patients with Brugada syndrome, *Circulation* 110(19):3017–3022, 2004.

83. Bengel FM, Ueberfuhr P, Hesse T, et al: Clinical determinants of ventricular sympathetic reinnervation after orthotopic heart transplantation, *Circulation* 106:831–835, 2002.

84. Schmitt C, Meyer C, Kosa I, et al: Does radiofrequency catheter ablation induce a deterioration in sympathetic innervation? A positron emission tomography study, *Pacing Clin Electrophysiol* 21:327–330, 1998.

85. Olgin JE, Sih HJ, Hanish S, et al: Heterogeneous atrial denervation creates substrate for sustained atrial fibrillation, *Circulation* 98:2608–2614, 1998.

86. Jayachandran JV, Sih HJ, Winkle W, et al: Atrial fibrillation produced by prolonged rapid atrial pacing is associated with heterogeneous changes in atrial sympathetic innervation, *Circulation* 101:1185–1191, 2000.

87. Allman KC, Stevens MJ, Wieland DM, et al: Noninvasive assessment of cardiac diabetic neuropathy by carbon-11 hydroxyephedrine and positron emission tomography, *J Am Coll Cardiol* 22:1425–1432, 1993.

88. Stevens MJ, Raffel DM, Allman KC, et al: Cardiac sympathetic dysinnervation in diabetes: Implications for enhanced cardiovascular risk, *Circulation* 98:961–968, 1998.

89. Stevens MJ, Raffel DM, Allman KC, et al: Regression and progression of cardiac sympathetic dysinnervation complicating diabetes: An assessment by C-11 hydroxyephedrine and positron emission tomography, *Metabolism* 48:92–101, 1999.

90. Schmid H, Forman LA, Cao X, et al: Heterogeneous cardiac sympathetic denervation and decreased myocardial nerve growth factor in streptozotocin-induced diabetic rats: Implications for cardiac sympathetic dysinnervation complicating diabetes, *Diabetes* 48:603–608, 1999.

91. Stevens MJ, Dayanikli F, Raffel DM, et al: Scintigraphic assessment of regionalized defects in myocardial sympathetic innervation and blood flow regulation in diabetic patients with autonomic neuropathy, *J Am Coll Cardiol* 31:1575–1584, 1998.

92. Di Carli MF, Bianco-Batlles D, Landa ME, et al: Effects of autonomic neuropathy on coronary blood flow in patients with diabetes mellitus, *Circulation* 100:813–819, 1999.

93. Pop-Busui R, Kirkwood I, Schmid H, et al: Sympathetic dysfunction in type-1 diabetes association with impaired myocardial blood flow reserve and diastolic dysfunction, *J Am Coll Cardiol* 44:2368–2374, 2004.

94. Bengel FM, Ueberfuhr P, Schäfer D, et al: Effect of diabetes mellitus on sympathetic neuronal regeneration studied in the model of transplant reinnervation, *J Nucl Med* 47:1413–1419, 2006.

95. Mancini D: Surgically denervated cardiac transplant. Rewired or permanently unplugged, *Circulation* 96:6–8, 1997.

96. Schwaiger M, Hutchins GD, Kalff V, et al: Evidence for regional catecholamine uptake and storage sites in the transplanted human heart by positron emission tomography, *J Clin Invest* 87:1681–1690, 1991.

97. Bengel FM, Ueberfuhr P, Ziegler SI, et al: Serial assessment of sympathetic reinnervation after orthotopic heart transplantation. A longitudinal study using PET and C-11 hydroxyephedrine, *Circulation* 99:1866–1871, 1999.

98. Uberfuhr P, Ziegler S, Schwaiblmair M, et al: Incomplete sympathetic reinnervation of the orthotopically transplanted human heart: Observation up to 13 years after heart transplantation, *Eur J Cardiothorac Surg* 17:161–168, 2000.

99. Odaka K, von Scheidt W, Ziegler SI, et al: Reappearance of cardiac presynaptic sympathetic nerve terminals in the transplanted heart: Correlation between PET using ^{11}C-hydroxyephedrine and invasively measured norepinephrine release, *J Nucl Med* 25:1011–1016, 2001.

100. Uberfuhr P, Frey AW, Ziegler S, et al: Sympathetic reinnervation of sinus node and left ventricle after heart transplantation in humans: Regional differences assessed by heart rate variability and positron emission tomography, *J Heart Lung Transplant* 19:317–323, 2000.

101. Ziegler SI, Frey AW, Uberfuhr P, et al: Assessment of myocardial reinnervation in cardiac transplants by positron emission tomography: Functional significance tested by heart rate variability, *Clin Sci (Lond)* 91(Suppl):126–128, 1996.

102. Di Carli MF, Tobes MC, Mangner T, et al: Effects of cardiac sympathetic innervation on coronary blood flow, *N Engl J Med* 336:1208–1215, 1997.

103. Bengel FM, Ueberfuhr P, Ziegler SI, et al: Noninvasive assessment of the effect of cardiac sympathetic innervation on metabolism of the human heart, *Eur J Nucl Med* 27:1650–1657, 2000.

104. Bengel FM, Ueberfuhr P, Schiepel N, et al: Myocardial efficiency and sympathetic reinnervation after orthotopic heart transplantation: A noninvasive study with positron emission tomography, *Circulation* 103:1881–1886, 2001.

105. Bengel FM, Ueberfuhr P, Karja J, et al: Sympathetic reinnervation, exercise performance and effects of β-adrenergic blockade in cardiac transplant recipients, *Eur Heart J* 25:1726–1733, 2004.

106. Bengel FM, Ueberfuhr P, Schiepel N, et al: Effect of sympathetic reinnervation on cardiac performance after heart transplantation, *N Engl J Med* 345:731–738, 2001.

107. Tipre DN, Goldstein DS: Cardiac and extracardiac sympathetic denervation in Parkinson's disease with orthostatic hypotension and in pure autonomic failure, *J Nucl Med* 46(11):1775–1781, 2005.

108. Berding G, Schrader CH, Peschel T, et al: [N-methyl^{11}C]meta-hydroxyephedrine positron emission tomography in Parkinson's disease and multiple system atrophy, *Eur J Nucl Med Mol Imaging* 30:127–131, 2003.

109. Goldstein DS, Holmes CS, Dendi R, et al: Orthostatic hypotension from sympathetic denervation in Parkinson's disease, *Neurology* 58:1247–1255, 2002.

110. Goldstein DS, Imrich R, Peckham E, et al: Neurocirculatory and nigrostriatal abnormalities in Parkinson disease from *LRRK2* mutation, *Neurology* 69:1580–1584, 2007.

111. Li ST, Dendi R, Holmes C, et al: Progressive loss of cardiac sympathetic innervation in Parkinson's disease, *Ann Neurol* 52:220–223, 2002.

112. Raffel DM, Koeppe RA, Little R, et al: PET measurement of cardiac and nigrostriatal denervation in Parkinsonian syndromes, *J Nucl Med* 47(11):1769–1777, 2006.

113. Goldstein DS, Imrich R, Peckham E, et al: Neurocirculatory and nigrostriatal abnormalities in Parkinson disease from *LRRK2* mutation, *Neurology* 69:1580–1584, 2007. Goldstein DS, Holmes C, Cannon RO III, et al: Sympathetic cardioneuropathy in dysautonomias, *N Engl J Med* 336:696–702, 1997.

114. Goldstein DS, Holmes C, Frank SM, et al: Cardiac sympathetic dysautonomia in chronic orthostatic intolerance syndromes, *Circulation* 106:2358–2365, 2002.

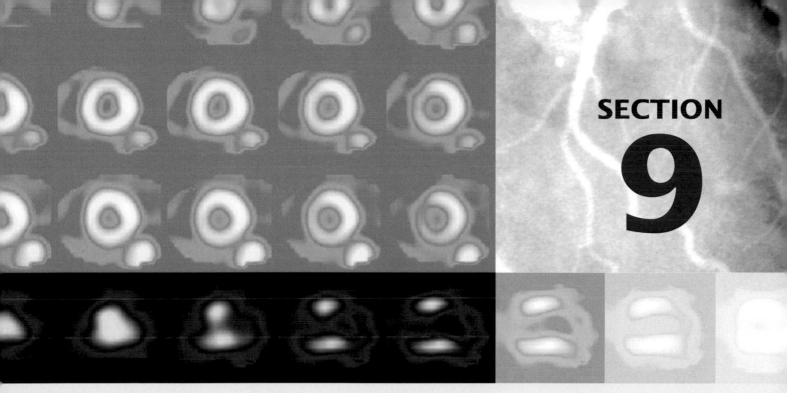

New Molecular Approaches

Molecular Imaging Approaches for Evaluation of Myocardial Pathophysiology: Angiogenesis, Ventricular Remodeling, Inflammation, and Cell Death

ALAN R. MORRISON AND ALBERT J. SINUSAS

INTRODUCTION

Molecular imaging is a targeted approach to noninvasively assess biological (both physiologic and pathologic) processes in vivo. The penultimate goal of molecular imaging is not just to provide diagnostic and prognostic information, but rather to guide individually tailored pharmacologic, cell-based, or genetic therapeutic regimens. This chapter will review recent myocardial molecular imaging tools in the context of our current understanding of the cardiovascular processes of angiogenesis, ventricular remodeling, inflammation, and apoptosis. The focus will be on radiotracer-based molecular imaging modalities. Imaging of these myocardial processes may have significant clinical utility in the areas of acute and chronic ischemia, acute myocardial infarction, congestive heart failure, or more global inflammatory and immune-mediated responses in the heart such as myocarditis and allogeneic cardiac transplant rejection.

By understanding the complex molecular interactions that take place within the cardiovascular system under physiologic conditions as well as in the development of pathologic states, physician-scientists have an opportunity to design more precise and effective medical therapies. This evolution of truly individualized health care will require enough knowledge of an individual's genome and proteome to model molecular interactions from levels of gene expression to the complex milieu and kinetics of protein expression and posttranslational modification. To detect and monitor both the disease and the therapeutic interventions in hopes of optimizing care and minimizing the burden of side effects and invasive injuries, a parallel engineering of tools to image specific molecular events must take place that allows in vivo serial assessment of the patient.

The application of imaging using biologically targeted markers (i.e., molecular imaging) has a number of requirements.[1] A molecular target that adequately represents the process being studied is critical to the specificity of any imaging approach. The target must then lend itself to a readily synthesizable probe(s) that will bind to the target molecule with a high degree of specificity. Lastly, an imaging technology that provides the best combination of sensitivity and resolution (both spatial and temporal) to identify and localize the probe within the target organ system needs to be immediately available and economically feasible. Molecular imaging approaches are currently being developed for most of the imaging modalities, including nuclear, magnetic resonance, x-ray computed tomography (CT), optical fluorescence, bioluminescence, and ultrasound.[2] Though each modality carries strengths and weaknesses, it is likely that the practical limitations of cost and widespread availability will determine which modalities become adapted for clinical use.

Single-photon emission computed tomography (SPECT) and positron emission tomography (PET) are imaging techniques that make use of radiolabeled probes and have been used for over 3 decades. Radiolabeling has the unique advantage of augmenting low signal-intensity objects. For example, PET can detect picomolar and nanomolar concentrations of a molecule of interest.[2] Though SPECT offers the advantage of decreased cost and widespread availability, PET offers the advantages of increased sensitivity in conjunction with the ability to quantitate as well as repetitively image using tracers with ultrashort half-lives. In the past, nuclear imaging modalities have been limited by attenuation artifacts from soft tissue and partial volume effects. More recent systems combining CT imaging with either SPECT or PET have allowed for attenuation correction, leading to improved imaging quantification and registration.

This chapter will review several important areas of active cardiovascular research in which nuclear-based molecular imaging have been used: *angiogenesis, ventricular remodeling, inflammation,* and *apoptosis.* Key molecular events or signaling proteins involved in each process that were identified through basic research have served as targets for imaging tools. It is important to keep in mind that some molecular signals can overlap between biological processes, which emphasizes the significance of understanding the complex setting in which any molecular event takes place.

ANGIOGENESIS

Atherosclerosis is a chronic inflammatory disease that leads to the progression of lipid-laden vascular plaques.[3,4] Monocyte adhesion and transendothelial migration result in activation and differentiation, with amplifying production of cytokines/chemokines, as well as foam cell development when these subendothelial macrophages endocytose oxidized lipid. The progression of atherosclerotic disease can lead to the development of chronic ischemia in areas of myocardium, secondary to poor perfusion through narrowed blood vessels. Subsequent signals in response to the ischemia may stimulate angiogenic and arteriogenic responses to restore perfusion.

Angiogenesis is defined as the process of sprouting new capillaries from preexisting microvessels.[5] There is a great deal of interest in understanding the processes of angiogenesis in order to design therapeutic treatments that allow revascularization through an iatrogenic-stimulated angiogenic response. This angiogenic process often occurs in association with arteriogenesis, which represents a remodeling of larger preexisting vascular channels or collateral vessels feeding the new

microvascular network. The goal for any myocardial revascularization strategy would be to initiate angiogenesis and arteriogenesis in manner that improves tissue perfusion. There is a large body of literature devoted to understanding these phenomena.[6-8]

Angiogenesis is stimulated by external processes such as ischemia, hypoxia, inflammation, and shear stress. Endothelial cells, smooth muscle cells, blood-derived macrophages, and circulating stem cells all play distinctive roles in the angiogenic process. There is the careful interaction of these cells with each other as well as within the tissue of extracellular matrix proteins. The process itself consists of a series of endothelial cell responses to angiogenic stimulation, such as degradation of extracellular matrix (ECM), budding from parent vessels, proliferation, migration, tube formation, and ultimately maturation and maintenance of the new vessel.[9] Figure 43-1 outlines a schematic representation of the process of angiogenesis on an endothelial cellular level.

Hypoxia, the imbalance between oxygen delivery and demand in a given tissue, is a potent stimulator of angiogenesis.[10] Hypoxic conditions such as myocardial ischemia from atherosclerotic disease or acute myocardial infarction (MI) result in up-regulation of the transcriptional activator hypoxia-inducible factor 1 (HIF-1).[11] HIF-1 is a heterodimeric protein composed of alpha and beta subunits. It is continuously expressed and degraded through oxygen-dependent proline hydroxylation of the alpha subunit and subsequent ubiquitination by von Hippel-Lindau E3 ligase for degradation in the proteosome.[12] Hypoxia stabilizes the HIF-1 protein by preventing the proline hydroxylation and ultimately the ubiquitination and degradation in the proteosome. This up-regulation of HIF-1 protein leads to the transcription of a number of hypoxia-inducible genes, including the key angiogenic mediators vascular endothelial growth factor (VEGF), platelet-derived growth factor (PDGF) and TGF-β, and the VEGF receptors, Flt-1 (VEGFR-1) and FLK-1 (VEGFR-2).[10,13-16]

When VEGF binds to its receptors on the surface of endothelial cells, a signal is transduced through their tyrosine kinase activity. This initiates a series of processes that results in endothelial cell proliferation, migration, survival, and angiogenesis.[17] Early work in this field generated enthusiasm for the prospect of therapeutic angiogenesis utilizing angiogenic proteins like VEGF or fibroblast growth factor 2 (FGF-2). In fact, a number of trials had been designed to attempt therapeutic angiogenesis, with the goals of stimulating new blood vessel growth and improving myocardial perfusion in ischemic heart disease. With relatively invasive measures to assess efficacy of treatment, preclinical studies in animal models had shown some benefit to therapeutic angiogenesis, supporting the transition to human trials.[18] Based on the early results, clinical trials were designed and initiated.

The FGF-2 Initiating Revascularization Support Trial (FIRST) randomized patients with chronic angina (class III-IV) to three doses of bFGF protein intracoronary injection versus placebo.[19] The study demonstrated no significant differences between the groups in exercise

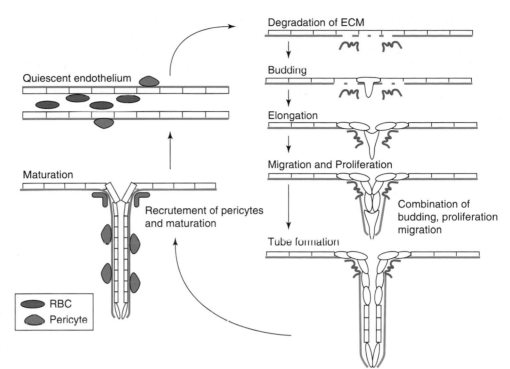

Figure 43-1 Schematic diagram of angiogenesis on a cellular level. This figure explains angiogenic progression, which starts with degradation of extracellular matrix (ECM) and is followed by survival and budding of activated endothelial cells, migration, and proliferation. By recruiting smooth muscle cells, such as pericytes, maturation proceeds. *(From Dufraine J, Funahashi Y, Kitajewski J: Notch signaling regulates tumor angiogenesis by diverse mechanisms, Oncogene 27: 5132–5137, 2008. Reprinted with permission.)*

time, nuclear perfusion, or quality of life at 90 days. The Angiogenic Gene Therapy Trial (AGENT) randomized patients to a single escalating intracoronary dose of replication-defective adenovirus containing the *FGF4* gene.[20] There was no significant difference in exercise treadmill time at 4 and 12 weeks.

In contrast, the VEGF in Ischemia for Vascular Angiogenesis (VIVA) Trial randomized patients with inducible ischemia on myocardial perfusion imaging to receive two (low- or high-dose) intracoronary injections of VEGF-1 protein versus placebo, followed by three more injections on days 3, 6, and 9.[21] There were no differences in exercise time or anginal class between the groups at 60 days, but anginal class was improved at 120 days in the high-dose group. There were no differences in myocardial perfusion throughout all the groups. The Randomized Evaluation of VEGF for Angiogenesis in Severe Coronary Disease (REVASC) Trial involved intramyocardial injection of replication-defective adenovirus containing the VEGF_{121} gene.[22] This study demonstrated a clinical improvement in the gene-therapy patients that was sustained from 3 to 6 months. Patients had significant improvements in exercise treadmill time to an additional 1 mm of ST depression, exercise time to angina, and angina class; however, nuclear perfusion imaging supported the control group, with the caveat that the treated group achieve higher workloads overall. More recently, the Euroinject One phase 2 clinical trial involved intramyocardial injections of plasmid containing VEGF in patients with Canadian Class 3 and 4 angina.[23] The study revealed no differences in perfusion abnormalities, but there were improvements in regional ventricular wall-motion disturbances and functional anginal class.

Unfortunately, these trials have met with mixed results. Clinical end points like anginal symptoms,

exercise tolerance, or perfusion imaging were largely used to measure outcomes, but there was little in the way of sensitive imaging modalities that could confirm and/or optimize the efficacy of therapeutic delivery of agents. This may in part reflect some of the differences between these trials and the earlier animal studies that used highly invasive measures to assess efficacy of treatment. The data suggest a need to develop concomitant imaging modalities that assess the efficacy of any angiogenic therapy. Moreover, there has recently been a shift in thought regarding mechanisms of angiogenesis, based largely on tumor angiogenesis research, resulting in a larger appreciation for the complexity of mechanisms that regulate VEGF and its receptors. Understanding these mechanisms may play an important role in developing a more effective therapeutic angiogenesis regimen.

One important signaling molecule is tie-2, a receptor tyrosine kinase, primarily expressed on vascular endothelium. Tie-2 has two major ligands: angiopoietin-1, which plays an agonistic signaling role, and angiopoietin-2, which appears to play an antagonistic signaling role.[24,25] In conjunction with VEGF, this signaling mechanism appears to help stabilize and mature new capillaries as they develop, providing an important dimension to endothelial signaling and effective therapeutic angiogenesis. Preliminary, animal studies support utilizing this multipronged approach to VEGF angiogenesis therapy to obtain a more functional vasculature.[26]

Another significant signaling system is that of the Notch–Delta-like ligand pathway. The Notch receptor is a single-pass transmembrane protein consisting of an extracellular domain that is responsible for ligand interaction, a transmembrane domain that is involved in receptor activation, and an intracellular signaling domain.[9] Signaling through Notch requires cell to cell contact through binding of its ligand, which is also a cell-surface protein. The ligands are members of the Jagged and Delta-like ligand family. Of interest to vascular endothelial cells are Notch 1 and Notch 4, as well as their ligands, Jagged1, Delta-like ligand 1 (Dll1), and Delta-like ligand 4 (Dll4). Dll4 is found exclusively on endothelial cells. Murine gene disruption experiments have revealed that Notch-Dll4 signaling is crucial to normal embryonic vascular development.[27] Blocking the Notch-Dll4 interaction can paradoxically lead to an increase in angiogenesis and new vessel budding, but the new vessels appear to function in an abnormal manner, which compromises blood flow and oxygenation to the area of interest.[28-30] It appears that VEGF up-regulates Dll4 in endothelial cells in a manner that creates a complex feedback loop to help achieve functional new blood vessels (Fig. 43-2). This argues for the importance of understanding what molecular switches are being activated in any attempt at therapeutic angiogenesis.

Endothelial signaling through VEGF and its concomitant receptor pathways is not the only molecular event undertaken during angiogenesis. There is also up-regulation and activation of molecules like integrins

that aid in the cell-cell signaling and ultimately extracellular remodeling process. Integrins are a family of heterodimeric ($\alpha\beta$) cell-surface receptors that mediate divalent, cation-dependent, cell-cell, and cell-matrix adhesion and signaling through tightly regulated interactions with their respective ligands.[31] During angiogenesis, endothelial cells make use of integrins to adhere to one another and the extracellular matrix to construct and extend new vessels. Peak expression of one integrin in particular, $\alpha_v\beta_3$ integrin, has been shown to occur 12 to 24 hours after initiation of angiogenesis with FGF2.[32] Integrins are capable of mediating an array of cellular processes, including cell adhesion, migration, proliferation, differentiation, and survival via a number of signal transduction pathways (Fig. 43-3).[33,34] Activation of c-Jun NH2-terminal kinase (JNK) and extracellular signal-regulated kinase (ERK) may lead to endothelial cell–induced remodeling of the ECM in response to mechanical stimuli. Specifically, the endothelial cell integrin $\alpha_v\beta_3$ allows cells to interact with the ECM in a way that aids in endothelial cell migration.[35] Through outside-in signaling, integrin $\alpha_v\beta_3$ also plays a critical roll in the survival of cells undergoing angiogenesis.[32]

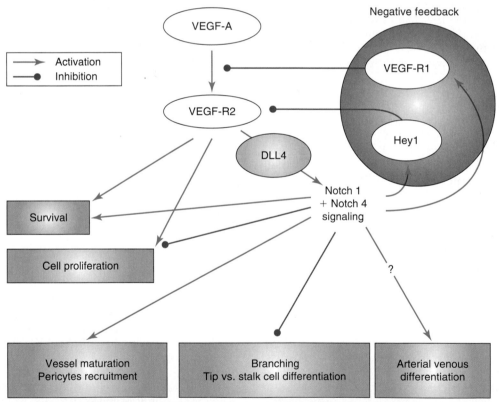

Figure 43-2 Delta-like ligand 4 signaling acts downstream of vascular endothelial growth factor (VEGF) signaling to prevent excessive angiogenesis and to trigger terminal differentiation of newly forming vessels. VEGF-A is a prime regulator of vessel elongation, acting through the activation of endothelial cell (EC) proliferation and EC survival. Activation of VEGF-R2 by VEGF-A occurs early during sprouting angiogenesis. Concomitantly, VEGF-A up-regulates Notch signaling locally through the activation of Dll4 expression. Dll4 in turn signals through Notch 1 and Notch 4 to block excessive branching by preventing the tip cell phenotype. Finally, Dll4 regulates vessel maturation through inhibition of EC proliferation, recruitment of mural cells, and potentially through arterial-venous differentiation. Dll4-dependent activation of Notch signaling also acts through a negative feedback mechanism to block VEGF signaling through induction of VEGF-R1 and repression of VEGF-R2. *(From Sainson RC, Harris AL: Anti-Dll4 therapy: Can we block tumour growth by increasing angiogenesis? Trends Mol Med 13:389–395, 2007. Reprinted with permission.)*

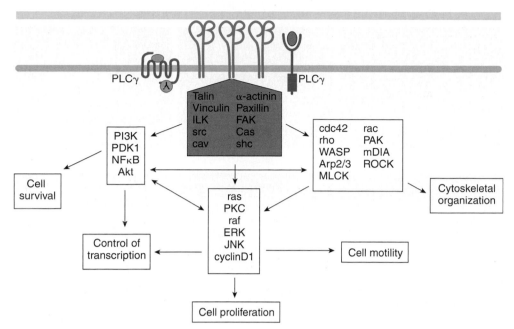

Figure 43-3 Integrin signaling. The major signal transduction pathways associated with the cellular processes mediated by integrins are shown. The integrin signaling often acts in concert with G protein–coupled or kinase receptor pathways. The major submembranous, integrin-associated links between the transmembrane clustered integrins and the transduction pathways are within the *pink-purple pentagon. (From Hynes RO: Integrins: Bidirectional, allosteric signaling machines, Cell 110:673–687, 2002. Reprinted with permission.)*

Several other molecules have been identified in this schema of endothelial cell activation. Syndecan-4 is a transmembrane heparan sulfate–carrying core protein that promotes binding of VEGF to VEGFR, resulting in activation of protein kinase C and downstream signaling.[36] CD13 is a cell-surface antigen that is expressed in endothelial cells as an aminopeptidase—in other words, a membrane-bound metalloproteinase that appears to be essential for capillary tube formation.[37] Degradation of the extracellular matrix involves up-regulation of matrix metalloproteinases, as well, to allow budding and expansion of the new vessel. Other molecular events include platelet-derived growth factor receptor signaling in response to HIF-1. This activates cell types like the perivascular pericytes or vascular smooth muscle cells, playing a crucial role in the new blood vessel development.[38]

RADIOTRACER-BASED IMAGING OF ANGIOGENESIS

Potential targets for molecular imaging of angiogenesis have been traditionally divided into three major categories: non-endothelial targets like molecules associated with monocytes, macrophages, and stem cells; endothelial cell targets like vascular endothelial growth factor (VEGF), integrins, CD13, and syndecan-4; and extracellular matrix proteins.[39] Despite the wide array of molecules available as potential imaging targets for angiogenesis in response to ischemia, there are just two real active areas of research: imaging VEGF receptors via labeled VEGF and imaging the $\alpha_v\beta_3$ integrin via ligand-like analogs.

Vascular Endothelial Growth Factor Receptors

VEGF receptors have been targeted for imaging techniques in models of ischemia-induced angiogenesis. Radiolabeled $VEGF_{121}$ has been used to effectively identify angiogenesis in a rabbit model of hindlimb ischemia.[40] In this study, KDR and Flt-1 receptor expression was increased in the immunohistochemistry analysis of the skeletal muscle, supporting the theoretical hypoxic-driven angiogenic response. Biodistribution of the radiotracer raises concern for the practical application of this system in humans. The biodistribution was 20-fold higher levels in critical organs (liver, kidneys) compared with ischemic limb and is presumably related to relative VEGFR density in these organ systems.

A PET tracer, copper-64-labeled (^{64}Cu)-6DOTA-$VEGF_{121}$, was recently developed for imaging angiogenesis in a rat model of MI (Fig. 43-4).[41] Rats underwent ligation of the left coronary artery and subsequent PET imaging at various time points after MI. The investigators hypothesized that this tracer would detect early angiogenic signals because ischemia drives VEGFR expression. Co-registration of images was carried out using CT, and the zone of infarct was demonstrated using fluorine-18-labeled fluorodeoxyglucose (^{18}F-FDG) uptake. The study demonstrated that ^{64}Cu-6DOTA-$VEGF_{121}$– specific signal was present in the infarct region and peaked on day 3, consistent with the changing levels of VEGFR expression in the tissue as analyzed by immunofluorescence microscopy. The same group has also published experiments supporting the use of ^{64}Cu-6DOTA-$VEGF_{121}$ for imaging of VEGFR-2 in a murine model of hindlimb ischemia-induced angiogenesis.[42]

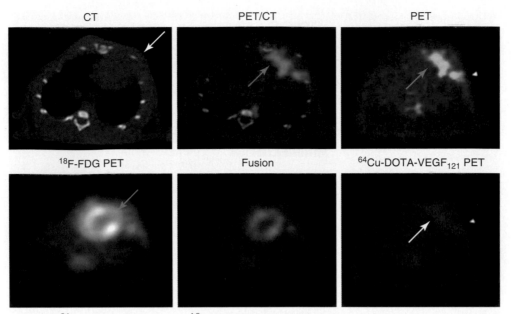

Figure 43-4 Myocardial ^{64}Cu-DOTA-VEGF$_{121}$ and ^{18}F-FDG PET/CT imaging after MI. *Upper images* demonstrate co-registered images of microCT *(left)*, PET *(right)*, and fused PET/CT image *(center)* in a representative animal after myocardial infarction. The ^{64}Cu-DOTA-VEGF$_{121}$ signal is detected by PET in the anterolateral myocardium (PET and fused images, *red arrow*). Intercostal muscle layer is designated on microCT image with a *white arrow*. There is some increased uptake in area of surgical wound (PET image, *arrowhead*). *Lower images* demonstrate ^{64}Cu-DOTA-VEGF$_{121}$ *(right)*, ^{18}F-FDG *(left)*, and ^{64}Cu-DOTAVEGF$_{121}$/^{18}F-FDG fused image *(middle)*. ^{18}F-FDG scan shows that coronary artery ligation resulted in development of a scar by lack of ^{18}F-FDG uptake *(red arrow)* and that uptake of ^{64}Cu-DOTA-VEGF$_{121}$ occurs in the region of that scar *(turquoise arrow)*. Fusion of both scans results in complementation of ^{18}F-FDG and ^{64}Cu-DOTA-VEGF$_{121}$ signals. Again, increased uptake in area of surgical wound is designated with an *arrowhead*. *(From Rodriguez-Porcel M, Cai W, Gheysens O, et al: Imaging of VEGF receptor in a rat myocardial infarction model using PET, J Nucl Med. 49:667–673, 2008. Reprinted with permission.)*

Another type of cardiac-specific reporter has been developed as a gene expression system for use in rats, with microPET imaging (see Chapter 45 for specific details).[43] Briefly, the system involves adenovirus delivery of mutated thymidine kinase under the control of a cytomegalovirus promoter driving expression in myocardial cells. The reporter probe is ^{18}F-labeled fluoro-3-hydroxy-methyl-butylguanine (^{18}F-FHBG), which crosses the myocardial membrane and gets phosphorylated by the thymidine kinase. Phosphorylation essentially traps the ^{18}F-FHGB in the myocardium for subsequent microPET imaging. Early studies revealed that the localized site of the mutated thymidine kinase, HSV1-sr39tk, corresponded closely with that defined by postmortem autoradiography, histology, and immunohistochemistry.[44] Other studies have demonstrated the feasibility of utilizing a similar reporter system in pigs using a clinical PET scanner.[45] The reporter system was then linked to VEGF to assess feasibility of developing an approach that links therapy and imaging.[46] Early experiments with rat embryonic cardiomyocytes revealed a strong correlation in that both the mutated thymidine kinase and VEGF were expressed in the same cells. Further studies involved injection of the VEGF/thymidine kinase reporter system in models of ischemia. Using microPET, cardiac transgene expression was assessed and the in vivo imaging correlated well with ex vivo tissue studies for gamma counting, thymidine kinase activity, and VEGF levels. There appeared to be increased capillaries and small blood vessels in the VEGF-treated myocardium; however, there

was no improvement in perfusion assessed by nitrogen-13 (^{13}N)-ammonia imaging or metabolism assessed with ^{18}F-FDG imaging. These studies suggest that a reporter system can be developed to help visualize the effectiveness of delivering VEGF gene therapies for stimulation of angiogenesis.

Integrin $\alpha_v\beta_3$

Imaging angiogenic vessels through targeting of $\alpha_v\beta_3$ integrin was first proposed through a series of magnetic resonance imaging studies using a monoclonal antibody to $\alpha_v\beta_3$ integrin tagged with a paramagnetic contrast agent.[47] The studies were complicated by poor clearance of the tracer from the blood pool. Later studies made use of a number of $\alpha_v\beta_3$ antagonists that were radiolabeled.[48,49] The experiments took advantage of the arginine-glycine-aspartate (RGD) binding sequence on integrins by synthesizing various RGD analogs.

An indium-111 (^{111}In)-labeled quinolone (^{111}In-RP748) revealed high affinity and selectivity for $\alpha_v\beta_3$ integrin in adhesion assays.[50] Subsequent studies using a cy3-labeled homolog of ^{111}In-RP748 demonstrated preferential binding to activated $\alpha_v\beta_3$ integrins on endothelial cells in culture, with localization to cell-cell contact points.[51] Initial studies with this agent focused on imaging tumor angiogenesis, although the first imaging of ischemia-induced myocardial angiogenesis using ^{111}In-RP748 was carried out in rat and canine models of infarction.[52] In these studies, ^{111}In-RP748 demonstrated favorable kinetics for in vivo SPECT imaging of ischemia-induced angiogenesis of the heart. Relative ^{111}In-RP748 activity was markedly increased in the infarcted region acutely and persisted for at least 3 weeks post reperfusion.[52,53] Therefore, targeted imaging with ^{111}In-RP748 has demonstrated integrin $\alpha_v\beta_3$ activation early post infarction, suggesting a role for this technique in early detection of angiogenesis as well as for detection of chronic ischemia (Fig. 43-5).[53]

Other experiments, utilizing a technetium-99m (^{99m}Tc)-labeled peptide, NC100692, in the rodent model of hindlimb ischemia for targeting of $\alpha_v\beta_3$ integrin have also been carried out and support the value of integrin imaging in models of peripheral arterial disease.[54] The recent imaging of $\alpha_v\beta_3$ integrin by the PET imaging tracer ^{18}F-galakto-RGD in a 35-year-old patient with a transmural MI 2 weeks prior demonstrates the feasibility of detecting angiogenesis in the myocardium in humans (Fig. 43-6).[55]

Recently, a new biodegradable positron-emitting nanoprobe targeted at $\alpha_v\beta_3$ integrin has been designed for noninvasive imaging of angiogenesis with a PET-based system (Fig. 43-7).[56] The nanoprobe has a core-shell architecture that allows radiolabeling with radiohalogens that are linked to the core to protect them from dehalogenation. The terminal ends of the outer shell are covalently linked to cyclic-RGD peptides to confer specificity to $\alpha_v\beta_3$ integrin. This nanoprobe revealed enhanced binding of $\alpha_v\beta_3$ integrin using in vitro and cellular assays. The nanoprobe demonstrated favorable biodistribution when compared with untargeted probe in rodents, with a slight increase in uptake in phagocytic-rich organs like the spleen, liver, and kidneys. Using a bromine-76 ([76]Br)-labeled derivative of the nanoprobe, the investigators targeted $\alpha_v\beta_3$ integrin in a murine model of hindlimb ischemia. In vivo PET imaging revealed specificity of the probe to the ischemic limb, using the nonischemic limb and a version of the probe lacking the cyclic RGD peptides for controls. Ex vivo imaging and histologic analysis allowed for quantification of the radioactivity, leading to further association of the probe to areas of increased $\alpha_v\beta_3$ integrin expression and new vessel formation. The application of nanotechnology to angiogenesis imaging is an exciting new area of research, but further studies will be required to assess the feasibility of applying this system to the in vivo imaging of angiogenesis in the myocardium.

VENTRICULAR REMODELING

Ventricular remodeling is a complex biological process that involves inflammation, angiogenesis, repair, and healing, with specific biochemical and structural alterations in the myocardial infarct and periinfarct regions as well as remote regions (Fig. 43-8).[57,58] The process is one of adaptation to form a scar that allows a degree of mechanical stability. The remodeling process involves several key cell types and structural elements, including myocardial cells, endothelial cells, inflammatory cells, and the extracellular matrix. Early in the first weeks after an MI, an innate immune response initiates a complex process of wound healing in the necrotic tissue. This

process evolves into a more chronic remodeling process that can involve hypertrophy, chamber dilation, and (depending on the success of healing or lack thereof) heart failure.

Matrix metalloproteinases (MMPs) are a family of zinc-containing enzymes that play a key role in ventricular remodeling by degradation of the extracellular matrix.[59,60] There are over 25 types of MMPs, and each can be distributed into subgroups based on substrate specificity and molecular structure.[61] Despite apparent differences between various MMPs, there is often substrate overlap among the subgroups. Moreover, the zinc-binding motif sequence homology provides fairly conserved structure to the catalytic regions of all the family members. Because of the overlap's substrate specificity, regulation of the various MMPs is critical to preventing pathologic phenomena. As such, MMPs are tightly regulated on several levels via transcriptional, posttranscriptional, and posttranslational mechanisms (Fig. 43-9). These regulatory mechanisms may serve as potential targets for disrupting MMP expression or activity. With regard to ventricular remodeling, MMPs appear to play an integral role in infarct expansion and left ventricular dilation. Gene deletion of MMPs has been demonstrated to have some cardioprotective effects from ventricular dilation and rupture post-infarct.[62] Pharmacologic inhibition of MMPs has also been shown to decrease left ventricular dilation in infarct models.[63–65]

Another enzyme, factor XIII, has been shown to be crucial in organizing the new matrix of the scar by involvement with extracellular matrix turnover and regulation of inflammatory cascades.[66,67] Mice with decreased levels of factor XIII demonstrate increased ventricular dilation and postinfarct rupture. Patients with infarct rupture were demonstrated to have lower levels of factor XIII in their myocardium. Factor XIII is activated by thrombin and often decreased in the setting of acute MI in part because of therapeutic inhibition of thrombin. It has been hypothesized that supplementing factor XIII activity may have a beneficial role in postinfarct remodeling.

A critical system that is locally activated during ventricular remodeling and contributes to the progression to heart failure is the renin-angiotensin system (Fig. 43-10).[68,69] As healing and remodeling are unsuccessful in the failing heart, there is increased expression of prorenin, renin, and angiotensin-converting enzyme (ACE). Activation of this system through signaling pathways mediated by the angiotensin II type I receptor (AT1) leads to myocyte hypertrophy, interstitial and perivascular collagen deposition, and myocyte apoptosis.[68] Inhibition of this pathway has been demonstrated to reverse the functional abnormalities associated with this negative remodeling.

RADIOTRACER-BASED IMAGING OF LEFT VENTRICULAR REMODELING

MMPs

By radiolabeling molecules that target MMPs, like pharmacologic inhibitors that specifically bind to the

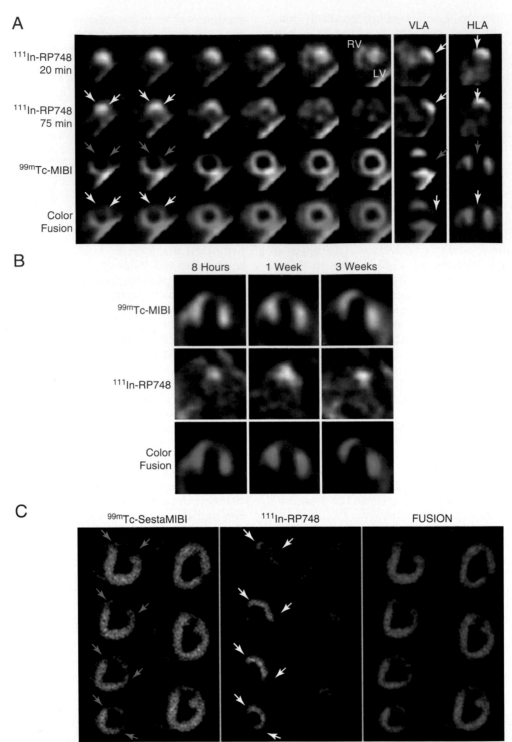

Figure 43-5 In vivo and ex vivo ^{111}In-RP748 and ^{99m}Tc-sestamibi (^{99m}Tc-MIBI) images from dogs with chronic infarction. (**A**) Serial in vivo ^{111}In-RP748 SPECT short-axis, vertical long-axis (VLA), and horizontal long-axis (HLA) images in a dog 3 weeks after LAD infarction at 20 minutes and 75 minutes after injection in standard format (Fig. 43-5A). ^{111}In-RP748 SPECT, images were registered with ^{99m}Tc-MIBI perfusion images *(third row)*. The 75-minute ^{111}In-RP748 SPECT images were colored red and fused with MIBI images *(green)* to better demonstrate localization of ^{111}In-RP748 activity within the heart *(color fusion, bottom row)*. Right ventricular (RV) and left ventricular (LV) blood pool activity are seen at 20 minutes. *White arrows* indicate region of increased ^{111}In-RP748 uptake in anterior wall. This corresponds to the anteroapical ^{99m}Tc-MIBI perfusion defect *(orange arrow)*. (**B**) Sequential ^{99m}Tc-MIBI *(top row)* and ^{111}In-RP748 in vivo SPECT HLA images at 90 minutes after injection *(middle row)* from a dog at 8 hours (Acute), and 1 and 3 weeks after LAD infarction (Fig. 43-5B). Increased myocardial ^{111}In-RP748 uptake is seen in anteroapical wall at all three time points, although appears to be maximal at 1 week post infarction. Color fusion ^{99m}Tc-MIBI *(green)* and ^{111}In-RP748 *(red)* images *(bottom row)* demonstrate ^{111}In-RP748 uptake within ^{99m}Tc-MIBI perfusion defect. Ex vivo ^{99m}Tc-sestamibi *(left)* and ^{111}In-RP748 *(center)* images of myocardial slices from a dog 3 weeks after LAD occlusion, with color fusion image on *right* (Fig. 43-5C). (**C**) Short-axis slices are oriented with anterior wall on top, RV on left. *Orange arrows* indicate anterior location of nontransmural perfusion defect region, and *white arrows* indicate corresponding area of increased ^{111}In-RP748 uptake. *(From Meoli DF, Sadeghi MM, Krassilnikova, S et al: Noninvasive imaging of myocardial angiogenesis following experimental myocardial infarction, J Clin Invest 113:1684–1691, 2004. Reprinted with permission.)*

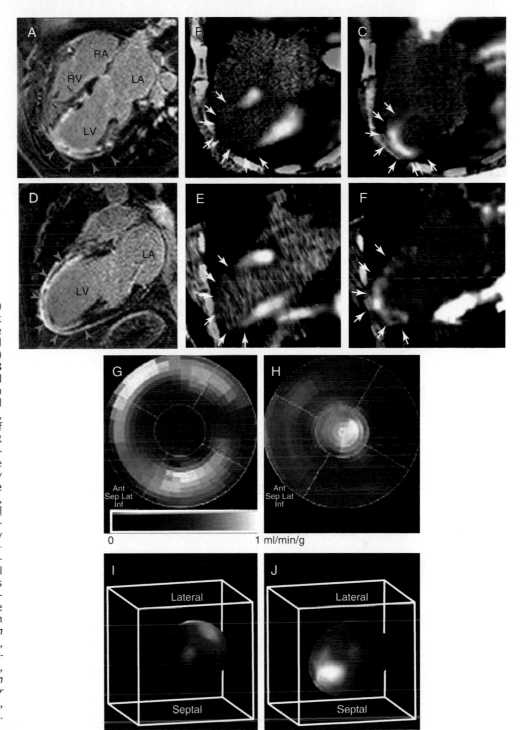

Figure 43-6 Cine-MRI (CMR) with delayed enhancement *(arrows)* extending from the anterior wall to the apical region in the four-chamber **(A)** and two-chamber **(D)** views. **B** and **E**, Identically reproduced location and geometry with severely reduced myocardial blood flow using ^{13}N-ammonia, corresponding to the regions of delayed enhancement by CMR *(arrows)*. **C** and **F**, Focal ^{18}F-RGD signal co-localized to the infarcted area. This signal may reflect angiogenesis within the healing area *(arrows)*. **G** and **I**, Polar map (I: 3D) of myocardial blood flow assessed by ^{13}N-ammonia, indicating severely reduced flow in the distal LAD-perfused region. **H** and **J**, Co-localized ^{18}F-RGD signal corresponding to the regions of severely reduced ^{13}N-ammonia flow signal, reflecting the extent of the $\alpha_v\beta_3$ expression within the infarcted area. *(From Makowski MR, Ebersberger U, Nekolla S, et al: In vivo molecular imaging of angiogenesis, targeting alpha$_v$beta$_3$ integrin expression, in a patient after acute myocardial infarction, Eur Heart J 29:2201, 2008. Reprinted with permission.)*

catalytic domain, MMP activation post infarct can be visualized in vivo (Fig. 43-11).[70] Initial studies involved nonimaging techniques with ^{111}In-labeled broad-spectrum MMP inhibitor (RP782), a molecule that selectively targets activated MMPs. This MMP-targeted agent demonstrated a favorable biodistribution in a murine model of MI. One week after MI, ^{111}In-RP782 localized primarily within the infarct region, although a lesser increase in retention was seen in the remote noninfarcted regions of the heart, consistent with global MMP activation and remodeling.

Further imaging studies were carried out utilizing a ^{99m}Tc-labeled analog of RP782 (^{99m}Tc-RP805) and hybrid SPECT/CT imaging with a dual-isotope protocol involving ^{99m}Tc-RP805 imaging and adjunctive thallium-201 perfusion imaging. The dual-isotope imaging studies revealed MMP activation within the perfusion defect region. This suggests that MMP activation is taking place primarily within the sites of injury and supports the concept that molecules that target MMP activation might be utilized to evaluate ventricular remodeling. An area of future investigation would be to address

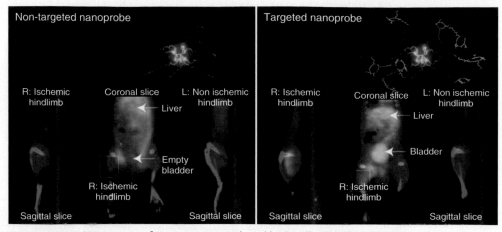

Figure 43-7 Noninvasive PET/CT images of angiogenesis induced by hindlimb ischemia in a murine model. Molecular models of the dendritic nanoprobe structures are shown in the *top right inset* in each set of images. Nontargeted dendritic nanoprobe *(left set of images)*. Uptake of $\alpha_v\beta_3$-targeted dendritic nanoprobes *(right set of images)* was higher in ischemic hindlimb (right limbs) as compared with control hindlimb (left limbs). *(From Almutairi A, Rossin R, Shokeen M, et al: Biodegradable dendritic positron-emitting nanoprobes for the noninvasive imaging of angiogenesis, Proc Natl Acad Sci U S A 106:685–690, 2009. Reprinted with permission.)*

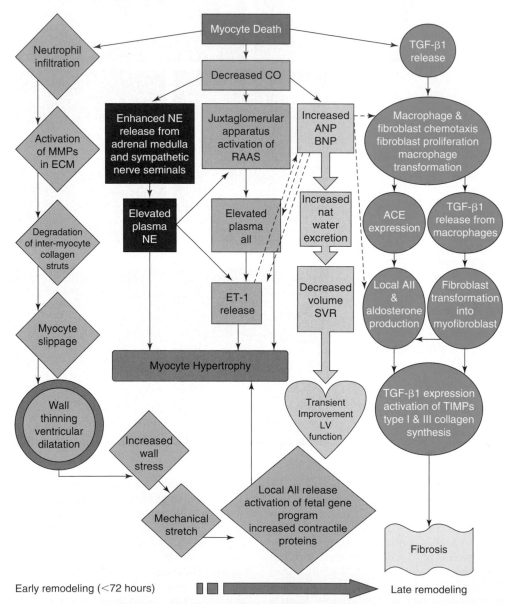

Figure 43-8 Diagrammatic representation of the many factors involved in the pathophysiology of ventricular remodeling. AII, angiotensin II; CO, cardiac output; ECM, extracellular matrix; LV, left ventricular; RAAS, renin-angiotensin-aldosterone system; SVR, systemic vascular resistance. *(From Sutton MG, Sharpe N: Left ventricular remodeling after myocardial infarction: Pathophysiology and therapy, Circulation 101:2981–2988, 2000. Reprinted with permission.)*

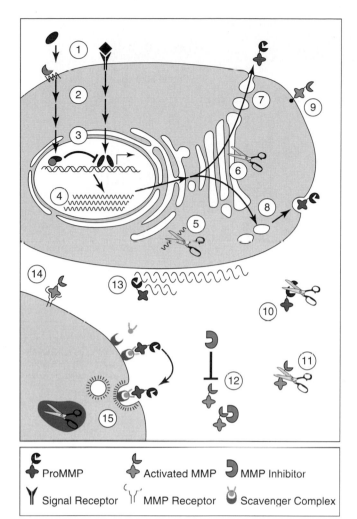

Figure 43-9 Regulation of the MMPs. MMP regulatory mechanisms include inductive and suppressive signaling (1), intracellular signal transduction (2), transcriptional activation and repression (3), posttranscriptional mRNA processing (4), mRNA degradation (5), intracellular activation of furin-susceptible MMPs (6), constitutive secretion (7), regulated secretion (8), cell surface expression (9), proteolytic activation (10), proteolytic processing and inactivation (11), protein inhibition (12), ECM localization (13), cell surface localization (14), and endocytosis and intracellular degradation (15). *(From Sternlicht MD, Werb Z: How matrix metalloproteinases regulate cell behavior, Annu Rev Cell Dev Biol 17:463–516, 2001. Reprinted with permission.)*

- ProMMP
- Activated MMP
- MMP Inhibitor
- Signal Receptor
- MMP Receptor
- Scavenger Complex

whether pharmacologic interventions known to favorably affect remodeling (e.g., ACE inhibitors) might influence MMP levels, allowing prognostication of an individual's response to therapy.

Factor XIII

^{111}In-DOTA-FXIII is a radiolabeled glutaminase factor XIII substrate analog that factor XIII cross-links to extracellular matrix proteins (Fig. 43-12).[67] ^{111}In-DOTA-FXIII has been shown to accumulate in areas of increased factor XIII activity, using microSPECT/CT imaging in a murine model of MI. Mice treated with factor XIII intravenously exhibited increased factor XIII activity as reflected by ^{111}In-DOTA-FXIII in the infarct zone. The

mice also demonstrated more rapid inflammatory turnover of neutrophils and increased recruitment of macrophages to the site of infarction. There was also increased collagen synthesis and capillary density in the factor XIII–treated animals, suggesting improved healing after infarction. The ^{111}In-labeled peptide substrate was demonstrated to be decreased in myocardial infarcts of animals treated with the direct thrombin inhibitor dalteparin. Moreover, dalteparin treatment increased the risk of infarct rupture. These experimental studies suggest there may be a role to image for factor XIII activity in an individual with MI and to therapeutically supplement activity where indicated to assist with positive ventricular remodeling, although further study is needed.

ACE Inhibitors and AT1 Antagonists

A number of ACE inhibitors and AT1 antagonists have been radiolabeled for molecular imaging techniques.[69] In a study of explanted hearts from patients with ischemic cardiomyopathy, ^{18}F-fluorobenzoyl-lisinopril was used to assess ACE levels in infarcted myocardium and fibrosed tissue (Fig. 43-13).[71] The study demonstrated that the radiolabeled ACE inhibitor bound with some degree of specificity to areas adjacent to the infarct. Other studies using AT1 antagonists have demonstrated a differential between ACE activity and AT1 levels.[72] In an ovine model of heart failure, ACE activity was primarily in the vascular endothelium while AT1 was up-regulated in the myofibroblasts of the infarct region. In a murine model of acute MI, a ^{99m}Tc-labeled AT1 receptor peptide analog was developed and demonstrated specificity to the myofibroblasts that localized to the infarct region in the weeks following the infarction. These early studies suggest the changes in the renin-angiotensin system that take place within an infarction may be utilized to identify those at risk for developing significant heart failure after MI. Much more work is needed to assess the feasibility of these agents for imaging of post-infarction remodeling in clinical trials.

Integrin $\alpha_v\beta_3$

Because collagen deposition and fibrosis in the failing heart appear to be mediated by myofibroblasts, markers that indicate increased myofibroblast recruitment and activity are of interest to the field.[73] Myofibroblasts demonstrate an up-regulation of angiotensin receptors as mentioned above; however, they demonstrate an up-regulation of integrin moieties as well.[72,74] Taking advantage of this molecular event, a recent study used the ^{99m}Tc-labeled cy5.5-RGD peptide analog, CRIP, to image up-regulated $\alpha_v\beta_3$ integrins in a murine model of MI (Fig. 43-14).[75] Fluorescence imaging and histologic analysis of explanted hearts revealed that CRIP co-localized to areas of myofibroblasts in the infarct region. Utilizing CT for registration, in vivo microSPECT analysis confirmed localization of the CRIP to the infarct and border zones. Maximum signal intensity was in the first 2 weeks post-infarction and then tapered at 4 and 12 weeks. A scrambled CRIP analog did not show uptake

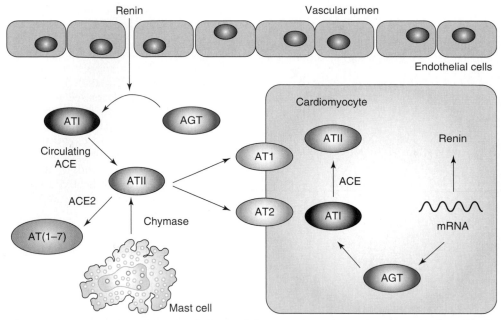

Figure 43-10 Schematic representation of the circulating and tissue renin-angiotensin system (RAS) within the heart is shown. Angiotensinogen (AGT) is cleaved by renin to form angiotensin I (ATI), which is converted by angiotensin-converting enzyme (ACE) to angiotensin II ATII. ATII in turn activates the angiotensin II type 1 (AT 1) and type 2 (AT 2) receptors. ATII may also be generated by an alternate pathway, mast-cell-derived chymase. *(From Aras O, Messina SA, Shirani J, et al: The role and regulation of cardiac angiotensin-converting enzyme for noninvasive molecular imaging in heart failure, Curr Cardiol Rep 9:150–158, 2007; and Shirani J, Dilsizian V: Imaging left ventricular remodeling: Targeting the neurohumoral axis, Nat Clin Pract Cardiovasc Med 5 Suppl 2:S57-S62, 2008. Reprinted with permission.)*

in the region, supporting the specificity of the CRIP for $\alpha_v\beta_3$ integrin binding. Moreover, a subgroup of animals were treated with either captopril or a combination of captopril and losartan in an attempt to positively affect ventricular remodeling and visualize the effect on the CRIP–$\alpha_v\beta_3$ integrin signal. Echocardiography supported smaller infarct size and improved ejection fraction in the treated animals. Ex vivo SPECT imaging of CRIP revealed lower signal intensity images in the treated hearts. This preliminary study suggests not only that critical changes in the ventricular myocardium after MI can be imaged using a molecular approach, but that a response to remodeling therapy may also be assessed.

INFLAMMATION

Inflammation is a broad reaction that involves a multifaceted interaction carried out through various forms of signaling between myocardial cells, the extracellular matrix, vascular cells, and immigrant cells like lymphocytes, neutrophils, and macrophages. The ultimate goal of the inflammatory reaction is removal of damaging or harmful substances and subsequent healing. As such, it is understandable that inflammation plays an important role in many cardiovascular processes, including MI, reperfusion injury, angiogenesis, apoptosis, cardiac allograft rejection, and myocarditis.

Initial attempts to image inflammatory processes involved radiolabeling leukocytes with ^{99m}Tc or [111]In. These techniques require removal of blood and in vitro labeling prior to reinjection into the blood stream for

imaging.[76,77] The concern over this in vitro labeling approach is the labeling often results in nonspecific activation of the cells, which in turn may interfere with cellular localization in vivo. Gallium-67-labeled, citrate has also been used but carries the same concerns regarding nonspecificity.[78] ^{18}F-FDG PET imaging takes advantage of increased metabolic activity of inflammatory cells, but changes in glucose uptake can be associated with other tissues and disease processes including tumors.[79,80] Thus, there is a tremendous amount of interest in developing more-specific noninvasive imaging techniques to detect inflammation in myocardium.

RADIOTRACER-BASED IMAGING OF INFLAMMATORY-MEDIATED PROCESSES

Antimyosin Antibodies

Injury to myocytes in the setting of inflammation leads to the disruption of cellular membranes and the release of myosin heavy chain. In order to take advantage of this extracellular exposure of myosin in the setting of inflammation and necrosis, monoclonal antibody to myosin was generated in hopes of applying this for imaging. Early attempts to visualize myosin utilized ^{111}In-labeled antimyosin antibodies to visualize myocyte damage in MI.[81] Other studies utilized ^{99m}Tc-labeled monoclonal antibody fragments to quantitate the degree of myosin exposure in patients in the setting of acute MI and correlate it with necrosis.[82] Inflammation associated with myocarditis, an inflammatory

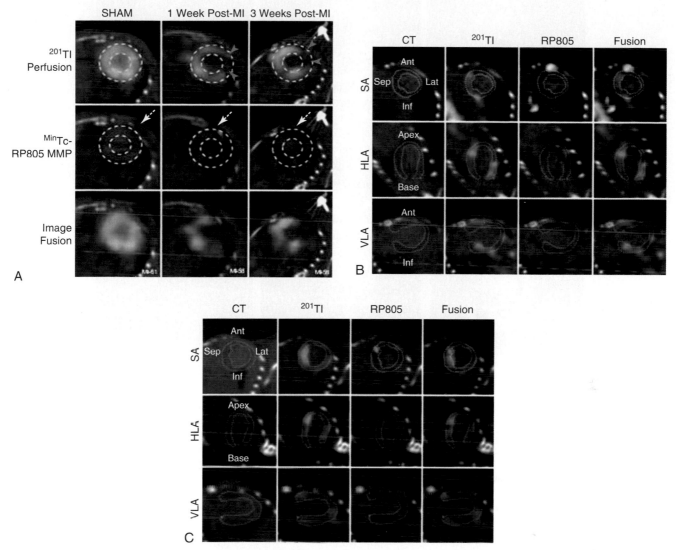

Figure 43-11 Imaging of matrix metalloproteinase (MMP) activity postinfarction. Hybrid micro-SPECT/CT reconstructed short-axis images were acquired without x-ray contrast (**A**) in control sham-operated mouse *(left)* and selected mice at 1 week *(middle)* and 3 weeks *(right)* after MI, after injection of ^{201}Tl *(top row, green)*, and ^{99m}Tc-RP805 *(middle row, red)*. A black-and-white and multicolor fusion image is shown on bottom. Control heart demonstrates normal myocardial perfusion and no focal ^{99m}Tc-RP805 uptake within the heart, although some uptake is seen in chest wall at the thoracotomy site *(white dotted arrows)*. All post-MI mice have a large anterolateral ^{201}Tl perfusion defect *(red arrows)* and focal uptake of ^{99m}Tc-RP805 in defect area. A *white dotted circle* is drawn around the heart to demonstrate localization of ^{99m}Tc-RP805, the MMP radiotracer, within the infarcted area of the heart. Some activity is also seen in the periinfarct border zone. Additional microSPECT/CT images were acquired by use of a higher-resolution SPECT detector after the administration of x-ray contrast at 1 week (**B**) and 3 weeks (**C**) after MI. The contrast agent permitted better definition of the LV myocardium, which is highlighted by *white dotted line*. Representative short-axis (SA), horizontal long-axis (HLA), and vertical long-axis (VLA) images are shown. Focal uptake of ^{99m}Tc-RP805 is seen within the central infarct and periinfarct regions, which again corresponds to ^{201}Tl perfusion defect. *(From Su H, Spinale FG, Dobrucki LW, et al: Noninvasive targeted imaging of matrix metalloproteinase activation in a murine model of postinfarction remodeling, Circulation 112:3157–3167, 2005. Reprinted with permission.)*

process not associated with ischemia, was also carried out using ^{111}In-anti-myosin antibodies.[83,84] Utilizing anti-myosin antibody imaging, patients with dilated cardiomyopathy and lower ejection fractions revealed positive studies, suggesting a role for this for stratifying appropriate patients for cardiac transplantation. Though these initial studies showed promise, the background antibody binding to necrotic debris in the cell was high, and therefore the specificity of ^{111}In-labeled anti-myosin antibody turned out to be very low (25% to 50%).[85]

Antitenascin-C Antibody

A monoclonal antibody against the extracellular matrix protein, tenascin-C, which appears to be involved in wound healing and inflammation, has been identified as another potential imaging agent for detection of inflammation. In rodent models of myocarditis, ^{111}In-labeled anti-tenascin-C localizes to the sites of myocardial inflammation.[86] Using a dual-isotope SPECT approach with ^{111}In-anti-tenascin-C and ^{99m}Tc-sestamibi, the antibody is localized to the injured septal

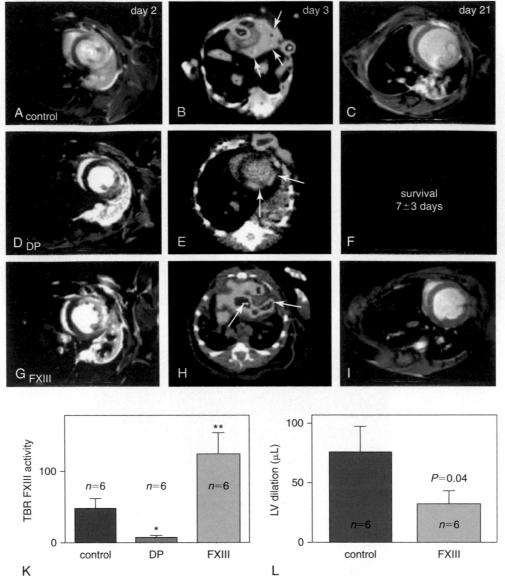

Figure 43-12 In vivo molecular imaging of transglutaminase factor XIII (FXIII) activity predicts survival and evolution of heart failure. **A-I**, Longitudinal imaging study (MRI day 2, SPECT/CT day 3, second MRI day 21). On day 2 (**A, D, G**), late enhancement MRI showed similar infarct size in all groups. FXIII treatment led to higher SPECT signal (**H, K**). In dalteparin-treated mice, the SPECT signal was lower (**E, K**). Serial MRI showed attenuated left ventricular (LV) dilation in FXIII-treated mice (**L**). Due to reduced survival in dalteparin (DP)-treated mice, the second MRI on day 21 was not acquired (**F**). $^*P < 0.05$, $^{**}P < 0.001$. *(From Nahrendorf M, Aikawa E, Figueiredo JL, et al: Transglutaminase activity in acute infarcts predicts healing outcome and left ventricular remodelling: Implications for FXIII therapy and antithrombin use in myocardial infarction, Eur Heart J 29:445–454, 2008. Reprinted with permission.)*

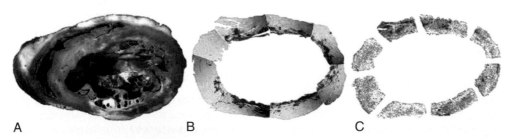

Figure 43-13 Presence and distribution of ACE activity in relation to collagen replacement as assessed by picrosirius red stain in human heart tissue removed from cardiac transplant recipient with ischemic cardiomyopathy. Gross pathology of midventricular slice (**A**), with corresponding contiguous midventricular slices stained with picrosirius red stain (**B**) and ^{18}F-FBL autoradiographic images (**C**), is shown. FBL binding to ACE is nonuniform in infarcted, periinfarcted, and remote, noninfarcted segments. Increased FBL binding can be seen in segments adjacent to collagen replacement. *(From Dilsizian V, Eckelman WC, Loredo ML, et al: Evidence for tissue angiotensin-converting enzyme in explanted hearts of ischemic cardiomyopathy using targeted radiotracer technique, J Nucl Med. 48:182–187, 2007. Reprinted with permission.)*

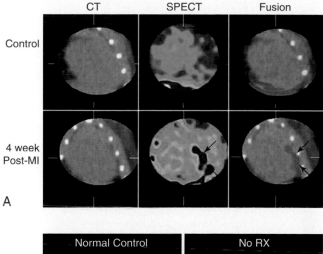

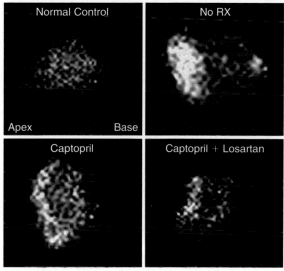

Figure 43-14 A, No uptake of technetium-labeled cy5.5 RGD imaging peptide (^{99m}Tc-CRIP) was observed in the unmanipulated animal *(top row)*. On the other hand, intense anterior uptake is seen in the infarcted mouse *(bottom row)*. The cardiac localization is confirmed in the computed tomography (CT) fusion image. MI, myocardial infarction; SPECT, single-photon emission computed tomography. **B,** In 4-week post-myocardial infarction (MI) animals, captopril treatment alone and in combination with losartan demonstrates significantly lower radiotracer uptake, as observed in gamma images of the explanted hearts. *(From van den Borne SW, Isobe S, Verjans JW, et al: Molecular imaging of interstitial alterations in remodeling myocardium after myocardial infarction, J Am Coll Cardiol 52:2017–2028, 2008. Reprinted with permission.)*

wall by in vivo imaging. More recently, ^{111}In-antitenascin-C monoclonal antibody fragments have been used in a dual-isotope SPECT imaging approach with ^{99m}Tc-MIBI to study in vivo expression of tenascin-C in a rodent model of MI (Fig. 43-15).[87] In this study, ^{111}In-antitenascin-C activity was associated with the ^{99m}Tc-MIBI perfusion defect, although not in sham animals, supporting this agent as a possible marker for inflammation associated with MI. Though much work is needed, the authors postulate that quantifying tenascin binding using a similar approach might allow for the evaluation of ventricular repair.

LTB$_4$ Receptor

LTB$_4$ is a lipid mediator synthesized from arachidonic acid and secreted by neutrophils, macrophages, and endothelial cells as a potent chemotactic agent.[88,89] The LTB$_4$ receptor can be found on neutrophils, and signaling through this receptor stimulates endothelial adhesion and superoxide production. Recently a radiolabeled LTB$_4$ receptor antagonist, ^{99m}Tc-RP517, was developed for in vivo imaging of inflammation.[90,91] ^{99m}Tc-RP517 localized to sites of inflammation induced by *Staphylococcus aureus* and *Escherichia coli* infection and chemical (phorbol ester)-induced bowel inflammation.

When prepared with human peripheral whole blood in vitro, fluorinated RP517 localized to neutrophils by fluorescence-activated cell sorter (FACs) analysis.[92] This confirmed the potential to specifically label human blood neutrophils with ^{99m}Tc-labeled RP517. In an attempt to characterize the in vivo imaging ability of ^{99m}Tc-RP517, a canine model of postischemic myocardial inflammation was utilized. ^{99m}Tc-RP517 was injected into open-chest dogs before occlusion and reperfusion. There was an inverse relationship between radiotracer uptake and occlusion flow, suggesting localization of the imaging agent to the site of ischemic inflammation (Fig. 43-16). Ex vivo segment analysis revealed that ^{99m}Tc-RP517 correlated with the neutrophil enzyme myeloperoxidase. Intramyocardial injection of tumor necrosis factor α (TNF-α) also correlated with ^{99m}Tc-RP517 uptake and concomitant myeloperoxidase activity, again supporting localization to the site of inflammation. One concern regarding the application of ^{99m}Tc-RP517 is the lipophilic nature of the molecule, resulting in high hepatobiliary clearance and thus large amounts of gastrointestinal uptake. To overcome this, alternative constructs of the LTB$_4$ antagonist are currently being evaluated.[93]

CELL DEATH

Apoptosis Versus Necrosis

Apoptosis is the physiologic process of programmed cell death whereby organisms selectively target cells to be eliminated when they are no longer needed. The cardiovascular pathologies of cardiomyopathy, heart failure, myocarditis, and MI are associated with increased levels of apoptosis, particularly in the myocyte. There is a subset of cell death that occurs as an outcome of these pathologic processes considered to be outside of programmed cellular mechanisms, termed *necrosis*. A recent study evaluating a role of apoptosis and necrosis in the setting of acute MI revealed a potential therapeutic role for cyclosporine.[94] The intervention is hypothesized to minimize periinfarct, reperfusion-related cell death that takes place in the setting of revascularization. It is estimated that 30% of cardiomyocytes in the injured myocardium become apoptotic as a result of ischemia, reperfusion injury, and animal models of acute infarction demonstrate that up to 50% of the final size of the infarct can be related to lethal reperfusion

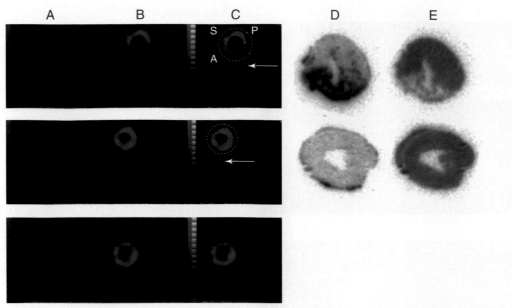

Figure 43-15 Comparison of SPECT imaging between ^{111}In-anti-TNC-Fab and ^{99m}Tc-MIBI. Transverse dual-isotope SPECT images (**A-C**) and autoradiographs of the same rats (**D, E**). The uptake of ^{111}In-anti-TNC-Fab *(red in A, C, D)* and ^{99m}Tc-MIBI *(green in B, C, E)* in acute MI heart *(upper panels)*, in sham-operated heart *(middle panels)*, and in normal rat heart *(lower panels)*. A, indicates anterior left ventricular wall; L, lateral left ventricular wall; P, posterior left ventricular wall; S, septal wall. *Red* color indicates the uptake of ^{111}In-anti-TNC-Fab and *green* color, the uptake of ^{99m}Tc-MIBI. *Yellow broken lines* circle myocardium. *White arrows* indicate sutured incision of the left intercostal space just below the myocardium. *(From Odaka K, Uehara T, Arano Y, et al: Noninvasive detection of cardiac repair after acute myocardial infarction in rats by ^{111}In-Fab fragment of monoclonal antibody specific for tenascin-C, Int Heart J 49:481–492, 2008. Reprinted with permission.)*

injury.[95,96] Other animal studies demonstrate that inhibition of apoptosis with caspase-inhibitors is cardioprotective.[97–99] There are also data that suggest early apoptosis may be the pathologic substrate leading from ischemia to necrosis.[100] An ability to assess cell death anywhere along the spectrum of apoptosis to necrosis would allow investigators to fine-tune a therapeutic regimen and optimize clinical outcome. In targeting these pathologies for new interventions, it is apparent that better in vivo imaging techniques for detection of apoptosis are required.

The earliest studies of apoptosis evolved around histologic assessment of the cells undergoing cell death. These descriptions included the microscopic visualization of chromatin condensation, dissolution of nuclear membrane, nuclear shrinkage, and formation of apoptotic bodies that were cleared by phagocytic cells.[101–103] Over time, it became evident that programmed cell death is central to the development and maintenance of homeostasis for any multicellular organism (Fig. 43-17).[104,105] In addition, cell death appears to play a role in the pathology of various disease states.[106] Depending on the initiating signals, there are two major pathways for cell death: intrinsic and extrinsic.[105] The intrinsic pathway is generated from within the cell through DNA damage, mitochondrial signals, and oncogene activation, leading to activation of caspase enzymes, cysteine proteases that cleave after aspartate residues. The extrinsic pathway is initiated through extracellular signals that target cell membrane receptors like Fas, a death receptor. The culmination of this event through either pathway is the activation of a key effector, caspase-3.[107]

Soon after the activation of caspase-3, the energy-dependent asymmetric distribution of phospholipids that enables the definition of various subregions within the lipid bilayer of cell membranes is lost. This leads to increased phosphatidyl serine (PS) on the outer cell membrane from its typical location on the inner cell membrane.[108] In part, this is the result of increased calcium levels and decreased amounts of ATP that block the translocase enzyme responsible for maintenance of PS. The exposure of PS on the surface of the cell makes it a target for binding the protein annexin V.[109] Annexin V binds to PS in a calcium-dependent manner. This has lead to an in vitro assay of Fas-ligand-initiated cell death through binding of annexin V.[108,110]

The first application of annexin binding to identify phosphatidyl serine on the surface of cells in a cardiovascular model came from a mouse model of acute MI.[111] In this study, the left anterior descending coronary artery of a series of mice was ligated shortly after the injection of biotinylated annexin V. Immunohistochemical analysis of the tissue distal to the site of ligation revealed annexin A5 binding in an area of cell death. DNA laddering confirmed programmed cell death to be occurring in the same region as the annexin A5 binding.

As myocardial ischemia or infarction persists, cells move from early apoptotic signals to complete necrosis. Breakdown of mitochondrial respiration and loss of membrane potential lead to the accumulation of calcium in the mitochondria of infarcted or severely injured myocardium.[112,113] With loss of membrane potential, cellular structures also begin to dissipate. Positively charged histones and other organelle proteins are

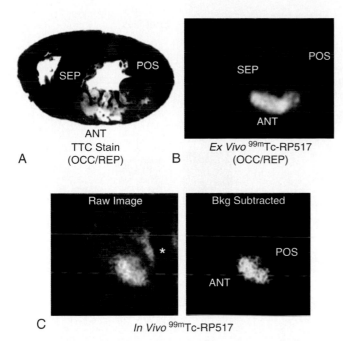

Figure 43-16 Imaging ischemic inflammation with the LTB$_4$ receptor antagonist RP517. TTC-stained heart slice (**A**) and ex vivo ^{99m}Tc-RP517 image (**B**) of the same heart slice. **C**, Raw *(left)* and background subtracted *(right)* in vivo ^{99m}Tc-RP517 images acquired from a dog 60 minutes after reperfusion. Background subtraction was performed to eliminate the surgically related tracer uptake in the field of view. The shadow on the raw image denoted by an *asterisk* is the metal rib spreader. Note that focal ^{99m}Tc-RP517 uptake was readily observed in the inflamed anteroseptal region of the heart on both ex vivo and in vivo images. Tracer uptake was negligible in the normal posterior wall. *(From Riou LM, Ruiz M, Sullivan GW, et al: Assessment of myocardial inflammation produced by experimental coronary occlusion and reperfusion with ^{99m}Tc-RP517, a new leukotriene B4 receptor antagonist that preferentially labels neutrophils in vivo, Circulation 106:592–598, 2002. Reprinted with permission.)*

exposed from the protection of their membrane barriers. These changes in early necrotic tissue have been utilized for imaging techniques that seek to identify early necrosis in acute MIs and are discussed in more detail below.

RADIOTRACER-BASED IMAGING IN APOPTOSIS AND NECROSIS

Annexin V

Initial studies utilized ^{99m}Tc-labeled annexin A5 for imaging the distribution of cells expressing PS noninvasively with a standard gamma camera. Radiolabeling involved derivatization of annexin A5 with hydrazinonicotinamide (HYNIC), which binds to reduced ^{99m}Tc.[114] The initial studies were carried out in mice with fulminant hepatic apoptosis through the injection of an anti-Fas antibody, which initiates an apoptotic cascade, particularly in hepatocytes.[115] Concomitant TUNEL studies confirmed localization of annexin A5 with apoptotic cells.

^{99m}Tc-labeled annexin V was subsequently utilized in humans to detect in vivo cell death in patients presenting with MI (Fig. 43-18).[116] Patients presenting with their first MI within 6 hours of symptom onset underwent standard revascularization with percutaneous intervention. Within 2 hours of revascularization, SPECT imaging was performed utilizing ^{99m}Tc-MIBI annexin V. This was followed by perfusion imaging 6 to 8 weeks after discharge using ^{99m}Tc-sestamibi. Regional retention of ^{99m}Tc-labeled annexin V correlated with the perfusion defect identified 6 to 8 weeks after discharge, providing a proof of concept that annexin V imaging can be utilized for noninvasive detection of myocardial cell death.

Heart transplant rejection is characterized by perivascular and interstitial mononuclear inflammatory infiltrates associated with myocyte apoptosis and necrosis.[117] In a study of 18 patients undergoing apoptotic imaging within 1 year of cardiac transplantation, annexin V retention correlated with the severity of rejection.[118] Patients with a negative scan had a concomitant negative biopsy. Of the five patients with a positive scan, three patients demonstrated regional uptake while two patients demonstrated diffuse uptake. The annexin V scans correlated with the degree of severity of rejection by biopsy specimens. The authors suggested that serial annexin V imaging for apoptotic cells could be used as a surrogate for detection of allograft rejection in place of serial biopsies in patients following heart transplantation.

Myocarditis is another pathologic condition where apoptosis is known to occur.[119] In a rat model of autoimmune myocarditis, ^{99m}Tc-labeled annexin V retention corresponded to histologic TUNEL staining for areas of myocardial apoptosis. Interestingly, ^{99m}Tc-labeled annexin V–positive areas could be differentiated from areas of inflammation identified by carbon-14 (^{14}C)-labeled deoxyglucose, reflecting foci of inflammation. This suggests that one could potentially differentiate between inflammation and active apoptosis with dual-isotope molecular imaging. To date, no studies have attempted to employ this technique in conjunction with FDG PET in human cases of myocarditis.

Caspase Inhibitors

Because phosphatidyl serine can be exposed on the surface of cells in physiologic conditions other than apoptosis, there is interest in developing more-specific apoptosis tracers. Recently, caspase-3 inhibitors have been synthesized and labeled with ^{18}F as potential PET tracers for in vivo imaging of apoptosis (see Fig. 43-17).[120,121] These caspase-3-targeted tracers have shown favorable biodistribution and clearance. MicroPET imaging in a murine model of hepatic apoptosis has shown specificity of the tracer to the liver; however, more studies are needed to assess binding relative to activated caspase density. In addition, further analysis in cardiovascular models will be necessary to determine feasibility of utilizing this new class of tracers for cardiac applications in humans.

Pyrophosphate and Glucarate

The in vivo noninvasive detection MI will allow for early diagnosis and treatment in patients when

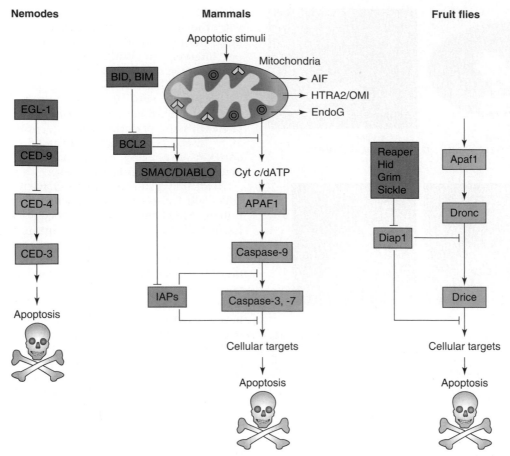

Nemodes

Mammals

Fruit flies

Figure 43-17 A conserved apoptotic pathway in nematodes, mammals, and fruit flies. Functional homologs of caspases and caspase regulators across species are indicated by the same color. Caspase-9 in mammals and Dronc in the fruit fly, *Drosophila melanogaster*, are initiator caspases, whereas caspase-3 and -7 in mammals and Drice in fruit flies belong to the class of effector caspases. CED-3 (cell-death abnormality-3) in the nematode worm, *Caenorhabditis elegans*, functions both as an initiator and effector caspase. The inhibitor of apoptosis (IAP) proteins suppresses apoptosis by negatively regulating the caspases, whereas SMAC (second mitochondria-derived activator of caspases)/DIABLO (direct IAP-binding protein with low pI) in mammals and the RHG proteins, Reaper, Hid, Grim, and Sickle, in fruit flies can remove the IAP-mediated negative regulation of caspases. AIF, apoptosis-inducing factor; APAF1, apoptotic-protease-activating factor-1; Cyt *c*, cytochrome *c*; EndoG, endonuclease G; HTRA2, high-temperature-requirement protein A2. *(From Riedl SJ, Shi Y: Molecular mechanisms of caspase regulation during apoptosis, Nat Rev Mol Cell Biol 5:897–907, 2004. Reprinted with permission.)*

electrocardiographic changes may not be evident, or when biomarkers may not distinguish between ischemic injury associated with acute plaque rupture that may be treatable with mechanical revascularization versus unstable angina and demand-related ischemia. In addition to visualizing apoptosis, several studies have demonstrated that certain agents allow for the visualization of ongoing myocardial necrosis as a mechanism of identifying acute infarction, potentially even in the presence of prior MI. ^{99m}Tc-labeled pyrophosphate has been shown to bind to areas of necrosis and is thought to bind exposed mitochondrial calcium.[112,113] ^{99m}Tc-pyrophosphate has a moderate degree of sensitivity for acute infarction, depending on the presence of Q-wave infarction or a non-ST-elevation infarction.[122] The specificity for acute MI is considered to be between 60% and 80%. The primary reason why ^{99m}Tc-pyrophosphate has not gained widespread clinical use is the limitation in the detection of early infarction. In fact, depending on the residual degree of perfusion to the infarct zone, the test may not be positive for the first 24 hours.

[99m]Tc-glucarate imaging provides an alternative to ^{99m}Tc-pyrophosphate imaging for the detection of acute infarction.[113] ^{99m}Tc-glucarate enters the necrotic cells by passive diffusion following breakdown of the sarcolemma, then binds to exposed histones in the nucleus of the myocytes. Canine models for ischemia and infarction reveal a high affinity of ^{99m}Tc-glucarate for necrotic tissue over ischemic but viable myocardium.[123] Moreover, establishing partial reperfusion did not inhibit the ability to detect acute infarct in canines (Fig. 43-19).[124] In a rabbit model of infarction, ^{99m}Tc-glucarate did not accumulate in areas of ischemia and could be imaged in areas of infarction as early as 10 minutes after reperfusion and within 30 to 60 minutes in nonreperfused zones.[125] Initial data in patients revealed that ^{99m}Tc-glucarate is able to noninvasively diagnose MI in patients presenting with chest pain, with a sensitivity that is dependent on the onset of symptoms, specifically within the first 9 hours of symptom onset.[126] ^{99m}Tc-glucarate also demonstrates rapid blood clearance and good target-to-background signal. ^{99m}Tc-glucarate

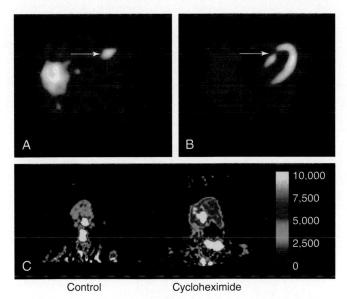

Figure 43-18 In vivo imaging of apoptosis. **A-B**: Transverse tomographic images of acute anteroseptal infarction in a patient. **A**, *Arrow* shows increased ^{99m}Tc-labeled annexin V uptake in the anteroseptal region 22 hours after reperfusion. **B**, Perfusion scintigraphy with sestamibi 6 to 8 weeks after discharge shows an irreversible perfusion defect that coincides with the area of increased ^{99m}Tc-labeled annexin V uptake *(arrow)*. **C**, *(lower panel)* Whole-body MicroPET images of caspase-3-specific inhibitor, ^{18}F-WC-II-89, distribution in a control rat *(left)* and cycloheximide-treated rat *(right)*. Images were summed from 10 to 60 minutes after intravenous injection of approximately 150 µCi of ^{18}F-WC-II-89. *(**A, B** from Hofstra L, Liem IH, Dumont EA, et al: Visualisation of cell death in vivo in patients with acute myocardial infarction, Lancet 356:209–212, 2000. **C** from Zhou D, Chu W, Rothfuss J, et al: Synthesis, radiolabeling, and in vivo evaluation of an ^{18}F-labeled isatin analog for imaging caspase-3 activation in apoptosis, Bioorg Med Chem Lett 16:5041–5046, 2006. Reprinted with permission.)*

imaging is currently under investigation as a tool to detect early infarction in a number of clinical trials.

CONCLUSIONS

Molecular imaging represents a targeted approach to noninvasively assess biological processes of the myocardium in vivo. The goal of molecular imaging is to develop an approach to studying not only the disease process but, more important, the efficacy of an individually tailored therapeutic regimen. The relatively high sensitivity of radiotracer-based imaging systems such as SPECT and PET has been of great use in the practical application of molecular imaging techniques. Research has demonstrated the feasibility of targeted imaging approaches in the evaluation of angiogenesis, ventricular remodeling, inflammation, and apoptosis. Studies in humans are actively being pursued in several of these areas. By combining nuclear and CT imaging modalities, issues of attenuation artifact or partial volume effect are being overcome. There is also improvement in the quantitative accuracy of these hybrid systems. In addition to the evolution of hybrid imaging systems, imaging protocols that include application of dual isotopes for monitoring physiologic parameters (metabolism or perfusion) with targeted molecular probes show promise in the areas of MI and angiogenesis. Tailoring gene therapy with PET reporter constructs is an active area of research with regard to the optimization of therapeutic angiogenesis. A role for apoptotic imaging in understanding reperfusion injury and the effects of therapeutic interventions, or in identifying the presence and severity of graft rejection following cardiac transplantation without the need for biopsy, shows some promise.

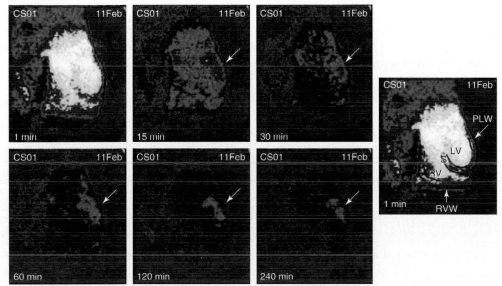

Figure 43-19 In vivo serial gamma camera ^{99m}Tc-glucarate scintigraphic images of a single heart, acquired at 1, 15, 30, 60, 120, and 240 minutes after tracer injection. A hot spot is clearly visualized involving the lateral wall at 30 minutes and persists to 240 minutes *(arrow)*. The schematic diagram at the *far right* shows the location of the right ventricular cavity (RV), septal wall (S), left ventricular cavity (LV), right ventricular free wall (RVW), and left ventricular posterolateral wall (PLW). *(From Johnson G III, Okada CC, Hocherman SD, et al: (99m)Tc-glucarate imaging for the early detection of infarct in partially reperfused canine myocardium, Eur J Nucl Med Mol Imaging 33:319–328, 2006. Reprinted with permission.)*

Imaging the activation of matrix metalloproteinases, active factor XIII, or the levels of renin-angiotensin system during ventricular remodeling may guide therapeutic regimens that could help positively influence outcomes post-infarction. There are early data in this regard using ACE inhibitor therapy and integrin imaging. In summary, targeted radiotracer-based molecular imaging is rapidly becoming feasible and will likely play a more important role in the evaluation and management of cardiovascular disease, including the future investigation of novel genetic or cell-based therapeutic interventions.

REFERENCES

1. Pichler A, Piwnica-Worms D: Overview of cardiovascular molecular imaging. In Gropler RJ, Glover DK, Sinusas AJ, et al: *Cardiovascular molecular imaging*, New York, 2007, Informa Healthcare U.S.A., Inc, pp 1–8.
2. Sinusas AJ, Bengel F, Nahrendorf M, et al: Multimodality cardiovascular molecular imaging, Part I, *Circ Cardiovasc Imaging* 1:244–256, 2008.
3. Hansson GK: Inflammation, atherosclerosis, and coronary artery disease, *N Engl J Med* 352:1685–1695, 2005.
4. Weber C, Zernecke A, Libby P: The multifaceted contributions of leukocyte subsets to atherosclerosis: lessons from mouse models, *Nat Rev Immunol* 8:802–815, 2008.
5. Fam NP, Verma S, Kutryk M, et al: Clinician guide to angiogenesis, *Circulation* 108:2613–2618, 2003.
6. Cai W, Chen X: Multimodality molecular imaging of tumor angiogenesis, *J Nucl Med* 49(Suppl 2):113S–128S, 2008.
7. Kerbel RS: Tumor angiogenesis, *N Engl J Med* 358:2039–2049, 2008.
8. Sasayama S, Fujita M: Recent insights into coronary collateral circulation, *Circulation* 85:1197–1204, 1992.
9. Dufraine J, Funahashi Y, Kitajewski J: Notch signaling regulates tumor angiogenesis by diverse mechanisms, *Oncogene* 27:5132–5137, 2008.
10. Shweiki D, Itin A, Soffer D, et al: Vascular endothelial growth factor induced by hypoxia may mediate hypoxia-initiated angiogenesis, *Nature* 359:843–845, 1992.
11. Lee SH, Wolf PL, Escudero R, et al: Early expression of angiogenesis factors in acute myocardial ischemia and infarction, *N Engl J Med* 342:626–633, 2000.
12. Semenza GL: Life with oxygen, *Science* 318:62–64, 2007.
13. Brogi E, Schatteman G, Wu T, et al: Hypoxia-induced paracrine regulation of vascular endothelial growth factor receptor expression, *J Clin Invest* 97:469–476, 1996.
14. Banai S, Jaklitsch MT, Shou M, et al: Angiogenic-induced enhancement of collateral blood flow to ischemic myocardium by vascular endothelial growth factor in dogs, *Circulation* 89:2183–2189, 1994.
15. Li J, Brown LF, Hibberd MG, et al: VEGF, flk-1, and flt-1 expression in a rat myocardial infarction model of angiogenesis, *Am J Physiol* 270:H1803–H1811, 1996.
16. Hu CJ, Iyer S, Sataur A, et al: Differential regulation of the transcriptional activities of hypoxia-inducible factor 1 alpha (HIF-1alpha) and HIF-2alpha in stem cells, *Mol Cell Biol* 26:3514–3526, 2006.
17. Ferrara N, Gerber HP, LeCouter J: The biology of VEGF and its receptors, *Nat Med* 9:669–676, 2003.
18. Giordano FJ, Ping P, McKirnan MD, et al: Intracoronary gene transfer of fibroblast growth factor-5 increases blood flow and contractile function in an ischemic region of the heart, *Nat Med* 2:534–539, 1996.
19. Simons M, Annex BH, Laham RJ, et al: Pharmacological treatment of coronary artery disease with recombinant fibroblast growth factor-2: double-blind, randomized, controlled clinical trial, *Circulation* 105:788–793, 2002.
20. Grines CL, Watkins MW, Helmer G, et al: Angiogenic Gene Therapy (AGENT) trial in patients with stable angina pectoris, *Circulation* 105:1291–1297, 2002.
21. Henry TD, Annex BH, McKendall GR, et al: The VIVA trial: Vascular endothelial growth factor in Ischemia for Vascular Angiogenesis, *Circulation* 107:1359–1365, 2003.
22. Stewart DJ, Hilton JD, Arnold JM, et al: Angiogenic gene therapy in patients with nonrevascularizable ischemic heart disease: a phase 2 randomized, controlled trial of AdVEGF(121) (AdVEGF121) versus maximum medical treatment, *Gene Ther* 13:1503–1511, 2006.
23. Kastrup J, Jorgensen E, Ruck A, et al: Direct intramyocardial plasmid vascular endothelial growth factor-A165 gene therapy in patients with stable severe angina pectoris A randomized double-blind placebo-controlled study: the Euroinject One trial, *J Am Coll Cardiol* 45:982–988, 2005.
24. Hanahan D: Signaling vascular morphogenesis and maintenance, *Science* 277:48–50, 1997.
25. Oliner J, Min H, Leal J, et al: Suppression of angiogenesis and tumor growth by selective inhibition of angiopoietin-2, *Cancer Cell* 6:507–516, 2004.
26. Zacchigna S, Tasciotti E, Kusmic C, et al: In vivo imaging shows abnormal function of vascular endothelial growth factor-induced vasculature, *Hum Gene Ther* 18:515–524, 2007.
27. Gale NW, Dominguez MG, Noguera I, et al: Haploinsufficiency of delta-like 4 ligand results in embryonic lethality due to major defects in arterial and vascular development, *Proc Natl Acad Sci U S A* 101:15949–15954, 2004.
28. Lobov IB, Renard RA, Papadopoulos N, et al: Delta-like ligand 4 (Dll4) is induced by VEGF as a negative regulator of angiogenic sprouting, *Proc Natl Acad Sci U S A* 104:3219–3224, 2007.
29. Noguera-Troise I, Daly C, Papadopoulos NJ, et al: Blockade of Dll4 inhibits tumour growth by promoting non-productive angiogenesis, *Nature* 444:1032–1037, 2006.
30. Sainson RC, Harris AL: Anti-Dll4 therapy: can we block tumour growth by increasing angiogenesis?*Trends Mol Med* 13:389–395, 2007.
31. Xiong JP, Stehle T, Diefenbach B, et al: Crystal structure of the extracellular segment of integrin alpha$_v$beta$_3$, *Science* 294:339–345, 2001.
32. Brooks PC, Montgomery AM, Rosenfeld M, et al: Integrin alpha v beta 3 antagonists promote tumor regression by inducing apoptosis of angiogenic blood vessels, *Cell* 79:1157–1164, 1994.
33. Schwartz MA, Schaller MD, Ginsberg MH: Integrins: emerging paradigms of signal transduction, *Annu Rev Cell Dev Biol* 11:549–599, 1995.
34. Hynes RO: Integrins: bidirectional, allosteric signaling machines, *Cell* 110:673–687, 2002.
35. Clyman RI, Mauray F, Kramer RH: Beta 1 and beta 3 integrins have different roles in the adhesion and migration of vascular smooth muscle cells on extracellular matrix, *Exp Cell Res* 200:272–284, 1992.
36. Li J, Brown LF, Laham RJ, et al: Macrophage-dependent regulation of syndecan gene expression, *Circ Res* 81:785–796, 1997.
37. Bhagwat SV, Lahdenranta J, Giordano R, et al: CD13/APN is activated by angiogenic signals and is essential for capillary tube formation, *Blood* 97:652–659, 2001.
38. Bergers G, Song S, Meyer-Morse N, et al: Benefits of targeting both pericytes and endothelial cells in the tumor vasculature with kinase inhibitors, *J Clin Invest* 111:1287–1295, 2003.
39. Lake Tahoe invitation meeting 2002: *J Nucl Cardiol* 10:223–257, 2003.
40. Lu E, Wagner WR, Schellenberger U, et al: Targeted in vivo labeling of receptors for vascular endothelial growth factor: approach to identification of ischemic tissue, *Circulation* 108:97–103, 2003.
41. Rodriguez-Porcel M, Cai W, Gheysens O, et al: Imaging of VEGF receptor in a rat myocardial infarction model using PET, *J Nucl Med* 49:667–673, 2008.
42. Willmann JK, Chen K, Wang H, et al: Monitoring of the biological response to murine hindlimb ischemia with ^{64}Cu-labeled vascular endothelial growth factor-121 positron emission tomography, *Circulation* 117:915–922, 2008.
43. Wu JC, Inubushi M, Sundaresan G, et al: Positron emission tomography imaging of cardiac reporter gene expression in living rats, *Circulation* 106:180–183, 2002.
44. Inubushi M, Wu JC, Gambhir SS, et al: Positron-emission tomography reporter gene expression imaging in rat myocardium, *Circulation* 107:326–332, 2003.
45. Bengel FM, Anton M, Richter T, et al: Noninvasive imaging of transgene expression by use of positron emission tomography in a pig model of myocardial gene transfer, *Circulation* 108:2127–2133, 2003.
46. Wu JC, Chen IY, Wang Y, et al: Molecular imaging of the kinetics of vascular endothelial growth factor gene expression in ischemic myocardium, *Circulation* 110:685–691, 2004.
47. Sipkins DA, Cheresh DA, Kazemi MR, et al: Detection of tumor angiogenesis in vivo by alphaVbeta3-targeted magnetic resonance imaging, *Nat Med* 4:623–626, 1998.
48. Haubner R, Wester HJ, Weber WA, et al: Noninvasive imaging of alpha(v)beta(3) integrin expression using 18F-labeled RGD-containing glycopeptide and positron emission tomography, *Cancer Res* 61:1781–1785, 2001.
49. Haubner R, Wester HJ, Burkhart F, et al: Glycosylated RGD-containing peptides: tracer for tumor targeting and angiogenesis imaging with improved biokinetics, *J Nucl Med* 42:326–336, 2001.
50. Harris TD, Kalogeropoulos S, Nguyen T, et al: Design, synthesis, and evaluation of radiolabeled integrin alpha v beta 3 receptor antagonists for tumor imaging and radiotherapy, *Cancer Biother Radiopharm* 18:627–641, 2003.
51. Sadeghi M, Krassilnikova S, Zhang J, et al: Imaging of avb3 integrin in vascular injury: Does this reflect increased integrin expression or activation? *Circulation* 108:404, 2008.

52. Meoli DF, Sadeghi MM, Krassilnikova S, et al: Noninvasive imaging of myocardial angiogenesis following experimental myocardial infarction, *J Clin Invest* 113:1684–1691, 2004.

53. Kalinowski L, Dobrucki LW, Meoli DF, et al: Targeted imaging of hypoxia-induced integrin activation in myocardium early after infarction, *J Appl Physiol* 104:1504–1512, 2008.

54. Su H, Hu X, Bourke B, et al: Detection of myocardial angiogenesis in chronic infarction with a novel technetium-99m labeled peptide targeted at avb3 integrin, *Circulation* 108:278–279, 2003.

55. Makowski MR, Ebersberger U, Nekolla S, et al: In vivo molecular imaging of angiogenesis, targeting alphavbeta3 integrin expression, in a patient after acute myocardial infarction, *Eur Heart J* 29:2201, 2008.

56. Almutairi A, Rossin R, Shokeen M, et al: Biodegradable dendritic positron-emitting nanoprobes for the noninvasive imaging of angiogenesis, *Proc Natl Acad Sci U S A* 106:685–690, 2009.

57. Weber KT: Extracellular matrix remodeling in heart failure: a role for de novo angiotensin II generation, *Circulation* 96:4065–4082, 1997.

58. Sutton MG, Sharpe N: Left ventricular remodeling after myocardial infarction: pathophysiology and therapy, *Circulation* 101:2981–2988, 2000.

59. Creemers EE, Cleutjens JP, Smits JF, et al: Matrix metalloproteinase inhibition after myocardial infarction: a new approach to prevent heart failure? *Circ Res* 89:201–210, 2001.

60. Spinale FG: Matrix metalloproteinases: regulation and dysregulation in the failing heart, *Circ Res* 90:520–530, 2002.

61. Sternlicht MD, Werb Z: How matrix metalloproteinases regulate cell behavior, *Annu Rev Cell Dev Biol* 17:463–516, 2001.

62. Ducharme A, Frantz S, Aikawa M, et al: Targeted deletion of matrix metalloproteinase-9 attenuates left ventricular enlargement and collagen accumulation after experimental myocardial infarction, *J Clin Invest* 106:55–62, 2000.

63. Rohde LE, Ducharme A, Arroyo LH, et al: Matrix metalloproteinase inhibition attenuates early left ventricular enlargement after experimental myocardial infarction in mice, *Circulation* 99:3063–3070, 1999.

64. Lindsey ML, Gannon J, Aikawa M, et al: Selective matrix metalloproteinase inhibition reduces left ventricular remodeling but does not inhibit angiogenesis after myocardial infarction, *Circulation* 105:753–758, 2002.

65. Yarbrough WM, Mukherjee R, Escobar GP, et al: Selective targeting and timing of matrix metalloproteinase inhibition in post-myocardial infarction remodeling, *Circulation* 108:1753–1759, 2003.

66. Nahrendorf M, Hu K, Frantz S, et al: Factor XIII deficiency causes cardiac rupture, impairs wound healing, and aggravates cardiac remodeling in mice with myocardial infarction, *Circulation* 113:1196–1202, 2006.

67. Nahrendorf M, Aikawa E, Figueiredo JL, et al: Transglutaminase activity in acute infarcts predicts healing outcome and left ventricular remodelling: implications for FXIII therapy and antithrombin use in myocardial infarction, *Eur Heart J* 29:445–454, 2008.

68. Aras O, Messina SA, Shirani J, et al: The role and regulation of cardiac angiotensin-converting enzyme for noninvasive molecular imaging in heart failure, *Curr Cardiol Rep* 9:150–158, 2007.

69. Shirani J, Dilsizian V: Imaging left ventricular remodeling: targeting the neurohumoral axis, *Nat Clin Pract Cardiovasc Med* 2(Suppl 5):S57–S62, 2008.

70. Su H, Spinale FG, Dobrucki LW, et al: Noninvasive targeted imaging of matrix metalloproteinase activation in a murine model of postinfarction remodeling, *Circulation* 112:3157–3167, 2005.

71. Dilsizian V, Eckelman WC, Loredo ML, et al: Evidence for tissue angiotensin-converting enzyme in explanted hearts of ischemic cardiomyopathy using targeted radiotracer technique, *J Nucl Med* 48:182–187, 2007.

72. Shirani J, Narula J, Eckelman WC, et al: Early imaging in heart failure: exploring novel molecular targets, *J Nucl Cardiol* 14:100–110, 2007.

73. Cleutjens JP, Blankesteijn WM, Daemen MJ, et al: The infarcted myocardium: simply dead tissue, or a lively target for therapeutic interventions, *Cardiovasc Res* 44:232–241, 1999.

74. Asano Y, Ihn H, Yamane K, et al: Increased expression of integrin alpha(v)beta3 contributes to the establishment of autocrine TGF-beta signaling in scleroderma fibroblasts, *J Immunol* 175:7708–7718, 2005.

75. van den Borne SW, Isobe S, Verjans JW, et al: Molecular imaging of interstitial alterations in remodeling myocardium after myocardial infarction, *J Am Coll Cardiol* 52:2017–2028, 2008.

76. Peters AM, Danpure HJ, Osman S, et al: Clinical experience with 99mTc-hexamethylpropylene-amineoxime for labelling leucocytes and imaging inflammation, *Lancet* 2:946–949, 1986.

77. Peters AM, Saverymuttu SH: The value of indium-labelled leucocytes in clinical practice, *Blood Rev* 1:65–76, 1987.

78. Lavender JP, Lowe J, Barker JR, et al: Gallium 67 citrate scanning in neoplastic and inflammatory lesions, *Br J Radiol* 44:361–366, 1971.

79. Mochizuki T, Tsukamoto E, Kuge Y, et al: FDG uptake and glucose transporter subtype expressions in experimental tumor and inflammation models, *J Nucl Med* 42:1551–1555, 2001.

80. Kubota R, Yamada S, Kubota K, et al: Intratumoral distribution of fluorine-18-fluorodeoxyglucose in vivo: high accumulation in macrophages and granulation tissues studied by microautoradiography, *J Nucl Med* 33:1972–1980, 1992.

81. Johnson LL, Seldin DW, Becker LC, et al: Antimyosin imaging in acute transmural myocardial infarctions: results of a multicenter clinical trial, *J Am Coll Cardiol* 13:27–35, 1989.

82. Khaw BA, Gold HK, Yasuda T, et al: Scintigraphic quantification of myocardial necrosis in patients after intravenous injection of myosin-specific antibody, *Circulation* 74:501–508, 1986.

83. Yasuda T, Palacios IF, Dec GW, et al: Indium 111-monoclonal antimyosin antibody imaging in the diagnosis of acute myocarditis, *Circulation* 76:306–311, 1987.

84. Dec GW, Palacios I, Yasuda T, et al: Antimyosin antibody cardiac imaging: its role in the diagnosis of myocarditis, *J Am Coll Cardiol* 16:97–104, 1990.

85. Narula J, Khaw BA, Dec GW, et al: Diagnostic accuracy of antimyosin scintigraphy in suspected myocarditis, *J Nucl Cardiol* 3:371–381, 1996.

86. Sato M, Toyozaki T, Odaka K, et al: Detection of experimental autoimmune myocarditis in rats by 111In monoclonal antibody specific for tenascin-C, *Circulation* 106:1397–1402, 2002.

87. Odaka K, Uehara T, Arano Y, et al: Noninvasive detection of cardiac repair after acute myocardial infarction in rats by 111In Fab fragment of monoclonal antibody specific for tenascin-C, *Int Heart J* 49:481–492, 2008.

88. Ford-Hutchinson AW: Regulation of leukotriene biosynthesis, *Cancer Metastasis Rev* 13:257–267, 1994.

89. Yokomizo T, Izumi T, Shimizu T: Leukotriene B4: metabolism and signal transduction, *Arch Biochem Biophys* 385:231–241, 2001.

90. Serhan CN, Prescott SM: The scent of a phagocyte: Advances on leukotriene b(4) receptors, *J Exp Med* 192:F5–F8, 2000.

91. Brouwers AH, Laverman P, Boerman OC, et al: A 99Tcm-labelled leukotriene B4 receptor antagonist for scintigraphic detection of infection in rabbits, *Nucl Med Commun* 21:1043–1050, 2000.

92. Riou LM, Ruiz M, Sullivan GW, et al: Assessment of myocardial inflammation produced by experimental coronary occlusion and reperfusion with 99mTc-RP517, a new leukotriene B4 receptor antagonist that preferentially labels neutrophils in vivo, *Circulation* 106:592–598, 2002.

93. van Eerd JE, Oyen WJ, Harris TD, et al: A bivalent leukotriene B(4) antagonist for scintigraphic imaging of infectious foci, *J Nucl Med* 44:1087–1091, 2003.

94. Piot C, Croisille P, Staat P, et al: Effect of cyclosporine on reperfusion injury in acute myocardial infarction, *N Engl J Med* 359:473–481, 2008.

95. Fliss H, Gattinger D: Apoptosis in ischemic and reperfused rat myocardium, *Circ Res* 79:949–956, 1996.

96. Yellon DM, Hausenloy DJ: Myocardial reperfusion injury, *N Engl J Med* 357:1121–1135, 2007.

97. Yaoita H, Ogawa K, Maehara K, et al: Attenuation of ischemia/reperfusion injury in rats by a caspase inhibitor, *Circulation* 97:276–281, 1998.

98. Dumont EA, Reutelingsperger CP, Smits JF, et al: Real-time imaging of apoptotic cell-membrane changes at the single-cell level in the beating murine heart, *Nat Med* 7:1352–1355, 2001.

99. Hayakawa Y, Chandra M, Miao W, et al: Inhibition of cardiac myocyte apoptosis improves cardiac function and abolishes mortality in the peripartum cardiomyopathy of Galpha(q) transgenic mice, *Circulation* 108:3036–3041, 2003.

100. Thimister PW, Hofstra L, Liem IH, et al: In vivo detection of cell death in the area at risk in acute myocardial infarction, *J Nucl Med* 44:391–396, 2003.

101. Wyllie AH: Glucocorticoid-induced thymocyte apoptosis is associated with endogenous endonuclease activation, *Nature* 284:555–556, 1980.

102. Kerr JF, Wyllie AH, Currie AR: Apoptosis: a basic biological phenomenon with wide-ranging implications in tissue kinetics, *Br J Cancer* 26:239–257, 1972.

103. Wyllie AH, Kerr JF, Currie AR: Cell death: the significance of apoptosis, *Int Rev Cytol* 68:251–306, 1980.

104. Danial NN, Korsmeyer SJ: Cell death: critical control points, *Cell* 116:205–219, 2004.

105. Riedl SJ, Shi Y: Molecular mechanisms of caspase regulation during apoptosis, *Nat Rev Mol Cell Biol* 5:897–907, 2004.

106. Green DR, Kroemer G: The pathophysiology of mitochondrial cell death, *Science* 305:626–629, 2004.

107. Tait JF: Imaging of apoptosis, *J Nucl Med* 49:1573–1576, 2008.

108. Martin SJ, Reutelingsperger CP, McGahon AJ, et al: Early redistribution of plasma membrane phosphatidylserine is a general feature of apoptosis regardless of the initiating stimulus: inhibition by overexpression of Bcl-2 and Abl, *J Exp Med* 182:1545–1556, 1995.

109. Koopman G, Reutelingsperger CP, Kuijten GA, et al: Annexin V for flow cytometric detection of phosphatidylserine expression on B cells undergoing apoptosis, *Blood* 84:1415–1420, 1994.

110. van Engeland M, Ramaekers FC, Schutte B, et al: A novel assay to measure loss of plasma membrane asymmetry during apoptosis of adherent cells in culture, *Cytometry* 24:131–139, 1996.

111. Dumont EA, Hofstra L, van Heerde WL, et al: Cardiomyocyte death induced by myocardial ischemia and reperfusion: measurement with recombinant human annexin-V in a mouse model, *Circulation* 102:1564–1568, 2000.

112. Khaw BA: The current role of infarct avid imaging, *Semin Nucl Med* 29:259–270, 1999.

113. Flotats A, Carrio I: Non-invasive in vivo imaging of myocardial apoptosis and necrosis, *Eur J Nucl Med Mol Imaging* 30:615–630, 2003.

114. Blankenberg FG, Katsikis PD, Tait JF, et al: In vivo detection and imaging of phosphatidylserine expression during programmed cell death, *Proc Natl Acad Sci U S A* 95:6349–6354, 1998.

115. Ogasawara J, Watanabe-Fukunaga R, Adachi M, et al: Lethal effect of the anti-Fas antibody in mice, *Nature* 364:806–809, 1993.

116. Hofstra L, Liem IH, Dumont EA, et al: Visualisation of cell death in vivo in patients with acute myocardial infarction, *Lancet* 356:209–212, 2000.

117. Laguens RP, Meckert PM, Martino JS, et al: Identification of programmed cell death (apoptosis) in situ by means of specific labeling of nuclear DNA fragments in heart biopsy samples during acute rejection episodes, *J Heart Lung Transplant* 15:911–918, 1996.

118. Narula J, Acio ER, Narula N, et al: Annexin-V imaging for noninvasive detection of cardiac allograft rejection, *Nat Med* 7:1347–1352, 2001.

119. Tokita N, Hasegawa S, Tsujimura E, et al: Serial changes in ^{14}C-deoxy-glucose and ^{201}Tl uptake in autoimmune myocarditis in rats, *J Nucl Med* 42:285–291, 2001.

120. Faust A, Wagner S, Law MP, et al: The nonpeptidyl caspase binding radioligand (S)-1-(4-(2-[^{18}F]Fluoroethoxy)-benzyl)-5-[1-(2-methoxy-methylpyrrolidinyl)s ulfonyl]isatin ([^{18}F]CbR) as potential positron emission tomography-compatible apoptosis imaging agent, *Q J Nucl Med Mol Imaging* 51:67–73, 2007.

121. Zhou D, Chu W, Rothfuss J, et al: Synthesis, radiolabeling, and in vivo evaluation of an ^{18}F-labeled isatin analog for imaging caspase-3 activation in apoptosis, *Bioorg Med Chem Lett* 16:5041–5046, 2006.

122. Corbett JR, Lewis M, Willerson JT, et al: ^{99m}Tc-pyrophosphate imaging in patients with acute myocardial infarction: comparison of planar imaging with single-photon tomography with and without blood pool overlay, *Circulation* 69:1120–1128, 1984.

123. Orlandi C, Crane PD, Edwards DS, et al: Early scintigraphic detection of experimental myocardial infarction in dogs with technetium-99m-glucaric acid, *J Nucl Med* 32:263–268, 1991.

124. Johnson G III, Okada CC, Hocherman SD, et al: (99m)Tc-glucarate imaging for the early detection of infarct in partially reperfused canine myocardium, *Eur J Nucl Med Mol Imaging* 33:319–328, 2006.

125. Narula J, Petrov A, Pak KY, et al: Very early noninvasive detection of acute experimental nonreperfused myocardial infarction with ^{99m}Tc-labeled glucarate, *Circulation* 95:1577–1584, 1997.

126. Mariani G, Villa G, Rossettin PF, et al: Detection of acute myocardial infarction by ^{99m}Tc-labeled D-glucaric acid imaging in patients with acute chest pain, *J Nucl Med* 40:1832–1839, 1999.

Radionuclide Imaging of Inflammation in Atheroma

H. WILLIAM STRAUSS, JOHAN W.H. VERJANS, BARRY L. ZARET
AND JAGAT NARULA

INTRODUCTION

Over 16 million people in the United States[1] are afflicted with coronary artery disease. Approximately 785,000 of these individuals will experience a sudden coronary event in 2009, and about 152,000 will succumb to the acute process. Although identification of each person at risk is the ultimate clinical goal, it is most desirable to definitively identify the subset of patients who are most likely to suffer an acute coronary event. In 60% to 80% of patients, the acute event is caused by thrombotic occlusion of the vessel due to rupture of an atheroma in the coronary artery; in a minority (especially patients < 50 years old and smokers), the occlusion results from erosion of endothelial cells overlying the plaque (likely due to apoptosis of endothelial cells, exposing thrombogenic proteoglycans and microparticulates[2]). Lesions undergoing plaque rupture occupy a significant fraction of the circumference of the vessel, contain numerous inflammatory cells in the necrotic core, have a thin cap (<65 μm) separating the atheroma from blood in the vessel lumen, and have a marked increase in vasa vasorum.[3] Diagnostic targeting strategies should identify plaques vulnerable to rupture or endothelial erosion.

EVOLUTION OF ATHEROSCLEROTIC LESIONS

The American Heart Association (AHA) classifies atherosclerotic lesions from type I through VI based on the severity of the disease (Fig. 44-1).[4] Type I plaque is an adaptive lesion consisting mostly of smooth muscle cells (SMC) with or without scattered macrophage infiltration. Type II plaque is a fatty streak consisting of foam cell infiltration. Type III plaque shows pools of extracellular lipid, but no

necrotic core is formed; the extracellular matrix predominantly consists of proteoglycans. Type IV plaque has a well-defined necrotic core with overlying fibrous cap consisting of SMC and evolving collagenous matrix. Type V lesions demonstrate a thick fibrous cap consisting of a predominantly fibrotic lesion (type Vc) with calcification (type Vb) or deep-seated necrotic core (type Va). Type VI is a classic plaque rupture that shows a region of fibrous cap disruption that allows continuation between the necrotic core and overlying luminal thrombus. Although this histologic classification has neat groupings, clinically, patients do not progress linearly from types I to VI. To make the classification more relevant, several authors have proposed modifications to this classification system. One such classification suggested by Virmani and colleagues[5] classifies lesions based on the morphologic description of the fibrous cap and neointima and their progression to complicated lesions. They have categorized atherosclerotic plaques as "intimal thickening" (equivalent to AHA type I), "intimal xanthoma" (type II), "pathologic intimal thickening" (type III), and "fibrous cap atheroma" (similar to types IV and V). The unique features of the Virmani classification include linking of pathologic intimal thickening (SMC + proteoglycan-rich lesions, equivalent to AHA type III) to acute coronary syndromes associated with plaque erosion, and description of an entity referred to as *thin fibrous cap atheroma*. The latter is a precursor of plaque rupture–related acute coronary syndromes. This classification has incorporated repeated cycles of healing on plaque ruptures and erosions toward development of more advanced lesions. On the other hand, the newer classification also assigns significance to calcific nodules in predisposition to the luminal thrombus. The morphologic characteristics of the atherosclerotic lesions described in the new classification are compared with the AHA classification in Figure 44-1.

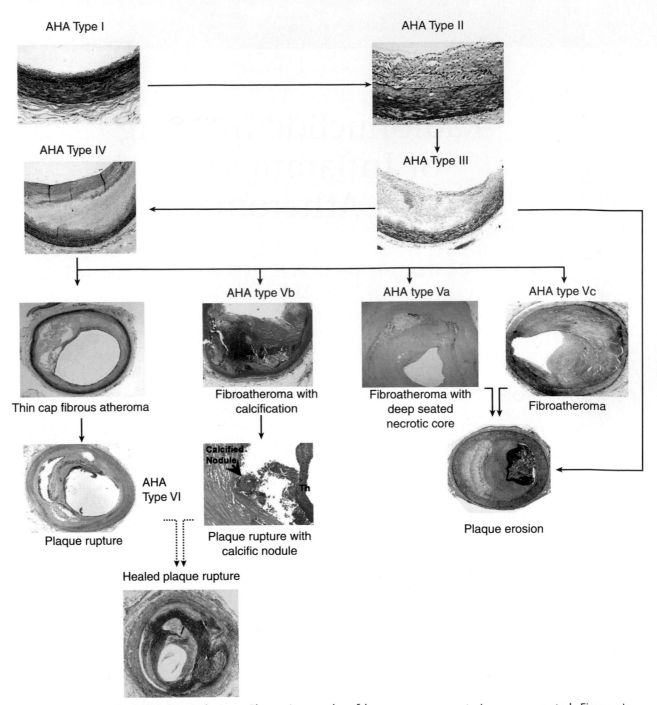

AHA Type I

AHA Type II

AHA Type IV

AHA Type III

AHA type Vb

AHA type Va

AHA type Vc

Thin cap fibrous atheroma

Fibroatheroma with calcification

Fibroatheroma with deep seated necrotic core

Fibroatheroma

Plaque rupture

AHA Type VI

Calcified Nodule

Th

Plaque rupture with calcific nodule

Plaque erosion

Healed plaque rupture

Figure 44-1 Pathology of atherosclerotic lesions. Photomicrographs of human coronary arteries are presented. Figure also represents the possible sequence of evolution of lesions and association of complications with underlying disease. More descriptive terms have been used in recently suggested classification by Virmani et al. *(Microphotographs courtesy of Dr. Renu Virmani.)*

PATHOGENETIC BASIS OF INFLAMMATION IN ATHEROSCLEROSIS

Atherosclerosis involves both an inflammatory response to lipid deposition in the vessel wall and an immunologic response of the endothelium to the injury. Damage to the vascular intima is initiated by various factors, including shear stress and, most important, hyperlipidemia.[6-8] Endothelial damage causes expression of selectins and adhesion molecules by the endothelial cell. These chemotactic factors cause recruitment of circulating monocytes to the region of injury; these cells migrate into the subendothelial layer. There, the short-lived monocytes are transformed into long-lived macrophages.[9] The macrophages phagocytize and start to metabolize low-density lipoprotein (LDL) cholesterol. In the process of metabolism, oxidative products are generated, leading to the formation of oxidized LDL cholesterol, both in the intracellular and extracellular environment. Oxidized LDL cholesterol causes greater inflammation, is difficult to metabolize, and in high concentration is toxic to the macrophages. Modified (mainly oxidized) LDL enters the macrophages through scavenger LDL receptors, which are not inhibited by the intracellular lipid contents, allowing the cells to continue gorging themselves on this relatively indigestible irritant. As large quantities of LDL cholesterol and oxidized LDL cholesterol accumulate in the macrophages, they become lipid-laden foam cells. Large quantities of intracellular oxidized LDL cholesterol causes death of the macrophages, in part by apoptosis[10] and in part due to necrosis. Part of the process of apoptosis is production of caspase-1 by the mitochondria of the macrophage. Caspase-1 production is associated with increased production of matrix metalloproteinases, resulting in degradation of stromal tissue containing the lesion.[11] These foam cells are restricted from moving away from the subintimal space. Concurrent with the release of selectins and attraction of monocytes to the site of injury, the injured endothelium releases substances that induce phenotypic alteration of medial SMC from contractile cells to the proliferating phenotype. The transformed smooth muscle cells migrate to the neointima.

The macrophage infiltration in the vessel wall follows a systematic process that includes reversible adhesion of the monocytes to the injured endothelium, followed by monocytic activation, leading to a more permanent binding and eventual subendothelial migration of monocytes (Fig. 44-2).[12] The initial injury to endothelial cells induces expression of integrin molecules such as E-selectin or P-selectin. Corresponding integrin moieties on the monocytes, such as L-selectin, facilitate interdigitating interaction between the endothelium and circulating monocytes that slows the monocytes as they

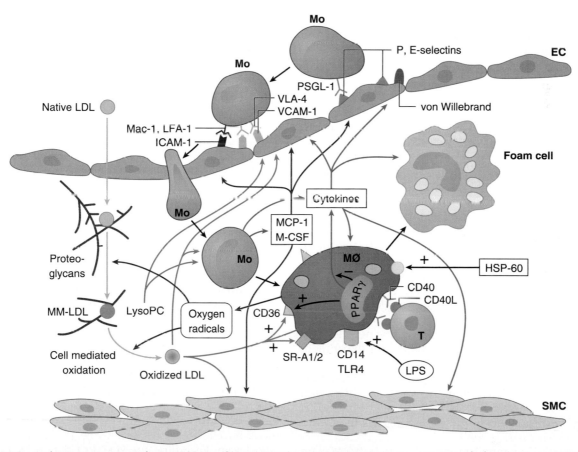

Figure 44-2 Multistage monocyte/macrophage infiltration in the atherosclerotic lesion. Stages include selectin molecule–based adherence of monocytes to endothelium, followed by firm engagement secondary to monocyte chemoattractant protein interaction and adhesion molecules expression. Passage to subintima is affected by cadherins, and resident monocytes develop novel receptors (CD36 and SR-A) for modified low-density lipoprotein (LDL). Macrophages are ultimately turned into foam cells. This process may be accelerated by macrophage colony stimulating factor (M-CSF), by lipopolysaccharide (LPS) via the receptor CD14 in conjunction with toll-like receptor 4 (TLR4), by heat shock protein (HSP-60) via CD14, and by platelet-activating factor and cytokines released from macrophages in an autocrine loop. Peroxisome proliferator-activated receptor-γ (PPARγ) is activated by LDL, leading to up-regulation of CD36 and down-regulation of cytokine release. Cytokines are released from macrophages; T lymphocytes are acting in concert on foam cells and on smooth muscle cells and endothelial cells (EC). T-cell mobilization and activation leads to secretion of the cytokine interferon-γ, which primes the macrophages, rendering them more susceptible to TLR-dependent activation. Activated T cells also express CD40 ligand (CD40L), which ligates its receptor CD40 on macrophages. Chemoattractants released from LDL, macrophages, and foam cells (MCP-1) promote further monocyte recruitment to the intima. Foam cells derived from smooth muscle cells, together with those derived from macrophages, generate the fatty lesion. (From Österud B, Bjorklid E: Role of monocytes in atherogenesis, Physiol Rev 83:1069–1112, 2003.)

start to roll along the vessel wall. Chemotactic peptides cause the monocytes to adhere to the injured endothelium. In the absence of chemoattractants, the selectins are shed, and the monocytes roll back to the bloodstream. The interaction of the endothelial chemoattractants and their receptors on monocytes lead to activation of β_1- or β_2-integrins (such as LFA-1, VLA-4, or Mac-1). These integrins bind firmly to endothelial expression of adhesion molecules of an immunoglobulin gene superfamily such as intercellular adhesion molecule 1 (ICAM-1), ICAM-2, and VCAM-1. The multipronged attachment of the monocytes to the endothelium commits monocytes to permeate through the endothelial cell junctions, mediated by co-adherins. In addition to the monocyte/macrophage infiltration, both PMNs and mast cells appear to play important roles in plaque rupture. Immune histology studies demonstrated that mast cells localize in the shoulders and cap of the plaque, suggesting a role for these cathepsin G–producing cells in plaque rupture.[13]

APPROACHES TO IMAGING ATHEROMA

There have been multiple radionuclide approaches to imaging atheroma:

1. Platelets radiolabeled with indium-111 (^{111}In) (1978)[14] identify actively forming thrombi on atheroma. This approach identifies lesions in their late phase and has limited clinical utility.
2. Low density lipoprotein radiolabeled with iodine-125 (^{125}I) (1983)[15] and technetium-99m (^{99m}Tc),[16] as well as oxidized LDL labeled with ^{99m}Tc (1996),[17] define the exchange of lipoproteins within the lesions. Despite their large size, these molecules diffuse into the lesions, reaching equilibrium in about 2 days.
3. Radiolabeled antibody recognizing a unique epitope expressed when vascular smooth muscle changes from the contractile to the proliferative phenotype in the atheroma (1995),[18] (1998).[19] This change in epitope occurs in advanced lesions, making this agent a useful marker for experimental studies.
4. Increased expression of receptors for chemoattractant peptides such as monocyte chemoattractant peptide-1[20] (2001). The receptors, called *CCR2*, are up-regulated on mononuclear cells in regions of atheroma (Fig. 44-3).[21]
5. Increased metabolism of inflammatory cells in atheroma (1996),[22] (2001),[23] (2002),[24] (2004),[25] (2005),[26,27] (2008).[28] This approach utilizes the glucose analog FDG (fluorine-18-labeled [^{18}F] fluorodeoxyglucose) and positron emission tomography (PET). Macrophages in atheroma require exogenous glucose for their metabolism, hence the localization of this glucose analog at sites of moderate to severe vascular inflammation. The integration of PET and computed tomography (CT) allows more precise localization of the lesions for evaluation of their metabolism.
6. Apoptosis of inflammatory cells in the plaque (2003),[29] (2009).[30] This approach will likely identify advanced lesions. Although laboratory studies have identified significantly greater concentration of radiolabeled annexin in experimental atheroma, the small but significant concentration of the tracer in adjacent background structures will make reliable imaging in humans challenging.
7. Metabolically active atheromas express high levels of matrix metalloproteinase (MMP). Radiolabeled MMP inhibitors have been advocated to identify MMP in the lesions (2008).[31]

Since inflammation is a major component of vulnerability, determining the metabolic activity of the lesion may be the most effective approach to specifically identifying vulnerable plaque with high specificity. An additional advantage of evaluating metabolic activity in a plaque with FDG is the technical benefit of the resolution of PET. Current PET imaging devices have a spatial resolution of under 4 mm, approximately twice the resolution of SPECT. In addition, the count density of PET images is about 10-fold greater than SPECT images, allowing greater certainty of lesion identification.

IMAGING INFLAMMATION IN CORONARY ATHEROMA

Even with PET technology, imaging inflammation in coronary atheroma is technically difficult. Histologic studies suggest that the average length of a necrotic core in atheromas of patients dying from an acute coronary event is about 8 mm, and the lesion typically occupies less than half of the 3- to 4-mm diameter circumference of the vessel.[32,33] The spatial resolution of a state-of-the-art PET scanner is approximately 4 mm. As a result, the combination of small lesion size and limited spatial resolution (without considering approaches to eliminate respiratory and cardiac motion) make coronary atheroma inflammation imaging a substantial challenge. In spite of the resolution problem(s), the technique works because of the extremely high concentration of the metabolic tracer achieved in the highly activated cells. The primary energy source of activated macrophages in the lesion is glucose. The glucose is delivered to the macrophages both by vasa vasorum and less efficiently by diffusion from extracellular fluids. The numerous activated macrophages in the core concentrate a sufficient amount of the glucose analog, FDG, following intravenous injection of the tracer to be readily visualized on a PET scan. Recording the FDG PET data with a contemporaneous CT scan for anatomic localization provides the most precise information (Fig. 44-4). Although imaging the coronaries is the goal of vascular inflammation imaging, most investigators are applying FDG vascular imaging in vessels of larger diameter, such as the aorta, carotids, and iliac arteries, in part as a surrogate for coronary imaging.

The feasibility of FDG imaging of experimental atheroma was reported by Vallabhajosula and Fuster in 1996 and 1997.[34,35] Subsequent observations demonstrated multiple focal sites of FDG uptake in the aorta of

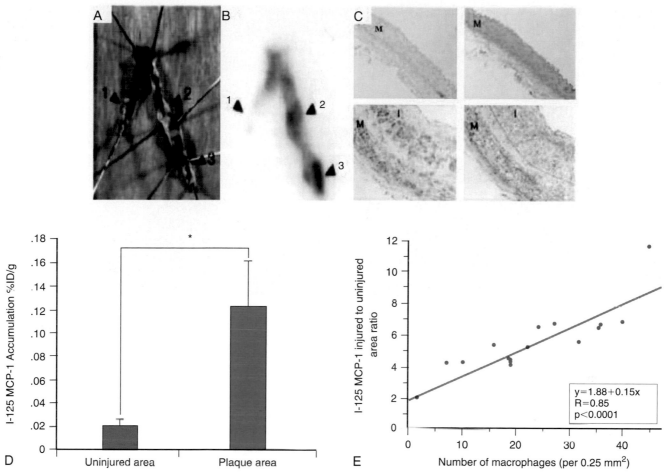

Figure 44-3 Localization of intraplaque inflammation by noninvasive imaging for macrophage (MCP) receptor up-regulation. In the injured regions, three levels of radioactivity are seen (*left*). The regions with most intense accumulation of iodine-125 (I-125) MCP-1 radioactivity (region 3) demonstrated intense macrophage infiltration. The areas of moderate radioactivity (region 2) had moderate macrophage infiltration, and the regions with least activity showed no inflammation. The maximum lesion/normal vessel ratio of I-125 MCP-1 in the damaged arterial wall was 45:1 (6.55 ± 2.26 versus 4.34 ± 1.43 optical density/pixel, $P < 0.05$). The accumulation of I-125 MCP-1 correlated ($r = 0.85$, $P < 0.0001$) with the number of macrophages per unit area (*right*). (*From Ohtsuki K, Hayase M, Akashi K, et al: Detection of monocyte chemoattractant protein-1 receptor expression in experimental atherosclerotic lesions: An autoradiographic study, Circulation 104:203–208, 2001.*)

humans,[36] where the intensity and number of sites of uptake correlated with risk factors.[37,38] Similarly, sites of aortic FDG uptake were correlated with sites of calcification.[39–41] Based on the pathology of calcified and noncalcified atheromas, it is not surprising that there was little overlap between the inflammatory and "tombstone" markers. Correlation between sites of aortic calcification and foci of FDG uptake were observed in 7% of patients in one series[33] and in less than 2% of patients in another series[35] when a criteria of greater than 130 Hounsfield units was employed as the CT criteria for calcification.

A study by Rudd et al., in eight patients undergoing carotid endarterectomy, reports the results of FDG scans and CT scans of their necks prior to surgery. The preoperative scan results were correlated with histology of the carotid specimens.[42] These investigators demonstrated significant uptake of FDG in the lesions associated with more clinical symptoms. These lesions also demonstrated histologic evidence of inflammation. The investigators also performed an autoradiographic study,

incubating endarterectomy specimens from three symptomatic patients with tritiated deoxyglucose. Autoradiographs of these specimens demonstrated uptake in macrophage-rich areas, with little uptake in other areas. FDG uptake in inflammation in carotid lesions was verified in a larger group of endarterectomy patients,[43] where FDG uptake correlated with CD68 (macrophage-specific) staining of the endarterectomy specimen. Following these reports, studies to validate the short-term (2 weeks) and longer-term (>6 months) stability reproducibility of vascular FDG uptake were performed. Nineteen patients with carotid and iliofemoral atheromas had two FDG PET scans performed within 2 weeks.[44] An intraclass correlation > 0.8 was observed. Another group of subjects had FDG studies of the carotids and aorta performed 2 weeks apart.[45] Uptake in the carotid arteries had intraclass correlation, $r > 0.9$, while the stability of aortic uptake was lower, $r = 0.7$. Other investigators have applied the technique of FDG carotid imaging to compare the effect on carotid inflammation of simvastatin therapy to dietary therapy alone.[46]

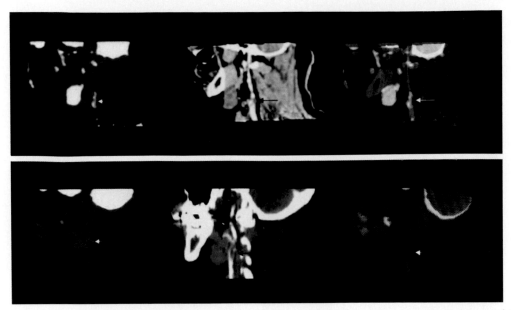

Figure 44-4 Images of positron emission tomography (PET), contrast computed tomography (CT), and merged PET/CT images, respectively. *Upper row* shows sagittal plane in a hemiparesis patient with a stenosis of her right internal carotid artery. The *white arrow* shows fluorine-18-deoxyglucose (FDG) uptake in the plaque, confirmed by the CT image (*black arrow*). The merged images precisely define the lesion localization. The *lower row* shows an asymptomatic carotid artery with lower FDG uptake. The black arrow in the CT image reveals a stenosis, but the white arrow demonstrates minimal FDG accumulation at this site. High FDG uptake was shown in brain, jaw muscles, and facial soft tissues, as expected. In a recent report by Rudd et al., eight patients with symptomatic carotid atherosclerosis were imaged. Symptomatic carotid plaques were visible in FDG PET images acquired 3 hours after FDG injection; the estimated net radiotracer accumulation rate (plaque/integral plasma) in symptomatic lesions was 27% higher than in contralateral asymptomatic lesions. There was no measurable FDG uptake in normal carotid arteries. Autoradiography of excised plaques confirmed accumulation of deoxyglucose in macrophage-rich areas of the plaque. *(From Rudd JH, Warburton EA, Fryer TD, et al: Imaging atherosclerotic plaque inflammation with [^{18}F]-fluorodeoxyglucose positron emission tomography, Circulation 105:2708–2711, 2002.)*

The investigators identified 43 cancer patients with FDG uptake in the carotid arteries. They randomized 21 subjects to receive simvastatin (dose range 5 to 20 mg) and 22 to diet therapy. Three months later, follow-up FDG PET/CT scan demonstrated a significant decrease in carotid uptake in the simvastatin group but no significant change in the group treated with diet alone.

The longer-term stability of FDG uptake is less certain.[47] Fifty patients had PET/CT studies performed 8 to 26 months apart. Of the lesions with FDG uptake and no calcification, 48% demonstrated a changing pattern on the second scan, where the site of FDG was no longer seen, or a new site of FDG uptake was observed. A second study in 100 patients undergoing serial FDG PET/CT scans for cancer surveillance identified changes in 45% of sites on two FDG scans performed 6 months apart.[48]

There are still major hurdles for FDG vascular imaging to overcome to make the procedure clinically useful. In view of the number of sites of FDG vascular uptake in major vessels, it is apparent that vascular inflammation is present at many sites at the same time. Based on autopsy observations, healed plaque ruptures were observed in 61% of hearts in patients who subsequently died suddenly.[49] This observation suggests that the number of ruptures is higher than the number of clinical events. As a result, FDG vascular inflammation imaging may have a very high sensitivity but a low predictive value for clinical outcome. There is a need to standardize data acquisition and analysis to produce both a score by individual lesion and a total score for each patient.

Most patients have multiple sites of uptake (>10 in the aorta alone)[34] associated with different levels of intensity, suggesting that there is variation in lesion size and/or variation in the number of activated macrophages within a lesion. It is logical that the more intense and larger the region of uptake, the more likely the lesion is to rupture. However, this relationship requires a large clinical study for validation.

TARGETING OF APOPTOSIS IN ATHEROMA

A strikingly high prevalence of apoptosis has recently been demonstrated in plaque rupture in the coronary arteries of victims of sudden cardiac death.[50] These apoptotic cells surrounded the ruptured plaque site (Fig. 44-5). On the other hand, apoptotic cells were only occasionally observed in the regions of the same plaque remote from the site of rupture, such as in the shoulder triangle or deeper in the intima; similarly, relatively few apoptotic cells were observed in the stable plaques. The ultrastructural examination and immunohistochemical staining for the identification of cell type revealed that the apoptotic cells at the rupture site were predominantly macrophages; apoptotic smooth muscle or T cells were only occasionally seen.

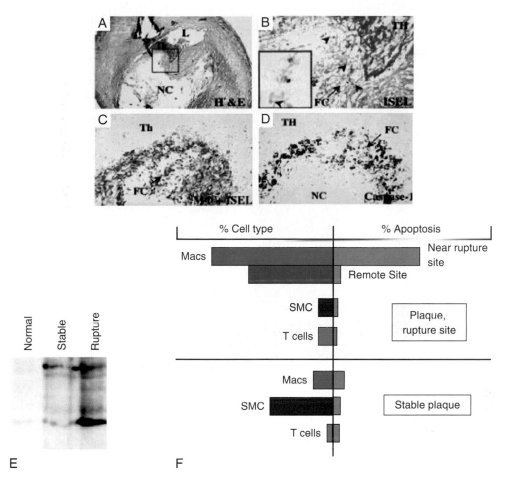

Figure 44-5 A, A micrograph of a cross-section of an epicardial coronary artery, showing a plaque rupture with an acute luminal thrombus (L), represented by a connection between luminal platelet-fibrin thrombus and the necrotic core (NC) through the fibrous cap disruption (hematoxylin-eosin, ∞30). **B**, Serial section of **A**, after DNA fragmentation staining by in situ end labeling (ISEL) at the site of plaque rupture and adjoining thin fibrous cap in the *magnified boxed area*. Numerous apoptotic cells (blue nuclear staining) are identified at the plaque rupture site (eosin counterstain ∞150). **C**, Further characterization demonstrated that the apoptotic cells in the culprit lesions were stained for combination of ISEL (dark-brown reaction product) and specific antibody for macrophages (KP-1/CD68, red reaction product). **D**, Further, immunohistochemical and biochemical characterization revealed that the apoptotic macrophages predominantly expressed caspase-1, or ICE (stained brown, ∞150). **E**, Immunoblot studies of the plaques demonstrated cleaved active band of ICE in the ruptured plaques. Only unprocessed ICE was present in stable plaques; processed and unprocessed ICE bands were not seen in normal vessel wall. **F**, Apoptotic cells were predominantly observed at the rupture site and only occasionally encountered in the regions of the same plaque remote from the site of rupture; stable plaques also demonstrated minimal evidence of apoptotic cells. Finally, quantitative assessment of the cell population demonstrated predominance of macrophages in the fibrous cap (*left*), most of which were apoptotic at the site of rupture and not away from there (*right*). (*From Kolodgie FD, Narula J, Burke AP, et al: Localization of apoptotic macrophages at the site of plaque rupture in sudden coronary death, Am J Pathol 157:1259–1268, 2000.*)

Immunohistochemical characterization revealed[44] that the apoptotic macrophages predominantly expressed caspase-1; caspase-3 staining was less intense. Immunoblot studies of the plaques demonstrated active caspase-1 in the ruptured plaques (see Fig. 44-5). In contrast to the rupture site, fibrous caps of stable plaques demonstrated lower prevalence of macrophages and higher numbers of SMC; stable plaques showed a much lower frequency of apoptotic cells. In the stable plaque, the occasional positive apoptotic cell also co-localized with both caspase-1 and caspase-3; only unprocessed caspase-1 was present in stable plaques.

Since apoptosis may contribute to plaque vulnerability, we tested the ability of exogenous radiolabeled annexin V to detect atherosclerosis in vivo in a rabbit model.[51] Animals were injected intravenously with 0.5 to 1 mg of annexin V labeled with 7 to 10 mCi of ^{99m}Tc for in vivo imaging studies, and after 3 hours there was clear delineation of radiolabeled annexin V within the abdominal aorta by in vivo gamma imaging (Fig. 44-6). In contrast, in vessels without plaques, at 3 hours after administration there was no localization of radiotracer within the normal vessel wall.

The accumulation of annexin V in atherosclerotic lesions was approximately 9-fold greater than in the corresponding control abdominal aortic region. The mean + SEM %ID/g uptake in the specimens with lesions (0.054% ± 0.0095%) was significantly higher than the background activity in the normal specimens (0.0058 ± 0.001; $P < 0.000$). Aortic sections from atherosclerotic animals demonstrated microscopically

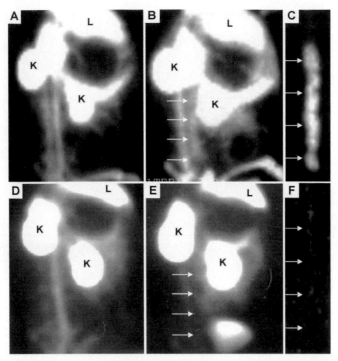

Figure 44-6 Left lateral oblique gamma images of experimental atherosclerotic (**A-C**) and control (**D-F**) rabbits injected with technetium (Tc)-99m-annexin V. Liver (L) and kidney (K) activities are marked. Images at the time of injection (*A, D*) and at 2 hours after injection (*B, E*) are shown. While blood pooling is seen at the time of injection, tracer uptake is clearly visible in the abdominal aorta at 2 hours (*B*). *C*, Ex vivo image of *B* shows intense ^{99m}Tc annexin V uptake in the arch and abdominal region. The annexin-positive areas were confirmed to contain atherosclerotic plaque by histology. *D to F* demonstrate corresponding images in the control animals. Note the aorta is indistinguishable from background at 2 hours after injection. *F*, Ex vivo aortic image of *E*, demonstrating the absence of ^{99m}Tc annexin V uptake. *(From Kolodgie FD, Petrov A, Virmani R, et al: Targeting of apoptotic macrophages and experimental atheroma with radiolabeled annexin V: A technique with potential for noninvasive imaging of vulnerable plaque, Circulation 108:3134–3139, 2003.)*

detectable plaques displaying various lesion types. Approximately 20% of plaques were classified as intimal xanthoma (AHA type II), 30% pathologic intimal thickening (AHA type III), and 50% fibrous cap atheroma (AHA type IV). Total SMC and macrophage burden in the various lesion types were quantified. There were no significant differences in SMC burden among the three lesion types: intimal xanthoma, pathologic intimal thickening, and fibrous cap atheroma (0.54 ± 0.24 mm^2, 0.64 ± 0.09 mm^2, and 0.56 ± 0.14 mm^2, respectively). In contrast, total macrophage burden was increased approximately twofold in fibrous cap atheroma (3.2 ± 0.93 mm^2) compared with intimal xanthoma (1.6 ± 1.2 mm^2) and lesions displaying pathologic intimal thickening (1.3 ± 0.73 mm^2). The annexin V uptake was dependent on lesion severity (Fig. 44-7); the mean %ID/g uptake was significantly higher in aortic segments with fibrous cap atheroma (0.034 ± 0.006) than with intimal xanthoma (0.013 ± 0.002; $P = 0.02$) or lesions with pathologic intimal thickening (0.0169 ± 0.0032; $P = 0.03$). Differences in radiotracer uptake between intimal xanthoma and lesions with pathologic intimal thickening were not significant. Regression analyses of a combined sample of aortic sections from all lesion types demonstrated a positive correlation between the overall macrophage burden of the plaque and uptake of radiolabeled tracer ($r = 0.47$, $P = 0.04$). In contrast, there was no association between SMC burden and radiotracer uptake ($r = 0.08$, $P = 0.73$). Thus, it appears that annexin V has an affinity for macrophage-rich areas within the plaque.[45]

FUTURE OF ATHEROSCLEROSIS IMAGING

Nuclear plaque imaging is clearly in its infancy. Early work in a variety of animal models has indicated proof of principle and investigative efficacy. It is now time to consider the next phase of improved imaging technology, which will permit reliable identification of lesions in the coronary arteries, as well additional biological tracers, as a prelude to early investigation in man. Preliminary studies describing FDG uptake in the carotid arteries appear particularly promising. Before embracing the technology as a marker of clinical disease, these studies require additional validation in larger groups of patients with longer follow-up. Nevertheless, it is clear that contrast angiography or any approach that solely evaluates the arterial lumen will be inadequate for identifying the biological and clinical relevance of disease in the arterial wall. Such information can only be determined by an understanding of the underlying principles of vascular and cell biology and their subsequent application to the imaging of vascular lesions. In such an arena, molecular nuclear imaging should clearly shine.

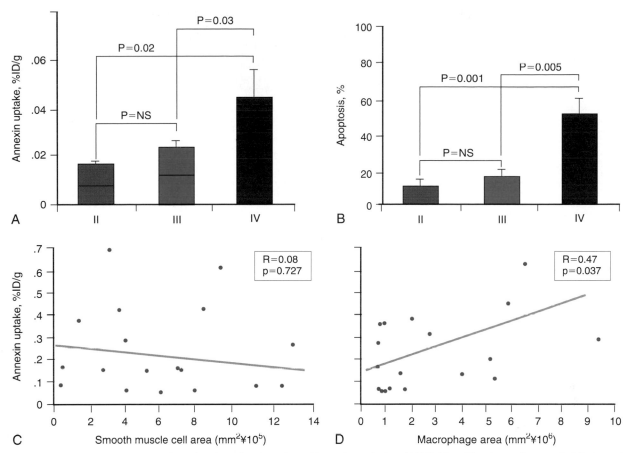

Figure 44-7 Lesion type was assigned using the American Heart Association (AHA) classification scheme. **A**, The uptake or radiolabel was significantly higher in AHA type IV lesions. **B**, Bar graph showing apoptotic index relative to lesion type; there was a significant increase in the prevalence of apoptosis in AHA type IV lesions. **C**, Simple regression analyses of smooth muscle cells (SMC) with ^{99m}Tc-annexin V uptake demonstrated no significant relationship between SMC, but a directly proportional relationship to macrophage burden (**D**). *(From Kolodgie FD, Petrov A, Virmani R, et al: Targeting of apoptotic macrophages and experimental atheroma with radiolabeled annexin V: A technique with potential for noninvasive imaging of vulnerable plaque, Circulation 108:3134–3139, 2003.)*

REFERENCES

1. American Heart Association: Heart disease and stroke statistics 2009: Update, Accessed at <http://circ.ahajournals.org/cgi/content/full/119/2/e21>.
2. Leroyer AS, Isobe H, Lesèche G, Castier Y, Wassef M, Mallat Z, Binder BR, Tedgui A: Boulanger CM.Cellular origins and thrombogenic activity of microparticles isolated from human atherosclerotic plaques, *J Am Coll Cardiol* 49(7):772–777, 2007.
3. Moreno P, Purushothaman KR, Fuster V, Echverri D, Truszcynska H, Sharma SK, Badimon JJ, O'connor WN: Plaque neovascularization is increased I nruptured atherosclerotic lesions of human aorta: Implication for plaque vulnerability, *Circulation* 110:2032–2038, 2004.
4. Stary HC, Chandler AB, Glagov S, et al: A definition of initial, fatty streak, and intermediate lesions of atherosclerosis. A report from the Committee on Vascular Lesions of the Council on Arteriosclerosis, American Heart Association, *Circulation* 89:2462–2478, 1994.
5. Virmani R, Kolodgie FD, Burke AP, Farb A, Schwartz SM: Lessons from sudden coronary death: a comprehensive morphological classification scheme for atherosclerotic lesions, *Arterioscler Thromb Vasc Biol* 20 (5):1262–1275, 2000.
6. Pasternak RC, Abrams J, Greenland P, et al: 34th Bethesda Conference: Task force #1-Identification of coronary heart disease risk: Is there a detection gap? *J Am Coll Cardiol* 41:1863–1874, 2003.
7. Ridker PM, Libby P. Risk factors for atherothrombotic disease. In *Braunwald's heart disease: A textbook of cardiovascular medicine*, 8th ed, Philadelphia, 2007, Saunders, pp 1004–1026.
8. Greenland P, Knoll MD, Stamler J, et al: Major risk factors as antecedents of fatal and nonfatal coronary heart disease events, *JAMA* 290:891–897, 2003.
9. Mitchell RN, Schoen FJ: Acute and chronic inflammation. In Kumar V, Abbas A, Fausto N, Aste JC, editors: *Robbins & Cotran Pathologic Basis of Disease*, 8th ed, Philadelphia, 2010, Saunders, pp 496–506.
10. Laufer EM, Reutelingsperger C, Narula J, Hofstra L: Annexin A5: an imaging biomarker of cardiovascular risk, *Basic Res Cardiol* 103: 95–104, 2008.
11. Haider N, Hartung D, Fujimoto S, et al. Dual molecular imaging for targeting MMP activity and apoptosis in atherosclerosis: molecular imaging facilities understanding of pathogenesis, *J Nucl Cardiol* 16:753–762, 2009.
12. Osterud B, Bjorklid E: Role of monocytes in atherogenesis, *Physiol Rev* 83:1069–1112, 2003.
13. Mäyränpää MI, Heikkilä HM, Lindstedt KA, Walls AF, Kovanen PT: Desquamation of human coronary artery endothelium by human mast cell proteases: implications for plaque erosion, *Coron Artery Dis* 17(7):611–621, 2006.
14. Davis HH, Heaton WA, Siegel BA, Mathias CJ, Joist JH, Sherman LA, Welch MJ: Scintigraphic detection of atherosclerotic lesions and venous thrombi in man by indium-111-labelled autologous platelets, *Lancet* 1(8075):1185–1187, 1978.
15. Lees RS, Lees AM, Strauss HW: External imaging of human atherosclerosis, *J Nucl Med* 24:154–156, 1983.
16. Lees AM, Lees RS, Schoen FJ, Isaacsohn JL, Fischman AJ, McKusick KA, Strauss HW: Imaging human atherosclerosis with ^{99m}Tc-labeled low density lipoproteins, *Arteriosclerosis* 8:461–470, 1988.
17. Iuliano L, Signore A, Vallabajosula S, Colavita AR, Camastra C, Ronga G, Alessandri C, Sbarigia E, Fiorani P, Violi F: Preparation and biodistribution of 99m technetium labelled oxidized LDL in man, *Atherosclerosis* 126:131–141, 1996.
18. Narula J, Petrov A, Bianchi C, Ditlow CC, Lister BC, Dilley J, Pieslak I, Chen FW, Torchilin VP, Khaw BA: Noninvasive localization of experimental atherosclerotic lesions with mouse/human chimeric Z2D3 F(ab')2 specific for the proliferating smooth muscle cells of human atheroma. Imaging with conventional and negative charge-modified antibody fragments, *Circulation* 92:474–484, 1995.
19. Carrio I, Pieri PL, Narula J, Prat L, Riva P, Pedrini L, Pretolani E, Caruso G, Sarti G, Estorch M, Berna L, Riambau V, Matias-Guiu X,

Pak C, Ditlow C, Chen F, Khaw BA: Noninvasive localization of human atherosclerotic lesions with indium 111-labeled monoclonal Z2D3 antibody specific for proliferating smooth muscle cells, *J Nucl Cardiol* 5:551–557, 1998.

20. Ohtsuki K, Hayase M, Akashi K, Kopiwoda S, Strauss HW: Detection of monocyte chemoattractant protein-1 receptor expression in experimental atherosclerotic lesions: an autoradiographic study, *Circulation* 104:203–208, 2001.

21. Oliveira RT, Mamoni RL, Souza JR, Fernandes JL, Rios FJ, Gidlund M, Coelho OR, Blotta MH: Differential expression of cytokines, chemokines and chemokine receptors in patients with coronary artery disease, *Int J Cardiol* 136:16–17, 2009.

22. Vallabhajosula S, Machac J, Knesaurek K: Imaging atherosclerotic macrophage density by positron emission tomography using F-18-fluorodeoxyglucose (FDG), *J Nucl Med* 37:38P, 1996.

23. Yun M, Yeh D, Araujo LI, Jang S, Newberg A, Alavi A: F-18 FDG uptake in the large arteries: a new observation, *Clin Nucl Med* 26(4):314–319, 2001.

24. Rudd JH, Warburton EA, Fryer TD, Jones HA, Clark JC, Antoun N, Johnstrom P, Davenport AP, Kirkpatrick PJ, Arch BN, Pickard JD, Weissberg PL: Imaging atherosclerotic plaque inflammation with [18F]-fluorodeoxyglucose positron emission tomography, *Circulation* 105:2708–2711, 2002.

25. Ogawa M, Ishino S, Mukai T, Asano D, Teramoto N, Watabe H, Kudomi N, Shiomi M, Magata Y, Iida H, Saji H: 18F-FDG Accumulation in Atherosclerotic Plaques: Immunohistochemical and PET Imaging Study, *J Nucl Med* 45:1245–1250, 2004.

26. Tawakol A, Migrino RQ, Hoffmann U, Abbara S, Houser S, Gewirtz H, Muller JE, Brady TJ, Fischman AJ: Noninvasive in vivo measurement of vascular inflammation with F-18 fluorodeoxyglucose positron emission tomography, *J Nucl Cardiol* 12:294–301, 2005.

27. Dunphy MP, Freiman A, Larson SM, Strauss HW: Association of vascular 18F-FDG uptake with vascular calcification, *J Nucl Med* 46(8):1278–1284, 2005.

28. Zhao Y, Kuge Y, Zhao S, Strauss HW, Blankenberg FG, Tamaki N: Prolonged high-fat feeding enhances aortic 18F-FDG and 99mTc-annexin A5 uptake in apolipoprotein E-deficient and wild-type C57BL/6J mice, *J Nucl Med* 49(10):1707–1714, 2008.

29. Kolodgie FD, Petrov A, Virmani R, Narula N, Verjans JW, Weber DK, Hartung D, Steinmetz N, Vanderheyden JL, Vannan MA, Gold HK, Reutelingsperger CP, Hofstra L, Narula J: Targeting of apoptotic macrophages and experimental atheroma with radiolabeled annexin V: a technique with potential for noninvasive imaging of vulnerable plaque, *Circulation* 108:3134–3139, 2003.

30. Laufer EM, Winkens HM, Corsten MF, Reutelingsperger CP, Narula J, Hofstra L: PET and SPECT imaging of apoptosis in vulnerable atherosclerotic plaques with radiolabeled annexin A5, *Q J Nucl Med Mol Imaging* 53(1):26–34, 2009.

31. Fujimoto S, Hartung D, Ohshima S, Edwards DS, Zhou J, Yalamanchili P, Azure M, Fujimoto A, Isobe S, Matsumoto Y, Boersma H, Wong N, Yamazaki J, Narula N, Petrov A, Narula J: Molecular imaging of matrix metalloproteinase in atherosclerotic lesions: resolution with dietary modification and statin therapy, *J Am Coll Cardiol* 52(23):1847–1857, 2008.

32. Narula J, Garg P, Achenbach S, Motoyama S, Virmani R, Strauss HW: Arithmetic of vulnerable plaque for non-invasive imaging, *Nature Clin Prac CV Med* Suppl 2:S2–10, 2008.

33. Davies JR, Rudd JH, Weissberg PL, Narula J: Radionuclide imaging for the detection of inflammation in vulnerable plaques, *J Am Coll Cardiol* 47(Suppl 8):C57–C68, 2006.

34. Vallabhajosula I, Machac K, Knesaurek J, et al: Imaging atherosclerotic macrophage density by positron emission tomography using F-18-fluorodeoxyglucose (FOG), *J Nucl Med* 37:38, 1996.

35. Vallabhajosula S, Fuster V: Atherosclerosis: imaging techniques and the evolving role of nuclear medicine, *J Nucl Med* 38(11):1788–1796, 1997.

36. Yun M, Yeh D, Araujo LI, Jang S, Newberg A, Alavi A: F-18 FDG uptake in the large arteries: a new observation, *Clin Nucl Med* 26(4):314–319, 2001.

37. Yun M, Jang S, Cucchiara A, Newberg AB: Alavi A. 18F FDG uptake in the large arteries: a correlation study with the atherogenic risk factors, *Semin Nucl Med* 32(1):70–76, 2002.

38. Tatsumi M, Cohade C, Nakamoto Y, Wahl RL: Fluorodeoxyglucose uptake in the aortic wall at PET/CT: possible finding for active atherosclerosis, *Radiology* 229(3):831–837, 2003.

39. Ben-Haim S, Kupzov E, Tamir A, Israel O: Evaluation of 18F-FDG uptake and arterial wall calcifications using 18F-FDG PET/CT, *J Nucl Med* 45(11):1816–1821, 2004.

40. Ben-Haim S, Kupzov E, Tamir A, Frenkel A, Israel O: Changing patterns of abnormal vascular wall F-18 fluorodeoxyglucose uptake on follow-up PET/CT studies, *J Nucl Cardiol* 13(6):791–800, 2006.

41. Dunphy MP, Freiman A, Larson SM, Strauss HW: Association of vascular 18F-FDG uptake with vascular calcification, *J Nucl Med* 46(8):1278–1284, 2005.

42. Rudd JH, Warburton EA, Fryer TD, Jones HA, Clark JC, Antoun N, Johnstrom P, Davenport AP, Kirkpatrick PJ, Arch BN, Pickard JD, Weissberg PL: Imaging atherosclerotic plaque inflammation with [18F]-fluorodeoxyglucose positron emission tomography, *Circulation* 105(23):2708–2711, 2002.

43. Tawakol A, Migrino RQ, Bashian GG, Bedri S, Vermylen D, Cury RC, Yates D, LaMuraglia GM, Furie K, Houser S, Gewirtz H, Muller JE, Brady TJ, Fischman AJ: In vivo 18F-fluorodeoxyglucose positron emission tomography imaging provides a noninvasive measure of carotid plaque inflammation in patients, *J Am Coll Cardiol* 48(9):1818–1824, 2006.

44. Rudd JH, Myers KS, Bansilal S, Machac J, Pinto CA, Tong C, Rafique A, Hargeaves R, Farkouh M, Fuster V, Fayad ZA: Atherosclerosis inflammation imaging with 18F-FDG PET: carotid, iliac, and femoral uptake reproducibility, quantification methods, and recommendations, *J Nucl Med* 49(6):871–878, 2008.

45. Rudd JH, Myers KS, Bansilal S, Machac J, Pinto CA, Tong C, Rafique A, Hargeaves R, Farkouh M, Fuster V, Fayad ZA: Atherosclerosis inflammation imaging with 18F-FDG PET: carotid, iliac, and femoral uptake reproducibility, quantification methods, and recommendations, *J Nucl Med* 49(6):871–878, 2008.

46. Tahara N, Kai H, Ishibashi M, Nakaura H, Kaida H, Baba K, Hayabuchi T.Imaizumi T.Simvastatin attenuates plaque inflammation: evaluation by fluorodeoxyglucose positron emission tomography, *J Am Coll Cardiol* 48(9):1825–1831, 2006.

47. Ben-Haim S, Kupzov E, Tamir A, Frenkel A, Israel O: Changing patterns of abnormal vascular wall F-18 fluorodeoxyglucose uptake on follow-up PET/CT studies, *J Nucl Cardiol* 13(6):791–800, 2006.

48. Meirrelles G, Larson S, Strauss H: Fluorodeoxyglucose uptake and calcifications in the vascular wall at PET/CT: Assessment of frequency, stability over time and association with cardiovascular risk factors [abstract], *J Nucl Med* (Suppl 1):126, 2006.

49. Burke AP, Kolodgie FD, Farb A, Weber DK, Malcom GT, Smialek J, Virmani R: Healed plaque ruptures and sudden coronary death: evidence that subclinical rupture has a role in plaque progression, *Circulation* 103(7):934–940, 2001.

50. Kolodgie FD, Narula J, Burke AP, et al: Localization of apoptotic macrophages at the site of plaque rupture in sudden coronary death, *Am J Pathol* 157:1259–1268, 2000.

51. Kolodgie FD, Petrov A, Virmani R, et al: Targeting of apoptotic macrophages and experimental atheroma with radiolabeled annexin V: A technique with potential for noninvasive imaging of vulnerable plaque, *Circulation* 108:3134–3139, 2003.

Molecular Imaging of Gene Expression and Cell Therapy

JOSEPH C. WU AND SANJIV SAM GAMBHIR

INTRODUCTION

In 1953, Watson and Crick elucidated the structure of deoxyribonucleic acid (DNA) in a 2-page letter published in the journal *Nature*.[1] Over the next 50 years, advances in genomic science and molecular medicine have resulted in a better understanding of the pathophysiology of many diseases. Recently, another revolution has been taking place. A new set of technologies, as part of a new field termed *molecular imaging*, is now being developed to noninvasively examine the integrative functions of molecules, cells, and organs in intact whole-body systems.[2,3] The field remains in its infancy at present and to a large extent is limited to the laboratory environment. Notable exceptions are in the disciplines of oncology, neurology, and cardiology, which have started to make the transition from basic science to clinical application. Cardiac imaging modalities such as computed tomography (CT), magnetic resonance imaging (MRI), single-photon emission computed tomography (SPECT), positron emission tomography (PET), and ultrasound have seen major advances over the past decades. In the clinical setting, these modalities can provide outstanding data regarding organ structure and physiologic function. This chapter serves as an introduction to the field of cardiovascular molecular imaging, with specific emphasis on its utility in evaluating gene and cellular therapy. Because the field may be new to many, we have purposely simplified much of the discussion on technical details to make the context more appealing to a broad range of readers with different backgrounds.

FUNDAMENTALS OF GENE EXPRESSION

The central dogma of molecular biology states that genetic information flows from DNA to ribonucleic acid (RNA) to protein. The human genome has 23 pairs of chromosomes containing approximately 3 billion base pairs of DNA and ~23,000 genes.[4,5] Each gene consists of sequences of four different nucleotides: adenine (A), guanine (G), cytosine (C), and thymine (T). The flow of information from DNA to RNA within the cell nucleus is termed *transcription*. Each messenger RNA (mRNA) is composed of intron and exon sequences. Introns are intervening sequences that are spliced out and removed. Exons are sequences that exit the nucleus to the cytoplasm to serve as templates for protein synthesis in a process called *translation*. The proteins are formed from a combination of 20 different units called *amino acids*. Proteins are considered the workhorse of cell machinery, performing activities ranging from gene regulation to cell integrity to receptor signaling. The versatility of molecular biology cloning techniques allows both the DNA and RNA to be manipulated. For example, restriction enzymes can be used to cleave the DNA of interest at specific sites to generate discrete gene fragments.[6] They are named after the bacteria from which they were isolated (e.g., Eco RI from *Escherichia coli* and Hind III from *Haemophilus influenza*) and serve originally as part of the bacterial immune arsenal to protect itself against invasion by cleaving the DNA of foreign vectors. These techniques have been used to "cut and paste" therapeutic genes and reporter genes, as will be discussed later. For an in-depth discussion on the basics of molecular biology and genomics, please refer to a recent review article.

BACKGROUND OF CARDIOVASCULAR MOLECULAR IMAGING

Traditionally, researchers have monitored cardiac gene transfer by using reporter constructs such as β-galactosidase (β-gal),[7] green fluorescent protein (GFP),[8] and chloramphenicol-acetyl transferase (CAT).[9] Cellular transplant therapies have employed similar techniques as well as newer approaches such as TaqMan reverse transcriptase polymerase chain reaction (RT-PCR),[10] Y-chromosome paint probes,[11] and antibodies specific to various stem cell types.[12] All of these established traditional techniques, however, require invasive biopsies and/or postmortem tissue sampling for analysis. Molecular imaging offers distinct advantages by allowing for noninvasive, quantitative, and repetitive imaging of targeted macromolecules and biological processes in living organisms.[2] Although a vast array of molecular imaging techniques are available, they all require two fundamental elements: (1) a molecular probe that can signal confirmation of gene expression by detecting messenger ribonucleic acid (mRNA) transcripts or proteins and (2) a method to monitor these probes or events. Presently, the two most widely used strategies are direct and indirect imaging.

Direct molecular imaging involves direct probe-target interaction. Targets can include receptors, enzymes, or mRNA. For *probe-receptor* imaging, radiolabeled monoclonal antibodies binding to tumor cell-specific surface antigens have been used for the past 2 decades.[13] Recent examples of cardiac application involved imaging $\alpha_v\beta_3$ integrin receptor[14] or vascular endothelial growth factor (VEGF) receptor[15] expressed during angiogenesis after myocardial infarction (MI). For *probe-enzyme* imaging, the most well-known cardiac application is fluorine-18 (^{18}F)-labeled-fluorodeoxyglucose (FDG), used to assess for myocardial tissue viability. After transport across an intact cell membrane, the ^{18}F-labeled glucose analog undergoes phosphorylation by hexokinase and is retained intracellularly in proportion to the rate of cellular glycolysis.[16] The radioactive ^{18}F undergoes positron annihilation into two high-energy γ rays (511 keV), which can be detected as coincidence events by PET. For *probe-mRNA* imaging, radiolabeled antisense oligonucleotide (RASON) probes can be used.[17,18] RASON probes are typically 12 to 35 nucleotides long and are complementary to a small segment of the target mRNA. However, the RASON approach is limited at this point due to (1) low number of target mRNA (~1000 copies) per cell compared to proteins (>10,000 copies); (2) limited tracer penetration across the cell membrane; (3) poor intracellular stability; (4) slow washout of unbound oligonucleotide probes; and (5) low target-to-background ratios. On the other hand, direct imaging of DNA (two copies) within the nuclear membrane has proven exceedingly difficult and is not yet feasible. In addition, knowing the *activity* of gene expression (as reflected in mRNA transcripts or protein levels) rather than the *number* of DNA copies is more relevant for biological research. The main disadvantage of direct imaging is that it requires synthesizing a customized probe for the product (e.g., receptor, enzyme, or mRNA) of every therapeutic gene of interest, which can be time-consuming and is not generalizable to most applications.

Indirect molecular imaging using reporter genes has only been recently validated. The concept of imaging reporter gene expression is illustrated in Figure 45-1. A reporter gene is first introduced into target tissues by viral or nonviral vectors. Using molecular biology techniques, the promoter or regulatory regions of genes can be cloned into different vectors to drive reporter gene

mRNA transcription. Promoter activity can be "constitutive" (always on), "inducible" (turned on or off), or "tissue specific" (expressed only in the heart, liver, or other organs). Translation of mRNA leads to a reporter protein that can interact with the reporter probe. This interaction may be enzyme based or receptor-based. Probe signals can then be detected by various imaging modalities such as an optical charged coupled device (CCD) camera, PET, SPECT, or MRI.

Clearly, the main advantage of the reporter gene system is its flexibility and multiplexing capacity.[19] By altering various components, the reporter gene can provide information about the regulation of DNA by upstream promoters, intracellular protein trafficking, and the efficiency of vector transduction on cells. Likewise, the reporter probe itself does not have to be changed in order to study a new biological process, saving time and resources required for synthesis, testing, and validation of new reagents. However, the main disadvantage of indirect imaging is that it remains a surrogate marker for the physiologic/biochemical process of interest, as opposed to directly measuring receptor density, mRNA copies, or intracellular enzymatic activity, which might be more clinically relevant. It should be noted that in the case of monitoring stem cell fate, this is less of a concern, since the focus is on detecting the presence of a population of cells. Finally, the ideal reporter gene and/or reporter probe should have the following characteristics:

1. The chromosomal integration or episomal expression of reporter gene should not adversely affect the cellular metabolism or physiology.
2. The reporter gene product should not elicit a host immune response.
3. The size of the promoter/enhancer elements and reporter gene should be small enough to fit into a delivery vehicle.
4. Transfection (e.g., plasmid or adeno-associated virus) or transduction (e.g., lentivirus or retrovirus) using the delivery vector should not be cytotoxic to the cells.
5. The reporter probe should be stable in vivo and reach the target site despite natural biological barriers (e.g., blood vessel wall or blood-brain barrier).
6. The reporter probe should only accumulate within cells that express the reporter gene to yield a high signal-to-background ratio.
7. Afterward, the reporter probe should clear rapidly from the circulation to allow repetitive imaging within the same living subject.
8. The reporter probe or its metabolites should not be cytotoxic to the cells.
9. The image signals should correlate well with true levels of reporter gene mRNA and protein in vivo.
10. The reporter gene and reporter probe should be potentially applicable for human imaging in the future.

At present, no single reporter gene and/or reporter probe assay meets all of these criteria. Thus, the optimal choice of which reporter gene and probe assay to

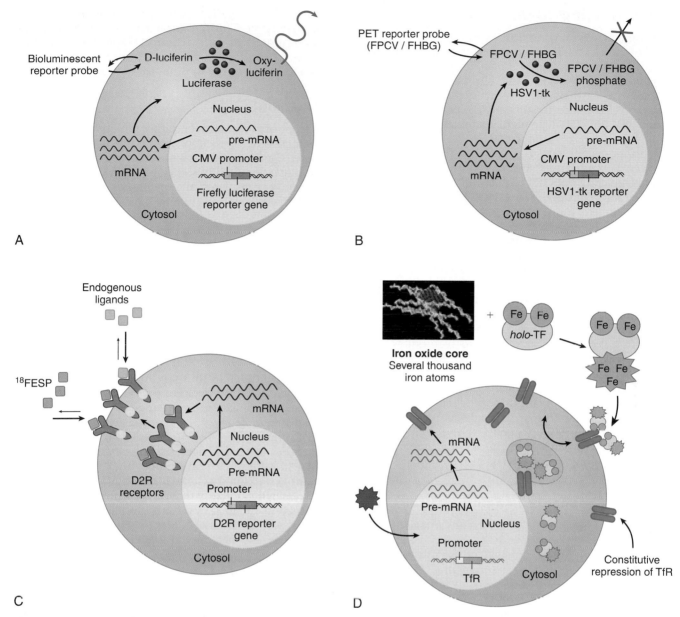

Figure 45-1 Four different strategies of imaging reporter gene/reporter probe. **A**, Enzyme-based bioluminescence imaging. Expression of the firefly luciferase reporter gene leads to the firefly luciferase reporter enzyme, which catalyzes the reporter probe (D-luciferin) that results in a photochemical reaction. This yields low levels of photons that can be detected, collected, and quantified by a charge-coupled device (CCD) camera. **B**, Enzyme-based PET imaging. Expression of the herpes simplex virus type 1 thymidine kinase (HSV1-tk) reporter gene leads to the thymidine kinase reporter enzyme (HSV1-TK), which phosphorylates and traps the reporter probe [^{18}F]-FHBG intracellularly. Radioactive decay of ^{18}F isotopes can be detected using PET. **C**, Receptor-based PET imaging. The [^{18}F]-FESP is a reporter probe that interacts with the dopamine 2 receptor (D2R) to result in probe trapping on or in cells expressing the D2R gene. **D**, Receptor-based MRI imaging. Overexpression of engineered transferrin receptors (TfR) results in increased cell uptake of the transferrin-monocrystalline iron oxide nanoparticles (Tf-MION). These changes result in a detectable contrast change on MRI.

use will depend on the particular application, organ system, and imaging modality available at a given institution.

IMAGING TECHNIQUES

Of the numerous molecular imaging modalities available for monitoring genetic and cellular activity, radionuclide-based assays (e.g., PET, SPECT, planar scintigraphy) are the most useful clinically. There are a number of other devices being used to monitor biological processes in animal models of diseases. Considerable efforts have been made towards the development of miniaturized, small-animal imaging systems such as CCD cameras for bioluminescence/fluorescence, ultrasound, SPECT, PET, and MRI. Given the vast array of imaging tools available for biological research, a brief discussion highlighting the strengths and weaknesses of each modality is warranted.

Optical Imaging

Bioluminescence imaging utilizes the photogenic properties of various luciferase genes cloned from different organisms, such as firefly (*Photinus pyralis*), jellyfish (*Aequorea*), coral (*Renilla*), and dinoflagellates (*Gonyaulax*). In the case of the firefly, the firefly luciferase enzyme (FL) converts its substrate (D-luciferin) to oxyluciferin via an ATP-dependent pathway. This process emits low levels of photons (2 to 3 eV) that can be detected and counted by a cooled CCD camera (e.g., Xenogen IVIS system).[20] Unlike bioluminescence, fluorescence imaging does not require injection of a reporter substrate but relies upon an excitation wavelength that produces an emission wavelength for measurement.[21] Recent technologic advances (e.g., eXplore Optix system) has allowed the measurement, quantification, and visualization of fluorescence intensity in small living animals using the time domain approach.[22] In general, optical-based imaging is a relatively low-cost endeavor (i.e., typically $100 to $200K versus $500K to $1 million for small-animal PET and MRI systems) with the capacity for high throughput (i.e., several mice can be scanned at once). However, the aforementioned techniques suffer from low spatial resolution, inability to monitor multiple physiologic processes, and photon attenuation/scatter within deep tissues.[23] Moreover, optical imaging has yet to be extrapolated into clinical usage. Use of novel intravascular catheter devices capable of detecting bioluminescence and/or fluorescence signals from deeper tissues or organs may be possible, but the general practicality of "invasive imaging" remains to be seen.[24]

Magnetic Resonance Imaging

Unlike optical imaging, MRI has the advantage of a very high spatial resolution (25 to 100 μm) and the ability to measure more than one physiologic parameter at once by using different radiofrequency pulse sequences.[25] This makes MR a very attractive option for imaging reporter gene expression. The imaging signal is generated as a result of spin relaxation effects, which can be altered by atoms with high magnetic moments (e.g., gadolinium and iron). One particularly useful MR imaging signal amplification system is based on the cellular internalization of superparamagnetic probes such as monocrystalline iron oxide nanoparticles (MION) and crosslinked iron oxide (CLIO).[26] MIONs or CLIOs can be linked to a variety of biomolecules to produce injectable probes for targets such as hematopoietic and neural progenitor cells,[27,28] activated thrombotic factor XIII,[29] and endothelial cell surface markers such as E-selectin.[30] These studies hold promise for in vivo imaging in humans, given the widespread availability of clinical MR scanners, nontoxic and biodegradable properties of intravenous superparamagnetic particles, and the precedent of similar preparations already in clinical use.[31] However, persisting residual signals from superparamagnetic particles may hinder the capacity for quantitative and repetitive imaging. MR is also several log of orders less sensitive (10^{-3} to 10^{-5} Molar) for detection of reporter probes compared to optical bioluminescence imaging (10^{-15} to 10^{-17}) or PET (10^{-11} to 10^{-12}) imaging.[2] Therefore, further strategies for robust signal amplification will be necessary before this modality can be of practical use for imaging cardiac gene expression and detecting small numbers of transplanted cells.

Ultrasound

The scope of ultrasound for cardiac molecular imaging has seen increasing applications over the past decade.[32–34] Targeted contrast agents have been constructed by linking ligands of interest to liposomes, perfluorocarbon nanoparticles, and encapsulated microbubbles,[35] but these agents are relatively large, precluding their extravasation from the vasculature. While ultrasound-based molecular imaging may play an increasing role in endothelial imaging,[36] its utility as a molecular cardiac imaging modality to track gene expression or cell therapy remains to be seen. Newer techniques in photoacoustic molecular imaging where the molecular imaging agents can extravasate from blood vessels may hold a potential solution to limitations of conventional ultrasound.[37]

Computed Tomography

CT is quite limited in its application as a true molecular imaging modality. Development of radiopaque probes that can accumulate in sufficient quantities for meaningful assessment of physiologic processes has proven difficult. Compared to MRI, CT-based images exhibit poor soft-tissue contrast, necessitating iodinated contrast media in addition to any probes that might be used. Presently, CT is best reserved for use as an adjunct anatomic imaging modality that can complement functional information obtained by other molecular imaging techniques, as will be discussed later. In the future, improved probes may also increase the applicability of CT imaging.

Radionuclide Imaging (See Chapter 11)

Radionuclide probes are the first example of molecular probes used in the clinical setting, and this technology represents the evolutionary roots of molecular imaging as it is known today. PET, SPECT, and planar scintigraphy have all been used to detect radionuclide-labeled probes. However, PET exhibits several advantages compared to other modalities. First, PET is more sensitive compared to SPECT and MRI for detection of probe activity, as already discussed. This may allow monitoring of gene delivery by vectors with relatively low transfection efficiencies (e.g., plasmid) or weak promoters (e.g., tissue specific), as well as detection of low numbers of cells (e.g., cardiac stem cell transplants). Second, PET imaging is more quantitative (unlike MRI) and allows for dynamic imaging with tracer kinetic modeling for analysis of rate constants underlying the biochemical processes.[38] Third, inasmuch as many PET tracers have a short half-life (e.g., ~110 minutes for ^{18}F), daily repetitive imaging of tracer retention by targeted tissues is possible. Fourth, PET imaging is tomographic (unlike two-dimensional (2D) images from optical imaging), so a relatively precise location of probe signal can be identified within the heart. This is especially apt in the basic research environment, because current generations of small-animal PET scanners have a resolution of 1^3 to 2^3 mm^3 compared to around 6^3 mm^3 for clinical PET scanners.[39] Finally, studies performed in these small-animal PET scanners can potentially be scaled up to human patients using clinical PET scanners with relative ease.[3]

IMAGING CARDIAC GENE THERAPY

Gene transfer has been heralded as the most promising therapy of molecular medicine in the 21st century. It is usually defined as the transfer and expression of DNA to somatic cells of an individual, with a resulting therapeutic effect (see Fundamentals of Gene Expression section). In cardiovascular diseases, gene therapy offers an exciting new approach to express the therapeutic factors locally in the myocardium.[40] In general, the successful application of gene therapy requires three essential elements: (1) a vector for gene delivery, (2) delivery of the vector to the target tissue, and (3) a therapeutic gene to be expressed in a particular patient population.

An ideal vector should enable efficient gene delivery to the target tissue, have minimal local or systemic toxicity, deliver enough concentration and duration to induce a therapeutic effect, and cause no germline transmission to the offspring. No single vector has all of these attributes, so the type of vector chosen will need to be tailored to the specific clinical applications. Vectors can be divided into viral vectors and nonviral vectors. Common viral vectors include adenovirus, adeno-associated virus, gutless adenovirus, and lentivirus. Nonviral vectors include plasmids, minicircles, naked DNA, and liposomes. The technique of vector delivery to the heart also depends on the intended target area, but in general can be categorized as: (1) direct epicardial injection, (2) endocardial injection, (3) intracoronary infusion, (4) retrograde coronary sinus infusion, and (5) pericardial injection.

Likewise, the choice of a therapeutic gene to be expressed is often driven by the intended application. In animal studies, successful gene therapy has been demonstrated for:

1. Treatment of coronary artery disease (CAD) using angiogenic factors such as VEGF,[41] fibroblast growth factor (FGF),[42] and hypoxia-inducible factor-1α (HIF-1α)[43]
2. Reduction of restenosis after angioplasty by inhibiting smooth muscle cell proliferation by suicide gene therapy using thymidine kinase[44]
3. Improvement of congestive heart failure by gene transfer of calcium ATPase pump (SERCA2a)[45]
4. Inhibition of atherosclerosis by overexpression of HDL receptor[46]
5. Reduction of hypoxia-induced apoptosis of cardiomyocytes[47]

These encouraging results have led to the initiation of several clinical trials, beginning in the 1990s. Of the 509 ongoing gene therapy trials in the United States, 46 are related to cardiovascular diseases. The majority of these are aimed at testing the safety and efficacy of therapeutic angiogenesis and, to a lesser extent, examining restenosis. In the late 1990s, several phase-1 open-labeled trials involving small numbers of patients with myocardial ischemia and peripheral vascular disease uniformly showed positive results.[48–50] However, recent phase-2 randomized, double-blind, placebo-controlled trials have yielded conflicting, if not disappointing, results. The Vascular Endothelial Growth Factor in Ischemia for Vascular Angiogenesis (VIVA),[51] FGF Initiating Revascularization Trial (FIRST),[52] Adenovirus Fibroblast Growth Factor Angiogenic Gene Therapy (AGENT),[53,54] and Kuopio Angiogenesis Trial (KAT)[55] tested gene therapy using either VEGF or FGF. Unfortunately, these trials failed to show any consistent improvement in various parameters such as symptomatic improvement, ejection fraction, wall motion scores, myocardial perfusion, and restenosis rate.

Nonetheless, important lessons can be learned from these trials. They showed that angiogenesis is a complex process regulated by the interaction of various growth factors and may be difficult to stimulate using a single protein or gene injection. The ideal injection method, delivery vector, and patient population remain to be determined. The pharmacokinetics and pharmacodynamics of therapeutic gene expression will need to be defined first before gene therapy can proceed further to widespread clinical usage, similar to the research and development of experimental drugs.[56] Finally, since there is no available method of assessing gene expression in vivo, the investigators are unable to determine whether the lack of symptomatic improvement is due to poor injection technique, insufficient gene expression, host inflammatory response, or an inappropriate therapeutic gene.

Imaging of cardiac transgene expression has been established in several proof-of-principle studies involving injection of various reporter genes into the myocardium and following the kinetics of transgene expression over time, using optical bioluminescence, microPET, and clinical PET imaging.[57–61] The feasibility of linking a PET reporter gene to a therapeutic gene was also demonstrated in two separate studies.[62,63] In this case, an adenovirus containing two constitutive cytomegalovirus promoters driving a VEGF$_{121}$ therapeutic gene and an HSV1-sr39tk PET reporter gene separated by polyadenine sequences was constructed (Ad-CMV-VEGF$_{121}$-CMV-HSV1-sr39tk). Wu et al. injected the construct into the myocardium of a rat in a myocardial infarction model.[63] Reporter gene expression (which indirectly reflects the VEGF$_{121}$ therapeutic gene expression) persisted for only about 2 weeks, owing to host immune response against the adenovirus. At 2 months, there were no significant improvements in myocardial contractility, perfusion, or metabolism, as measured by echocardiography, nitrogen-13-labeled ammonia (^{13}N-NH$_3$), and FDG imaging, between study and control groups (Fig. 45-2). Thus, this study highlights the importance of monitoring the pharmacokinetics of gene expression. It also demonstrates the proof of principle that any other cardiac therapeutic genes of interest

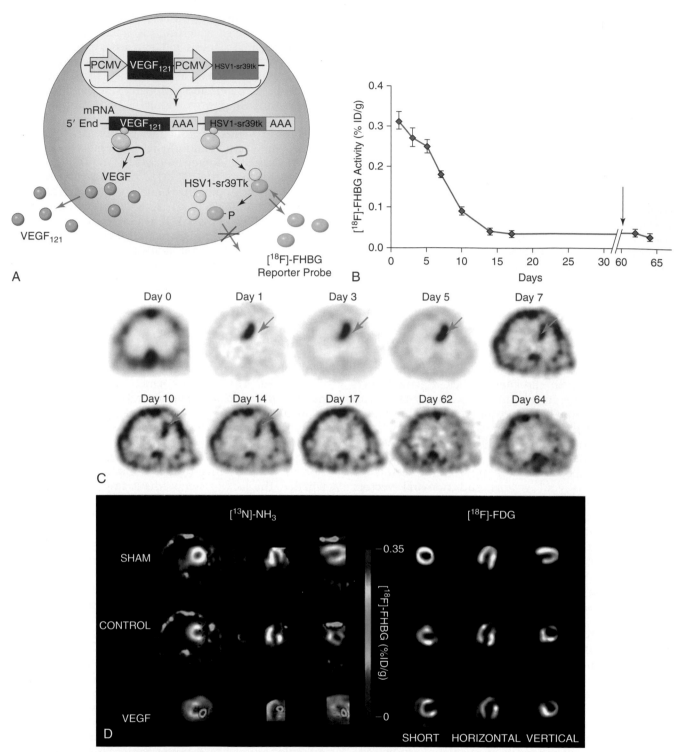

Figure 45-2 PET imaging of cardiac angiogenic gene therapy. **A,** Schematic of Ad-CMV-VEGF$_{121}$-CMV-HSV1-sr39tk–mediated gene expression. Two separate gene cassettes with CMV promoters driving the expression of a VEGF$_{121}$ therapeutic gene and an HSV1-sr39tk reporter gene separated by polyA tails. The translated product of VEGF$_{121}$ is soluble and excreted extracellularly, whereas the translated product of HSV1-sr39tk (HSV1-sr39Tk) traps ^{18}F-FHBG intracellularly by phosphorylation. **B,** Noninvasive imaging of the kinetics of cardiac transgene expression. Gene expression peaked at day 1 and rapidly decreased thereafter. A second injection *(arrow)* of Ad-CMV-VEGF$_{121}$-CMV-HSV-sr39tk at day 60 yielded no detectable signal on day 62 and day 64. *Error bars* represent mean ± SEM. **C,** A representative rat scanned longitudinally with transaxial ^{18}F-FHBG PET images shown at similar slice levels of the chest cavity. The gray scale is normalized to the individual peak activity of each image. In this rat, myocardial [^{18}F]-FHBG accumulation was visualized at the anterolateral wall *(arrow)* from day 1 to day 14 but not days 17, 62, or 64. **D,** In vivo gene, perfusion, and metabolism imaging with PET. At day 2, representative images showing normal perfusion ([^{13}N]-NH$_3$) and metabolism ([^{18}F]-FDG) in a sham rat, anterolateral infarction in a control rat (Ad-null), and anterolateral infarction in a VEGF-treated study rat (Ad-CMV-VEGF$_{121}$-CMV-HSV1-sr39tk) in short, vertical, and horizontal axis (gray scale). The color scale is expressed as %ID/g for [^{18}F]-FHBG uptake. As expected, both the sham and control animals had background ^{18}F-FHBG signal only (blue color) that outlined the shape of the chest cavity. In contrast, the study rat showed robust HSV1-sr39tk reporter gene activity near the site of injection. *(From Wu JC, Chen IY, Wang Y, et al: Molecular imaging of the kinetics of vascular endothelial growth factor gene expression in ischemic myocardium, Circulation 110:685–691, 2004. Reproduced with permission.)*

(e.g., HIF-1α, SERCA2a, heat shock protein, or endothelial nitric oxide synthase) can likewise be coupled to a PET reporter gene for subsequent noninvasive monitoring.

The feasibility of transferring imaging results from a small-animal PET scanner to a clinical PET scanner (ECAT EXACT scanner, Siemens/CTI) has been demonstrated in porcine models as well. Bengel et al. showed that myocardial tissues infected with adenovirus expressing HSV1-tk had significantly higher iodine-124-labeled 2'-fluoro-2'-deoxy-1-beta-D-arabinofuranosyl-5-iodouracil (^{124}I-FIAU) retention during the first 30 minutes following injection.[60] The FIAU uptake correlated with ex vivo images, autoradiography, and immunohistochemistry for reporter gene product after euthanasia. However, the signal-to-background ratio at the site of HSV1-tk injection was only around 1.25 during the first 30 minutes following delivery. Afterwards, there was significant washout at 45 to 120 minutes post injection, and the ^{124}I-FIAU retention became similar to control myocardial regions. Recently, Rodriquez-Porcel et al. also demonstrated the feasibility of imaging HSV1-tk reporter gene expression with fluorine-18-labeled fluoro-3-hydroxymethyl butylguanine (^{18}F-FHBG) reporter probe in a porcine model. Following endomyocardial injection using a Biocardia catheter, myocardial gene expression activity was quantified by clinical PET-CT system (Fig. 45-3). The best myocardial

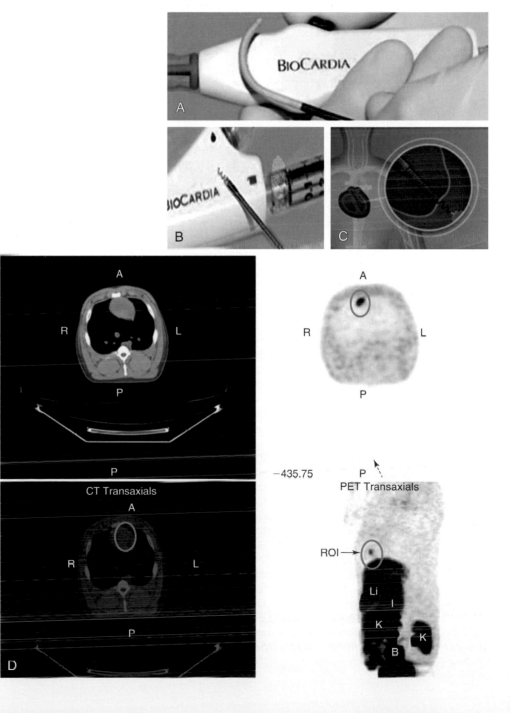

Figure 45-3 Imaging of HSV-1tk/[^{18}F]FHBG in preclinical large-animal model. Percutaneous delivery system consisting of (**A**) steerable guiding catheter and (**B**) helical needle infusion catheter. A steerable catheter provides maximum flexibility, allowing catheter positioning in virtually any area of the left ventricular cavity. The infusion catheter is used first to confirm intramyocardial positioning of the catheter and then for the delivery of therapeutic material. **C**, The infusion catheter is "screwed" inside the myocardium. **D**, Representative PET/CT image 48 hours after percutaneous gene delivery. A, anterior; B, bladder; CL, contralateral; I, intestines; K, kidney; L, left; Li, liver; LV, left ventricular; P, posterior; R, right. (*From Rodriguez-Porcel M, Brinton TJ, Chen IY, et al: Reporter gene imaging following percutaneous delivery in swine moving toward clinical applications, J Am Coll Cardiol 51:595-597, 2008. Reproduced with permission.*)

signal-to-background (left ventricular) ratio was obtained 3 hours post-injection (180 minutes, 4.63 ± 1.4, versus 90 minutes, 1.78 ± 0.6; $P < 0.05$). Autoradiography and microPET confirmed the increased ^{18}F-FHBG uptake in the anteroseptum. Overall, these studies suggest that the combination of HSV1-tk/FHBG may be superior to HSV1-tk/FIAU for imaging cardiac transgene expression.[64]

In the future, it will also be useful to have the following arsenals for cardiac gene therapy: (1) non-immunogenic vectors such as non-viral minicircle plasmids that can prolong transgene expression in the myocardium,[65] (2) cardiac tissue-specific promoter (e.g., myosin light chain kinase or troponin) that can diminish unwanted extracardiac activity,[66] (3) development of novel gene therapy approaches such as short hairpin RNA interference,[67] and (4) multimodality molecular imaging approaches that can monitor the location, magnitude, and duration of transgene expressions, as well as their downstream functional effects.[56]

IMAGING CARDIAC CELL DELIVERY

In recent years, research in stem cell therapy has rivaled or even surpassed gene therapy as a promising treatment for ischemic heart disease. In fact, stem cell therapy now occupies the lion's share of scientific presentations, media attention, and the public imagination. By most accounts, this field "started" in 2001 when Orlic et al. published a seminal (albeit still controversial to date) study showing that a particular type of bone marrow cells (lin⁻/c-kit⁺) could form de novo myocardium occupying 68% of the infarcted left ventricle just 9 days after transplantation in a mouse model.[68] At present, there are many studies reporting the efficacy of fetal and neonatal cardiomyocytes,[69] skeletal myoblasts,[70,71] bone marrow cells (BMCs),[68] and embryonic stem cell derivatives[72] for myocardial repair. As with any type of therapy, each cell type also has its own merits and pitfalls.[73]

Fetal and neonatal cardiomyocytes have been regarded as promising candidates for cell replacement therapy,[69] but their restricted availability and ethical dilemma render widespread clinical application impractical. Autologous skeletal myoblasts were the first cell type to be used clinically for cell-based cardiac repair.[70] Skeletal myoblasts are attractive candidates because they can be cultured and expanded ex vivo from muscle biopsies, and they survive well after transplantation because of their strong resistance to ischemia. Skeletal myoblast transplantation has been shown to provide functional benefit in animal models of infarction, but a large placebo-controlled, randomized trial in humans did not demonstrate sustained efficacy as defined by the primary end point of left ventricular ejection fraction (LVEF).[74] Furthermore, the increased number of early postinjection arrhythmic events after skeletal myoblast transplantation raises serious concerns and warrants further investigation. By contrast, transplantation of BMCs has been shown to improve heart function in animal

studies, and no serious complications have been reported in clinical trials to date. However, results from three large clinical trials published in 2006 in the *New England Journal of Medicine* showed inconsistent benefits that at best led to short-term but no long-term improvement.[75-77] In the accompanying editorial, the author urges the scientific community to "guard against both premature declarations of victory and premature abandonment of a promising therapeutic strategy" and that "this strategy is likely to depend on continued and effective coordination of rigorous basic and clinical investigations."[78] More recently, isolation of resident cardiac stem cells from human biopsy samples has been demonstrated.[79] Whether these cells can promote cardiac regeneration and improve heart function in humans following transplantation will need to be addressed in future clinical trials.

One of the main limitations of cardiac stem cell therapy is the lack of available methods to assess stem cell survival. In clinical studies, changes in myocardial perfusion, viability, and perfusion are assessed by echocardiography, nuclear SPECT and PET imaging, or MR imaging. These parameters measure the therapeutic effects but do not actually detect the presence or absence of transplanted stem cells. This is an important distinction because most patients also undergo concurrent coronary artery bypass grafting (CABG) or percutaneous coronary intervention (PCI), and it is not clear whether the improvement is due to these procedures or to the transplanted stem cells. Likewise, in animal studies, analysis of stem cell survival is based on postmortem histology, which is invasive and precludes longitudinal monitoring. Thus, the ability to study stem cells in the context of the intact whole-body system rather than by *indirect* (clinical trials) or *invasive* (animal studies) means will give better insight into the underlying biology and physiology of stem cells. Several investigators have started addressing this issue via different approaches, including radionuclide labeling, ferromagnetic labeling, and reporter gene labeling (Fig. 45-4).[73]

Radionuclide Labeling

This technique requires the transplanted cells to be directly labeled with a radioisotope prior to transplantation. The advantages are high sensitivity and immediate translation to clinical practice because indium-111 (^{111}In)-oxine and ^{18}F-FDG are approved by the U.S. Food and Drug Administration (FDA) as clinical radiotracers. The technique has demonstrated utility for tracking cell homing in, on infarcted myocardium and distribution following injection. Aicher et al. demonstrated that ^{111}In-oxine-labeled endothelial and hematopoietic progenitor cells accumulated in infarcted rat myocardium after intraventricular injection.[80] However, by 96 hours postinjection, only about 5% of the injected dose of radioactivity was found in the heart. This highlights the sensitivity of the method, because although only a few cells persisted in the heart, they were nevertheless detectable. An inherent limitation of radionuclide labeling is the short half-life of the radioactive probes, which precludes long-term imaging. For radiotracers with a

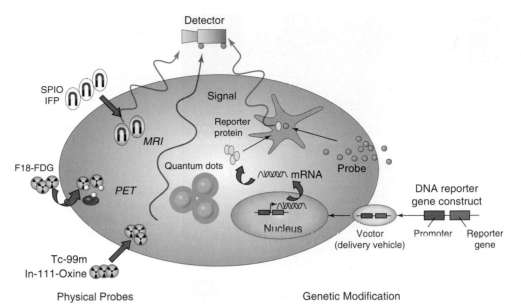

Figure 45-4 Overview of techniques used for noninvasive imaging of stem cell fate. The four different techniques include magnetic particle labeling, radionuclide labeling, quantum dot labeling, and reporter gene labeling. IFP, iron fluorescent particles; SPIO, superparamagnetic iron oxide. *(From Zhang SJ, Wu JC: Comparison of imaging techniques for tracking cardiac stem cell therapy, J Nucl Med 48:1916–1919, 2007. Reproduced with permission.)*

shorter half-life (e.g., ^{18}F-FDG is 110 minutes), one can follow those cells at most, out to 1 day. Even for radiotracers that have longer half-lives (e.g., copper-64 [^{64}Cu], 12.7 hrs; [^{111}In], 67.3 hours; thallium-201 [^{201}Tl], 74 hours; [^{124}I], 96 hours), the longest time period of imaging would still be limited to within the first 1 to 2 weeks. Furthermore, the radiotracer itself has other concerns, specifically potential adverse effects of the tracer on stem cell viability and differentiation and the leakage of the tracer from the labeled cells, which can provide a false-positive signal.[81]

Nanoparticle Labeling

Semiconductor quantum dots (QDs) are a new class of fluorescent probes that have been used in noninvasive imaging in recent years.[82,83] This technique makes use of fluorescent semiconductor nanocrystals to detect membrane molecules of interest. The excitation wavelengths of the QDs can be manipulated, ranging from ultraviolet to near-infrared ranges. Depending on the size and composition of these probes, they can be designed to emit different wavelengths of light. The photostability of QDs, as seen in their resistance to photobleaching and long-lasting fluorescence, makes them appealing for tracking stem cells in vivo.[84] However, the effects of QDs on stem cell proliferation and differentiation remain unclear; mixed results have been reported using different origins of stem cells or experimental protocols.[82,85] Finally, several other obstacles, including the tendency for aggregation of QDs in the cytosol, difficulty in delivery of QDs into cells, and nonspecific binding to multiple molecules,[86] must be overcome before QDs can realize their full potential in clinical imaging. More recently, Raman nanoparticles have also started to be imaged in small living subjects and may provide as much as 100-fold greater sensitivity than QD-based approaches.[87,88]

Iron Particle Labeling

Compared to radionuclide imaging, the main advantage of MRI is its capacity for high anatomic resolution. In general, MRI techniques can be divided into two classes based on the contrast agent being used. Lanthanide gadolinium (Gd^{3+}) is applied for T1-weighted contrast enhanced images, and superparamagnetic iron oxide (SPIO) particles are applied for T2-weighted images. Gadolinium-enhanced images have been used in previous studies to track human neural and mesenchymal stem cells for up to 6 weeks.[89] However, SPIO particles are favored and more widely used for stem cell imaging because a lower concentration (5–10 μm/L) is required. The immediate translation of SPIO to clinical studies is feasible because certain superparamagnetic formulations have already been approved by the FDA and found to be biocompatible, safe, and nontoxic. Recent studies have demonstrated the utility of MRI for long-term tracking of bone-marrow-derived mesenchymal stem cells (MSCs). Amado et al. labeled porcine MSCs with iron oxide, induced a myocardial infarct (MI) by balloon occlusion of the left anterior descending (LAD) artery, and then injected MSCs intramyocardially 3 days after MI.[90] The iron oxide–labeled cells created hypoenhanced regions. Interestingly, relative to the intensity of hypoenhancement at 2 days posttransplantation, approximately 42% of the signal still remained at 8 weeks. Similarly, Kraitchmen et al. magnetically labeled porcine MSCs with iron oxide, injected the cells into adult swine following MI, and demonstrated that the cells could be tracked for up to 3 weeks using MRI.[91] MRI showed that the cell survival trend correlated with proximity to the infarct; specifically, cells injected into the infarct zone had more robust survival than those injected into healthy myocardium. In a related study, Kraitchmen et al. compared the sensitivity of SPECT to MRI to detect MSCs injected intravenously following MI in canines (Fig. 45-5).[92] MSCs were

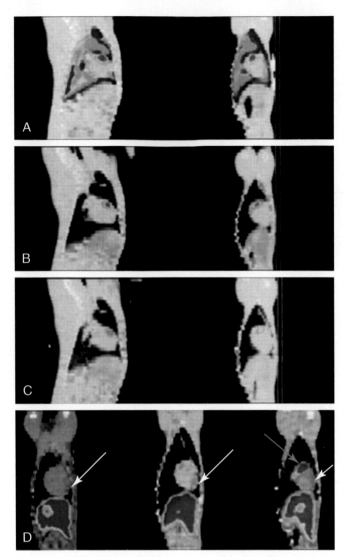

Figure 45-5 Radionuclide imaging of mesenchymal stem cells following intravenous injection. Sagittal *(left)* and coronal *(right)* views of fused SPECT/CT images on days 1 (**A**), 2 (**B**), and 7 (**C**) in an animal that demonstrated focal uptake in the anterior midventricular region of the heart. At the last imaging time point on days 5 to 8 (**D**), an anterior apical region of MSC uptake *(arrow)* is shown in three representative animals in the coronal view. This more anterior apical distribution was present independent of whether an early focal hot spot was observed *(yellow arrowhead)*. *(From Kraitchman DL, Tatsumi M, Gilson WD, et al: Dynamic imaging of allogeneic mesenchymal stem cells trafficking to myocardial infarction, Circulation 112:1451–1461, 2005. Reproduced with permission.)*

co-labeled with [^{111}In]-oxine and iron oxide, thus enabling SPECT and MRI tracking, respectively. SPECT demonstrated MSCs homing and engrafting to the heart for up to 7 days, whereas MRI was insufficiently sensitive to detect the cells in the heart or any other organ. In summary, MRI currently lacks the sensitivity of radionuclide-based labeling (SPECT/PET), which limits its ability to detect small numbers of cells in the heart ($>10^5$ cells are needed to be detectable).[92] In addition, the ferromagnetic probe may become diluted with cell

division, making it difficult to quantify proliferating cells. Last, the detected signal does not necessarily indicate whether the cells are viable. This is because iron particles can remain internalized in nonviable cells, and the iron particle may be engulfed by tissue macrophages, both events creating a false-positive signal.[93,94]

Reporter Gene Labeling

In contrast to physical labeling (radionuclide and iron particles), reporter gene labeling requires genetic modification of the stem cells. In the first proof-of-principle study using reporter genes to track cardiac cell survival, Wu et al. transfected rat H9c2 embryonic cardiomyoblasts with adenovirus carrying either firefly luciferase or HSV1-sr39tk reporter gene before injection into the rat myocardium.[95] Cell survival was monitored noninvasively by optical bioluminescence or small-animal PET imaging. Cell signal activity was quantified in units of photons per second per square centimeter per steradian (photons/sec/cm^2/sr) or percentage injected dose of ^{18}F-FHBG per gram tissue (%ID/g), respectively. In both cases, drastic reductions in signal activity were seen within the first 1 to 4 days due to acute donor cell death from inflammation, ischemia, and apoptosis. Interestingly, this pattern of cell death was consistent with other reports using traditional ex vivo assays such as TUNEL apoptosis,[96] classical histology,[97] and TaqMan RT-PCR.[10] However, all of these ex vivo techniques required large numbers of animals to be sacrificed at different time points.

Given that several types of reporter genes and reporter probes are now available, it should be possible in the future to perform multimodality imaging of stem cell transplantation. For example, the feasibility of imaging murine embryonic stem cells transplanted into the rodent myocardium has been demonstrated (Fig. 45-6).[98] These cells were genetically manipulated to express a triple-fusion reporter that consists of red fluorescence protein (RFP) for fluorescence activated cell sorting (FACS) analysis and single cell fluorescence microscopy, firefly luciferase (Fluc) for high throughput bioluminescence imaging, and herpes simplex virus thymidine kinase (HSVtk) for small-animal PET imaging. Imaging analysis revealed significant intracardiac and extracardiac teratoma formation with transplantation of undifferentiated embryonic stem cells. Thus, future efforts will need to involve differentiated derivatives such as embryonic stem cell–derived endothelial cells[99] or cardiomyocytes[100] for myocardial repair while avoiding the tumorigenicity issues.[101] Follow-up studies have also been demonstrated in a large-animal model using clinical PET/CT imaging of porcine MSCs stably transduced with *Renilla* luciferase, red fluorescent protein, and herpes simplex virus truncated thymidine kinase (RL-RFP-HSVttk) (Fig. 45-7).[102] In addition, several studies have used transgenic mice that constitutively express reporter genes to understand the spatiotemporal kinetics of bone marrow stem cell homing,[103] the optimal adult stem cell type for improving cardiac function,[104] the efficacy of different biomatrices capable of improving cell survival,[105] the fate of resident stem cells isolated

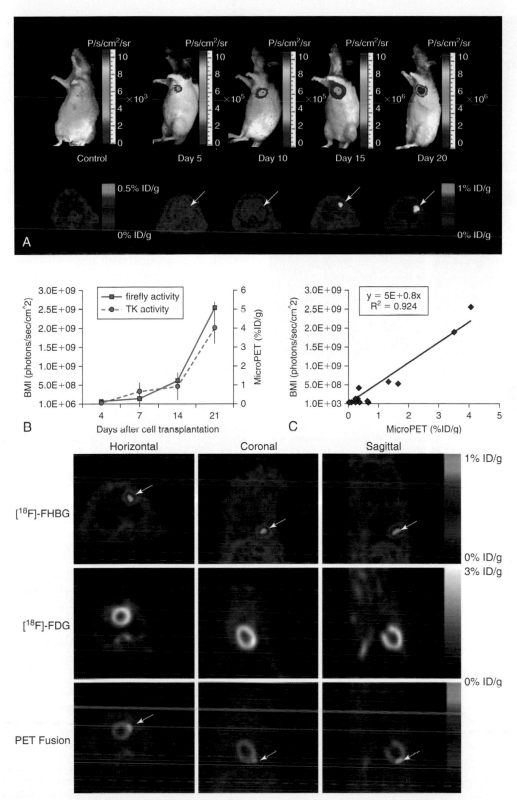

Figure 45-6 Reporter gene imaging of embryonic stem cells expressing triple-fusion reporter gene. **A,** To assess longitudinal cell survival, animals were imaged for 4 weeks. A representative study animal injected with ES-TF cells showed significant bioluminescence *(top)* and PET *(bottom)* signals at day 4, week 1, week 2, week 3, and week 4. In contrast, control animals had background activities only. **B,** Quantification of imaging signals showed a drastic increase of fluc and ttk activities from week 2 to week 4. Extracardiac signals were observed during subsequent weeks. **C,** Quantification of cell signals showed a robust in vivo correlation between bioluminescence and PET imaging ($r^2 = 0.92$). BLI indicates bioluminescence. **D,** After cell transplant, animals underwent [^{18}F]-FHBG reporter probe imaging *(top row)* for detection of cell survival and [^{18}F]-FDG imaging *(middle row)* for assessment of myocardial metabolic activity. Note background bone uptake of free fluoride is seen in both images. Fusion of the two images *(bottom row)* shows the exact location of transplanted embryonic stem cells carrying the triple-fusion reporter gene *(arrow)* at the anterolateral wall. The small-animal PET imaging provides horizontal, coronal, and sagittal views. Similar studies should be feasible using human clinical PET scanners in the future. *(From Cao F, Lin S, Xie X, et al: In vivo visualization of embryonic stem cell survival, proliferation, and migration after cardiac delivery. Circulation 113:1005–1014, 2006. Reproduced with permission.)*

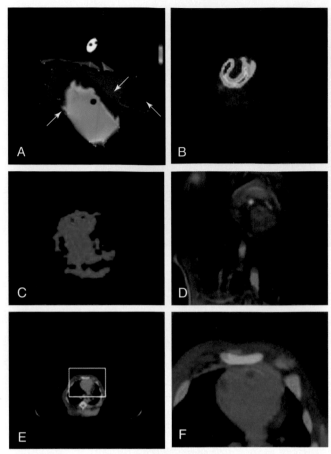

Figure 45-7 Reporter gene of stem cell therapy in a large-animal preclinical model. **A**, Endocardial mapping of a pig heart 16 days after myocardial infarction. Voltage map with sites *(black points)* of NOGA-guided intramyocardial injections of LV-RL-RFP-tTK-MSC *(white arrows* at border zone of infarction) and nontransfected mesenchymal stem cells (MSCs) *(yellow arrow* at noninfarcted posterior wall). Normal viability is represented by blue and pink colors. Yellow and green color represents decreased viability in the mid-distal anterior wall, and red, nonviability at the heart apex. **B**, $[^{13}N]$-NH$_3$ PET with transmission scan of the pig heart (supine position) 16 days after acute myocardial infarction, indicating perfusion defect in the anterior wall and apex. **C**, $[^{18}F]$-FHBG tracer uptake in the two injected points, representing the location of the LVRL-RFP-tTK-MSC 8 hours after cell delivery into the myocardium (PET transmission scan, pig in supine position). No activity in the posterior wall, where the nontransfected MSCs were injected. **D**, Fusion image of MRI (grayscale) and $[^{18}F]$-FHBG-PET (hot scale) indicating tracer accumulation in the sites only where LV-RL-RFP-tTK-MSCs were intramyocardially injected. **E**, $[^{18}F]$-FHBG-PET-CT hybrid image for localization of the injected cells in the anterior wall. *(From Gyongyosi M, Blanco J, Marian T, et al: Serial non-invasive in vivo positron emission tomographic (PET) tracking of percutaneously intramyocardially injected autologous porcine mesenchymal stem cells modified for transgene reporter gene expression, Circ Cardiovasc Imaging 1:94–103, 2008. Reproduced with permission.)*

Clinical Imaging

The first steps toward using molecular imaging technology to track cardiac cell therapy in humans have already been undertaken. In a recent study by Hofmann et al., PET imaging was used to track $[^{18}F]$-FDG-labeled autologous bone marrow cells for treatment of patients following acute MI (Fig. 45-8).[108] Unselected bone marrow cells were radiolabeled with 100 MBq $[^{18}F]$-FDG and infused into the infarct-related coronary artery (3 patients), or injected into the antecubital vein (3 patients). In an additional group of 3 patients, a CD34$^+$-enriched population of bone marrow cells was delivered by intracoronary infusion. In all groups, cells were administered 5 to 10 days following coronary stenting, and PET imaging was carried out 50 to 75 minutes after the procedure. PET successfully detected $[^{18}F]$ signals in all groups, with higher intramyocardial signal in the intracoronary versus intravenous delivery groups. Of the two groups receiving intracoronary infusion, the CD34$^+$-enriched population had a higher myocardial signal than unselected BMSCs (1.3% to 2.6% versus

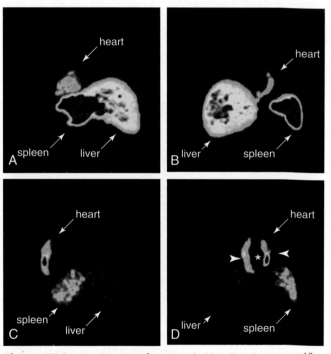

Figure 45-8 Monitoring of myocardial biodistribution of ^{18}F-FDG-labeled BMC in humans. Left posterior oblique (**A**) and left anterior oblique (**B**) views of the chest and upper abdomen of a patient, 65 minutes after transfer of ^{18}F-FDG-labeled, unselected bone marrow cells into the left circumflex coronary artery. BMC homing is detectable in the lateral wall of the heart (infarct center and border zone), liver, and spleen. Left posterior oblique (**C**) and left anterior oblique (**D**) views of the chest and upper abdomen of another patient, 70 minutes after transfer of ^{18}F-FDG-labeled, CD34-enriched bone marrow cells into the left anterior descending coronary artery. Homing of CD34$^+$-enriched cells is detectable in the anteroseptal wall of the heart, liver, and spleen. CD34$^+$ cell homing is most prominent in the infarct border zone *(arrowheads)* but not in the infarct center *(asterisk). (From Hofmann M, Wollert KC, Meyer GP, et al: Monitoring of bone marrow cell homing into the infarcted human myocardium, Circulation 111:2198–2202, 2005. Reproduced with permission.)*

from the heart,[106] and the effect of acute versus chronic infarction on stem cell viability.[107] These multi-reporter gene approaches may be helpful for evaluating other issues relevant to stem cell biology, such as imaging stem cell survival, proliferation, and differentiation using tissue-specific promoters.

14% to 39%, $P < 0.005$), suggesting enhanced homing to the injured myocardial milieu associated with CD34$^+$ stem cells (see Fig. 45-8). Although conducted in a small number of patients, this study demonstrates nicely a potential means to track stem cell therapy on a short-term basis. The fact that differing myocardial signal between groups was observed is encouraging insofar as it helps validate the sensitivity of clinical PET scanning for tracking cellular delivery and homing. As mentioned earlier, the major limitation of this technique is its inability to track long-term survival kinetics and cellular trafficking following therapy, given the half-life of ^{18}F-FDG is only around 110 minutes. Furthermore, radiolabeled cell signals do not provide information regarding cell proliferation, because the radiotracers cannot be "passed on" from mother to daughter cells. It would be most useful, for example, to observe changes in myocardial stem cell populations over weeks and correlate their late-phase survival or proliferation with functional improvement. In the future, genetically engineered constructs integrated into the transplanted stem cells may allow for such measurements, using a variety of molecular imaging techniques discussed here. Very recently, the feasibility of imaging CD8$^+$ T cells genetically engineered to express the HSV1-tk and imaged with ^{18}F-FHBG PET has been performed, and this sets the stage for human imaging of cell populations.[109] However, significant challenges remain to be overcome. From the imaging standpoint, the main obstacles are understanding the lowest number of detectable stem cells in the heart and the use of other reporter genes (e.g., human dopamine 2 receptor or human sodium iodide symporter or humanized HSVtk) that may be less immunogenic compared to the viral HSV1 tk.[61,110,111]

CONCLUSION

In summary, various approaches for monitoring cardiac gene and cell therapy have been discussed. Molecular imaging has emerged as a valuable tool for monitoring gene delivery and, more recently, following cellular therapy. Although the field is in its infancy, molecular imaging in humans is likely to grow rapidly as "molecular medicine" tailored to individual patients becomes a clinical reality in the future. Without a doubt, successful therapies will be predicated on a sound understanding of the pharmacokinetics, functional, and biological aspects of gene therapy and cellular delivery. Cardiac molecular imaging is an important tool that can help achieve these goals. The next 5 years should witness great excitement and progress as it has been for the past 5 years.

REFERENCES

1. Watson JD, Crick FH: Molecular structure of nucleic acids; a structure for deoxyribose nucleic acid, *Nature* 171:737–738, 1953.
2. Massoud TF, Gambhir SS: Molecular imaging in living subjects: seeing fundamental biological processes in a new light, *Genes Dev* 17:545–580, 2003.
3. Phelps ME: Inaugural article: positron emission tomography provides molecular imaging of biological processes, *Proc Natl Acad Sci U S A* 97:9226–9233, 2000.
4. International Human Genome Sequencing Consortium: Finishing the euchromatic sequence of the human genome, *Nature* 431 (7011):931–945, 2004.
5. International Human Genome Sequencing Consortium: Initial sequencing and analysis of the human genome, *Nature* 409 (6822):860–921, 2001.
6. Tefferi A: Genomic basics: DNA structure, gene expression, cloning, genetic mapping, and molecular tests: *Semin Cardiothorac Vasc Anesth* 10(4):282–290, 2006.
7. Schröder G, Risch K, Nizze H, et al: Immune response after adenoviral gene transfer in syngeneic heart transplants: effects of anti-CD4 monoclonal antibody therapy, *Transplantation* 70:191–198, 2000.
8. Hajjar RJ, Schmidt U, Matsui T, et al: Modulation of ventricular function through gene transfer in vivo, *Proc Natl Acad Sci U S A* 95:5251–5256, 1998.
9. Kass-Eisler A, Falck-Pedersen E, Alvira M, et al: Quantitative determination of adenovirus-mediated gene delivery to rat cardiac myocytes in vitro and in vivo, *Proc Natl Acad Sci U S A* 90:11498–11502, 1993.
10. Muller-Ehmsen J, Whittaker P, Kloner RA, et al: Survival and development of neonatal rat cardiomyocytes transplanted into adult myocardium, *J Mol Cell Cardiol* 34:107–116, 2002.
11. Herzog EL, Chai L, Krause DS: Plasticity of marrow-derived stem cells, *Blood* 102:3483–3493, 2003.
12. Shim WS, Jiang S, Wong P, et al: Ex vivo differentiation of human adult bone marrow stem cells into cardiomyocyte-like cells, *Biochem Biophys Res Commun* 324:481–488, 2004.
13. Verel I, Visser GW, van Dongen GA: The promise of immuno-PET in radioimmunotherapy, *J Nucl Med* 46(Suppl 1):164S–171S, 2005.
14. Meoli DF, Sadeghi MM, Krassilnikova S, et al: Noninvasive imaging of myocardial angiogenesis following experimental myocardial infarction, *J Clin Invest* 113:1684–1691, 2004.
15. Rodriguez-Porcel M, Cai W, Gheysens O, et al: Imaging of VEGF receptor in a rat myocardial infarction model using PET, *J Nucl Med* 49: 667–673, 2008.
16. Schelbert HR: 18F-deoxyglucose and the assessment of myocardial viability, *Semin Nucl Med* 32:60–69, 2002.
17. Shi N, Boado RJ, Pardridge WM: Antisense imaging of gene expression in the brain in vivo, *Proc Natl Acad Sci U S A* 97:14709–14714, 2000.
18. Tavitian B, Terrazzino S, Kuhnast B, et al: In vivo imaging of oligonucleotides with positron emission tomography, *Nat Med* 4:467–471, 1998.
19. Wu JC, Yla-Herttuala S: Human gene therapy and imaging: cardiology, *Eur J Nucl Med Mol Imaging* 32(2):S346–57, 2005.
20. Contag PR, Olomu IN, Stevenson DK, et al: Bioluminescent indicators in living mammals, *Nat Med* 4:245–247, 1998.
21. Lippincott-Schwartz J, Patterson GH: Development and use of fluorescent protein markers in living cells, *Science* 300:87–91, 2003.
22. Ramjiawan B, Ariano RE, Mantsch HH, et al: Immunofluorescence imaging as a tool for studying the pharmacokinetics of a human monoclonal single chain fragment antibody, *IEEE Trans Med Imaging* 21:1317–1323, 2002.
23. Wu JC, Sundaresan G, Iyer M, et al: Noninvasive optical imaging of firefly luciferase reporter gene expression in skeletal muscles of living mice, *Mol Ther* 4:297–306, 2001.
24. Funovics MA, Weissleder R, Mahmood U: Catheter-based in vivo imaging of enzyme activity and gene expression: feasibility study in mice, *Radiology* 231:659–666, 2004.
25. Bogdanov A, Weissleder R: In vivo imaging of gene delivery and expression, *Trends Biotechnol* 20:S11–S18, 2002.
26. Weissleder R, Moore A, Mahmood U, et al: In vivo magnetic resonance imaging of transgene expression, *Nat Med* 6:351–355, 2000.
27. Kircher MF, Allport JR, Graves EE, et al: In vivo high resolution three-dimensional imaging of antigen-specific cytotoxic T-lymphocyte trafficking to tumors, *Cancer Res* 63:6838–6846, 2003.
28. Lewin M, Carlesso N, Tung CH, et al: Tat peptide-derivatized magnetic nanoparticles allow in vivo tracking and recovery of progenitor cells, *Nat Biotechnol* 18:410–414, 2000.
29. Jaffer FA, Tung CH, Wykrzykowska JJ, et al: Molecular imaging of factor XIIIa activity in thrombosis using a novel, near-infrared fluorescent contrast agent that covalently links to thrombi, *Circulation* 110:170–176, 2004.
30. Kang HW, Josephson L, Petrovsky A, et al: Magnetic resonance imaging of inducible E-selectin expression in human endothelial cell culture, *Bioconjug Chem* 13:122–127, 2002.
31. Bulte JW, Kraitchman DL: Iron oxide MR contrast agents for molecular and cellular imaging, *NMR Biomed* 17:484–499, 2004.
32. Kaufmann BA, Lewis C, Xie A, et al: Detection of recent myocardial ischaemia by molecular imaging of P-selectin with targeted contrast echocardiography, *Eur Heart J* 28:2011–2017, 2007.
33. Kaufmann BA, Sanders JM, Davis C, et al: Molecular imaging of inflammation in atherosclerosis with targeted ultrasound detection of vascular cell adhesion molecule-1, *Circulation* 116:276–284, 2007.
34. Pascotto M, Leong-Poi H, Kaufmann B, et al: Assessment of ischemia-induced microvascular remodeling using contrast-enhanced

ultrasound vascular anatomic mapping, *J Am Soc Echocardiogr* 20: 1100–1108, 2007.

35. Dayton PA, Ferrara KW: Targeted imaging using ultrasound, *J Magn Reson Imaging* 16:362–377, 2002.

36. Kaufmann BA, Lindner JR: Molecular imaging with targeted contrast ultrasound, *Curr Opin Biotechnol* 18:11–16, 2007.

37. de la Zerda A, Zavaleta C, Keren S, et al: Carbon nanotubes as contrast agents for photoacoustic imaging of living mice, *Nat Nanotechnol* 3:557–562, 2008.

38. Schelbert HR, Inubushi M, Ross RS: PET imaging in small animals, *J Nucl Cardiol* 10:513–520, 2003.

39. Tai YC, Chatziioannou AF, Yang Y, et al: MicroPET II: design, development and initial performance of an improved microPET scanner for small-animal imaging, *Phys Med Biol* 48:1519–1537, 2003.

40. Yla-Herttuala S, Alitalo K: Gene transfer as a tool to induce therapeutic vascular growth, *Nat Med* 9:694–701, 2003.

41. Takeshita S, Pu LQ, Stein LA, et al: Intramuscular administration of vascular endothelial growth factor induces dose-dependent collateral artery augmentation in a rabbit model of chronic limb ischemia, *Circulation* 90:II228–II234, 1994.

42. Brogi E, Wu T, Namiki A, et al: Indirect angiogenic cytokines upregulate VEGF and bFGF gene expression in vascular smooth muscle cells, whereas hypoxia upregulates VEGF expression only, *Circulation* 90:649–652, 1994.

43. Shyu KG, Wang MT, Wang BW, et al: Intramyocardial injection of naked DNA encoding HIF-1alpha/VP16 hybrid to enhance angiogenesis in an acute myocardial infarction model in the rat, *Cardiovasc Res* 54:576–583, 2002.

44. Steg PG, Tahlil O, Aubailly N, et al: Reduction of restenosis after angioplasty in an atheromatous rabbit model by suicide gene therapy, *Circulation* 96:408–411, 1997.

45. Miyamoto MI, del Monte F, Schmidt U, et al: Adenoviral gene transfer of SERCA2a improves left-ventricular function in aortic-banded rats in transition to heart failure, *Proc Natl Acad Sci U S A* 97:793–798, 2000.

46. Kozarsky KF, Donahee MH, Glick JM, et al: Gene transfer and hepatic overexpression of the HDL receptor SR-BI reduces atherosclerosis in the cholesterol-fed LDL receptor-deficient mouse, *Arterioscler Thromb Vasc Biol* 20:721–727, 2000.

47. Matsui T, Li L, del Monte F, et al: Adenoviral gene transfer of activated phosphatidylinositol 3′-kinase and Akt inhibits apoptosis of hypoxic cardiomyocytes in vitro, *Circulation* 100:2373–2379, 1999.

48. Rosengart TK, Lee LY, Patel SR, et al: Angiogenesis gene therapy: phase I assessment of direct intramyocardial administration of an adenovirus vector expressing VEGF121 cDNA to individuals with clinically significant severe coronary artery disease, *Circulation* 100:468–474, 1999.

49. Symes JF, Losordo DW, Vale PR, et al: Gene therapy with vascular endothelial growth factor for inoperable coronary artery disease, *Ann Thorac Surg* 68:830–836, 1999 discussion 836–837.

50. Vale PR, Losordo DW, Milliken CE, et al: Left ventricular electromechanical mapping to assess efficacy of phVEGF(165) gene transfer for therapeutic angiogenesis in chronic myocardial ischemia, *Circulation* 102:965–974, 2000.

51. Henry TD, Annex BH, McKendall GR, et al: The VIVA trial: Vascular endothelial growth factor in Ischemia for Vascular Angiogenesis, *Circulation* 107:1359–1365, 2003.

52. Simons M, Annex BH, Laham RJ, et al: Pharmacological treatment of coronary artery disease with recombinant fibroblast growth factor-2: double-blind, randomized, controlled clinical trial, *Circulation* 105:788–793, 2002.

53. Grines CL, Watkins MW, Mahmarian JJ, et al: A randomized, double-blind, placebo-controlled trial of Ad5FGF-4 gene therapy and its effect on myocardial perfusion in patients with stable angina, *J Am Coll Cardiol* 42:1339–1347, 2003.

54. Grines CL, Watkins MW, Helmer G, et al: Angiogenic Gene Therapy (AGENT) trial in patients with stable angina pectoris, *Circulation* 105:1291–1297, 2002.

55. Hedman M, Hartikainen J, Syvanne M, et al: Safety and feasibility of catheter-based local intracoronary vascular endothelial growth factor gene transfer in the prevention of postangioplasty and in-stent restenosis and in the treatment of chronic myocardial ischemia: phase II results of the Kuopio Angiogenesis Trial (KAT), *Circulation* 107: 2677–2683, 2003.

56. Pislaru S, Janssens SP, Gersh BJ, et al: Defining gene transfer before expecting gene therapy: putting the horse before the cart, *Circulation* 106:631–636, 2002.

57. Wu JC, Inubushi M, Sundaresan G, et al: Positron emission tomography imaging of cardiac reporter gene expression in living rats, *Circulation* 106:180–183, 2002.

58. Wu JC, Inubushi M, Sundaresan G, et al: Optical imaging of cardiac reporter gene expression in living rats, *Circulation* 105:1631–1634, 2002.

59. Inubushi M, Wu JC, Gambhir SS, et al: Positron-emission tomography reporter gene expression imaging in rat myocardium, *Circulation* 107:326–332, 2003.

60. Bengel FM, Anton M, Richter T, et al: Noninvasive imaging of transgene expression by use of positron emission tomography in a pig model of myocardial gene transfer, *Circulation* 108:2127–2133, 2003.

61. Chen IY, Wu JC, Min JJ, et al: Micro-positron emission tomography imaging of cardiac gene expression in rats using bicistronic adenoviral vector-mediated gene delivery, *Circulation* 109:1415–1420, 2004.

62. Anton M, Wittermann C, Haubner R, et al: Coexpression of herpesviral thymidine kinase reporter gene and VEGF gene for noninvasive monitoring of therapeutic gene transfer: an in vitro evaluation, *J Nucl Med* 45:1743–1746, 2004.

63. Wu JC, Chen IY, Wang Y, et al: Molecular imaging of the kinetics of vascular endothelial growth factor gene expression in ischemic myocardium, *Circulation* 110:685–691, 2004.

64. Miyagawa M, Anton M, Haubner R, et al: PET of cardiac transgene expression: comparison of 2 approaches based on herpesviral thymidine kinase reporter gene, *J Nucl Med* 45:1917–1923, 2004.

65. Huang M, Chen ZY, Hu S, Jia F, Li Z, Hoyt G, Robbins RC, Kay MA, Wu JC: Novel minicircle vector for gene therapy in murine myocardial infarction, *Circulation* 120:S230–S237, 2009.

66. Boecker W, Bernecker OY, Wu JC, et al: Cardiac-specific gene expression facilitated by an enhanced myosin light chain promoter, *Mol Imaging* 3:69–75, 2004.

67. Huang M, Chan DA, Jia F, Xie X, Li Z, Hoyt G, Robbins RC, Chen X, Giaccia AJ, Wu JC: Short hairpin RNA interference therapy for ischemic heart disease, *Circulation* 118:S226–S233, 2008.

68. Orlic D, Kajstura J, Chimenti S, et al: Bone marrow cells regenerate infarcted myocardium, *Nature* 410:701–705, 2001.

69. Soonpaa MH, Koh GY, Klug MG, et al: Formation of nascent intercalated disks between grafted fetal cardiomyocytes and host myocardium, *Science* 264:98–101, 1994.

70. Menasche P, Hagege AA, Vilquin JT, et al: Autologous skeletal myoblast transplantation for severe postinfarction left ventricular dysfunction, *J Am Coll Cardiol* 41:1078–1083, 2003.

71. Taylor DA, Atkins BZ, Hungspreugs P, et al: Regenerating functional myocardium: improved performance after skeletal myoblast transplantation, *Nat Med* 4:929–933, 1998.

72. Laflamme MA, Chen KY, Naumova AV, et al: Cardiomyocytes derived from human embryonic stem cells in pro-survival factors enhance function of infarcted rat hearts, *Nat Biotechnol* 25:1015–1024, 2007.

73. Zhang SJ, Wu JC: Comparison of imaging techniques for tracking cardiac stem cell therapy, *J Nucl Med* 48(12):1916–1919, 2007.

74. Menasche P, Alfieri O, Janssens S, et al: The Myoblast Autologous Grafting in Ischemic Cardiomyopathy (MAGIC) trial: first randomized placebo-controlled study of myoblast transplantation, *Circulation* 117:1189–1200, 2008.

75. Assmus B, Honold J, Schachinger V, et al: Transcoronary transplantation of progenitor cells after myocardial infarction, *N Engl J Med* 355:1222–1232, 2006.

76. Lunde K, Solheim S, Aakhus S, et al: Intracoronary injection of mononuclear bone marrow cells in acute myocardial infarction, *N Engl J Med* 355:1199–1209, 2006.

77. Schachinger V, Erbs S, Elsasser A, et al: Intracoronary bone marrow-derived progenitor cells in acute myocardial infarction, *N Engl J Med* 355:1210–1221, 2006.

78. Rosenzweig A: Cardiac cell therapy: Mixed results from mixed cells, *N Engl J Med* 355:1274–1277, 2006.

79. Smith RR, Barile L, Cho HC, et al: Regenerative potential of cardiosphere-derived cells expanded from percutaneous endomyocardial biopsy specimens, *Circulation* 115:896–908, 2007.

80. Aicher A, Brenner W, Zuhayra M, et al: Assessment of the tissue distribution of transplanted human endothelial progenitor cells by radioactive labeling, *Circulation* 107:2134–2139, 2003.

81. Adonai N, Nguyen KN, Walsh J, et al: Ex vivo cell labeling with ^{64}Cu-pyruvaldehyde-bis(N_4-methylthiosemicarbazone) for imaging cell trafficking in mice with positron-emission tomography, *Proc Natl Acad Sci U S A* 99:3030–3035, 2002.

82. Dubertret B, Skourides P, Norris DJ, et al: In vivo imaging of quantum dots encapsulated in phospholipid micelles, *Science* 298:1759–1762, 2002.

83. Jaiswal JK, Mattoussi H, Mauro JM, et al: Long-term multiple color imaging of live cells using quantum dot bioconjugates, *Nat Biotechnol* 21:47–51, 2003.

84. Lin S, Xie X, Patel MR, et al: Quantum dot imaging for embryonic stem cells, *BMC Biotechnol* 67, 2007.

85. Hsieh SC, Wang FF, Lin CS, et al: The inhibition of osteogenesis with human bone marrow mesenchymal stem cells by CdSe/ZnS quantum dot labels, *Biomaterials* 27:1656–1664, 2006.

86. Jaiswal JK, Simon SM: Potentials and pitfalls of fluorescent quantum dots for biological imaging, *Trends Cell Biol* 14:497–504, 2004.

87. Keren S, Zavaleta C, Cheng Z, et al: Noninvasive molecular imaging of small living subjects using Raman spectroscopy, *Proc Natl Acad Sci U S A* 105:5844–5849, 2008.

88. Zavaleta C, de la Zerda A, Liu Z, et al: Non-invasive Raman spectroscopy in living mice for evaluation of tumor targeting with carbon nanotubes, *Nano Lett* 8:2800–2805, 2008.

89. Bulte JW, Douglas T, Witwer B, et al: Magnetodendrimers allow endosomal magnetic labeling and in vivo tracking of stem cells, *Nat Biotechnol* 19:1141–1147, 2001.

90. Amado LC, Saliaris AP, Schuleri KH, et al: Cardiac repair with intramyocardial injection of allogeneic mesenchymal stem cells after myocardial infarction, *Proc Natl Acad Sci U S A* 102:11474–11479, 2005.

91. Kraitchman DL, Heldman AW, Atalar E, et al: In vivo magnetic resonance imaging of mesenchymal stem cells in myocardial infarction, *Circulation* 107:2290–2293, 2003.

92. Kraitchman DL, Tatsumi M, Gilson WD, et al: Dynamic imaging of allogeneic mesenchymal stem cells trafficking to myocardial infarction, *Circulation* 112:1451–1461, 2005.

93. Li Z, Suzuki Y, Huang M, et al: Comparison of reporter gene and iron particle labeling for tracking fate of human embryonic stem cells and differentiated endothelial cells in living subjects, *Stem Cells* 26:864–873, 2008.

94. Chen IY, Greve JM, Gheysens O, Willmann JK, Rodriguez-Porcel M, Chu P, Sheikh AY, Faranesh AZ, Paulmurugan R, Yang PC, Wu JC, Gambhir SS: Comparison of optical bioluminescence reporter gene and superparamagnetic iron oxide MR contrast agent as cell markers for noninvasive imaging of cardiac cell transplantation, *Mol Imaging Biol* 11(3):178–187, 2009.

95. Wu JC, Chen IY, Sundaresan G, et al: Molecular imaging of cardiac cell transplantation in living animals using optical bioluminescence and positron emission tomography, *Circulation* 108:1302–1305, 2003.

96. Zhang M, Methot D, Poppa V, et al: Cardiomyocyte grafting for cardiac repair: graft cell death and anti-death strategies, *J Mol Cell Cardiol* 33:907–921, 2001.

97. Murry CE, Wiseman RW, Schwartz SM, et al: Skeletal myoblast transplantation for repair of myocardial necrosis, *J Clin Invest* 98:2512–2523, 1996.

98. Cao F, Lin S, Xie X, et al: In vivo visualization of embryonic stem cell survival, proliferation, and migration after cardiac delivery, *Circulation* 113:1005–1014, 2006.

99. Li Z, Wu JC, Sheikh AY, et al: Differentiation, survival, and function of embryonic stem cell derived endothelial cells for ischemic heart disease, *Circulation* 116:I46–I54, 2007.

100. Cao F, Wager RA, Wilson KD, et al: Transcriptional and functional profiling of human embryonic stem cell-derived cardiomyocytes, *PLoS ONE* e3474, 2008.

101. Cao F, Li Z, Lee A, et al: Noninvasive de novo imaging of human embryonic stem cell-derived teratoma formation, *Cancer Res* 69:2709–2713, 2009.

102. Gyongyosi M, Blanco J, Marian T, et al: Serial non-invasive in vivo positron emission tomographic (PET) tracking of percutaneously intramyocardially injected autologous porcine mesenchymal stem cells modified for transgene reporter gene expression, *Circ Cardiovasc Imaging* 1:94–103, 2008.

103. Sheikh AY, Lin SA, Cao F, et al: Molecular imaging of bone marrow mononuclear cell homing and engraftment in ischemic myocardium, *Stem Cells* 25:2677–2684, 2007.

104. van der Bogt KE, Sheik AY, Schrepfer S, et al: Comparison of different adult stem cell types for treatment of myocardial ischemia, *Circulation* 118:S121–S129, 2008.

105. Cao F, Sadrzadeh Rafie AH, Abilez OJ, et al: In vivo imaging and evaluation of different biomatrices for improvement of stem cell survival, *J Tissue Eng Regen Med* 1:465–468, 2007.

106. Li Z, Chun H, Xie X, et al: Imaging survival and function of transplanted cardiac stem cells, *J Am Coll Cardiol* 53:1229–1240, 2009.

107. Swijnenburg RJ, Govaert JA, Stein W, et al: Effect of timing of bone marrow cell delivery on cell viability and cardiac recovery following myocardial infarction [abstract], *Circulation* 118:S_790, 2008.

108. Hofmann M, Wollert KC, Meyer GP, et al: Monitoring of bone marrow cell homing into the infarcted human myocardium, *Circulation* 111:2198–2202, 2005.

109. Yaghoubi S, Jensen MC, Satyamurthy N, et al: Non-invasive detection of therapeutic cytolytic T cells with [18F]FHBG positron emission tomography in a glioma patient, *Nat Clin Pract Oncol* 6(1):53–58, 2009.

110. Ponomarev V, Doubrovin M, Shavrin A, et al: A human-derived reporter gene for noninvasive imaging in humans: mitochondrial thymidine kinase type 2, *J Nucl Med* 48:819–826, 2007.

111. Terrovitis J, Kwok KF, Lautamaki R, et al: Ectopic expression of the sodium-iodide symporter enables imaging of transplanted cardiac stem cells in vivo by SPECT or PET, *J Am Coll Cardiol* 52(20):1650–1660, 2008.

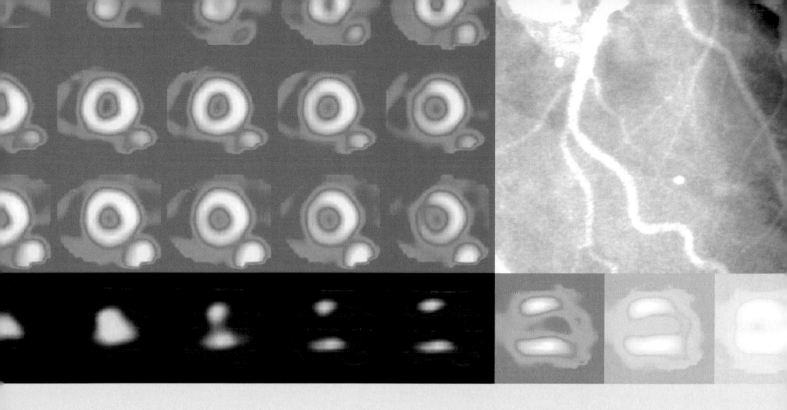

Atlas of Cases

CASE 1

A 68-year-old man with a history of hypertension presented to the emergency department for evaluation of new-onset weakness and diaphoresis. He denied chest pain. He had no other coronary disease risk factors.

Laboratory examination was normal except for leukocytosis (WBC = 22,000). He left against medical advice but returned 2 days later for persistent symptoms. Exercise SPECT MPI was requested.

Baseline ECG

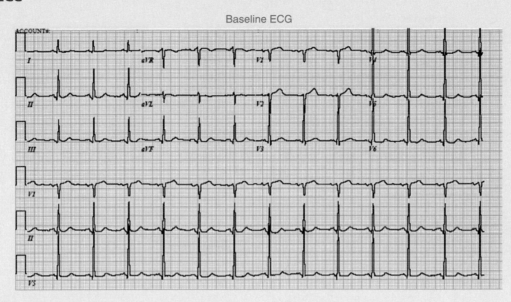

Baseline ECG

The baseline ECG shows normal sinus rhythm with slightly increased QRS voltage consistent with left ventricular hypertrophy.

Exercise Parameters

He exercised on a Bruce protocol for 6:32 minutes, achieving an estimated workload of 7.7 METs.

The peak exercise heart rate was 146 beats/min (96% of maximum age-predicted heart rate). No chest pain was reported, and the blood pressure response to exercise was normal.

Peak Exercise ECG

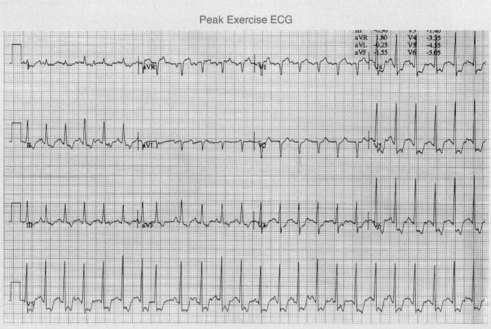

Peak Exercise ECG

The peak exercise ECG demonstrated sinus tachycardia with 4 mm of downsloping ST-segment depression suggestive of ischemia.

Raw Planar Images

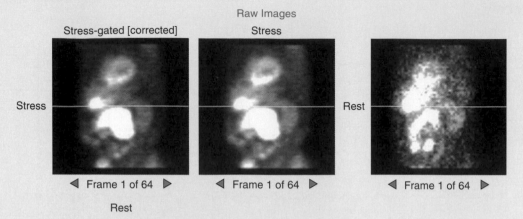

Raw Images

Stress-gated [corrected]   Stress

Stress

◀ Frame 1 of 64 ▶   ◀ Frame 1 of 64 ▶   ◀ Frame 1 of 64 ▶

Rest

Rest

The postexercise *(above)* and resting *(below)* raw images are shown. Image quality appears adequate.

Short-Axis Tomograms

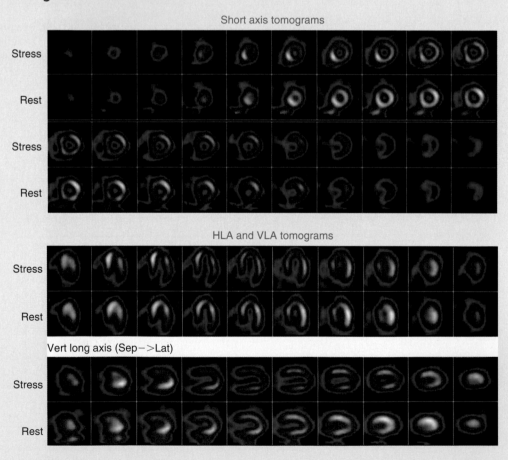

Short axis tomograms

Stress

Rest

Stress

Rest

HLA and VLA tomograms

Stress

Rest

Vert long axis (Sep−>Lat)

Stress

Rest

SPECT Tomographic Slices

The poststress images demonstrate a mild defect in the anterior and anterolateral regions and a moderately severe defect in the apical region. Resting images demonstrate nearly complete defect reversibility.

Polar Map

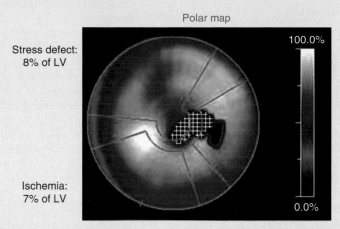

Polar map

Stress defect:
8% of LV

100.0%

Ischemia:
7% of LV

0.0%

Quantitative Polar Map

On comparison of the patient's perfusion pattern to a male-specific normal database, the apical perfusion is deemed to be abnormal (the apical defect involves 8% of the left ventricular myocardium). On comparison to resting images, significant defect reversibility is evident (7% of the left ventricular myocardium).

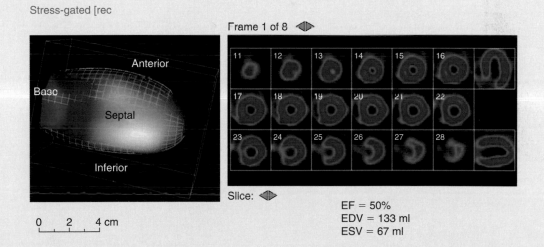

Stress-gated [rec

Frame 1 of 8

Anterior

Base

Septal

Inferior

Slice:

0   2   4 cm

EF = 50%
EDV = 133 ml
ESV = 67 ml

Gated SPECT Images

Postexercise gated SPECT images demonstrated low-normal global left ventricular systolic function (LVEF = 50%) with borderline increased left ventricular end-diastolic (normal < 120 mL) and end-systolic (normal < 70 mL) volumes.

Patient Management

The SPECT MPI results were reviewed in the clinical context of the patient's presenting symptoms. The presentation was atypical for an acute coronary syndrome and more consistent with an infectious etiology. The SPECT MPI results suggested the presence of inducible ischemia, though the perfusion abnormality appeared to be confined to a small portion (<10%) of the left ventricle. Medical therapy for CAD was therefore contemplated as a reasonable approach. However, the exercise ECG parameters suggested that the patient may be at high risk for cardiac events. The computed Duke treadmill score (DTS) was −13 (high-risk category). The DTS was calculated as: (7 min exercise) − (5 × 4 mm ST depression) − (4 × 0 anginal index*) = 13. Because of the high-risk DTS, he was referred for coronary angiography.

Coronary Angiography

The coronary angiogram revealed 80% stenosis of the distal left main artery (LM), with mild (10%) diffuse stenoses in the LAD, LCX, and RCA. Coronary artery bypass grafting was recommended.

Detection of Left Main Stenosis

This case illustrates the detection of isolated LM stenosis by SPECT MPI. The sensitivity of contemporary SPECT MPI for detecting isolated LM stenosis is low (<50%). Frequently, LM disease is detected "fortuitously" because there is a second focal stenosis present in a remote coronary artery that produces a perfusion defect and leads to diagnostic coronary angiography. Patients with isolated LM stenosis (who lack an additional flow-limiting stenosis elsewhere) frequently have minimal to no perfusion defect detected on SPECT MPI.

Several imaging (and nonimaging) markers have been proposed to enhance detection of LM stenosis with SPECT MPI. These markers include:

- A decline in blood pressure with exercise
- Severe exercise-induced ST depression at a low heart rate and/or low exercise workload
- ST depression during pharmacologic stress
- Increased stress/rest left ventricular cavity ratio (also known as *transient ischemic dilation*)
- Increased lung tracer activity on poststress images
- Increased right ventricular activity (relative to left ventricular activity) on poststress images

In this patient, clues to the presence of left main stenosis included marked ST depression and an increase in stress/rest LV cavity ratio (1.49; normal < 1.22). In the future, it is hoped that routine measurement of absolute (rather than relative) myocardial blood flow with rubidium-82 PET MPI may improve our ability to detect isolated LM stenosis (and other conditions in which "balanced" myocardial hypoperfusion occurs during stress).

CASE 2

A 45-year-old man is urged by his wife to have a cardiac risk assessment. He has no cardiac symptoms.

His only coronary risk factor is dyslipidemia (LDL = 143 mg/dL, HDL = 35 mg/dL).

National Cholesterol Education Program (NCEP) Adult Treatment Panel III

National Cholesterol Education Program (NCEP)
Adult Treatment Panel III

2 "non-LDL" risk factors: Age (men ≥ 45 years)
Low HDL (< 40 mg/dl)

⬇

Determine Framingham risk score

Circulation 2004; 110:227-239.

According to the NCEP Adult Treatment Panel III, he has two "non-LDL" risk factors. The next step is to determine his Framingham Risk Score (FRS).

Framingham Risk Score

Age: 45
Gender: Male
Total Cholesterol: 240 mg/dL
HDL Cholesterol: 35 mg/dL
Smoker: No
Systolic BP: 135 mm Hg
BP Medication: No
Risk Score: 6% over 10 years (low risk)

NCEP Adult Treatment Panel III

NCEP Adult Treatment Panel III

Low CHD risk (Framingham risk score < 10%)

⬇

Goal LDL < 160 mg/dl

⬇

Threshold for drug therapy: LDL ≥ 190 mg/dl

Because his FRS is "low risk" and his target LDL is < 160 mg/dL, no treatment with cholesterol-lowering medications would be recommended. No other diagnostic testing is recommended.

Proposed Management Strategy for Asymptomatic Patients

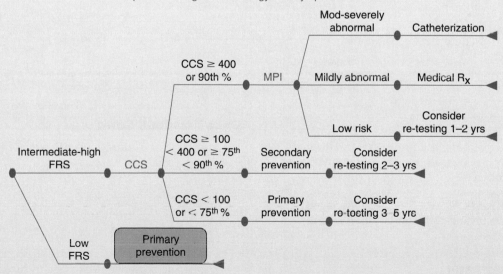

Proposed Management Strategy for Asymptomatic Patients

Because his FRS is "low risk," the proposed treatment algorithm would suggest that he be managed according to primary prevention guidelines.

However, the patient's wife requested that he have a coronary calcium score (CCS). According to published appropriateness criteria, CCS would be considered inappropriate (median score = 1) in this man with a low (<10% event rate over 10 years) FRS. However, at the urging of his wife, the CCS was obtained. (Refer to Hendel et al. J Am Coll Cardiol 48:1475-1497, 2006.)

Coronary Calcium Score

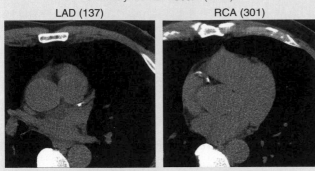

Coronary Calcium Score (CCS)

LAD (137)   RCA (301)

CCS = 137 + 301 = 438 (> 90th %)

Calcified plaque was detected in the LAD (137) and RCA (301), with a total CCS of 438 (>90th percentile for age and gender).

Clinical Questions

1. Does he have coronary artery disease (CAD), and would he benefit from aggressive risk-factor modification? Yes. Despite his low-risk FRS, the presence of extensive coronary calcification confirms the presence of atherosclerosis and warrants aggressive risk-factor modification according to secondary prevention guidelines.
2. Would he benefit from coronary revascularization? At this point, we cannot answer this question. The presence of coronary atherosclerosis by CCS does not imply the presence of flow-limiting CAD that might benefit from revascularization.

Proposed Management Strategy for Asymptomatic Patients

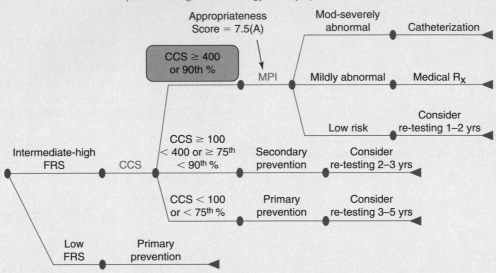

Proposed Management Strategy for Asymptomatic Patients

Adapted from Shaw LJ, et. *J Nuc Cardiol 2005*; 12:131-142.

According to the proposed management strategy for asymptomatic patients, the finding of an elevated CCS (>400 or >90th percentile for age and gender) is an appropriate indication for stress MPI (median appropriateness score = 7.5). Regardless of the stress MPI results, his risk factors should be managed aggressively according to secondary prevention guidelines.

Exercise SPECT MPI

He exercised on a Bruce protocol for 14:30 minutes (17 METs). No symptoms were reported, and his hemodynamic response was normal. He had 1 mm horizontal ST depression at peak exercise that resolved <1 minute into recovery.

Duke Treadmill Score

(14 min) − (5 × 1 mm) − (4 × 0 index*) = +9

Score	Risk	5-yr Survival
<−10	High	<75%
−10 to 4	Intermediate	95%
>4	Low	99%

Despite the presence of exercise-induced ST-segment depression, his excellent exercise capacity and lack of anginal symptoms resulted in a computed Duke treadmill score of +9 (>4 = low risk).

*Angina index: 0 = none, 1 = nonlimiting, 2 = limiting

SPECT Images

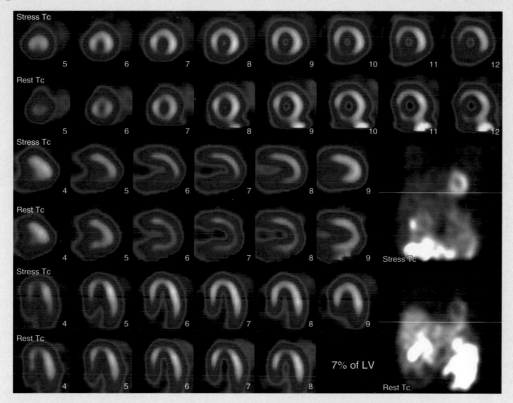

On poststress images, there was a mild to moderate focal perfusion defect noted in the inferior and inferobasilar regions. Resting images demonstrated defect reversibility consistent with inducible ischemia. Interpretation was complicated by GI tracer interference.

Gated SPECT Images

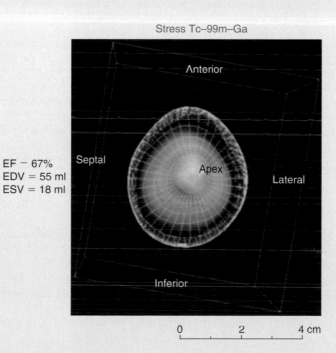

On poststress gated SPECT images, there was normal myocardial systolic thickening in all myocardial regions, with a normal computed left ventricular ejection fraction of 67%.

ASNC Management Strategy for Asymptomatic Patients

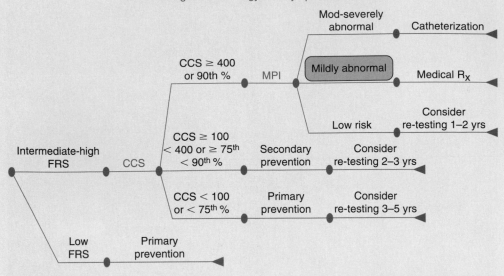

ASNC Management Strategy for Asymptomatic Patients

Shaw LJ, et. *J Nuc Cardiol 2005*; 12:131-142. (slide courtesy of Dr. Mieres)

This exercise stress SPECT MPI study would be classified as mildly abnormal based on the mild (localized) inducible ischemia at a high exercise workload and normal left ventricular systolic function. According to the proposed management algorithm for asymptomatic patients, medical therapy is the recommended treatment for patients with mildly abnormal MPI studies.

Recommendations

1. Aggressive medical therapy (secondary prevention guidelines) was recommended.
2. Coronary angiography could be considered if the patient develops angina symptoms or shows evidence of progression of disease on subsequent testing.

However, the patient's wife convinced his cardiologist to perform coronary angiography.

Coronary Angiography

- Left main: normal
- LAD: mild diffuse plaque
- LCX: normal
- RCA: 60% proximal, 70% mid

The coronary angiogram demonstrated mild diffuse atheromatous plaque in the LAD and sequential moderate (60% proximal and 70% mid) stenoses in the RCA. The coronary angiogram results were consistent with the CCS (plaque was confirmed in the LAD and

RCA territories). The angiogram results were also consistent with the SPECT MPI study (mild inferior and inferobasilar ischemia at a high exercise workload is consistent with moderate sequential stenoses in the RCA). Given the absence of angina and the excellent exercise capacity, no coronary revascularization was performed, and medical therapy was recommended.

Teaching Points (See Chapters 20 and 22)

This case demonstrates the complementary roles of MPI and CCS.

The CCS demonstrated the presence of coronary atherosclerosis and guided the aggressiveness of medical therapy for his coronary risk factors. The invasive coronary angiogram did not add additional information in this regard. CCS is the test of choice when the clinical question is, "Does this patient have coronary atherosclerosis and would he/she benefit from aggressive risk-factor modification?"

The MPI study demonstrated mild inducible ischemia at a high exercise workload, suggesting the presence of flow-limiting coronary stenosis but a favorable prognosis. The invasive coronary angiogram confirmed the MPI findings. MPI is the test of choice when the clinical question is, "Would this patient derive benefit from coronary revascularization?"

The CCS and MPI results provide complementary information and are used to answer distinct clinical questions.

CASE 3

A 60-year-old woman was referred for SPECT MPI for evaluation of chest pain. The chest pain description was consistent with atypical angina. Her coronary risk factors included hyperlipidemia, hypertension, and a family history of premature coronary artery disease (CAD).

Resting ECG was normal.

According to published appropriateness criteria, stress MPI would be appropriate (median score = 7) in a patient with chest pain, an interpretable ECG, and an intermediate pretest probability of CAD based on presenting symptoms, age, and gender.

Exercise Data

She exercised to a maximal workload of 10 METs, achieving a peak heart rate of 150 beats/min (94% of maximum age-predicted heart rate). No chest pain was reported during exercise, and the blood pressure and ECG responses were normal.

SPECT Images

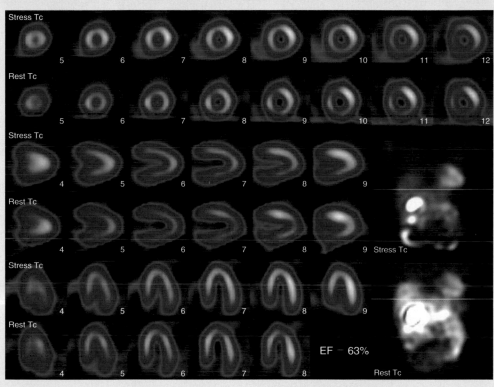

SPECT MPI demonstrated normal uniform uptake of ^{99m}Tc-sestamibi in all myocardial regions. Gated SPECT demonstrated normal myocardial systolic thickening in all myocardial regions, with a computed left ventricular ejection fraction (LVEF) of 63%.

Clinical Questions

1. Would she benefit from coronary revascularization? No. The absence of inducible ischemia at an adequate exercise workload and the presence of normal left ventricular function suggest a low short-term risk for myocardial infarction or cardiac death.
2. Does she have coronary artery disease, and would she benefit from aggressive risk-factor modification? At this point, we cannot answer this question. The finding of normal myocardial perfusion on MPI does not exclude the presence of nonobstructive coronary atherosclerosis.

Framingham Risk Score

Age: 60
Gender: Female
Total Cholesterol: 210 mg/dL
HDL Cholesterol: 45 mg/dL
Smoker: No
Systolic BP: 155 mm Hg
BP Medication: Yes
Risk Score: 6% over 10 years

Based on her age, gender, lipid values, blood pressure, and smoking status, her calculated Framingham Risk Score is 6% (10-year risk). This places her in a low-risk category. Primary prevention guidelines would apply.

Coronary Calcium Score (CCS)

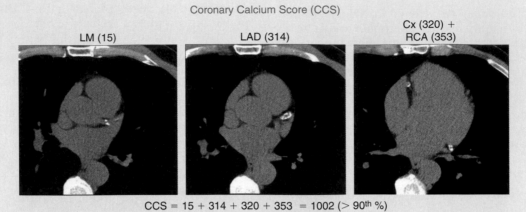

Coronary Calcium Score (CCS)

| LM (15) | LAD (314) | Cx (320) + RCA (353) |

CCS = 15 + 314 + 320 + 353 = 1002 (> 90th %)

Coronary calcium scoring (CCS) was performed to further assess her risk for coronary events. Calcified plaque was detected in the left main (15), LAD (314), left circumflex (320), and RCA (353), with a total CCS of 1002 (>90th percentile for age and gender). These findings confirm the presence of extensive coronary atherosclerosis and suggest that she is at increased long-term risk for cardiac events.

Observation studies have shown that over 50% of patients with normal MPI studies have evidence of clinically significant coronary atherosclerosis (CCS > 100). Therefore, CCS may be used to further define long-term coronary risk in patients with normal MPI results.

However, CCS is *not* appropriate following a normal MPI study in patients who already qualify for aggressive risk-factor modification, such as those with:

1. Known coronary artery disease (prior MI, PCI, or CABG)

2. Coronary heart disease risk equivalents (carotid disease, peripheral arterial disease, abdominal aortic aneurysm, diabetes)

Patient Management

Based on the normal MPI results and the markedly elevated CCS, aggressive medical therapy would be appropriate (according to secondary prevention guidelines). However, the managing cardiologist was concerned that the normal SPECT MPI results might represent a "false-negative" study due to balanced myocardial ischemia. Coronary angiography was therefore performed. The angiogram demonstrated mild diffuse coronary artery disease (<20% stenoses in all three major coronary arteries). Thus, the coronary angiogram added no additional information in this case. The angiogram simply confirmed the findings of mild diffuse CAD (already documented on CCS) and the absence of flow-limiting stenosis (already documented on MPI).

CASE 4

A 56-year-old man with no prior cardiac history was referred for SPECT MPI for evaluation of dyspnea.

Exercise parameters: 10:00 Bruce protocol (11.7 METs), peak HR 169 beats/min (102% of maximum age-predicted HR), no symptoms, normal BP response, abnormal ECG response (>1 mm ST depression)

Baseline 12-Lead ECG

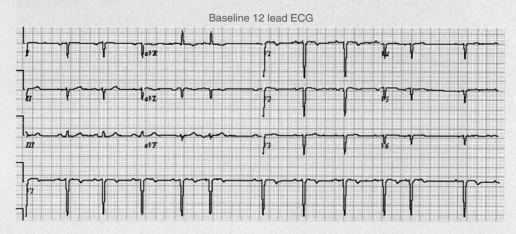

Baseline 12 lead ECG

The baseline ECG demonstrates an abnormal P-wave axis, premature supraventricular complexes, and right-axis deviation of the QRS complexes. There is abnormal R wave progression in the precordial leads. The constellation of findings is suggestive of dextrocardia.

Raw Planar Images

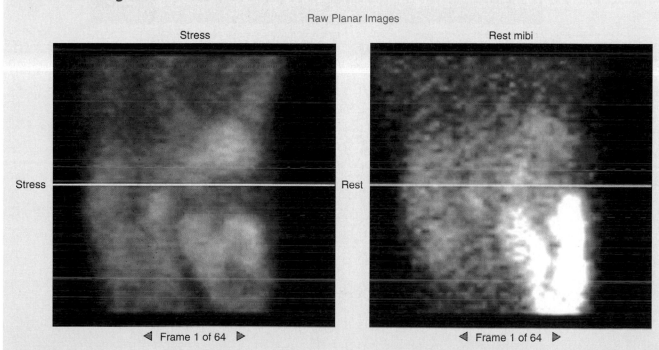

Raw Planar Images

The images were acquired over 180 degrees from the 45-degree right posterior oblique to 45-degree left anterior oblique orientations. Note that the heart is located in the right side of the chest, consistent with dextrocardia. The liver is located on the left, consistent with situs inversus.

SPECT Tomographic Slices

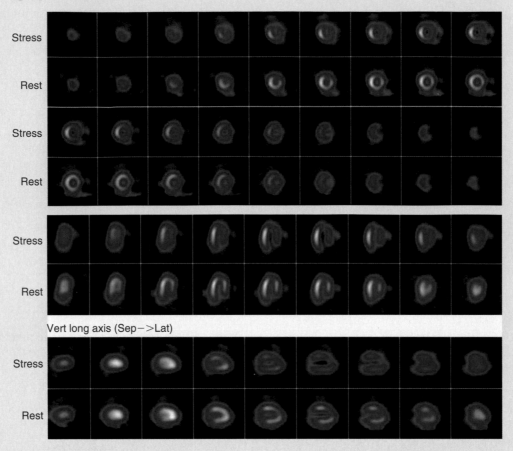

Stress

Rest

Stress

Rest

Stress

Rest

Vert long axis (Sep−>Lat)

Stress

Rest

SPECT images are displayed in the standard short-axis, horizontal long-axis, and vertical long-axis orientations. Note that the left and right ventricles are reversed from their usual locations. The appearance is consistent with dextrocardia. Severe inducible ischemia is also present.

Polar Maps

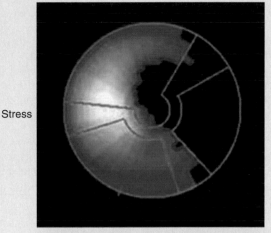

Stress

Defect blackout map

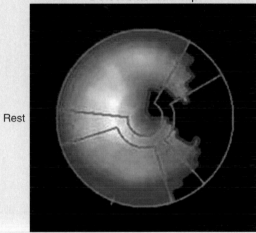

Rest

Defect blackout map

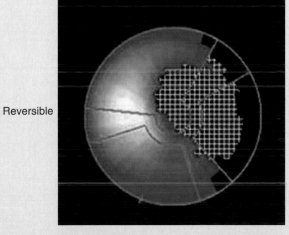

Reversible

The polar maps suggest that the reversible perfusion defect is located in the anterolateral region, and the perfusion defect corresponds to the territory of the left circumflex coronary artery. Actually, the defect is located in the anteroseptal region and is due to left anterior descending disease. The polar maps are displayed in their normal format and are not corrected for the patient's dextrocardia.

Poststress Gated SPECT MPI

Stress-gated [rec

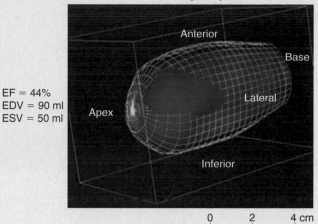

EF = 44%
EDV = 90 ml
ESV = 50 ml

0   2   4 cm

The poststress gated SPECT images demonstrate moderately reduced myocardial systolic thickening in the anteroseptal region, with a computed LVEF of 44%. The regional hypokinesis and reduced LVEF may be due to postischemic myocardial stunning or an imaging artifact created by the severe perfusion defect (leading to an inaccurate tracking of the endocardial border by the automated gated SPECT algorithm).

Cardiac Catheterization

Cardiac Cathotorization

Lossy compression - not intended for diagnosis

Lossy compression - not intended for diagnosis

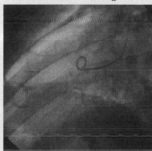
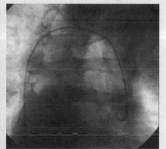

At cardiac catheterization, the heart and aorta demonstrated mirror-image reversal of the normal left-right orientation, consistent with dextrocardia.

Coronary Angiography

Coronary Angiography

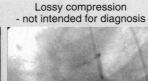

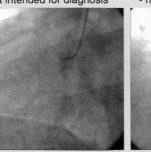

Lossy compression - not intended for diagnosis   Lossy compression - not intended for diagnosis

As expected, coronary angiography demonstrated severe LAD stenosis, which was treated with PCI.

Mirror-Image Dextrocardia with Situs Inversus

This patient had mirror-image dextrocardia with situs inversus. This condition has a prevalence of 1 in 10,000. In 25% of cases, there is associated sinusitis and bronchiectasis (Kartagener's syndrome).

It is crucial to review the raw planar images, paying attention to both the location and orientation of the heart and the liver. If the condition is suspected prior to imaging, the images should be acquired from left anterior oblique to right posterior oblique.

Unless the images are reoriented (left-right reversed), the quantitative polar maps cannot be used to localize perfusion defects or to correctly compare the patient's tracer distribution to a normal gender-specific database.

CASE 5

A 65-year-old man with chronic cigarette smoking but no prior cardiac history was referred for exercise SPECT MPI for evaluation of exertional dyspnea.

Raw Planar Images and SPECT Tomograms

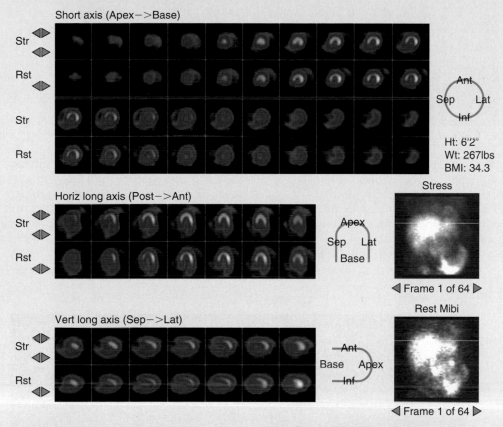

Ht: 6'2"
Wt: 267lbs
BMI: 34.3

The raw planar images demonstrate soft-tissue attenuation and GI tracer activity in close proximity to the heart. Based on the patient's height and weight, his body mass index is 34.3 (>30 = obese). Patient motion is also noted.

SPECT images demonstrate a severe and extensive inferior perfusion defect. Because of GI tracer interference, it is difficult to discern if defect reversibility is present.

Quantitative Polar Map

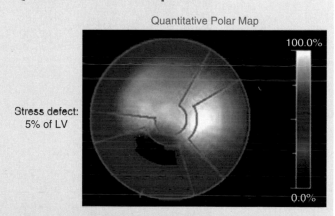

When the perfusion pattern of this patient was compared to a male-specific normal database, the inferior-wall stress perfusion defect was judged to be abnormal by quantitative criteria. This suggests that the defect may not be entirely related to soft-tissue attenuation artifact and GI tracer interference.

Gated SPECT Images

Frame 1 of 8

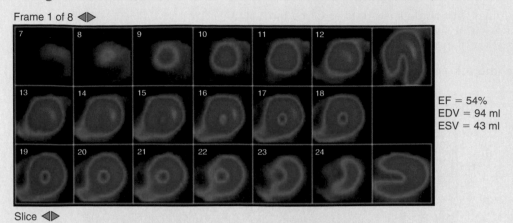

EF = 54%
EDV = 94 ml
ESV = 43 ml

Slice

Gated SPECT images show normal myocardial systolic thickening in all regions, with a normal computed LVEF (54%). However, the presence of normal myocardial systolic thickening cannot be used to confidently exclude inducible myocardial ischemia when defect reversibility is evident.

The patient was referred for rubidium-82 (^{82}Rb) PET MPI.

The SPECT study results were equivocal, owing to the partly reversible perfusion defect in the presence of coexisting soft-tissue attenuation artifact and GI tracer interference. Therefore, confirmatory diagnostic testing was needed. He was subsequently referred for dipyridamole stress ^{82}Rb gated PET MPI.

PET Tomograms

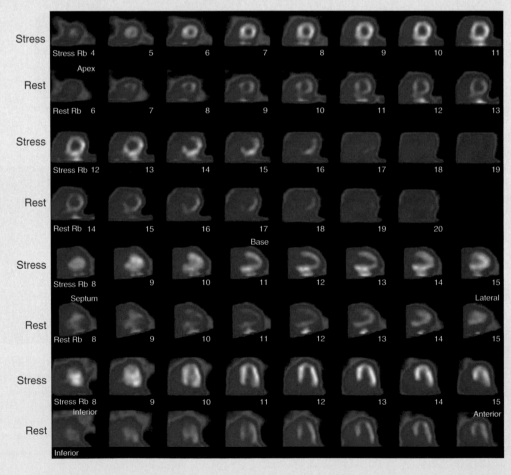

The ^{82}Rb PET images demonstrate normal myocardial perfusion in all regions, including the inferior wall. PET images are routinely corrected for soft-tissue attenuation, and therefore PET MPI provides a more reliable assessment of regional myocardial perfusion, irrespective of gender or body habitus.

Note that GI tracer activity is present on the peak stress and resting ^{82}Rb perfusion images. However, because of the superior spatial resolution of PET (compared to SPECT), the GI tracer activity does not result in problems with PET image interpretation.

Gated PET Images

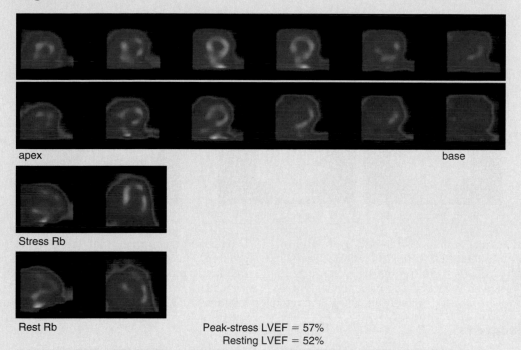

apex

base

Stress Rb

Rest Rb

Peak-stress LVEF = 57%
Resting LVEF = 52%

The ^{82}Rb PET images are gated both at rest and at peak stress. The ability to measure regional and global left ventricular systolic function at peak stress is a unique advantage of PET MPI. In this case, the LVEF was normal (52%) on resting gated PET images, and the LVEF increased to 57% at peak stress. An increase in computed LVEF is frequently observed during dipyridamole stress in patients without coronary artery disease. An appropriate increase in gated PET LVEF (from rest to peak stress) can be used to exclude the presence of left main or severe multivessel coronary artery disease.

CASE 6

A 69-year-old woman was referred for adenosine stress SPECT MPI for evaluation of dyspnea and chest pressure. She had a history of stent placement in the mid-LAD 3 years previously.

Adenosine was infused at 140 mcg/kg/min over 4 minutes. She was unable to perform low-level treadmill exercise during the infusion. No symptoms were reported during the adenosine infusion, and her blood pressure and ECG responses to adenosine were normal.

Raw Images

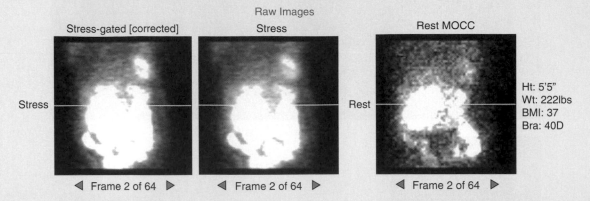

Raw Images

Stress-gated [corrected]   Stress   Rest MOCC

Stress   Rest

Ht: 5'5"
Wt: 222lbs
BMI: 37
Bra: 40D

◄ Frame 2 of 64 ▶   ◄ Frame 2 of 64 ▶   ◄ Frame 2 of 64 ▶

The raw planar images demonstrate moderate photon attenuation by the left breast (the bra cup size is 40 D). There is chest-wall adipose tissue present, resulting in further soft-tissue attenuation. The patient's body mass index is 37 (>30 = obese). In addition, there is marked hepatic and gastrointestinal (GI) tracer activity in close proximity to the heart. GI tracer interference is frequently problematic with pharmacologic stress, particularly when the patient is unable to perform low-level treadmill exercise during the infusion.

SPECT Tomograms

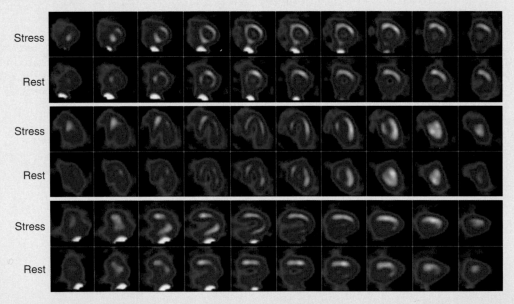

Stress

Rest

Stress

Rest

Stress

Rest

SPECT images demonstrate a mild defect in the distal anteroseptal region, with very mild defect reversibility on resting images. The defect could be consistent with breast attenuation artifact, though the mild defect reversibility raises concern for ischemia (possibly in the territory of the prior LAD stent placement). There is also a mild defect in the inferior and inferolateral regions, and subtle defect reversibility is evident on resting images. This stress defect (and the subtle defect reversibility evident on resting images) might be entirely due to GI tracer interference. Ischemia cannot be confidently excluded.

Quantitative Polar Map

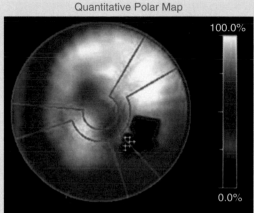

Quantitative Polar Map

Stress defect:
4% of LV

Ischemia:
1% of LV

100.0%

0.0%

When the perfusion pattern of this woman was compared to a female-specific normal database, the distal anteroseptal defect was judged to be within normal limits. Female-specific normal databases take into account the expected reduction in tracer activity in this region, owing to breast attenuation. However, the inferior/inferolateral wall stress perfusion defect was judged to be abnormal by quantitative criteria, and subtle defect reversibility was detected, suggesting the presence of inducible ischemia.

Gated SPECT Images

Frame 1 of 8 ◁▷

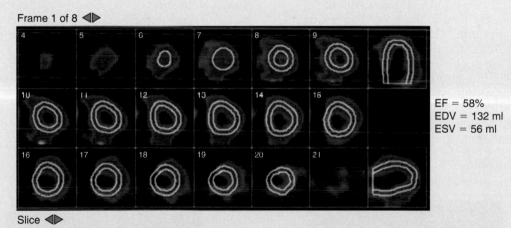

EF = 58%
EDV = 132 ml
ESV = 56 ml

Slice ◁▷

Gated SPECT images show normal myocardial systolic thickening in all regions, with a normal computed LVEF (58%). In the setting of nonreversible perfusion defects, the assessment of myocardial systolic thickening is useful for distinguishing defects caused by soft-tissue attenuation from defects caused by myocardial infarction. However, in the setting of completely or partially reversible defects, the presence of normal myocardial systolic thickening cannot be used to confidently exclude the presence of inducible myocardial ischemia.

She was referred for rubidium-82 (^{82}Rb) PET MPI.

Because there was significant diagnostic uncertainty present after SPECT MPI, the patient was subsequently referred for dipyridamole stress ^{82}Rb PET MPI.

PET Tomograms

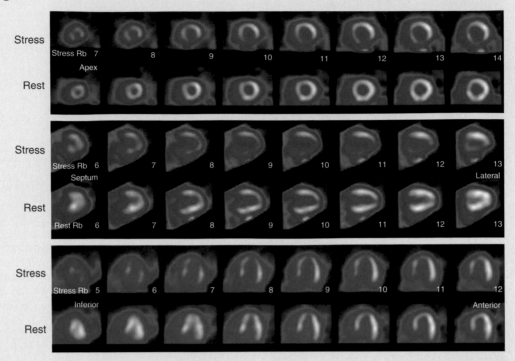

The peak stress ^{82}Rb PET images demonstrate a severe perfusion defect in the inferior region, extending from the base to the apex. The resting images show uniform ^{82}Rb activity in all myocardial regions, including the distal anteroseptal region (where breast attenuation was noted on the SPECT MPI study). PET images are routinely corrected for soft-tissue attenuation, and therefore PET MPI provides a more reliable assessment of regional myocardial perfusion, irrespective of gender or body habitus. Note that mild GI tracer activity is present on the peak stress and resting ^{82}Rb perfusion images. However, because of the superior spatial resolution of PET (compared to SPECT), the GI tracer activity does not result in problems with PET image interpretation.

Also note that the left ventricular cavity appears larger on peak stress images compared to resting images. An increased peak stress-to-rest left ventricular cavity ratio is frequently observed on PET MPI in the setting of inducible ischemia. This finding is seen more frequently with PET MPI than with SPECT MPI.

Gated PET Images

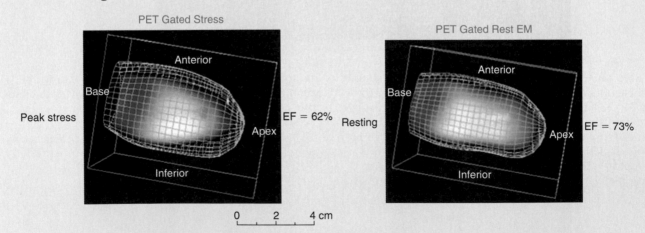

The ^{82}Rb PET images are gated both at rest and at peak stress. The ability to measure regional and global left ventricular systolic function at peak stress is a unique advantage of PET MPI. In this case, the LVEF was normal (73%) on resting gated PET images, but the LVEF decreased to 62% at peak stress. A decrease in computed LVEF is frequently observed during dipyridamole stress in patients with extensive coronary artery disease and inducible myocardial ischemia. A decline in LVEF from rest to peak stress is an additional marker of ischemia on gated PET MPI. This marker is especially useful in detecting balanced myocardial ischemia due to multivessel coronary artery disease. In such cases, the peak stress myocardial blood flow may appear homogeneous due to similarly decreased blood flow reserve in all myocardial regions.

Coronary Angiography

Coronary Angiography

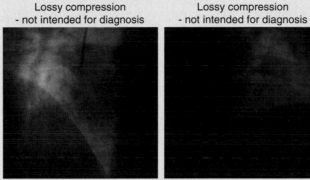

The coronary angiogram confirmed that the LAD stent remained widely patent. However, the right coronary artery (RCA) was totally occluded, and the RCA territory was fed by collateral vessels. The presence of RCA disease was confidently and accurately predicted by the PET MPI study, while the SPECT MPI study was equivocal for ischemia in this region.

CASE 7

A 39-year-old woman with a history of hypertension, chronic renal failure (creatinine = 3.1), and remote cocaine abuse was admitted for evaluation of nonexertional dull chest pain. She had a normal coronary angiogram 4 years previously for similar symptoms.

Initial Diagnostic Evaluation

Laboratory data: troponin T = 0.375 ng/mL (normal < 0.040), CK = 38 U/L

ECG: NSR, LVH with nonspecific ST-T abnormalities

Echocardiogram: moderate concentric LVH, no regional wall-motion abnormalities, EF = 50%

Referred for adenosine stress ^{99m}Tc sestamibi SPECT MPI

5-Minute adenosine infusion without supplemental low-level treadmill exercise, peak HR = 91 beats/min, normal BP response

Baseline ECG

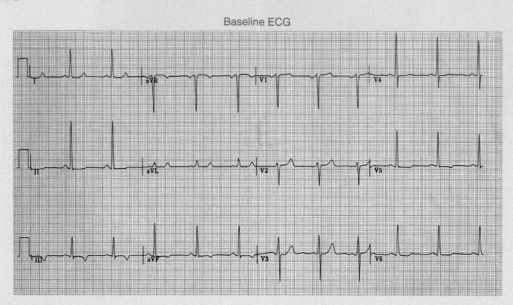

Baseline ECG

The baseline ECG demonstrates increased QRS voltage consistent with left ventricular hypertrophy (LVH), with nonspecific ST-T abnormalities possibly related to LVH.

4:50 Adenosine (Mild Chest Pain)

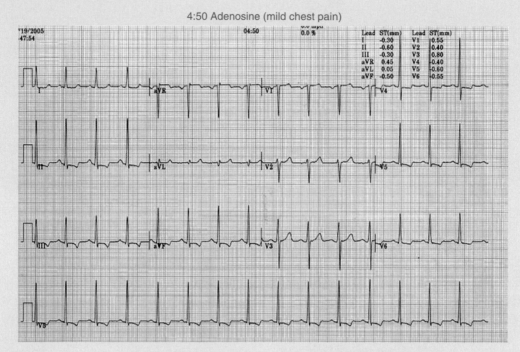

The patient complained of mild chest pain near the completion of the adenosine infusion. The ECG tracing obtained at 4 minutes, 50 seconds of the adenosine infusion demonstrated more prominent ST-T abnormalities with T-wave inversions suspicious for (but not diagnostic for) myocardial ischemia. This finding is common in patients with baseline LVH.

5:50 Recovery (Persistent Chest Pain)

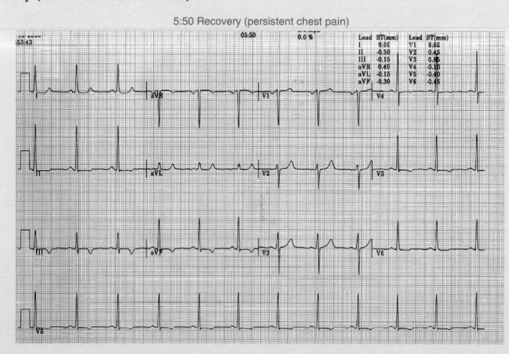

The patient described persistent chest pain nearly 6 minutes after completion of the adenosine infusion. This is highly unusual; the side effects of adenosine are typically very short-lived, owing to the very short half-life of adenosine (<10 seconds). An ECG tracing was obtained and demonstrated persistent nonspecific ST-T abnormalities.

9:00 Recovery (Worsening Chest Pain)

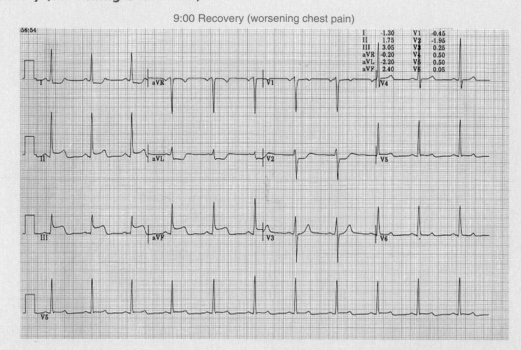

9:00 Recovery (worsening chest pain)

The patient described worsening chest pain 9 minutes after completion of the adenosine infusion. A repeat ECG tracing was obtained and demonstrated ST-segment elevation in the inferior leads (II, III, and aVF) and ST depression in V2 (suggestive of inferior and posterior injury, respectively), associated with reciprocal ST depression in leads I and aVL.

14:50 Recovery (No Chest Pain)

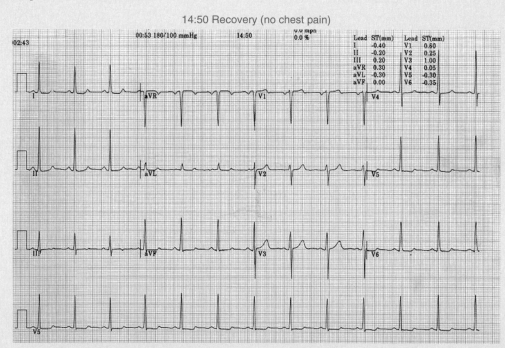

14:50 Recovery (no chest pain)

Sublingual nitroglycerin was administered, and the patient's chest pain resolved. An ECG tracing performed at 14 minutes, 50 seconds after the adenosine infusion demonstrated resolution of the inferior-posterior injury pattern, with mild residual nonspecific ST-T abnormalities.

Rotating Raw Planar Images

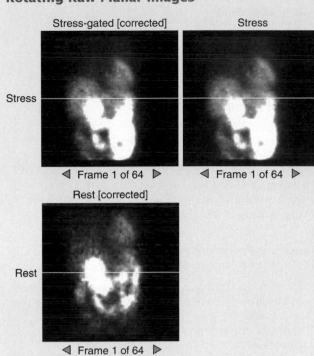

Stress-gated [corrected] Stress

Stress

◁ Frame 1 of 64 ▷   ◁ Frame 1 of 64 ▷

Rest [corrected]

Rest

◁ Frame 1 of 64 ▷

The rotating raw images demonstrate moderately severe subdiaphragmatic ^{99m}Tc sestamibi activity on both the poststress and resting images. The finding of subdiaphragmatic tracer activity on poststress images is common when pharmacologic stress is employed without supplemental low-level exercise. Subtle localized tracer activity is also noted on the anterior chest wall on poststress images, likely due to a small amount of tracer contamination of the chest wall or the patient's gown.

SPECT Images

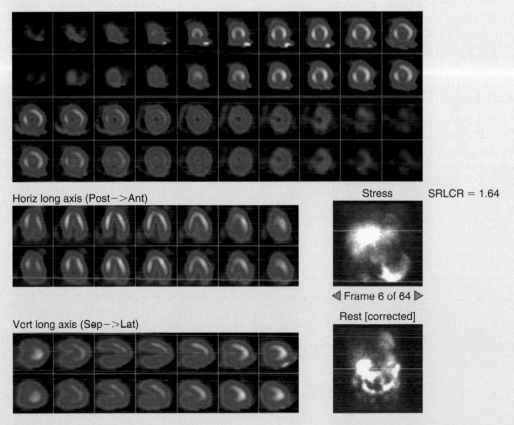

Horiz long axis (Post–>Ant)

Stress   SRLCR = 1.64

◁ Frame 6 of 64 ▷

Vert long axis (Sep–>Lat)

Rest [corrected]

The poststress SPECT images demonstrate a mild perfusion defect involving the inferior and inferoapical regions. Interpretation of perfusion in the inferior wall was complicated by adjacent GI tracer activity. There is minimal defect reversibility evident on resting images, which is equivocal for ischemia. Also note that the left ventricular cavity appears larger on poststress images, with a computed stress/rest LV cavity ratio (SRLVCR) of 1.64 (normal < 1.22 with the same-day, low-dose rest, high-dose stress ^{99m}Tc sestamibi protocol).

Gated SPECT Images

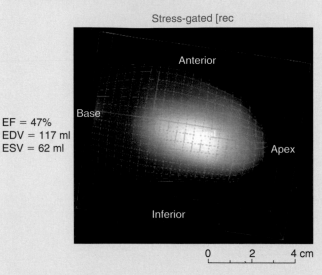

Stress-gated [rec

Anterior

Base

EF = 47%
EDV = 117 ml
ESV = 62 ml

Apex

Inferior

0   2   4 cm

The poststress gated SPECT images demonstrated mild global left ventricular hypokinesis, with a computed left ventricular ejection fraction (LVEF) of 47%. The left ventricular end-diastolic volume (LVEDV) and left ventricular end-systolic volume (LVESV) were borderline increased at 117 and 62 mL, respectively.

Patient Management

Though the stress perfusion abnormalities were subtle (and interpretation was complicated by GI tracer interference), the presence of the inferior-posterior injury pattern on ECG following adenosine stress raised suspicion for a high-grade coronary stenosis. The patient was therefore referred for urgent coronary angiography.

Coronary Angiography

- RCA: 60% distal
- LAD: mild diffuse
- LCX: 40% distal

Medical therapy was recommended by the interventional cardiologist.

Coronary Angiography

- RCA: 80% distal PCI (DES)
- LAD: mild diffuse
- LCX: 40% distal

After further consideration of the implications of the stress ECG findings, the angiogram was reviewed more closely, and the RCA lesion was felt to be more severe. A drug-eluting stent was placed.

Teaching Points: Stress-Induced ST-Segment Elevation

1. Exercise-induced ST-segment elevation (in absence of baseline Q waves) suggests transmural ischemia and predicts severe (usually > 95%) coronary stenosis in the artery supplying the region with ST elevation.
2. If ST elevation is detected, inject the isotope, terminate exercise, and have a low threshold to admit the patient to the hospital for urgent coronary angiography.
3. If the patient is not admitted, perform a recovery ECG to confirm resolution of ST elevation before permitting the patient to leave the nuclear laboratory.
4. There have been a few case reports of ST elevation during recovery after adenosine stress (as in the present case report). The mechanism of ST elevation following adenosine stress is not known. In the cases reported thus far, coronary angiography has not demonstrated severe coronary artery disease. Nonetheless, until much more experience has accumulated, coronary angiography is advisable.

CASE 8

A 51-year-old man with hyperlipidemia was referred for exercise SPECT MPI for evaluation of nonexertional localized chest pain.

He exercised for 8:54 minutes on a Bruce protocol, achieving an estimated workload of 10 METs.

No exercise-induced symptoms were reported, and the blood pressure and ECG responses were normal.

SPECT Images

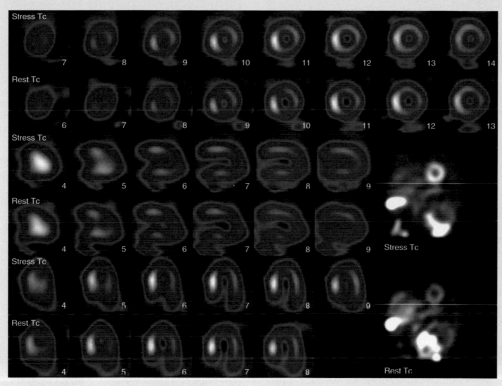

The SPECT images demonstrate a mild, nonreversible reduction in tracer activity in the lateral, anterior, inferior, and apical regions (relative to the septum). This perfusion pattern (highest myocardial tracer activity in the septum) is abnormal. In men, the highest myocardial tracer activity is typically found in the anterolateral region, since this region is least susceptible to photon attenuation. The observed perfusion pattern in this patient could represent multivessel coronary artery disease (CAD) with extensive subendocardial infarction, severe soft-tissue attenuation artifact, or increased septal wall thickness. Because of the limited spatial resolution of the SPECT camera, the apparent tracer activity in a myocardial region is directly related to the thickness of the myocardial wall. This is referred to as the "partial volume effect."

Defect Severity Polar Maps

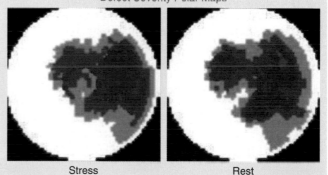

Defect Severity Polar Maps

Stress   Rest

When the tracer distribution is compared to a male-specific normal database, there is a fixed reduction in tracer activity in the lateral, anterior, and apical regions. The mild inferior defect does not exceed normal limits compared to a male-specific normal database.

Gated SPECT Images

Diastole   Systole

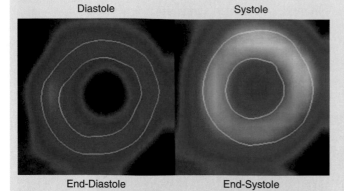

End-Diastole   End-Systole

Estimated % thickening

> 40%
25% => 40%
10% => 25%
0% => 10%
−10% => 0%
< −10%

EF = 61%   EDV = 94 ml   ESV = 36 ml

The relationship between regional wall thickness and apparent tracer activity (the "partial volume effect") is used to measure regional myocardial systolic wall thickening on gated SPECT images. The gated images in this patient demonstrate normal regional systolic thickening in the regions with reduced tracer activity. This finding argues against extensive subendocardial infarction as the cause for the observed fixed perfusion defects.

The septal wall demonstrates mildly reduced regional systolic thickening (see color-coded thickening polar map at *bottom*). An apparent reduction in regional systolic thickening can occur due to increased diastolic wall thickness. The relationship between regional wall thickness and apparent tracer activity (the "partial volume effect") does not apply when the wall thickness approaches the spatial resolution of the detector. Therefore, regional systolic wall thickening will be underestimated in myocardial regions with markedly increased wall thickness.

Echocardiography

Echocardiography

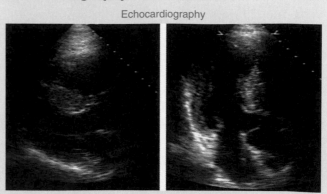

Hypertrophic cardiomyopathy with severe asymmetric septal hypertrophy (23 mm)

Hypertrophic cardiomyopathy (HCM) with severe asymmetric septal hypertrophy (23 mm).

Echocardiography demonstrated asymmetric septal hypertrophy (23 mm; normal = 7 to 12 mm) consistent with hypertrophic cardiomyopathy.

Echocardiogram-SPECT Correlation

Echocardiogram–SPECT Correlation

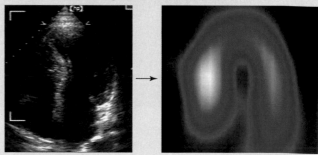

Side-by-side comparison of the apical four-chamber view on echocardiography *(left)* and the horizontal long-axis SPECT image *(right)* is shown. The area of increased septal tracer activity on SPECT correlates with the region of increased septal wall thickness on echocardiography. The apparent increase in tracer activity is therefore consistent with the "partial volume effect."

Teaching Points: MPI in Hypertrophic Cardiomyopathy

1. Quantitative perfusion polar maps compare regional tracer activity to a "normal" database, and patients with HCM will appear to have perfusion defects in myocardial regions with less hypertrophy (relative to regions with more severe hypertrophy).

2. Myocardial regions with severe hypertrophy will demonstrate an apparent reduction of regional systolic wall thickening due to the decreasing impact of the "partial volume effect" (relationship between wall thickness and apparent tracer activity).

3. Ischemia can be seen in HCM even in the absence of epicardial CAD, presumably due to myocardial fibrosis and "microvascular" disease. Therefore, specificity for diagnosis of CAD is reduced in patients with HCM.

4. Sensitivity of SPECT MPI is preserved in HCM. Therefore, the absence of reversible perfusion defects is useful for excluding ischemia. Normal SPECT MPI studies are associated with a more favorable prognosis in patients with HCM.

CASE 9

A 56-year-old woman with diabetes and a family history of coronary artery disease (CAD) was referred for exercise SPECT MPI for evaluation of exertional chest pain. The resting ECG was normal.

She exercised for 9:20 on a Bruce protocol, achieving an estimated workload of 10 METs. The peak heart rate was 144 beats/min (88% of maximum age-predicted heart rate). She described severe (9/10) chest pain at peak exercise, and there was greater than 1 mm ST depression at peak exercise. The blood pressure response was normal.

SPECT Images

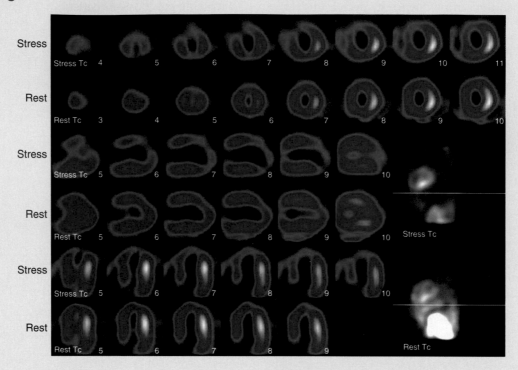

The SPECT images demonstrate a severe and extensive, partially reversible perfusion defect involving the anterior, anteroseptal, apical, and inferoapical regions. The perfusion pattern suggests proximal left anterior descending (LAD) disease.

In addition, the left ventricular cavity appears larger on poststress images compared to resting images. This finding (sometimes termed *transient ischemic dilatation*) is suggestive of extensive ischemia and is a marker of increased risk for future cardiac events. Note that the increased stress/rest LV cavity ratio (SRLVCR) is apparent on the vertical and horizontal long-axis images. Be wary of commenting on increased SRLVCR if the finding is only visually evident on the short-axis images. Misalignment of the short-axis slices may result in artifactual elevated SRLVCR. Misalignment of the long-axis slices will result in apparent increased SRLVCR on only half of the slices, while the reverse (decreased SRLVCR) will be evident on the other half of the slices.

Polar Map

Polar Map

46% of LV
26% of defect is reversible

When the tracer distribution is compared to a female-specific normal database, there is an extensive (46% of the left ventricle), partially reversible (26% of the defect) perfusion defect in the anterior, anteroseptal, apical, and inferoapical regions. The partial (rather than complete) defect reversibility is suggestive of infarction with residual ("border zone") inducible ischemia.

Viability Polar Map

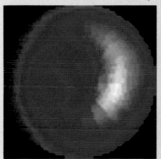
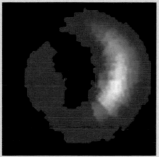

Viability Polar Map

Resting image, 50% threshold

Using a 50% reduction in resting regional ^{99m}Tc-sestamibi activity as an arbitrary threshold for myocardial viability, the resting tracer distribution suggests that a significant portion of the defect zone is composed of infarcted (nonviable) myocardium.

Poststress Gated SPECT Images

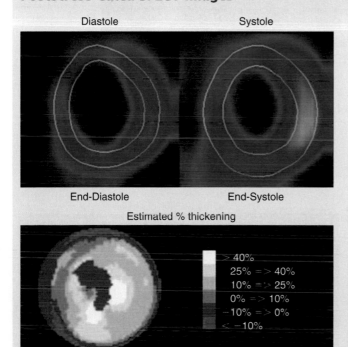

Diastole   Systole

End-Diastole   End-Systole

Estimated % thickening

> 40%
25% => 40%
10% => 25%
0% => 10%
−10% => 0%
< −10%

EF = 39%   EDV = 160 ml   ESV = 99 ml

The poststress gated SPECT images demonstrate severely reduced regional systolic thickening in the anterior, anteroseptal, apical, and inferoapical regions, with moderately reduced global left ventricular systolic function (LVEF = 39%). The computed left ventricular volumes are mildly increased (left ventricular end-diastolic and end-systolic volumes = 160 and 99 mL, respectively). Reduced regional systolic thickening on poststress images can be caused by infarction, postischemic myocardial stunning, or an artifactual underestimation of wall thickening due to a severe perfusion defect.

Coronary Angiography

- LVEF − 55% normal wall motion
- LAD: 95% proximal PCI (DES)
- LCX: 10% diffuse
- RCA: 10% diffuse

As expected, coronary angiography demonstrated severe (95%) stenosis of the proximal left anterior descending (LAD) coronary artery. The stenosis was treated with a drug-eluting stent.

Interestingly, the left ventriculogram demonstrated normal myocardial systolic thickening in all regions with a normal left ventricular ejection fraction (55%). This suggests that the severely reduced regional systolic thickening on poststress gated SPECT images was not due to infarction. The reduced regional systolic thickening on gated SPECT could represent postischemic myocardial stunning or an artifactual underestimation of wall thickening by the gated SPECT algorithm caused by the severe perfusion defect.

Myocardial Stunning or Imaging Artifact?

Myocardial Stunning or Imaging Artifact?

Ejection fraction

Rest   Stress   30   60   90   120
Time (min)

Using only a single poststress gated SPECT acquisition, it is not possible to distinguish postischemic myocardial stunning from an artifactual underestimation of wall thickening by the gated SPECT algorithm. If myocardial stunning is responsible, the regional systolic dysfunction would be expected to resolve over time, and improvement would be detected on serial poststress gated SPECT acquisitions. If an artifactual underestimation of wall thickening by the gated SPECT algorithm is responsible, the regional dysfunction would be expected to persist over time (because the perfusion defect responsible for the artifact would persist).

Clinical Follow-Up

The patient returned 8 months later for follow-up exercise ^{99m}Tc sestamibi SPECT MPI. She denied chest pain since the PCI.

She exercised for 10:50 minutes on a Bruce protocol (13.1 METs). Peak heart rate was 154 beats/min (94% of maximal age-predicted heart rate). No exercise-induced symptoms were reported, and the blood pressure and ECG responses were normal.

SPECT Images 8 Months Later

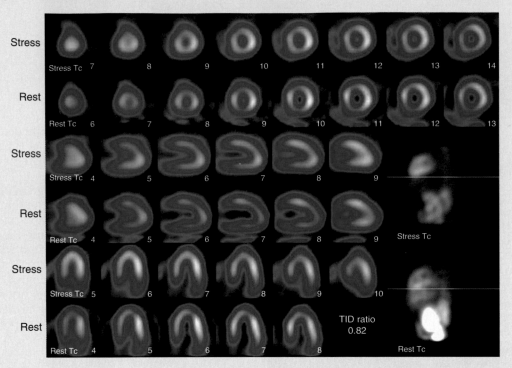

The SPECT images demonstrate normal homogeneous myocardial perfusion in all regions. Inducible ischemia is no longer present in the territory of the left anterior descending coronary artery (LAD). The previously noted resting perfusion defect (suggestive of infarction, based on resting defect zone tracer activity < 50% of maximal tracer activity) is no longer present.

The stress/rest LV cavity ratio is now normal (0.82).

Gated SPECT Images 8 Months Later

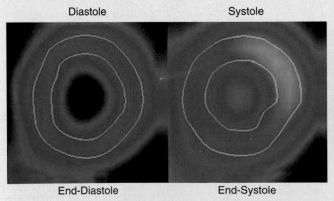

Diastole | Systole

End-Diastole | End-Systole

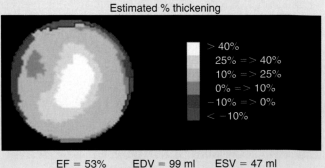

Estimated % thickening

> 40%
25% => 40%
10% => 25%
0% => 10%
−10% => 0%
< −10%

EF = 53%   EDV = 99 ml   ESV = 47 ml

The gated images demonstrate normal myocardial systolic thickening in all regions, with normal global left ventricular systolic function (LVEF = 53%). The computed left ventricular volumes are normal (left ventricular end-diastolic and end-systolic volumes = 99 and 47 mL, respectively).

Comparison of Resting SPECT Images at Baseline and 8 Months After PCI

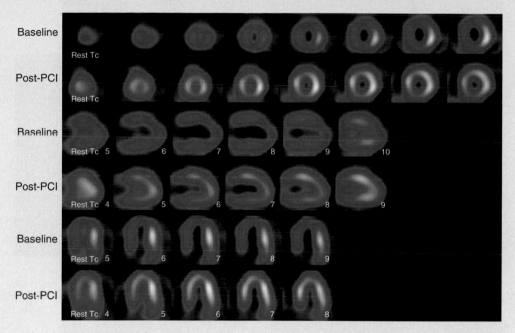

There is a marked change in the resting SPECT perfusion images following PCI of the LAD. Homogeneous myocardial perfusion is now present, and the left ventricular cavity size is smaller. In retrospect, the severe resting perfusion abnormality (on the initial baseline study) was entirely due to ischemia. No infarction is evident on follow-up imaging.

Teaching Point

Be cautious in diagnosing infarction in the presence of severe inducible ischemia, *even if incomplete defect reversibility is present and regional myocardial systolic thickening is reduced*. It is more appropriate to emphasize ischemia on the report. The presence (and extent) of infarction can be overestimated in the setting of severe ischemia.

CASE 10

A 45-year-old woman was referred for exercise ^{99m}Tc-sestamibi SPECT MPI because of an abnormal ECG. She denied cardiac symptoms.

She exercised for 5:16 minutes on a Bruce protocol (7 METs). Peak heart rate was 158 beats/min (90% of maximal age-predicted heart rate). No exercise-induced symptoms were reported, and the blood pressure and ECG responses were normal.

Short-Axis SPECT Images

Short-axis SPECT images

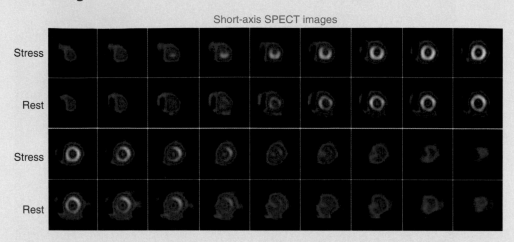

The short-axis SPECT images demonstrate a mild reversible defect in the anterior and anteroapical regions. The defect location and appearance are consistent with breast attenuation artifact, but the presence of defect reversibility is suggestive of ischemia.

Rotating Raw Planar Images

Rotating Raw Planar Images

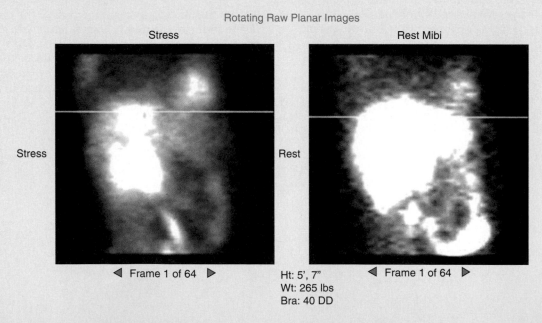

Ht: 5', 7"
Wt: 265 lbs
Bra: 40 DD

The rotating raw planar images demonstrate a prominent shadow due to photon attenuation by the left breast. Note that the position of the left breast shadow is higher on the poststress images (the breast shadow eclipses only the upper half of the heart). The preferential attenuation of photons emitted from the anterior wall of the left ventricle results in an anterior perfusion defect. The breast shadow is lower on the resting images and eclipses the entire heart. The resulting uniform photon attenuation does not create a perfusion defect. Therefore, shifting breast position can cause a reversible anterior wall defect that can be misinterpreted as anterior wall inducible ischemia.

The position of the breast can vary depending on the extent to which the patient's arms are raised above the head during image acquisition. Consistent arm positioning is important to ensure consistent breast position and high-quality SPECT images.

Teaching Points: "Shifting" Breast Attenuation (See Chapter 5)

1. A change in breast position (from resting to poststress images) can result in a reversible anterior-wall perfusion defect suggestive of ischemia.
2. Careful review of raw planar images can identify the "shifting" breast attenuation pattern.
3. Be cautious in attributing a reversible perfusion defect to "shifting breast attenuation artifact," especially if other markers of ischemia are present (e.g., exercise-induced chest pain or ST-segment depression). For confirmation, this patient underwent rubidium-82 PET MPI, which demonstrated normal homogeneous rubidium-82 uptake in all myocardial regions. PET MPI studies employ robust attenuation correction, and therefore breast attenuation (and other soft-tissue attenuation) artifacts are less problematic.

CASE 11

A 36-year-old man with a history of hypertension presented to the ED with the sudden onset of left-sided weakness. He also described a 6-month history of exertional dyspnea and leg edema. He had stopped taking his antihypertensive medications several months ago. He admitted to consuming a "moderate" amount of alcohol on a daily basis.

Baseline ECG

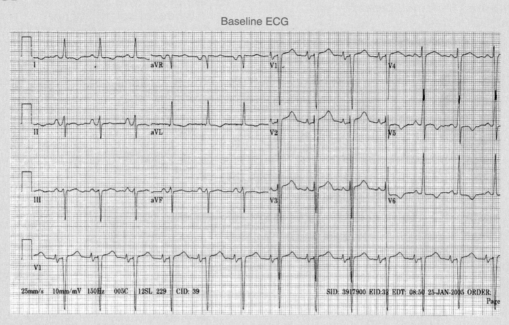

Baseline ECG

The baseline ECG demonstrates sinus rhythm, increased QRS voltage consistent with left ventricular hypertrophy (LVH), and nonspecific ST-T abnormalities possibly related to LVH. There is also evidence of biatrial conduction abnormality.

Echocardiogram

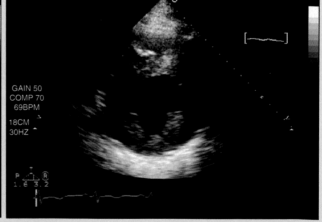

Echocardiogram

Echocardiogram

Parasternal long-axis and short-axis images demonstrate left ventricular dilation, increased left ventricular wall thickness, and severe global left ventricular systolic dysfunction with an estimated left ventricular ejection fraction of 20% to 25%. These findings are consistent with ischemic or nonischemic cardiomyopathy.

He was referred for adenosine stress ^{99m}Tc-sestamibi SPECT MPI to evaluate for ischemic cardiomyopathy as the cause for the left ventricular systolic dysfunction.

He underwent a 4-minute adenosine infusion without supplemental low-level treadmill exercise. No adenosine-induced symptoms were reported. Baseline blood pressure was elevated, but the blood pressure response to adenosine was normal. The ECG response was nondiagnostic owing to baseline LVH and ST-T abnormalities.

Raw Planar Images

Raw planar images

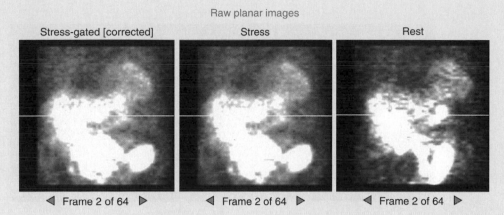

The rotating raw planar images demonstrate left ventricular enlargement. Lateral projections demonstrate reduced inferior wall tracer activity possibly due to diaphragmatic attenuation artifact.

SPECT Images

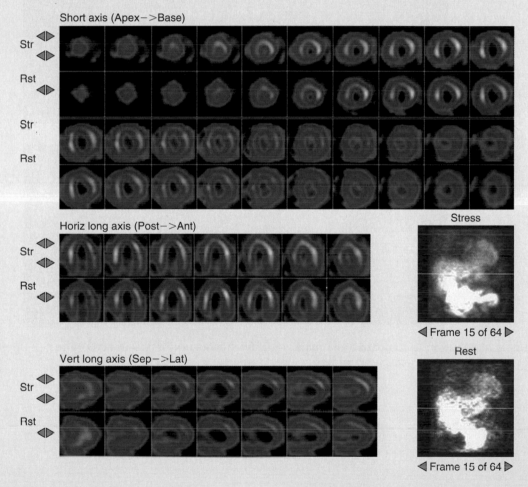

The SPECT images demonstrate left ventricular enlargement. There is a moderate to severe fixed inferior perfusion defect extending from the base to the apex. These findings could be consistent with inferior infarction or nonischemic cardiomyopathy with inferior wall attenuation artifact. The inferior wall attenuation artifact in nonischemic cardiomyopathy is typically attributed to diaphragmatic attenuation, though photons emitted by the inferior region may be attenuated by the enlarged heart itself. "Heart attenuation" may be the predominant mechanism of the inferior wall artifact.

Polar Maps

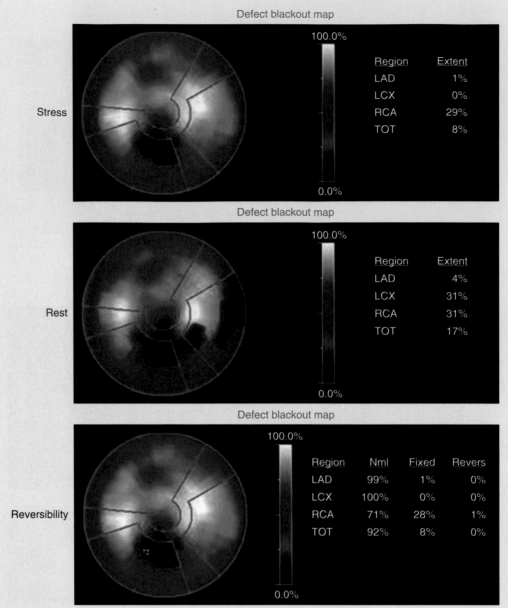

When the tracer distribution is compared to a male-specific normal database, there is a predominantly fixed reduction in tracer activity in the inferior and inferoapical regions.

Gated SPECT Images

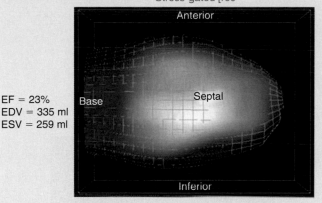

Stress-gated [rec

Anterior

EF = 23%
EDV = 335 ml
ESV = 259 ml

Base   Septal

Inferior

0   2   4 cm

The poststress gated SPECT images demonstrate severe global left ventricular hypokinesis, with a computed left ventricular ejection fraction (LVEF) of 23%. The left ventricular end-diastolic volume (LVEDV) and left ventricular end-systolic volume (LVESV) were markedly increased at 335 and 259 mL, respectively.

Teaching Points

SPECT MPI in Cardiomyopathy *(See Chapter 30)*

1. In this case, the left ventricular systolic dysfunction was more severe than the observed perfusion abnormalities. These findings favor nonischemic cardiomyopathy, with untreated hypertension and alcohol abuse as possible etiologies. Medical therapy for cardiomyopathy and abstinence from alcohol were recommended.
2. Patients with nonischemic cardiomyopathy frequently demonstrate fixed inferior wall perfusion defects due to attenuation by the enlarged heart.
3. Reversible perfusion defects are occasionally observed in patients with nonischemic cardiomyopathy, presumably due to myocardial fibrosis and microvascular disease. Perfusion abnormalities can also be seen in other "noncoronary heart diseases," including hypertrophic cardiomyopathy, sarcoidosis, scleroderma, myocarditis, Duchenne's muscular dystrophy, cardiac lymphoma, left bundle branch block, and right ventricular pacing.

CASE 12

A 65-year-old woman presents with recent onset of nonexertional chest pain. She has no coronary disease risk factors. She is referred for SPECT MPI.

She exercised on a Bruce protocol to a maximal workload of 10 METs. Peak heart rate was 155 beats/min (100% of maximal age-predicted heart rate). No exercise-induced symptoms were reported, and the blood pressure and ECG responses were normal.

Raw Planar Images

Raw Planar Images

Stress Tc–99m

Rest Tc–99m

Stress

Rest

◀ Frame 1 of 64 ▶

◀ Frame 1 of 64 ▶

Ht: 5', 3"
Wt: 153 lbs
BMI: 27.1

The rotating raw planar images demonstrate a prominent shadow produced by the right breast, but no left breast shadow is present. This patient has a history of breast cancer, and her prior treatment included left mastectomy. Mild patient motion is also present, and moderate GI tracer interference is evident on resting images.

SPECT Images

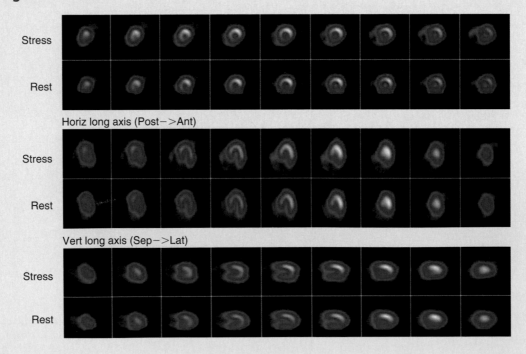

Stress

Rest

Horiz long axis (Post–>Ant)

Stress

Rest

Vert long axis (Sep–>Lat)

Stress

Rest

The poststress SPECT images demonstrate a mild defect in the inferior and inferolateral regions. Minimal defect reversibility is evident on resting images, suggestive of ischemia (but possibly the result of GI tracer interference). The perfusion pattern (highest tracer activity in the anterior and anterolateral regions, with relatively reduced activity in the inferior region) is a typical pattern in men. However, this perfusion pattern is not typical for a normal woman.

Quantitative Polar Maps

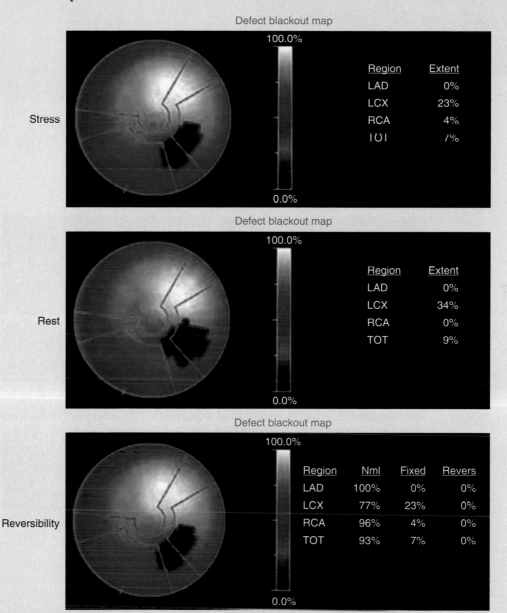

When the perfusion pattern is compared to a female specific normal database, the perfusion in the inferior and inferolateral regions is identified as abnormal. Despite visually apparent defect reversibility, no significant reversibility was identified by quantitative assessment. The predominantly fixed perfusion defects could be consistent with prior infarction or soft-tissue attenuation artifact.

Gated SPECT Images

Frame 1 of 16 ◄▷

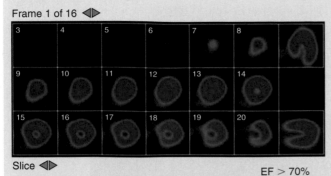

Slice ◄▷

EF > 70%
EDV = 56 ml
ESV = 15 ml

The poststress gated SPECT images demonstrate normal myocardial systolic thickening in all regions,

with a computed LVEF of > 70%. These findings favor soft-tissue attenuation artifact (rather than infarction) as the cause of the observed inferior and inferolateral defects.

Teaching Points: Left Mastectomy

1. In women with left mastectomy, absence of the anterior attenuation produced by the left breast results in a male perfusion pattern (unopposed "diaphragmatic attenuation").
2. Review of the raw planar images is important for identifying the absence of the left breast shadow.
3. Technologists should alert the interpreting physician to the history of left mastectomy.
4. In women with left mastectomy, use a male database for quantitative perfusion assessment.

Quantitative Polar Maps

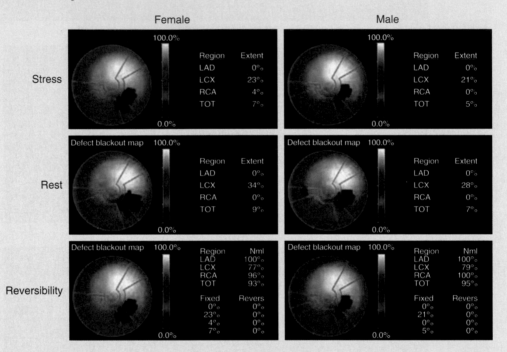

When the perfusion pattern is compared to a male-specific normal database *(right)*, the perfusion defects in the inferior and inferolateral regions are less extensive than the defects identified by comparison to the female-specific normal database *(left)*.

However, even compared to a male-specific normal database, the perfusion pattern remains mildly abnormal. Because of residual diagnostic uncertainty, confirmatory testing was performed (rubidium-82 PET MPI).

Quality-Control Display

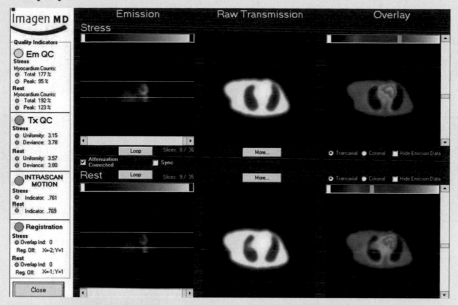

The PET MPI quality-control display shows the rubidium-82 emission images *(left)*, the germanium rod source transmission images *(center)*, and an overlay of the emission and transmission images *(right)* to confirm proper registration (alignment). Note that the right breast is clearly identified on the transmission images, but the left breast is absent.

Dipyridamole Stress PET Images

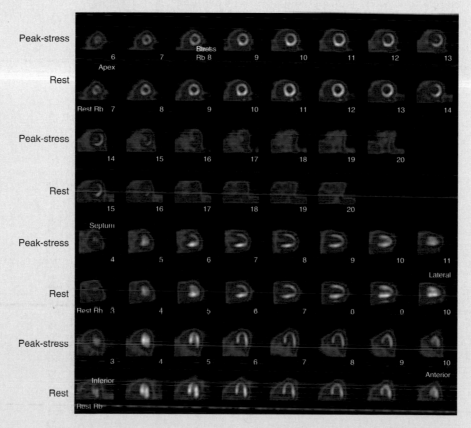

The peak stress and resting PET images demonstrate normal rubidium-82 activity in all myocardial regions, including the inferior and inferolateral regions. PET MPI interpretation is less likely to be complicated by soft-tissue attenuation artifacts, because 100% of PET MPI studies are attenuation corrected.

Gated PET Images

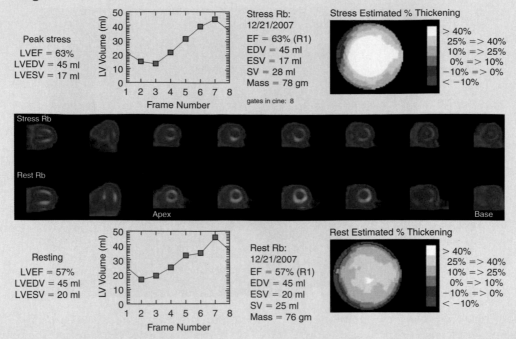

Peak stress
LVEF = 63%
LVEDV = 45 ml
LVESV = 17 ml

Stress Rb:
12/21/2007
EF = 63% (R1)
EDV = 45 ml
ESV = 17 ml
SV = 28 ml
Mass = 78 gm

gates in cine: 8

Stress Estimated % Thickening
> 40%
25% => 40%
10% => 25%
0% => 10%
−10% => 0%
< −10%

Stress Rb

Rest Rb

Apex   Base

Resting
LVEF = 57%
LVEDV = 45 ml
LVESV = 20 ml

Rest Rb:
12/21/2007
EF = 57% (R1)
EDV = 45 ml
ESV = 20 ml
SV = 25 ml
Mass = 76 gm

Rest Estimated % Thickening
> 40%
25% => 40%
10% => 25%
0% => 10%
−10% => 0%
< −10%

The gated PET images demonstrate normal myocardial systolic thickening in all regions. The resting and peak stress LVEF was 57% and 63%, respectively. An increase in LVEF at peak dipyridamole stress (compared to resting LVEF) is commonly observed on gated PET imaging in the absence of ischemia. The ability to measure LVEF at rest and at *peak* stress (rather than *after* stress, as is done with gated SPECT) is a major advantage of PET MPI.

CASE 13

A 74-year-old man with hypertension and diabetes was referred for preoperative assessment prior to bladder surgery. He reports a "normal" stress test 14 years ago.

He describes severely reduced functional capacity (<4 METs), but he denies angina. Dipyridamole PET MPI was requested for preoperative risk assessment.

12-Lead ECG

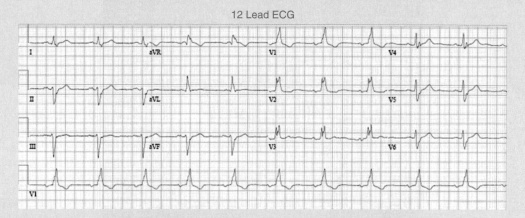

The baseline ECG demonstrates normal sinus rhythm, right bundle branch block, and left anterior fascicular block.

PET Images

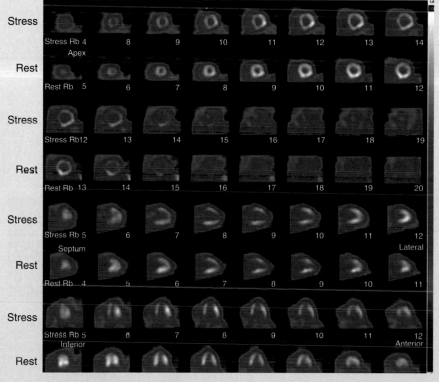

Ht: 5', 3"
Wt: 189 lbs
BMI: 33.5
SRLVCR = 1.39

The peak stress PET images demonstrate a mild defect in the apical region. Mild defect reversibility is evident on resting images, suggestive of ischemia. Also note that the left ventricular cavity is much larger on peak stress images compared to resting images, with a computed stress/rest left ventricular cavity ratio (SRLVCR) of 1.39.

Quantitative Polar Map

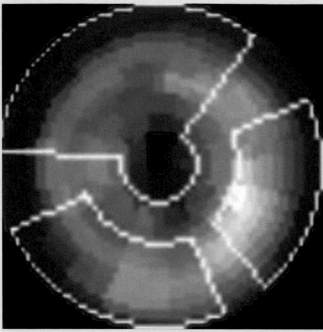

Stress Defect
(1% of LV)

When the perfusion pattern is compared to a normal rubidium-82 (^{82}Rb) perfusion database, the perfusion defect in the apical region is identified as abnormal. However, the extent of the perfusion abnormality is extremely limited, confined to only 1% of the LV myocardium. Quantitative measurements of absolute myocardial blood flow (e.g., in mL/min/g) were not performed on this study.

Gated PET Images

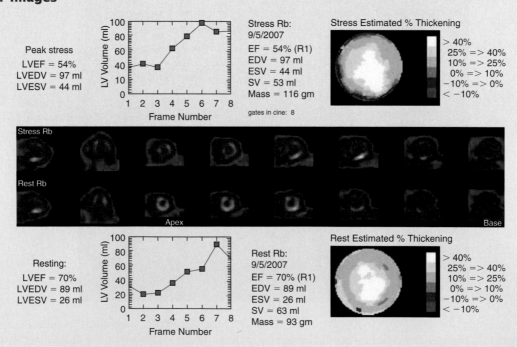

The gated PET images demonstrate normal myocardial systolic thickening in all regions. The resting and peak stress LVEF was 70% and 54%, respectively. A decrease in LVEF at peak dipyridamole stress (compared to resting LVEF) is an abnormal finding on gated PET imaging; it is commonly observed in patients with severe single-vessel disease, multivessel disease, or left main disease.

Despite the limited extent of ischemia detected by perfusion imaging, the elevated SRLVCR and the abnormal decline in LVEF at peak dipyridamole stress prevented the study from being designated as a "low-risk" abnormal study. Therefore, coronary angiography was recommended.

Coronary Angiography

Coronary Angiography

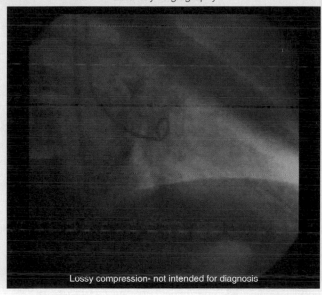

Lossy compression- not intended for diagnosis

Cardiac Catheterization

Contrast left ventriculography showed normal left ventricular systolic function.

Coronary Angiography

Coronary Angiography

| Lossy compression - not intended for diagnosis | Lossy compression - not intended for diagnosis |

Coronary angiography revealed mild diffuse left main disease, moderate diffuse LAD stenoses, 80% proximal circumflex stenosis, 50% ostial RCA stenosis, and 30% mid-RCA stenosis. Percutaneous intervention of the proximal circumflex artery stenosis was recommended by the interventional cardiologist, but drug-eluting stent placement was deferred until after bladder surgery (to avoid the risk of stent thrombosis if interruption of clopidogrel therapy would be required perioperatively).

Teaching Points: Detection of Balanced Ischemia

1. The presence of multivessel CAD (and the extent and severity of ischemia) can be underestimated by techniques that measure only "relative" myocardial perfusion.
2. Elevated stress/rest left ventricular cavity ratio (SRLVCR) is a marker of extensive ischemia. Elevated SRLVCR is an important "high-risk" marker on PET MPI.
3. A decline in LVEF from rest to peak stress on gated PET images is a marker of extensive ischemia and predicts the presence of severe (often multivessel or left main) CAD.
4. Measurement of absolute myocardial blood flow with ^{82}Rb PET will improve our ability to identify patients with balanced ischemia due to diffuse multivessel disease.

CASE 14

A 62-year-old man with a history of left bundle branch block (LBBB) diagnosed 25 years earlier is now referred for cardiology consultation because of an abnormal gated SPECT MPI at an outside facility. By report, there are fixed inferior and septal defects suggestive of infarction, as well as severe LV systolic dysfunction (LVEF = 14%).

He has no cardiac symptoms despite vigorous physical activity. He has no coronary artery disease (CAD) risk factors. His mother had an "enlarged heart."

12-Lead ECG

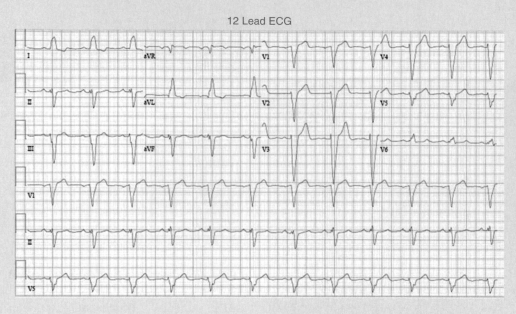

12 Lead ECG

The baseline ECG demonstrates normal sinus rhythm, left-axis deviation, and LBBB.

Following are options for identification of cardiomyopathy due to CAD (ischemic cardiomyopathy):
  A. Dobutamine echo
  B. Vasodilator stress PET MPI
  C. Coronary CT angiography
  D. Invasive coronary angiogram

The patient preferred to avoid invasive coronary angiography. After discussion of the available options, he elected to undergo coronary CT angiography.

Functional (Gated) CT Left Ventricular Angiogram

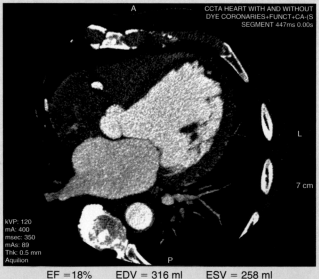

EF = 18%   EDV = 316 ml   ESV = 258 ml

The left ventricular cavity volumes were markedly elevated, and left ventricular systolic function was severely reduced, with a computed LVEF of 18%. Severe global hypokinesis was observed, consistent with ischemic or nonischemic cardiomyopathy.

Coronary Calcium Score (CCS)

- LM = 9
- LAD = 120
- LCX = 15
- RCA = 805
- CCS = 949 (>90th %)

The total calcium score was 949 (>90th percentile for his age and gender). Coronary calcification was noted in the left main and all three major coronary arteries. The right coronary artery (RCA) showed the most extensive calcification.

Coronary CTA of Left Main

Left Main

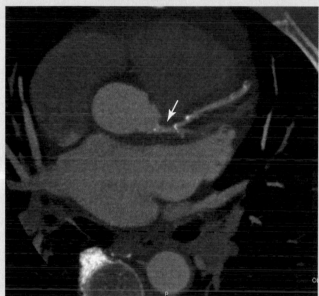

The left main demonstrated calcified nonobstructive plaque.

Coronary CTA of Left Anterior Descending

LAD

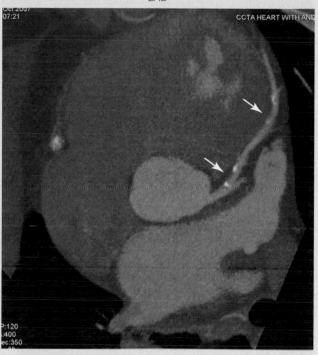

The LAD demonstrated diffuse mixed (calcified and noncalcified) nonobstructive plaque.

Coronary CTA of Left Circumflex

Circumflex

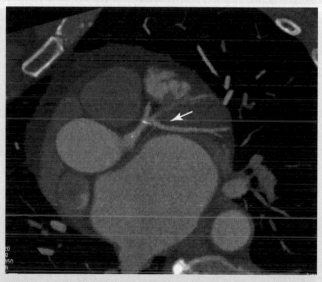

The LCX demonstrated mild (nonobstructive) plaque.

Proximal Right Coronary Artery

Proximal RCA

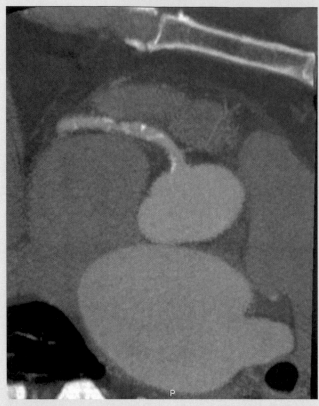

Mid-RCA

Mid RCA

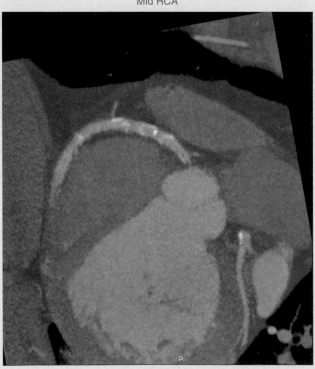

Coronary CTA of Right Coronary Artery

The proximal and mid-RCA demonstrated diffuse calcified (nonobstructive) plaque.

Clinical Questions

1. Does he have ischemic cardiomyopathy? Probably not. His severe left ventricular systolic dysfunction is out of proportion to the mild (nonobstructive) CAD identified by CTA. The constellation of findings (LBBB, severe global left ventricular hypokinesis, nonobstructive CAD) are most consistent with nonischemic cardiomyopathy.
2. Is he likely to benefit from coronary revascularization? No. There was no inducible ischemia reported on SPECT MPI (and he has no evidence of obstructive CAD by CTA).
3. Would he benefit from aggressive risk-factor modification? Yes. There is diffuse coronary atherosclerosis confirmed by CTA. This information would not have been available if a physiologic test (e.g., dobutamine echocardiography or PET MPI) rather than an anatomic test (CTA) had been performed to evaluate for ischemic cardiomyopathy.

MPI	CTA
Physiology	Anatomy
Myocardial perfusion	Coronary plaque
Short-term (2-year) risk	Long-term (10-year) risk
Revascularization?	Secondary Prevention?

Complementary Roles of MPI and CTA (See Chapter 22)

This case illustrates the complementary roles of myocardial perfusion imaging (MPI) and coronary CT angiography (CTA). If the clinical question is, "Will the patient benefit from coronary revascularization?", MPI is the test of choice. The extent and severity of ischemia (and presence of myocardial viability) is the most reliable predictor of benefit from revascularization. If the clinical question is, "Does the patient have CAD and would he/she benefit from aggressive (secondary prevention) risk-factor modification?", CTA (or calcium scoring) is the test of choice.

CASE 15

A 66-year-old man with known severe three-vessel coronary artery disease (CAD) and ischemic cardiomyopathy was referred for myocardial viability assessment.

Heart catheterization demonstrated severe left ventricular systolic dysfunction (left ventricular ejection fraction [LVEF] = 15% to 20%) and severe three-vessel CAD (75% proximal left anterior descending [LAD], 80% proximal circumflex, 80% mid–first obtuse marginal [OM1], 100% proximal right coronary artery [RCA]).

12-Lead ECG

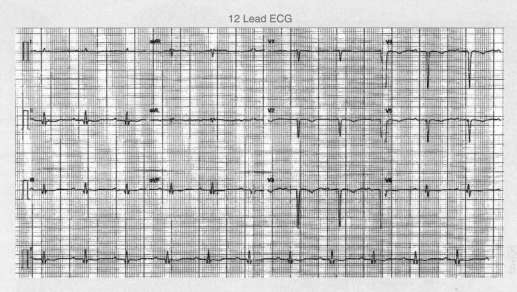

12 Lead ECG

The baseline ECG demonstrates normal sinus rhythm, first-degree AV block, and Q waves suggestive of extensive anterior (and possibly inferior) infarction.

Perfusion and Glucose Metabolism

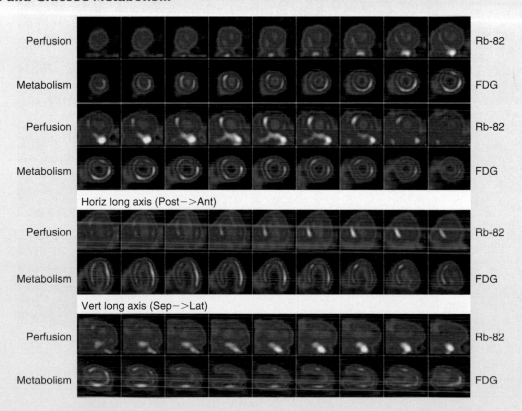

Rubidium-82 (^{82}Rb) PET MPI demonstrates moderately severe and extensive perfusion defects in the anterior, anteroapical, and anterolateral regions. [^{18}F] Fluorodeoxyglucose (^{18}FDG) PET images demonstrate a mild localized area of reduced glucose metabolism in the anteroapical region. The "perfusion-metabolism mismatch" is consistent with preserved myocardial viability and predicts improvement of left ventricular systolic function with revascularization.

Semiquantitative Assessment of Myocardial Perfusion and Glucose Metabolism

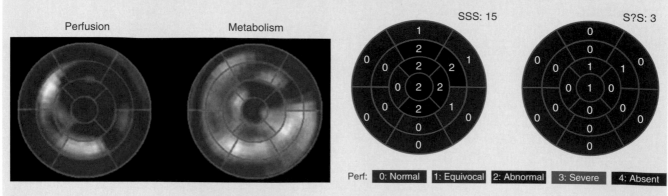

The polar plots and 17-segment scoring results confirm that the regional reduction in myocardial perfusion (^{82}Rb) is more severe and extensive than the reduction in glucose metabolism (^{18}FDG).

Peak stress Perfusion and Glucose Metabolism

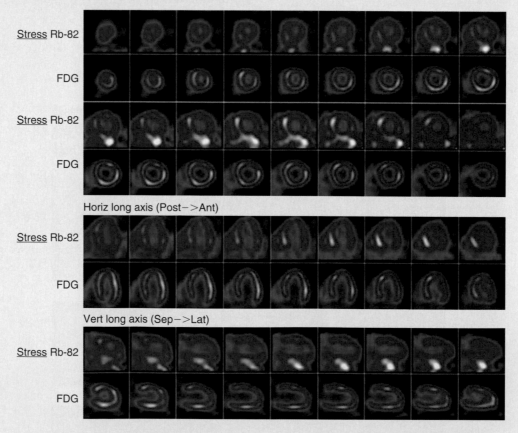

The perfusion-metabolism images (shown earlier and shown here again) were actually comparing *peak stress* myocardial perfusion (using dipyridamole stress) and resting glucose metabolism (^{18}FDG).

Resting Perfusion and Glucose Metabolism

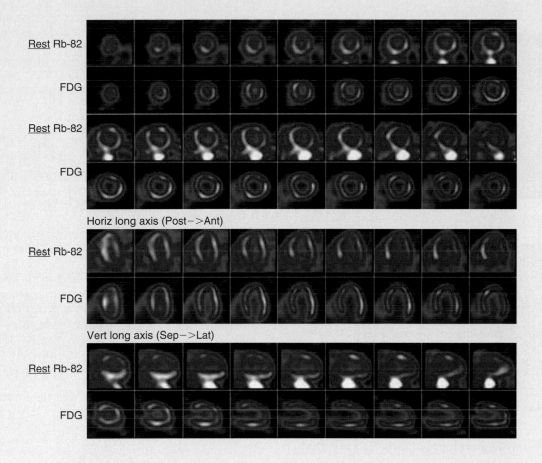

The images shown here depict resting myocardial perfusion (^{82}Rb) and resting glucose metabolism (^{18}FDG). This is the more conventional display used for assessment of myocardial viability. Note that the resting perfusion defect is much less severe and extensive than the peak stress perfusion defect (shown previously). The resting perfusion defect is comparable in extent and severity to the resting glucose metabolism defect. This pattern (matched reduction in perfusion and glucose metabolism) implies absence of hibernating myocardium and suggests that the patient is unlikely to benefit from myocardial revascularization. The conclusion derived using the resting ^{82}Rb myocardial perfusion images is completely opposite to the conclusion derived using the peak stress ^{82}Rb perfusion images.

Peak stress and Resting Gated PET Images

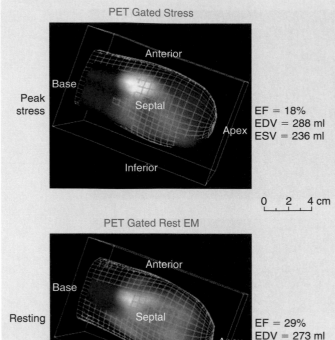

PET Gated Stress

Peak stress

Base
Anterior
Septal
Apex
Inferior

EF = 18%
EDV = 288 ml
ESV = 236 ml

0   2   4 cm

PET Gated Rest EM

Resting

Base
Anterior
Septal
Apex
Inferior

EF = 29%
EDV = 273 ml
ESV = 193 ml

Comparison of the peak stress and resting gated PET images also revealed evidence of inducible myocardial ischemia. The computed LVEF declined from 29% at rest to 18% at peak stress. A decline in LVEF at peak stress is an abnormal response to dipyridamole infusion, and it implies the presence of extensive inducible ischemia. The decline in LVEF at peak stress occurred primarily due to an increase in left ventricular end-systolic volume (LVESV). The LVESV increased from 193 mL at rest to 236 mL at peak stress.

Practical Approach to Assessment of Myocardial Viability (See Chapters 37 and 38)

1. Preserved resting perfusion (thallium-201 [^{201}Tl], technetium-99m [^{99m}Tc], rubidium-82 [[82]Rb], nitrogen-13-labeled ammonia [[13]NH$_3$]) implies myocardial viability.
2. Assessment for inducible ischemia (when clinically feasible) should be included as part of the routine assessment of myocardial viability. The presence of inducible ischemia implies viability and predicts benefit from revascularization. In the present case, the resting and peak stress [82]Rb perfusion images and gated PET images demonstrated extensive inducible ischemia (and therefore viability). The [18]FDG metabolism images confirmed the presence of viability but added no additional clinical information.
3. In cases in which there is no detectable ischemia in the myocardial region of interest, [18]FDG PET can be helpful.

An Example in Which [18]FDG Imaging Adds Important Incremental Information to the Assessment of Myocardial Viability

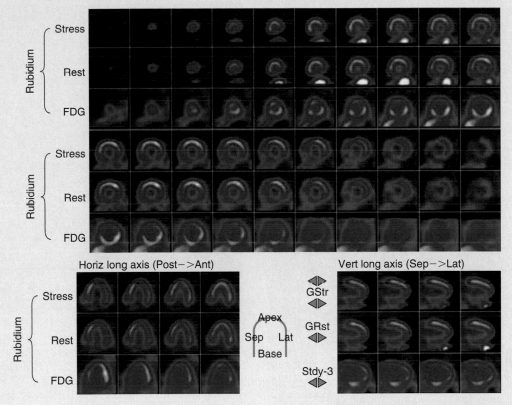

This patient has a severe and extensive nonreversible perfusion defect in the inferior and inferolateral regions (by [82]Rb). Based on the perfusion findings alone, this region would appear to be composed of predominantly irreversibly injured (infarcted) myocardium. However, normal myocardial uptake of [18]FDG throughout the defect zone implies preserved glucose metabolism and viable myocardium. In cases such as this (in which there is no detectable ischemia in the myocardial region of interest), [18]FDG PET is especially helpful for clinical decision making.

CASE 16

A 76-year-old male with known coronary artery disease (CAD) and multiple myocardial infarctions (MIs) and congestive heart failure (CHF) in the past was admitted to the hospital because of chest pain and worsening heart failure. He underwent cardiac catheterization, which showed 100% occlusion of the right coronary artery (RCA) and left circumflex (LCX) and 80% narrowing of the left anterior descending (LAD). Left ventriculogram showed severely impaired left ventricular ejection fraction (LVEF) of 15%.

(Video 1)

Left side coronary arteries

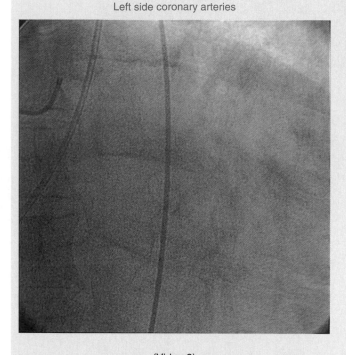

(Video 2)

Right coronary artery

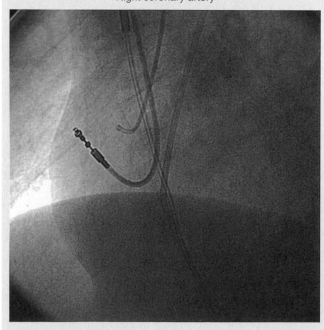

Left ventriculogram

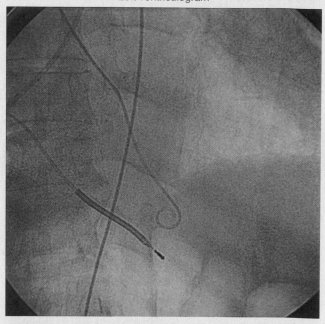

He was referred for a viability study to decide the further course of management and possible revascularization. A dose of 3.2 mCi of thallium-201 was injected at rest, followed by gated SPECT imaging 15 minutes and 4 hours later (Videos 4 and 5 and Figures 1 and 2). What is your interpretation of this study?

(Video 4a)

Rest   Redistribution

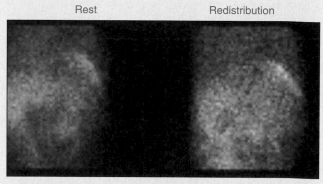

Rest   Redistribution

(Video 4b)

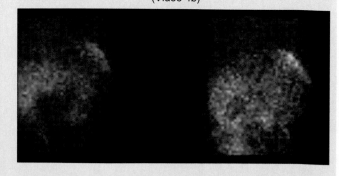

(Fig. 1a)

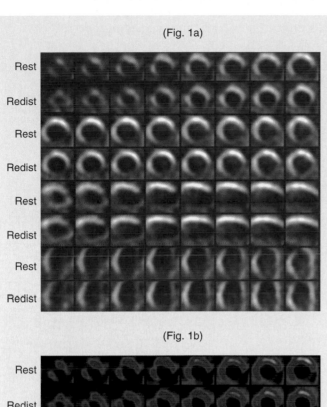

Rest
Redist
Rest
Redist
Rest
Redist
Rest
Redist

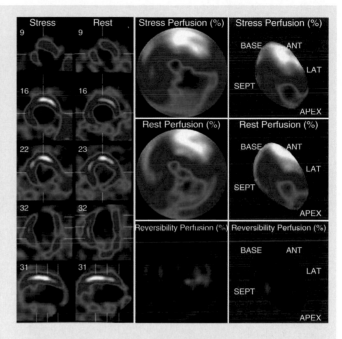

Stress   Rest   Stress Perfusion (%)   Stress Perfusion (%)
9   9
16   16   BASE   ANT
22   23   LAT
32   32   SEPT
31   31   APEX
Rest Perfusion (%)   Rest Perfusion (%)
BASE   ANT
LAT
SEPT
APEX
Reversibility Perfusion (%)   Reversibility Perfusion (%)
BASE   ANT
LAT
SEPT
APEX

(Fig. 1b)

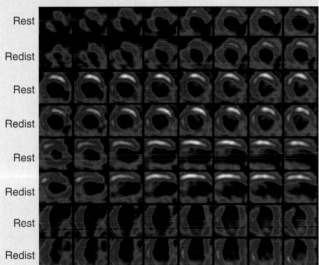

Rest
Redist
Rest
Redist
Rest
Redist
Rest
Redist

Rest   Redistribution
(Video 5)

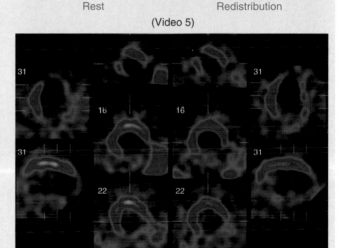

31   31
16   16
31   31
22   22

(Fig. 1c)

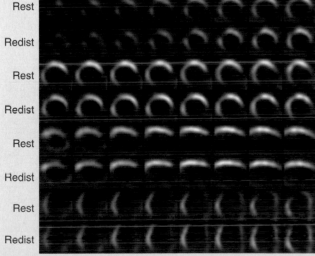

Rest
Redist
Rest
Redist
Rest
Redist
Rest
Redist

The left ventricle (LV) is massively enlarged. There is a very large, dense area of perfusion abnormality involving the inferior and lateral walls and apex, which does not change on delayed images. The tracer uptake in septum is decreased, which does not change on delayed imaging. Tracer uptake is normal in the anterior wall. The LV is severely hypokinetic and LVEF is depressed at 7%. This study indicated dense scar involving the inferior and lateral walls and apex with no evidence of viability. The septum shows an admixture of scar and viable myocardium, and the anterior wall is normally perfused.

This study reveals a very large, dense scar with no evidence of viability involving the inferior and lateral walls and apex, which correspond to completely occluded RCA and LCX. The septum and anterior wall show viability. These walls are perfused by a severely narrowed LAD. Revascularization of the LAD may improve the perfusion and possibly the function of the septum and anterior wall. However, the revascularization of the LAD in this case would be a very high-risk procedure, and global LVEF may not show any improvement, given the presence of a very large, dense scar involving the inferior and lateral walls.

The patient opted to be treated medically without any revascularization. His heart failure continued to worsen, and he died of refractory heart failure.

FURTHER READING

1. Perrone-Filardi P, Chiariello M, Underwood R: The assessment of myocardial viability and hibernation using resting thallium imaging [review], *Clin Cardiol* 23:719–722, 2000.
2. Travin MI, Bergmann SR: Assessment of myocardial viability [review], *Semin Nucl Med* 35:2–16, 2005.

CASE 17

A 53-year-old male with a history of diabetes, hypertension, hyperlipidemia, and end-stage renal disease (ESRD) presented to the hospital with chest pain and ruled-in non-ST-elevation myocardial infarction (NSTEMI). He had a renal transplant 3 years earlier, and his transplanted kidney is rejecting, with high serum urea (67 mg/dL) and creatinine levels (7 mg/dL), but he is still not on dialysis. Coronary angiography could not be done because of renal function impairment. He was treated medically and sent for rest and adenosine stress myocardial perfusion imaging (MPI) for risk stratification.

Medications: Aspirin, diltiazem, metoprolol, cyclosporine, Rapamune, calcitrol, prednisone, folic acid.

Pharmacologic stress test with 5-minute adenosine infusion is performed ^{99m}Tc-sestamibi was injected during adenosine infusion. HR changes from 55 to 71 beats/min and BP from 202/101 to 176/86 mm Hg. He has no chest pain or ST depression.

Resting ECG shows normal sinus rhythm with left axis deviation, flat T waves in leads II, III, aVF, and V4-6, with no change on adenosine infusion.

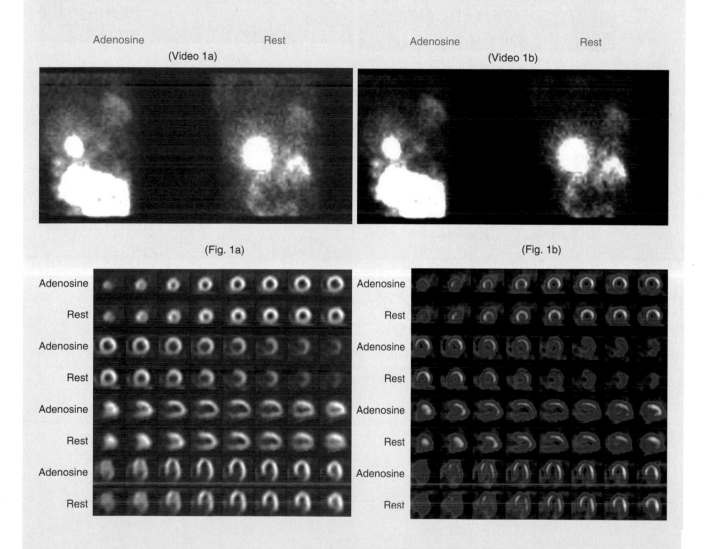

Adenosine   Rest
(Video 1a)

Adenosine   Rest
(Video 1b)

(Fig. 1a)

(Fig. 1b)

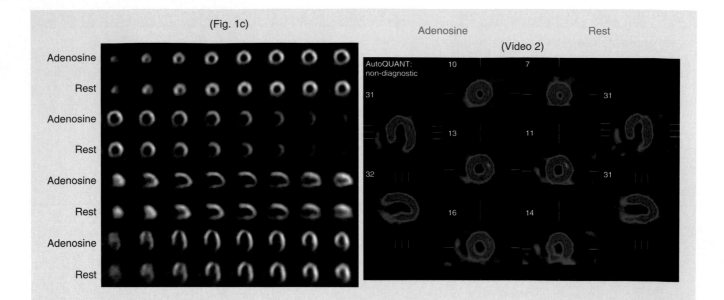

(Fig. 1c)

Adenosine | Rest

(Video 2)

Myocardial perfusion imaging shows a small area of perfusion abnormality involving the inferior wall, with minimal reversibility on the rest images. The inferior wall is hypokinetic and the left ventricular ejection fraction (LVEF) is mildly depressed at 45%. There is transient poststress LV dilation with transient ischemic dilation (TID) of 1.44.

Chronic kidney disease (CKD) is an independent risk factor for obstructive coronary artery disease, and patients with CKD have higher cardiovascular mortality (See Chapter 16). Another important management factor to consider in this patient is tighter BP control. The patient will need to undergo coronary angiography after he starts hemodialysis. If he receives another renal transplant, he will need catheterization prior to the surgery.

FURTHER READING

1. Cook JR, Dillie KS, Hakeem A, et al: Effectiveness of anemia and chronic kidney disease as predictors for presence and severity of coronary artery disease in patients undergoing stress myocardial perfusion study, *Am J Cardiol* 102:266–271, 2008.
2. Chonchol M, Whittle J, Desbien A, et al: Chronic kidney disease is associated with angiographic coronary artery disease, *Am J Nephrol* 28:354–360, 2008.
3. Rabbat CG, Treleaven DJ, Russell JD, et al: Prognostic value of myocardial perfusion studies in patients with end-stage renal disease assessed for kidney or kidney-pancreas transplantation: A meta-analysis, *J Am Soc Nephrol* 14:431–439, 2003.

CASE 18

A 54-year-old woman with inadequately controlled hypertension for the last several years complains of exertional angina at the outpatient office and is referred for pharmacologic stress/rest perfusion imaging. She is on oral atenolol 50 mg per day.

She underwent 2-day rest/stress ^{99m}Tc-sestamibi perfusion imaging using 5-minute adenosine infusion as an outpatient study. Her heart rate increased from 83 to 93 beats/min and blood pressure from 185/99 to 179/98 mm Hg. She developed anginal chest pain during adenosine infusion. Her baseline and peak stress ECGs are shown. What is your interpretation?

(Fig.1a)

Baseline ECG

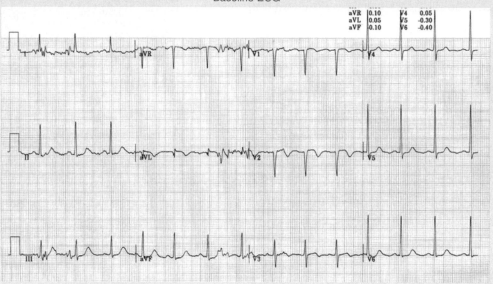

(Fig. 1b)

During Adenosine infusion

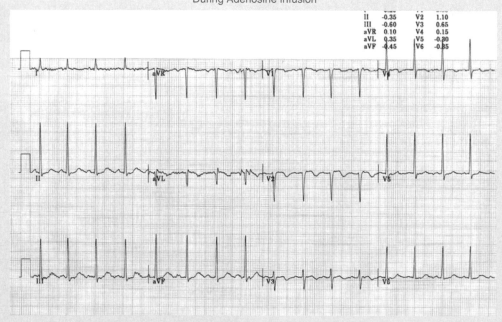

There is normal sinus rhythm with Q waves in aVL and V2, with T-wave inversion in leads aVL and V2-3.

There is left ventricular hypertrophy. There is no ST-segment depression with adenosine infusion.

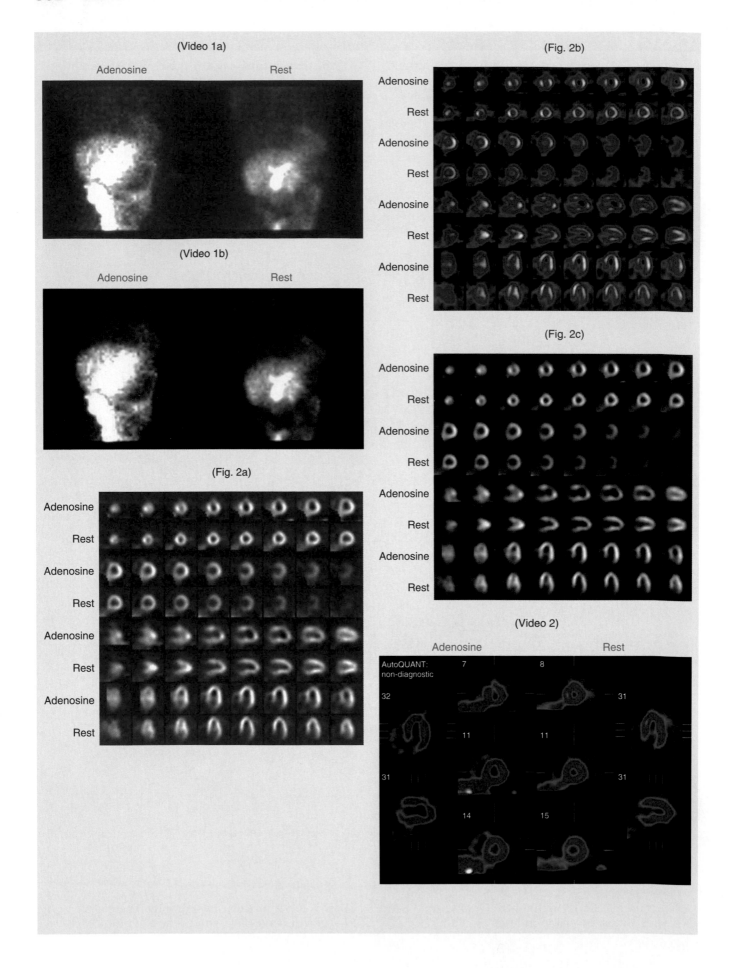

(Video 1a)

Adenosine   Rest

(Video 1b)

Adenosine   Rest

(Fig. 2a)

Adenosine
Rest
Adenosine
Rest
Adenosine
Rest
Adenosine
Rest

(Fig. 2b)

Adenosine
Rest
Adenosine
Rest
Adenosine
Rest
Adenosine
Rest

(Fig. 2c)

Adenosine
Rest
Adenosine
Rest
Adenosine
Rest
Adenosine
Rest

(Video 2)

Adenosine   Rest

AutoQUANT:
non-diagnostic

Perfusion imaging shows a large area of ischemia involving the anterior wall and apex. There is transient hypokinesia involving the anterior wall and apex, which normalizes at rest. LVEF is 51% on the poststress images and 59% on the rest images. This is a high-risk abnormal study.

What should the nuclear cardiology laboratory do about this patient?

She is at high risk for developing adverse cardiac events in the short term as well as the long term. Apart from sending the printed test report, to avoid any delays in communication, the interpreting physician should immediately communicate personally by phone call with the referring physician regarding the test result. This was done in this case. Her antianginal medication was increased, and she was brought back to the hospital 1 day later for cardiac catheterization.

She underwent cardiac catheterization, which showed single-vessel coronary artery disease (CAD). There was smooth, 60% narrowing in the distal segment of the left anterior descending (LAD) coronary artery.

However, there was anterolateral wall akinesia that could not be explained by angiographic disease. Although angiographically noncritical, due to her symptoms of angina and evidence of inducible ischemia, intervention was undertaken with percutaneous transluminal coronary angioplasty (PTCA) and a drug-eluting stent.

If there is no prior evidence of ischemia, during catheterization, fractional flow reserve (FFR) can be used to guide intervention in noncritical intermediate coronary stenosis.

FURTHER READING

1. Coiera E: Communication systems in healthcare, *Clin Biochem Rev* 27:89–98, 2006.
2. Lippi G, Fostini R, Guidi GC: Quality improvement in laboratory medicine: Extra-analytical issues, *Clin Lab Med* 28:285–294, 2008.
3. Magni V, Chieffo A, Colombo A: Evaluation of intermediate coronary stenosis with intravascular ultrasound and fractional flow reserve: Its use and abuse, *Catheter Cardiovasc Interv* 73:441–448, 2008.

CASE 19

A 65-year-old man had abnormalities on his electrocardiogram (ECG) at a routine outpatient office visit with his primary physician. He was referred for exercise stress/rest myocardial perfusion imaging.

He exercised for 9 minutes, 15 seconds, achieving 10 METs with Bruce protocol. His heart rate changed from 55 beats/min to 135 beats/min (achieving 87% target) and blood pressure from 150/70 to 190/90 mm Hg. Resting ECG showed sinus rhythm with left anterior fascicular block and nonspecific ST-T changes in limb leads. No chest pain or ST-segment change occurred on stress. Patient underwent stress-rest ^{99m}Tc-sestamibi perfusion imaging.

(Video 1a)

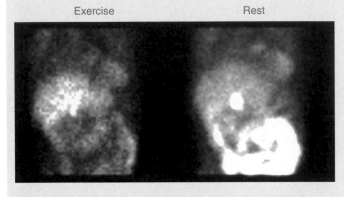

(Video 1b)

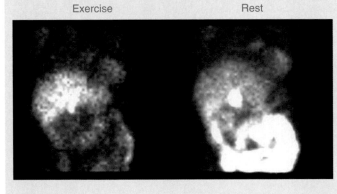

(Fig. 1)

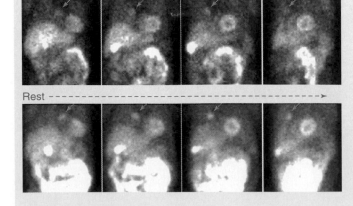

(Fig. 2a)

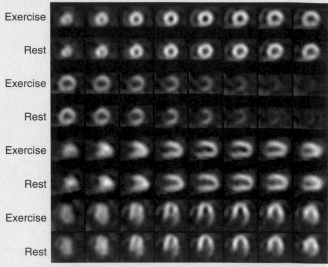

(Fig. 2b)

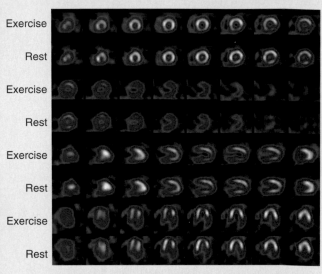

(Fig. 2c)

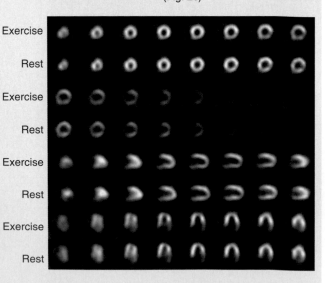

(Video 2a)

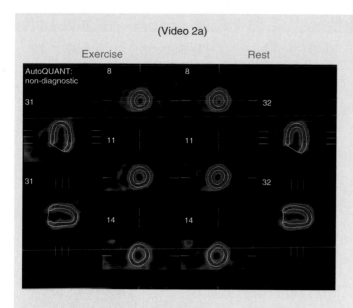

(Video 2b)

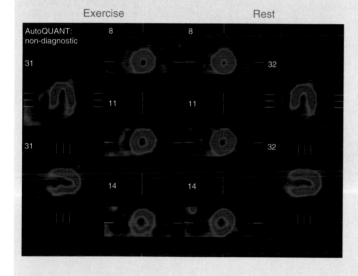

Perfusion imaging showed a small area of perfusion abnormality involving the inferolateral wall, which was reversible on rest images. Left ventricular ejection fraction (LVEF) was 61%. There was a large nodular area of radiotracer uptake in the right lung in the mediastinum, which was suspicious for thymoma, ectopic thyroid tissue, or some other malignant mass such as lymphoma.

Coronary angiogram showed bilateral coronary calcifications, with luminal irregularities in distal left anterior descending (LAD) and proximal large first obtuse marginal, and focal 50% stenosis in proximal right coronary artery (RCA).

Computed tomography scan of the patient's chest showed an anterior mediastinal mass measuring 3.8 × 2.5 cm. He underwent thoracotomy and excision of the mediastinal mass, which proved to be a thymoma.

CASE 20

A 43-year-old woman is admitted to the hospital for evaluation of chest pain. She had a prior history of hypertension, peripheral vascular disease, coronary artery disease, congestive heart failure, and defibrillator implant for primary prevention. She underwent coronary artery bypass grafting and pericardial stripping 12 years earlier. The details of this surgery and the indication are not available. Six years earlier, she underwent multivessel angioplasty in another hospital. She also had end-stage renal disease and was on hemodialysis. During her current admission to the hospital with chest pain, acute myocardial infarction was ruled out, and she was sent for pharmacologic stress perfusion imaging. She was on diltiazem, carvedilol, and pantoprazole. She underwent 2-day rest/stress perfusion imaging using 25 mCi of ^{99m}Tc-sestamibi on both days.

Pharmacologic stress was carried out using 5-minute adenosine infusion protocol. Her heart rate remained unchanged at 86 beats/min, and blood pressure changed from 144/64 to 122/63 mm Hg. There was no chest pain with adenosine infusion.

(Fig. 1)

Baseline ECG

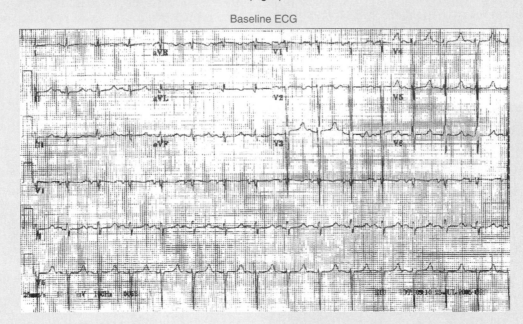

Her baseline electrocardiogram showed normal sinus rhythm. There was poor R-wave progression from V1 to V3, suspicious of an old anteroseptal myocardial infarction, and there were Q-waves in leads I and aVL, indicative of old lateral wall infarction. Electrocardiogram did not show changes from baseline with adenosine infusion.

(Video 1b)

Stress   Rest

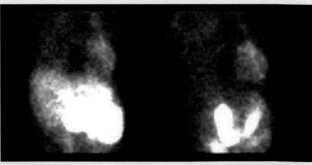

(Video 1a)

Stress   Rest

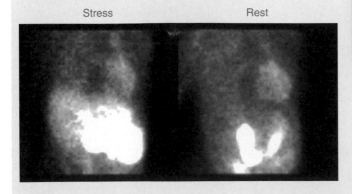

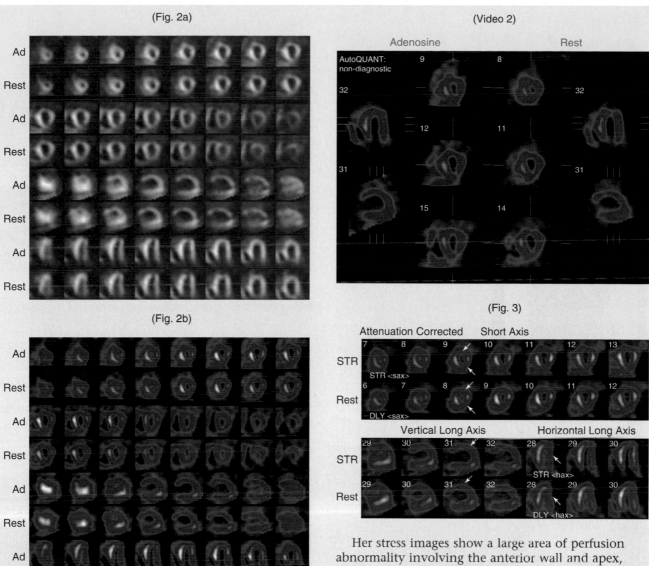

(Fig. 2a)

(Video 2)

(Fig. 2b)

(Fig. 2c)

(Fig. 3)

Her stress images show a large area of perfusion abnormality involving the anterior wall and apex, which does not change on rest images. There is another moderate-sized area of perfusion abnormality involving the inferolateral wall, which also does not change on rest images. On gated SPECT imaging, the anteroapical wall is akinetic, and the remaining left ventricle is hypokinetic. The left ventricular ejection fraction is depressed at 29%. There is significant tracer activity in the gut on stress images, that is close to the heart. Nevertheless, the inferolateral perfusion abnormality does not appear to be contributed by gut activity alone. The patient was unable to lift her left arm above her head, and the left arm does result in attenuation artifact.

In addition, there is a large photopenic area in the left side of her chest involving the lower two-thirds of the hemithorax, raising suspicion of a large loculated left pleural effusion, a large bullous lesion, or a very large mass in the left hemithorax. This lesion seems to be pushing the mediastinum to the right and compressing on the lateral wall of the heart. The right lung is clear.

(Fig. 3a)

Emission   Scatter

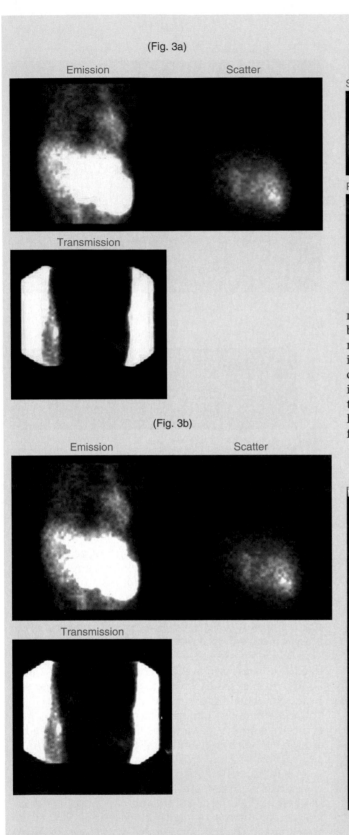

Transmission

(Fig. 3b)

Emission   Scatter

Transmission

(Fig. 4)

Raw images

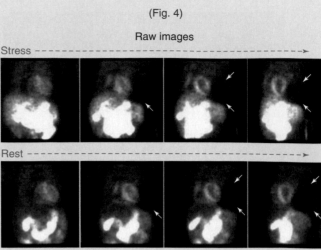

Stress --->

Rest --->

The raw transmission images indicate this to be radiodense lesion, excluding the possibility of a large bullous lesion. This dense mass could have also resulted in an attenuation artifact involving the inferior and lateral defects. However, the attenuation-corrected stress and rest images are not different from images not attenuation corrected. Therefore, it appears that despite the presence of a large thoracic mass and her left arm on her side, both anterior and inferolateral fixed perfusion abnormalities are real.

(Fig. 5)

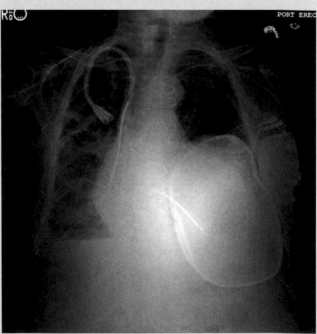

This study raises a question about the nature of her left thoracic mass. Her chest x-rays show a very large calcified mass in the left lower hemithorax extending into the upper abdomen. The patient suffered from massive left hemothorax in the past following pericardial stripping surgery, which resolved slowly over a long period and resulted in a large calcified mass in her left lung.

Discussion

In this case, the raw images reveal an interesting thoracic abnormality. The large photopenic area in the left lung can be due to a large mass, cyst, fluid in the pleural cavity, or a bullous lesion. A careful examination of the rotating raw emission and transmission images can help to differentiate these conditions. A bullous lesion can be readily differentiated from the solid or fluid-filled lesions in the transmission images. The former lesion appears bright on the transmission images, whereas the latter images appear dark, as in this case. Free fluid in the pleural cavity generally tracks the pleural space and is more obvious in the subpulmonary, posterior, and lateral aspects of the chest, since SPECT images are acquired in the supine position. Mass lesions and loculated fluid-filled lesions appear more localized. Malignant mass lesions may show increased radiotracer uptake, since myocardial perfusion tracers also accumulate in malignant lesions. The scintigraphic appearance of this lesion in the patient's left hemithorax was highly suspicious of a loculated fluid or some nonmalignant mass lesion.

(Fig. 6)

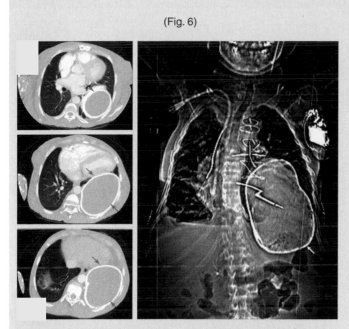

Computed tomography scan of the patient's chest shows a large, peripherally calcified hematoma measuring 14 × 14 × 10 cm. Echocardiography showed global hypokinesia, with left ventricular ejection fraction 25%. There is a reverberation echo artifact, noted on the lateral wall of the left ventricle from the calcified mass.

FURTHER READING

1. Williams KA, Hill KA, Sheridan CM: Noncardiac findings on dual-isotope myocardial perfusion SPECT, *J Nucl Cardiol* 10:395–402, 2003.
2. Raza M, Meesala M, Panjrath G, et al: Abnormal photopenic area on nuclear perfusion imaging, *J Nucl Cardiol* 12:607–609, 2005.
3. Raza M, Panjrath G, Jain D: Unusual retrocardiac radiotracer uptake on sestamibi perfusion images, *J Nucl Cardiol* 11: e1–e2, 2004.
4. Meesala M, Raza M, Yaganti V, et al: Bilateral photopenic areas in the lungs on SPECT imaging, *J Nucl Cardiol* 13:728–730, 2006.
5. Hendel RC, Gibbons RJ, Bateman TM: Use of rotating (cine) planar images in the interpretation of a tomographic myocardial perfusion study, *J Nucl Cardiol* 6:234–240, 1999.
6. Panjrath GS, Narra K, Jain D: Myocardial perfusion imaging in a patient with chest pain, *J Nucl Cardiol* 11:515–517, 2004.

(Fig. 7)

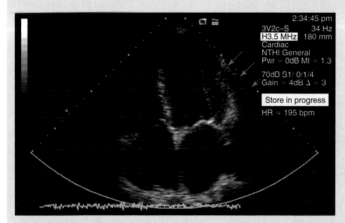

This patient was treated medically for heart failure. She subsequently succumbed to gangrene of her legs due to peripheral vascular disease followed by amputations. She died 2 years later of fulminant sepsis from nonhealing stump ulcers.

CASE 21

A 45-year-old Caucasian male who is a truck driver and hauls sand and stones started experiencing palpitations and shortness of breath 2 months previously, which progressively worsened to four-pillow orthopnea. He is a heavy drinker (6 to 12 beers per day) and chronic smoker. He was admitted to an outside hospital in frank pulmonary edema, where he underwent catheterization after diuresis.

(Video 1)

LCA

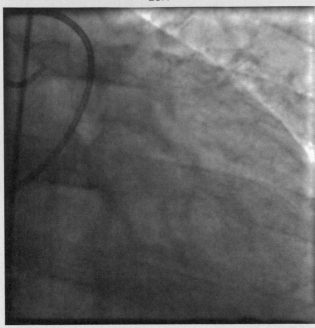

(Video 2)

RCA

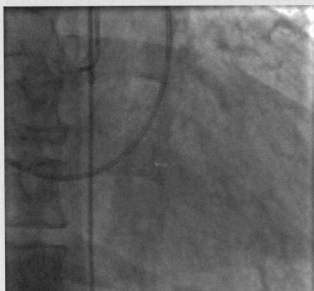

(Video 3)

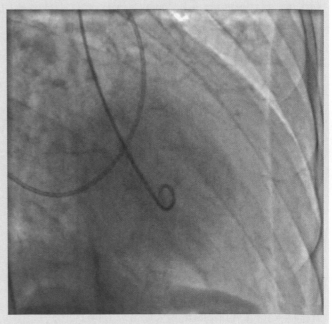

He was found to have complete occlusion of the LCX, severe disease of the D1 and D2, normal RCA, and aneurysm of the lateral wall. He was referred to our hospital for further evaluation and surgical treatment.

(Video 4a)

Rest	Redistribution

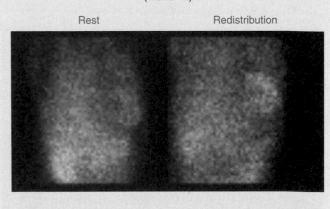

(Video 4b)

Rest	Redistribution

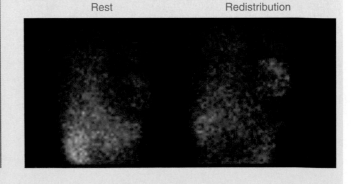

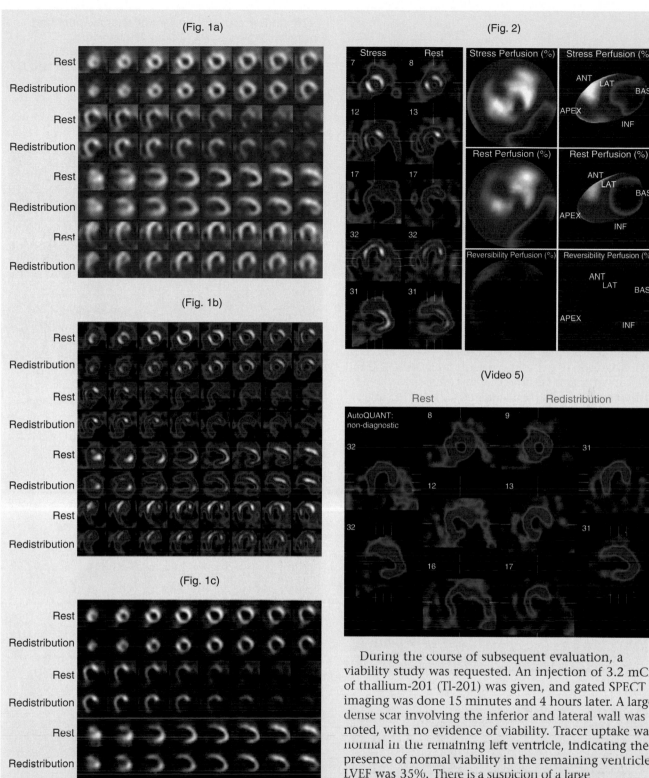

(Fig. 1a)

Rest
Redistribution
Rest
Redistribution
Rest
Redistribution
Rest
Redistribution

(Fig. 1b)

Rest
Redistribution
Rest
Redistribution
Rest
Redistribution
Rest
Redistribution

(Fig. 1c)

Rest
Redistribution
Rest
Redistribution
Rest
Redistribution
Rest
Redistribution

(Fig. 2)

Stress   Rest

Stress Perfusion (%)   Stress Perfusion (%)
ANT LAT   BASE
APEX   INF

Rest Perfusion (%)   Rest Perfusion (%)
ANT LAT   BASE
APEX   INF

Reversibility Perfusion (%)   Reversibility Perfusion (%)
ANT LAT   BASE
APEX   INF

(Video 5)

Rest   Redistribution

AutoQUANT:
non-diagnostic

During the course of subsequent evaluation, a viability study was requested. An injection of 3.2 mCi of thallium-201 (Tl-201) was given, and gated SPECT imaging was done 15 minutes and 4 hours later. A large dense scar involving the inferior and lateral wall was noted, with no evidence of viability. Tracer uptake was normal in the remaining left ventricle, indicating the presence of normal viability in the remaining ventricle. LVEF was 35%. There is a suspicion of a large pseudoaneurysm arising from the lateral wall on this study, because of the presence of a large dense photopenic area adjoining the lateral wall. He underwent MUGA scan.

(Video 6a)

Ant   LAO   L Lat

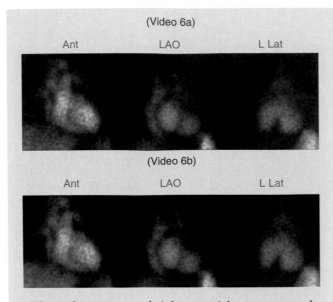

(Video 6b)

Ant   LAO   L Lat

The right atrium and right ventricle were normal, but MUGA showed a massive pseudoaneurysm arising from the lateral and inferobasal walls. The remaining LV contracts normally and vigorously. The EF of the LV after exclusion of the pseudoaneurysm is 36%. TEE and CT scan with and without contrast were performed to further evaluate the pseudoaneurysm prior to surgery. Contrast CT showed large mural thrombi within the pseudoaneurysm.

(Fig. 3)

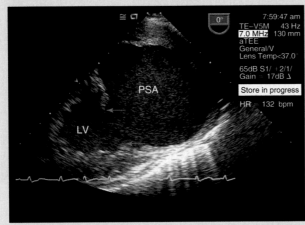

(Fig. 4)

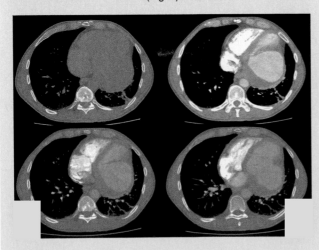

He underwent surgery for aneurysmectomy and coronary bypass grafts. A large lateral wall pseudoaneurysm was excised. The lateral wall required a patch, MV was replaced, and OM1, OM2, D1, and D2 bypassed. He had an uneventful postoperative recovery.

(Fig. 5a)

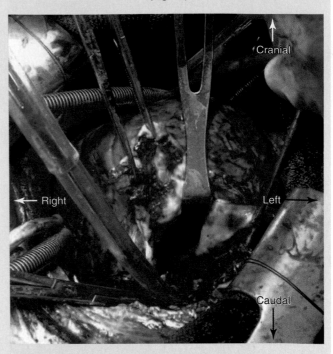

(Fig. 5b)

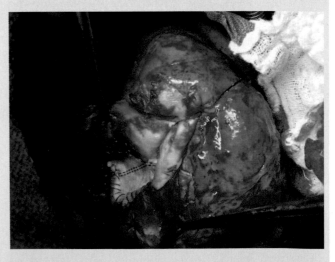

(Video 7a)

Ant   LAO   L Lat

(Video 7b)

Ant   LAO   L Lat

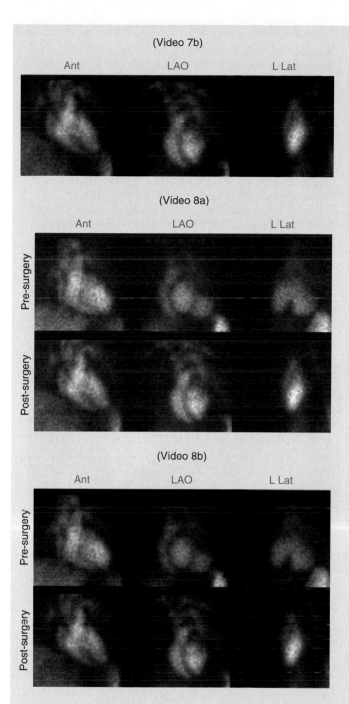

(Video 8a)

Ant   LAO   L Lat

Pre-surgery

Post-surgery

(Video 8b)

Ant   LAO   L Lat

Pre-surgery

Post-surgery

(Fig. 6)

Chest X-Rays

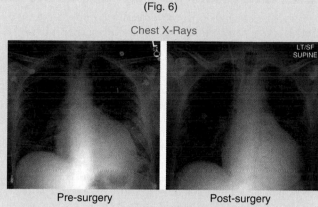

LT/SF
SUPINE

Pre-surgery   Post-surgery

Left ventricular pseudoaneurysm is a rare complication following Ac myocardial infarction. This follows rupture of infarcted myocardium, which is contained by adherent pericardium. This is more common in inferior, lateral, and apical infarctions, whereas true aneurysms are more common with anterior infarcts. Untreated pseudoaneurysms carry a high risk of spontaneous rupture. MUGA is a highly reliable technique for the detection of pseudoaneurysm of the LV.

FURTHER READING

1. Brown SL, Gropler RJ, Harris KM: Distinguishing left ventricular aneurysm from pseudoaneurysm. A review of literature, *Chest* 111:1403–1409, 1997.
2. Frances C, Romero A, Grady G: Left ventricular pseudoaneurysm, *J Am Coll Cardiol* 32:557–561, 1998.

CASE 22

A 66-year-old male with hypertension, hyperlipidemia, and known coronary artery disease presented to the hospital with worsening angina over the last few weeks. He had suffered a myocardial infarction and underwent coronary artery bypass grafting in the past (1982 and 1992). He presented with angina in October 2004, and coronary angiography showed proximal complete occlusion of all three native vessels. Left internal mammary graft to the left anterior descending coronary artery was patent, but there was 70% narrowing distal to the left internal mammary artery touchdown. SVGs to the RCA and D1 were occluded. SVGs to the OM2 and OM3 had 95% occlusion. He underwent PCI and stenting of the SVGs to OM2 and OM3.

During this admission, acute myocardial infarction was ruled out, but the patient was found to be severely anemic. His hemoglobin was 5.7 g/dL, white count was 5100/μL, with a differential of N-49%, L-31%, M-17%, E-2%, Blasts-1%, and a platelet count of 93,000/μL.

He was transfused with multiple units of blood, and his hemoglobin increased to 10 g/dL. He was scheduled to undergo upper and lower gastrointestinal endoscopy to look for any possible sources of blood loss. He had no evidence of hemolytic anemia.

He was referred for pharmacologic stress perfusion imaging for cardiac evaluation prior to the endoscopy procedures.

He underwent 2-day rest/stress perfusion imaging using 25 mCi of ^{99m}Tc-sestamibi on each day. With 5-minute adenosine infusion, his heart rate changed from 57 to 66 beats/min, and blood pressure changed from 168/83 to 155/84 mm Hg. He complained of chest tightness during adenosine infusion. His electrocardiogram showed normal sinus rhythm with intraventricular conduction delay and nonspecific ST-T changes. There was further 1-mm ST depression during adenosine infusion.

(Video 1a)

(Video 1b)

Stress   Rest   Stress   Rest

(Fig. 1a)

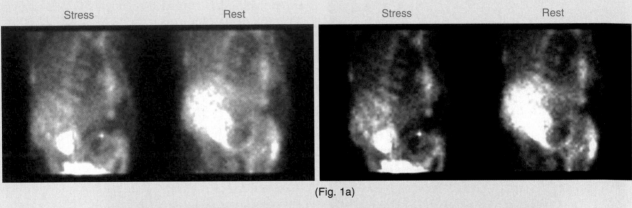

(Fig. 1b)

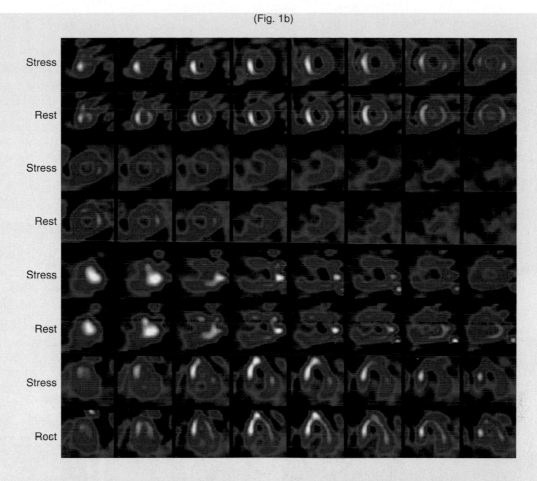

(Fig. 1c)

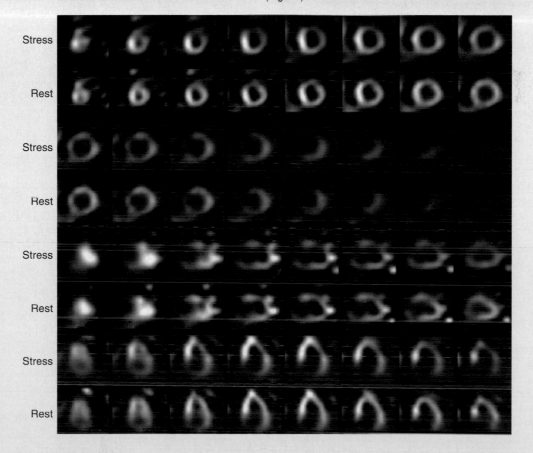

(Video 2a)

Stress   Rest

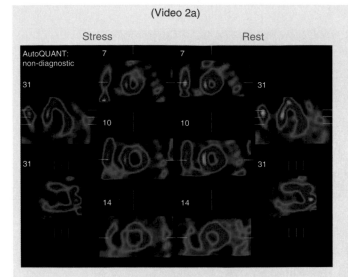

(Video 2b)

Stress   Rest

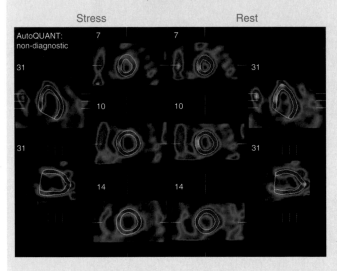

The representative raw images and processed stress and rest slices in the short, vertical, and horizontal long axes show marked tracer uptake in the ribs, sternum, vertebrae, and scapulae on both stress and rest images. Bone uptake interferes to some extent with the image interpretation. There is a large area of perfusion abnormality involving the anterior and lateral walls, which is predominantly reversible on the rest imaging. There is transient poststress anterior wall hypokinesia and transient poststress LV dilation. TID was calculated as 1.22 (upper limit of normal 1.16). Left ventricular ejection fraction was 49% (poststress) and 55% (rest).

This patient turned out to have high-risk abnormal images. However, extensive skeletal radiotracer uptake was quite intriguing. Prompted by the observation of marked skeletal uptake noted on the first day of imaging, whole-body images were acquired following the stress images on the second day. The whole body images showed abnormal tracer uptake predominantly in the flat bones and proximal ends of long bones.

(Fig. 2)

Whole Body Images

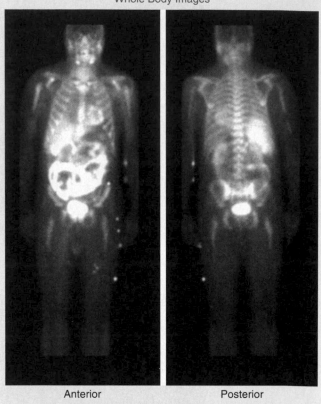

Anterior   Posterior

On reexamination, he denied any symptoms of bone pain, and there was no skeletal tenderness anywhere.

He had a whole-body bone scan, which was negative.

He underwent skeletal survey, which showed rounded lytic lesions in the calvarium. The rest of the x-rays did not show any abnormality. He also underwent extensive biochemical and hematologic workup, including bone marrow biopsy.

(Fig. 3)

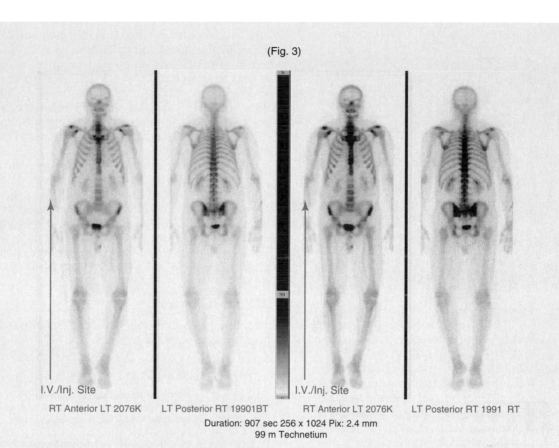

I.V./Inj. Site

RT Anterior LT 2076K   LT Posterior RT 19901BT

I.V./Inj. Site

RT Anterior LT 2076K   LT Posterior RT 1991 RT

Duration: 907 sec 256 x 1024 Pix: 2.4 mm
99 m Technetium

(Fig. 4)

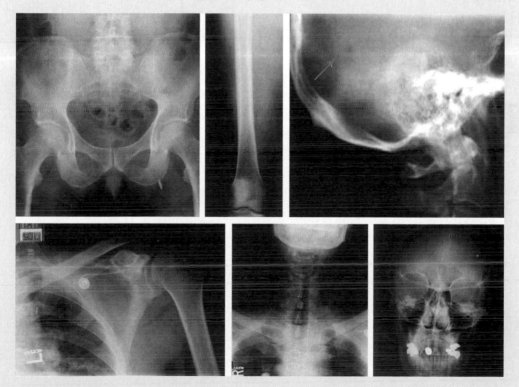

His bone marrow biopsy showed diffuse infiltration by neoplastic plasma cells, and this picture was consistent with plasma cell myeloma. Flow cytometry showed approximately 70% atypical plasma cells with kappa light-chain restriction.

(Fig. 5)

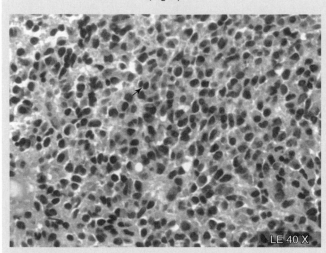

LE 40 X

His serum protein electrophoresis showed elevated total protein 11.6 g/dL (normal range: 6.0 to 8.0 g/dL) with predominantly alpha$_1$ globulin 0.4 g/dL (normal range: 0.15 to 0.35 g/dL) and gamma immunoglobulins 5.5 g/dL (normal range: 0.7 to 1.5 g/dL). Albumin 3.8 mg/dL (normal range: 3.5 to 5.5 g/dL), alpha$_2$ globulin -1 g/dL (normal range: 0.5 to 1.0 g/dL) and beta globulin 1 g/dL (normal range: 0.7 to 1.5 g/dL) were in the normal range. Beta$_2$ microglobulin level, which is a poor prognostic indicator, was elevated to 12.07 mg/L (normal range 0 to 3.0 mg/L).

In the quantitative immunoglobulin panel, there was high level of IgG 8430 mg/dL (normal range: 751 to 1560 mg/dL) and low levels of IgA 26 mg/dL (normal range: 82 to 453 mg/dL) and IgM 29 mg/dL (normal range: 46 to 306 mg/dL). Serum immunofixation showed an electrophoretic pattern consistent with monoclonal gammopathy of IgG kappa type.

Although sestamibi is primarily a myocardial perfusion radiotracer, it is also taken up by various tumors. ^{99m}Tc-sestamibi has also been used quite successfully as a tumor imaging agent. The mechanism of sestamibi concentration in malignant tissue is still uncertain. The strong electronegative mitochondrial and plasma membrane potentials are considered relevant factors. Alterations in cell metabolism could affect the membrane potential, favoring sestamibi accumulation in plasma cells As suggested in some reports, the patterns of technetium uptake in patients with multiple myeloma are related to both the clinical state and stage of the disease; the presence of intense diffuse uptake is suggestive of active and advanced-stage disease. It also correlates with the amount of monoclonal component and the percentage of bone marrow plasma cells.

It could be a very useful technique in identifying patients with active disease, and hence guide selection of patients who need treatment and follow-up of patients after chemotherapy. This becomes very important, especially since bone scan is not sensitive in detecting myeloma lesions, and radiologic lesions would not be useful in indicating whether it is an active disease.

Acknowledgment

This case has been borrowed (with permission) from a case report by Gowda A et al.[1]

FURTHER READING

1. Gowda A, Peddington L, Shandilya V, Gavriluke A, Jain D: Abnormal intense skeletal radiotracer uptake on myocardial perfusion imaging with Tc-99m sestamibi, *J Nucl Cardiol* 13:427–431, 2006.
2. Fonti R, Del Vecchio S, Salvatore M: Bone marrow uptake of ^{99m}Tc-MIBI in patients with multiple myeloma, *Eur J Nucl Med* 28:214–220, 2001.
3. Pace L, Catalano L, Salvatore M: Different patterns of technetium-99m sestamibi uptake in multiple myeloma, *Eur J Nucl Med* 25:714–720, 1998.
4. Lette J, Cerino M, Demaria S, et al: Serendipitous diagnosis of multiple myeloma during sestamibi myocardial perfusion imaging, *Clin Nucl Med* 27:832–833, 2002.
5. Fisher C, Vehec A, Kashlan B, et al: Incidental detection of skeletal uptake on sestamibi cardiac images in a patient with previously undiagnosed multiple myeloma, *Clin Nucl Med* 25:213–214, 2000.
6. Yi A, Jacobs M: Skeletal tetrofosmin uptake in a patient undergoing myocardial perfusion imaging with subsequent diagnosis of multiple myeloma, *Clin Nucl Med* 29:327–328, 2004.
7. Schömäcker K, Schicha H: Use of myocardial imaging agents for tumour diagnosis—a success story? *Eur J Nucl Med* 27:1845–1863, 2000.

CASE 23

A 61-year-old male with hypertension, hyperlipidemia, and known coronary artery disease was admitted to the hospital with worsening congestive heart failure. He suffered from a myocardial infarction in the past, for which he underwent percutaneous transluminal coronary angioplasty (PTCA). He was referred for pharmacologic stress perfusion imaging prior to consideration for a biventricular pacing ICD.

Medications: aspirin, furosemide, lisinopril, carvedilol, atorvastatin, spironolactone, and digoxin.

He underwent pharmacologic stress using 5-minute adenosine infusion protocol. His heart rate changed from 63 to 90 beats/min and blood pressure from 115/71 to 133/76 mm Hg. There was no chest pain. Baseline and peak stress ECGs are shown next. What is your interpretation?

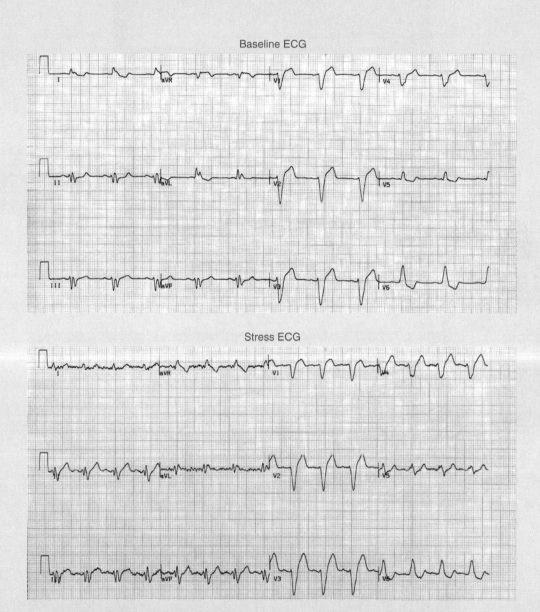

Baseline ECG

Stress ECG

There is normal sinus rhythm with left bundle branch block and markedly prolonged QRS. QRS measures more than 180 msec. There is no change with adenosine infusion.

His ^{99m}Tc-sestamibi stress and rest images are shown next. What is your interpretation?

(Video 1a)

Adenosine   Rest

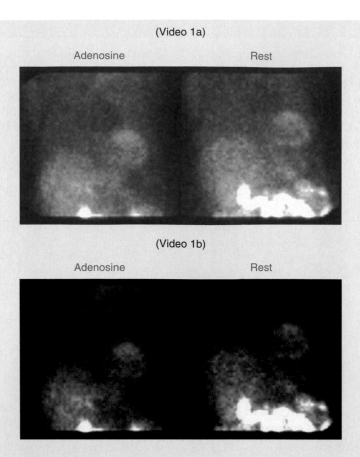

(Video 1b)

Adenosine   Rest

(Fig. 1a)

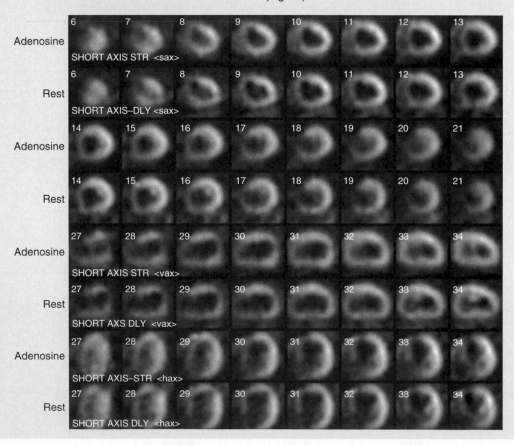

(Fig. 1b)

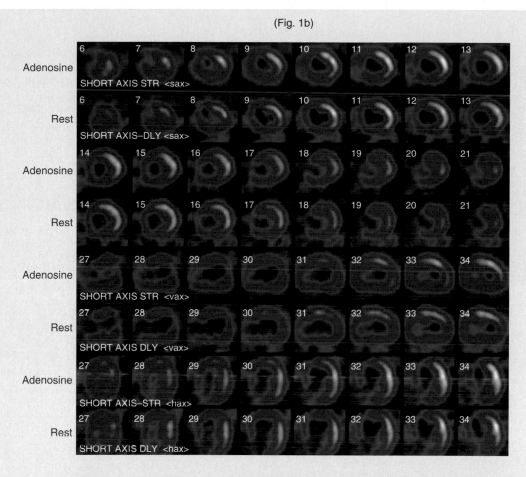

(Fig. 1c)

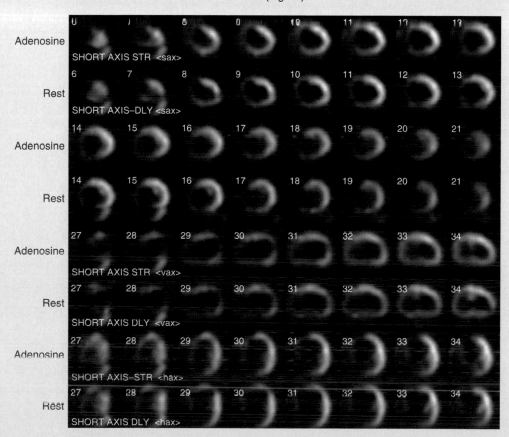

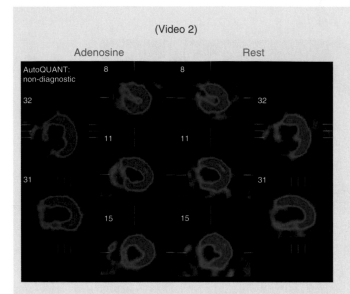

(Video 2)

Adenosine   Rest

AutoQUANT:
non-diagnostic

The LV is massively enlarged. There is a large, dense area of perfusion abnormality involving the septum and part of the inferior wall and anterior wall. There is no change on rest images. On gated SPECT images, the septum is dyskinetic, and the remaining LV is severely hypokinetic. LVEF is severely reduced at 23%.

He received BiV-ICD for ischemic cardiomyopathy. During subsequent outpatient follow-ups, his heart failure has remained stable.

FURTHER READING

1. Tang AS, Wells GA, Arnold M, et al: Resynchronization/ defibrillation for ambulatory heart failure trial: Rationale and trial design, *Curr Opin Cardiol* 24:1–8, 2009.
2. Reynolds MR, Josephson ME: MADIT II (second Multicenter Automated Defibrillator Implantation Trial) debate: Risk stratification, costs, and public policy, *Circulation* 108:1779–1783, 2003.

CASE 24

A 76-year-old male with known CAD and prior myocardial infarction was admitted to the hospital with worsening heart failure. He was referred for rest-redistribution thallium-201 (^{201}Tl) imaging for the detection of myocardial viability. An injection of

3.3 mCi of ^{201}Tl was given intravenously at rest, and this was followed by gated SPECT imaging 15 minutes and 4 hours later. The images are shown next. What is your interpretation?

(Fig. 1)

Baseline ECG

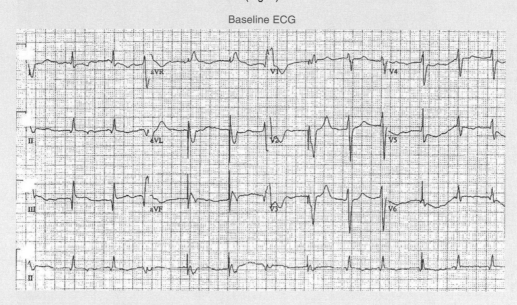

Atrial fibrillation with intermittent BiV paced beats. There are Q waves noted in inferior leads and V6 in the nonpaced beats.

(Video 1a)

Rest   Redistribution

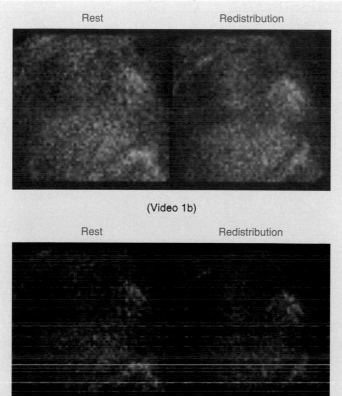

(Video 1b)

Rest   Redistribution

(Fig. 2a)

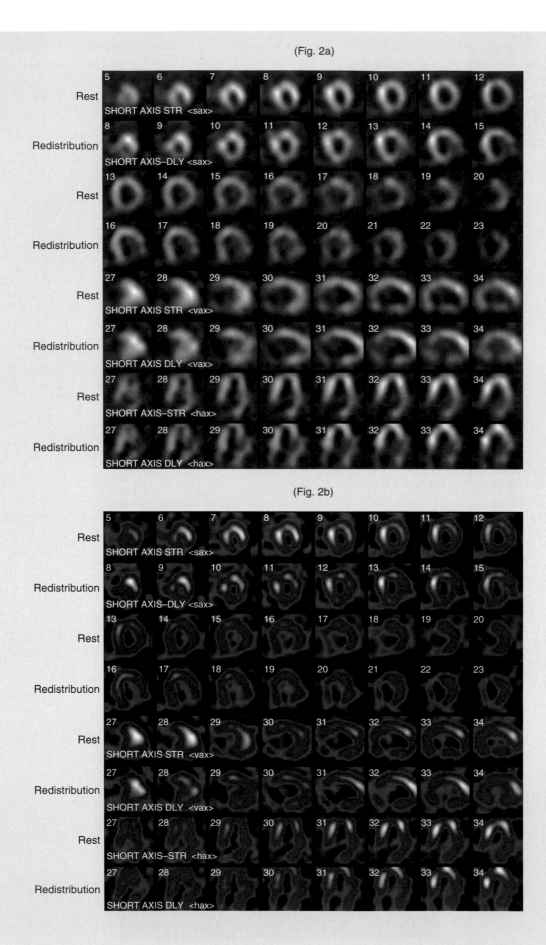

(Fig. 2b)

(Fig. 2c)

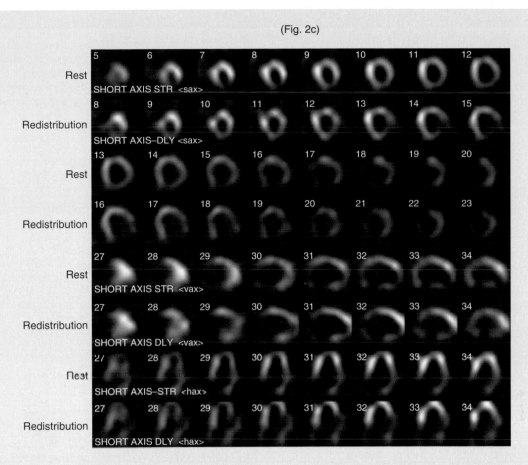

(Video 2)

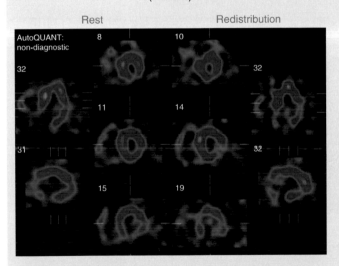

and severely hypokinetic. There is increased lung thallium uptake. However, importantly, there is a very large pleural effusion on the right side. It is likely that this effusion is contributing substantially to the patient's symptoms.

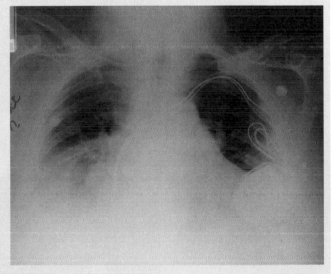

The left ventricle is enlarged, and there is a large area of perfusion abnormality involving the inferior and lateral walls, which does not show any reversibility on the delayed images. There is evidence of reverse redistribution in these areas of perfusion abnormality. There is global hypokinesia of the left ventricle, and left ventricular ejection fraction is severely impaired at 24%. The right ventricle is also massively enlarged

CASE 25

A 42-year-old male with hypertension and end-stage renal disease complains of chest pain. Medications: hydrochlorothiazide, amlodipine, metoprolol, clonidine, and hydralazine.

A 5-minute adenosine infusion stress test was performed. ^{99m}Tc-sestamibi was used for stress and rest images are shown next. His heart rate changed from 71 to 87 beats/min and blood pressure from 183/87 to 206/85 mm Hg. There was no chest pain. ECG showed normal sinus rhythm, generalized nonspecific ST-T changes, and no further change with adenosine infusion.

(Fig. 1a)

Baseline ECG

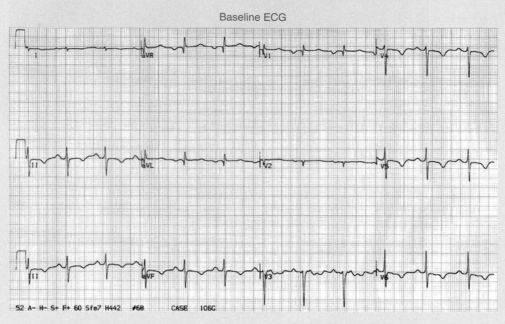

(Video 1a)

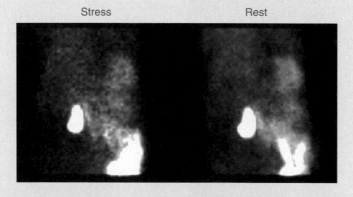

Stress   Rest

(Video 1b)

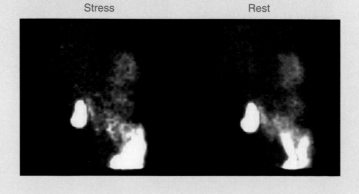

Stress   Rest

(Fig. 2a)

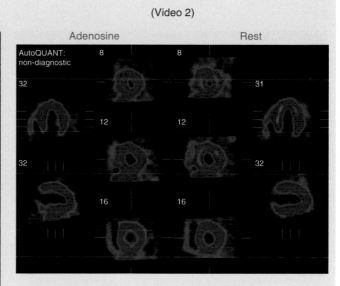

Stress

Rest

Stress

Rest

Stress

Rest

Stress

Rest

(Fig. 2b)

Stress

Rest

Stress

Rest

Stress

Rest

Stress

Rest

(Fig. 2c)

Stress

Rest

Stress

Rest

Stress

Rest

Stress

Rest

(Video 2)

Adenosine   Rest

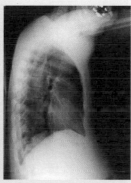

Left ventricle is enlarged and hypertrophied, but there is no regional perfusion abnormality. Left ventricular ejection fraction is marginally impaired at 47%. Myocardial perfusion imaging (MPI) findings are consistent with hypertensive heart disease, but there is no evidence of coronary artery disease. There are large photopenic masses in both flanks of the abdomen. These are consistent with polycystic kidney disease. The diaphragm is pushed superiorly, and intestinal loops are pushed toward the midline. The patient was cleared for renal transplant based upon no perfusion abnormalities on MPI.

(Fig. 3)

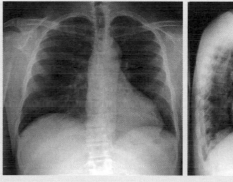

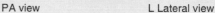

PA view   L Lateral view

(Fig. 4)

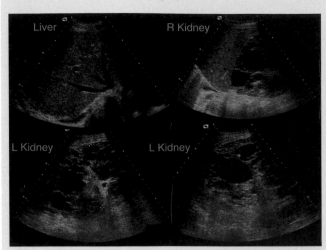

Ultrasound of the abdomen showed that the liver and pancreas were unremarkable, but the kidneys were enlarged and had numerous cysts of various sizes, consistent with polycystic kidney disease. Six months later, the patient required bilateral nephrectomy because of persistent abdominal discomfort and pain from massively enlarged native kidneys. Histopathology of kidneys was consistent with polycystic kidney disease.

FURTHER READING

Ghanbarinia A, Chandra S, Chhabra K, Jain D: Renal abnormalities as incidental findings on myocardial single-photon emission computed tomography perfusion imaging, *Nucl Med Commun* 29(7):588–592, 2008.

CASE 26

A 49-year-old African American woman with hypertension, hyperlipidemia, and smoking suffered from an anterior wall myocardial infarction (MI). She was transferred from a small community hospital and presented to our hospital via MedEvac. She underwent urgent cath, which showed large left anterior descending (LAD) with a large diagonal branch that was completely occluded in the mid-part. The occluded LAD was opened and stented, with no residual lesion. The left circumflex (LCX) was a small nondominant vessel with 50% lesion in the mid-vessel. The right coronary artery (RCA) was also a medium-caliber vessel, with a focal 80% lesion in the mid-segment, followed by 50% narrowing. The LCX and RCA were not angioplastied. She recovered from her MI and was referred for adenosine stress and rest myocardial perfusion imaging 6 weeks later to determine whether she needs revascularization of the RCA lesion.

Medications: lisinopril, Coreg, aldactone, Lipitor, iron, aspirin, and Plavix.

Results of the 5-minute adenosine infusion were changes in heart rate from 68 to 80 beats/min and blood pressure from 151/100 to 135/85 mm Hg. No chest pain was reported.

(Fig. 1a)

PABL Baseline ECG

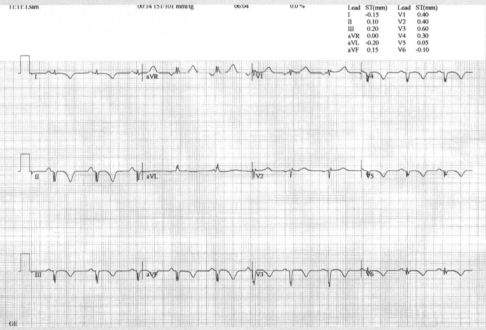

Lead	ST(mm)	Lead	ST(mm)
I	-0.15	V1	0.40
II	0.10	V2	0.40
III	0.20	V3	0.60
aVR	0.00	V4	0.30
aVL	-0.20	V5	0.05
aVF	0.15	V6	-0.10

(Fig. 1b)

PABL Adenosine ECG

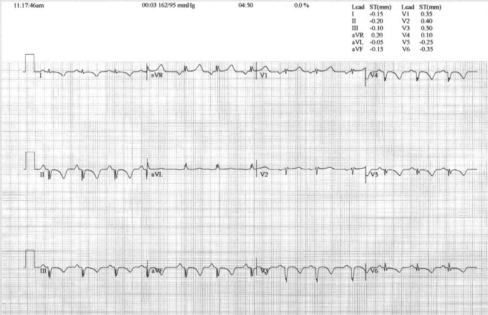

Lead	ST(mm)	Lead	ST(mm)
I	-0.15	V1	0.35
II	-0.20	V2	0.40
III	-0.10	V3	0.50
aVR	0.20	V4	0.10
aVL	-0.05	V5	-0.25
aVF	-0.15	V6	-0.35

Normal sinus rhythm with Q waves in precordial leads and in leads II, III, and aVF. No change with adenosine.

(Video 1a)

(Video 1b)

(Fig. 2a)

(Fig. 2b)

(Fig. 2c)

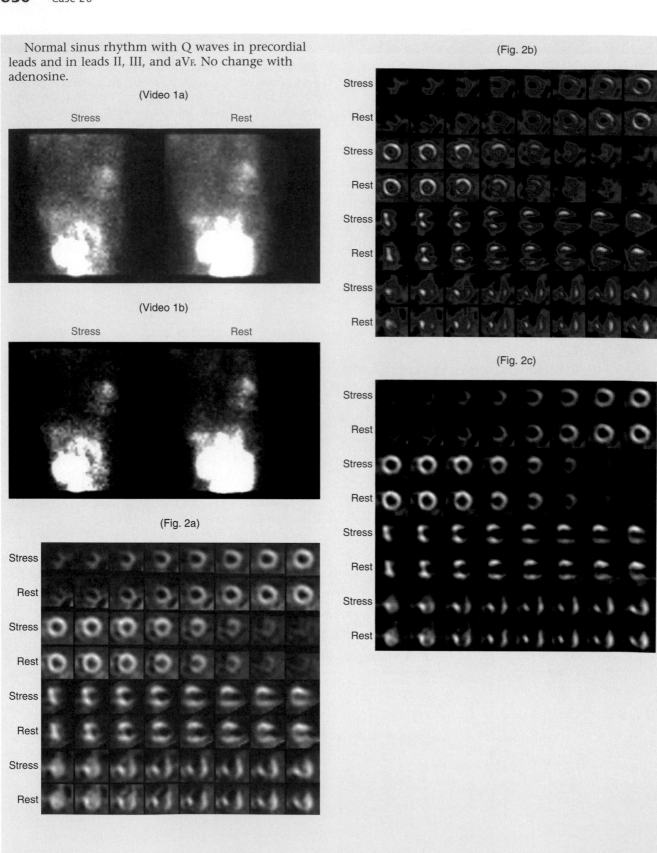

(Fig. 3a)

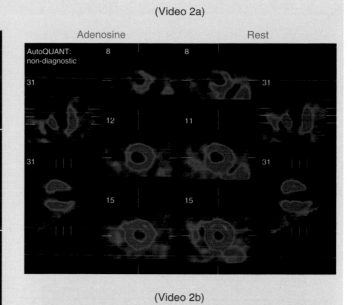

(Video 2a)

(Video 2b)

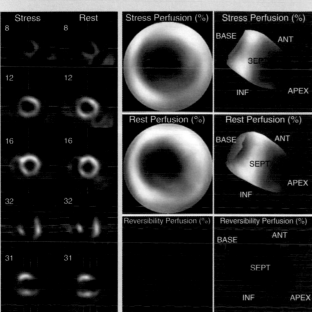

(Fig. 3b)

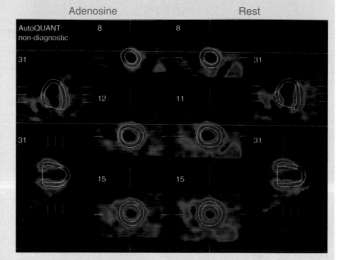

There is a large dense area of perfusion abnormality involving the distal part of the anterior wall, septum, apex, and contiguous inferior wall. The anterior wall and septum are hypokinetic, and the apex is dyskinetic. Left ventricular ejection fraction (LVEF) is impaired at 39%.

Months later, the patient presented with recurrence of chest pain and was ruled in for a small non-ST-segment elevation MI. Repeat coronary angiography showed 40% in-stent narrowing of the LAD, and RCA had 90% mid-narrowing and 100% distal narrowing. Both lesions were successfully angioplastied and stented.

Her LVEF was impaired at 25%. She also received an implantable cardioverter defibrillator (ICD) for primary prevention of sudden cardiac death.

CASE 27

A 64-year-old male with idiopathic dilated cardiomyopathy (angiographically normal coronary arteries) is undergoing cardiac transplant evaluation. He is admitted with severe biventricular failure and treated with aggressive medical management that includes milrinone. An equilibrium radionuclide angiocardiography and dynamic first-pass imaging study were performed to assess his left and right ventricular function.

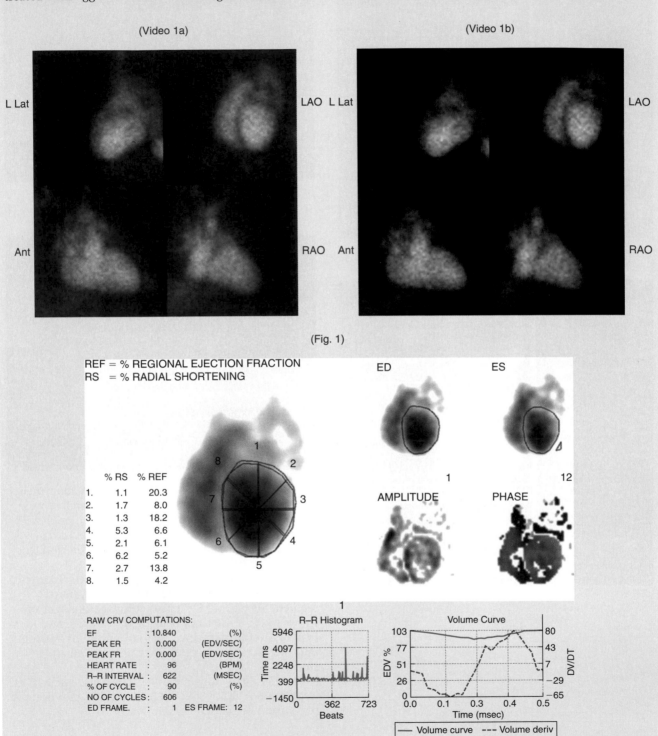

(Video 1a)

(Video 1b)

(Fig. 1)

REF = % REGIONAL EJECTION FRACTION
RS = % RADIAL SHORTENING

	% RS	% REF
1.	1.1	20.3
2.	1.7	8.0
3.	1.3	18.2
4.	5.3	6.6
5.	2.1	6.1
6.	6.2	5.2
7.	2.7	13.8
8.	1.5	4.2

ED   ES

AMPLITUDE   PHASE

RAW CRV COMPUTATIONS:

EF	: 10.840	(%)
PEAK ER	: 0.000	(EDV/SEC)
PEAK FR	: 0.000	(EDV/SEC)
HEART RATE	: 96	(BPM)
R–R INTERVAL :	622	(MSEC)
% OF CYCLE	: 90	(%)
NO OF CYCLES :	606	
ED FRAME.	: 1	ES FRAME: 12

R–R Histogram

Volume Curve

— Volume curve   --- Volume deriv

On first-pass imaging, RA and RV are enlarged, and RVEF is 19% with suspicion of severe tricuspid incompetence. On multiple gated acquisition (MUGA), LV is massively enlarged with global severe hypokinesia, and LVEF is 11%.

Right heart catheterization during this admission showed: RA pressure = 20 mm Hg, RV = 55/20 mm Hg, PA = 56/26 mm Hg, PCWP = 33 mm Hg, PA Saturation = 41%, C.I = 1.42 L/min/m^2.

He underwent heart transplant and had an uneventful postoperative recovery.

(Fig. 2)

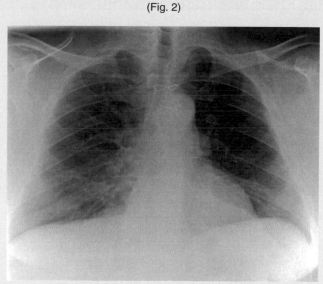

Chest x-ray PA view after cardiac transplant

CASE 28

The patient is an 81-year-old male with type 2 diabetes, hypertension, hyperlipidemia, and myocardial infarction 30 years earlier. He did not consent to cardiac catheterization and never underwent catheterization or revascularization. He is currently doing well and is physically active with normal exercise tolerance. He was referred for a routine stress/rest ^{99m}Tc-sestamibi perfusion imaging study.

Medications: pravastatin, nadolol, lisinopril, nifedipine, aspirin, and metformin.

Pharmacologic stress perfusion imaging using 5-minute adenosine infusion was performed, and the following changes were noted: heart rate rose from 60 to 70 beats/min and blood pressure dropped from 130/90 to 125/61. The patient reported no chest pain.

Baseline ECG shows normal sinus rhythm, first degree AV block left atrial enlargement, and possibly old inferior wall infarction and generalized ST-T changes. With adenosine infusion, there is 1.5-mm ST-segment depression in leads V4-5, which recovers within 3 minutes of termination of the infusion. Given the baseline ECG changes, this is a nonspecific ST-segment change.

(Fig. 1a)

ECG at rest

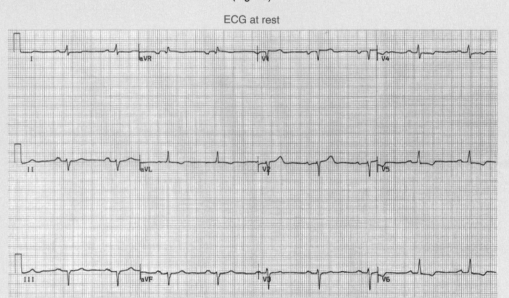

(Fig. 1b)

ECG during Adenosine infusion

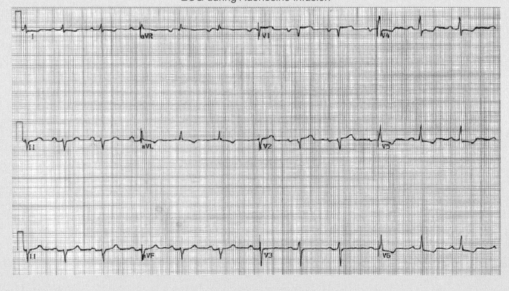

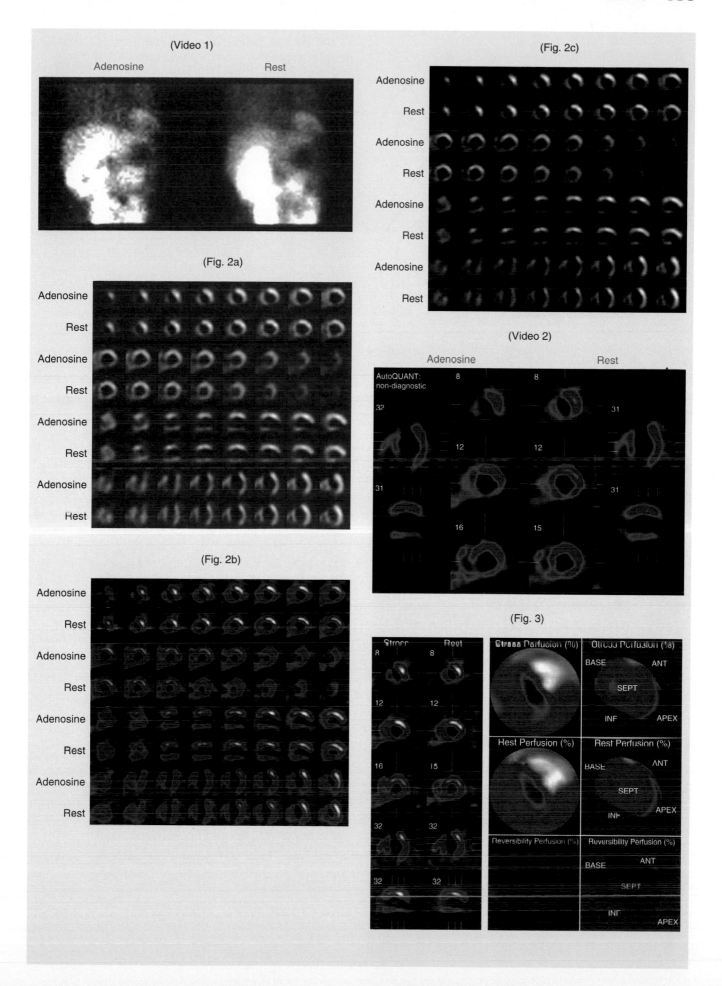

(Video 1)

Adenosine   Rest

(Fig. 2a)

Adenosine

Rest

Adenosine

Rest

Adenosine

Rest

Adenosine

Hest

(Fig. 2b)

Adenosine

Rest

Adenosine

Rest

Adenosine

Rest

Adenosine

Rest

(Fig. 2c)

Adenosine

Rest

Adenosine

Rest

Adenosine

Rest

Adenosine

Rest

(Video 2)

Adenosine   Rest

AutoQUANT:
non-diagnostic

(Fig. 3)

(Fig. 4)

ROWH

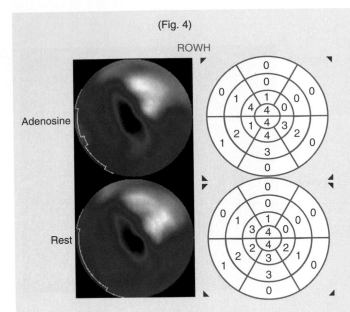

Adenosine

Rest

The left ventricle is enlarged, and there is a large, dense scar involving the septum, apex, inferior wall, and contiguous lateral wall, with no reversibility. The septum and inferior wall are severely hypokinetic, and LVEF is depressed at 34%.

Despite a large scar, the patient is doing quite well. He is on optimal medical management.

CASE 29

A 53-year-old male with a medical history of type 2 diabetes mellitus, hypertension, hepatitis C infection, end-stage liver disease, and end-stage renal disease, and on chronic hemodialysis is referred for stress testing as a part of a cardiac evaluation prior to consideration for liver and renal transplant.

Adenosine stress/rest Cardiolite imaging was performed. His heart rate increased from 80 to 84 beats/min, and blood pressure changed negligibly from 91/56 to 92/55 mm Hg. He reported no chest pain.

(Fig. 1a)

ECG Baseline

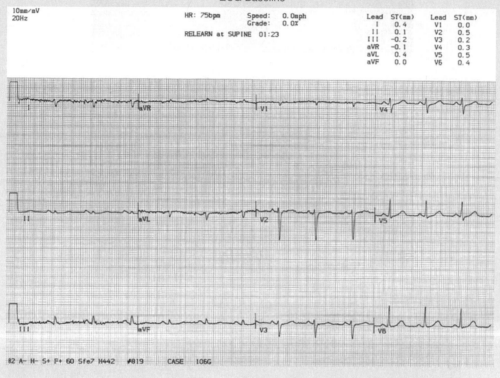

(Fig. 1b)

ECG with Adenosine

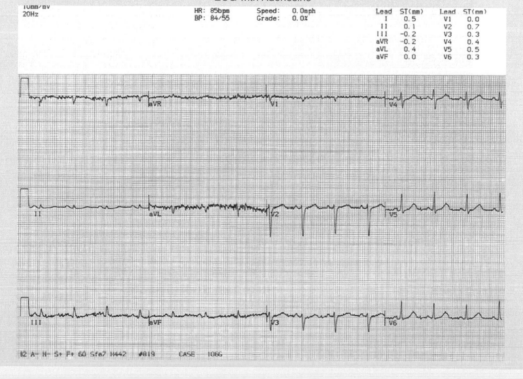

(Video 1a)

Stress   Rest

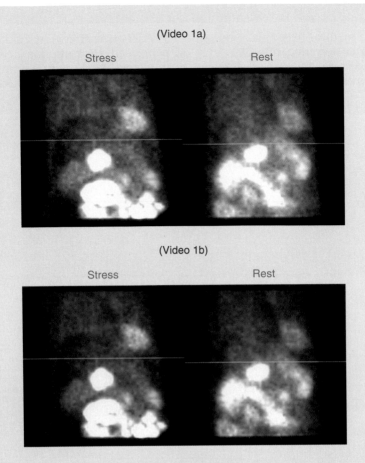

(Video 1b)

Stress   Rest

(Fig. 2a)

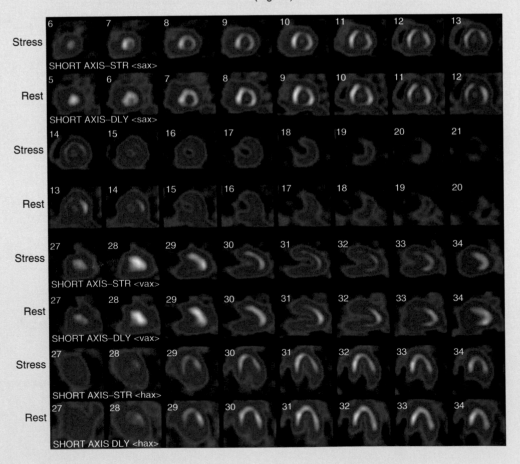

(Fig. 2b)

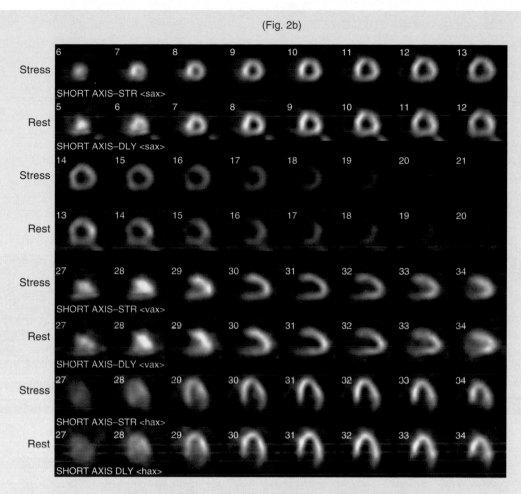

(Video 2)

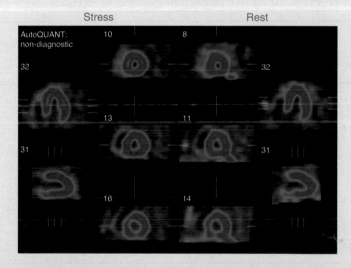

Perfusion imaging showed massive ascites, splenomegaly, and a small shrunken liver. There was no abnormality in myocardial perfusion. Left ventricular wall motion and left ventricular ejection fraction were normal (62% poststress images, 70% rest).

Variable degrees of ascites, splenomegaly, and enlarged or shrunken liver are common incidental findings in patients with end-stage liver disease. Readers should be familiar with the scintigraphic appearance of these abnormalities.

CASE 30

A 61-year-old overweight male (6 feet tall, weight 280 pounds) presented with a history of progressively worsening shortness of breath over the last month. At admission, he was found to be in atrial fibrillation. He had a remote history of smoking and recent heavy drinking. He was referred for a pharmacologic stress test. He was taking heparin, aspirin, and digoxin.

He underwent 2-day imaging protocol because of his overweight. Rest imaging was done on the first day, using 30 mCi of technetium-99-sestamibi.

He underwent pharmacologic stress using 5-minute adenosine infusion protocol on the second day. His heart rate changed from 101 to 89 beats/min and blood pressure from 178/100 to 189/100. He did not complain of chest pain. His ECG showed atrial fibrillation, left axis deviation, and nonspecific T-wave flattening. There was no further change with adenosine infusion.

His stress and rest images are shown next. What is your interpretation?

(Video 1a)

Adenosine   Rest

(Video 1b)

Adenosine   Rest

(Fig. 1a)

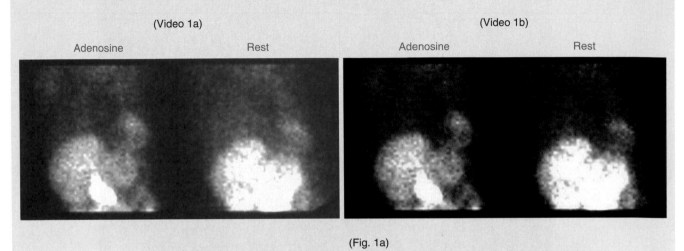

(Fig. 1b)

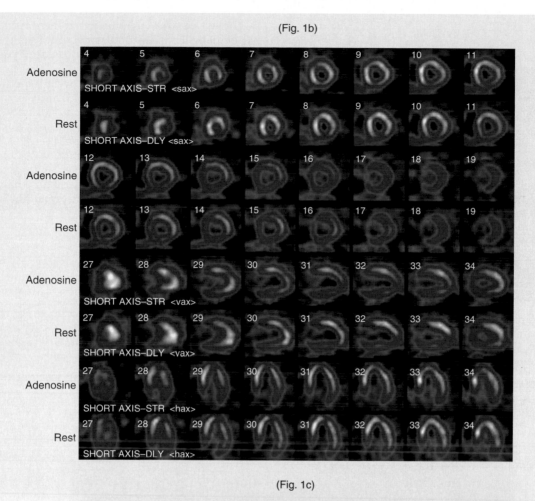

(Fig. 1c)

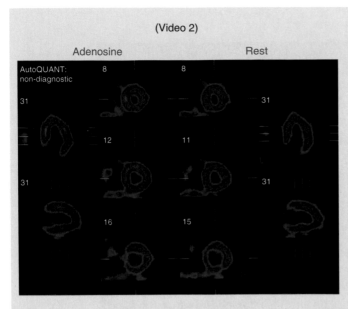

(Video 2)

Adenosine   Rest

AutoQUANT:
non-diagnostic

The left ventricle is enlarged, hypertrophied, and hypokinetic. Left ventricular ejection fraction is impaired at 36%, but there is no regional perfusion abnormality.

These findings are consistent with hypertensive heart disease. However, the long history of alcohol abuse and atrial fibrillation with uncontrolled heart rate may have contributed to the LV dysfunction.

He was DC-cardioverted and put on medical therapy with angiotension-converting enzyme (ACE) inhibitors, digoxin, and β-blockers. With good rate control, blood pressure control, and abstinence from alcohol, one should expect improvement in his cardiac function.

CASE 31

A 19-year-old African American woman who had a normal vaginal delivery 3 weeks earlier developed progressive shortness of breath after delivery. She was found to be in severe heart failure at admission and was diagnosed with postpartum heart failure.

(Fig. 1)

Resting ECG shows sinus tachycardia with generalized non-specific T wave changes and significant QTc prolongation

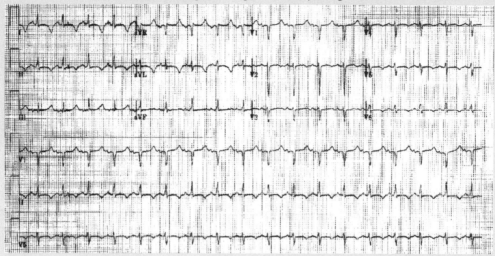

(Fig. 2a)

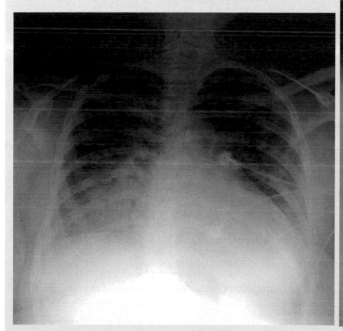

Chest x-ray at admission

(Fig. 2b)

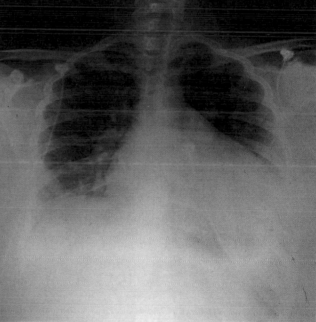

Chest x-ray 5 days later

She improved with treatment and is being prepared for discharge. A multiple gated acquisition (MUGA) scan and first-pass imaging were carried out prior to discharge. ECG showed sinus tachycardia with generalized nonspecific T-wave changes and significant QTc prolongation.

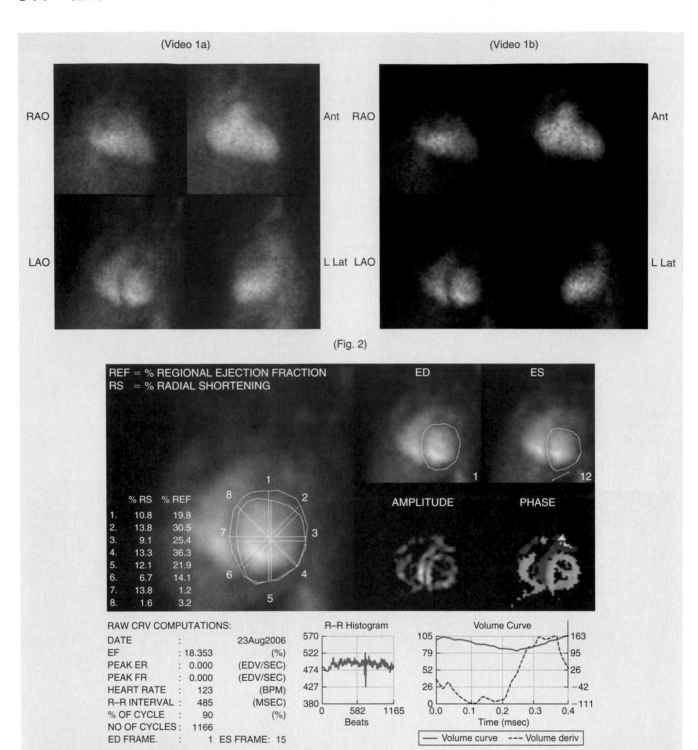

(Video 1a)

RAO

Ant

LAO

L Lat

(Video 1b)

RAO

Ant

LAO

L Lat

(Fig. 2)

REF = % REGIONAL EJECTION FRACTION
RS = % RADIAL SHORTENING

	% RS	% REF
1.	10.8	19.8
2.	13.8	30.5
3.	9.1	25.4
4.	13.3	36.3
5.	12.1	21.9
6.	6.7	14.1
7.	13.8	1.2
8.	1.6	3.2

ED   ES

AMPLITUDE   PHASE

RAW CRV COMPUTATIONS:

DATE	: 23Aug2006	
EF	: 18.353	(%)
PEAK ER	: 0.000	(EDV/SEC)
PEAK FR	: 0.000	(EDV/SEC)
HEART RATE	: 123	(BPM)
R–R INTERVAL	: 485	(MSEC)
% OF CYCLE	: 90	(%)
NO OF CYCLES	: 1166	
ED FRAME.	: 1 ES FRAME: 15	

R–R Histogram

Volume Curve

Volume curve --- Volume deriv

On dynamic first imaging, the right atrium and right ventricle are enlarged and severely hypokinetic, and right ventricular ejection fraction is depressed at 12%. On MUGA, right atrium and right ventricle are markedly enlarged and severely hypokinetic, and left ventricle is massively enlarged and severely hypokinetic. Left ventricular ejection fraction is severely impaired at 18%.

The patient was discharged home and continued to improve after discharge. Echocardiogram 2 years later showed a significant reduction in LV and RV size, and LVEF improved to 40%.

(Video 2)

Follow-up Echo After 2 Years

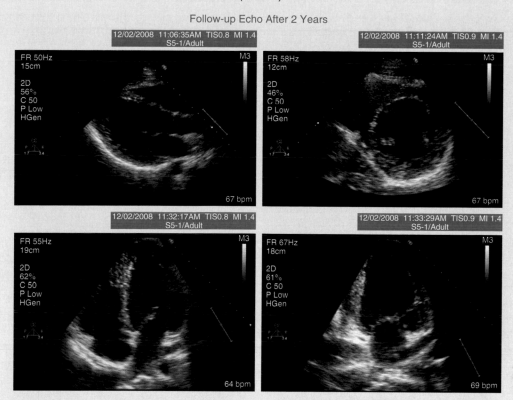

Peripartum cardiomyopathy generally occurs in the last month of pregnancy or within 5 months of delivery, and its incidence is reported to be 1 in 4000 to 15,000 deliveries in the United States. Clinical course is variable, with 50% to 60% of patients showing significant improvement within the next 6 months; the remaining 40% to 50% show no improvement or deterioration over time.

FURTHER READING

1. Ntusi NB, Mayosi BM: Aetiology and risk factors of peripartum cardiomyopathy: A systematic review, *Int J Cardiol* 131:168–179, 2009.
2. Hilfiker-Kleiner D, Sliwa K, Drexler H: Peripartum ardiomyopathy: Recent insights in its pathophysiology. *Trends Cardiovasc Med* 18:173–179, 2008.

CASE 32

A 65-year-old male with end-stage liver disease awaiting liver transplant underwent adenosine stress perfusion imaging as part of his preoperative evaluation.

Heart rate changed from 78 to 89 beats/min, and blood pressure from 182/86 to 148/69 mm Hg.

(Fig. 1a)

ECG at rest

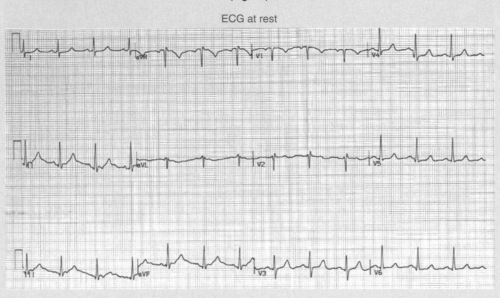

(Fig. 1b)

ECG during Adenosine infusion

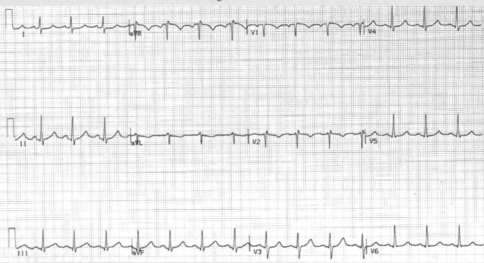

(Video 1)

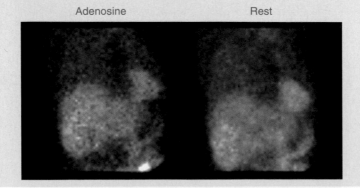

Adenosine   Rest

(Fig. 2a)

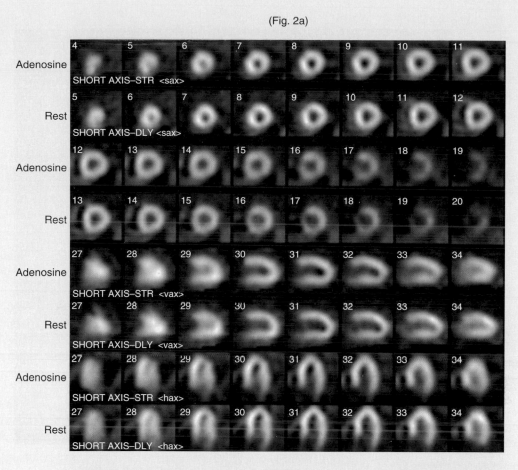

(Fig. 2b)

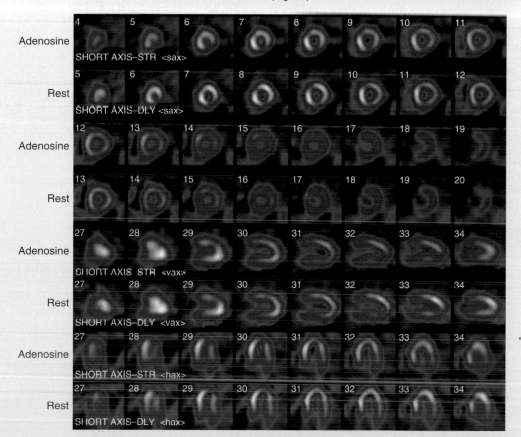

(Fig. 2c)

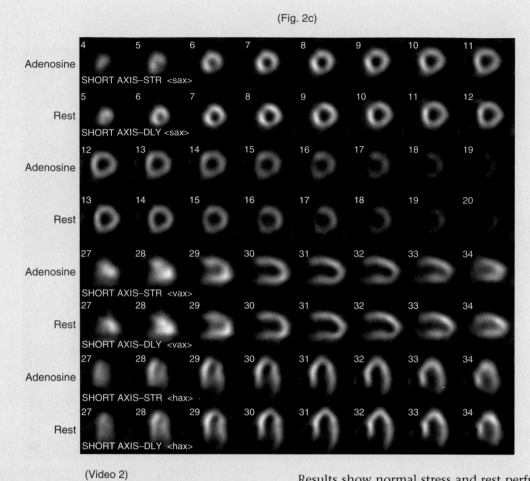

(Video 2)

Results show normal stress and rest perfusion imaging with left ventricular ejection fraction of 60%. Incidentally, a very large spleen is seen in raw images.

CASE 33

A 60-year-old male with coronary artery disease suffered from an inferior wall myocardial infarction 2 years earlier and underwent staged percutaneous coronary intervention (PCI) of the completely occluded left circumflex and right coronary arteries. He presents now with complaints of chest pain.

Medications: ramipril, isosorbide mononitrate, aspirin, atorvastatin, and clopidogrel.

Pharmacologic stress test was performed with 5-minute adenosine infusion. His heart rate changed from 74 to 80 beats/min and blood pressure from 100/60 to 90/60 mm Hg. He had no chest pain or ST changes. He had Q waves in inferior leads, with no change with adenosine infusion. ^{99m}Tc-sestamibi was used for stress-rest perfusion imaging.

(Video 1a)

Stress   Rest

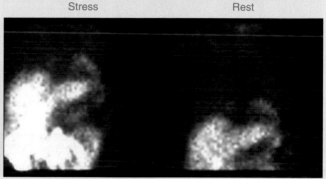

(Video 1b)

Stress   Rest

(Fig. 1a)

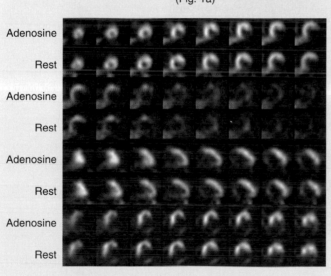

(Fig. 1b)

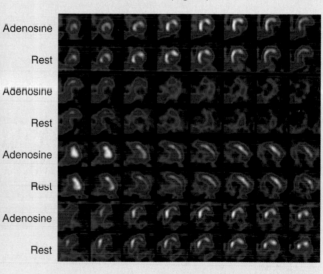

(Fig. 1c)

(Video 2)

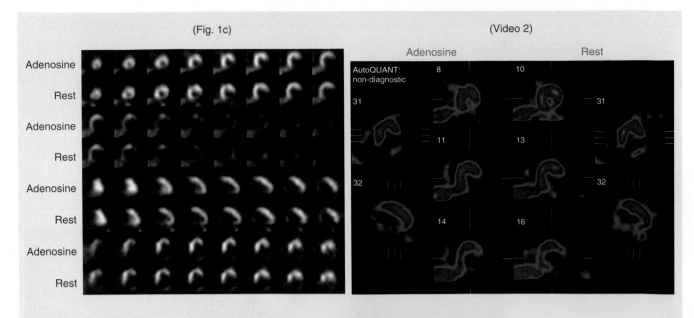

(Fig. 2)

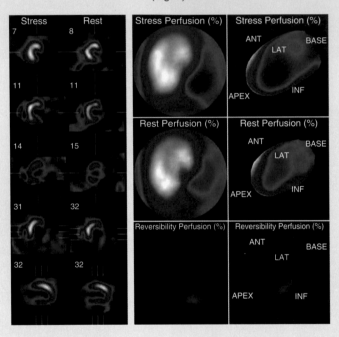

Myocardial perfusion imaging shows a large, dense scar involving the inferior and lateral walls. Left ventricular ejection fraction is 37%. Inferior and lateral walls are akinetic.

This patient underwent successful PCI of the left circumflex and the right coronary arteries. However, there is a large dense scar involving these vascular territories.

CASE 34

A 75-year-old male with hypertension, hyperlipidemia, and old myocardial infarction (26 years earlier) presented with complaints of occasional exertional angina. He never underwent cardiac catheterization, and he was treated medically.

Medications: lisinopril, isosorbide dinitrate, atorvastatin, and aspirin.

He was referred for exercise-rest myocardial perfusion imaging study.

He underwent symptom-limited treadmill exercise using Bruce Protocol. He exercised for 6:30 minutes, achieving an estimated workload of 7 METs. His heart rate increased from 75 to 144 beats/min, and blood pressure increased from 116/64 to 130/60 mm Hg. He developed no chest pain on exercise.

(Fig. 1a)

Rest

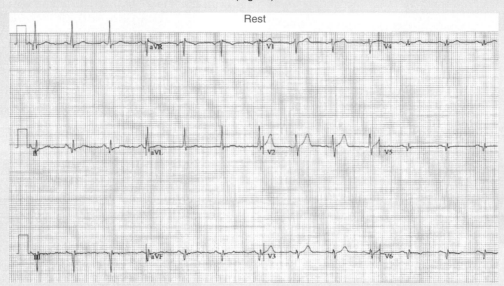

(Fig. 1b)

Peak exercise

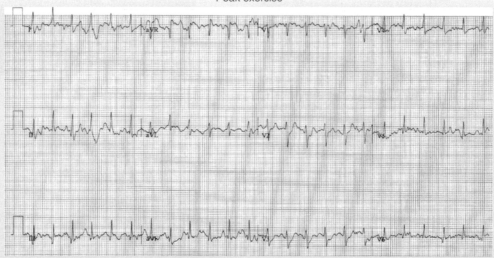

The test was terminated due to shortness of breath and fatigue. Baseline electrocardiogram shows normal sinus rhythm and Q waves in inferior and lateral leads, with no further ST-segment change on exercise.

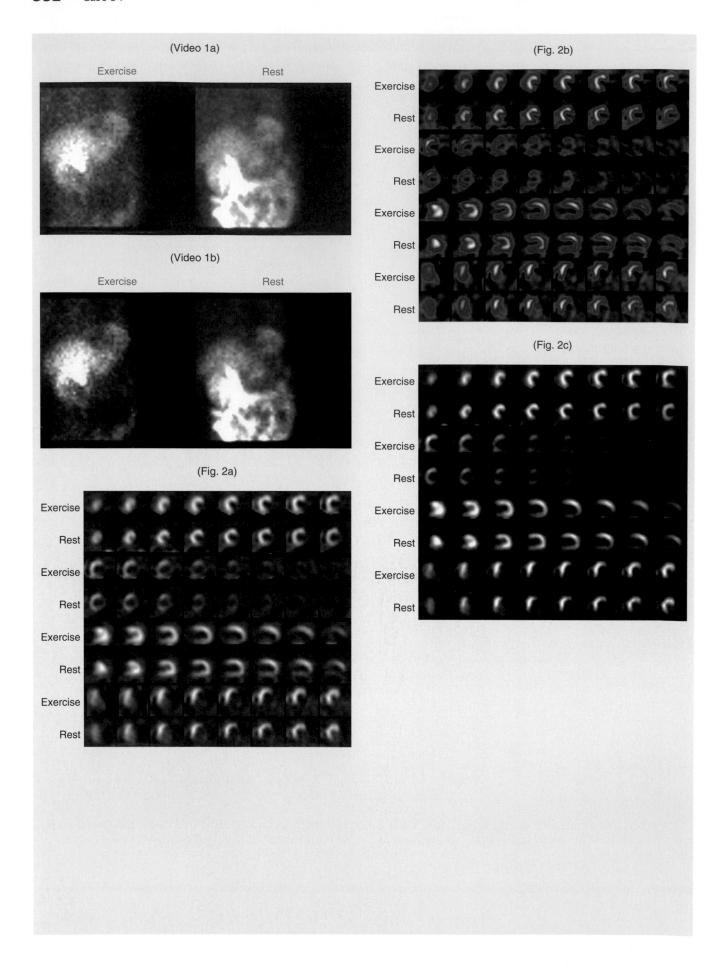

(Video 1a)

Exercise   Rest

(Video 1b)

Exercise   Rest

(Fig. 2a)

Exercise
Rest
Exercise
Rest
Exercise
Rest
Exercise
Rest

(Fig. 2b)

Exercise
Rest
Exercise
Rest
Exercise
Rest
Exercise
Rest

(Fig. 2c)

Exercise
Rest
Exercise
Rest
Exercise
Rest
Exercise
Rest

(Video 2)

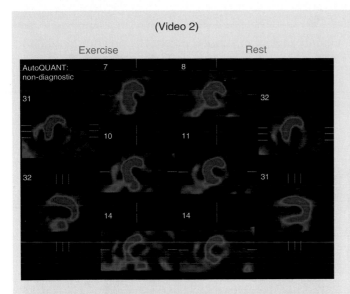

(Fig. 3)

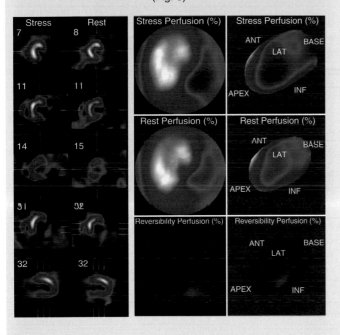

Exercise-rest perfusion imaging study shows a very large area of perfusion abnormality involving the inferior wall, lateral wall, and apex, with minimal reversibility in the inferior wall. The lateral wall is akinetic, and left ventricular ejection fraction is 34%.

Based upon the presence of a large scar involving the inferior and lateral wall, with only minimal ischemia involving the inferior wall, medical management was continued in this patient.

No coronary angiography was performed in this case.

CASE 35

A 53-year-old African American male was admitted to the hospital with complaints of shortness of breath and dizziness. He was diagnosed with hypertension 4 to 5 years earlier and is receiving treatment. He also has hyperlipidemia and remote history of smoking. He has history of palpitations since childhood. There is family history of sudden death. His one brother died suddenly at age 43 years. ECG showed normal sinus rhythm with marked left ventricular hypertrophy, generalized ST-segment depression, and deep T-wave inversions in precordial as well as limb leads. His ECG is shown next. What is your interpretation?

(Video 1)

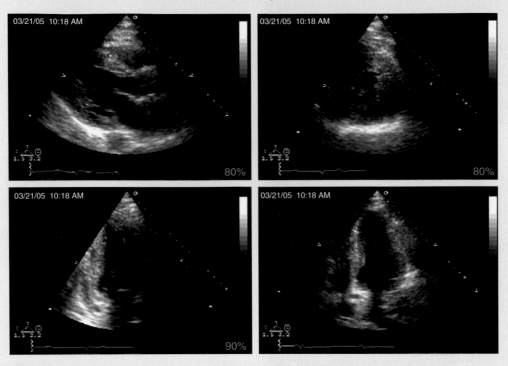

Echo shows severe left ventricular hypertrophy (LVH). Left ventricular ejection fraction (LVEF) is 65% to 70%, without evidence of regional wall-motion abnormalities.

He was ruled out for acute myocardial infarction, but because of a very abnormal echocardiogram, he underwent cardiac catheterization and coronary angiography. This is shown next.

(Video 2)

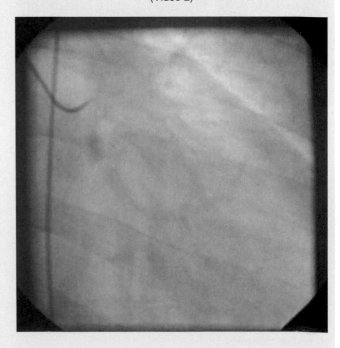

(Video 3)

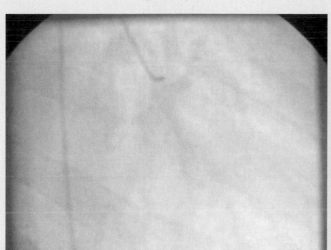

(Video 4)

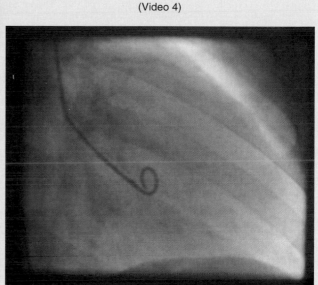

Coronary arteries are normal with no luminal obstruction. LV cavity is small, and the LV is hyperdynamic, with cavity obliteration in the distal part of the LV during systole.

He was referred for exercise perfusion imaging to detect any exercise-induced arrhythmias and exercise-induced perfusion abnormalities. He was receiving verapamil.

He underwent symptom-limited treadmill exercise using modified Bruce Protocol. He exercised for only 8:09 minutes, achieving an estimated workload of 4 METs. His heart rate increased from 80 to 98 beats/min and blood pressure from 100/70 to

120/80 mm Hg. He complained of tiredness and fatigue on exercise. His resting and peak exercise ECGs show is normal sinus rhythm with occasional premature ventricular beats. There is marked LVH with generalized ST-segment depression and deep symmetric T-wave inversion, and prolonged QTc. There is no arrhythmia with exercise. There is no change in ST-T with exercise. QT narrows with exercise, but QTc remains prolonged. There is alternans of T waves on the ECG.

His stress and rest images are shown next. What is your interpretation?

(Fig. 1a)

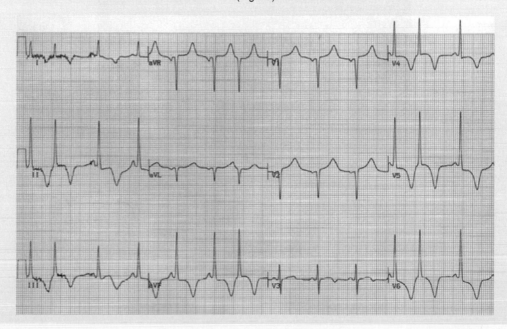

(Fig. 1b)

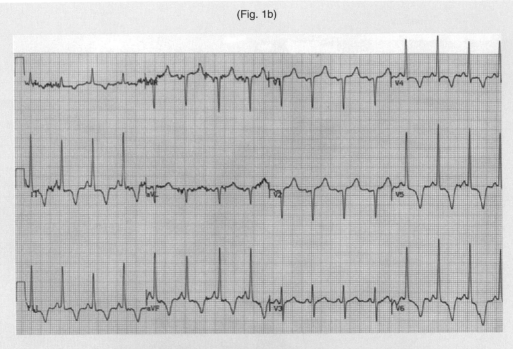

(Video 5a)

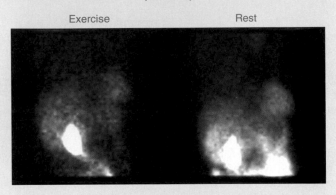

Exercise   Rest

(Video 5b)

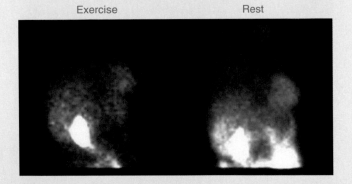

Exercise   Rest

(Fig. 2a)

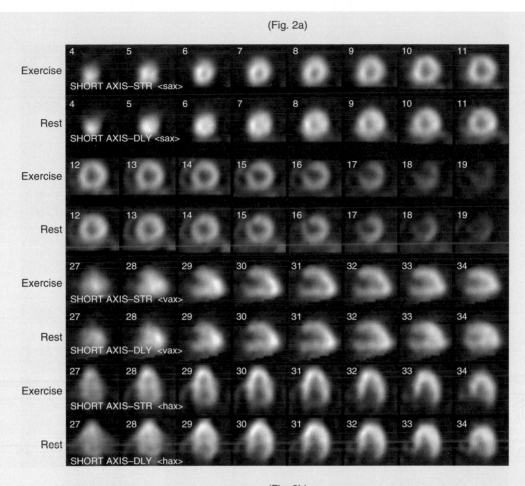

(Fig. 2b)

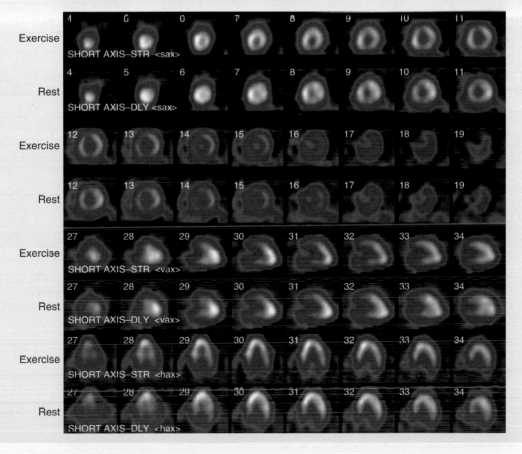

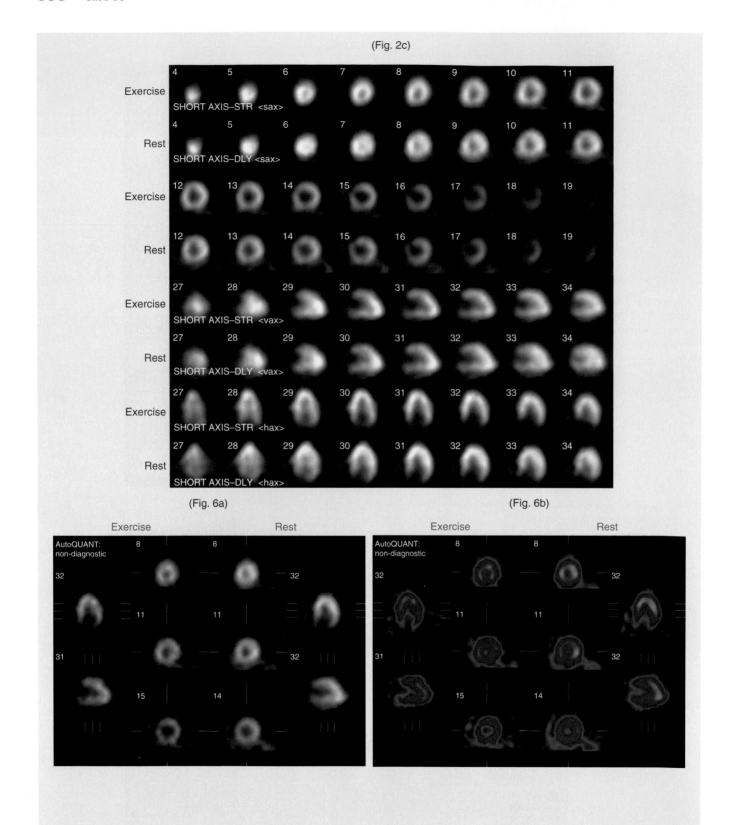

(Fig. 2c)

(Fig. 6a)

(Fig. 6b)

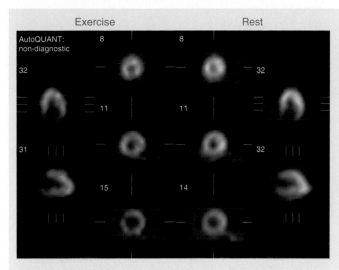

There is marked LVH with small left ventricular cavity. The hypertrophy appears to be more pronounced in the apical part of the LV. There is no regional perfusion abnormality. Interestingly, one can notice that the LV cavity is slightly bigger on the poststress images compared to the rest images. TID ratio was calculated at 1.24. The calculated LVEF is 31% on the poststress images and 36% on the rest images.

This case highlights the difficulties in calculation of LVEF by the automated gated SPECT programs. Generally, there is underestimation of the LVEF by these programs in hypertrophied ventricles secondary to the difficulties in reliably tracking the contours of the LV myocardium. These programs tend to assume only fixed thickness of the myocardium, as shown in the next images where LV contour is tracked by the myocardium. This results in underestimation of the LVEF.

This case also highlights another interesting phenomenon. Generally, transient dilation of the LV on the poststress images has been shown to be an indicator of severe multivessel coronary artery disease. However, it appears to be somewhat less specific in patients with LVH.

This patient has marked LVH, with normal coronary arteries and normal myocardial perfusion and function. Although the patient does have longstanding hypertension, the degree of LVH is disproportionate to what could be attributed to hypertensive heart disease. This raises the issue of hypertrophic cardiomyopathy, but in the absence of localized areas of hypertrophy in the LV, it is quite difficult to diagnose this condition.

In view of the history of dizziness, family history of sudden cardiac death, prolonged QTc, and T-wave alternans on the resting ECG, he underwent cardioverter-defibrillator (ICD) implantation.

INDEX

. . . .